Advance Praise for

Textbook of Psychiatry, 7th Edition

"For all mental health practitioners, all medical practitioners concerned with behavioral health and its integration into holistic care, and for consumers of mental health services, the seventh edition of APA Publishing's *Textbook of Psychiatry* is an indispensable tool and reference to inform practice, lifelong learning, and shared decision-making. Comprehensive in scope, this volume reflects admirably the enormous breadth of psychiatric, neuropsychiatric, and behavioral sciences that have continued to evolve. The *Textbook of Psychiatry* bridges contemporary scientific streams and practice in a balanced and forward-looking way that is rarely achieved. Praise is due to the senior editor, Laura Roberts, for the vision she has brought to this undertaking, fully in keeping with, and furthering, the scholarly tradition launched by the inaugural editors, Robert Hales and Stuart Yudofsky. The volume reminds us all how fortunate we are to have so many authors that represent our profession at its best—as clinicians, educators, and researchers."

Charles F. Reynolds III, M.D., Distinguished Professor of Psychiatry and UPMC Endowed Professor in Geriatric Psychiatry emeritus, University of Pittsburgh School of Medicine

"In this outstanding new seventh edition of *The American Psychiatric Association Publishing Textbook of Psychiatry*, Laura Roberts has brought together many of the field's luminaries to provide students and practitioners in all branches of the mental health professions the best currently available single volume textbook spanning the entire field. Covering the broad scope of our rapidly changing scientific and clinical domains, following the tradition of its esteemed predecessors, the chapters in this edition offer novices and experts the most contemporary perspectives, frameworks, and evidence necessary to assure intellectual mastery and best clinical practices."

Joel Yager, M.D., Professor, Department of Psychiatry, University of Colorado School of Medicine; Professor Emeritus, Department of Psychiatry and Biobehavioral Sciences, David Geffen School of Medicine, UCLA

"Bigger and better. The seventh edition of APA Publishing's *Textbook of Psychiatry* has added seven new chapters to its immediate predecessor. These additional chapters, along with timely revisions of carry-over chapters, provide the reader with a readable yet comprehensive and up-to-date resource for students, trainees, clinicians, and clinical scholars alike. The goals of the seventh edition, to "elucidate the essentials of sound psychiatric practice and to illuminate the future directions of our field," are handily met. The two new chapters I immediately went to were the ones on "Assessment of Suicide Risk in the Psychiatric Interview" and "Standardized Assessment and Measurement-Based Care." Both were thoughtful, evidence based, and clinically focused and added to my understanding of these important topics. Other new chapters, such as ones on social determinants of mental health, precision psychiatry, e-health strategies, and complementary and integrative care, represent critical contemporary topics not yet addressed in most other psychiatry texts. They are a welcome and thought-provoking addition. Throughout the textbook, the selection of chapter authors skillfully blends many of the leading scholars in the field with a refreshing mix of next-generation stars as co-authors. The overall result is an outstanding resource that belongs on the work desk of students, trainees, and clinicians learning about, or treating, mental disorders. If I had to select just one textbook for any of these groups, this would be the one. Congratulations to Dr. Laura Roberts and the many contributors for a job well done."

Sidney Zisook, M.D., Distinguished Professor, Department of Psychiatry, UC San Diego

The American Psychiatric Association Publishing

TEXTBOOK OF

PSYCHIATRY

SEVENTH EDITION

Editorial Board

The American Psychiatric Association Publishing

TEXTBOOK OF

PSYCHIATRY

SEVENTH EDITION

EDITED BY

Laura Weiss Roberts, M.D., M.A.

WITH FOREWORD BY

Robert E. Hales, M.D., M.B.A.
Stuart C. Yudofsky, M.D.

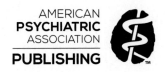

AMERICAN
PSYCHIATRIC
ASSOCIATION
PUBLISHING

If you wish to buy 50 or more copies of the same title, please go to www.appi.org/specialdiscounts for more information.

Copyright © 2019 American Psychiatric Association Publishing
ALL RIGHTS RESERVED

Manufactured in the United States of America on acid-free paper
23 22 21 20 19   5 4 3 2 1
Seventh Edition

American Psychiatric Association Publishing
800 Maine Avenue S.W., Suite 900
Washington, DC 20024
www.appi.org

Library of Congress Cataloging-in-Publication Data
Names: Roberts, Laura Weiss, editor. | American Psychiatric Association
    Publishing, issuing body.
Title: The American Psychiatric Association Publishing textbook of psychiatry
    / edited by Laura Weiss Roberts ; with foreword by Robert E. Hales, Stuart
    C. Yudofsky.
Other titles: American Psychiatric Publishing textbook of psychiatry. |
    Textbook of psychiatry
Description: Seventh edition. | Washington, D.C. : American Psychiatric
    Association Publishing, [2019] | Preceded by American Psychiatric
    Publishing textbook of psychiatry / edited by Robert E. Hales, Stuart C.
    Yudofsky, Laura Weiss Roberts. Sixth edition. 2014. | Includes
    bibliographical references and index.
Identifiers: LCCN 2019011542 (print) | LCCN 2019012800 (ebook) | ISBN
    9781615372560 (ebook) | ISBN 9781615371501 (hardcover : alk. paper)
Subjects: | MESH: Mental Disorders | Psychiatry
Classification: LCC RC454 (ebook) | LCC RC454 (print) | NLM WM 100 | DDC
    616.89—dc23
LC record available at https://lccn.loc.gov/2019011542

British Library Cataloguing in Publication Data
A CIP record is available from the British Library.

For Eric

Contents

PART I
Foundations

PART III
Treatments

PART IV
Caring for Special Populations

Contributors

Tarek Adam, M.D., M.Sc.
Attending Psychiatrist, Traditions Behavioral Health; Consultant Psychiatrist, New York University Langone Hospital–Brooklyn, Brooklyn, New York

Neil Krishan Aggarwal, M.D., M.B.A., M.A.
Assistant Professor of Clinical Psychiatry, Columbia University, and Research Psychiatrist, New York State Psychiatric Institute, New York, New York

W. Stewart Agras, M.D.
Professor of Psychiatry, Emeritus, Stanford University, Stanford, California

Jon G. Allen, Ph.D.
Clinical Professor, Department of Psychiatry and Behavioral Sciences, Baylor College of Medicine, Voluntary Faculty, Houston, Texas

Jonathan Avery, M.D.
Director of Addiction Psychiatry, Associate Professor of Clinical Psychiatry, Assistant Dean of Student Affairs, Weill Cornell Medical College, New York–Presbyterian Hospital, New York, New York

Tali M. Ball, Ph.D.
Instructor, Stanford University School of Medicine, Stanford, California

Richard Balon, M.D.
Professor of Psychiatry and Anesthesiology and Associate Chair for Education and Faculty Affairs, Department of Psychiatry and Behavioral Neurosciences, Wayne State University School of Medicine, Detroit, Michigan

John W. Barnhill, M.D.
DeWitt Wallace Senior Scholar and Professor of Clinical Psychiatry; Director, House Staff Mental Health Program; Psychiatric Liaison, Perkin Center for Heart Failure; Chief, Division of Psychiatry, Hospital for Special Surgery; and Vice Chair, Consultation–Liaison Psychiatry, Weill Cornell Medicine I New York–Presbyterian, New York, New York

Aaron T. Beck, M.D.
University Professor Emeritus of Psychiatry, Department of Psychiatry, Perelman School of Medicine, University of Pennsylvania, Philadelphia, Pennsylvania

Donna S. Bender, Ph.D.
Director, Counseling and Psychological Services (CAPS), and Clinical Professor of Psychiatry and Behavioral Sciences, Tulane University, New Orleans, Louisiana

Mahendra T. Bhati, M.D.
Clinical Associate Professor, Department of Psychiatry and Behavioral Sciences and Department of Neurosurgery, Stanford University, Stanford, California

Dan G. Blazer, M.D., Ph.D.
J.P. Gibbons Professor Emeritus, Department of Psychiatry and Behavioral Sciences, Duke University Medical Center, Durham, North Carolina

Kevin M. Bozymski, Pharm.D.
Assistant Professor of Clinical Sciences, Medical College of Wisconsin School of Pharmacy, Milwaukee, Wisconsin

Jack D. Burke, M.D., M.P.H.
Professor of Psychiatry, Harvard Medical School, Boston, Massachusetts

Vivien K. Burt, M.D., Ph.D.
Professor Emeritus of Psychiatry, Geffen School of Medicine at UCLA, Los Angeles, California

Eve Caligor, M.D.
Clinical Professor of Psychiatry, Columbia University Vagelos College of Physicians and Surgeons; Director, Psychotherapy Division, Columbia University Center for Psychoanalytic Training and Research, New York, New York

Steven Z. Chao, M.D., Ph.D.
Staff Neurologist, VA Palo Alto Health Care System, Palo Alto, California; Clinical Associate Professor (Affiliated), Department of Neurology and Neurological Science, Stanford University School of Medicine, Stanford, California

John F. Clarkin, Ph.D.
Clinical Professor of Psychology in Psychiatry and Co-Director, Personality Disorders Institute, Weill Cornell Medical College, New York, New York

Michael T. Compton, M.D., M.P.H.
Professor of Clinical Psychiatry, Columbia University College of Physicians and Surgeons, New York

Deborah S. Cowley, M.D.
Professor, Department of Psychiatry and Behavioral Sciences, University of Washington, Seattle, Washington

Ericka L. Crouse, Pharm.D.
Associate Professor, Department of Pharmacotherapy and Outcomes Science, Virginia Commonwealth University School of Pharmacy, Richmond, Virginia

Mantosh J. Dewan, M.D.
Distinguished Service Professor, Department of Psychiatry and Behavioral Sciences, SUNY Upstate Medical University, Syracuse, New York

Darin D. Dougherty, M.D., M.M.Sc.
Director, Division of Neurotherapeutics, Department of Psychiatry, Massachusetts General Hospital, Charlestown; Associate Professor of Psychiatry, Harvard Medical School, Boston, Massachusetts

Jonathan Downar, M.D., Ph.D.
Director, MRI-Guided rTMS Clinic, Centre for Mental Health and Krembil Research Institute, University Health Network; Associate Professor, Department of Psychiatry, University of Toronto, Toronto, Ontario, Canada

Jack Drescher, M.D.
Clinical Professor of Psychiatry, Columbia University, New York, New York; and Adjunct Professor, New York University, New York, New York

Laura B. Dunn, M.D.
Professor of Psychiatry and Behavioral Sciences, Department of Psychiatry and Behavioral Sciences, Stanford University, Stanford, California

Amit Etkin, M.D., Ph.D.
Professor, Department of Psychiatry and Behavioral Sciences, Wu Tsai Neuroscience Institute, Stanford University, Stanford, California; Veterans Affairs Palo Alto Healthcare System, and the Sierra Pacific Mental Illness, Research, Education, and Clinical Center (MIRECC), Palo Alto, California

Peter Fonagy, Ph.D., F.B.A., F.Med.Sci., FAcSS
Professor of Contemporary Psychoanalysis and Developmental Science, and Head, Division of Psychology and Language Sciences, UCL, London, UK; Chief Executive, Anna Freud National Centre for Children and Families, London, UK; Adjunct Professor of Psychiatry, Baylor College of Medicine, Houston, Texas; Clinical Professor of Psychiatry, Yale University School of Medicine, New Haven, Connecticut

Lawrence K. Fung, M.D., Ph.D.
Clinical Assistant Professor, Department of Psychiatry and Behavioral Sciences, Stanford University, Stanford, California

Patricia L. Gerbarg, M.D.
Assistant Clinical Professor in Psychiatry, New York Medical College, Valhalla, New York

Karen Gilmore, M.D.
Clinical Professor of Psychiatry, Columbia University Medical Center, New York, New York

John F. Greden, M.D.
Rachel Upjohn Professor of Psychiatry and Clinical Neurosciences; Research Professor, Molecular and Behavioral Neurosciences; Founder and Executive Director, University of Michigan Comprehensive Depression Center; Founding Chair, National Network of Depression Centers; Chair Emeritus, Department of Psychiatry, University of Michigan, Ann Arbor, Michigan

Roger P. Greenberg, Ph.D.
Distinguished Professor and Head, Psychology Division, Department of Psychiatry and Behavioral Sciences, SUNY Upstate Medical University, Syracuse, New York

Robert E. Hales, M.D., M.B.A.
Joe P. Tupin Chair, Emeritus, and Distinguished Professor of Clinical Psychiatry, Emeritus, Department of Psychiatry and Behavioral Sciences, University of California Davis School of Medicine, Sacramento, California

Thomas A. Hammeke, Ph.D., ABPP-CN
Professor Emeritus, Department of Psychiatry and Behavioral Medicine, Medical College of Wisconsin, Milwaukee, Wisconsin

Antonio Hardan, M.D.
Professor, Department of Psychiatry and Behavioral Sciences, Stanford University, Stanford, California

Nicholas M. Hatzis, M.D.
Clinical Instructor, Department of Psychiatry and Behavioral Sciences, Northwestern University Feinberg School of Medicine, Chicago, Illinois

John Hearn, M.D.
Senior Instructor, University of Colorado Denver Anschutz Medical Campus, Aurora, Colorado

Eric Hollander, M.D.
Professor of Psychiatry and Behavioral Sciences and Director, Autism and Obsessive-Compulsive Spectrum Program and Anxiety and Depression Program, Albert Einstein College of Medicine and Montefiore Medical Center, Bronx, New York

David S. Hong, M.D.
Assistant Professor, Department of Psychiatry and Behavioral Sciences, Stanford University, Stanford, California

Sandra A. Jacobson, M.D.
Research Associate Professor, Department of Psychiatry, University of Arizona College of Medicine, Phoenix, Arizona

Michael A. Jenike, M.D.
Director Emeritus, OCD and Related Disorders Program, Department of Psychiatry, Massachusetts General Hospital, Charlestown; Professor of Psychiatry, Harvard Medical School, Boston, Massachusetts

Margery R. Johnson, M.D.
Assistant Professor, Department of Psychiatry and Behavioral Sciences, Northwestern University Feinberg School of Medicine, Chicago, Illinois

Amandeep Jutla, M.D.
Whitaker Scholar in Developmental Neuropsychiatry, Division of Child and Adolescent Psychiatry, Columbia University, New York, New York

Corey Keller, M.D., Ph.D.
Resident and Postdoctoral Fellow, Department of Psychiatry and Behavioral Sciences, Wu Tsai Neuroscience Institute, Stanford University, Stanford, California; Veterans Affairs Palo Alto Healthcare System, and the Sierra Pacific Mental Illness, Research, Education, and Clinical Center (MIRECC), Palo Alto, California

Michael Kelly, M.D.
Senior Psychiatrist Supervisor, Forensic Services Division, Coalinga State Hospital, Coalinga, California

Otto F. Kernberg, M.D.
Professor of Psychiatry and Director, Personality Disorders Institute, Weill Cornell Medical College, New York, New York

Catherine L. Kircos, M.A.
Research Coordinator, Stanford University School of Medicine, Stanford, California

Helena C. Kraemer, Ph.D.
Professor of Biostatistics in Psychiatry (Emeritus), Department of Psychiatry and Behavioral Sciences, Stanford University, Palo Alto, California

Clete A. Kushida, M.D., Ph.D.
Professor of Psychiatry and Behavioral Sciences, Stanford University, Stanford, California

Ryan E. Lawrence, M.D.
Assistant Professor of Psychiatry, Department of Psychiatry, Columbia University Medical Center and New York–Presbyterian Hospital, New York, New York

James L. Levenson, M.D.
Rhona Arenstein Professor of Psychiatry, and Professor of Internal Medicine and Surgery, Virginia Commonwealth University, Richmond, Virginia

Petros Levounis, M.D., M.A.
Professor and Chair, Department of Psychiatry, Rutgers New Jersey Medical School; Chief of Service, University Hospital, Newark, New Jersey

Jeffrey A. Lieberman, M.D.
Lawrence C. Kolb Professor and Chairman of Psychiatry, Columbia University College of Physicians and Surgeons, New York State Psychiatric Institute; Psychiatrist-in-Chief, New York–Presbyterian Hospital and Columbia University Medical Center, New York, New York

Steven E. Lindley, M.D., Ph.D.
Director of Outpatient Mental Health, Veterans Affairs Palo Alto Health Care System, Menlo Park; Associate Professor, Department of Psychiatry and Behavioral Sciences, Stanford University School of Medicine, Stanford, California

James Lock, M.D., Ph.D.
Professor of Child Psychiatry and Pediatrics, Department of Psychiatry and Behavioral Sciences, and Director, Eating Disorder Program for Children and Adolescents, Stanford University School of Medicine, Stanford, California

José R. Maldonado, M.D., F.A.P.M., F.A.C.F.E.
Professor of Psychiatry and Behavioral Sciences (General Psychiatry and Psychology–Adult) and, by courtesy, of Emergency Medicine and of Medicine at the Stanford University Medical Center and, by courtesy, of Law, Stanford, California

Lila Massoumi, M.D., ABOIHM
Assistant Clinical Professor in Psychiatry, Michigan State University, Detroit, Michigan

Anne McBride, M.D.
Assistant Clinical Professor, Department of Psychiatry and Behavioral Sciences, University of California, Davis, Sacramento, California

Pamela Meersand, Ph.D.
Associate Professor of Medical Psychology, Columbia University Medical Center, New York, New York

Edwin J. Mikkelsen, M.D.
Associate Professor of Psychiatry, Harvard Medical School, Boston, Massachusetts

Shefali Miller, M.D.
Clinical Assistant Professor, Department of Psychiatry and Behavioral Sciences, Stanford University, Stanford, California

Erin Murphy-Barzilay, M.D.
Assistant Professor of Health Sciences, Geffen School of Medicine at UCLA, Los Angeles, California

Philip R. Muskin, M.D., M.A.
Professor of Psychiatry, Columbia University Irving Medical Center, New York, New York

Uma Naidoo, M.D.
Director of Nutritional and Lifestyle Psychiatry, Massachusetts General Hospital, Boston, Massachusetts

John M. Oldham, M.D.
Distinguished Emeritus Professor, Menninger Department of Psychiatry and Behavioral Sciences, Baylor College of Medicine, Houston, Texas

Michael Ostacher, M.D.
Associate Professor, Department of Psychiatry and Behavioral Sciences, Stanford University, Stanford, California

Sagar V. Parikh, M.D.
Professor, Department of Psychiatry, University of Michigan, Ann Arbor, Michigan

Roger K. Pitman, M.D.
Professor, Department of Psychiatry, Harvard Medical School; Psychiatrist, Massachusetts General Hospital, Boston, Massachusetts

Sonya Rasminsky, M.D.
Associate Clinical Professor of Psychiatry, Geffen School of Medicine at UCLA, Los Angeles, California

Martin Reite, M.D.
Clinical Professor of Psychiatry, University of Colorado School of Medicine, Aurora, Colorado

Michelle B. Riba, M.D., M.S.
Professor, Department of Psychiatry, University of Michigan, Ann Arbor, Michigan

Laura Weiss Roberts, M.D., M.A.
Chairman and Katharine Dexter McCormick and Stanley McCormick Memorial Professor, Department of Psychiatry and Behavioral Sciences, Stanford University School of Medicine, and Chief, Psychiatry Service, Stanford Hospital and Clinics, Stanford, California; Editor-in-Chief, Books, American Psychiatric Association Publishing

Allyson C. Rosen, Ph.D., ABPP-CN
Clinical Associate Professor (Affiliated), Palo Alto VA Health Care System/Department of Psychiatry, Stanford University School of Medicine, Stanford, California

Craig S. Rosen, Ph.D.
Acting Director, National Center for PTSD Dissemination and Training Division, Veterans Affairs Palo Alto Health Care System, Menlo Park; Associate Professor, Department of Psychiatry and Behavioral Sciences, Stanford University School of Medicine, Stanford, California

M. David Rudd, Ph.D., A.B.P.P.
President, Distinguished University Professor of Psychology, University of Memphis, Memphis, Tennessee

Jitender Sareen, M.D., F.R.C.P.C.
Professor and Head, Department of Psychiatry; Professor, Departments of Psychology and Community Health Sciences, Max Rady College of Medicine, University of Manitoba, Winnipeg, Manitoba, Canada

Lorin M. Scher, M.D.
Associate Professor, and Director, Emergency Psychiatry and Integrated Behavioral Health Services, Department of Psychiatry & Behavioral Sciences, University of California, Davis, School of Medicine, Sacramento, California

Danya Schlussel, B.A.
Research Associate, Autism and Obsessive-Compulsive Spectrum Program, Albert Einstein College of Medicine and Montefiore Medical Center, Bronx, New York

Ruth S. Shim, M.D., M.P.H.
Luke and Grace Kim Professor in Cultural Psychiatry and Associate Professor, Department of Psychiatry and Behavioral Sciences, University of California, Davis, School of Medicine, Sacramento, California

Jay Shore, M.D., M.P.H.
Professor, Department of Psychiatry and Family Medicine, School of Medicine, Centers for American Indian and Alaska Native Health, Colorado School of Public Health, University of Colorado Anschutz Medical Campus, Denver, Colorado

Erik Shwarts, M.D.
Assistant Clinical Professor (Volunteer Faculty), Department of Psychiatry and Behavioral Sciences, University of California, Davis, School of Medicine, Sacramento, California

Naomi M. Simon, M.D., M.Sc.
Professor, Department of Psychiatry, New York University School of Medicine, New York, New York

Andrew E. Skodol, M.D.
Research Professor of Psychiatry, University of Arizona College of Medicine, Tucson, Arizona

David Spiegel, M.D., F.A.P.A.
Jack, Lulu, and Sam Willson Professor and Associate Chair, Department of Psychiatry and Behavioral Sciences, and Director, Center on Stress and Health and Center for Integrative Medicine, Stanford University School of Medicine, Stanford, California

Brett N. Steenbarger, Ph.D.
Teaching Professor of Psychiatry and Behavioral Sciences, SUNY Upstate Medical University, Syracuse, New York

David C. Steffens, M.D., M.H.S.
Birnbaum/Blum Professor and Chair, Department of Psychiatry, University of Connecticut School of Medicine, Farmington, Connecticut

Murray B. Stein, M.D., M.P.H., F.R.C.P.C.
Distinguished Professor of Psychiatry and of Family Medicine and Public Health, and Vice Chair for Clinical Research in Psychiatry, University of California San Diego, La Jolla, California; Staff Psychiatrist, Veterans Affairs San Diego Healthcare System, San Diego, California

Shannon Wiltsey Stirman, Ph.D.
Acting Deputy Director, National Center for PTSD Dissemination and Training Division, Veterans Affairs Palo Alto Health Care System, Menlo Park, California; Associate Professor, Department of Psychiatry and Behavioral Sciences, Stanford University School of Medicine, Stanford, California

Frederick J. Stoddard Jr., M.D.
Professor, Department of Psychiatry, Harvard Medical School; Psychiatrist, Massachusetts General Hospital, Boston, Massachusetts

T. Scott Stroup, M.D., M.P.H.
Professor of Psychiatry, Department of Psychiatry, Columbia University Medical Center and New York–Presbyterian Hospital, New York, New York

Mark Sullivan, M.D.
PGY-3, Cornell Psychiatry, Department of Psychiatry, Weill Cornell Medicine, New York, New York

Trisha Suppes, M.D., Ph.D.
Professor, Department of Psychiatry and Behavioral Sciences, Stanford University, Stanford, California

Rita Suri, M.D.
Clinical Professor of Psychiatry, Geffen School of Medicine at UCLA, Los Angeles, California

Bonnie P. Taylor, Ph.D.
Assistant Professor of Psychiatry and Behavioral Sciences, Autism and Obsessive-Compulsive Spectrum Program, Albert Einstein College of Medicine and Montefiore Medical Center, Bronx, New York

Gabrielle Termuehlen, B.A.
Department of Psychiatry and Behavioral Sciences, Stanford University, Stanford, California

Michael E. Thase, M.D.
Professor of Psychiatry, Department of Psychiatry, Perelman School of Medicine, University of Pennsylvania, Philadelphia, Pennsylvania

Ramanpreet Toor, M.D.
Assistant Professor, Department of Psychiatry and Behavioral Sciences, University of Washington, Seattle, Washington

Michael Weissberg, M.D.
Professor of Psychiatry (retired), University of Colorado School of Medicine, Aurora, Colorado

Elisabeth A. Wilde, Ph.D.
Associate Professor, Department of Neurology, University of Utah School of Medicine, Salt Lake City, Utah

Sabine Wilhelm, Ph.D.
Director, OCD and Related Disorders Program, Department of Psychiatry, Massachusetts General Hospital, Charlestown; Professor of Psychiatry, Harvard Medical School, Boston, Massachusetts

Leanne M. Williams, Ph.D.
Professor, Stanford University School of Medicine, Stanford, California

Arnold Winston, M.D.
Chairman Emeritus, Department of Psychiatry, Mount Sinai Beth Israel Medical Center, New York

Jesse H. Wright, M.D., Ph.D.
Professor and Kolb Endowed Chair for Outpatient Psychiatry and Director, University of Louisville Depression Center, Department of Psychiatry and Behavioral Sciences, University of Louisville, Louisville, Kentucky

Eric Yarbrough, M.D.
New York, New York

Peter Yellowlees, M.B.B.S., M.D.
Professor of Psychiatry and Vice Chair for Faculty Development, Department of Psychiatry, University of California, Davis, Sacramento, California

Frank E. Yeomans, M.D., Ph.D.
Clinical Assistant Professor of Psychiatry and Director of Training, Personality Disorders Institute, Weill Cornell Medical College, New York, New York

Stuart C. Yudofsky, M.D.
Distinguished Professor Emeritus, Menninger Department of Psychiatry and Behavioral Sciences, Baylor College of Medicine, Houston, Texas; Director, Medical Research Grant Program, and Chairman, Scientific Advisory Board, Brockman Foundation, Hamilton, Bermuda

Disclosure of Interests

The following contributors to this textbook have indicated a financial interest in or other affiliation with a commercial supporter, manufacturer of a commercial product, and/or provider of a commercial service as listed below:

Neil Krishan Aggarwal, M.D., M.B.A., M.A.   Dr. Aggarwal receives grant funding from the National Institute of Mental Health to study the effects of the DSM-5 Cultural Formulation Interview vs. standard care on patient and clinician outcomes (MH102334).

Aaron T. Beck, M.D.   *Royalties:* Guilford Press.

Mahendra T. Bhati, M.D.   *Advisory Board:* Psychiatric Disease Steering Committee, Focused Ultrasound Foundation.

Peter Fonagy, Ph.D., F.B.A., F.Med.Sci., FAcSS   Dr. Fonagy is Chief Executive of the Anna Freud National Centre for Children and Families, which benefits from short courses and training programs it provides in relation to a range of mentalization-based treatments. Dr. Fonagy also holds research grants on mentalizing at University College London, which bring research income to the university.

Shefali Miller, M.D.   *Research Grants:* Merck, Sunovion.

Michael Ostacher, M.D.   *Consultant:* Johnson & Johnson, H. Lundbeck A/S, Otsuka, Sunovion, Supernus; *Research Funding:* Palo Alto Health Sciences.

Laura Weiss Roberts, M.D., M.A.   Dr. Roberts serves as Chairman and Katharine Dexter McCormick and Stanley McCormick Memorial Professor in the Department of Psychiatry and Behavioral Sciences at the Stanford University School of Medicine. Dr. Roberts has received federal funding for competitive, peer-reviewed research grants. These grants or contracts are awarded to Stanford University. Dr. Roberts owns a small company that develops science-based educational products, Terra Nova Learning Systems. This company competes for peer-reviewed small business grants and contracts. The key stakeholders, such as Stanford University and the National Institutes of Health, are fully aware of this arrangement and have given prior approval for this set of professional commitments.
In addition, Dr. Roberts:

- Serves as Editor-in-Chief, Books, for American Psychiatric Association Publishing. Funds associated with these duties are provided to Stanford University.
- Gives academic and public/community talks, for which she sometimes receives honoraria.
- Serves as the Editor-in-Chief for the journal *Academic Psychiatry*. She does not receive income for this role.
- Serves on the Advisory Board of the Bucksbaum Institute for Clinical Excellence and receives modest compensation for this role.
- Has published books and receives royalties. These royalties represent a very small proportion of Dr. Roberts' overall income.

Dr. Roberts does not receive direct funding from pharmaceutical companies for her work, and she is not on any "Speakers' Bureaus" of any kind.

Trisha Suppes, M.D., Ph.D.   In the past 12 months, Dr. Suppes has reported the following: *Grants:* National Institutes of Health, National Institute of Mental Health, National Institute on Drug Abuse, Palo Alto Health Sciences, Pathway Genomics, Stanley Medical Research Institute, VA Cooperative Studies Program; *Consultant:* Sunovion; *CME and Honoraria:* CMEology, Global Medical Education, Medscape Education; *Royalties:* Jones & Bartlett, UpToDate; *Travel Reimbursement:* CMEology, Global Medication, Sunovion.

Michael E. Thase, M.D.   During the past 3 years, Dr. Thase has reported the following: *Advisor/Consultant:* Acadia, Akili, Alkermes, Allergan (Forest, Naurex), AstraZeneca, Biohaven, Boehringer-Ingelheim, Cerecor, Clexio, Eli Lilly, Fabre-Kramer, Genomind, Gerson Lehrman Group, Guidepoint Global, Johnson & Johnson (Janssen, Ortho-McNeil), Lundbeck, MedAvante, Merck, Moksha8, Nestlé (Pamlab), Novartis, Otsuka, Pfizer, Shire, Sunovion, Takeda; *Grant Support:* Acadia, Agency for Healthcare Research and Quality, Alkermes, Avanir, Forest, Intracellular, Janssen, National Institute of Mental Health, Otsuka, Patient Centered Outcomes Research Institute (PCORI), Takeda; *Royalties:* American Psychiatric Association Publishing, Guilford Publications, Herald House, W.W. Norton & Company; *Employment (spouse):* Diane M. Sloan, Pharm.D., is a Senior Medical Director for Peloton Advantage, which does business with a number of pharmaceutical companies.

Jesse H. Wright, M.D., Ph.D.   *Equity Interest:* Empower Interactive, Mindstreet; *Royalties:* American Psychiatric Association Publishing, Guilford Press, Simon & Schuster.

The following contributors stated that they had no competing interests during the year preceding manuscript submission:

Tarek Adam, M.D., M.Sc.; W. Stewart Agras, M.D.; Jonathan Avery, M.D.; Richard Balon, M.D.; Donna S. Bender, Ph.D.; Dan G. Blazer, M.D., Ph.D.; Nicholas M. Hatzis, M.D.; Eric Hollander, M.D.; Sandra A. Jacobson, M.D.; Margery R. Johnson, M.D.; Amandeep Jutla, M.D.; Michael Kelly, M.D.; Petros Levounis, M.D., M.A.; Steven E. Lindley, M.D., Ph.D.; James Lock, M.D., Ph.D.; Lila Massoumi, M.D., ABOIHM; Edwin J. Mikkelsen, M.D.; Philip R. Muskin, M.D., M.A.; John M. Oldham, M.D.; Michelle B. Riba, M.D., M.S.; Craig S. Rosen, Ph.D.; Ruth S. Shim, M.D., M.P.H.; Andrew E. Skodol, M.D.; David Spiegel, M.D., F.A.P.A.; David C. Steffens, M.D., M.H.S.; Shannon Wiltsey Stirman, Ph.D.; Frederick J. Stoddard Jr., M.D.; Mark Sullivan, M.D.; Bonnie P. Taylor, Ph.D.

Foreword

Transitions and Perspectives

Robert E. Hales, M.D., M.B.A.
Stuart C. Yudofsky, M.D.

Transitions

For each of the six prior editions of *The American Psychiatric Publishing (APP) Textbook of Psychiatry* (the *Textbook*), we have had the privilege of collaborating with extraordinary chapter authors and gifted staff from American Psychiatric Publishing on nearly every aspect the book. This collaboration included the choice of chapter topics, innumerable communications with chapter authors, and the line-by-line and word-by-word editing of submitted chapter texts, tables, and references by us and the APP staff. We did this for over thirty years, along with editing six editions of the companion textbook, *The APP Textbook of Neuropsychiatry and Clinical Neurosciences*.

For the Sixth Edition of the *Textbook*, we enthusiastically invited Dr. Laura Weiss Roberts to join us as an editor. We wished to include her extraordinary talents and experience as an excellent author of many scientific articles, books, and book chapters. Dr. Roberts also provides a sturdy bridge to a new generation of chapter authors of the *Textbook*. Working with her on the previous edition was an absolute delight, and we were confident that under her editorial leadership, the Seventh Edition would continue to excel in the education of medical students, psychiatry residents, practicing psychiatrists, and colleagues in other subspecialties of medicine, as well as other mental health professionals. Upon reading the "galleys" of all the chapters of the Seventh Edition of the *Textbook*, we realized that our very high expectations for the future of the *Textbook* had been surpassed.

If it is true that (in many ways) "past is prelude," we believe that comparing the First Edition of the *Textbook* (Talbot et al. 1988) with the Seventh Edition (Roberts 2019) might provide some useful insights into how our field has remained the same in certain respects and how and why it has changed in other ways over the past 30 years. Given the understandable word limitations, we will touch upon only what we deem to be certain highlights in this consideration.

Perspectives

Similarities

When we compared the two books, we were surprised at how little has changed in the organizational structure over the seven editions of the *Textbook*.

The First Edition was divided into the following sections:

- Theoretical Foundations
- Assessment
- Psychiatric Disorders
- Psychiatric Treatments
- Special Topics

In the Seventh Edition, Theoretical Foundations and Assessment were collapsed into a single section, resulting in the following streamlined structure:

- Foundations
- Psychiatric Disorders
- Treatments
- Caring for Special Populations

Despite this change, even the most cursory comparison of the Contents of the First and Seventh Editions of the *Textbook* shows that the overall topical organization of the two books is essentially the same. We attribute this similarity to the current editor's steadfast adherence to our conscious decision—from the beginning—to pattern the *Textbook* on other major textbooks of the day in internal medicine, surgery, and pediatrics. Another goal was to create a textbook that was useful clinically to the busy practitioner, regardless of medical specialty or discipline.

Over the first half of the twentieth century, psychiatry strayed from its roots as a subspecialty of medicine, which diminished the respect of our colleagues from other medical specialties. At the time of the publication of the First Edition of the *Textbook*, Melvin Sabshin, M.D., the Medical Director of the American Psychiatric Association, wrote the following:

> The combination of psychiatry's boundary expansion [beyond medicine], the predominance of ideology over science, and the field's demedicalization began to produce a vulnerability. Many decision makers became skeptical about psychiatrists' capacity to diagnose and treat patients. (Sabshin 1990, p. 1270)

This demedicalization was reflected in the organizational structure and contents of some of the psychiatry textbooks of the era. Hence, our emphasis from the beginning was on basic neuroscience, genetics, epidemiology, nosology, clinical assessment, psychiatric disorders, and the full range of treatments. We applaud the decision of the editor of the new edition to retain this emphasis, as we believe that it will help to keep psychiatry squarely within the mainstream of medicine.

Other similarities in the two editions of the *Textbook* relate to the specific conditions and syndromes conceptualized as "Psychiatric Disorders." The decision not to extend the boundaries of psychiatric disorders confirms that our field has learned from the past about the dangers of overextending to areas that do not serve our profession or our patients well.

Although there is general overlap between diagnostic considerations of the two editions, one example of an exception is "Trauma- and Stressor-Related Disorders," which was not considered as a separate chapter in the First Edition. This difference is likely due to the extraordinary advances that psychiatry has made in the diagnosis and treatment of posttraumatic stress disorder (PTSD), acute stress disorder, and other trauma- and stressor-related disorders. PTSD did not become an official psychiatric diagnosis until it was included in DSM-III in 1980. Subsequently, there has been substantial research into traumatic conditions and disorders—encompassing epidemiology, genetics, neurobiology, psychosocial issues, and therapies. These topics and others are considered and covered masterfully in Chapter 15 of the Seventh Edition *Textbook* by Drs. Fred Stoddard, Naomi Simon, and Roger Pitman. We recommend this chapter as a timely, interesting, and clinically useful presentation and review of a psychiatric disorder that is particularly challenging to understand and treat.

Also similar in both editions are the exceptional expertise and reputations of the chapter authors. The primary chapter authors in the First Edition represented a veritable who's who of psychiatrists from around the world. Additionally, many of the First Edition's chapter coauthors have gone on to become major leaders in the field, and to publish influential works on the subjects of their chapters.

The uniformly high quality of the First Edition's chapter authors also applies to the authors of the Seventh Edition. We especially look forward to following the academic accomplishments and careers of the more junior chapter authors over the years to come. Finally, not only is each author a leading authority in his or her particular field, but each is also broadly based with regard to his or her approach to etiology, pathophysiology, and treatment. Thus, the biopsychosocial model pervades and prevails in both editions of the *Textbook*.

Differences

Perhaps the most dramatic difference between the two editions of the *Textbook* is found in the Treatments section. For example, the First Edition had only seven chapters in this section, while this edition of the *Textbook* features twelve. Only one chapter—"Individual Psychotherapies"—was allotted to psychotherapeutic treatments in the First Edition, whereas four chapters—"Brief Psychotherapies," "Psychodynamic Psychotherapy," "Cognitive-Behavior Therapy," and "Supportive Psychotherapy"— are needed to adequately cover these treatments in the Seventh Edition. Furthermore, in this edition of the *Textbook*, five new chapters are devoted to novel treatment approaches: "Mentalizing in Psychotherapy," "Hybrid Practitioners and Digital Treatments," "Complementary and Integrative Psychiatry," "Integrated and Collaborative Care," and "Standardized Assessment and Measurement-Based Care." These differences reflect the astounding progress in the realm of treatment that our field has made over the past quarter of a century.

Research advances have enabled us to understand much more about the psychiatric disorders that afflict our patients and how best to treat our patients with evidence-based care that is specific to the individual. This progress is emphasized in the introductory paragraph of the first chapter in the section on Treatments in the Seventh Edition of the *Textbook*, titled "Precision Psychiatry" and written by Drs. Leanne Williams, Tali Ball, and Catherine Kircos, which captures the prowess of the present and the promise of the future:

> A revolution is under way in psychiatry. We are witnessing the emergence of precision medicine for psychiatry: "precision psychiatry." Precision psychiatry is an integrative approach, one that pulls together the scientific foundations of the discipline and recent technological advances and directs them toward closing the gap between discovery and clinical translation.

Similarly, whereas in the First Edition of the *Textbook*, somatic treatments were covered in a single chapter—"Psychopharmacology and Electroconvulsive Therapy"—in which a scant 5 pages were allotted to electroconvulsive treatment, the Seventh Edition features a separate large, profusely illustrated chapter—titled "Brain Stimulation Therapies" and written by Drs. Corey Keller, Mahendra Bhati, Jonathan Downar, and Amit Etkin—devoted to this burgeoning treatment modality. Once more, an excerpt from the opening paragraph of this chapter captures the exciting state of innovation in electrical-based treatments today and the robust possibilities for tomorrow:

> In the past 20 years, brain stimulation therapies have undergone a revolution with the development of a number of novel brain stimulation interventions. Many of these new therapies have emerged from progress in neuroimaging and brain stimulation technology, and some are entering routine clinical use. Brain stimulation interventions represent a novel and expanding approach to understanding and treating psychiatric disorders.

Another important change from the First Edition of the *Textbook* to the Seventh Edition is the increased emphasis on populations whose specific concerns have been historically underappreciated in American psychiatry. In this edition, for example, the chapter titled "The Social Determinants of Mental Health," by Drs. Ruth Shim and Michael Compton, helps illuminate factors influencing mental health needs and barriers to care among special patient populations:

> Social determinants of mental health are defined as societal, environmental, and economic conditions that influence and affect mental health outcomes at the population level. In considering the current state of psychiatry as well as future directions for the field, the importance of social factors that contribute to mental health should not be underestimated. These factors are primarily responsible for disparities and inequities in mental health services access, treatment quality, and outcomes seen within and between population groups.

Conclusion

In conclusion, we have carefully read and enjoyed each chapter of the Seventh Edition of the *Textbook* and have learned a great deal in the process. We recommend this edition highly and without reservation to our students, residents, and clinical colleagues. We are deeply grateful to Dr. Roberts and the chapter authors for doing such a spectacular job of vitalizing and carrying forward the torch of this *Textbook*, which was our privilege to ignite 30 years ago and which we continue to hold closely to our hearts.

References

Roberts LW (ed): The American Psychiatric Association Publishing Textbook of Psychiatry, 7th Edition. Washington, DC, American Psychiatric Association Publishing, 2019

Talbott JA, Hales RE, Yudofsky SC (eds): The American Psychiatric Press Textbook of Psychiatry. Washington, DC, American Psychiatric Press, Inc., 1988

Sabshin M: Turning points in twentieth-century American psychiatry. Am J Psychiatry 147(10):1267–1274, 1990 2205113

Preface

With advances in basic, translational, clinical, and population sciences, the field of psychiatry is undergoing positive, transformational change. The practice of psychiatry is evolving to incorporate deeper understanding of mechanisms of disease, novel therapeutic approaches, richer evidence-based clinical approaches, and adaptive systems and models of care. Clinical assessment and treatment approaches are oriented toward recovery, well-being, and the restoration of health, rather than the simple elimination of debilitating symptoms. Stigma toward people living with mental health issues is unraveling, and it is increasingly recognized that mental disorders, which affect every age and gender, every community, and all nations, represent one of the greatest threats to public health worldwide. Psychiatrists now work shoulder to shoulder with colleagues across the health professions and the sciences and with stakeholders across society to bring about better health outcomes for the millions of people affected by mental disorders and related conditions.

A sense of great anticipation and demonstrable progress in the care of people living with or at risk for mental disorders accompanies the publication of this new Seventh Edition of *The American Psychiatric Association Textbook of Psychiatry*. Our authors have sought to put so much, with so much momentum and great care, between the covers of this book. The Seventh Edition seeks to elucidate the essentials of sound psychiatric practice and to illuminate the future directions of our field. The *Textbook* is proffered with the intentions of sharing knowledge for the benefit of our patients and our students, of dismantling health disparities, and of stimulating inquiry, so that we are not satisfied with the answers of the present day but continue to seek to meet the imperative of improving health for all people.

The *Textbook* is organized, as in the past, in four sections (Parts I through IV). Each of these sections features new authors and new content, with attention to age-related, cultural, societal, and population considerations in the practice of psychiatry.

Part I covers knowledge foundational to the practice of psychiatry, with chapters on psychiatric interviewing, diagnostic formulation, developmental assessment, laboratory testing and neuroimaging, and ethical and legal aspects of clinical psychiatry. This section also includes two new chapters on timely and highly important topics in our field, suicide risk assessment and social determinants of mental health.

Part II is focused on psychiatric disorders in alignment with DSM-5. Each of the 19 chapters in this section outlines the major diagnostic characteristics and clinical features of a specific disorder category and includes general information on the approach to the care and treatment of patients with those conditions.

Part III offers an overview of treatment strategies and methods in present-day psychiatry, a combination of evidence-based biological interventions and psychotherapies, and gives a clear sense of exciting new directions in psychiatric therapeutics. This section features contributions from true luminaries in the fields of psychiatry and psychology and proffers five rich new chapters on topics such as precision psychiatry, e-health strategies in psychiatry and mental health, complementary and integrative therapies, integrated and collaborative care, and standardized assessment and measurement-based care.

Part IV, the final section of the *Textbook,* is focused on special patient populations, including the care of women; children and adolescents; lesbian, gay, bisexual, and transgender individuals; older adults; and culturally diverse people. With these four sections, the *Textbook* offers a valuable grounding for practicing clinicians and clinical trainees in psychiatry and related mental health disciplines.

Textbooks are meant to be read, and they are meant to be read in context. Built at a particular moment in the development of a field, textbooks provide an overview of the observations, approaches, and lessons of the past and guide the reader to anticipate the discoveries, innovations, and practices of the future. In other words, textbooks provide a perspective on an academic discipline at one point in its evolution. One hopes that much of the information conveyed in a textbook will be sound and enduring, but it is certain that what is accepted as knowledge today will be informed, and revised, by new findings and novel frameworks for understanding that will arise over time. For these reasons, readers of this *Textbook* are encouraged to be rigorous in their thinking and to nurture efforts to continue learning from their scientific and clinical colleagues—and, perhaps most importantly, from their patients.

The authors of this *Textbook* have endeavored to include only accurate and up-to-date information and guidance that is in keeping with current standards of psychiatric and medical practice. Information and standards will change as medicine advances. In addition, because this *Textbook* provides a broad overview of knowledge in the field of psychiatry, the specific needs and circumstances of individual patients may not be fully addressed. This *Textbook* serves as a resource for clinical care, but diagnostic and therapeutic approaches for individual patients must be undertaken with professional judgment.

One final note: this *Textbook* is big. It is more than 1,300 pages in length and has six more chapters than appeared the Sixth Edition. In light of this new material, to keep the book readable and reasonably sized, we asked our chapter authors to focus on key features of the psychiatric disorders, and we did not reprint verbatim all of the DSM-5 diagnostic criteria. Readers are referred to DSM-5 and to companion resources, such as the Study Guide for DSM-5, for details on the DSM-5 classification.

I wish to thank my outstanding colleagues and dear friends, Robert Hales and Stuart Yudofsky, who edited earlier versions of this *Textbook* so beautifully and who invited my participation as a coeditor of the Sixth Edition, published in 2014. I offer my sincere appreciation to Ann Tennier, Senior Editor and Publishing Projects Manager, who managed this project with her usual wisdom, professionalism, and eye for detail, and to Gabrielle Termuehlen, who provided expert copyediting and logistical support for the project. The excellence of the American Psychiatric Association Publishing team merits special recognition, and I would like to thank Greg Kuny, Managing Editor, Rebecca Richters, Senior Editor, Susan Westrate, Production Manager, and Judy Castagna, Assistant Director of Production Services, for their invaluable assistance. John McDuffie, Publisher, runs an outstanding organization, and I am grateful for the privilege of having worked with him in the publishing arena for 25 years.

Laura Weiss Roberts, M.D., M.A.
Stanford, California

PART I

Foundations

CHAPTER 1

The Psychiatric Interview and Mental Status Examination

John W. Barnhill, M.D.

The psychiatric interview involves the development of a history of the patient's present illness, a mental status examination (MSE), an assessment of dangerousness and substance use, and a differential diagnosis and treatment plan. Developmental, family, and social histories are also part of the initial interview, as is a history of prior psychiatric treatments and co-occurring medical conditions. A therapeutic alliance and a therapeutic effect are both reasonable expectations, as is some sort of psychological understanding of the patient. This information is generally compiled within an often-clunky electronic medical record. Such efforts are a challenge, especially when the clinician is also expected to be kind, tactful, patient, and friendly.

The goal of this chapter is to simplify and clarify the interview process so that the clinician can confidently approach this foundational psychiatric skill. The chapter will begin with a discussion of ways in which the clinician might prepare for doing the interview, including the development of a psychiatric attitude, a biopsychosocial approach, and an ever-evolving fund of psychiatric knowledge. The second section focuses on the performance of the interview, including an outline of the phases of the typical interview and a roster of core interviewing techniques. The third section explores common clinical situations and types of patients. The chapter concludes with a discussion of ways in which goals focus and simplify the actual interview.

General Preparation

Setting the Stage

Effective psychiatric interviews can be done under almost any conditions. One interview with an agitated patient might last for a few moments in a hallway surrounded by patients, staff, and security guards. Another interview might consist of an hour-long session in a calm, quiet, uncluttered outpatient office. A third might feature a patient and trainee being observed as part of a 30-minute oral examination. Although the details vary, an underlying goal of all interviews is to provide a safe and respectful opportunity for the patient to tell his or her story. Regardless of whether the interview takes a minute or an hour, each interview has a similar underlying structure that involves observation, interaction, assessment, and plan.

Clinicians who work in an emergency department or a consultation-liaison service or who are in training generally interview everyone they are assigned. Other clinicians often decline outpatient evaluations because of a lack of expertise in a specific subspecialty area, such as substance abuse or child psychiatry. After agreeing to conduct the interview, the clinician might clarify to herself the initial goals of the patient and/or referring clinician. Clarity can ensure that the presenting issues are adequately addressed. In addition, hints of violence or other special difficulties should help steer inexperienced staff and students away from dangerous encounters.

A quick perusal of the patient's medical records, either before or after the initial interview, can inform the overall assessment by providing cross-sectional MSEs, medication lists, contact numbers, and an array of co-occurring medical and psychiatric diagnoses. Such information can suggest issues that might not otherwise be addressed in the interview.

> **Tip:** Outside information warrants appreciative skepticism. Such data can be very helpful. On the other hand, the patient's situation and diagnosis may have evolved, and the prior evaluation may have been incomplete or misguided.

Clinicians vary in the extent to which they take notes during the interview. Some only write down hard-to-remember facts, such as medication dosages and dates of hospitalizations. Others jot down reminders to themselves. For example, if an anxious patient mentions binge drinking early in the interview but is in the midst of an emotionally charged story, the interviewer might write down "alcohol" to trigger a more thorough discussion later in the session. Some interviewers bring with them an outline of an initial write-up and jot down brief notes as pertinent material comes up. Whether the interviewer is using paper and pencil or a computer, the goal is to avoid letting the recording device interfere with the development of an alliance or with the interviewer's ability to pay attention to nonverbal behavioral and interpersonal clues.

Prior to seeing the patient, the interviewer may discover that relatives and/or friends expect to be involved, either by sitting in on the interview or via an open communication with the interviewer. Some outpatient clinicians hardly ever talk to relatives. When family members are going to be involved in the eventual treatment and/or possess pertinent historical information, they are often brought into the interview. For example, family members are routinely involved in the evaluation of children and of patients who have a developmental disorder or a dementia. In addition, patients from most of the world anticipate that family members will be involved in their medical evaluations and treatment. The American emphasis on individuality and privacy can be seen as idiosyncratic to an immigrant family that presents en masse for a psychiatric evaluation. At the same time, adults are generally allowed to refuse access to relatives. States vary somewhat in regard to privacy legislation, but they generally restrict the psychiatrist's right to contact relatives over patient objection to situations that involve acute risk. Even in emergency situations, the interviewer aims to elicit information from the family without giving up unnecessary or confidential information.

Interviewer Attitude

The preferred clinical attitude combines a host of desirable emotions, such as warmth and spontaneity. Of course, interviewing styles vary, but in general, interviewers try to maintain an attitude of respectful curiosity.

Interviewers listen differently. In interviewing a patient who presents with prominent anxiety, one psychiatrist might listen with an ear for symptom clusters that fit DSM-5 (American Psychiatric Association 2013) criteria for disorders that often co-occur with anxiety: substance use, trauma, obsessions/compulsions, or one of the anxiety disorders. A more psychodynamically oriented therapist might look for factors that contributed to the anxiety; for example, unreliable early caregivers might lead to an inhibited ability to express anger, associated with a variety of defenses (e.g., denial, undoing, reaction formation) that reduce efficacy and perpetuate the baseline anxiety (Auchincloss 2015). A couples counselor might hear the same anxiety but listen for maladaptive patterns of interpersonal behavior, focusing less on the individual and more on the couple. A therapist with a cognitive-behavioral perspective might listen for cycles of thinking and behavior that could contribute to and exacerbate the presenting symptoms (Beck 2011). Most interviewers learn to listen in ways that conform to the needs of the patient and situation as well as their own training and theoretical and personal biases.

Biopsychosocial Approach

Without having a broad working knowledge of psychiatry, the interviewer will be awash in unanalyzed data and will be unable to develop a coherent narrative that explains the patient's situation. Sherlock Holmes is the quintessential interviewer-observer. Underestimated, however, is the amount of background information available to him. He might notice mud on shoes, for example, and conclude that the victim (or perpetrator) had spent time in a particular quarry in the north of England. Although anyone might notice the muddy shoes, Holmes notices the relevance both because he is observant and because he maintains a vast fund of knowledge. Even with the Internet readily available, the modern interviewer needs to be able to spontaneously recognize a wide variety of triggers that should prompt further investigation.

Clinicians who study only the areas that interest them risk making systematic errors throughout their careers. Practice may make perfect, as the saying goes, but practice also makes permanent; without diligently studying the entire field, the interviewer will miss unappreciated details.

There are several ways for the interviewer to develop and maintain a knowledge base. The first is to read and study broadly via journals, texts, conferences, and review courses (Muskin and Dickerman 2016; Roberts and Louie 2014). Another is to read pertinent information prior to seeing a particular patient. Some interviewers jot notes during the interview that can later trigger an Internet or textbook search. Such a process can improve the quality of the interviewer's understanding of the patient and—

when the search is explained to the patient at the next meeting—lay the groundwork for a deepening of the therapeutic alliance.

The types of information sought can be subdivided into three categories, conforming to the biopsychosocial model of psychiatry (Engel 1980). Although the three pillars will not be equally pertinent in each clinical situation, there are few psychiatric interviews that can afford to completely neglect any one component of the biopsychosocial model.

Biological

Interviewers do not need to be psychopharmacologists, but the mention of venlafaxine, for example, may prompt the clinician to wonder if some physician had diagnosed the patient with depression. Venlafaxine, however, is also used for anxiety and panic, is frequently used for pain, and—as is true for all medications—is sometimes mistakenly prescribed. If the patient then mentions having diabetes, the interviewer would want to spontaneously recognize the interrelationship between depression, psychiatric medication, and diabetes. When the interviewer then asks whether the patient gained weight on psychiatric medications or whether the patient has troublesome diabetic neuropathy (which might have been the trigger for choosing venlafaxine), the story of the illness becomes more coherent, and the patient is implicitly reassured of the interviewer's competence (Goldberg and Ernst 2012; Levenson and Ferrando 2016).

Similarly, the interview is simplified and strengthened when the interviewer recognizes the relevance when the patient indicates that he has been dutifully taking 25 mg/day (or 225 or 375 mg/day) of venlafaxine for the past 2 months, or when he mentions that he only takes it on the days he feels especially symptomatic, or when he casually mentions that he ran out of pills several days earlier and has been feeling sick ever since. Without quite a lot of practical knowledge about all of the pertinent medications, the interviewer will not know whether the patient's story includes a therapeutic trial or whether the patient's symptoms might be attributable to side effects from a high dosage or side effects from withdrawal. In other words, the mention of a drug like venlafaxine or an illness like diabetes may prompt the interviewer to consider a broad array of topics, including depression, anxiety, panic, pain, metabolic syndrome, medication adherence, and medication withdrawal effects. Such recognition simplifies and strengthens the interview by bringing together seemingly disparate bits of information and by helping to guide the direction of the interview.

Psychological

The psychological understanding of patients can be separated into diagnostic descriptions (e.g., DSM-5 criteria) and narrative descriptions that are heavily informed by psychotherapeutic schools of thought (e.g., psychodynamics, cognitive-behavioral therapy [CBT], interpersonal therapy).

The currently dominant model in American psychiatry is descriptive. In the descriptive model, which is featured in DSM-5 and other medical nomenclatures such as the *International Classification of Diseases*, 10th Revision (ICD-10; World Health Organization 1992), symptoms are clustered into recognizable disorders. For example, people with schizophrenia do not all have the same symptoms, but they generally do have a history of psychosis, cognitive problems, and psychosocial dysfunction. One or two of these variables (e.g., long-standing homelessness and poor functioning) might trigger an efficient search for commonly co-occurring symptoms (Black and Grant 2014; First 2014).

> **Tip:** All combinations of information can yield a differential diagnosis that can evolve with additional information.

For example, "car wreck + 20-year-old man" might prompt inquiry into substance abuse and impulse-control problems, whereas "new-onset depression + hospitalization + elderly" might prompt a focused inquiry into delirium as well as depression. An understanding of typical symptom constellations improves the interviewer's efficiency and thoroughness and simplifies the process of doing the interview.

Interviews are prone to systematic error. For example, we might have a tendency to repeatedly see the same diagnosis, finding, say, mood instability or trauma in almost every patient. Such "confirmation bias" may reflect a training or personal bias or an unconscious defense against the complexity and ambiguity of psychiatry and medicine. Confirmation bias may also allow the clinician to make use of a preferred therapeutic modality (a mood stabilizer for bipolar disorder, for example, or perhaps CBT for posttraumatic stress disorder [PTSD]). Another common bias relates to the "loudness" of a disorder. Obvious and potentially dangerous complaints are generally recognized, whereas less-obvious diagnoses (e.g., obsessive-compulsive disorder, avoidant personality disorder) can get ignored. Evidence increasingly points to the reality that treatments are more successful when they address all pertinent psychiatric disorders (e.g., substance use and depression) rather than addressing diagnoses sequentially (Avery and Barnhill 2018).

Description may be the dominant psychiatric paradigm, but much of the field also relies on narrative. Data-gathering in psychiatry, unlike that in other medical fields, involves information that is filtered through a patchwork of complex and uncomfortable wishes, fears, and memories. Such complexity presumably underlay Jerome Groopman's decision to specifically exclude psychiatrists from his best-selling book *How Doctors Think*. As he wrote, "How psychiatrists think was beyond my abilities" (Groopman 2007, p. 7).

The psychiatric interviewer will frequently encounter *resistance*, which refers to anything that prevents the patient from talking openly to the interviewer. *Conscious resistance* occurs when the patient knowingly neglects, distorts, or makes things up. *Unconscious resistance* leads to similarly incomplete stories, but the mechanism is assessed to be outside of the patient's awareness. Sigmund Freud focused much of his work on this process of keeping material out of awareness (i.e., *repression*), although later psychoanalysts focused on delineating a variety of other defenses.

Sublimation and *humor* are considered to be healthy defenses, and they can contribute to alliance building and treatment decisions. Other defenses are more likely to derail a successful interview. For example, a paranoid patient may *project* malevolent thoughts onto the interviewer, and the interviewer may accept and internalize such projections in a process known as *projective identification*. In such a situation, the clinician may find him- or herself behaving with uncharacteristic hostility. By recognizing his or her own internal reaction, the clinician can better maintain equilibrium while also gaining greater insight into the patient (Gabbard 2014; Yudofsky 2005).

Unconscious processes also contribute to the development of *transference*, which is defined as the redirection of feelings from one relationship to another; most classically, the transference grows out of an early relationship (such as with a parent) onto the therapist. *Positive transference* allows patients to trust strangers with their life stories. Such automatic reactions are generally not discussed in an extended therapy, much less in a single interview, but without them, the interview would likely remain superficial (Viederman 2011). Transference is more often discussed when it interferes with the interview, such as when the patient has a *negative transference*. Although some so-called difficult patients may be manifesting negative transference, others are manifesting generic hostility. In either event, the initial interview is rarely the time for the clinician to try to explicitly interpret the transference to the patient. More typically, the interviewer silently identifies the defense (e.g., devaluation or projection), prompting both a deeper understanding of the patient and maintenance of a professional, helpful attitude toward a patient who might otherwise be experienced as difficult.

The interviewer may also want to monitor his or her own reactions to patients, especially when these reactions feel unusual. This recognition of one's own reactions—generally described as *countertransference*—can help the interviewer maintain a professional attitude under trying circumstances and can also provide crucial insight into the patient's interpersonal world. For example, if the interviewer feels an uncharacteristic aversion to a particular patient, she might wonder if this patient has pushed a particular historical button (perhaps an overbearing patient is reminiscent of the interviewer's overbearing parent). If so, the silent recognition of her own countertransference reaction can be a personal "Aha!" moment for the clinician and allow her to proceed more robustly with the interview. In addition, the interviewer's sense of aversion provides a visceral understanding of the patient's world when he says that he is lonely and people always avoid him.

Social

The "social" aspect of *biopsychosocial* refers to the sociological, religious, spiritual, ethnic, and racial issues that may be pertinent to patients. Some of this information may seem like "common knowledge," but exploring specifics will often lead to a discussion that can inform an understanding of the patient (Lewis-Fernández et al. 2016; Lim 2014).

For example, a 20-year-old woman might come in with a chief complaint of sadness after a loss. If the patient is also a lesbian African American college student, the interviewer has choices. One option is to dutifully write down these demographic details in the section for "identifying information" and then forget them, perhaps in an effort to see the patient as an individual rather than as some sort of reductionistic stereotype. This option may, however, be a mistake, because it might ignore clues that help make sense of the patient's situation (Gara et al. 2012).

Instead of passing over these demographic variables, the preferable action for the interviewer is to mull over possible links and listen for clues to their possible relevance. For example, what is this particular patient's perspective on being lesbian? In what phase of the coming out process is she? To what extent is she ambivalent about her orientation? Has she told her family? Is she dating (Levounis et al. 2012)? Similar questions might arise regarding her being African American. Although an interviewer from the dominant subculture (e.g., white in many areas of the United States) may view America as being beyond racial issues, such a view is not shared by many people who belong to marginalized subcultures. For them, discrimination remains an ongoing threat to mental health (Chae et al. 2011). Alternatively, if the clinician is also black or gay (or both), then shared, unanalyzed assumptions can lead to other kinds of blind spots and errors.

When interviewing people from differing backgrounds, the interviewer need not become either de-skilled or a cultural anthropologist. If "sadness after a loss" is the patient's chief complaint, cultural factors may or may not be especially pertinent to an initial assessment. It is difficult for the interviewer to know in advance which aspects of the patient's life might have significantly triggered or complicated the presenting constellation of symptoms. When in doubt, the interviewer can simply ask for the patient's perspective.

Performance of the Interview

The psychiatric interview begins with observation, but the interviewer needs to recall that first impressions work both ways. At the same time that the clinician is silently creating and discarding potential diagnoses, the patient is likely formulating questions of her own. Does the interviewer seem pleasant? Respectful? Trustworthy? Knowledgeable? It would be difficult to overstate the importance of nonverbal communication to the psychiatric interview.

For purposes of discussion, the interview is divided into three phases (for an overview of the structure of an interview, see Table 1–1). The *initial phase* allows the patient to voice his or her chief concern, whereas the *later phase* will become increasingly driven by efforts to clarify the history, MSE, and DSM-5 diagnoses. The interview concludes with a period of *negotiation and summary*. Information from all phases of the interview will inform the overall assessment of the patient. Distillation of many types of information into a straightforward note is integral to the process of completing an interview (discussed in the section "Structure of the Write-Up of the Psychiatric Interview").

Following discussion of these three interview phases, this section of the chapter concludes with a roster of interview *techniques*.

Initial Phase: The Patient's Chief Concern

The initial phase of the interview has two main goals. The first is to understand and explore the patient's current chief concern. The second is to give the interviewer the time and the information to begin to make a set of tentative hypotheses about the patient. This phase allows the patient to tell her own story.

While the patient is talking, the clinician might consciously consider how she is dressed; how she moves, speaks, and interacts; and what she chooses to discuss. Such observations can lead almost immediately to tentative theories about the patient and the beginnings of a differential diagnosis.

An opening, nondirective question might be "Tell me about what brought you here today." The initial interview is not, however, the moment to become a caricature of a mid-twentieth-century psychoanalyst—that is, a silent, dour, and impassive observer. Even silence is active; nonverbal encouragements can include nods of the

TABLE 1–1.	Performance of the interview

Initial phase

   Patient's chief concern

Later phase

   Active development of the story

   Mental status examination

Negotiation and summary

   Patient preferences

   Treatment plan

head, appropriate amounts of eye contact, and body language that conveys attentive concern. Short requests can help—for example, "Tell me more about what you mean"—as can specifically going back to a point that the patient made moments earlier. An empathic stance is surprisingly difficult to maintain, however, and the interviewer may feel tempted to quickly shift the interview to fit her own agenda and associations. Under most circumstances, the interviewer preserves this initial phase for the patient's point of view.

When given an opportunity to speak freely, some patients will present a crystalline story that fits exactly what the interviewer is looking for. Others will spin a story that may be internally consistent but barely touches on the issues that brought the patient in for the evaluation. Still others will founder and either drift across seemingly unrelated life events or grind to a halt within a few moments. While "saying what comes to mind" is a central tenet in psychoanalysis, a diagnostically oriented interviewer pays consistent attention to his or her goals. Even early on, the interviewer may flexibly and tactfully bring the patient back to the reason he or she has appeared for the interview. One way to accomplish this redirection is to ask the patient why he called for an appointment on that particular day or to speculate on what has led others to be concerned about him (e.g., "Do you have any thoughts about what might have prompted your wife to call the ambulance?").

While providing the patient with the opportunity to speak freely, the interviewer continues to develop a tentative differential diagnosis and history of present illness. The rest of the interview will be devoted to gathering additional information and testing hypotheses that spring from these initial observations.

> **Tip:** While developing a differential diagnosis, consciously consider diagnoses that span multiple DSM-5 chapters (e.g., anxiety, depression, obsessive-compulsive disorder) before investigating any one of them.

Techniques vary during this early phase. Open-ended questions are most often recommended (see subsection "Techniques" following discussion of phases), but some patients do best with "warm-up" questions that are intended to yield straightforward demographic information and yes/no answers. Some people prefer to begin with small talk, while others resent discussion that does not refer specifically to their most pressing issues. Patients generally allow attentive and well-meaning interviewers the opportunity to try out different approaches to determine what works best.

Later Phase: Deepening the Understanding

By the end of the initial phase of the interview, the clinician will have a sense of likely diagnoses as well as a tentative understanding of the patient. Much of the rest of the interview consists of completing three tasks that were begun during the initial phase: 1) further development of the history of present illness, 2) collection of other aspects of the patient's history, and 3) performance of the MSE.

A core goal of this later phase is for the interviewer to make a conscious effort to shift the patient's concerns and complaints into the interviewer's story of the patient's present illness. To do so, the interviewer considers silent hypotheses, likely comorbidities, and the breadth of possible diagnoses. While remaining attentive to various points of view (including that of the patient), the clinician begins to fashion a narrative that is his own.

A working alliance underlies this data acquisition. Attentive, kindly curiosity goes a long way, especially when the patient is being asked by a near stranger to explore behaviors, thoughts, and feelings that she might prefer to avoid. A clinician armed with a lot of excellent questions (or validated rating tools) and a harsh manner is likely to compile data that are incomplete and misleading. In contrast, the creation of a strong initial working alliance can be therapeutic in itself, encouraging transparency and smoothing the transition when the interviewer wants to shift to a more active, direct assessment of symptoms or history.

The interviewer should elicit a significant amount of other information, including psychiatric, medical, family, developmental, and social histories. As described later in the section "Components of the Psychiatric Write-Up," historical information may not be directly related to the presenting complaint but may play a crucial role in an understanding of the person and the development of a treatment plan.

The MSE is a cross-sectional evaluation of the patient and is a core aspect of every psychiatric contact. It includes assessments of the patient's general appearance, mood, affect, speech, thought process, thought content (including suicidality and homicidality), perceptions, cognition, and executive functioning. Mental status is assessed throughout the interview, although some aspects of the MSE, such as cognition and memory, tend to be more formally assessed toward the end of the interview. See the section titled "Mental Status Examination" later in the chapter for definitions and a more thorough discussion of these terms.

The later phase of the interview features an increasing number of closed-ended questions that seek clear-cut answers. Approving nods and tactful eye contact can help maintain the alliance during this period of data acquisition. It is fine for the clinician to explicitly explain the situation, saying, for example, "We are short on time, so let's move on to talk about your work," or "It sounds like the situation at work has been rough, but let's shift gears to talking about your family." Transitions can often be smoothly effected by making use of any topics or words that the patient has recently used. If, for example, the patient has been talking about her family at length, the interviewer might say, "You mentioned that your husband has been having some 'senior moments.' Have you been having problems with your own memory?" Regardless of the answer to that question, the interviewer can then shift to a more formal cognitive assessment.

Prior to ending this phase, the interviewer may want to ask the patient if there is anything else he or she would like the clinician to know.

Negotiation and Summary Phase

The interview is generally incomplete without some discussion of diagnosis and treatment. This conversation might take place at the end of the initial session, or it might occur during an ensuing session after the interviewer has had a chance to obtain more information, seen the patient for a second (or third) visit, or received supervision. This phase of the process is not part of the standard oral examinations taken by trainees and may seem superfluous to the interviewer, but to the patient it is often the key element of the evaluation. Active patient participation is strategically crucial because cooperation and adherence are central to treatment success, and patient preference plays a critical role in treatment success (van Schaik et al. 2004).

The negotiation phase is also the time for psychoeducation, referral to another clinician or clinic, and gaining a sense of whether the patient has been satisfied with the assessment process. Before the interview ends, the interviewer might ask the most relevant clinical question of all: "Do you think you will follow through with the recommended treatment?"

Techniques

Verbal and nonverbal communications are central to the psychiatric interview. These communications can be divided into three overlapping types: nonspecific, nondirective, and directive. *Nonspecific* interview techniques are used throughout the interview to enhance the patient's experience and lay the groundwork for an alliance and a more productive interview. *Nondirective* techniques encourage the patient to continue on a train of thought. *Directive* techniques narrow the focus, perhaps to a factual answer or a topic change. Table 1–2 lists these core interview techniques.

There are many ways to develop interview skills. Observation is the classic method, and the novice interviewer will quickly see that senior interviewers have a variety of styles. Trainees may practice with each other, sometimes interviewing actual patients and sometimes interviewing each other. Other interviewers read guidebooks (e.g., Evans et al. 2010). Knowledge of core techniques and the avoidance of derailing errors can improve all aspects of the interaction.

Tact and timing are central to the interview. For example, a patient might say, "I've been so sad since my mother died." In response to that poignant piece of information, the interviewer has choices. For example, she might decide to explore the patient's emotional reaction to the mother's death by looking directly at the patient, appearing warmly interested, and saying, "Could you tell me more about it?" An attentive, open-ended approach can allow the patient to express reactions to the death that are more complex than relatively straightforward sadness. If the patient then discusses ambivalence or relief, the interviewer might decide to tactfully make use of a confrontation (e.g., "It sounds like you've been very sad since your mother's death, and that her death after so many years of suffering has also felt like a relief"). On the other hand, time might be short or the patient may be especially dramatic or tangential, and

TABLE 1–2.	Core interviewing techniques

Nonspecific techniques

Attentive listening involves tactful eye contact and encouraging body language that demonstrate attention, as well as questions and comments that indicate that the patient has been heard.

Confidentiality allows patients to speak more freely. Clarification of what will—and what will not—be shared with others enhances the therapeutic alliance.

Neutrality is a psychoanalytic dictum that technically means working equidistant from the id, the ego, and the superego. This stance discourages the interviewer from moralizing, intellectualizing, and launching into prematurely zealous therapy.

The *therapeutic alliance* develops as the patient and clinician work together to understand the presenting problem and create a treatment plan.

The *therapeutic effect* often develops in a diagnostic interview after the patient feels heard.

An *uninterpreted positive transference* is a basic trust in the benevolence of the clinician. It allows for the rapid development of a therapeutic alliance.

Nondirective techniques

Open-ended questions usually elicit an extensive response.

"Could you tell me more about your marriage?"

"What brought you to the hospital today?"

Open-ended sounds are often accompanied by an encouraging facial expression and body language.

"Mm-hmm."

Open-ended encouragement serves a similar purpose to open-ended sounds.

"Go on…."

"Please explain what you mean."

Reflecting content and feelings reinforces that the patient has been heard and encourages continued discussion.

"It sounds like you've been really depressed."

Repetition and restatement are more specific ways to encourage the patient to continue.

Patient: I feel like no one ever listens to me.

Interviewer: So it seems like no one is listening….

Directive techniques

Closed-ended questions elicit short answers. They get facts.

"How long have you been married?"

Confrontations communicate discrepancies to the patient. They can help assess the patient's ability to work with conflictual information, model the recognition of such discrepancies, and potentially deepen the relationship. *Confrontation* is not a synonym for *attack*.

"You mention you were abandoned by your boyfriend,…and…you also said that you kicked him out and changed the locks."

Limit setting and transitions make it clear that the interviewer is changing gears.

"I'd like to hear more about your family, but I'm going to need to learn more about your depression."

the pursuit of an emotional story could distract from the goals of that phase of the interview. The clinician might then choose to use closed-ended questions to inquire more specifically about depressive symptoms or to explore specific historical details about the mother's death.

Other interviewing behaviors are more likely to be derailing errors—comments and questions that tend to reduce clinical effectiveness (Table 1–3). For example, the interviewer might respond to the news about the patient's mother's death with her own discomfort, perhaps from a countertransference reaction to the topic of parental mortality. This might lead the clinician to psychologically back away from the patient, becoming silent and distant, perhaps by ducking behind a laptop to take notes. Alternatively, clinician discomfort might lead to excessive personal disclosure (e.g., "I know how you feel. My own mother died a few months ago, and I'm a wreck.") or to premature advice (e.g., "How about a support group?"). Although such behaviors and comments might negatively affect the interview, patients generally rebound quickly from the derailment if they perceive the interviewer to be flexible and well-meaning. And when used judiciously, self-disclosure and supportive suggestions can deepen the alliance and/or help the patient.

Interviewing strategies depend heavily on the goals of the particular phase of the clinical interaction. Two other variables that significantly influence the interviewer's minute-to-minute decisions are the *type of situation* and the *type of patient*.

Types of Situations

Although all interviews include a safety assessment and a differential diagnosis, there are many types of interviews, each with a different goal and a different primary concern (Table 1–4).

For example, an elderly man is being evaluated in the emergency department for cognitive decline, agitation, and depression. While such a patient may evoke a variety of thoughts and concerns among members of the treatment team, the primary evaluation goals are always the same: *safety* (determining whether the patient is suicidal, homicidal, or unable to care for himself) and *triage* (considering whether the patient is to be admitted, discharged, transferred to medicine, or held overnight). If the interviewer decides that the patient has mild cognitive decline, a serious depression, *and* an inability to care for himself, the patient is likely to be admitted to psychiatry. If that same patient is deemed to be safe—perhaps because of excellent social supports—but with the same psychiatric diagnoses, he will likely be discharged to outpatient treatment. In that setting, definitive diagnosis becomes less pivotal than the social assessment.

When that same patient is admitted to the adjacent *inpatient psychiatric unit*, the next clinician's interview will have a different mandate. On the unit, dangerousness is again assessed, but the focus is on making the most accurate possible diagnosis and fine-tuning a treatment strategy. Those clinicians will focus on whether the patient has a dementia, and if so, which kind. They will look for a major depression, a history of successful or unsuccessful treatments, and any comorbidities. The inpatient clinicians will also aggressively seek out old records, collateral sources, and any other pieces of information that can help clarify the situation.

That same patient may then agree to take part in an *oral examination* that is performed annually in all psychiatric residencies accredited by the Accreditation Council

---

TABLE 1–3.   **Derailing errors**

Double questions are problematic because they generally warrant multiple answers.

"Have you been depressed or had trouble with substance abuse?"

False reassurance differs from a reassuring attitude by not being true.

"It is great to meet you. I'm sure we'll fix you up in no time."

Judgmental questions inhibit responses.

"Do you realize suicide is a sin?" (said with implied disapproval)

Nonverbal disapproval also inhibits responses.

"How long have you been a disappointment to your parents?" (said with a squinted eye and critical tone)

Poor eye contact is one of many ways the interviewer can express a lack of interest.

Premature advice involves making suggestions prior to developing a solid understanding of the situation (e.g., proposing behavioral changes within minutes of meeting a patient).

"I'm sorry to hear about the breakup, but you'll feel better if you meet someone new. Maybe you should join a couple of dating websites."

Premature closure involves accepting a diagnosis before it is fully verified (e.g., immediately assuming that a sad patient has major depression). It is one of many types of cognitive errors that can mislead the interviewer.

Psychiatric jargon is likely to confuse patients.

TABLE 1–4.   **Types of situations**

Interview type/location	Primary goal	Primary concern
Emergency department	Triage (geographical)	Suicide/injury
Inpatient psychiatric unit	Diagnosis/treatment	Suboptimal treatment
Psychotherapist office	Triage (choice of therapy)	Suboptimal therapy
Nontherapeutic (e.g., capacity) interview	Evaluation	Balancing safety and autonomy

for Graduate Medical Education. In many ways, the oral examination has become the prototypical psychiatric interview. In it, an examiner observes while an interviewer conducts a 30-minute interview with a patient; after the patient leaves, the interviewer is asked to present and discuss the case with the examiner. Evaluation is focused on ensuring competency in about 25 areas in five major categories (physician–patient relationship, psychiatric interview, case presentation, differential diagnosis, and treatment plan). The goal of this examination is to demonstrate broad competence. This situation is typical in some ways (talking to a patient for half an hour) but quite unique in others (a silent observer, no collateral information, no follow-up, and no actual treatment relevance aside from the possibility of a therapeutic effect of the interview itself). Most pertinent to this discussion, the primary goal is demonstration of overall competency (i.e., examination success), and generally speaking, the primary concern is inability to demonstrate broad competency (i.e., examination failure).

While that patient is hospitalized, his son might recognize his own caretaker stress from being the primary patient's only living relative. The son might then seek a consultation in an outpatient psychotherapist's office. The outpatient therapist might recognize that although the son does not have a major mental illness, he is exhausted and worried. That interviewer-therapist might devote a modest amount of time to diagnosis, minimal time to dangerousness, and extensive time to issues that may be justifiably given short shrift in an emergency department or inpatient unit. For example, a psychodynamically oriented clinician might do an initial screen and then focus on topics such as psychotherapy history, relationship stability, psychological mindedness, empathy, ability to trust, intelligence, school or work history, and impulse control. In the clinician's choice of treatment options, these variables can play as large a role as the DSM-5 diagnosis. By the end of the evaluation, the son may have decided two things: that he is interested in seeking psychotherapy and that he is unwilling to have his father live with him.

The inpatient clinician may decide that the father has a dementia and an improving depression and begin treatment. If the patient improves psychiatrically but insists on returning home despite a marginal ability to safely live alone, the team might call for a *nontherapeutic* interview to assess capacity. In this interview, a clinician would assess the patient's ability to discuss the risks and benefits of the proposed disposition. Diagnosis would play a role in this assessment, but capacity does not hinge on diagnosis (i.e., people with a diagnosis of schizophrenia or dementia often retain capacity). As is the case in all forensic evaluations, this interviewer is functioning in the role of evaluator, not of therapist, a distinction that has ethical, legal, and practical implications.

Types of Patients

Interviews are affected by the type of patient as well as the type of situation. Excellent texts discuss how diagnosis affects the clinical interview (e.g., MacKinnon et al. 2015), but tailoring of the interview to the specific patient presupposes knowledge of the diagnosis. For the purposes of this chapter, I subdivide patients into four groups—revved up, down, odd, and evasive—based on what can generally be observed within a few minutes.

Revved-Up Patient

Revved-up patients appear excited or high and tend to display psychomotor agitation. Likely diagnoses include mania, psychosis, hyperactive delirium, and substance withdrawal or intoxication.

Evaluation of the revved-up patient involves two focal concerns. The first is safety. The interviewer might station himself near the doorway to ensure a quick exit in case of a threat, and he might ensure the availability of helpful staff members, security guards, and sedating medications. In addition to being watchful for dangers to the staff, the interviewer must remain alert to the possibility that the revved-up patient could hurt herself or could be withdrawing from a substance such as alcohol. Pursuit of more routine information generally is deferred when safety is at stake.

Second, the interviewer will need to be primed to shift to an unusually active approach (Freed and Barnhill 2019). Instead of offering a wide-open time for the agitated, threatening patient to clarify her complaints, the interviewer will likely shift to a series of binary choices: "You are too excited now to be safe, so I would like to offer you a choice. Would you like to go to your room and remain quiet, or would you like medication?" This question would likely be followed by, "Would you like to take these medications by mouth or by a shot?"

The interview is also adapted for revved-up patients who are not dangerous. Revved-up patients tend to calm when talking to an interviewer who is clear, soft-spoken, and pleasantly firm. The patient might pull for humor and banter—and these can be used judiciously to develop an alliance—but they can further rev up the patient and distract the interview. The revved-up presentation also calls for exploration of likely diagnoses (e.g., mania, substance use, delirium), potentially at the expense of other aspects of the interview.

Down Patient

The "down" patient appears depressed and/or speaks little. Shrugs abound. While interviews often begin with a period of "free speech," the down patient may manage only a few monotonous words. This behavior can be disheartening to the interviewer, but, as in working with the revved-up patient who veers immediately away from talking about pertinent information, the interview of the down patient is adapted to the patient.

Appearing constricted and quiet can reflect depression, of course, but it can also reflect anxiety, a neurocognitive disorder, a developmental delay, or a variety of disorders that can involve wariness and a concern about how the individual is perceived (e.g., body dysmorphic disorder, PTSD, psychosis, avoidant personality disorder). In other words, the differential diagnosis of the down patient should extend beyond the DSM-5 "Depressive Disorders" chapter.

Different sorts of down patients warrant different interviews. For example, the deeply depressed patient may be quiet because he feels that his situation is hopeless. The psychotically paranoid patient may be quiet because she does not trust the interviewer. The depressed patient tends to feel isolated and abandoned, so the interviewer might sit a bit closer and amp up the warmth. The interviewer might also comment on the patient's appearance (e.g., "You look very sad"). The paranoid patient—who fears attack—often responds best to an interview style that is notably sober minded and in which the interviewer sits a few inches further away than usual. It would probably be a tactical error for the interviewer to sit with a silent, frightened, paranoid patient and start off by saying, "Your biggest worry is that people can read your mind." Although this statement may perhaps be accurate, the patient may feel that his core paranoid concern has just come true. Stated later and more tactfully, such a communication can help the patient trust the situation.

There are, of course, multiple variations of paranoia and depression, and the alert interviewer will look attentively for patterns. In the emergency department, a paranoid man who is clean but disheveled might prompt a concern for acute stimulant intoxication, whereas more chronic signs of self-neglect (e.g., grimy fingernails) might point toward long-standing substance abuse or a chronic psychosis such as schizophrenia.

Anxiety—either acute and situational or long-standing—can often lead to a stymied interview. Like the depressed or paranoid patient, the anxious patient is often more able to relax with an interviewer whose words and style directly counterbalance the patient's primary concerns. In other words, anxiety can be diminished by tactful, calm reassurance.

Odd Patient

Initially odd or idiosyncratic behavior involves a broad differential diagnosis. Many psychotic and manic patients present with odd or disorganized speech, but so do people with substance use disorders and those with several types of neuropsychiatric problems (e.g., aphasias, neurocognitive disorders).

So-called odd patients may not make complete sense. Such patients can frustrate the interviewer who is seeking a sturdily explanatory psychiatric narrative, marked by a crisp roster of symptoms. Interview adaptations focus on helping structure the patient, serving as an external "container" for the disorganization. Tactful interruptions are commonly used (e.g., "I know you have much to tell me, but I would like to shift to getting some basic information"). Similarly, while the patient may want to give a "complete" answer, efficient interviewing may involve asking questions that pull for brief answers (e.g., "I see you've thought a lot about the previous treatment team, but could you tell me when you had that last hospitalization?").

Evasive Patient

Many patients evade meaningful content. An obsessional patient is liable to focus on relatively trivial or dry details, for example, and the interviewer might try to "follow the affect" by picking up on scraps of emotionally laden content. A histrionic patient may talk at length but not provide the sort of meaningful narrative that helps with the diagnosis; the interviewer will likely need to shift gears and "follow the content" in order to gather a sufficient amount of concrete detail.

Other evasive patients are deceptive or self-deceptive. For example, many people underreport substance use, which complicates diagnosis and treatment. Motivational interviewing may reduce deception by nonjudgmentally exploring the patient's substance use and interest in treatment (Levounis et al. 2017; Miller and Rollnick 1991). Transparency about so-called toxic habits can remain elusive, however, and clinicians who seek a substance use history often combine information from the interview with collateral information and suggestive lab results. It is also common practice to double the self-estimated substance use and move on with other aspects of the history.

People may appear evasive for a variety of reasons. Dissociative patients provide incomplete histories because of memory gaps, whereas patients with PTSD steer away from relevant material to avoid painful memories and feelings. Malingering patients consciously lie, whereas patients with factitious disorder know that they are creating an untrue story but do not know why. Patients with somatic symptom and related disorders tend to answer psychological inquiries with physical symptoms and a lack of insight.

Evasive patients can demoralize and anger their interviewers. Steady professionalism may be easier to maintain when we recognize that it is often very difficult to distinguish between the types of evasive patients, and most of them are not deliberately lying or trying to undercut the interview.

Local Cultures

Psychiatric subcultures vary across regions, hospitals, and even different services within the same institution. Often unspoken and incompletely clarified, these cultural/institutional differences dramatically affect the interviewer. The following is a sampling of questions affected by local cultures: Should a male interviewer wear a tie? When interviewing a 25-year-old woman, should the clinician call her "Ms." or "Miss," use her first name, or just avoid calling her anything? What should the patient be expected to call the clinician? Generally speaking, dress code and name conventions are gauged so as not to interfere with the work; clinicians who choose to assert their individuality against the locally prevailing professional custom are likely to encounter difficulty.

In comparison with local conventions regarding professional appearance and accepted ways of addressing patients, the locally prevailing model of the mind will be more variable and less visible. As with other variations from expectations, culturally dystonic models of the mind are likely to lead to conflict. For example, one inpatient service might expect a psychodynamic life narrative to be provided for every patient (Perry et al. 1987; Summers 2003). A different service might expect every case discussion to include a careful review of DSM-5 symptom clusters, specifiers, and co-occurring diagnoses. A third team—even on the same physical unit—might instead expect an approach that explicitly draws from several different models and modes of explanation (McHugh and Slavney 1998). Medical and neurological inquiries may be standard, or they may be exceptional. As part of a biopsychosocial assessment, the Cultural Formulation Interview (CFI) might be conducted with every patient (see the "Cultural Formulation" chapter in DSM-5 Section III ["Emerging Measures and Models"]). Alternatively, no one on another unit might have ever heard of the CFI. Does the local culture encourage an attempt to "do it all"? Or does the local culture encourage the pursuit of only the most pertinent components of the evaluation? Does the culture encourage dissent?

Many U.S. clinicians work outside of an institution, but few work completely outside the reach of organizations such as Medicaid and Medicare. These bureaucracies do not intrude into the subtleties of the interview, but their rules directly affect reimbursement, malpractice, documentation, and ultimately the expected interview.

Structure of the Write-Up of the Psychiatric Interview

Write-up expectations inform the actual interview. Although interviews vary widely in terms of duration and structure, all initial psychiatric notes include the same basic categories (Table 1–5).

Interviewers who do not anticipate these expectations will not be able to elicit enough specific information. At the same time, the amount of required information can seem daunting and can lead the interviewer to feel like a rushed interrogator. Integration of these expectations will be discussed throughout this chapter.

Although longhand writing is still used by some clinicians, the electronic medical record (EMR) has revolutionized note creation. The resulting write-up generally mirrors the categories listed in Table 1–5. This information can be a gold mine for clinical care, both at the time of the interview and into the future.

The EMR can be problematic. For example, some systems afford the option of clicking boxes for much of the write-up, allowing the development of a multipage document without writing a sentence. This electronic reality can lead the interviewer to a

TABLE 1–5.	Outline of the interview write-up

1. Identifying information
2. Chief complaint
3. History of present illness
4. Past psychiatric history
5. Past medical history
6. Family history
7. Developmental and social history
8. Mental status examination
9. Differential diagnosis and list of diagnoses
10. Assessment and formulation
11. Treatment plan

single-minded quest to obtain information that may be superficial or unprocessed. The EMR may also contain a vast amount of medical information or a series of psychiatric notes. This can lead the interviewer to accept the medical team's history of present illness (HPI) as the psychiatric HPI (when, presumably, the psychiatric and medical illnesses are different). Extensive psychiatric note-taking can lead to time-saving cutting and pasting, but it can also lead to passivity; repetition of unprocessed, inaccurate, and outdated information; and administrative difficulties when notes are compared using widely available software. Perhaps most relevant, time spent typing is time not spent meeting with patients.

Components of the Psychiatric Write-Up

Identifying information varies dramatically. An urgent evaluation might yield "35M," whereas other services might identify that same person as "35-year-old separated engineer with two children, a recent history of stimulant use disorder and social isolation, and a remote history of alcohol use disorder, school truancy, and ADHD [attention-deficit/hyperactivity disorder]." Still other services ask the interviewer to list a few identifiers and avoid highlighting demographics that are not directly related to the presenting problems.

The *chief complaint* is intended to be the patient's primary psychiatric concern and is generally written as a quotation. It is, therefore, not the spouse's biggest complaint, or the prior therapist's biggest concern, or the interviewer's assessment of what *should be* the chief complaint. This brief section belongs to the patient. Quoting nonsensical or tangential responses can provide an excellent window into the patient's mental status. Clearly marking the patient's priority lays the groundwork for later adherence and an effective treatment plan.

The *history of present illness* is the interviewer's integrated narrative of the patient's current psychiatric illness. The development of an accurate and effective HPI can be deceptively difficult. The present illness needs to be identified, and the clinician might need to attend, for example, to a 35-year-old man's report of having become hopelessly lonely after being abandoned by his girlfriend 3 months earlier, to the girl-friend's report that she left him after he had become violent while abusing crystal methamphetamine, to the emergency department doctor's report that the patient was admitted after an acetaminophen overdose the day before, and to the patient's mother's report that her son had been difficult for the prior three decades. After weighing the available information, the first sentence of the HPI might become: "Asked to assess for depression and suicidality in this 35-year-old man after he was admitted to the emergency department with an acetaminophen overdose in the context of crystal methamphetamine abuse, a relationship breakup 3 months earlier with subsequent dysphoria and social isolation, and chronic interpersonal difficulties."

Once the actual illness has been clarified, the HPI becomes a narrative that de-scribes precipitants as well as the onset, duration, and intensity (and extent of the as-sociated debility) of symptoms. Commonly associated comorbidities and symptoms can be specifically included or excluded.

A model for the HPI is provided by news journalism. The newspaper headline fo-cuses the story, as does the first sentence of the HPI. Ensuing sentences explain and flesh out the details. When the newspaper suggests that the reader turn to page 19A, the reader can be assured that the initial thesis of the story will not be refuted on the later page. "Don't bury the lead" is a central demand of journalism, and it pushes the reporter to focus her story so that she does not mislead her audience. A similar liter-ary technique stems from an assertion generally attributed to the playwright Anton Chekhov over a century ago: If a gun appears in the first act, it needs to be fired by the end of the play. In a psychiatric HPI, the buried lead or unfired gun would be pieces of information that are accurate but do not contribute to a focused understand-ing of the patient's present illness.

> **Tip:** The HPI is the primary opportunity for the interviewer to argue her specific point of view about the patient's current illness. The search for a point of view focuses and simplifies the actual interview.

The journalistic approach to the HPI contrasts with another common HPI style, that of the essay. An "essay" type of HPI builds to a point eventually, but too often it reflects interviewer uncertainty. Such an HPI might begin with a lengthy description of identifiers that may or may not be relevant to the HPI, followed by the chief com-plaint, followed by the beginnings of a story of the illness, the clinician's obstacles in the pursuit of that perspective, quotations from the interview with the patient, and collateral and historical information that is true but not immediately relevant. At that point, the presenter often looks up, waiting for questions—or, if it is a written HPI, the note simply progresses to other aspects of the write-up. This approach may be the expectation in certain hospital cultures—and trainees do need to be attentive to ex-pectations—and it makes particular sense for situations such as case conferences, in which the audience is expected to think along with the clinician in the pursuit of un-derstanding the patient. Nevertheless, the "essay" form of HPI encourages the reader/listener to develop his or her own perspective on the case, and that leads to errors, extra effort, and unnecessary ambiguity. In addition, without the expectation of a focused HPI, the interviewer may become distracted, fail to develop a working narrative, and perhaps incorrectly conclude that all true information is equally valid.

The *past psychiatric history* focuses on data that can guide current and future evaluations. Ideally, historical diagnoses are accompanied by a list of pertinent symptoms and potential co-occurring disorders, such as substance abuse. In discussing hospitalizations, the clinician might include the name of the institution, the reason for admission, the discharge diagnosis, the treatment, and its efficacy. Listing medication or psychotherapy trials is more informative when accompanied by an estimate of duration, intensity, adverse effects, level of adherence, and effect. Collateral information can inform patient recall, which is often flawed (Simon et al. 2012). Furthermore, whereas psychiatric dysfunction tends to be chronic, specific diagnoses often develop or shift over time (Bromet et al. 2011).

Substance use disorders are so common that even their apparent absence might be specifically mentioned in the HPI and/or the past psychiatric history section. Repetition can be warranted. For example, the HPI, past psychiatric history, and MSE might all include assessments of psychosis, suicidality, and homicidality.

Past medical history is pertinent because psychiatric and nonpsychiatric medical conditions frequently co-occur. Over-the-counter and complementary medications may have direct effects and interactions with prescribed medications. Inquiry into healthy behaviors demonstrates that the clinician is interested in the patient's strengths and may increase the likelihood of the patient's participation in potentially therapeutic behaviors such as exercise, yoga, and meditation. Interviewers who know little about "alternative" treatments might use a few minutes of the interview to tactfully ask what makes these treatments important to their patients.

> **Tip:** Nonpsychiatric medical information informs the psychiatric assessment. The very thick medical chart requires the interviewer to make a series of judgments about relevance. The absence of a medical chart does not mean that medical issues are irrelevant.

Family history refers to pertinent disorders found in biological relatives (e.g., schizophrenia in a brother). Diabetes in a first-degree relative may also be pertinent, especially given the link between metabolic syndrome and many psychiatric medications, and between diabetes and depression. Parental divorce and depression in a stepmother belong, on the other hand, in social history.

The *developmental and social history* will vary significantly in relevance. For children and adolescents and for any patient whose primary diagnosis appears in the DSM-5 chapter "Neurodevelopmental Disorders," much of the interview might focus on developmental and social issues. For other patients, this section is fairly irrelevant to a relatively brief evaluation and is unlikely to affect the eventual differential diagnosis. Cursory or careless reviews can lead to missing many types of pertinent findings, however, and even a "normal" childhood will be filled with experiences that bear on an understanding of the patient. A thorough developmental and social history informs both the assessment and the eventual treatment plan.

Mental Status Examination

To a psychiatrist, the MSE is equivalent to the internist's physical examination. As a relatively objective cross-sectional evaluation, the MSE shapes and informs the history, labs, collateral information, and eventual treatment strategy. The assessment of mental status begins the moment the interviewer sees the patient, and most of it can be accomplished casually and outside the patient's awareness.

> **Tip:** The MSE does not require the patient's cooperation or the interviewer's ability to read minds. The MSE is based on an interview-long snapshot of what the patient says and does.

When reviewed days, months, or even years later, an effective MSE informs a longitudinal perspective. MSEs include a basic set of information, as listed in Table 1–6.

Regarding *general appearance and behavior,* the interviewer notes the patient's level of consciousness, behavior, dress, grooming, and attitude toward the examiner. A well-considered assessment of appearance can, therefore, contribute heavily to the development of a differential diagnosis. For example, a disheveled, distracted, hypoactive elderly hospitalized patient presents a differential diagnosis that centers on delirium even before the interviewer or patient says a word. Level of cooperation can contribute directly to an understanding of the patient and inform aspects of the interview that require motivation (e.g., the history, cognitive testing).

> **Tip:** The interviewer pays attention to details that do not quite fit the rest of the story. Appearance "idiosyncrasies" might include prominent tattoos on an otherwise "buttoned-down" businessman.

Mood and *affect* are often linked within the MSE. *Mood* refers to the patient's predominant emotional state during the interview, whereas *affect* is the expression of those feelings. The interviewer infers mood from the patient's posture and appearance as well as the patient's own account of his or her mood. Affect is described in multiple ways, including range (e.g., labile or constricted), appropriateness to the situation, congruency with the thought content, and intensity (e.g., blunted).

A second way to assess mood is to quote directly from the patient's self-report. In this model, the interviewer's assessment of the patient's interior affective state is defined as *affect.* Putting mood in quotations readily identifies the patient's perspective and reduces the need for the interviewer to infer mood. This version of mood/affect is akin to quoting the patient's self-report of his or her chief complaint. In both instances, the reader gets a window into the patient's perspective, even if what we hear bears little resemblance to a literal chief complaint or mood. There are downsides to this mood/affect paradigm. Often, the stated mood is clearly inaccurate. While the quotation "fine" reveals something about the patient's level of insight into her mood and psychiatric situation, it may not address her actual mood (Serby 2003).

A third model likens *mood* to *climate* (long-standing emotions) and *affect* to the more changeable *weather* (see the DSM-5 "Glossary of Technical Terms"). One problem with this definition is that the interviewer will be tempted to shift from having a cross-sectional perspective on the patient (i.e., based on an assessment of the patient's mood at the time of the interview) to making an estimate of the patient's mood during the entire course of his or her illness. In so doing, the interviewer's assessment of mood and affect has shifted from being a component of the cross-sectional MSE to being the more longitudinal HPI.

These two latter definitions of mood and affect can be confusing to trainees, at least partly because they do not conform to standard English. The mood-as-climate, affect-

TABLE 1–6.   Mental status examination
General appearance and behavior
Level of consciousness (alert, sleepy)
Dress and grooming (casual, disheveled)
Idiosyncrasies (unusual tattoos, unusual dress)
Attitude (cooperative, hostile)
Psychomotor agitation and retardation
Mood (depressed, euphoric)
Patient quotations ("depressed," "great") OR
Examiner inferences (dysphoric, euphoric)
Affect
Range (constricted, flat)
Appropriateness to interview topics
Speech
Rate (slow, pressured, difficult to interrupt)
Volume (loud, soft)
Quality (fluent, idiosyncratic)
Thought process
Goal directed, tangential
Thought content
Preoccupations, delusions, suicidality, homicidality
Perceptions
Illusions, hallucinations, derealization, depersonalization
Cognition
Orientation
Memory (immediate recall, short-term memory, long-term memory)
Concentration and attention
Insight
Judgment

as-weather dichotomy is often misremembered by trainees, whereas quoting a patient's perspective on her own mood often requires the interviewer to list a mood state that is clearly inaccurate.

> **Tip:** Local customs and expectations guide the interview. Expectations for the HPI, the MSE, and even words like *mood* and *affect* will vary across different clinical services at the same institution, as well as across different institutions, regions, and countries.

Speech patterns are a window into the patient's *thought process.* For example, rate, volume, and organization of speech should be observed throughout the interview. Pressured, tangential speech is often found in mania. Slow speech with impoverished content is often found in depression, schizophrenia, and delirium. Guarded, withholding speech can accompany paranoia.

> **Tip:** Based on patterns of communication, diagnoses can often be tentatively made within moments of meeting a patient.

The evaluation of *thought content* focuses on unusual, preoccupying, or dangerous ideas. *Delusions* are common in psychosis, for example, whereas *ruminations of guilt* are common in depression. Both delusions and ruminations can be "fixed and false," but the two symptoms are associated with different diagnoses and treatments.

Suicidality and *homicidality* are integral to the evaluation of thought content. For both, the interviewer assesses for ideation, intent, and plan, as well as access to weapons. Interviewers will sometimes shy away from such exploration, perhaps fearing that introduction of the topic will cause the patient to become offended or impulsive or that the mere presence of suicidal or homicidal ideation will inevitably lead to psychiatric admission. Such concerns are generally unwarranted. Passive suicidal and homicidal thoughts are common, and discussion can often lead to a deepening of the alliance. Furthermore, most such thoughts do not lead to involuntary treatment. At the same time, people who do eventually kill themselves or others have often sent out clear warnings beforehand. Manualized suicide assessment screens are increasingly being used by mental health practitioners as well as general medical services and schools. All assessments are imperfect, but a tactful and attentive interview is an effective time to identify people at risk (Fowler 2012).

As with other aspects of the MSE, the suicide and homicide assessment is intended to focus on the patient's current thought content. If the patient is denying all suicidal ideation the day after a clear suicide attempt, the MSE might indicate the following: "Denies all suicidal ideation, intent, and plan (but did overdose yesterday; see HPI)."

Perceptions refer to any perceptual abnormalities, including hallucinations, illusions, derealization, and depersonalization. Diagnosis and treatment depend on distinguishing between these types of misperceptions.

Hallucinations have the clarity and impact of true perceptions but without the pertinent sensory input (see the DSM-5 "Glossary of Technical Terms"). For example, a person who "hears voices" is hearing a voice coming from outside her head that generally consists of meaningful sentences or phrases. Hallucinations that occur just prior to falling sleep and just prior to waking are termed *hypnagogic* and *hypnopompic*, respectively, and are considered normal. Talking to oneself is not considered an auditory hallucination (even if so labeled by the patient), nor is misinterpretation of actual voices from the hallway (those are often misperceptions and/or reflections of paranoia). Auditory hallucinations have long been associated with schizophrenia, but they are also present in psychoses related to mania, depression, delirium, substance abuse, and dementia. Hallucinations can occur in any of the five senses, although nonauditory hallucinations tend to be symptoms of neuropsychiatric and/or systemic medical disease.

Illusions are misperceptions of actual sensory inputs. For example, a delirious patient might misinterpret the shadows on a television screen as crawling bugs.

Depersonalization refers to a sense of being detached from one's own thoughts, body, or actions, whereas *derealization* refers to detachment from one's own surroundings. They often co-occur. These symptoms are less often explored than hallucinations or illusions; if found, however, they can trigger further search into often comorbid conditions that range from substance abuse to PTSD to dissociative disorders.

Assessment of *cognition* can be an uncomfortable part of the MSE. The same interviewers who freely ask their patients about sex, money, and a broad panoply of toxic behaviors often become sheepishly apologetic when faced with doing a formal cognitive assessment. Straightforward is good. Explain that a cognitive assessment is part of the interview, ask a few questions, do a Montreal Cognitive Assessment (Nasreddine et al. 2005) and/or a clock drawing test (Samton et al. 2005), and make the preliminary assessment. For patients with no risk factors or signs of cognitive decline, a cognitive screen can be done quickly, and experience with normal cognitive examinations is helpful when faced with abnormal examinations. For patients with apparent neuropsychiatric dysfunction, a working knowledge of typical symptom clusters and disorders can help make sense of the functional decline (Yudofsky and Hales 2012).

Orientation is generally assessed by the patient's accurate recitation of name, location, and date (i.e., orientation to person, place, and time). Some texts refer to a fourth dimension, the situation, whereas others probe more deeply into specifics (e.g., orientation to person requires not only a knowledge of one's name but also one's address, phone number, age, occupation, and marital status). The inability to correctly state the exact date and location is fairly common and may not reflect problems with orientation but rather with memory, motivation, or situation (e.g., a lengthy hospitalization).

A brief MSE screens for three types of *memory* dysfunction. *Immediate recall* is essentially an assessment of attention and is most often tested by asking patients to repeat the names of three unrelated objects (e.g., apple, table, penny). *Recent* or *short-term memory* is typically tested by asking the patient to recall, after a few minutes, the three objects repeated as part of the test for immediate recall. If the patient was unable to repeat the objects in the first place, the inability to recall after 3–5 minutes does not necessarily indicate the loss of short-term memory but could instead reflect inattention or amotivation. *Long-term memory* is generally assessed during the course of the interview through the patient's ability to accurately recall events in recent months and throughout the course of a lifetime. Many patients with dementia will retain long-term memory, whereas patients with a dissociative disorder often present with clinically relevant memory gaps. Distortions and embellishments of the past may be psychologically motivated and not indicative of cognitive decline and would therefore not be addressed in this category. Confabulations, on the other hand, are false memories that are created to fill in memory gaps; they are linked to neurocognitive disorders and therefore are included in the MSE.

Attention refers to the ability to sustain interest in a stimulus, whereas *concentration* involves the ability to maintain mental effort. Counting backward by sevens (serial 7s) requires that the patient retain interest in the task, recall the last number, subtract seven from it, and then continue to the next number. The task also requires competence at math. Spelling *world* backward is a similarly good screening test of attention and concentration, but only for people who are fairly good spellers. For other patients, it is preferable to use a test that is less dependent on education, such as reciting the months backward.

> **Tip:** All formal cognitive assessments demand some awareness of the patient's cultural and educational background and any variables that could impact performance, such as motivation, anxiety, or pain.

Disturbances of orientation, memory, attention, and concentration often cluster to-gether and may reflect a wide range of diagnoses, including dementia, depression, at-tention-deficit/hyperactivity disorder, and dissociative disorders. Disturbances may prompt a more detailed screening. Brief, validated tools for cognitive assessment in-clude the Montreal Cognitive Assessment (Nasreddine et al. 2005) and the clock drawing test (Samton et al. 2005). Each has its strengths and weaknesses and is avail-able free on the Internet. No single assessment is diagnostic, however, and a thorough assessment of the patient will require integration of the findings from the MSE with the rest of the interview.

Abstract reasoning can generally be assessed during the course of the interview. Proverb interpretation is often used as an adjunctive assessment. For example, the in-terviewer might ask, "How would you explain the following to a child: 'You can't judge a book by its cover'?" Patients with mania often respond with a tangential riff, whereas many other types of patients respond with concreteness and a lack of imag-ination. Proverbs are notoriously bound to cultural and educational norms, however, so many clinicians have dispensed with this traditional part of the MSE.

Insight and *judgment* are often linked within the MSE because both are part of in-terrelated skills and behaviors that include such executive functions as reasoning, im-pulsivity, initiation, organization, and self-monitoring. Various types of executive dysfunction underlie or accompany most psychiatric disorders.

Insight refers to how well the patient understands his or her own current psychiatric situation; it does not refer to insightful perspectives on politics, sports, or the inter-viewer. *Judgment* is often extrapolated from recent behavior or assessed by asking such questions as "If you were in a movie theater and smelled smoke, what would you do?"

The assessments of insight and judgment depend heavily on context, and the struc-tured calm of the interview setting can lead many patients to appear healthier than their recent history might suggest. For example, a clinician might be interviewing, for the fourth time in as many weeks, a patient whose previous four visits involved the same sequence of relationship conflict, illicit substance use, and sublethal suicide at-tempt. Even if this patient can describe his situation insightfully and is able to indicate what he might do in the burning theater, few clinicians would be content to describe his insight and judgment as being "intact." However, an interviewer who notes, in the MSE, that the patient has poor insight and judgment based on recent history is inter-mingling the HPI (which extends over recent days, weeks, or months) with the MSE (which is intended to be a cross-sectional snapshot). One option for reconciling this dilemma is to explicitly distinguish between the longitudinal and the cross-sectional types of assessments within the MSE (e.g., "Judgment: currently able to reasonably discuss choices and situation [recent judgment, however, has been poor; see HPI]").

Assessment and Plan

The psychiatric interview often has multiple goals, but its ultimate focus is the devel-opment of an integrated assessment and treatment plan.

Expectations for an assessment vary dramatically. A DSM-5 diagnosis is a minimum requirement. The concluding assessment might include a brief narrative of the patient's story, but it need not rehash the whole HPI. Wordy assessments are unlikely to be read.

The concluding plan aims to be brief and biopsychosocially complete. In other words, "sertraline 50 mg in the morning" is not a plan if it is not accompanied by some reference to who is going to write that prescription, whether psychotherapy is recommended, and whether there is a recommendation to adapt the patient's environment in some way.

The interviewer may be expected to provide, in addition to the write-up, a brief written or oral summary of the patient. The particulars of the summary will depend very much on the situation. For example, insurance companies and other institutions will probably want the summary to be limited to codes for diagnosis and procedure; the clinician will then need to be prepared, of course, in case they request access to the full written evaluation.

For clinical purposes, most curbside discussions between colleagues will feature a focused version of the history, assessment, and plan. For example: "This is a 27-year-old man who presented with hallucinations and paranoid delusions that began a month ago in the context of some marijuana use and insomnia, as well as a lengthy prodrome of declining function and odd behavior. Our tentative assessment is schizophrenia, but we will need to specifically evaluate for substance-induced psychosis. Our plan is to admit him to psychiatry, get more collateral information, provide support and structure, ensure sleep, and begin antipsychotic medication." Such a summary is too brief to satisfy all needs, but it provides a framework for further exploration.

Conclusion

Taught to students and trainees in every mental health discipline, the initial interview is fundamental to the practice of psychiatry. At the same time, the successful interview weaves together a tapestry of complex threads: differential diagnosis and common comorbidities, the link between assessment and treatment, the use of tact and timing to shift between different components of the exam, the tendency to form premature and incomplete conclusions, and the development of a therapeutic alliance. While taught to beginners, the psychiatric interview and mental status exam encapsulate much of the complexity of modern psychiatry.

Key Clinical Points

- Interview tools include nonverbal communication and observation.
- Without a strong fund of knowledge, the interviewer is lost.
- Information is useful only when interpreted.
- Not all information is relevant.
- The interviewer adapts to fit the patient and the situation.
- The history of present illness is a creation of the interviewer.
- The history of present illness is longitudinal.

- The mental status examination is cross-sectional.
- The psychiatric interview is enriched by the active cultivation of such interpersonal characteristics as curiosity and warmth.

References

American Psychiatric Association: Diagnostic and Statistical Manual of Mental Disorders, 5th Edition. Arlington, VA, American Psychiatric Association, 2013

Auchincloss EL: The Psychoanalytic Model of the Mind. Washington, DC, American Psychiatric Publishing, 2015

Avery JD, Barnhill JW: Co-occurring Mental Illness and Substance Use Disorders: A Guide to Diagnosis and Treatment. Washington, DC, American Psychiatric Publishing, 2018

Beck JS: Cognitive Behavior Therapy: Basics and Beyond, 2nd Edition. New York, Guilford, 2011

Black DW, Grant JE: DSM-5 Guidebook: The Essential Companion to the Diagnostic and Statistical Manual of Mental Disorders, 5th Edition. Washington, DC, American Psychiatric Publishing, 2014

Bromet EJ, Kotov R, Fochtmann LJ, et al: Diagnostic shifts during the decade following first admission for psychosis. Am J Psychiatry 168(11):1186–1194, 2011 21676994

Chae DH, Lincoln KD, Jackson JS: Discrimination, attribution, and racial group identification: implications for psychological distress among black Americans in the National Survey of American Life (2001–2003). Am J Orthopsychiatry 81(4):498–506, 2011 21977935

Engel GL: The clinical application of the biopsychosocial model. Am J Psychiatry 137(5):535–544, 1980 7369396

Evans DR, Hearn MT, Uhlemann MR, et al: Essential Interviewing: A Programmed Approach to Effective Communication, 8th Edition. Belmont, CA, Brooks/Cole, 2010

First MB: DSM-5 Handbook of Differential Diagnosis. Washington, DC, American Psychiatric Publishing, 2014

Fowler JC: Suicide risk assessment in clinical practice: pragmatic guidelines for imperfect assessments. Psychotherapy (Chic) 49(1):81–90, 2012 22369082

Freed PJ, Barnhill JW: Evaluating an emergency patient, in Approach to the Psychiatric Patient, 2nd Edition Edited by Barnhill JW. Washington, DC, American Psychiatric Publishing, 2019, pp 236–241

Gabbard GO: Psychodynamic Psychiatry in Clinical Practice, 5th Edition. Washington, DC, American Psychiatric Publishing, 2014

Gara MA, Vega WA, Arndt S, et al: Influence of patient race and ethnicity on clinical assessment in patients with affective disorders. Arch Gen Psychiatry 69(6):593–600, 2012 22309972

Goldberg JF, Ernst CL: Managing the Side-Effects of Psychotropic Medications. Washington, DC, American Psychiatric Publishing, 2012

Groopman J: How Doctors Think. New York, Houghton Mifflin, 2007

Levenson JL, Ferrando SJ: Clinical Manual of Psychopharmacology in the Medically Ill, 2nd Edition. Arlington, VA, American Psychiatric Publishing, 2016

Levounis P, Drescher J, Barber M (eds): The LGBT Casebook. Washington, DC, American Psychiatric Publishing, 2012

Levounis P, Arnaout B, Marienfeld C (eds): Motivational Interviewing for Clinical Practice. Arlington, VA, American Psychiatric Association Publishing, 2017

Lewis-Fernández R, Aggarwal NK, Hinton L, et al (eds): DSM-5 Handbook on the Cultural Formulation Interview. Washington, DC, American Psychiatric Publishing, 2016

Lim E: Clinical Manual of Cultural Psychiatry, 2nd Edition. Washington, DC, American Psychiatric Publishing, 2014

MacKinnon RA, Michels R, Buckley PJ: The Psychiatric Interview in Clinical Practice, 3rd Edition. Washington, DC, American Psychiatric Publishing, 2015

McHugh PR, Slavney PR: The Perspectives of Psychiatry, 2nd Edition. Baltimore, MD, Johns Hopkins University Press, 1998

Miller WR, Rollnick S: Motivational Interviewing: Preparing People for Change. New York, Guilford, 1991

Muskin PR, Dickerman AL (eds): Study Guide for the Psychiatry Board Examination. Washington, DC, American Psychiatric Publishing, 2016

Nasreddine ZS, Phillips NA, Bédirian V, et al: The Montreal Cognitive Assessment, MoCA: a brief screening tool for mild cognitive impairment. J Am Geriatr Soc 53(4):695–699, 2005 15817019

Perry S, Cooper AM, Michels R: The psychodynamic formulation: its purpose, structure, and clinical application. Am J Psychiatry 144(5):543–550, 1987 3578562

Roberts LW, Louie AK: Study Guide to DSM-5. Washington, DC, American Psychiatric Publishing, 2014

Samton JB, Ferrando SJ, Sanelli P, et al: The clock drawing test: diagnostic, functional, and neuroimaging correlates in older medically ill adults. J Neuropsychiatry Clin Neurosci 17(4):533–540, 2005 16387994

Serby M: Psychiatric resident conceptualizations of mood and affect within the mental status examination. Am J Psychiatry 160(8):1527–1529, 2003 12900321

Simon GE, Rutter CM, Stewart C, et al: Response to past depression treatments is not accurately recalled: comparison of structured recall and patient health questionnaire scores in medical records. J Clin Psychiatry 73(12):1503–1508, 2012 23290322

Summers RF: The psychodynamic formulation updated. Am J Psychother 57(1):39–51, 2003 12647568

van Schaik DJ, Klijn AF, van Hout HP, et al: Patients' preferences in the treatment of depressive disorder in primary care. Gen Hosp Psychiatry 26(3):184–189, 2004 15121346

Viederman M: The induction of noninterpreted benevolent transference as a vehicle for change. Am J Psychother 65(4):337–354, 2011 22329336

World Health Organization: International Statistical Classification of Diseases and Related Health Problems, 10th Revision. Geneva, World Health Organization, 1992

Yudofsky SC: Fatal Flaws: Navigating Destructive Relationships With People With Disorders of Personality and Character. Washington, DC, American Psychiatric Publishing, 2005

Yudofsky SC, Hales RE: Clinical Manual of Neuropsychiatry. Washington, DC, American Psychiatric Publishing, 2012

Recommended Readings

Barnhill JW (ed): DSM-5 Clinical Cases. Washington, DC, American Psychiatric Publishing, 2013

Barnhill JW (ed): Approach to the Psychiatric Patient, 2nd Edition. Washington, DC, American Psychiatric Association Publishing, 2018

Coverdale JH, Louie AK, Roberts LW: Arriving at a diagnosis: the role of the clinical interview, in Study Guide to DSM-5. Edited by Roberts LW, Louie AK. Washington, DC, American Psychiatric Publishing, 2015

MacKinnon RA, Michels R, Buckley PJ: The Psychiatric Interview in Clinical Practice, 3rd Edition. Washington, DC, American Psychiatric Publishing, 2015

CHAPTER 2

DSM-5 as a Framework for Psychiatric Diagnosis

Jack D. Burke, M.D., M.P.H.

Helena C. Kraemer, Ph.D.

In medicine and public health, diagnostic classification systems provide a framework for understanding and communicating about clinical conditions. They offer a systematic presentation of diagnostic categories, based on delineation of specific clinical conditions organized into meaningful groups. After examining patients, clinicians specify the diagnoses—that is, state which disorders they believe are present. This complex task demands skill in assessment as well as knowledge of the basis for defining and categorizing mental disorders.

Classification systems reflect the current state of scientific knowledge, so they need to be revised periodically. Besides research, classification systems are also influenced by their intended uses, prior history, and underlying concepts of illness (Moriyama et al. 2011; Sadler 2005; Zachar and Kendler 2007). Contemporary approaches are introducing efforts to apply dimensional measures to characterize clinical conditions more precisely (Helzer et al. 2008; Kraemer 2007).

Background

In the United States, the current classification system for psychiatric practice is the *Diagnostic and Statistical Manual of Mental Disorders,* 5th Edition (DSM-5; American Psychiatric Association 2013).

The "official" classification system for public health reporting is the *International Classification of Diseases and Related Health Problems* (ICD), developed and periodically revised by the World Health Organization (WHO). All member countries of WHO have agreed to use this system to report disease statistics to its surveillance system, although they may not adopt each updated version as soon as it is available. Each country does have the ability to make its own changes, for example, to include terms that are used locally or to add precision to the system. In the United States, the National Center for Health Statistics (NCHS) oversees this process, which produces a "clinical modification" of ICD (ICD-10-CM). The NCHS collaborates with specialty organizations such as the American Psychiatric Association (APA) to incorporate diagnostic categories used in the United States.

Challenges for Psychiatric Classification

The periodic table constitutes an ideal classification system. Chemical elements fit into an array based on their atomic numbers; this classification provides a clear, unduplicated placement for each element. The periodic table is exclusive, because each element fits into only one category; it is exhaustive, because every element can be classified within it; and it is discrete, because the defining characteristic, the atomic number, matches one integer or another, rather than one of the infinite real numbers between two integers. Its columns group elements by similar properties, and its rows demonstrate their electron structures (Kendell 1975).

If each illness could be shown to have just one cause, illnesses could be categorized on the basis of etiology and the associated mechanism of disease. Infectious diseases and nutritional deficiencies provide a model for this approach. Once an etiological agent or cause becomes established, researchers can study methods to cure the illness or prevent it. This model has been the accepted standard for thinking about diagnoses in medicine (Loscalzo 2011).

Defining illnesses, however, is challenging. Even with a single cause, a clinical condition can present with a variable mix of symptoms, as in myocardial infarction. In many conditions, especially psychiatric disorders, multiple biological, psychological, and environmental factors interact in complex ways over time to produce an illness. Specification of the way these factors interact is difficult because so many processes in medicine, especially in neuroscience and psychology, are complex and poorly understood (Loscalzo and Barabasi 2011). As a result, it is not possible to classify psychiatric illnesses as diseases based on etiology and mechanism, using a reductionistic, one-level explanation (Kendler 2012).

Diagnostic Entities

Clinical conditions are not freestanding entities like chemical elements, so the periodic table is an unrealistic model for classification in medicine. Even for medical conditions with a single known etiology, types of causes—such as infectious agents, chromosomal abnormalities, or neoplasms—vary considerably. There is no single defining characteristic, like an atomic number, to govern their classification (Kendler 2008). Even a single defining characteristic of a disease may produce ambiguity in distinguishing between normality and disease; for example, an individual can be a carrier of an infectious agent, such as tubercle bacillus, without having an illness. The defining characteristics of some conditions are continuous measures, such as blood pressure or hormone levels, and require a threshold to be set for a category to be identified. Research on epigenomics, proteomics, and other aspects of systems biology will lead to even greater complexity of disease classification (Hyman 2010; Institute of Medicine 2012; Loscalzo 2011).

When a defining characteristic has not been established, clinical conditions are identified as syndromes. A *syndrome* is based on pattern recognition and comprises a characteristic set of signs and symptoms that usually occur together, have a typical prognosis, and may have a similar response to treatment. A syndrome, such as anemia, is usually anticipated to be heterogeneous in terms of causes; eventually specific diseases may be identified within the broad syndrome, such as thalassemia or hemorrhagic anemia. Clinical conditions can present with an incomplete symptom picture, and they can be confusing because the signs and symptoms are not exclusive to a single syndrome. Assessment of a patient can be challenging, because an individual may present with more than one condition or with a condition that does not fit any recognized syndromal pattern. Because of this reliance on syndromal diagnosis, the goal of producing a psychiatric classification that is exclusive, exhaustive, and based on discrete entities is not attainable without new knowledge and a paradigm shift (Kendler and First 2010).

In contemporary psychiatric classification systems, many categories derive from long-recognized syndromes that clinicians and researchers have refined over time based on experience, research, and shifts in their explanatory models of illness. In the past two centuries, syndromes have been introduced by leading figures in psychiatry such as Emil Kraepelin or Eugen Bleuler. Since 1952, classification systems have been developed by panels of experts who have been charged with reviewing evidence and developing refinements based on a consensus of opinion. The judgments that produce any given classification must balance widely varying concepts of psychiatric illness, such as the assumptions made about causation, the threshold for determining abnormality, and standards for interpreting research evidence (Fulford et al. 2006; Zachar and Kendler 2007).

Definition of Mental Disorder

Because the etiology and pathogenesis of so many psychiatric conditions are not yet established, contemporary classification systems describe the conditions being categorized as *disorders* rather than *diseases,* a term associated with conditions whose causes are known. Both DSM and the ICD section on mental disorders have acknowledged that *disorder* is a convenient but inexact term.

This imprecision in describing diagnostic categories has led critics to question how clinicians can distinguish mental disorders from reactions to normal life or problems in living. Over the past half-century, the task of identifying and classifying mental disorders has drawn attack as doing nothing more than labeling unwelcome social, political, or other behaviors as mental illnesses. These lingering criticisms have led to a more formal effort in recent DSM editions to offer a general definition of mental disorders, even though clinicians typically worry only about specific disorders and the rest of medicine is untroubled by the lack of rigorous definitions of disease and illness (Kendell 1975).

The introduction to DSM-IV acknowledged the imprecision of the concept: "it must be admitted that no definition adequately specifies precise boundaries for the concept of 'mental disorder'" (American Psychiatric Association 1994, p. xxi). The introduction went on to list the characteristics that the system used to conceptualize mental disorders:

- Behavioral or psychological syndrome occurring in an individual;
- Associated with
    1. Distress (e.g., painful symptom) or
    2. Disability (impaired functioning) or
    3. Increased risk of death, pain, disability, or loss of freedom

When there is no way to identify the causal factors or mechanisms of an illness, and the clinical presentation does not provide a clear division between normality and clinically relevant illness, specifying the point at which a syndrome crosses the boundary from normal to abnormal is one of the challenges for a classification system (Kendell and Jablensky 2003). In DSM-IV, this challenge was met by requiring that a syndrome be associated with distress, impairment, or risk of other harmful outcomes. More than 70% of the specific disorders in DSM-IV included distress or impairment among the required criteria for the condition. Despite the relevance of the third associated characteristic, "increased risk" of a harmful consequence, this factor was not included in DSM-IV's standard criterion of "clinically significant distress or impairment" (Lehman et al. 2002).

This pragmatic approach generated problems of its own. Terms such as *clinically significant* and *impairment* are not defined. Requiring impairment for diagnosis of a clinical disorder could preclude early intervention in preclinical phases of the disorder. Requiring that impairment be present could also complicate efforts to study the evolving relationship between the syndrome and any subsequent disability. Attempting to attribute distress or impairment to a particular disorder when more than one disorder is present would be difficult at best (Lehman et al. 2002; Sartorius 2009).

In DSM-5 (American Psychiatric Association 2013, p. 20), the definition of *mental disorder* is phrased in terms of dysfunctions and their underlying processes:

> A mental disorder is a syndrome characterized by clinically significant disturbance in an individual's cognition, emotion regulation, or behavior that reflects a dysfunction in the psychological, biological, or developmental processes underlying mental functioning. Mental disorders are usually associated with significant distress or disability in social, occupational, or other important activities.

This definition still does not provide operational guidance on specifying a threshold for diagnosis. The difficulty in determining when a dysfunction has produced a change from normal variation to pathology has meant that the coupling of the definition to "significant distress or impairment" could not be removed completely.

This definition in DSM-5 serves mainly as a guidepost to the future. DSM-5 introduced a new effort to apply dimensional measures to determine clinical significance, to identify preclinical conditions, or to assess heterogeneity among cases. This dimensional approach anticipates a time when "dysfunction" can be measured and its underlying processes can be identified (Hyman 2010; Insel and Wang 2010).

Multiple Uses

From the manual's first publication in 1952, its title—*Diagnostic and Statistical Manual*—has referred to dual purposes. DSM was intended to serve as both a diagnostic manual for clinicians and a guide to statistical reporting useful for hospital and public health officials. Trying to serve both purposes was another challenge for the experts developing the classification system.

For clinicians, DSM-I (American Psychiatric Association 1952) presented a list of diagnostic terms, to serve as a nomenclature. Although the terms could have been listed alphabetically, the list was presented according to the coding system in the then-current ICD-6 (World Health Organization 1949). DSM-I also provided a "definition of terms," with a brief description of each condition within a diagnostic category. The standardized terms for the diagnostic categories and the corresponding definitions were the essential elements of the manual for clinicians.

For institutional and public health officials, the manual explained how the classification could be used to report the number of cases seen in a clinical setting, usually a public mental hospital, over a given period of time. For this reporting process, coding clerks noted the diagnostic term used by a clinician and counted the patient in the appropriate category within a tabular aggregation of total cases. For the clerk's reporting effort, the definition of terms was irrelevant; instead, the code corresponding to the clinician's diagnosis was the key information used from the manual.

These two different uses highlighted conflicts that initially affected the way psychiatric diagnoses were made. The manual offered a classification of disorders; the statistical report offered a classification of cases, with numbers of cases in each given class of disorder presented in a table. For statistical reports, each person was counted only once, so the goal of limiting a patient's diagnosis to a single disorder influenced clinical practice, and this limitation became one of the major controversies addressed in the preparation of DSM-II (American Psychiatric Association 1968). A compromise allowed clinicians to document more than one disorder, with the understanding that one of these would be considered the "primary" diagnosis for statistical reporting.

A second problem arose from the tension between "splitting" and "lumping," a conflict that continues to be confronted in each revision of a classification. Clinicians wanted the conditions to be described at an appropriate level of precision to allow meaningful distinctions to be made. Statisticians needed to have a manageable number of categories, so they envisioned a system whose individual diagnostic classes could be collapsed into broader but still meaningful categories. They favored a hierarchical system that would allow such aggregation and still preserve the logic of a classification (American Psychiatric Association 1952, pp. 88–89).

Over time, these two conflicts have eased. DSM no longer expects the clinician to restrict the number of diagnoses artificially; in fact, one recent concern has centered on how many "comorbid" conditions are diagnosed in a given patient. Also, the classification no longer tries to construct a formal hierarchy of conditions but instead groups conditions by some perceived similarity. As these original conflicts among different types of uses have faded, additional problems have arisen, more recently from several nonclinical applications of DSM. In the United States, commercial and government payers have selectively applied DSM categorizations to determine which disorders would be covered by a beneficiary's insurance plan. Some disorders have also been further restricted by payers on the basis of the Global Assessment of Functioning (GAF) Scale scores introduced by DSM-III-R in 1987 (American Psychiatric Association 1987). Payers have determined in advance whether a GAF Scale score for some conditions justifies a certain level of service, such as hospitalization for a depressive episode. This approach uses the diagnostic manual as an indicator of "need for treatment" rather than presence of a disorder, thereby reducing the complicated problem of treatment planning to an arbitrary, nonclinical process. DSM-5 has emphasized that although a diagnosis can have clinical utility for clinicians, such as aiding them in developing treatment plans, a diagnosis does not by itself equate to a need for treatment. Need for treatment depends on multiple factors beyond diagnosis (American Psychiatric Association 2013, p. 20), such as any of the following:

- Symptom severity (e.g., suicidal ideation)
- Distress
- Disability
- Risk of progression
- Complications in managing other medical conditions

In other fields of medicine, a clinical condition often receives clinical attention even when the condition is not considered a disease, as with childbirth (Kendell 1975). Risk conditions, such as metabolic syndrome or intestinal polyps, have also been legitimate objects of clinical intervention even without a diagnosis of a disease state. DSM-5's distinction between a diagnosis and a need for treatment is intended to support the same flexible application of clinical judgment in psychiatric practice.

The diagnostic system has also been broadly used in judicial proceedings (e.g., to bolster a defense in a criminal trial), as well as in social welfare systems to justify claims for disability payments. However, DSM revisions have noted that a diagnosis can only be made by well-trained clinicians. DSM-5 (American Psychiatric Association 2013, p.20) has reiterated that the presence of a mental disorder does not substitute for these other judgments:

> This definition of mental disorder was developed for clinical, public health, and research purposes. Additional information is usually required beyond that contained in the DSM-5 diagnostic criteria in order to make legal judgments on such issues as criminal responsibility, eligibility for disability compensation, and competency.

Although these cautions are intended to prevent misuse of DSM-5 diagnoses, other users besides practitioners rely on the manual for legitimate purposes. Trainees in clinical disciplines benefit from the extensive descriptions provided for each diagnostic category. This breadth of content also makes the manual a useful resource for patients and their families, as well as for members of the public and policy makers.

Development of Psychiatric Classification Systems

In the nineteenth century, psychiatrists in Europe and the United States concentrated on identifying and describing individual disorders encountered in their hospitals or offices but had less concern about formulating an overall classification system to organize the full range of disorders found in a population. Not until the mid–twentieth century did the profession recognize the need for a system that incorporated diagnostic terms for a broad array of patients who were seen outside a public hospital (American Psychiatric Association 1952).

Classification Systems Reflecting Public Health Interests (1840–1943)

In the United States, public health concerns drove the initial efforts to classify mental disorders. Beginning in 1840 and continuing for the next century, components of the federal government enlisted leaders of the new specialty of psychiatry to help develop systems for classifying psychiatric illnesses for use in public health reporting (American Psychiatric Association 1952, 1968).

From 1840 through 1890, the U.S. Census Bureau attempted to count people who had a mental disorder, characterized as "insanity" or "idiocy." In 1880, a special census survey tried to apply a system with seven categories, but officials found it impossible to construct a list that would be endorsed by leaders of psychiatry and psychology (American Psychiatric Association 1952).

After 1890, the Census Bureau abandoned its effort to determine the prevalence of psychiatric illness in the population. In 1917, when the Census Bureau began planning a survey of individuals who resided in mental institutions, the bureau asked the precursor of the APA for assistance in developing a classification system for psychiatric illnesses. This system, revised periodically through consultation with the APA and the American Medical Association, was used to survey psychiatric patients residing in hospitals beginning in 1923 and continuing up to World War II.

Classification Systems Reflecting Clinical Practice (1943–1980)

When the United States entered World War II, the need to assess volunteers and to treat soldiers and veterans exposed the shortcomings of the existing system. "Military psychiatrists, induction station psychiatrists, and Veterans Administration psychiatrists found themselves operating within the limits of a nomenclature specifically not designed for 90% of the cases handled" (American Psychiatric Association 1952, p. vi).

To provide a more useful nomenclature, the U.S. Army's Office of the Surgeon General prepared a technical bulletin that provided a comprehensive set of diagnostic terms, explained by definitions and grouped into categories such as *psychoneurotic disorders, character and behavior disorders,* and *psychotic disorders.* Definitions of several of the categories (e.g., psychoneurotic disorders) reflected a psychodynamic orientation (Houts 2000).

After the war, the APA's Committee on Nomenclature and Statistics prepared a new classification based on the version created by the Army. The logic of the classification used in DSM-I applied the major viewpoints in American psychiatry:

- Major distinction: organic vs. nonorganic
- Within nonorganic section, psychoneurotic disorders defined in psychodynamic terms
- Within psychoneurotic disorders, specific "reactions" defined in Adolf Meyer's life-history terms

Despite the hope that the new manual would improve the basis for uniform application of diagnostic terms, clinicians' use of psychiatric diagnoses continued to vary widely within the United States and around the world. An international survey conducted for WHO found little agreement about concepts or even names to be used for the conditions. Its recommendation for increasing agreement was for future classification systems to rely on "operational" statements based on observation rather than prototypes developed locally (Stengel 1959). These results prompted WHO to expand the coverage of mental disorders in ICD as it began planning a new revision (ICD-8) in the mid-1960s.

In concert with this effort, the APA's Committee on Nomenclature and Statistics produced DSM-II in 1968. This second edition mirrored the format of DSM-I and continued a psychodynamic approach to psychoneurotic disorders. Reflecting the same lack of consensus found in the WHO survey a decade earlier, the committee members disagreed on the descriptions, and even the names to use, for conditions such as schizophrenia. Growing research evidence also demonstrated that agreement on clinical diagnosis of mental disorders remained low.

In an effort to understand the wide variations in diagnostic practice as shown in hospital statistical reports through the 1960s, a cross-national study examined patients hospitalized in New York and London. Investigators developed sets of explicit criteria for the disorders under study and then trained American and British psychiatrists to use a common set of data about each patient to assign a diagnosis based on these criteria. The patient data included results from systematic clinical interviews and historical information from case records. Using a consensus diagnosis, the study demonstrated that reported variations in the clinical diagnoses came from variations in practice, not from true variations in the patient mix (Cooper et al. 1972). Adopting a similar perspective, psychiatrists in St. Louis, Missouri, who wanted to pursue research on mental disorders developed explicit criteria sets for 16 disorders. They published these criteria sets so that other researchers who wanted to study similar groups of patients could use them (Feighner et al. 1972). Soon after, a multisite study of depression sponsored by the National Institute of Mental Health (NIMH) adopted this approach with modified criteria (Spitzer et al. 1978).

Classification Systems Reflecting Clinical Research and Practice (1980–2013)

Descriptive Approach of DSM-III

As this approach of specifying explicit criteria for individual disorders gained rapid acceptance among clinical researchers, WHO undertook another revision of ICD. In 1974, Robert Spitzer, one of the leaders in these efforts to improve reliability, became chair of the APA Task Force on Nomenclature and Statistics to prepare DSM-III in parallel with ICD-9). He recruited task force members largely from the growing clinical research community, and their commitment to enhance clinical and research diagnoses led to a new paradigm for classifying mental disorders (Klerman et al. 1984).

DSM-III (American Psychiatric Association 1980) provided an explicit set of criteria for each clinical disorder. These criteria specified characteristics that must be present in some combination ("inclusion criteria") and characteristics that would prevent the disorder from being diagnosed ("exclusion criteria"). The task force used inclusion criteria that were descriptive in terms of psychopathology, without any assumptions about etiology unless it had been clearly established. DSM-III dropped the concept of psychoneurotic disorders that had been introduced in the Army's nomenclature and continued in DSM-I and DSM-II. DSM-III also removed the term *neurosis* from the classification system. Rather than giving a brief one- or two-sentence definition of a disorder, DSM-III provided extensive information beyond the criteria sets in an effort to help clinicians understand the disorder; typically, each disorder also included a description of associated features, course of illness, and differential diagnosis (Spitzer et al. 1980).

Multiaxial Assessment in DSM-III

Besides developing criteria for specific disorders, the task force also provided clinicians with a framework to record nondiagnostic data about a patient's condition that would be relevant in planning treatment and gauging prognosis. DSM-III recommended that each diagnostic formulation should include five types, or "axes," of information. Axis IV, the severity of psychosocial stressors, and Axis V, the highest level of adaptive functioning in the past year, constituted novel additions to the traditional diagnostic assessment, to support a comprehensive evaluation (Spitzer and Williams 1994; Spitzer et al. 1980).

DSM-III–Revised

Because so many of the disorders in DSM-III had not been well studied before 1980, and because some aspects of the classification—such as its length and multiaxial structure—were new, the APA undertook a review process beginning in 1983 to examine points that needed refinement to improve ease of use or to reflect new research that had been stimulated by publication of DSM-III. The revised edition of DSM-III, referred to as DSM-III-R, was published in 1987 (American Psychiatric Association 1987). One of the principal changes was to remove many of the diagnostic hierarchies that had been introduced in DSM-III through its exclusion criteria; for example, DSM-III did not permit a diagnosis of panic disorder if the panic attacks occurred only in the course of a major depressive episode. Studies of clinical and epidemiological populations demonstrated that the use of hierarchies had prevented clinicians from assigning more than one diagnosis when multiple syndromes occurred in an episode. The particular pattern of exclusion criteria in DSM-III did not explain the co-occurrence of syndromes, so the exclusion criteria were simplified (American Psychiatric Association 1987, p. xxiv).

DSM-IV

In concert with preparation of ICD-10 by WHO in the late 1980s, the APA established the DSM-IV Task Force to produce the next edition of the classification, which was published in 1994 (American Psychiatric Association 1994). This group had the advantage of considerable research stimulated by DSM-III and DSM-III-R, enhanced by diagnostic interviews designed to provide systematic assessment of a respondent by DSM-III and DSM-III-R criteria.

After a thorough review of each disorder, consisting of literature reviews, reanalysis of existing data sets, and field trials of selected criteria, 13 work groups simplified, clarified, and sometimes modified the criteria and thresholds for diagnosis. Major changes in the system included the decision to drop "organic mental disorders," because the term implied that other mental disorders did not have an "organic" component. Similarly, "physical disorders," which had been used to refer to other medical conditions, was replaced by "general medical conditions" to remove the suggestion of a mind–body split for illness. The threshold for adding new disorders to the classification was raised from the threshold used in DSM-III; clinical relevance was generally not sufficient as a rationale, and some research on the disorder was required. For conditions that might need further study, such as binge-eating disorder, an appendix was created to present criteria sets for further study. Although Axes IV and V were refined in concept, their focus on aiding a comprehensive evaluation of the patient was maintained.

DSM-IV–Text Revision

To avoid any disruption in continuity for clinical researchers and to reduce the burden on clinicians of learning new criteria sets, the APA decided not to publish a major revision of DSM-IV until at least 2010. However, to keep the text descriptions current with research findings, and to correct any ambiguities or errors, the APA did publish a text revision of DSM-IV, referred to as DSM-IV-TR, in 2000 (American Psychiatric Association 2000). None of the criteria sets were modified, and no structural changes were undertaken.

Preparation of DSM-5

Principles Guiding Revision

In 2000, the APA sponsored a workshop to identify high-priority areas for study in preparation for DSM-5. A series of workshops over the next several years refined the issues to be addressed and led to formation of the DSM-5 Task Force. David Kupfer, M.D., was appointed chair, and Darrel A. Regier, M.D., M.P.H., became vice chair.

As with DSM-IV, guidelines for DSM-5 emphasized the importance of clinical relevance. This emphasis was coupled with a requirement that significant changes from DSM-IV should be based on empirical research. Although no changes from DSM-IV were precluded, the APA leadership also wanted to preserve continuity with DSM-IV whenever possible to minimize unnecessary disruptions for clinicians or researchers.

One concern arose from the growing worry that commercial and other interests might hope to influence the selection of disorders or the formulation of their criteria. To forestall possible conflicts of interest among the many experts who would be asked to participate in the deliberations about DSM-5, the APA Board of Trustees developed eligibility criteria to ensure the independence of participants in any level of the revision work. Some critics objected that the standards restricting financial support should have been even more stringent, but the APA leadership reiterated their commitment to the principle of independence, their confidence in the guidelines, and their acceptance of the fact that many leading experts in psychiatry and related disciplines had been excluded from any role in DSM-5 by virtue of their participation in industry-sponsored research or consultations.

The APA Board of Trustees also established three types of peer review groups to support the task force. One group monitored the extensive process of managing the effort to ensure that work proceeded efficiently and to guard against inadvertent conflicts of interest. A scientific review committee reviewed proposed changes to DSM-IV in terms of specific research findings on improvements in validity, when such data existed (Kendler 2013). For some conditions, a clinical and public health committee also reviewed proposals that were based on clinical or public health considerations or other scientific evidence beyond the correlation with validators (Yager and McIntyre 2014). Final recommendations were reviewed by leaders of the APA and ultimately its board of trustees.

Problems Considered for DSM-5

Work group members undertook extensive literature reviews and analyses of preexisting data sets as they reviewed DSM-IV criteria. They identified several types of problems:

- Some diagnoses had low reliability.
- Some diagnostic groups showed excessive use of the nonspecific residual category, labeled "not otherwise specified" (NOS) in DSM-IV.
- Some chapters had created distinct disorders in what may be better considered a single disorder with a range of presentations.
- Other chapters seemed to have gaps in coverage of clinical conditions, so that new disorders might need to be added to the classification.

The structure of the classification—both in the way it grouped disorders into chapters and in its overall use of a multiaxial system—was also examined (Regier et al. 2013a).

One problem for almost all of the conditions was determining proper diagnostic boundaries—that is, separating a specific disorder from other disorders and from normal, nonclinical variations. The difficulty of setting boundaries in prior DSM editions had led to high rates of reported comorbidity and to uncertainty about setting a threshold for diagnoses without using "distress or impairment" as indicators (Regier et al. 2009).

Key Changes in DSM-5

Structural Changes

Uniaxial Structure

In DSM-5, the multiaxial framework was eliminated. Although this framework had had the beneficial effect of encouraging clinicians to conduct a full-range evaluation, including personality disorders, intellectual development, other medical conditions, stressors, and level of functioning, the multiaxial system was not applied uniformly in practice. Other important factors, such as consideration of gender or cultural characteristics, also needed to be included in a comprehensive evaluation but did not have a separate axis. The development of a more robust and informative rating scale, the WHO Disability Assessment Schedule 2.0 (WHODAS II; Üstün et al. 2010), resulted in an instrument that could replace the GAF Scale that formed Axis V in DSM-III-R through DSM-IV-TR.

Grouping of Disorders

Grouping disorders into chapters conveys information that a simple alphabetical listing would not. For clinical use, the organizing principles should make the classification easy to use and logical in expressing some similarities among disorders. The organization may be helpful in guiding differential diagnosis and in stimulating research on closely related conditions.

In DSM-5, disorders are grouped by development over the life span, starting with the chapter "Neurodevelopmental Disorders," which includes intellectual disabilities, communication disorders, autism spectrum disorder, attention-deficit/hyperactivity disorder, specific learning disorder, and motor disorders such as Tourette's disorder. Within each chapter, disorders likely to occur in childhood are listed first. This approach made it possible to drop the earlier section on disorders usually arising in childhood and to integrate a life-span perspective into all the mental disorder chapters. Each chapter was placed in close proximity to chapters for disorders thought to be closely related, at least clinically; for example, "Bipolar and Related Disorders" follows "Schizophrenia Spectrum and Other Psychotic Disorders" and precedes "Depressive Disorders."

For certain diagnoses, the appropriateness of the disorder's placement within a particular chapter was also reevaluated in DSM-5. Gambling disorder, for example, was moved from the chapter "Impulse-Control Disorders Not Elsewhere Classified" in DSM-IV to "Substance-Related and Addictive Disorders" in DSM-5, reflecting more recent evidence about behavioral addictions. Conditions such as posttraumatic stress disorder (previously in the chapter "Anxiety Disorders") and adjustment disorders (previously in their own chapter) were aggregated into the new chapter "Trauma- and Stressor-Related Disorders."

Changes in Specific Disorders

Combining Disorders Into a Broader Category

In DSM-5, five disorders previously distinguished as separate categories were combined into a single autism spectrum disorder. The task force found that this broader disorder could be distinguished from normal development and other "nonspectrum" disorders in a reliable way, but that distinguishing among the individual disorders showed variation over time and across settings and was influenced by other factors, such as language level. This change prompted expressions of concern from advocacy groups, who feared that it would increase stigma for patients who had previously been diagnosed with Asperger's disorder, for example. However, the task force felt that stigma should be directly addressed as a problem on behalf of all of the patients with a condition in this spectrum.

For substance use disorders, the task force agreed to collapse the categories of abuse and dependence. In DSM-5, a dimensional approach is used to grade the severity of a substance use disorder.

Many somatoform disorders in DSM-IV relied on a determination of "medically unexplained symptoms." The task force found that this assessment could not be performed reliably and that distinctions among the individual disorders were unclear. In DSM-5, several of the DSM-IV somatoform disorders are now grouped into a single category, somatic symptom disorder, on the basis of their common features (i.e., somatic symptoms and cognitive distortions).

Separating Disorders

In DSM-IV, agoraphobia and panic disorder had been defined in relation to each other (panic disorder with agoraphobia, panic disorder without agoraphobia, and agoraphobia without panic disorder). The task force agreed to simplify this system by uncoupling the disorders and presenting two separate disorders defined without regard to the presence or absence of the other.

Extending Disorders

One change to criteria that generated public concern was the decision to eliminate the so-called bereavement exclusion in the criteria for major depressive disorder. The goal of this change was to make it possible for clinicians to determine when treatment might be needed for a major depressive episode occurring after a loss, when grief can resemble a depressive episode. After concerns were expressed about appearing to "medicalize" normal life reactions, the task force provided language to clarify that grief reactions are not automatically considered evidence of a major depressive disorder.

Adding Disorders

Binge-eating disorder was listed in Appendix B of DSM-IV as a disorder that needed more study before being included in the list of Axis I disorders. In DSM-5, the disorder was formally moved into the new chapter "Feeding and Eating Disorders." Although this move drew criticism as being an unwarranted expansion into diagnosis of normal behavior, the task force disagreed with this criticism for several reasons. As noted in reviews of eating disorders, the average proportion of patients given an NOS or "other disorder" designation using DSM-IV and ICD-10 (World Health Organization 1992) systems ranged from 40% to 60% of patients seen in different clinical settings. The use of more precise criteria for the narrowly defined categories, such as anorexia and bulimia, and the addition of binge-eating disorder ("bulimia without purging") were adopted for both DSM-5 and the draft ICD-11 (World Health Organization 2018).

Mild neurocognitive disorder (sometimes called "mild cognitive impairment") was added to DSM-5 because clinical and epidemiological data had demonstrated the existence of a clinical condition that did not reach the severity of major neurocognitive disorder but nevertheless required assessment, care, and follow-up. This condition can be produced by a varied set of underlying illnesses, including HIV-related cognitive changes and traumatic brain injury. The description of mild neurocognitive disorder reflects a new dilemma in the task of writing diagnostic criteria. In addition to reports of observable decline in intellectual functioning, formal neuropsychological testing is recommended for the diagnosis. The task force recognized that some clinical settings may not have access to this resource and acknowledged that an equivalent clinical evaluation might be required in many settings.

Removing Disorders and Subtypes

Personality disorders.　One area that posed a particular challenge was personality disorders. An initial review concluded that several of these categories had rarely been used by clinicians, and also that some had received little attention from researchers. Studies using DSM-IV criteria had demonstrated that most individuals with a personality disorder diagnosis met criteria for more than one personality disorder type and were usually given an NOS designation. However, even when people were given a specific diagnosis, those with the same diagnosis showed great heterogeneity. Furthermore, within a given diagnosis, there was little temporal stability, so that diagnoses changed over time. Some researchers also felt that the 10 personality types included in DSM-IV did not adequately cover the range of these disorders.

In reviewing these problems, the work group considered revising the DSM-5 approach to personality disorders by adopting a hybrid system that combined the traditional categorical model with a new model that used quantitative ratings of personality domains and traits. In this approach, 4 of the previous 10 personality disorder types would be eliminated from the classification. To assess a patient, the clinician would determine whether the individual had an impairment in either 1) self-identity/self-direction or 2) interpersonal functioning, as in intimacy and empathy. If so, and if one of the 6 remaining personality disorder types were present, a diagnosis for that specific disorder would be given; if not, a series of rating scales would be used to characterize the features of the disorder, designated as personality disorder—trait specified (PD-TS). This category would replace the NOS category and would provide specific information about the individual's characteristics. Because the PD-TS designation does not affect the judgment of whether a personality disorder is present, it serves as a way to characterize patients, not to establish a diagnostic threshold. However, the peer review committees felt that this approach was not well enough established to be incorporated into the manual for routine clinical use, and that removing any personality disorders was premature. Section III of DSM-5 contains this alternative model for personality disorders, which will need more study before being formally incorporated into the classification system.

Schizophrenia.　Along with making several revisions in the criteria for schizophrenia, such as removing the special significance given to bizarre delusions and Schneiderian first-rank hallucinations in DSM-IV, the task force deleted the five subtypes of schizophrenia. Evidence suggests that subtypes do not explain the heterogeneity of the disorder, and they do not correlate with longitudinal course or treatment outcome. Most of the subtypes have been used only infrequently. Replacing the subtypes is a new specification of psychotic dimensions, such as rating negative symptoms, which is expected to provide a better description of heterogeneity and of change over time.

Use of Dimensional Measures

Development of Cross-Cutting Measures

An early focus of the effort to introduce dimensional measures for use with DSM-5 was on the assessment of important aspects of psychopathology that should be evaluated in an ongoing way with almost all patients (Helzer et al. 2008; Hyman 2010). These measures cut across diagnostic boundaries; for example, anxiety, somatic concerns, and substance use would be assessed in patients with any diagnosis. These measures were expected to help identify changes in a patient during treatment, as well as indicate areas for more clinical assessment outside the criteria sets of the specific diagnostic category. These cross-cutting measures performed well in the field trials for reliability and for clinical usefulness as reported by patients and clinicians (Narrow et al. 2013). Before they can gain widespread use, however, more testing of their performance in tracking clinical change will be needed. The cross-cutting dimensional measures are included in Section III of DSM-5.

Dimensional Measures and Dimensional Diagnosis

In a classification system, the term *categorical* applies to a response that can be only one of two choices: yes or no. In the context of diagnosis, either the person is positive or negative for a particular diagnosis. The term *dimensional* means that the individual differences between persons in expression of a disorder are reflected in one or more ordinal scales (e.g., level of relevant symptoms). A dimensional approach can identify clinically important differences (e.g., symptom intensity, frequency, duration) among those persons who have a positive categorical diagnosis. Even more important, a dimensional approach is meant to detect such differences among persons who have a negative categorical diagnosis (such as subsyndromal or prodromal manifestations)—including patients given the NOS labels in the earlier DSM system.

Use of categorical diagnosis sacrifices power in testing and precision in estimation compared to dimensional diagnosis, resulting in slow progress in studies of the cause, course, or cure of psychiatric disorders. This problem arises because clinical research based on a categorical diagnosis assumes that everyone with a positive diagnosis is homogeneous, and that everyone with a negative diagnosis is also homogeneous, with regard to disorder status. In statistical analysis, ignoring individual differences within these two groups is regarded as producing "random error" (Kraemer et al. 2004).

A major issue in defining a categorical diagnosis is the choice of "cut point," which is used to identify individuals of interest. Setting a cut point with a dimensional scale offers more precision in making the diagnosis: the higher the dimensional diagnosis score, the more likely the patient is to have the categorical diagnosis and thus the disorder. The extremes of such a dimensional diagnostic scale would be 1) absolutely no probability of a positive diagnosis and 2) absolutely no probability of a negative diagnosis. Deciding where the optimal cut point should be placed depends on the intended use of the cut point. To screen for presence of a disorder, a lower cut point would reduce false-negative rates. To identify cases that might benefit from a specific treatment, a higher cut point would reduce false-positive rates. Other cut points would produce other placements of the threshold; for example, different cut points may be needed to distinguish those individuals for whom a particular treatment may be most effective or those who are likely to have onset at some future time. Indeed, it may be that different cut points should be established, depending on which particular treatment is being considered (e.g., a specific psychotherapy or a specific drug). An advantage of having a dimensional diagnosis is the possibility of setting different cut points for different clinical applications, with each cut point optimal for one clinical application (Kraemer 2007).

A dimensional *diagnosis* is one special case of a dimensional *measure*. In DSM-5, the cross-cutting measures are dimensional but are not specific to any disorder, as a dimensional diagnosis would be. Cross-cutting measures are meant to be used at periodic clinic visits, whereas dimensional diagnoses are used when a specific diagnosis needs to be established or reevaluated. Cross-cutting measures are expected to support longitudinal follow-up of patients, particularly for management purposes, whereas dimensional diagnoses capture a patient's clinical status at one time point to guide decision making in the next time span. Cross-cutting measures may sometimes remind clinicians to reevaluate certain diagnoses, but they are generally not intended for use as screening measures in themselves.

Dimensional diagnoses were not assessed in the DSM-5 field trials, given that the dimensional ratings were usually applied only after a categorical diagnosis was made. Thus, dimensional ratings were used as specifiers of severity, not as a way to facilitate finer distinctions between cases and noncases, or within noncases (Regier et al. 2013b).

Evaluating Diagnostic Classification Systems

Just after the earliest U.S. classification of psychiatric illness was used in the 1840 census, members of the newly formed American Statistical Association submitted to Congress a detailed critique of the system and its use. Even though the "system" used only two diagnostic terms, they had not been defined, the census enumerators had not been trained to use them, and no one tested whether the self-reports were reliable. The 1840 census results had remarkable internal inconsistencies and, when comparisons with external measures were possible, could be shown to have tremendous inaccuracies (Gorwitz 1974).

That experience indicates the need to demonstrate how well a classification serves its purpose.

Evaluating the System

In addition to the criteria for specific disorders, a classification system can be evaluated on several overall characteristics. One question is about feasibility, asking whether the classification is clear enough to be used by clinicians in their practice; for an international system such as ICD, feasibility includes the ease of translating its terms into local languages. Another characteristic to assess is the suitability of the system for patients seen in a clinical practice, through measures such as the use of residual diagnoses (e.g., "NOS" categories in DSM-IV).

Evaluating Criteria for Specific Disorders

Reliability and Validity

Several questions are important in considering the reliability and validity of diagnostic criteria:

- Do the criteria for a disorder provide a basis for high agreement between raters that a disorder is or is not present? This property of agreement constitutes the *reliability* of a given diagnosis.

- Do the criteria for a disorder provide the basis for making an accurate diagnosis? Because every clinician or researcher needs to assign a diagnosis based on assessing the patient or subject, evaluating the *validity of a diagnosis* is always important.
- Do the criteria for a disorder identify a "true disease"? Determining the *validity of the disorder* could rest, in the simplest model, on demonstrating a clear etiology and a straightforward pathogenic mechanism. In the absence of a definitive cause and mechanism, one proposal for validity is to show that a disorder has clear boundaries from other disorders and from normal variation (Kendell and Jablensky 2003).

Testing Reliability and Validity in a Population

A *disorder* is defined by its set of diagnostic criteria. In testing the reliability and validity of a given disorder, a study relies on a *diagnosis*, which is an expert opinion that a patient has a certain disorder. For any diagnosis, categorical or dimensional, the total variance (i.e., individual differences among subjects) in a particular population comprises three nonoverlapping parts:

- *Signal:* The characteristic the measure is intended to detect in the subject (i.e., the disorder)
- *Interference:* Characteristics of the subject unrelated to the disorder being tested (e.g., another disorder)
- *Noise:* Effects on the measure having nothing to do with the subject (e.g., rater inconsistency)

The *reliability* of a measure is the percentage of total variance free of noise, and *validity* is the percentage specifically from the signal, free of both noise and interference. Reliability is always at least as great as validity. Thus, a measure that is completely reliable may have zero validity, but a measure that has very poor reliability must also have very poor validity. For that reason, DSM-III and subsequent editions have taken reliability as an essential first goal for disorder specifications.

To measure reliability, investigators sample subjects from the population of interest and have each subject "blindly" evaluated several times over a period of time that is long enough to avoid carrying over noise from the first to the second diagnosis, but short enough that the disorder is unlikely to disappear in those who have it or to appear in those who do not. Agreement is measured as the percentage of variance without the noise component. The preferred reliability coefficients are the intraclass kappa for a categorical diagnosis and the intraclass correlation coefficient for a dimensional diagnosis.

Compared with measuring reliability, measuring validity is a greater challenge because of the difficulty of distinguishing between the signal and interference components of the total variance. In testing, the validity of the diagnosis and the validity of the underlying concept of a disorder are difficult to separate. One approach to testing the accuracy of a diagnosis would be to study a sample of subjects and correlate the diagnosis with a "gold standard" indication of the disorder. However, psychiatry has no "gold standard" to date. Some alternatives have relied on "best estimate" diagnoses from a panel of experts or on routine use of a standard interview to guide the diagnostic assessment.

A more robust approach would be to challenge validity in various ways. A diagnosis might be correlated with a diagnosis using another system of classification that has proved useful or with future outcomes known to be associated with the disorder. If the correlation is high, the results show convergent or predictive validity. The diagnosis might be correlated with the diagnosis of a different disorder, and if the correlation is low, the results show discriminative validity. The more such challenges a diagnosis can pass, the more likely it is to be valid. However, the process of documenting validity is long and tedious. In assessing the empirical evidence to make revisions for DSM-5, work group members considered both reliability and correlations with a set of validators derived from classic papers and prioritized by importance.

Progress in Psychiatric Diagnosis

Status and Implications of the Revisions in DSM-5

Disorder-Specific Changes

Although the DSM-5 Task Force and its work groups carefully reviewed each disorder and considered whether changes in the descriptions or criteria sets would be warranted, the reviews did not result in extensive changes from DSM-IV. This conservative outcome could be interpreted in two different ways:

1. Major categories of disorders continue to be viewed in a way similar to their earlier descriptions. This temporal stability of concepts confers a sense of reassurance about their usefulness.
2. The lack of changes reflects the limit of research on these conditions. Clinical research has often taken the specified criteria sets as a given, applying them in studies rather than testing alternative criteria or new formulations of disorders or groups of disorders. More basic research across a range of neuroscience or psychosocial fields has not yielded results that can be used to reconceptualize disorders or ways to identify them. Research on assessment, such as use of dimensional measures for diagnosing or monitoring patients, has not yet produced tools that can be used in the classification system.

The most extensive changes were proposed for personality disorders. With removal of a multiaxial structure, these conditions were placed on the same level as other mental disorders. Along with mild neurocognitive disorder and some sleep disorders, personality disorders were redefined using a combination of categorical and dimensional approaches. This change represented an effort to continue with a clinically useful structure in retaining six categorical diagnoses, even though personality researchers had proposed revising it more radically. Because this proposal represents the most ambitious use of dimensional ratings considered for DSM-5 and was questioned by the peer review committees, it will need more testing before clinicians can be asked to use it in routine practice settings.

Of the various changes envisioned for DSM-5 and its near-term revisions, the use of quantitative ratings may require the largest adjustment by clinicians. As with personality disorders, this effort demonstrates the tension that can arise between the desire to introduce changes based on research and the desire not to disrupt current clinical practice. This conflict will arise in the future as more research-based and quantitative measures are proposed for incorporation into the classification. In cases such as the proposal for personality disorders, task force members and the peer review groups disagreed about the nature and strength of evidence that should be applied in considering changes from DSM-IV criteria.

Dimensional Measures

The most immediate application of a dimensional approach is the use of cross-cutting measures to conduct ongoing evaluation of elements of psychopathology that are not tied to specific diagnostic criteria. The next step would be to develop dimensional measures to help set the threshold for diagnosis of an individual disorder. Initially, such a dimensional diagnosis may be tied to the criteria used for defining the category; with quantitative ratings, different cut points can be studied to determine where to place the threshold of diagnosis, as has been accomplished in hypertension or hyperlipidemia, for example (Hyman 2010; Kraemer 2007; Kupfer and Regier 2011).

Clinicians are likely to face increasing demands to use quantitative ratings as payers and public rating sites begin to focus on reported outcomes of treatment across medicine. These multiple demands may lead to redundant, contradictory, or cumbersome sets of instruments that are forced into clinical practice. If quantitative measures tied to the diagnostic system can be shown to be useful, it may be possible to simplify the expectations on practitioners even as the pressure to document outcomes increases. Ultimately, the use of quantitative ratings of underlying biological, psychological, and developmental processes may help in the clinical application of research findings on etiology and causal mechanisms, as forecast in the DSM-5 definition of mental disorders.

Future Classifications for Research and Clinical Use

Historically, medical classification approaches have reflected a tension between clinical and scientific needs for a diagnostic system. In 1874, in an influential discussion of these dual needs in the classification of epileptic disorders, John Hughlings Jackson (1985) contrasted these two separate needs:

> We are in medical art and science, as in other arts and sciences, obliged to make arbitrary divisions where there are no clear divisions in Nature.... There are two ways of investigating diseases, and two kinds of classification corresponding thereto, the empirical and scientific. The former is to be illustrated by the way in which a gardener classifies plants, the latter by the way in which a botanist classifies them. [The gardener's] object is the direct application of knowledge to utilitarian purposes.... The other kind of classification...is rather for the better organization of existing knowledge, and for discovering the relations of new facts; its principles are methodical guides to further investigation. It is of great utilitarian value, but not directly.... (pp. 190–192)

With the adoption of specified criteria linked to new diagnostic interviews, DSM-III allowed clinicians and researchers to use the same diagnostic classification system as a starting point for their work. This use of a common system provided the benefit of tying research findings to clinical diagnoses, in the hope that the classification could support both clinical utility and scientific progress.

As part of the DSM-5 revision process, concerns were expressed about the impact of using a unitary system intended for both clinical and research use. Some clinicians have felt that the fully specified criteria sets with inclusion and exclusion rules are too complicated for routine use; conversely, some researchers and funding agencies have worried that using the DSM or ICD categories as pre-established entities imposes a constraint on investigations. These concerns are reflected in the different priorities given to clinical utility in the current formulation of the eleventh revision of ICD by WHO, now under way, and to scientific investigation in the Research Domain Criteria (RDoC) project, initiated by NIMH.

ICD-11

WHO develops and maintains the ICD to serve multiple purposes: 1) providing a coding system for public health reporting on mortality and morbidity, and 2) offering clinicians in different settings and researchers a standard, globally recognized system for categorizing illnesses and other reasons for contact with a health system. When the eleventh revision is adopted by the World Health Assembly, as is scheduled to occur in May 2019, WHO will release different versions of the overall classification system—statistical, clinical specialty, primary care, and research—so that these different uses can be served directly. This approach had been introduced in ICD-10, which included two different versions: the first manual of clinical descriptions and diagnostic guidelines (CDDG), and a more fully specified set of diagnostic criteria for research on mental disorders.

The ICD-11 version to be used for public health statistical reporting will be simpler than the clinical and research versions, with each entity coded in only one chapter. For example, in previous versions of ICD and in the clinical version of ICD-11, aspects of dementia appeared in both the chapter on mental disorders and the chapter on neurological disorders. In the ICD-11 statistical version, dementia will appear only in the neurology chapter.

For the ICD-11 clinical version, as with ICD-10, a CDDG manual will provide more guidance for clinicians, with less specificity than the criteria sets in DSM-5. A manual for research use, providing greater specificity in regard to number and duration of symptoms, is also expected.

Throughout development of these ICD-11 materials for mental disorders, emphasis has been placed on clinical utility as the most important priority of the revision. Early in the process, international surveys of psychiatrists, psychologists, and other clinicians demonstrated a consistent preference for reducing the number of diagnostic categories, diminishing the specificity of criteria (e.g., in terms of number and duration of symptoms), and lessening the occurrence of comorbid diagnoses. WHO must also provide a system that accommodates the wide range in specialty mental health and other health care resources available in its member nations (First et al. 2015; Keeley et al. 2016).

An explicit formulation developed by WHO (Reed et al. 2013) to guide the ICD revision process assesses clinical utility in terms of a classification's ability to facilitate the following objectives:

- Communication about clinical conditions
- Understanding of mental disorders
- Implementation by providers
- Planning of treatment and management
- Improvement in outcomes

To expand the definition of each disorder, the CDDG will delineate the following components:

- Essential features
- Boundary with normality
- Boundary with other conditions (differential diagnosis)
- Course of the disorder

Additional content not directly related to diagnostic decisions will provide information on issues such as variations in presentation, culture-related features, and developmental presentations (First et al. 2015; Gaebel et al. 2017).

As an example of the effort to prioritize clinical utility and to emphasize the role of clinical judgment, the draft version of ICD-11 (World Health Organization 2018) eliminated the categories and criteria for individual personality disorders and adopted a dimensional approach. Clinicians will use the overall definition to establish whether a personality disorder is present, and, if so, will rate it by severity (mild, moderate, severe) as the primary dimension of the diagnosis. Once a severity level has been identified, specific maladaptive personality traits can be recorded as appropriate, similar to the approach outlined in Section III of DSM-5. Other proposed changes to ICD-11 reflect the same reasoning used by the DSM-5 Task Force, such as introducing binge-eating disorder, collapsing disorders into an autism spectrum, and dropping the subtypes of schizophrenia (Gaebel et al. 2017).

Preliminary versions of the ICD-11 classification for mental disorders are being tested for use in both specialty and primary care settings (First 2016). An Internet-based resource, the Global Clinical Practice Network, has also been established by WHO's Department of Mental Health and Substance Abuse to provide draft versions of the criteria for comment (Reed et al. 2016).

Research Domain Criteria

Since 1980, each revision of DSM has had the goal of basing changes on the best evidence available. However, few studies have conducted formal comparisons of different sets of criteria. The prevailing research strategy for understanding mental disorders has been to examine associated characteristics, such as risk factors, familial patterns, treatment response, or biological markers. This "top-down" approach uses the prespecified disorder in a classification like DSM or ICD as the starting point for an investigation. That approach has not led to breakthroughs in identifying biomarkers or other validating factors for the disorders; instead, this routine application of pre-established criteria can lead to a reification of the existing categories (Cuthbert 2014; Hyman 2010).

A more open-ended approach would be to examine basic cognitive, psychological, social, or biological processes and then determine how any dysfunctions in them are expressed clinically. This "bottom-up" strategy, which corresponds to the scientific model described by Jackson (1985), might lead to new paradigms for specifying and classifying clinical disorders. In 2010, the RDoC project announced its intention to use this approach as an organizational framework for studying and classifying the genetic, neural, developmental, and behavioral features of mental disorders (Insel et al. 2010). Such an ambitious undertaking fits with the definition of mental disorder in

DSM-5 but will require much time and funding; it will span research from molecular genetics to neural circuitry to social interactions.

The basic structure of RDoC consists of five broad domains of functioning, each identified as a major neurobehavioral system serving the motivational and adaptive needs of the human organism, and each depending on an associated neurocircuitry network responsible for its implementation and functioning:

1. Negative valence systems (e.g., responding to aversive situations)
2. Positive valence systems (e.g., reward responsiveness)
3. Cognitive systems (e.g., attention)
4. Systems for social processes (e.g., affiliation and attachment)
5. Arousal and regulatory systems (e.g., sleep and wakefulness)

Each of these five domains of human behavior and functioning is composed of multiple dimensional constructs. For example, the domain "negative valence systems" incorporates the dimensions of 1) acute threat ("fear"), 2) potential threat ("anxiety"), 3) sustained threat, 4) loss, and 5) frustrative nonreward (Cuthbert 2014). For each of these dimensions, research strategies and findings are described at different levels of analysis: molecules, cells, circuits, physiology, behavior, and self-reports; genes will be considered in a later stage of the project once more information is available. For each element in this matrix, dimensional measures that can be used to assess the construct are identified. The entire project is presented on the NIMH website (National Institute of Mental Health 2017), with updates about findings and revisions. The long-term goal of this research initiative is to find more fundamental explanations of the mechanisms that lead to psychiatric disorders, so that prevention and treatment can be improved (Cuthbert 2014; Insel 2014; Yager and Feinstein 2017).

One assumption of this strategy is that classification systems such as DSM and ICD can someday be revised on the basis of this presumed broader understanding of etiology and pathogenesis to support better care for patients and those at risk of becoming ill. Initial descriptions of this aspiration seemed to many in the field to underestimate how long and difficult the journey would be to accomplish this goal. Labeling the project "Research Domain *Criteria*" rather than "Research Domain *Constructs*" probably amplified the concern. However, NIMH leaders have since acknowledged that RDoC is currently only a way to guide research and catalog findings: "At this point, however, RDoC is not a diagnostic system, it's merely a framework for organizing research. It begins with the humble realization that we do not know enough to develop a precision medicine approach to mental disorders" (Insel 2014, p. 396).

Other concerns have arisen from the complexity of the task of interpreting the huge matrix of domains versus units of analysis. Analyzing results from different levels of study across species and across different human samples, and across the life span, will be challenging. This daunting task will require integrating many different fields, such as molecular genetics, neuroscience, clinical assessment, biostatistics, and mathematical modeling (Institute of Medicine 2012; Kendler 2012; Kraemer 2015; Weinberger and Goldberg 2014). Analysis of interactions over time among multiple elements in a causal chain has been a focus of systems biology, which has shown the highly complex nature of even the apparently simplest cardiovascular diseases, for example (Loscalzo et al. 2007). As the analytic complexity grows, the application of network science to studying diseases has become highly relevant in systems biology. "Network medicine" may provide a way to interpret the most complex diseases of the brain, which likely involve a "network of networks" (Silbersweig and Loscalzo 2017).

Another risk with this directed research program appears to be that the most readily available areas that can support successful peer review to win research funding will be concentrated in only one or two of the domains, especially the more "biological" rather than social or environmental; an examination of the first 6 years of NIMH funding found that only two of the domains, negative valence and cognitive systems, were well represented in the pool of studies. Of even more importance is that most studies assessed constructs in only one domain, so the importance of interactions across all of these constructs could not be investigated (Barch 2017; Carcone and Ruocco 2017).

DSM as a "Living Document": The Continuing Evolution of DSM-5

Classification systems now have the advantage of appearing in an era when digital publication and wide access to information over the Internet allow incremental changes to be made in the classification without the full-scale effort required for preparation of an entirely new diagnostic manual. After publication of DSM-5, the APA established a Steering Committee to monitor its use and to consider changes to it when new findings emerge. This approach treats DSM-5 as a "living document" that can be updated as needed on a much smaller scale, and more frequently than the 10–20 years that have elapsed between earlier revisions of DSM.

The DSM-5 Steering Committee will consider three types of changes in this "continuous improvement" model of revision:

1. Changes within existing diagnostic categories, to improve validity, reliability, or clinical utility or to reduce deleterious consequences
2. Addition of a new category, subtype, or specifier
3. Deletion of an existing category, subtype, or specifier

While this approach promises more rapid introduction of changes in DSM-5 based on new knowledge, it also acknowledges that a total revision of the classification (DSM-6) could be needed to reflect future significant advances in fields such as neuroscience or molecular genetics (First et al. 2017).

DSM-5 maintained continuity with prior editions by retaining a basic reliance on categorical diagnosis. However, anticipating that new data will emerge from the RDoC project, the DSM-5 Steering Committee also identified the opportunity to incorporate a new approach in the future through early use of quantitative measures such as the following:

- Rating of personality traits.
- Developing reliable cross-cutting measures to assess standard elements of psychopathology more broadly than just those specified with an individual disorder's criteria set.
- Introducing new dimensional measures to establish the threshold for diagnosis without depending on the "distress and impairment" language of the past.

As findings emerge from the RDoC project, or perhaps from the implementation of ICD-11's CDDG outside the United States, the Steering Committee will consider when and how to incorporate them into DSM. At least two substantial challenges will face the Steering Committee as RDoC and other research projects produce new data:

1. An empirical approach cannot fully eliminate the need for some expert consensus. As shown in the DSM-5 deliberations about personality disorders, disagreements about the timing of change and about the necessary strength of research findings to support notable changes will likely occur. Even the most thoughtful peer review cannot compensate for a lack of research or overcome strong disagreements about the proper type of research to consider in reviewing proposed changes. Agreeing on the type of data to consider, and on when the data have reached a threshold for application clinically, will require deliberation among the committee members and other bodies that review and approve proposed changes.
2. Allowing for routine use in settings that have few resources to apply advanced assessment methods may require consideration of different tiers of confidence for a diagnosis. In preparation of DSM-5, for example, accommodations were needed for sites that do not have access to polysomnography for diagnosing several sleep disorders or to neuropsychological assessment for evaluating mild neurocognitive impairment (American Psychiatric Association 2013).

The APA's website hosts reference material on DSM-5, including guidance on the revision process and a summary of changes to the system. The earliest changes to DSM-5 since its publication have been technical ones, to improve correspondence with ICD codes.

Future of Psychiatric Diagnosis

Progress in understanding and classifying mental disorders is likely to be incremental, with improvements occurring through a process of successive approximations using the diverse approaches embodied in DSM, ICD, RDoC, and mathematical models that incorporate new quantitative measures. Unless an unforeseen breakthrough produces an entirely new paradigm for mental disorders, the process of improvement in the short term is likely to involve gradual accumulation of small bits of knowledge and integration of these bits in a piecemeal way to shape the evolution of DSM and other classification systems. Such deliberate, stepwise progress, rendered fully visible and readily accessible on the Internet, should make future revisions manageable for clinicians while serving the need for continued scientific advances.

Key Clinical Points

- *Mental disorders typically co-occur with each other and with other medical conditions.* Patients need a full clinical assessment at the initial examination and monitoring throughout the course of treatment.

- *Even beyond the complexity of creating treatment plans, arriving at a diagnosis requires a full-scale clinical examination.* Mental disorders result from a complex interplay of biological, psychological, and developmental factors. Diagnostic assessment includes a comprehensive, pluralistic approach to the patient, not simply a mechanical count of symptoms.

- *Diagnosis of a mental disorder is not equivalent to a need for treatment.* The threshold for diagnosis is still uncertain for many disorders, and the presence of distress or impairment may occur with subthreshold or preclinical conditions.

- *Judgments about competence for trial or disability for social benefits need distinct assessments of their own.* These judgments cannot rely simply on presence or absence of a mental disorder.

- *Clinicians need to develop strategies to continue learning about advances in psychiatric classification and diagnosis on a real-time basis.* Future changes based on new knowledge and technology will be introduced into DSM-5 on a piecemeal basis as appropriate, rather than all at once at long intervals.

- *Advances in DSM-5 in the future will likely include specification of quantitative clinical ratings or laboratory measurements.* These new measures will require clinicians to adopt new assessment strategies and acquire new technical skills over the course of their careers.

- *Future emphasis on assessing outcomes of medical interventions will produce a greater need for clinicians to develop skill in interpreting quantitative ratings of a patient's clinical status.* Clinicians will need to maintain a pluralistic perspective to avoid choosing a single model of explanation and dismissing aspects of clinical assessment that they find unfamiliar or less preferred. Limiting clinical approaches through a reductionistic mind-set will deprive patients of the full range of future advances in assessment and management.

- *Stigma is likely to continue in the future until the public understands that mental disorders have etiologies and pathogenic mechanisms similar to those of other medical conditions.* Popular conceptions about single etiologies and simple causal mechanisms of "real disease" will continue to impede understanding of complex conditions like mental disorders. Clinicians will continue to face the need to advocate for patients with mental disorders and their families, who will likely face discrimination in access to care, insurance coverage, employment, and other areas.

References

American Psychiatric Association: Diagnostic and Statistical Manual: Mental Disorders. Washington, DC, American Psychiatric Association, 1952

American Psychiatric Association: Diagnostic and Statistical Manual of Mental Disorders, 2nd Edition. Washington, DC, American Psychiatric Association, 1968

American Psychiatric Association: Diagnostic and Statistical Manual of Mental Disorders, 3rd Edition. Washington, DC, American Psychiatric Association, 1980

American Psychiatric Association: Diagnostic and Statistical Manual of Mental Disorders, 3rd Edition, Revised. Washington, DC, American Psychiatric Association, 1987

American Psychiatric Association: Diagnostic and Statistical Manual of Mental Disorders, 4th Edition. Washington, DC, American Psychiatric Association, 1994

American Psychiatric Association: Diagnostic and Statistical Manual of Mental Disorders, 4th Edition, Text Revision. Washington, DC, American Psychiatric Association, 2000

American Psychiatric Association: Diagnostic and Statistical Manual of Mental Disorders, 5th Edition. Arlington, VA, American Psychiatric Association, 2013

Barch DM: The neural correlates of transdiagnostic dimensions of psychopathology. Am J Psychiatry 174(7):613–615, 2017 28669209

Carcone D, Ruocco AC: Six years of research on the National Institute of Mental Health's Research Domain Criteria (RDoC) initiative: a systematic review. Front Cell Neurosci 11:46–53, 2017 28316565

Cooper JE, Kendell RE, Gurland BJ, et al: Psychiatric Diagnosis in New York and London: A Comparative Study of Mental Hospital Admissions. New York, Oxford University Press, 1972

Cuthbert BN: The RDoC framework: facilitating transition from ICD/DSM to dimensional approaches that integrate neuroscience and psychopathology. World Psychiatry 13(1):28–35, 2014 24497240

Feighner JP, Robins E, Guze SB, et al: Diagnostic criteria for use in psychiatric research. Arch Gen Psychiatry 26:57–63, 1972 5009428

First MB: The importance of developmental field trials in the revision of psychiatric classifications. Lancet Psychiatry 3(6):579–584, 2016 27133547

First MB, Reed GM, Hyman SE, et al: The development of the ICD-11 Clinical Descriptions and Diagnostic Guidelines for Mental and Behavioural Disorders. World Psychiatry 14(1):82–90, 2015 25655162

First MB, Kendler KS, Leibenluft E: The future of the DSM: implementing a continuous improvement model. JAMA Psychiatry 74(2):115–116, 2017 27851854

Fulford KWM, Thornton T, Graham G: Oxford Textbook of Philosophy and Psychiatry. New York, Oxford University Press, 2006

Gaebel W, Zielasek J, Reed GM: Mental and behavioural disorders in the ICD-11: concepts, methodologies, and current status. Psychiatr Pol 51(2):169–195, 2017 28581530

Gorwitz K: Census enumeration of the mentally ill and the mentally retarded in the nineteenth century. Health Serv Rep 89(2):180–187, 1974 4274650

Helzer JE, Wittchen H-U, Krueger RF, et al: Dimensional options for DSM-5: the way forward, in Dimensional Approaches in Diagnostic Classification: Refining the Research Agenda for DSM-5. Edited by Helzer JE, Kraemer HC, Krueger RF, et al. Arlington, VA, American Psychiatric Association, 2008, pp 115–127

Houts AC: Fifty years of psychiatric nomenclature: reflections on the 1943 War Department Technical Bulletin, Medical 203. J Clin Psychol 56(7):935–967, 2000 10902952

Hyman SE: The diagnosis of mental disorders: the problem of reification. Annu Rev Clin Psychol 6:155–179, 2010 17716032

Insel TR: The NIMH Research Domain Criteria (RDoC) Project: precision medicine for psychiatry. Am J Psychiatry 171(4):395–397, 2014 24687194

Insel TR, Wang PS: Rethinking mental illness. JAMA 303(19):1970–1971, 2010 20483974

Insel T, Cuthbert B, Garvey M, et al: Research domain criteria (RDoC): toward a new classification framework for research on mental disorders. Am J Psychiatry 167(7):748–751, 2010 20595427

Institute of Medicine: Evolution of Translational Omics: Lessons Learned and the Path Forward. Washington, DC, National Academies Press, 2012

Jackson JH: On the scientific and empirical investigation of epilepsies (1874), in Selected Writings of John Hughlings Jackson, Vol 1. Edited by Taylor J. London, Hodder & Stoughton, 1985

Keeley JW, Reed GM, Roberts MC, et al: Developing a science of clinical utility in diagnostic classification systems field study strategies for ICD-11 mental and behavioral disorders. Am Psychol 71(1):3–16, 2016 26766762

Kendell RE: The concept of disease and its implications for psychiatry. Br J Psychiatry 127:305–315, 1975 1182384

Kendell R, Jablensky A: Distinguishing between the validity and utility of psychiatric diagnoses. Am J Psychiatry 160(1):4–12, 2003 12505793

Kendler KS: Explanatory models for psychiatric illness. Am J Psychiatry 165(6):695–702, 2008 18483135

Kendler KS: Levels of explanation in psychiatric and substance use disorders: implications for the development of an etiologically based nosology. Mol Psychiatry 17(1):11–21, 2012 21670729

Kendler KS: A history of the DSM-5 scientific review committee. Psychol Med 43(9):1793–1800, 2013 23822994

Kendler KS, First MB: Alternative futures for the DSM revision process: iteration v. paradigm shift. Br J Psychiatry 197(4):263–265, 2010 20884947

Klerman GL, Vaillant GE, Spitzer RL, et al: A debate on DSM-III. Am J Psychiatry 141(4):539–553, 1984 6703133

Kraemer HC: DSM categories and dimensions in clinical and research contexts. Int J Methods Psychiatr Res 16 (suppl 1):S8–S15, 2007 17623398

Kraemer HC: Research Domain Criteria (RDoC) and the DSM—two methodological approaches to mental health diagnosis. JAMA Psychiatry 72(12):1163–1164, 2015 26559143

Kraemer HC, Noda A, O'Hara R: Categorical versus dimensional approaches to diagnosis: methodological challenges. J Psychiatr Res 38(1):17–25, 2004 14690767

Kupfer DJ, Regier DA: Neuroscience, clinical evidence, and the future of psychiatric classification in DSM-5. Am J Psychiatry 168(7):672–674, 2011 21724672

Lehman AF, Alexopoulos GS, Goldman H, et al: Mental disorders and disability: time to reevaluate the relationship? in A Research Agenda for DSM-5. Edited by Kupfer DJ, First MB, Regier DA. Washington, DC, American Psychiatric Association, 2002, pp 201–218

Loscalzo J: Systems biology and personalized medicine: a network approach to human disease. Proc Am Thorac Soc 8(2):196–198, 2011 21543801

Loscalzo J, Barabasi AL: Systems biology and the future of medicine. Wiley Interdiscip Rev Syst Biol Med 3(6):619–627, 2011 21928407

Loscalzo J, Kohane I, Barabasi A-L: Human disease classification in the postgenomic era: a complex systems approach to human pathobiology. Mol Syst Biol 3:124, 2007 17625512

Moriyama IM, Loy RM, Robb-Smith AHT, et al: History of the Statistical Classification of Diseases and Causes of Death. Hyattsville, MD, U.S. Department of Health and Human Services, Centers for Disease Control and Prevention, National Center for Health Statistics, 2011

Narrow WE, Clarke DE, Kuramoto SJ, et al: DSM-5 field trials in the United States and Canada, III: development and reliability testing of a cross-cutting symptom assessment for DSM-5. Am J Psychiatry 170(1):71–82, 2013 23111499

National Institute of Mental Health: NIMH Research Domain Criteria (RDoC), 2017. Available at: https://www.nimh.nih.gov/research-priorities/rdoc/index.shtml. Accessed August 4, 2017.

Reed GM, Roberts MC, Keeley J, et al: Mental health professionals' natural taxonomies of mental disorders: implications for the clinical utility of the ICD-11 and the DSM-5. J Clin Psychol 69(12):1191–1212, 2013 24122386

Reed GM, First MB, Elena Medina-Mora M, et al: Draft diagnostic guidelines for ICD-11 mental and behavioural disorders available for review and comment. World Psychiatry 15(2):112–113, 2016 27265692

Regier DA, Narrow WE, Kuhl EA, et al: The conceptual development of DSM-V. Am J Psychiatry 166(6):645–650, 2009 19487400

Regier DA, Kuhl EA, Kupfer DJ: The DSM-5: classification and criteria changes. World Psychiatry 12(2):92–98, 2013a 23737408

Regier DA, Narrow WE, Clarke DE, et al: DSM-5 field trials in the United States and Canada, part II: test-retest reliability of selected categorical diagnoses. Am J Psychiatry 170(1):59–70, 2013b 23111466

Sadler JZ: Values and Psychiatric Diagnosis. New York, Oxford University Press, 2005

Sartorius N: Disability and mental illness are different entities and should be assessed separately. World Psychiatry 8(2):86, 2009 19516925

Silbersweig D, Loscalzo J: Precision psychiatry meets network medicine: network psychiatry. JAMA Psychiatry 74(7):665–666, 2017 28514455

Spitzer RL, Williams JB: American psychiatry's transformation following the publication of DSM-III. Am J Psychiatry 151(3):459–460, 1994 8109673

Spitzer RL, Endicott J, Robins E: Research diagnostic criteria: rationale and reliability. Arch Gen Psychiatry 35:773–782, 1978 655775

Spitzer RL, Williams JB, Skodol AE: DSM-III: the major achievements and an overview. Am J Psychiatry 137(2):151–164, 1980 7188721

Stengel E: Classification of mental disorders. Bull World Health Organ 21:601–663, 1959 13834299

Ustün TB, Chatterji S, Kostanjsek N, et al: Developing the World Health Organization Disability Assessment Schedule 2.0. Bull World Health Organ 88(11):815–823, 2010 21076562

Weinberger DR, Goldberg TE: RDoCs redux. World Psychiatry 13(1):36–38, 2014 24497241

World Health Organization: Manual of the International Statistical Classification of Diseases, Injuries, and Causes of Death, 6th Revision. Geneva, World Health Organization, 1949

World Health Organization: International Statistical Classification of Diseases and Related Health Problems, 10th Revision. Geneva, World Health Organization, 1992

World Health Organization: International Statistical Classification of Diseases and Related Health Problems, 11th Edition (ICD-11), Draft Version. Geneva, World Health Organization, June 18, 2018. Available at: http://www.who.int/classifications/icd/en/. Accessed October 17, 2018.

Yager J, Feinstein RE: Potential applications of the National Institute of Mental Health's Research Domain Criteria (RDoC) to clinical psychiatric practice: how RDoC might be used in assessment, diagnostic processes, case formulation, treatment planning, and clinical notes. J Clin Psychiatry 78(4):423–432, 2017 28002661

Yager J, McIntyre JS: DSM-5 Clinical and Public Health Committee: challenges and considerations. Am J Psychiatry 171(2):142–144, 2014 24500457

Zachar P, Kendler KS: Psychiatric disorders: a conceptual taxonomy. Am J Psychiatry 164(4):557–565, 2007 17403967

Recommended Readings

Cooper JE, Kendell RE, Gurland BJ, et al: Psychiatric Diagnosis in New York and London: A Comparative Study of Mental Hospital Admissions. New York, Oxford University Press, 1972

Feighner JP, Robins E, Guze SB, et al: Diagnostic criteria for use in psychiatric research. Arch Gen Psychiatry 26(1):57–63, 1972

First MB: DSM-5 Handbook of Differential Diagnosis. Washington, DC, American Psychiatric Publishing, 2014

First MB, Skodol AE, Williams JBW, et al: Learning DSM-5 by Case Example. Arlington, VA, American Psychiatric Association Publishing, 2017

Loscalzo J, Barabasi AL, Silverman EK (eds): Network Medicine. Cambridge, MA, Harvard University Press, 2017

Redish AD, Gordon JA (eds): Computational Psychiatry. Cambridge, MA, MIT Press, 2016

Roberts LW, Louie AK (eds): Study Guide to DSM-5. Washington, DC, American Psychiatric Publishing, 2015

Robins E, Guze SB: Establishment of diagnostic validity in psychiatric illness: its application to schizophrenia. Am J Psychiatry 126(7):983–987, 1970

Spitzer RL, Endicott J, Robins E: Research diagnostic criteria: rationale and reliability. Arch Gen Psychiatry 35(6):773–782, 1978

CHAPTER 3

Normal Child and Adolescent Development

Karen Gilmore, M.D.

Pamela Meersand, Ph.D.

Theories of development, either explicit or implicit, are ubiquitous in scientific approaches to the human subject. Such theories have their own developmental process, because they reflect the contemporaneous zeitgeist and theoretical trends shared by neighboring disciplines. In the past half-century, dynamic systems theory has fully saturated a wide range of scientific disciplines and has come to inform the approach to change processes, from genetic expression to earth sciences. Most developmental theories of the present day eschew positivist and linear thinking and embrace the idea of change based on the activity and dynamic interface of multiple systems, both within the individual and within the environment.[1] As the level of inquiry moves from the molecular to cognitive development, personality development within families, or broad social outcomes (such as the appearance of new developmental challenges in the digital age), developmental processes are understood to arise from the nonlinear, transactional, and self-organizing interactions of component systems at multiple levels. An important fundamental premise of such an approach for human development is that each individual's evolution reflects a range of interacting systems embedded in a nested, hierarchical series of contexts that constitute each individual's social-ecological environment (Ungar et al. 2013). Such a layered and dynamic conceptualization makes self-evident that a search for singular causality is almost always misleading, because complexity operates at every level of organization when studying living organisms, especially people. Thus, despite their vastly different levels of analysis and value hierarchy, most contemporary disciplines view

---

[1] Examples of contemporary developmental theories include dynamic systems theory, developmental contextualism, probabilistic epigenesis, relational development systems model, and holistic–interactionistic theory.

causality as a (mostly) indeterminate, interactive process as an intrinsic feature of change, and transformation as inevitable.

Despite the fact that psychodynamic thinking has its origins in the linear and deterministic thinking of Freud and his followers, all of whom were powerfully influenced by the mechanistic scientific model of their time, psychodynamic thinking has gradually shifted toward a recognition of the complexity and nonlinearity of human development (Abrams 1983; Gilmore 2008). Most psychodynamic thinkers emphasize that developmental thinking is different from tracing conflicts and symptoms backward to their childhood roots (called the "genetic" viewpoint historically); instead, the developmental viewpoint looks forward toward the emergence of new capacities, new challenges, and new levels of adaptation. The two approaches can both "inform and misinform each other" (Abrams 1999, p. 3). Maintaining and coordinating the two viewpoints—the "genetic" and the developmental—are difficult challenges that are nonetheless crucial to any psychodynamic consideration of human personality development, given that each viewpoint constitutes a system in itself, with its own contributing systems. In this contemporary climate, the notion of linear causality has become outmoded, and etiology is now a complex narrative. The search for causes or reasons for a given outcome has been supplanted by the quest to understand the meanings and processes of change. Indeed, the evolution of the individual narrative "that provides coherence and social meaning" is considered an important treatment outcome (Hammack and Toolis 2014, p. 43).

However, we do agree with some critics (Berman 1996) who draw attention to the overzealous application of systems theory at the expense of certain fundamental principles: the existence of meaningful differential values, the impact of prior history, the recognition of individual responsibility as well as biological inevitability, and so on. As becomes clear in what follows, our proposals privilege some systems over others and recognize critical developmental moments: limits in potentialities are often predetermined by biological endowment or very early and usually irreversible interaction with the environment. Our lens is focused on development as an interface between physical maturation, emerging ego capacities, mental structure, the unconscious mind and its drives, and the interpersonal (and, more recently, the computer-mediated) world, as represented by and filtered through the family early in life and gradually including the society at large. Although developmental phases have been considered a problematic simplification of developmental complexity, we continue to utilize the categories of developmental phases, primarily as a convenient heuristic device to roughly identify maturational stage and environmental expectations, recognizing that the latter (and even the former, to some extent) are powerfully shaped by interfacing with culture, educational access and expectations, standard of living, diet, socioeconomic class, and so on.

We conceptualize psychological development as a series of hierarchically organized, individually unique, and yet recognizable mental organizations corresponding to the familiar divisions of childhood: infancy; toddlerhood; the oedipal phase; latency; pre-, early, mid-, and late adolescence; and emerging adulthood. We hope to show how the interaction of multiple systems, ranging from tangible physical maturation all the way to the intangible development of unconscious fantasy, produces infinite variations of the superficially identifiable (albeit profoundly individualized) phases traversed as children progress through life in a given society. Across the wide swath of cultural conditions, these phases seem to emerge and, in the language of systems theory, represent *attractor states*—that is, novel configurations individually and idiosyncratically composed out of multiple interacting systems but nonetheless recognizable across individuals in similar societies. These states self-organize by virtue of development in each contributing component; they replace each other sequentially by reconfiguring or discarding old elements as new capacities emerge and experience exerts its own influence. The results are quantum shifts in personality organization. Thus, periods such as latency or adolescence are differently shaped, paced, and experienced in each culture but are simultaneously identifiable within a given culture. Such a theoretical perspective ensures that fluidity, unpredictability, and dramatic shifts are expected in the context of recurrent tropes of the human developmental progression.

There are a few fundamental features that distinguish the orientation described herein from many other developmental perspectives (Table 3–1). Perhaps the most basic is our emphasis on the *subjective experience* of development, which forms the basis of the autobiographical narrative that is part of everyone's mental life, whether conscious or unconscious. This narrative usually becomes clear in the course of a psychodynamic therapy and is often radically revised during treatment. Subjective experience unites many of the features emphasized in a psychodynamic perspective.

Another fundamental theme is the *role of the body*. Indeed, mental life or consciousness is grounded in bodily function and experience, and the body propels development forward through its maturation. The normal process of growth varies in its pace within the individual during different phases, in addition to varying greatly among individuals. The *meaning* of these bodily transformations challenges the mind throughout development, because each new physical change, capacity, or limitation must be incorporated into the self-representation.

In the course of development, we also single out evolving *ego capacities* as a crucial feature. Ego capacities emerge from the interaction of endowment (in itself an unfolding contribution as new functions come online throughout the first two decades) and the environment; the experience emerging from this interaction interacts in turn with other developing systems. The concept of ego capacities includes aspects of cognition, self-regulation, defenses, emotional repertoire, object relations, and self-reflection that emerge in a roughly invariant (although highly individualized) program, provided that the environment offers the essential nutriment required for their appearance.

The last-mentioned provision is encompassed in the emphasis on *environment*, both human and cultural, in shaping the path of development. The impact of the environment on developmental experience and outcome is so idiosyncratic and variable that it is difficult to theorize, but nonetheless it is profound and far-reaching. On the larger scale, every society, from developing nations to fully digitalized cultures, produces a paced and sequential set of expectations as the individual matures and enters that specific society's form of adulthood. In the ideal circumstance, these expectations and demands are commensurate with children's maturing capacities, but they are rarely synchronous throughout development.

Nonetheless, the environment, in its interface with the developing organism, is also a source of supports that sustain positive adaptation despite stressors; one capacity arising from the interface has been called *resilience*, a term widely cited in developmental literature but elusive and difficult to define. Early conceptualizations of resilience placed emphasis on the child's genetic endowment or other intrinsic fac-

TABLE 3–1.	Core features of the psychodynamic developmental viewpoint

Human development is a multifactorial process, broadly encompassing endowment, environment, and experience, that progresses in a nonlinear fashion through a series of mental organizations.

These organizations correspond to familiar phases of childhood that are recognizable but infinitely variable and often unevenly achieved in any individual child at any given moment.

A psychodynamic approach to development considers subjective experience and narratives and privileges the role of the body, emerging ego capacities, the interpersonal world, unconscious fantasy, and the pull toward the next level of mental organization.

The environment exerts influence throughout development. With the exception of major upheavals or extreme circumstances such as war, totalitarian regimes, natural disasters, poverty, and the like, the family buffers and shapes the impact of the environment, usually until adolescence, when the child begins to negotiate the world independently.

tors. Currently, most studies of childhood resilience acknowledge a balance between genetic and environmental factors, the G×E equation. Among the environmental influences that may inoculate children in advance of or support them during adverse events, caretakers are generally considered the most immediate and powerful influences as sources of resilience. Whether the resulting balance produces resilience depends on the type of stressor studied and the type of supports available, in addition to variance in the genetic contributions (Rutter 2013).

The modern psychodynamic viewpoint embraces a bidirectional model whereby the interpersonal world, initially represented by the family and then expanded by a growing network of relationships and institutions as a child matures, acts on a given child's endowment; the maturing child in turn reciprocally acts on his or her environment. As noted, this exchange results in the emergence of the sequential mental organizations that characterize infancy, middle childhood, adolescence, and beyond and also contributes to unconscious fantasy and subjective experience. In terms of mental structure, we have already mentioned the *ego,* which we see as a broad collection of capacities, including *cognitive components, defenses,* and *self-regulatory functions.* In addition, we focus on *drives, impulses,* and *unconscious fantasy* and *the dynamic unconscious* (the *id*) as well as the emergence of the *superego.* We assess these features as we contemplate an individual at a given point in development while maintaining an awareness of potential resilience and a developmental engine that can self-correct and repair.

Infancy and the Beginning of Mental Structure

Psychological Life of the Parent

Well before their child is born, parents' early memories, relational history, and psychological conflicts begin to coalesce around the imagined and anticipated baby. During the latter stage of pregnancy, the mother's increasingly inward focus—the *primary maternal preoccupation*—prepares her for the arrival of the newborn, fostering an empathic identification with the baby's needs and nonverbal signals (Winnicott 1956). Fathers and expectant adoptive parents describe similar experiences as their mental lives center more and more on the baby's imminent arrival. Beginning at birth, the mother's and father's unconscious reactions to the neonate's sex, temperament, and developmental needs powerfully shape their handling of the child. Indeed, parental accounts of their own childhood experiences and their attitudes toward relationships have proven highly reliable predictors of the baby's eventual relational patterns (Fonagy et al. 1993).

The newborn is innately equipped for social responsiveness: remarkable capacities for self and other awareness and for the organization of interpersonal information have been well documented (e.g., Gergely and Watson 1996). Behaviors that are available at or soon after birth, such as sucking, crying, and smiling, help the baby seek and maintain proximity to the parent. These manifestations of a biologically based *attachment system* (Bowlby 1969) help ensure the infant's physical and emotional survival. The baby's relative helplessness and dependency lead to heavy reliance on parental ego capacities—in particular, adults' ability to mirror and modulate intense affects— for the gradual acquisition of internalized, autonomous self-regulatory functions.

For parents with psychiatric vulnerabilities or severe environmental stressors, the emotional and physical demands of the newborn can seem daunting. "Ghosts in the nursery"—unresolved childhood feelings, conflicts, and traumatic experiences—may compromise the adult's empathic responsiveness; the infant's signals of distress or bids for social interaction may elicit emotion-laden memories of the parent's past suffering and helplessness (Fraiberg et al. 1975). As a result, the baby's cries may be misinterpreted; under circumstances wherein the infant's natural feelings and self-expression are rebuffed or ignored, a *false self* (Winnicott 1960) may develop as the child, rather than the parent, learns to accommodate the other's needs.

First Months of Life, Parent–Child Bonding, and Foundations of Self-Regulation

The body is the chief conduit for the infant's earliest mental experiences. Bodily pleasures and discomforts, along with the parent's holding and feeding, give rise to the baby's first internal representations (Fonagy and Target 2007). Preverbal infants signal distress largely by fussing and crying; when *contingent responses*—caretaking behaviors that closely match the baby's signals and actions—are consistently received, the parent's comforting presence and interventions are gradually internalized. Over time, the infant's enhanced social and cognitive apparatus, along with the parent's reliable reactions, contribute to increasingly complex, organized representations of tension-reducing parent–child interactions. The result is a greater internal tolerance for momentary distress and a dawning capacity for self-regulation. Naturally occurring parental demonstrations of *marked affect* are particularly well-suited to infants' needs: these empathically attuned but slightly altered manifestations of infants' actual states (e.g., a playful, "mock" unhappy face) help babies internalize a modulated, less acute version of their own feelings (Gergely 2000).

Beginning at 2–3 months with the emergence of social smiling, the infant enters a period of intense social interest and availability. Dyadic face-to-face exchanges with the parent bring tremendous pleasure and excitement to both; these affectively reciprocal interactions are comprised of continuous, largely unconscious processes of mutual self-regulating shifts and gestures (Beebe 2000). Young infants' sensitivity to their parents' interactive style is illustrated in the *still face* experiment, wherein mothers are instructed to engage in normal face-to-face behavior, followed by a "still face" (i.e., an impassive, unresponsive expression). When confronted with a nonreactive parent, babies exhibit acute distress, frequently crying and averting their gazes (Tronick et al. 1978). The infant's internal representations of multiple caregiving and socialization experiences form the building blocks for *internal working models* (Bowlby 1969), mental depictions of self and other that will powerfully influence social and emotional functioning throughout the life span.

Hatching, Intersubjective Awareness, and Patterns of Attachment

By the middle of the first year of life, the infant begins to emerge from the parent–child "cocoon" and become increasingly aware of the world just beyond the dyad. Mahler refers to this emergence as the process of *hatching*, wherein the baby begins to realize that the parent and the self are separate, differentiated individuals (Mahler 1972). *Transitional objects*—often soft, familiar items from the infant's immediate environment—and other *transitional phenomena* (such as bits of ritually repeated songs that the infant may invoke when alone) provide comfort as the child copes with a novel sense of separateness and the subjective loss of parent–child intimacy (Winnicott 1960). The baby's growing interest in objects and active investigations of the physical world, enhanced by the parents' enthusiastic endorsement, are a critical source of learning: during the *sensorimotor stage of intelligence*, which extends from birth until 18 months of age, the child actively constructs information about the world via physical explorations and actions (Piaget and Inhelder 1969).

At 8–10 months of age, a momentous shift in the baby's social and emotional capacities becomes evident as he or she actively begins to seek a shared mental experience with the parent. For the first time, the infant engages in *joint attention*, gazing back and forth from the mother's face to an object of mutual focus (e.g., a toy). An emerging propensity for *social referencing*, the deliberate soliciting and use of the parent's emotional state, is demonstrated in the *visual cliff* experiment: in this paradigm, crawling infants are placed upon an apparent visual drop-off; when their mothers smile and beckon, the children cross the "cliff," but when their mothers manifest fear or alarm, the babies refuse to move (Sorce and Emde 1981). This remarkable capacity to use the mother's expression as a guide serves as an extension of the attachment system into more complex, distal exchanges.

Such manifestations of the infant's enhanced social awareness, ability to seek adult feedback for affect regulation, and early forays into the world demonstrate the use of the parent as a *beacon of orientation* (Mahler and McDevitt 1982). Similar to attachment theory's notion of the *secure base* (Bowlby 1969), this term refers to the infant's highly visible use of the parent's bodily presence and facial expressions for security and exploration. The crawling or newly upright baby repeatedly ventures a short distance from the parent's side, examines toys, looks back to share pleasure and interest, and returns to the adult for *emotional refueling*. The infant's enhanced and specific awareness of the mother frequently leads to distress around separations and the arrival of strangers, known respectively as *separation anxiety* and *stranger anxiety*.

Ainsworth's seminal research on patterns of attachment examined the *secure base* behaviors in 12- to 18-month-old children in order to assess the quality of the mother–infant relationship (Ainsworth et al. 1978). In the widely replicated Strange Situation experiment, mother and child are observed in a laboratory playroom as they are exposed to a sequence of 3-minute events that stress the infant's sense of security. After a period of playing and acclimating to the new environment, the dyad is joined by a stranger; then the mother departs. When the mother returns to the baby, particular attention is paid to the quality of their reunion, which is considered to be the most potent indicator of the quality of *attachment security.*

The original Strange Situation research yielded three distinct types of attachment. *Secure* babies acclimate to the unfamiliar room and explore comfortably while the mother is near, evidence distress during separation, and are comforted by the parent's return. In contrast, *avoidant* children appear less connected, and their expression of emotionality is muted; they pay little overt attention to the mother's comings and goings despite somatic evidence of distress. *Ambivalent/Resistant* babies manifest angry, upset, poorly regulated reactions: they are hard to settle even before the mother has left the room and fail to use her proximity for soothing and self-regulation. More recently, Main and Solomon (1990) identified children with *disorganized/disoriented* attachments whose inconsistent and incoherent reactions to separation indicated a particular vulnerability to poor self-regulation. These four relational patterns, established in the first year of life, have proved to be powerful predictors of lifelong trends and are highly correlated with the quality of attachment narratives in adulthood (Waters et al. 2000). For nonclinical middle-class samples, the proportions of attachment styles have been found to be fairly consistent and tend to fall in the following distribution: secure (62%), avoidant (15%), ambivalent/resistant (9%), and disorganized/disoriented (15%) (van Ijzendoorn et al. 1999).

Although studies on father–infant attachment are far less numerous than those on the maternal relationship, contemporary scholarship suggests a need for enhanced focus in this area. A meta-review of the past three decades of work reveals modest associations between paternal sensitivity during the early months of life and the ensuing security of father–infant attachment (Lucassen et al. 2011); however, existing measures of sensitive responsiveness may need to be adjusted in order to incorporate the unique interactions between fathers and babies (Fuertes et al. 2016). Moreover, some studies (e.g., Ramchandani et al. 2013) point to links between paternal disengagement during infancy and the early onset of young children's externalizing behaviors, implying a potentially critical role for male involvement in a child's later psychological development.

Despite the depth and importance of the parent–child bond, the drive to achieve upright mobility soon begins to eclipse the older infant's preoccupation with the mother's presence. The pursuit of walking mastery creates a temporary imperviousness to minor bumps and mishaps; many babies, caught up in the intense practicing and excitement of locomotion, temporarily seem to lose sight of the parent. The achievement of this major motor milestone brings infancy to a close and ushers in the next developmental phase.

Table 3–2 lists the main tasks of infancy.

TABLE 3–2.	Tasks of infancy (ages 0–12 months)

Manifest beginning self-regulatory capacities as representations of shifting psychosomatic states, along with the parent's holding and caretaking behaviors, are increasingly organized.

Develop greater awareness of self–other differentiation (*hatching*), fueled by cognitive and motor milestones.

Engage in dyadic *affective sharing and reciprocity,* such as social smiling, *joint attention,* and *social referencing.*

By the end of the first year, achieve stable *patterns of parent–infant attachment as internal working models* of self and other are consolidated.

Acquire basic concepts about the world through *sensorimotor* practice.

Toddlerhood, the Sense of Self, and Moral Development

Between the first and third birthdays, children's motoric and mental achievements transform their *sense of self* and relationship to the parents. The early months of the toddler phase are dominated by the recent mastery of walking: after a period of exhilaration, the child's mobility and enhanced self-knowledge fuel an increasing awareness of personal smallness and vulnerability. By the middle of the second year, the child has already begun to realize that the world is not "his oyster" (Mahler 1972, p. 494). Huge advances in language and emerging symbolic play enrich and expand the parent–child relationship but lessen the intense bodily closeness of infancy. Moreover, as parents sense their child's increasing capacities, they begin to impose limits and demands; expected standards of behavior are established via the powerful shaping influence of adult approval. The formation of *superego precursors* provides necessary structure for incipient autonomous self-regulation and bodily self-control.

Self-Awareness

As the baby enters the toddler period, he or she begins to acquire knowledge about the self as a separate, objective entity. Empirically, this major leap of self-awareness is illustrated via *mirror self-recognition,* a clever experiment wherein children are placed in front of a mirror after their noses are surreptitiously rouged; beginning at around 18 months, toddlers tend to smile and attempt to remove the marks from their own noses rather than merely pointing toward their reflections (Lewis and Brooks-Gunn 1979). At around the same point in development, self-referential play gestures (e.g., pretending to self-feed from an empty bowl) and language make an appearance.

The toddler's enhanced degree of self-awareness is accompanied by the emergence of *self-conscious emotions,* such as pride and shame. These novel emotional experiences, highly susceptible to parental demonstrations of love and approval or displeasure, are powerful motivators for learning and mastery. Importantly, maltreated toddlers evince self-recognition but manifest either neutral or negative affect when they encounter their reflections in the mirror (Schneider-Rosen and Cicchetti 1984); their lack of pleasure attests to the presence of self-feelings in this age group and suggests that these are deeply colored by the quality of the parent–child bond.

By around the age of 2 years, most children begin to acquire a *gendered sense of self.* They accurately label themselves as boy or girl; positive and negative self-feelings accrue to the toddler's notion of male and female. However, a full understanding of gender concepts—that is, of the link between one's sex and genitalia, the stability of one's sex, and the idiosyncratic but shared meanings of gender—is not grasped until several years later, toward the close of the oedipal phase (de Marneffe 1997). During the toddler years, children tend to associate a person's sex with tangible features, such as length of hair or manner of dress. One 2.5-year-old girl, after arriving at a play date and encountering her female friend's fresh short haircut, exclaimed to her mother, "Sarah's a boy!" Such concrete, *preoperational* thinking (Piaget and Inhelder 1969) and limited grasp of the permanence of sexual differences give rise to age-typical anxieties and envious feelings: for example, girls may express desire for a penis, and boys may exhibit concern over girls' "loss" of what feels to them like a fundamental bodily feature.

Rapprochement Crisis and Object Constancy

Junior toddlers' joyful absorption in walking and impervious attitude toward inevitable falls and minor mishaps soon yield to more sober realities. A physical ability to move farther from the parents and a growing awareness of the separate self give rise to a sense of personal smallness, powerlessness, and vulnerability. Such realizations often lead to an upsurge of separation anxiety and renewed efforts to reestablish the proximity of infancy. At the same time, the toddler is vigorously motivated toward autonomy, exploration, and mastery. These competing urges cause the child unfamiliar internal discomfort and confusion, often expressed via moodiness and tantrums; noting the toddler's intensified need for parental reassurance, Mahler referred to this period of relative negativity and contradictory behaviors (e.g., shadowing the parent and then darting away) as the *rapprochement crisis* (Mahler 1972).

The young child's distress and oppositionality—such as relentless use of the beloved word "no"—evoke strong reactions in parents, who then must manage their own aggression and frustration as well as the toddler's. Stable, empathic, and nonretaliatory parental responses are essential to support the child's growing tolerance of uncomfortable feelings and inner conflicts. The parents' capacity to reflect on the child's affective turmoil, label emotional experience, and refrain from angry responses helps the toddler modulate and integrate strong positive and negative affects. The gradual development of *object constancy*—a stable, internalized image of the self and others that is not vulnerable to shifting moods and situations—is a major accomplishment of early childhood. This extremely important intrapsychic capacity allows the child to retain an ongoing sense of the comforting parent even when in the throes of anger and aggressive outbursts and provides an essential foundation for autonomous self-regulation.

Superego Precursors, Internal Conflict, and Role of Toilet Training in Early Development

Beginning in the early years of childhood, morality is increasingly integrated into the child's sense of self (Kochanska et al. 2010). The toddler's enhanced symbolic capacities—language and playful imitation—are foundational for social learning. The parent's vocal praise and reproaches are progressively more meaningful, and mimicking parental behavior is a highly pleasurable activity. Moreover, the toddler's capacity for self-aware emotions and increased grasp of self–other boundaries and the novel pressure of parental discipline all contribute to the formation of *superego precursors* or internalizations of the parents' expectations and attitudes. Over time, these mental representations grow more stable, reliable, and organized; ultimately, they allow the child to achieve an autonomous internal "moral compass" that does not require the physical presence of the parent.

The toddler's awareness of behavioral standards and of the potential to incur parental displeasure gives rise to new anxieties. The concern about parental proximity is supplanted by the toddler's worries about *loss of the parent's love and approval;* once the adult's expectations are known and internalized, the young child's opposing desires—for example, to touch forbidden objects, pinch a sibling, or urinate on the floor—create *internal conflict.* Although painful, the toddler's inner discomfort, dread of shaming, and fears of parental irritation powerfully motivate him or her toward better self-control and emotional self-regulation.

Toilet training represents a crucial juncture in the parent–child relationship, as the toddler begins the lengthy process of assuming bodily control and responsibility (Furman 1992). The child's alternating compliant, teasing, and withholding behaviors arouse strong parental emotions and may evoke the parent's own *anal phase conflicts:* wishes to mess, control, withhold and expel, and resist compliance. These conflicts revive in the parent's urgent wishes to restrain the toddler, untoward levels of anger, and extreme distaste for the child's "dirtiness." The combined presence of adult expectations and compassion for the toddler's struggles helps children gradually relinquish dirty pleasures, strengthen their awareness of inner and outer boundaries, and increasingly identify with parental standards of cleanliness and self-management. A central defense employed in this process is *reaction formation,* which turns a given affect or impulse into its opposite: the wish to mess is replaced by extreme fastidiousness and orderliness, and the wish to oppose is transformed into compliance.

Table 3–3 outlines the important tasks of the toddler phase.

The Oedipal Phase, Its Significance in Development, and the Emerging Capacities of Early Childhood

Between 3 and 6 years of age, the child's inner and object relational life is transformed: a confluence of psychological, bodily, and familial factors gives rise to new mental structure as the world beyond the mother–child dyad is increasingly brought into awareness. Emotional complexity, born of the complicated force field of family love and rivalry and elaborated in the growing capacity to express the inner life in language and play, dominates the oedipal-age child's experience. By the time this developmental period draws to a close and the child enters the grade-school (latency) years, enduring self-fantasies, patterns of relating, and self-regulatory and self-monitoring capacities (*superego elements*) have begun to emerge.

Yet why identify this phase, generally called *early childhood,* by a term that may seem outmoded? We continue to think that there is value in Freud's original idea

TABLE 3–3.	Tasks of toddlerhood (ages 1–3 years)

Achieve an objective and separate sense of self, with rudimentary grasp of gender distinctions.

Enter the *preoperational* phase of cognitive development, marked by *object permanence* and more abstract symbolic functions, such as word combinations, deferred imitation, and early forms of pretense.

Develop capacity and tolerance for *internal conflict* (e.g., between personal impulses and desire for parental approval, or between competing wishes for autonomy and reinfantilization).

Begin the process of socialization (e.g., toilet training) via the establishment of *superego precursors*.

about human development and what he considered to be the most momentous period in early life. His reference to the timeless drama of intrafamilial conflict depicted in Sophocles' tragedy—neglect, abandonment, love, desire, hate, incest, parricide, shame, guilt, and reparations—highlights the intensity of emotion experienced by the oedipal-age child and adumbrates the profound impact this phase has on subsequent mental organization.

Although psychosexuality is by no means the sole force propelling oedipal development, the regular occurrence of an upsurge in sexual and aggressive drives, curiosity about parental intimacy and sexual relations, new emotions of jealousy and painful ambivalence, increased awareness of gender role identity and sexual orientation, and the emerging capacity to conform to social rules and experience shame and guilt repetitively cohere into a version of the oedipal narrative: desire for one parent and rivalry and hatred toward competitors, including the other parent and siblings. In our opinion, the regular appearance of these triangular force fields merits the continued use of this evocative terminology. The superego, that internal voice of conscience and moral standards, has been called the "heir of the Oedipus complex"; although its development begins much earlier, it predictably emerges as a coherent mental agency as this phase comes to a close, and it plays a key role in the transformation of the oedipal child into a more tractable and rule-observant school-age child.

Emerging Cognitive, Emotional, Social, and Self-Regulatory Capacities

Both psychodynamic and developmental theorists envision the years of early childhood as a foundational period of mental growth. An explosion of symbolic function, such as language and imaginary play, shifts concrete, perceptually bound thinking and communication toward increasing abstraction and complexity. The child's self-referential, *egocentric* viewpoint (Piaget and Inhelder 1969) is modified as distinctions between inner experience and outer reality become clearer, and the subjective mental states of others (i.e., private thoughts, feelings, and intentions) are increasingly grasped (Fonagy and Target 1996). Together, these multiple developments vastly improve the child's capacity to express inner states, share meanings, engage in social collaboration, and regulate the typically unruly urges and conflicts of the oedipal phase.

Although the child's interpersonal world is expanding, the role of the mother–child relationship provides the groundwork for key psychological advances. Elaborative mother–child discourse encourages the preschooler to tell meaningful, embellished stories. Children with insecure attachments demonstrate inhibited pretend play and narrative incoherence (Lyons-Ruth 2006). Moreover, maternal use of mental state language (terms such as "think," "want," "hope") is linked to the child's development of social and emotional competence (Ruffman et al. 2002).

Language Development

The ability to narrate experience and share meaningful stories is a major development of early childhood. Autobiographical narratives and age-salient stories, such as where babies come from, acquire special significance. Moreover, young children become fiercely attached to beloved literature and fairy tales; these frequently feature oedipal themes and plots, often with more satisfactory conclusions than in real life. Desirous and aggressive feelings toward parents are safely displaced onto fictional love-objects and rivals; forbidden wishes are given free rein and then punished, via *talion*-style justice (i.e., retributive justice, as in "an eye for an eye, a tooth for a tooth").

Theory of Mind

The acquisition of a *theory of mind*, or understanding of mental states, is a transformational process in development demonstrable by the age of 4 years. Once children achieve this cognitive-social-emotional capacity, they begin to grasp the difference between inner life and outer reality, the notion that people possess unique subjectivities, and the link between internal states and behavior (Fonagy and Target 1996). *False belief* tests are often used to assess whether children can successfully discern another person's point of view and then predict behavior based upon that individual's knowledge.

The ability to discern others' perspectives and see connections between mental states and behavior brings new meaning to the child's interpersonal world; one's own and others' actions seem more predictable. Not surprisingly, mental state knowledge is correlated with other essential developmental capacities, such as self-reflection, emotional self-regulation, and social competence (Denham et al. 2003). Research (e.g., Imuta et al. 2016) suggests a significant correlation between the acquisition of theory of mind and the emergence of prosocial behaviors, such as helping, cooperating, and comforting actions; indeed, children who demonstrate mental state knowledge at age 6 years score higher on assessments of social adjustment at age 10 years than those who lack this capacity (Devine et al. 2016).

At the same time, an enhanced awareness of others' inner lives exposes the child to new vulnerabilities, such as the dawning realization of the parents' private relationship and a keener sense of exclusion. The painful notion that others may withhold confidential thoughts and feelings or that peers may share bonds and play dates from which one is excluded enters the oedipal child's consciousness for the first time and becomes part of enduring psychological experience.

Imagination and Play

Pretend play is a natural, growth-promoting developmental capacity that provides a window into the child's inner life. Vygotsky (1978) noted that in play, "the child is always behaving beyond his age": narrative building, dialogue creation, social perspective taking, and elaborate planning are in evidence as the child acts out deeply satisfying imaginary roles and plots. Moreover, by age 4 or 5 years, social fantasy play is a core feature of peer relationships, encouraging the need to collaborate, verbally share intentions, and incorporate others' ideas and desires (Howe et al. 2005).

In addition to providing the opportunity to practice emerging cognitive and social skills, imaginary play provides a safe, nonconsequential outlet for the increased sexual and aggressive urges of the oedipal phase. Both narrative building and play facilitate the organization and expression of intense affects and help the child achieve mastery over impulses (Knight 2003). By attaching feelings and wishes to stories and playing them out, the child's inner experience is modulated: conflicts, anxieties, and impulses are elaborated, tempered, and then reintegrated. For example, the child who longs for adult roles and glorified romantic relationships is temporarily assuaged while playing mother or father, princess or superhero. For an illustration of imaginary play with oedipal themes, readers are referred to the video segment "Four-Year-Old Girl" that accompanies Chapter 4 in our book *Normal Child and Adolescent Development: A Psychodynamic Primer* (Gilmore and Meersand 2014).

Imaginary companions are a commonly observed phenomenon that begins during the oedipal years; a survey of children 5–12 years of age reported that 46% of children acknowledged an imaginary companion currently or in the past (Pearson et al. 2001). These invented creatures often serve as the repository of the child's unwanted impulses while providing their creators with a sense of control and power. For example, a preschooler wrestling with self-control and fears of bodily injury may find consolation in a friendly, domesticated, but nonetheless invincible lion or tiger that requires frequent admonishments and behavioral restrictions. Interestingly, children with access to this imaginary vehicle show richer narratives and greater communication skills. As is true with the transitional objects of infancy, parents instinctively tend to tolerate the companion's existence and refrain from challenging its basis in reality.

Emerging Capacities and Emotional Life

From a modern psychodynamic development point of view, the oedipal complex must be understood as a product of the interaction of multiple development strands occurring within a family system. Major components include the emerging capacities described earlier as well as the shift in the child's bodily focus toward the genitals. Increased sexual arousal and curiosity, expressions of aggression, and the growing capacity to regulate behavior interact with parental reactions and the family situation. Expanded interpersonal relations, including both parents and siblings, foment a proliferation of new or amplified emotions: love, desire, rivalry, hate, humiliation, and guilt. These elements are organized into recurrent but individualized oedipal configurations that structure the child's experience.

The variations of the oedipal configuration are infinite. It is nonetheless usually possible to recognize components of the classical "positive" configuration—the child's longings for the opposite-sex parent (daughter for father, son for mother) and rivalry with the same-sex parent—as well as elements of the so-called negative oedipal complex (son longing for father, daughter for mother; rivalry with the opposite-sex parent). Complications ensue from within the child (including prior development, constitutional endowment, environmental nutriment, and their interactions) and from current environmental factors (such as parental dynamics, divorce, adoption, sibling cohort, and so on). Thus, although everyone's oedipal constellation has similar elements—interpersonal triangles, competition and rivalry, elements of *primal scene imagery* (the child as onlooker to an exciting spectacle of parental union)—each one is unique. Some children focus their rivalry on the "new baby," whereas others might struggle with the conviction that their hostility toward one parent resulted in the parents' divorce.

Passage through the oedipal phase inevitably shapes the organization of development going forward despite infinite variability, new elements, and unpredictable impingements from the environment. There is no prescribed "normal" passage through this phase. Furthermore, it is clear that the origins of self-regulation are traceable all the way back to infancy, when the mother–infant interaction gradually inducts the infant's behavioral control and self-regulatory capacities (Blum and Blum 1990; Sheikh and Janoff-Bulman 2010). The coalescence of superego precursors into the relatively coherent mental agency that emerges toward the end of the oedipal phase requires contributions from a range of other developing systems, including receptive and expressive language, affect elaboration and affect tolerance, new defenses such as internalization, reaction formation and identification with the aggressor, the new capacity to mentalize, and a new cognitive organization of preoperational thinking. These developments all contribute to the relatively stable and coherent organization of superego activities, primarily *direction giving, limiting,* and *punishing/rewarding functions.* Although the superego evolves throughout development and is notoriously subject to corruption and inconsistency, its future shape is deeply imprinted by the end of the oedipal phase.

From an ego psychological point of view, the confluence of developmental strands that compose the oedipal complex is perhaps most noteworthy for its enduring impact on personality. The conflictual constellation or template of triadic relationships reverberates in the object-relational patterns of the developing child into adolescence and adulthood and contributes narrative content to masturbatory fantasies. Future sexual arousal, desire, competitive strivings, rivalries, tolerance of ambivalence, sensitivity to narcissistic mortification, and revenge motives are all affected by passage through this phase. It is for this reason that the oedipal phase is seen as a watershed in development in terms of defenses, anxiety tolerance, object relations, sublimatory channels, impulse control, and nature of superego integration; *preoedipal* implies poor anxiety tolerance, reliance on splitting as a predominant defense, superego pathology, and impulsivity.

The developmental literature has offered multiple supportive correlations for the updated oedipal drama. Children consolidate the connection between genital and biological sex at around 3 years (de Marneffe 1997), so that the emergence of genital anxieties corresponds to the new appreciation of their differences. Despite this correlation, young children do creatively imagine that anatomy is fluid for some time afterward, supporting the notion of bisexuality (Senet 2004). Children's sexual and aggressive behaviors peak at roughly age 5 years (Friedrich et al. 1998; Mayes and Cohen 1993) and then recede. The observed quiescence in the child's overt expression of impulses as he or she moves into latency corresponds to the emergence of self-control and the efficacy of parental moral education. Emotional complexity and moral reasoning, linked to acquisition of theory of mind, show a demonstrable increase from 4 to 6 years of age (Eisenberg-Berg and Roth 1980); similarly, theory of mind and emotional understanding facilitate awareness of others' psychological needs and the motivation to adhere to socially acceptable behaviors as children approach age 6 (Lane et al. 2010). As we shall see, the superego of early latency is relatively rigid and unbending; indeed, the superego requires the whole sweep of development to assume its mature form.

Table 3–4 contains a précis of the important accomplishments of the oedipal phase.

Latency Years and the Shift Toward Autonomy

During the grade-school years, roughly between ages 6 and 10 years, children's enormous gains in cognition and self-regulation allow them to move well beyond the familial circle and invest increasingly in the world of peers and learning. The latency child's industrious demeanor, cooperative attitudes, and capacity to absorb vast quantities of knowledge and skills are universally recognized. Originally, Freud (1905/ 1962) applied the term *latency* to this phase, bookended by the more turbulent oedipal and adolescent periods, in order to capture the relative dormancy of the child's sexual and aggressive urges. However, current thinking about latency acknowledges children's ongoing struggles with management of impulses and emotions and their vivid fantasy lives, even while documenting the achievement of momentous intellectual advances.

Central Role of Learning in the Latency Child's Life

The latency child is confronted with a dazzling array of developmental tasks and expectations: multiple academic and extracurricular skills are assimilated, practiced, and mastered under the scrutiny of adults and peers. After the typically unstructured and permissive atmosphere of preschool and kindergarten, the grade-school experience veers sharply toward specific assignments and relentless assessment. Learning and accruing skills play an increasingly central role in the child's self-concept; slow acquisition of basic academics or poor athletic proficiency pose substantial threats to the child's ongoing sense of pride, mastery, and competence.

When learning, both in and out of the classroom, is compromised as a result of innate cognitive or visual-motor weaknesses, the development of certain latency-phase defensive resources—for example, *sublimation* (the transformation of socially unacceptable impulses and feelings into structured activities such as academics and competitive sports) and *intellectualization* (the avoidance of intense feelings by a retreat to logic and rationality)—is also impeded. The redirection of the child's urges and affects into the beloved activities of grade-school children, such as school-based projects, sports, collecting, and other hobbies, is strengthened during the elementary years by environmental opportunities. These *sublimatory channels* help in the gradual attainment of emotional self-regulation; for example, the oedipal child's avid curiosity about bodies and sexuality is usefully converted into the grade-school student's intellectual inquisitiveness, scientific research, and fact gathering. The presence of language-based or attentional weakness not only affects learning and self-regulation but also contributes to difficulty with the absorption and internalization of behavioral standards, interferes with self-monitoring and self-control, impairs socialization, and subjects the child to external and internal overstimulation.

TABLE 3–4.   **Tasks of the oedipal phase (ages 3–6 years)**

Achieve the following crucial symbolic capacities: narrative building, fantasy, imaginative play, and *mentalization (theory of mind)*.

Use language, stories, and pretend play for purposes of emotional self-regulation.

Begin to grasp *triadic relationships* in which complex emotions flourish in the family context; tolerate and modulate rivalry, jealousy, narcissistic mortification, excitement and desire, hatred and love; experience ambivalence.

Manage the new emotion of guilt around moral transgressions, a manifestation of a functioning superego.

Contemporary viewpoints on learning differences are influenced by the concept of *neurodiversity,* a movement that originated in the 1990s and grew out of advocacy work for individuals with autistic spectrum and other developmental disorders. Proponents of neurodiversity advocate use of a less deficit-oriented model for categorizing such conditions, which they instead conceptualize as variations in normative development (Kapp et al. 2013; Masataka 2017). Within this perspective, the heterogeneity of the autistic spectrum is emphasized: for example, advocates point to the huge diversity within the autistic population, ranging from individuals whose language is severely impaired to those who demonstrate rich linguistic capacities and superior intelligence. Distinctive components of the autistic person's experience are conceptualized as essential aspects of personal identity rather than as signs and symptoms of a disorder.

The neurodiversity model has brought about a paradigm shift in educational policy, including increased awareness of autistic youngsters' special abilities (e.g., enhanced perception of certain details in the environment, facility with numbers). Indeed, some advocates have challenged the widespread use of behavioral treatments that aim to reduce nonharmful repetitive movements in individuals with autism spectrum disorder, asserting that such interventions are unnecessary. Instead, the overall goal is to promote a difference-oriented rather than a disease-based model for unique developmental presentations and to favor diverse treatments that promote coping and adaptation without necessarily seeking to normalize behavior.

The Phases of Latency

Early Phase: Cognitive Reorganization and the Child's Struggle for Self-Regulation

Between the ages of 6 and 8 years, the child's psychological functioning is dominated by recently acquired superego capacities: emotional self-regulation and behavioral self-control are fragile and easily disturbed by challenging circumstances. Although a "good citizen" deportment and growing capacity for sublimation are fundamental to the latency experience, the early elementary years remain somewhat tumultuous. Protests about perceived unfairness, tears about the difficulties of homework, or meltdowns over losing a board game are common manifestations. Such vulnerabilities of self-management contribute to the young child's rigid insistence on rules and to keen scrutiny and reporting of others' minor transgressions.

The child's entry into the cognitive period of *concrete operations* (Piaget and Inhelder 1969) at around the age of 7 years brings an increasing orientation to the reality-based world. Time and money concepts are mastered; collecting, sorting, and classifying materials are favored activities. More organized, coherent mental structures allow for internal, rather than action-oriented, problem solving; this momentous change has huge implications for the child's capacity to substitute thought for behavior and avoid impulsive reactions. Thinking becomes more logical, and the child is less likely to be deceived by the appearance of things; the process of *decentering*—that is, the shift away from highly subjective, egocentric thinking toward awareness of multiple perspectives—makes it possible to engage in abstract reasoning. This trend is beautifully illustrated by Piaget's *Tests of Conservation*, a series of experiments assessing children's ability to think beyond highly conspicuous physical features. For example, a child observes as water is poured from one beaker into a second with a notably wider shape; a researcher then queries the youngster about the quantity of liquid. The *preoperational* child, highly influenced by the beaker's concrete form, insists that the second beaker contains more liquid "because it is wider"; the concrete operational youngster, however, grasps that the volume of water is unchanged despite appearances.

Despite these myriad advances, the child's capacity for complex moral and social reasoning remains somewhat limited. The 6- or 7-year-old tends toward concrete, categorical judgments: behavior is good or bad, nice or mean. Notions about gender roles and characteristics are often rigid and highly conventional. Inward reflection and self-recrimination are often avoided; internal discomfort and conflict are *externalized,* and environmental rather than interior solutions are sought. For example, when painful feelings of guilt arise, children may elicit parental punishment via misbehaving rather than enduring internal guilty feelings. Although the early latency child's capacity for autonomy is expanding, key motivators for prosocial behavior remain tied to important adults; concern over parental or teacher disapproval and punishment, rather than appreciation for mutual regard and reciprocity, continue to guide the child's social thinking and reactions.

Later Phase: Use of Fantasy and the Increasing Importance of the Peer Group

The 8- to 10-year-old child is increasingly self-reliant. A confluence of enhanced self-control, smoother superego functioning, easier grasp of others' mental perspectives, more flexible social-emotional reasoning, and better planning capacities allows the older latency child to participate fully in complex peer interactions and rule-bound activities, such as group sports and clubs. Friendships and group memberships help children grapple with the sense of internal separation and loneliness that accompanies their greater autonomy and diminished dependence on the parents. The *family romance,* a universal latency fantasy, further compensates for the gradual de-idealization of parental figures and provides a safe outlet for the child's accompanying sense of loss and disappointment. The core of such fantasies, immortalized in well-known fiction such as the *Superman* story, is the theme of adoption: the child was born of royal or otherwise extraordinary lineage only to be separated from their family at birth and then raised by the real-life, ordinary parents; eventually, the special powers or status of the birthright will be restored.

Latency peer relations are foundational for a sense of companionship and belonging and for adolescent social, emotional, and behavioral adjustment (Pedersen et al. 2007). Those children who demonstrate a consistent capacity for emotional self-regulation and self-control are likely to enjoy good social adjustment in the grade-school years (Eisenberg et al. 1996). A substantial proportion of the child's social experience is conducted within same-sex groups, wherein gender identifications and roles are further reinforced and consolidated; as intimacy with the parents diminishes, membership in these groups provides an increasingly important source of social learning and self-esteem. Boys' groups tend toward exclusionary and competitive attitudes as well as hierarchical organizations; girls' groups are often somewhat more tolerant and less stratified (Friedman and Downey 2008). For examples of the thinking and socializing of normally developing latency-age children, readers are referred to the three video segments of latency-age children (a 7-year-old boy, a 7-year-old girl, and two 10-year-old boys interviewed together) that accompany Chapter 6 in our book *Normal Child and Adolescent Development: A Psychodynamic Primer* (Gilmore and Meersand 2014).

Table 3–5 summarizes the tasks and challenges of the latency years.

Preadolescence, Adolescence, and Emerging Adulthood

Adolescence became a legitimate development phase only at the turn of the twentieth century and was viewed as a cultural invention well into the 1950s. Today, developmental thinkers in Western postindustrial society view the years between age 11 and age 22 or 23 years as a rich period of transformation—of body, brain, cognition, interpersonal relationships, and emotional life—consisting of a preamble (preadolescence) and three phases—early, middle, and late—although the boundaries of these epochs vary within the developmental literature, within the culture, and among teenagers themselves. More recently, the idea of developmental transformation extending into the twenties, termed *emerging adulthood* (Arnett 2000), has been enthusiastically endorsed by a range of developmental thinkers. Arnett proposed that changes in society had brought the process of transitioning to adulthood into sharp relief; whether what he described represents a transient phenomenon related to a shift from the postindustrial to the fully technocultural society or a "true" developmental phase (i.e., associated with brain, body, and cognitive changes) continues to be debated (Arnett et al. 2011).

The massive developmental transformations of this entire period rival the astonishing developmental changes of infancy in terms of pace and extent. The anticipation of physical transformation, the associated intensification of drives, and the new psychological agenda of adolescence begin to preoccupy children as latency draws to a close. The onset of puberty, depending on definition, is usually clear: menarche and first nocturnal emission are commonly chosen as the definitive moments and assume major significance for the child. Wide variations in the timing and pace of development notwithstanding, both preadolescents and the adults around them are keenly aware that this momentous decade will take them from obedient childhood, in which parents both rule and protect them, to the status of adulthood (or emerging adulthood),

TABLE 3–5.   **Tasks of latency (ages 6–10 years)**

Achieve increasingly autonomous emotional self-regulation and superego functioning.

Begin to establish peer relationships and pursue group activities.

Enter the phase of *concrete operations* and begin to master multiple intellectual skills and an enormous fund of academic information.

Adjust to the self-regulatory, social, and cognitive demands of the learning environment.

Use fantasy and *sublimation* to deal with feelings and impulses.

hopefully accompanied by achievements in the arenas of autonomy, personal identity, sexuality, self-determined values, and professional aspirations. Along the way, teens must renegotiate their relationship to parents, grapple with a peer group of growing importance, integrate their sexual bodies and desires into their self-representations, and consolidate their identities, moral codes, and life goals. Whether these challenges inevitably create upheaval ("storm and stress") has been debated over the decades; today most adolescent scholars take a middle ground. They describe adolescence as a vulnerable period, due to the confluence of rapid growth and shifting psychosocial demands, where developmental conflict, risky behavior, and moodiness are common (Arnett 2000) and family relationships must be reconfigured (Granic et al. 2003).

Compounding the demand to integrate the radically changed body into the self-representation, the brain of the adolescent is also transforming. The adolescent brain undergoes massive synaptic pruning and proliferation of axonal connections, creating a leaner, more efficient organ (Hagmann et al. 2010); this process has been implicated in the asynchronous progression of impulses and sensation-seeking on the one hand and inhibitory controls on the other (Dahl 2004). This same neurobiological observation is often invoked to explain the uptick in *risky behaviors* in this age group, a finding that is clearly the result of many interacting systems. From a psychological perspective, this asynchrony correlates with renunciation of the internalized parental voice before the teenager is capable of consistent and self-determined modulation. Remarkably, there is a 200% jump in morbidity and mortality "due to *difficulties in the control of behavior and emotion*" in the adolescent (Dahl 2004, p. 3) compared with the grade-school child. These difficulties are manifested in alarming and even life-threatening acts, including substance abuse, carrying weapons, driving while intoxicated, unsafe sex, and suicide attempts. The action orientation has been understood as a counterphobic flight into risky behavior as teens become increasingly conscious of their own urges and their mortality while rebelling against parental restraint. In addition, adolescence is distinguished from earlier childhood by the onset of many serious psychiatric disorders, including eating disorders, personality disorders, mood disorders, and psychotic illnesses.

Preadolescence

During the brief but critical phase of preadolescence, roughly between the ages of 10 and 12 years, the latency period is brought to a close and children begin to experience the mental and physical transformations of prepuberty. The calm, industrious, and cooperative stance of the grade-school youngster shifts toward internal discomfort and outward restlessness as the changing body asserts itself. New sexual feelings and bodily preoccupations, in the context of familiar parent–child closeness, are disconcerting for the preadolescent; an urgent push toward independence, a rejection of infantile ties and dependency, and a powerful turn to the peer group propel the child out into the world beyond the family. A sense of loss of control and fears about the potential, unknowable outcomes of growth spurts, weight gains, and changing physical contours disrupt the latency child's recently acquired self-regulatory capacities and feelings of pride and mastery. Under the pressure of physical, psychological, and familial changes, children tend to regress and earlier phases of development are revived (Blos 1958).

During preadolescence, the child's struggle against regression makes dependence on the mother's *auxiliary ego functions*—her empathic mirroring, affect modulation, and support for the child's self-regulation—less tolerable. Parent–child conflicts are common as the adults' authority and the parent–child roles are reorganized and renegotiated. Such changes are often experienced by parents as sudden and bewildering; they are unprepared for the dissolution of previously intimate and harmonious bonds. Increased efforts to restore closeness may only lead to further rejections as the child veers sharply toward the world of peer socialization.

Attachment to gangs, posses, and cliques and the intimacy of the "best friend" relationship help mitigate the preadolescent's sense of separation and loneliness as the parent–child bonds are loosened. Social acceptance and popularity gain importance; the peer group increasingly functions as a source of self-esteem, companionship, and security. However, although preteen bonds appear intense, they are simultaneously superficial and mercurial: often apparently close friendships are easily dissolved and new identifications are rapidly substituted for previous ones.

Table 3–6 lists the developmental tasks of preadolescence.

Adolescence

Three major intrapsychic developments are central to the adolescent experience: *integration of the sexual self and romantic longings into the self-representation*, the *second individuation* (Blos 1967), and the *identity crisis* (Erikson 1968). Sexuality, gender identity, romantic love, individuation, and resolution of the adolescent identity crisis rely on new relationships, require new opportunities for growth, and are deeply shaped by the nature of the environmental context, demands, and responses.

Early Adolescence (Age 11 or 12 Through Age 14 Years), Middle School, and the Body

The preteen and young adolescent experience is fraught with transformation; for most pubertal children, the changes in their bodies are their primary focus. Beginning with the prepubertal growth spurt, the pace of change in terms of height, weight, and development of secondary sexual characteristics rivals the growth rate in infancy. As a consequence, self-consciousness, often with a negative valence, is a common feature of early adolescence.

Beginning in the preteen period, the child's enhanced social and intellectual capacities include an increased awareness of others' opinions and a greater tendency to incorporate external evaluations into the self-concept; these lead to heightened self-

TABLE 3–6.   **Tasks of preadolescence (ages 10–12 years)**

Begin adjusting to the subjective experience of heightened hormonal pressures and changing bodies.

Turn more powerfully away from parental intimacy and toward peer socialization.

Enter the cognitive period of *formal operations:* begin to think more abstractly about intellectual problems and social dilemmas.

scrutiny, anxiety about bodily appearance and personal attractiveness, a sharper sense of social status and popularity, and all-around harsher self-appraisals (Molloy et al. 2011). Delayed or precocious puberty is likely to be accompanied by great shame and self-consciousness and fears of being perceived by the all-important peer group as outside of the mainstream. Likewise, unusually early maturity and rapid rate of pubertal change have been linked to a variety of psychological risk factors, including depression and decline in the quality of peer relationships (Mendle et al. 2012).

The bodily transformation poses new demands, including unfamiliar hygienic regimens; unprecedented "accidents" related to menses and nocturnal emissions; unexpected, often humiliating indications of arousal; and other manifestations of "raging hormones" (Dahl 2004). Beyond the daunting challenge of integrating the actual sexual body into the self-representation, the young adolescent must also grapple with sexual fantasies and desires that disrupt many established patterns of his or her emotional life. A new sense of self as a sexual person—and even more challenging, a specific kind of sexual person (e.g., someone who is turned on by a person of the same sex or by a person who is unacceptable to one's family culture)—can be disturbing and disorienting. Masturbation, which provides a mostly safe opportunity to explore these sexual feelings and fantasies, can feel shameful to a young teenager who has yet to feel entitled to a sexual life. Shame complicates the emergence of romantic feelings and the interest in others for sexual experimentation. The desire to escape the physical self and renounce sexual and aggressive urges gives rise to novel defensive trends, such as *intellectuality* and *asceticism* (Sandler and Freud 1984). Seeking refuge in the life of the mind through books, ideas, and cognitive pursuits of all kinds or by pursuing abstemious practices, such as dieting or vegetarianism, provides a sense of control over internal feelings and impulses. The use of technology, such as social media, further allows an imagined, temporary escape from the corporeal world.

The culture of middle school is rigidly hierarchical, with a pecking order of cliques and crowds that typically affiliate around conventional similarities, such as academic performance and athleticism, and show intolerance of differences: "opposites detract" (Laursen et al. 2010). These exclusionary attitudes and cliques support the sense of identity and assuage the loneliness of the young adolescents who "belong"; those excluded can feel ostracized and bullied. Fortunately, a recent report (Waasdorp et al. 2017) on the rates of bullying shows a moderate decline since 2005, possibly due to greater public awareness.

Psychiatric disorders, especially those related to bodily transformation, begin to emerge in early to middle adolescence. Preoccupation with weight and diet has been linked to the young adolescent's struggle to control the body and postpone sexual maturation. Many dieters have subthreshold disorders that resolve over the course of adolescence.

Middle Adolescence (Age 14 or 15 Through Age 18 Years), High School, and Autonomy

Middle adolescence corresponds roughly to the high school years, the period made famous in media and literature. These teens are motivated by a desire to experience the world, augmented by their new privileges and opportunities; pocket money, cars, media input, Internet availability, opportunities for sexual experiences, and availability of illicit substances must all be managed while students are simultaneously competing strenuously to obtain entry to college. Focus on college shapes the high school experience of a majority of American youth: 69.7% of the 2016 class of graduating seniors in the United States were attending college in October of that year (Bureau of Labor Statistics 2017).

Middle adolescence is a peak conflictual moment in parent–child relationships as teenagers' increasing independence makes the task of knowing how and when to intervene, set limits, and guide behavior a tremendous challenge for parents. This tension corresponds to adolescents' ongoing intrapsychic process of disengaging from parental values and morals, which leaves them more susceptible to peer and media influences and more prone to risky behaviors. Emotional dysregulation is strongly associated with risk taking, including early sexual activity, substance abuse, and behavior problems.

Midadolescents are relatively settled into their maturing bodies but are still seeking to define their own version of their identified gender; the meaning of gender and sexuality continues to evolve in the midst of an onslaught of suggestive media messages. At the same time, a "midadolescence shift" toward romance has been described: teens ages 15–17 years choose partners based on personal compatibility as opposed to the conventional status features (e.g., clothing, looks, or possessions [Collins 2003]) more typical of middle schoolers, and they use texting and social media to communicate and sustain meaningful relationships. As noted, the reported time of first intercourse, a notoriously unreliable statistic, seems to occur toward the end of high school, earlier in girls than in boys, most often with a romantic partner among teens (75%; Furman and Shaffer 2011). For a sampling of the themes of middle adolescence, readers are referred to the video segment of a 15-year-old boy accompanying Chapter 8 in our book *Normal Child and Adolescent Development: A Psychodynamic Primer* (Gilmore and Meersand 2014). This self-reflective tenth grader describes the gamut of typical midadolescent concerns: love, risky behavior, and family relationships.

Late Adolescence (Age 18 Through Age 22 or 23 Years), College/Employment, and the Consolidation of Personality

Late adolescence begins with the transition from home to college and marks a significant shift in adolescents' relationship to family and their sense of autonomy and self-determination. Beginning in the senior year of high school, particularly after college applications are in, there is increasing anticipation of college life, which portends release from parental supervision and the opportunity to make independent choices about the future. A remarkable transformation occurs in many seniors as they contemplate the end of their high school chapter; the rigidity of their social world begins to dissolve, interesting personalities and relationships emerge as cliques fragment in anticipation of separation, and more egalitarian relationships with teachers develop. These changes are often deeply enjoyed by the graduating senior, who feels newly recognized as a unique freestanding individual and affirmed as a person with a future. Such shifts ideally launch the identity exploration of the coming years.

As a result of the "college for all" mandate, the majority of graduating seniors attend college, be it the local community college or an Ivy League university (Rosenbaum 2011). The years of college provide the breathing room for the intrapsychic transformation into more coherent and defined personalities as young people explore identities, refine their interests, stabilize their defensive organization and sublimatory channels, and develop relatively smooth and consistently patterned functioning. Although physical development is minimal compared with the early phases of adolescence, there is a sense of maturation and a deepening and specialization of cognitive capacities as the choice of college major and employment opportunities begin to shape the vision of adulthood in the adolescent's mind.

The struggle for identity in college is never fully independent of prior identity formation, but the geographical and psychological remove provides a clarity and perspective on family culture and the older adolescent's identity within it. For some, entry into college can be rocky due to the complete dismantling of parental controls, revealing unreliable and immature self-regulation. The search for self-selected "new developmental objects" (i.e., adults available for idealization and identification) such as a mentor facilitates the gradual *revision of the superego* that is the work of late adolescence. The grip of parental values diminishes as the older adolescent is exposed to a vastly expanded world; new identifications develop that are at least in part directed by self-selected interests and ideals. Of course, these identifications are both conscious and unconscious; the college student may actively strive to emulate an admired professor and, out of awareness, be deeply influenced by a charismatic roommate or the contemporary cultural idol.

As older adolescents develop more meaningful relationships, the *self-in-relationships* contributes to identity and sense of self. Falling in love, truly a universally occurring altered state with neurobiological underpinnings (Yovell 2008), is a developmental accomplishment that optimally both relies on and facilitates individuation from the family of origin and evolution of an identity. Indeed, the capacity for intimacy in late adolescence and emerging adulthood (see section that follows) seems correlated with both ego strength and relational identity assessed in middle adolescence (Beyers and Seiffge-Krenke 2010). This finding supports a multisystem view that recognizes that identity is composed of multiple "identity domains" and that the capacity for intimacy is a complex outcome of interacting developmental strands.

Readers are referred to the video segment of a 20-year-old that accompanies Chapter 9 in our book *Normal Child and Adolescent Development: A Psychodynamic Primer* (Gilmore and Meersand 2014). This young woman, who enjoyed a very close relationship with her family, is grappling with the conflict between autonomy and dependence.

Table 3–7 summarizes the tasks of adolescence.

Emerging Adulthood

A New Developmental Phase?

Just as adolescence was "discovered" in the twentieth century, so also the newly designated phase of *emerging adulthood*, variously placed somewhere between 18 and 30 years, was discovered and embraced in the twenty-first. Jeffrey Arnett (2000) pro-

TABLE 3–7. **Tasks of adolescence (ages 12 through 22 or 23 years)**

Manage transformation of the body and self-representation, especially in relation to peers.

Achieve formal operations, including higher executive function.

Move toward psychological differentiation and individuation from parents.

Contain and integrate sexuality to facilitate intimate relationships.

Develop foundation for identity consolidation.

Rework superego toward greater self-determination and autonomous standards.

posed the "theory of emerging adulthood," launching a field of study and research dedicated to understanding this population. Arnett observed that the contemporary generation of young people making the transition from adolescence to adulthood seems skeptical of the traditional markers—financial independence, separate domicile, marriage, parenthood, and career—that were the criteria in the past. Not only are many of those achievements now delayed until the mid- to late twenties, but they no longer suffice to confer the feeling of having arrived at adult status. Young adults today traverse an uncharted path distinguished by job changes, continued financial dependence, and the ongoing search for identity. The term "emerging adulthood" was meant to differentiate this phase from what was formerly called youth or young adulthood and to identify the twenties as a time of significant developmental progression in our society. Arnett asserted that there are important psychological transformations during this preadult interlude—in regard to cognition, emotions, and behavior. His five defining criteria for the stage, widely adopted in the literature, are weighted toward the challenge of identity formation in this extended moratorium: identity explorations, instability, self-focus, feeling in-between, and a widening of possibilities. Above all, he emphasized that *role exploration* was "the heart of emerging adulthood" (Arnett 2000).

Despite the vast popularity and scholarly exploration of these ideas and this population, there have been dissenting views. Some believe that "adult development" is a misnomer: development is a biologically driven process, manifested by quantum transformations of brain, mind, and body. This objection has been countered by brain studies showing anatomic changes in brain architecture—cortical changes and further gender differentiation—occurring throughout the twenties (Creze et al. 2014). A different group of detractors, primarily sociologists, highlight the dissolution of hallowed pathways to adulthood as the culture transforms; in the throes of global change, these young people cannot rely on adult guidance or time-honored cultural conduits to help them. Moreover, their financial circumstances (or other factors) often require a return to the parental home, which can prove problematic for forward momentum. In a Pew Research Center analysis of U.S. Census data from 2014, a remarkable 50% of 18- to 24-year-olds and 25% of 24- to 29-year-olds were living with parents (DeSilver 2016).

The coincidence of Arnett's discovery with the rise of the millennial generation has brought forth another group of critics who focus on the impact of digital culture. According to thinkers such as Twenge and Campbell (2009) and Turkle (2012, 2015), the proponents of emerging adulthood underestimate the role of rapid social change in producing this "in-between" generation (Arnett 2013; Twenge 2006). These critics decry the narcissism, entitlement (Twenge and Campbell 2009), and interpersonal alienation (Turkle 2012, 2015) associated with hours spent on social media. Surveys of the subjective state of this age group do indeed show self-focus, anxiety arising from on-going identity struggles (Arnett 2013), and a sense of being in-between (Horowitz and Bromnick 2007), but scholars differ on how to interpret these features: Do they represent a transient phenomenon associated with the first generations of digital natives? Do they herald a new developmental journey to the new adulthood of the twenty-first century? Or do they reflect the narcissism and isolation of our (digital) times? From a systems viewpoint, it is inevitable that culture in the throes of such momentous changes will influence the course of human development, especially the generation at the vanguard. The commentators who understand this population as a product of the digital revolution see the immersion in social media and associated narcissism as both defining features and psychological burdens—hence the monikers "Generation Me(dia)" and "Generation Me."

The Contemporary Challenges of Twenty-Somethings

The transition to adulthood may be further complicated by changing definitions of what it means to be an adult. When queried about their own views, emerging adults agree that financial independence is still key, but they also appear to believe that the true mark of adult status is taking responsibility and making independent decisions (Arnett 1998). These capacities are rarely linked to narcissism.

The idea of emerging adulthood rests on the observation that the conflicts assigned to adolescents currently have a biphasic dimension. In this society, after a period of exploration and stabilization in college, the search for identity is extended, revisited, and resized for the adult world of the twenty-first century. In the process, there is instability, confusion, self-focus, and an escalation of the risky behaviors, especially alcohol consumption, that historically were considered the result of the "college effect" (Arnett 2000). Career choices can seem serendipitous, intimate relationships feel premature without identity consolidation, and marriage is a crumbling institution. Moreover, twenty-something adults are haunted by their recognition that the solutions to developmental challenges introduced during this phase—whether premeditated or random, adaptive or maladaptive—can have profound effects on their future adjustment (e.g., see Tucker et al. 2005). Standing between adolescence and an uncertain adulthood, these young persons cannot be helped to find the way by "analog parents," whose career choices, values, and interpretations of gender roles may seem outmoded and irrelevant. In addition, the emerging adult's perspective on love and marriage may be colored by disappointment in the parental relationship; noteworthy is the fact that the divorce rate, which peaked in 1990, is now estimated to be about 42%–45% and is very gradually falling ("The true facts about divorce in the US" 2018). Indeed, some commentators believe that millennials are responsible for the decline in divorce rate (Miller 2018); despite the generational disavowal of marriage as a true marker of adulthood, married millennials seem to be reversing the divorce trend by staying married. The radical transformation of contemporary Western society has led to a rapid dissolution of centuries-old cultural institutions and categories, such as "traditional families" and "family values," gender and gender roles, and the hallowed one-word career paths of the twentieth century (doctor, lawyer, engineer, teacher). Is the confrontation of millennials with the technoculture that they helped to shape inevitably creating this "winding road to adulthood" (Arnett 2014)?

TABLE 3–8.	Tasks of emerging adulthood (ages 22 or 23 through 30 years)

Determine the personal importance of traditional adult milestones, including autonomous living, career, marriage, and child rearing.

Complete identity exploration to achieve a role in contemporary society.

Renegotiate family relationships toward equality.

Develop the capacity to love, commit to, and depend on a significant other.

Emerging Adulthood as a Preamble to a Different Pathway to Adulthood

The notion of universal developmental challenges in the third decade circles back to the more fundamental question about the relative contributions of intrinsic, biologically driven developmental transformation and contemporaneous society to the shape of the life course. Do the prolongation of identity issues and the decade of "emerging" reflect the intrapsychic experience of 20- to 30-year-olds, or have they been produced by the remarkable social changes that have radically altered the nature of adulthood? Or is it both? The swell of scholarly interest in this contemporary preamble to adulthood still leaves unanswered the crucial question: What kind of adulthood is it leading to? Is adulthood in the twenty-first century so transformed that, as the dimly perceived endpoint of the progression from early childhood until deep into the twenties, it will continue to revise the whole arc of development (Scott 2014)?

Table 3–8 presents the current consensus concerning the key tasks of emerging adulthood. Readers are also referred to the video segments of 25- and 26-year-old men accompanying Chapter 10 in our book *Normal Child and Adolescent Development: A Psychodynamic Primer* (Gilmore and Meersand 2014). These young men describe their efforts to find a path to an adult identity, each through the unique lens of his psychology and history.

Conclusion

Psychological development is a series of hierarchically organized, individually unique, and yet recognizable mental organizations corresponding to the familiar divisions of childhood: infancy; toddlerhood; the oedipal phase; latency; pre-, early, mid-, and late adolescence; and emerging adulthood. Developmental progression is driven by the interaction of multiple systems, both intrinsic and extrinsic, that yield a recognizable sequence of forms in any given society while nonetheless producing a vast range of variations. Phases should be understood as a convenient shorthand that acknowledges the age-stages imposed by social expectations and conventions, the biological unfolding of maturation in an array of systems (cognitive, socio-emotional, motoric, bodily), and the impact of environment and technology on these processes and the desired outcome. Any assessment of a child is constrained by how much variation is tolerated in a given culture and must always be contextualized.

Key Clinical Points

- Development is the process that integrates endowment, emerging capacities, environment, and experience and results in nonlinear sequential mental organizations.

- Developmental tasks are the specific challenges to the mind emanating from environmental expectations and individual maturation and their interaction in personal experience.

- A psychodynamic approach to development considers subjective experience and narratives and privileges the role of the body, the interpersonal world, unconscious fantasy, and the maturational pull toward the next level of mental organization.

- During the infancy period (ages 0–12 months) mental structure begins to form in the context of an ongoing dyadic relationship. Parental history and fantasies are crucial determinants of the baby's psychological development. The infant's shifting psychosomatic states, along with the parents' comforting presence and consistent care, are gradually internalized, leading to the formation of increasingly consolidated mental representations of self and other. Affective sharing and reciprocity are fundamental to the parent–infant bond; by the end of the first year, the dyad displays distinct styles of attachment.

- Toddlerhood (ages 1–3 years) commences with the baby's upright mobility, increased self-awareness, and emerging sense of separateness from the parent. An inward drive toward independence and exploration conflicts with a newfound sense of vulnerability, leading to ambivalence and negative moods. The toddler's self-conscious emotions (shame and pride) and increased capacity for verbal communication facilitate the gradual internalization of parental standards and expectations, such as toilet training.

- The oedipal phase (ages 3–6 years) is a rich period of development with a range of emerging capacities: complex language and narrative creation, imaginary fantasy, symbolic play, and the child's acquisition of a theory of mind are among the most essential. *Oedipal complex* is a term used to designate the coalescence of the child's expanding object relations, emotions, and sexual and aggressive drives into recurrent triadic dramas involving the family: love, desire, rivalry, murderous aggression, and narcissistic mortification are all part of this tumultuous period. The advance of the superego, in addition to the development of other systems, facilitates the gradual quiescence and repression of this force field, although its impact is evident in personality development going forward.

- The latency phase (ages 6–10 years) is marked by the child's vastly increased availability for learning, enhanced self-regulation, and expanding social horizons. In early latency, the ongoing process of superego integration contributes to rigidity and fragile self-control; in the later years, less concrete thinking and more reliable self-management facilitate a deeper immersion in the world of school, friendships, and group activities.

- Preadolescence is a brief but turbulent phase (ages 10–12 years) in which the child subjectively begins to experience the imminent psychological and bodily changes of puberty; these disrupt the calm, compliant attitude of the latency child and initiate a period of inner turmoil and regression.

- Adolescence is usually roughly divided into early (age 11 or 12 years through age 14 years), middle (age 14 or 15 through age 18 years), and late (age 18 years through age 22 or 23 years). Dramatic physical changes make the body the primary focus of young adolescents, and with that, sexuality, sexual identity, masturbation, and love pose associated challenges that extend into late adolescence. Renegotiation of family relationships is hastened by the emerging sexuality of the child, and the superego of latency is re-externalized in order to be reworked over the course of this entire period. Fighting with and distancing from parents (the overt part of *the second individuation*) augments the importance of peer group, which becomes a measure of self-esteem as well as a vital opportunity for new relationships. The *identity* crisis comes to a head in late adolescence, fostered by the psychosocial moratorium provided by college.

- Emerging adulthood (22–30 years) is newly recognized (in Western cultures) as a developmental phase with its own challenges. Arguably a response to the radical cultural shift to a techno-informational society, the proposal of a new phase of "emerging adulthood" highlights the extended period of intrapsychic and interpersonal identity formation that continues through the twenties, as young people forge pathways to the twenty-first-century version of adulthood.

References

Abrams S: Development. Psychoanal Study Child 38:113–139, 1983 6647649

Abrams S: How child and adult analysis inform and misinform one another. The Annual of Psychoanalysis 26–27:3–20, 1999

Ainsworth MDS, Blehar MC, Waters E, et al: Patterns of Attachment: A Psychological Study of the Strange Situation. Hillsdale, NJ, Erlbaum, 1978

Arnett JJ: Learning to stand alone: the contemporary American transition to adulthood in cultural and historical context. Human Development 41:295–315, 1998

Arnett JJ: Emerging adulthood. A theory of development from the late teens through the twenties. Am Psychol 55(5):469–480, 2000 10842426

Arnett JJ: The evidence for Generation We and against Generation Me. Emerging Adulthood 1(1):5–10, 2013

Arnett JJ: The Winding Road From the Late Teens Through the Twenties, 2nd Edition. New York, Oxford University Press, 2014

Arnett JJ, Kloep M, Hendry LB, et al: Debating Emerging Adulthood: Stage or Process? New York, Oxford University Press, 2011

Beebe B: Coconstructing mother-infant distress: the microsynchrony of maternal impingement and infant avoidance in the face-to-face encounter. Psychoanalytic Inquiry 20(3):421–440, 2000

Berman M: The shadow side of systems theory. Journal of Humanistic Psychology 36(1):27–55, 1996

Beyers W, Seiffge-Krenke I: Does identity precede intimacy? Testing Erikson's theory of romantic development in emerging adults of the 21st century. Journal of Adolescent Research 25(3):387–415, 2010

Blos P: Preadolescent drive organization. J Am Psychoanal Assoc 6(1):47–56, 1958 13502229

Blos P: The second individuation process of adolescence. Psychoanal Study Child 22:162–186, 1967 5590064

Blum EJ, Blum HP: The development of autonomy and superego precursors. Int J Psychoanal 71(Pt 4):585–595, 1990 2074146

Bowlby J: Attachment and Loss, Vol I. New York, Basic Books, 1969

Bureau of Labor Statistics: Economic news release: College enrollment and work activity of 2016 high school graduates. U.S. Department of Labor, Bureau of Labor Statistics, April 27, 2017. Available at: https://www.bls.gov/news.release/hsgec.nr0.htm. Accessed August 15, 2017.

Collins WA: More than myth: the developmental significance of romantic relationships during adolescence. Journal of Research on Adolescence 13(1):1–24, 2003

Creze M, Versheure L, Besson P, et al: Age- and gender-related regional variations of human brain cortical thickness, complexity, and gradient in the third decade. Hum Brain Mapp 35(6):2817–2835, 2014 24142374

Dahl RE: Adolescent brain development: a period of vulnerabilities and opportunities. Keynote address. Ann N Y Acad Sci 1021:1–22, 2004 15251869

de Marneffe D: Bodies and words: a study of young children's genital and gender knowledge. Gender and Psychoanalysis 2:3–33, 1997

Denham SA, Blair KA, DeMulder E, et al: Preschool emotional competence: pathway to social competence? Child Dev 74(1):238–256, 2003 12625448

DeSilver D: Increase in living with parents driven by those ages 25–34, non-college grads. Fac-Tank: News in the Numbers, June 8, 2016. Available at: http://www.pewresearch.org/fact-tank/2016/06/08/increase-in-living-with-parents-driven-by-those-ages-25-34-non-college-grads/. Accessed August 10, 2017.

Devine RT, White N, Ensor R, Hughes C: Theory of mind in middle childhood: longitudinal associations with executive function and social competence. Dev Psychol 52(5):758–771, 2016 26914214

Eisenberg N, Fabes RA, Guthrie I, et al: The relations of regulation and emotionality to problem behavior in elementary school children. Development and Psychopathology 8(1):141–162, 1996

Eisenberg-Berg N, Roth K: Development of young children's prosocial moral judgment: a longitudinal follow up. Development and Psychopathology 16(4):375–376, 1980

Erikson E: Identity: Youth and Crisis. New York, WW Norton, 1968

Fonagy P, Target M: Playing with reality, I: theory of mind and the normal development of psychic reality. Int J Psychoanal 77(Pt 2):217–233, 1996 8771375

Fonagy P, Target M: The rooting of the mind in the body: new links between attachment theory and psychoanalytic thought. J Am Psychoanal Assoc 55(2):411–456, 2007 17601099

Fonagy P, Steele M, Moran G, et al: Measuring the ghost in the nursery: an empirical study of the relation between parents' mental representations of childhood experiences and their infants' security of attachment. J Am Psychoanal Assoc 41(4):957–989, 1993 8282943

Fraiberg S, Adelson E, Shapiro V: Ghosts in the nursery. A psychoanalytic approach to the problems of impaired infant-mother relationships. J Am Acad Child Psychiatry 14(3):387–421, 1975 1141566

Freud S: Three essays on the theory of sexuality (1905), in The Standard Edition of the Complete Psychological Works of Sigmund Freud, Vol 7. Translated and edited by Strachey J. London, Hogarth Press, 1962, pp 123–246

Friedman RC, Downey JI: Sexual differentiation of behavior: the foundation of a developmental model of psychosexuality. J Am Psychoanal Assoc 56(1):147–175, 2008 18430706

Friedrich WN, Fisher J, Broughton D, et al: Normative sexual behavior in children: a contemporary sample. Pediatrics 101(4):E9, 1998 9521975

Fuertes M, Faria A, Beeghly M, et al: The effects of parental sensitivity and involvement in caregiving on mother-infant and father-infant attachment in a Portuguese sample. J Fam Psychol 30(1):147–156, 2016 26437145

Furman E: Toddlers and Their Mothers: A Study in Early Personality Development. Madison, CT, International Universities Press, 1992

Furman W, Shaffer L: Romantic partners, friends, friends with benefits, and casual acquaintances as sexual partners. J Sex Res 48(6):554–564, 2011 21128155

Gergely G: Reapproaching Mahler: new perspectives on normal autism, symbiosis, splitting and libidinal object constancy from cognitive developmental theory. J Am Psychoanal Assoc 48(4):1197–1228, 2000 11212188

Gergely G, Watson JS: The social biofeedback theory of parental affect-mirroring: the development of emotional self-awareness and self-control in infancy. Int J Psychoanal 77(Pt 6):1181–1212, 1996 9119582

Gilmore K: Psychoanalytic developmental theory: a contemporary reconsideration. J Am Psychoanal Assoc 56(3):885–907, 2008 18802135

Gilmore K, Meersand P: Normal Child and Adolescent Development: A Psychodynamic Primer. Washington, DC, American Psychiatric Publishing, 2014

Granic I, Hollenstein T, Dishion TJ, et al: Longitudinal analysis of flexibility and reorganization in early adolescence: a dynamic systems study of family interactions. Dev Psychol 39(3):606–617, 2003 12760527

Hagmann P, Sporns O, Madan N, et al: White matter maturation reshapes structural connectivity in the late developing human brain. Proc Natl Acad Sci USA 107(44):19067–19072, 2010 20956328

Hammack PL, Toolis E: Narrative and the social construction of childhood, in Rereading Personal Narrative and Life Course: New Directions in Child and Adolescent Development, No 145. Edited by Schiff B. San Francisco, CA, Wiley Periodicals, 2014, pp 43–56

Horowitz A, Bromnick R: "Contestable adulthood": variability and disparity in markers for negotiating the transition to adulthood. Youth and Society 39(2):209–231, 2007

Howe N, Petrakos H, Rinaldi CM, et al: "This is a bad dog, you know…": constructing shared meanings during sibling pretend play. Child Dev 76(4):783–794, 2005 16026496

Imuta K, Henry JD, Slaughter V, et al: Theory of mind and prosocial behavior in childhood: a meta-analytic review. Dev Psychol 52(8):1192–1205, 2016 27337508

Kapp SK, Gillespie-Lynch K, Sherman LE, et al: Deficit, difference, or both? Autism and neurodiversity. Dev Psychol 49(1):59–71, 2013 22545843

Knight R: Margo and Me, II: the role of narrative building in child analytic technique. Psychoanal Study Child 58:133–164, 2003 14982018

Kochanska G, Koenig JL, Barry RA, et al: Children's conscience during toddler and preschool years, moral self, and a competent, adaptive developmental trajectory. Dev Psychol 46(5):1320–1332, 2010 20822241

Lane JD, Wellman HM, Olson SL, et al: Theory of mind and emotion understanding predict moral development in early childhood. Br J Dev Psychol 28(Pt 4):871–889, 2010 21121472

Laursen B, DeLay D, Adams RE: Trajectories of perceived support in mother-adolescent relationships: the poor (quality) get poorer. Dev Psychol 46(6):1792–1798, 2010 21058837

Lewis M, Brooks-Gunn J: Social Cognition and the Acquisition of Self. New York, Plenum, 1979

Lucassen N, Tharner A, Van Ijzendoorn MH, et al: The association between paternal sensitivity and infant-father attachment security: a meta-analysis of three decades of research. J Fam Psychol 25(6):986–992, 2011 22004434

Lyons-Ruth K: Play, precariousness and the negotiation of shared meaning: a developmental research perspective on child psychotherapy. J Infant Child Adolesc Psychother 5(2):142–159, 2006

Mahler MS: On the first three subphases of the separation-individuation process. Int J Psychoanal 53(Pt 3):333–338, 1972 4499978

Mahler MS, McDevitt JB: Thoughts on the emergence of the sense of self, with particular emphasis on the body self. J Am Psychoanal Assoc 30(4):827–848, 1982 6927241

Main M, Solomon J: Procedures for identifying infants as disorganized/disoriented during the Ainsworth Strange Situation, in Attachment in the Preschool Years: Theory, Research, and Intervention. Edited by Greenberg MT, Cicchetti D, Cummings EM. Chicago, IL, University of Chicago Press, 1990, pp 121–160

Masataka N: Implications of the idea of neurodiversity for understanding the origins of developmental disorders. Phys Life Rev 20:85–108, 2017 27876343

Mayes LC, Cohen DJ: The social matrix of aggression. Enactments and representations of loving and hating in the first years of life. Psychoanal Study Child 48:145–169, 1993 8234549

Mendle J, Harden KP, Brooks-Gunn J, et al: Peer relationships and depressive symptomatology in boys at puberty. Dev Psychol 48(2):429–435, 2012 22103302

Miller RW: Add divorce to the list of things Millennials are killing. USA Today, September 26, 2018. Available at: https://www.usatoday.com/story/news/nation-now/2018/09/26/millennials-blame-lower-us-divorce-rate-study/1429494002/. Accessed January 4, 2019.

Molloy LE, Ram N, Gest SD: The storm and stress (or calm) of early adolescent self-concepts: within- and between-subjects variability. Dev Psychol 47(6):1589–1607, 2011 21928883

Pearson D, Rouse H, Doswell S, et al: The prevalence of imaginary companions in a normal child population. Child Care Health Dev 27(1):13–22, 2001 11136338

Pedersen S, Vitaro F, Barker ED, et al: The timing of middle-childhood peer rejection and friendship: linking early behavior to early adolescent adjustment. Child Dev 78(4):1037–1051, 2007 17650124

Piaget J, Inhelder B: The Psychology of the Child. New York, Basic Books, 1969

Ramchandani PG, Domoney J, Sethna V, et al: Do early father-infant interactions predict the onset of externalising behaviours in young children? Findings from a longitudinal cohort study. J Child Psychol Psychiatry 54(1):56–64, 2013 22808985

Rosenbaum J: The complexities of college for all: beyond fairy-tale dreams. Sociology of Education 84(2):113–117, 2011

Ruffman T, Slade L, Crowe E: The relation between children's and mothers' mental state language and theory-of-mind understanding. Child Dev 73(3):734–751, 2002 12038548

Rutter M: Annual research review: resilience—clinical implications. J Child Psychol Psychiatry 54(4):474–487, 2013 23017036

Sandler J, Freud A: Discussions in the Hampstead Index on "The ego and the mechanisms of defense," XIII: instinctual anxiety during puberty. Bulletin of the Anna Freud Centre 7:79–104, 1984

Schneider-Rosen K, Cicchetti D: The relationship between affect and cognition in maltreated infants: quality of attachment and the development of visual self-recognition. Child Dev 55(2):648–658, 1984 6723453

Scott AO: The death of adulthood in American culture. New York Times Magazine: The Culture Issue, September 11, 2014. Available at: https://www.nytimes.com/2014/09/14/magazine/the-death-of-adulthood-in-american-culture.html?_r=0. Accessed August 19, 2017.

Senet NV: A study of preschool children's linking of genitals and gender. Psychoanal Q 73(2):291–334, 2004 15108403

Sheikh S, Janoff-Bulman R: Tracing the self-regulatory bases of moral emotions. Emotion Review 2(4):386–396, 2010

Sorce J, Emde R: Mother's presence is not enough: effect of emotional availability on infant experience. Developmental Psychology 17(6):737–745, 1981

Tronick E, Als H, Adamson L, et al: The infant's response to entrapment between contradictory messages in face-to-face interaction. J Am Acad Child Psychiatry 17(1):1–13, 1978 632477

"The true facts about divorce in the U.S." Divorce Lawyers for Men (blog). 2018. Available at: https://www.divorcelawyersformen.com/blog/divorce-rate-us-2018/. Accessed January 4, 2019.

Tucker JS, Ellickson PL, Orlando M, et al: Substance use trajectories from early adolescence to emerging adulthood: a comparison of smoking, binge drinking, and marijuana use. Journal of Drug Issues 35(2):307–332, 2005

Turkle S: Alone Together: Why We Expect More From Technology and Less From Each Other. New York, Basic Books, 2012

Turkle S: Reclaiming Conversation: The Power of Talk in a Digital Age. New York, Penguin Books, 2015

Twenge JM: Generation Me: Why Today's Young Americans Are More Confident, Assertive, Entitled—and More Miserable Than Ever Before. New York, Free Press, 2006

Twenge JM, Campbell WK: The Narcissism Epidemic: Living in the Age of Entitlement. New York, Atria Paperback, 2009

Ungar M, Ghazinour M, Richter J: Annual Research Review: What is resilience within the social ecology of human development? J Child Psychol Psychiatry 54(4):348–366, 2013 23215898

van Ijzendoorn MH, Schuengel C, Bakermans-Kranenburg MJ: Disorganized attachment in early childhood: meta-analysis of precursors, concomitants, and sequelae. Dev Psychopathol 11(2):225–249, 1999 16506532

Vygotsky L: Mind in Society: The Development of Higher Psychological Processes. Cambridge, MA, Harvard University Press, 1978

Waasdorp TE, Pas ET, Zablotsky B, Bradshaw CP: Ten-year trends in bullying and related attitudes among 4th- to 12th-graders. Pediatrics 139(6), 2017 28562260

Waters E, Merrick S, Treboux D, et al: Attachment security in infancy and early adulthood: a twenty-year longitudinal study. Child Dev 71(3):684–689, 2000 10953934

Winnicott DW: The primary maternal preoccupation, in From Pediatrics to Psychoanalysis: Collected Papers. New York, Basic Books, 1956, pp 300–305

Winnicott DW: The theory of the parent-infant relationship. Int J Psychoanal 41:585–595, 1960 13785877

Yovell Y: Is there a drive to love? Neuro-psychoanalysis 10:117–144, 2008

Recommended Readings

Arnett J: Emerging Adulthood: The Winding Road From the Late Teens Through the Twenties. New York, Oxford University Press, 2006

Fonagy P, Gergely G, Jurist E, et al: Affect Regulation, Mentalization, and the Development of the Self. New York, Other Press, 2000

Fraiberg SH: The Magic Years: Understanding and Handling the Problems of Early Childhood. New York, Scribner, 1996

Gilmore K, Meersand P: Normal Child and Adolescent Development: A Psychodynamic Primer. Washington, DC, American Psychiatric Publishing, 2013

The Guttmacher Institute: In Brief: Facts on American Teens' Sexual and Reproductive Health. Washington, DC, The Guttmacher Institute, February 2012. Available at: http://www.guttmacher.org/pubs/FB-ATSRH.html.

Sroufe LA, Egeland B, Carlson E, et al: The Development of the Person: The Minnesota Study of Risk and Adaptation From Birth to Adulthood. New York, Guilford, 2005

Recommended Novels

Kincaid J: Annie John. New York, Farrar Strauss and Giroux, 1997
McCullers C: The Member of the Wedding. Boston, MA, Houghton Mifflin, 1946
Mitchell D: Black Swan Green. New York, Random House, 2006
Salinger JD: Catcher in the Rye. New York, Little Brown, 1951

CHAPTER 4

Assessment of Suicide Risk

M. David Rudd, Ph.D., A.B.P.P.

Laura Weiss Roberts, M.D., M.A.

Suicide is one of the leading preventable causes of premature mortality among young people, elders, and other special populations and the proximal cause of death for many mental and physical disorders. The Centers for Disease Control and Prevention (CDC) recently reported that suicide rates in the United States have risen nearly 30% since 1999, with increases affecting both men and women (Stone et al. 2018). Nearly 1 million people die each year by suicide throughout the world, and yet clinicians may consider patient suicide to be a rare event in the context of psychiatric practice and training. Assessment of acute suicide risk is very complex and lacks a robust standard of care (Simon 2012). Every patient has a different degree of risk, and a patient's risk may change dramatically and quickly. Standardized suicide risk scales cannot predict which patients will die by suicide. Similarly, self-administered scales for patients are sensitive but not specific. For these reasons, learning to assess suicide risk and maintaining an up-to-date skill set in the context of a clinical interview are both very important and very difficult.

The stated desire to die may be a form of problem solving to eliminate what feels like overwhelming and unrelenting psychological pain (Chiles et al. 2019). A thorough psychiatric interview will cover these issues in detail, as well as other aspects of the patient's presentation. The CDC's recent suicide study revealed that approximately half of suicide decedents in the National Violent Death Reporting System did not have a known preexisting psychiatric diagnosis (Stone et al. 2018). Empirical efforts have led to greater appreciation of how the following factors contribute to completed suicide: 1) the presence of acute distress, commonly but not always associated with an existing mental disorder, combined with 2) an acute sense of loss or rupture in feelings of belonging, along with 3) access to means of committing suicide (Joiner et al. 2009). A review of 22 clinical practice guidelines and resource documents in suicide prevention and risk management (Bernert et al. 2014) revealed that best practices include 1) evaluation of risk factors and warning signs associated with risk, including static and dynamic risk factors such as diagnostic, demographic, and psychosocial factors, plus protective factors; 2) evaluation of the degree of suicidal intent and planning; 3) consideration of evidence-based approaches for management of suicide risk; and 4) proactive efforts to restrict access to means of self-harm. Suicide risk assessment also should take into consideration a continuum of suicidality: acute, chronic, chronic high-risk, and chronic high-risk with acute exacerbation (Bryan and Rudd 2006).

To perform a thorough, attuned, and accurate psychiatric interview in line with best practices, focusing on evaluating and managing suicide risk, it is essential that the psychiatrist create a milieu of safety and a basis for therapeutic engagement with the patient. The patient may be greatly distressed, frightened, volatile, or withdrawn. The patient may feel trapped and out of control. The patient may seem unreachable, challenging, or even dangerous. The psychiatrist, when faced with the at-risk patient, may experience a range of emotions, from empathetic to overwhelmed. While seeking to understand the patient's experience, the psychiatrist should monitor his or her own feelings carefully to ensure that they do not interfere with his or her ability to establish and sustain a positive alliance with the patient. A positive physician–patient alliance is helpful in improving the accuracy of the clinician's evaluation and may be especially valuable in helping the patient to clarify the symptoms, stressors, and challenges that led to the situation in which a suicide assessment was warranted.

The basis for future therapeutic work is established in the first interaction with the patient. The crisis team may not have a role in the patient's ongoing care, but the patient's future expectations will be shaped by the crisis encounter—even if it is short or only one episode among dozens in the patient's care. The interaction may affect whether the patient steps forward, with a sense of hope, to receive necessary care willingly or resists the recommendations of the clinical team.

Many patients identify suicide as a solution to unrelenting and severe emotional pain. Some severely thought-disordered patients may be experiencing command hallucinations or delusions that make suicide feel necessary. These patients are truly fighting for their lives. It is critical that the clinician keep the patient's symptoms in mind and remember that the patient may have difficulties with emotional regulation, concentration, communication, memory, and/or cognition that interfere with the interview.

To establish an alliance with the patient, it is vital that the clinician use clear, unambiguous language and pay full attention to the patient's concerns (the patient, not the electronic health record, should be the focus). It is important for the clinician to reassure the patient and try to make the patient comfortable (e.g., offering juice or a snack to a patient who has not eaten). The clinician should recognize and explicitly acknowledge the patient's painful struggle and, when possible, should attempt to normalize the distress that the patient is experiencing. For example, it may be appropriate to talk about natural feelings of anxiety, guilt, and self-doubt when speaking with a veteran who has recently returned from difficult wartime experiences overseas. It may be appropriate to discuss the overwhelming pain of losing a spouse when speaking with a widower who experiences suicidal thoughts.

It is important for all clinicians to understand that raising the issue of suicide does not lead to new suicidal thoughts or in some way motivate a patient toward suicide.

Evidence suggests that engaging with patients explicitly, and with a therapeutic approach, will reduce risk in the immediate situation or near term (Gould et al. 2005). Careful and fine-grained, highly specific questions, when offered in a gentle and supportive manner, facilitate a good therapeutic connection with the patient. Detailed questioning can communicate positive therapeutic intent and support for the patient's efforts in being fully open and detailed with the clinician.

The clinician should clarify that the goal of the interview is to help the patient recover a sense of personal agency, safety, control, and hope. If the patient has been contemplating suicide for a while, it is helpful to positively acknowledge any ambivalence and to express support for whatever efforts the patient has made in self-care and in staying alive. If the patient gives the clinician an opening, the clinician can take a few minutes to explore reasons for the patient to stay alive. The clinician can acknowledge the patient's distress, comment on how the patient's symptoms are influencing the patient's feelings, and clarify that his or her intent is to collaborate with the patient toward a safe solution. Providing accurate information about how suicidal feelings can be managed and how mental health issues can be addressed will help to establish trust and may serve to inspire hope for the distressed patient contemplating self-harm.

Because fear and shame may dominate the thinking of suicidal individuals (Rudd et al. 2004), the clinician must avoid comments that may be experienced as threatening or judgmental. This concern is especially important when the patient has experienced a sudden sense of loss or rupture in his or her feelings of belonging. Intensifying the fear and shame will cause the patient to disengage and may rupture the physician–patient alliance that is so valuable in determining and working with the patient's suicidality in a therapeutic manner. Without positive intervention, feelings of fear and shame may lead the patient to hide or deny important symptoms or stressors influencing the crisis.

Feelings of fear and shame are perhaps most salient in the care of a person newly experiencing suicidal thoughts and having an initial encounter with a psychiatrist or other mental health professional. A young college student with first-episode psychosis, for example, may be scared of the voices or intrusive thoughts he is experiencing. He may be worried that others will reject him or "lock him up," and because of these fears, his thoughts of suicide may intensify. In this situation, it is ideal if the psychiatrist can first reassure the patient, address his fears as natural under the circumstances, offer nonjudgmental support, and introduce some basic information about mental disorders and the system of care. The clinician may then be able to turn to the task of assessing more deeply the differential diagnosis, precipitating factors, and the student's context, strengths, relevant safety issues, and resources.

In a crisis situation, clinicians must anticipate and prepare for patients who become irritable, provocative, hostile, or aggressive and are unable to connect therapeutically. The patient may have experienced trauma in the past and may feel that he must protect himself. The patient may have severe psychopathology that is difficult to control and that manifests in a dangerous manner. The patient may have personality pathology and an opportunity for secondary gain, and the behavior may be intentional, although this scenario is less common. The clinician should work to ensure that the environment is safe. Then, to the extent possible, the clinician should acknowledge the patient's hardships and intense emotions and return the patient to the tasks of assessment and treatment planning, emphasizing the collaboration between the clinician and clinical team and the patient. As illustrated by Rudd (2012), the clinician could say:

> I can understand why you'd be so upset. You've had some very painful things happen in the past several weeks. We can take a few minutes and talk more about some of those things if you'd like, but in the next 5 or 10 minutes I'm going to need to ask you some questions and get some information so that we can make a decision about how to respond today and over the next several days. We will come back to some of the things that have happened to you after we make a decision about what is best to do right now.

Exploring modifiable and treatable risk factors that may be influencing the situation is an important focus of the initial assessment. Examples of such risk factors include the presence, diagnostically, of depression, anxiety, panic attacks, psychosis, sleep disruption or sleep disorders, medication side effects, and substance abuse or withdrawal. The potential contributions of impulsivity, agitation, physical illness, or psychosocial stressors such as divorce or loss of employment are also crucial to the initial evaluation.

Assessment of suicide risk can be a challenging, complex, and high-stakes task, especially in a busy clinical setting. Remaining empathic and nonjudgmental while learning about the patient's experience is important, as are establishing a therapeutic connection, proffering accurate information, and creating a sense of safety and hope. The evaluation is also predicated on an astute psychiatric and medical assessment as well as a psychosocial inventory of contributing stressors. Such efforts will improve the quality and accuracy of the assessment and strengthen the likelihood that the patient will engage in recommended care willingly.

Evaluating Suicidal Cognitions and Behaviors

Evaluating suicidal cognitions and behaviors, with a focus on suicidal intent and means, requires a careful and thorough approach. Such an approach should be guided by a larger framework, introduced below, that allows the clinician to keep track of a wide number of issues with bearing on the patient's situation. The framework aids the clinician in developing a more precise understanding of the patient and of the patient's level of risk.

A number of systematic measures have been recommended in clinical practice guidelines for suicide assessment and prevention, including the Beck Scale for Suicidal Ideation, the Beck Depression Inventory, the Beck Hopelessness Scale, the Child-Adolescent Suicidal Potential Index, and the Columbia Teen Screen (Bernert et al. 2014). Some of these measures are administered by clinicians, whereas others may be self-administered and incorporated into a more comprehensive clinical interview. It is important to note that these measures have not been demonstrated to accurately predict suicide. They cannot, alone, formally determine suicide risk. They can, however, supplement a careful psychiatric assessment in the context of a clinical interview.

A valuable framework for the clinical interview is provided in Figure 4–1 in the form of a flowchart with six steps and related questions. The flowchart is the result of iterative conceptual and empirical work by one of us (M.D.R.) over many years (Rudd 2006, 2012). The flowchart includes elements and dimensions that are present in guidelines developed by the American Psychiatric Association (Jacobs et al. 2010) as well as in other guidelines and resource documents (Bernert et al. 2014). Following this systematic approach will help to clarify the precise character and seriousness of suicidal cognitions and behaviors and will help the clinician to arrive at a formulation of suicidal intent.

The first step of the flowchart in Figure 4–1 is to determine the presence of suicidal thoughts. The clinician should ask the patient the following straightforward question: *Have you had thoughts about suicide, thoughts of killing yourself?* The question should be asked in a neutral, nonjudgmental, and gentle manner. If the patient has difficulty answering, it may help for the clinician to say something that destigmatizes the topic, such as, *You mentioned that you have been feeling so hopeless and down and depressed. It is not unexpected for people who are depressed to have thoughts of dying. Is this something you have been thinking about? Have you been looking into ways to end your life?*

This initial step of asking about suicidal thoughts then leads to further inquiries, structured in a hierarchical and sequential fashion to support a clinical interview. Transitioning from past suicidal episodes to emphasize the present situation after a set of initial screening questions reduces the anxiety and resistance of the distressed patient. The patient's response will vary depending on the chronicity of suicidality. For some patients, the interview will focus on the immediate situation. For others, the interview will entail a discussion of a number of past suicidal episodes.

It is important to differentiate among three constructs of suicidal cognitions: suicidal thoughts, morbid ruminations, and thoughts of self-harm (Rudd 2012). *Suicidal thoughts* are thoughts of intentionally ending one's life—of killing oneself. *Morbid ruminations* are thoughts about death, dying, ending up dead, or nonexistence, without active thoughts about killing oneself. *Thoughts of self-harm* may have little to do with a desire to die and are typically motivated as a strategy for emotional regulation and problem solving, or for a reason other than seeking death, such as avoiding embarrassment, feelings of unrelenting guilt, dealing with a stigmatizing event, or managing serious interpersonal conflict.

When attempting to differentiate between morbid ruminations and suicidal thoughts, the clinician must engage in a careful, detailed review of the patient's history of suicidal thoughts and behaviors, even when the patient is not currently endorsing such thoughts. As noted in Figure 4–1, morbid ruminations carry lower risk than suicidal thoughts. Morbid ruminations are viewed by some suicidologists as being passive suicidal thoughts, but it is not known whether all morbid ruminations could progress to active suicidal thoughts, as implied by this conceptualization. Patients can rapidly progress (or move back and forth) from morbid ruminations to suicidal thoughts, which is especially worrisome in the context of patients with a history of previous suicide attempts. The transition from morbid ruminations to suicidal thinking can be used as an easily recognized warning sign. The patient can learn to recognize the differences among the three types of thoughts and openly divulge when morbid ruminations become suicidal thoughts. This newly developed self-awareness can also be integrated into the therapeutic and safety management plan (Wenzel et al. 2008). Keeping the three constructs—suicidal thoughts, morbid ruminations, and thoughts of self-harm—in mind, the clinician may document different kinds of cognitions and potential warning signs in a manner that will allow them to be tracked over time.

Differentiating among suicidal thoughts, morbid ruminations, and thoughts of self-harm is important for the patient and the clinician. Knowing that having thoughts

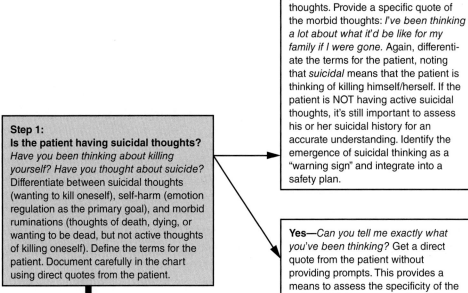

Step 1:
Is the patient having suicidal thoughts?
Have you been thinking about killing yourself? Have you thought about suicide? Differentiate between suicidal thoughts (wanting to kill oneself), self-harm (emotion regulation as the primary goal), and morbid ruminations (thoughts of death, dying, or wanting to be dead, but not active thoughts of killing oneself). Define the terms for the patient. Document carefully in the chart using direct quotes from the patient.

No—Indicate in the chart that the patient did not manifest acute suicidal thoughts. Provide a specific quote of the morbid thoughts: *I've been thinking a lot about what it'd be like for my family if I were gone.* Again, differentiate the terms for the patient, noting that *suicidal* means that the patient is thinking of killing himself/herself. If the patient is NOT having active suicidal thoughts, it's still important to assess his or her suicidal history for an accurate understanding. Identify the emergence of suicidal thinking as a "warning sign" and integrate into a safety plan.

Yes—*Can you tell me exactly what you've been thinking?* Get a direct quote from the patient without providing prompts. This provides a means to assess the specificity of the patient's thinking, one marker of intent. Explore each individual method separately. Always question for "multiple methods."

Step 2:
Reduce resistance and anxiety surrounding suicidal thinking by exploring the patient's suicide history before examining the current episode in detail. This will reduce anxiety and resistance by helping the patient become more comfortable with the general topic of suicide. *Before we go into detail about what's going on now, can you tell me about the first time you ever thought about or attempted suicide? Tell me about what was going on at the time. What was the outcome? Were you injured? Did you get medical care? How did you end up at the hospital? Why did you want to die? Did you think [method] would kill you? How did you feel about surviving? Did you learn anything from the previous attempt? How many suicide attempts have you made? Have you thought about suicide in the past year or the past month?* For those with multiple attempts, target only two previous attempts, the "first" and "worst," with the patient subjectively defining "worst."

Step 3:
Transition back to the current suicidal crisis. *OK, we've talked about some of the previous crises; let's talk in more detail about what brought you here today.* **Assess specificity of thinking, including frequency, intensity, and duration (and access). You can use the acronym F-I-D.** *How have you been thinking about killing yourself? Have you decided when and where? How often do you have the thoughts: daily, more than once a day, weekly, monthly? Can you tell me how intense or severe the thoughts are for you? How long do the thoughts last: a few seconds, minutes, or longer? How much time do you spend thinking about suicide in an average day/week/month? Do you have access to [method] or have you taken steps to get access? Have you thought about any other method of suicide?* It's important to ask the multiple method question until the patient says no.

> **Step 4:**
> **Assess subjective intent, including reasons for dying.** *What are your reasons for dying? Why do you want to kill yourself? Do you have any intention of acting on your thoughts? Can you rate your intent on a scale of 1 to 10, with 1 being "no intent at all" and 10 being "certain that you'll act on your thoughts as quickly as you can"?*

> **Step 5:**
> **Assess objective intent.** *Have you taken steps to act on your suicidal thoughts? Have you done anything in preparation for your death (e.g., life insurance, letters to loved ones, research on the Internet)? Have you in any way rehearsed your suicide? In other words, have you gotten your [method] out and gone through the steps of what you'd do to kill yourself?*

> **Step 6:**
> **Assess protective factors, including reasons for living.** *What are your reasons for living? What keeps you going in difficult times like this?*

FIGURE 4–1. Hierarchical approach to identifying and exploring suicidal thoughts.

Source. Reprinted from Rudd MD: "The Clinical Risk Assessment Interview," in *The American Psychiatric Publishing Textbook of Suicide Assessment and Management,* 2nd Edition. Edited by Simon RI, Hales RE. Washington, DC, American Psychiatric Publishing, 2012, pp 57–74. © 2012 American Psychiatric Publishing. Used with permission.

about death is not the same as being actively suicidal may ease the anxiety of a patient with morbid ruminations. Developing a shared language and set of definitions will help both the patient and the clinician and will allow them to track the symptom pattern over time. Furthermore, one of us (M.D.R.) has suggested that use of precise and shared definitions can itself serve as a clinical intervention, affording the patient a heightened sense of control in efforts to self-monitor and effectively regulate affective states (see, e.g., Rudd et al. 2004).

Evaluating Suicidal Intent

There is no foolproof way to predict suicide, and accordingly, there is currently no clear standard of care in suicide assessment. In assessing intent, the clinician should look for the following: 1) a combination of sources of preexisting distress, 2) an event or experience that led to a rupture in the patient's sense of place or belonging, and 3) access to means of committing suicide (Joiner et al. 2009; Lane-McKinley 2018).

In seeking to assess suicidal intent, clinicians should encourage patients to describe their thoughts in their own words. The clinician may ask, for example, *What have you been thinking about? What is happening—what are the thoughts going through your head? Have you been looking at the topic of suicide or how to commit suicide on the Internet?* Direct quotes from the patient, elicited at the beginning of the interview, provide a measure to assess the specificity of the patient's thoughts about suicide. Behavioral intent to commit suicide has both subjective (a patient's stated intent) and objective (the patient's demonstrated intent) elements (Rudd 2006). Greater specificity in describing suicidal thoughts and behaviors points to increased behavioral intent to commit suicide.

Asking about frequency, intensity, and duration (FID) may help in clarifying the features of any past suicidal thoughts or behaviors. The length of time that the patient has engaged in suicidal thought, any associated behaviors such as preparation or rehearsals or Internet research, past suicide attempts, and access to methods of committing suicide are all important to examine and document in the medical record. As noted by Joiner (2005), the patient's capacity to complete suicide builds with exposure to previous suicidal behavior, self-harm, trauma, and interpersonal violence. The clinician should find out whether the patient has been writing goodbye letters, updating his or her will, revising life insurance arrangements, calling suicide hotlines, talking with friends about the idea, or researching methods for suicide. The clinician should also explore whether the patient has made suicide attempts or has been rehearsing or preparing for a suicide method.

If the patient has made past attempts, it is crucial to learn the details and assess the potential lethality and the overall pattern of the patient's behavior. Understanding the patient's emotional reactions to past suicide attempts is also very important. Was the patient glad to have survived the attempt? Did he or she regret surviving the attempt? What did the patient learn from the experience? Increasing evidence of objective intent often means that the patient has evolved from considering suicide to actively implementing a suicide plan. This progression is an indication not only of greater intent but also of heightened risk. The patient's emotional reactions to previous attempts can help the clinician to identify the persistence of what has been called "residual" intent (e.g., patient answers such as "I learned that next time I need to use a gun") (Rudd 2006).

Engaging the patient in the exercise of examining reasons for living and reasons for dying, as noted in the flowchart in Figure 4–1, may be very helpful in assessing intent and finding a therapeutic foothold with the patient. An imbalance between identified reasons for living and reasons for dying provides a metric for either intent or ambivalence (e.g., many reasons for dying and few reasons for living may signify that the intent is more heavily weighted toward death). On the other hand, reasons for living may be few but powerful, such as family relationships, cultural values, or religious beliefs.

The clinician should also ask the patient about suicide as a "solution" to his or her current problems. The clinician could ask, *How does suicide address the problems you are facing? How effective would suicide be in solving your problems, on a scale of 1 to 5, where 1 is not effective and 5 is very effective? Why? Can you tell me more about this? What other solutions have you considered?* The patient may feel a sense of relief when such questions are asked simply and directly and with kindness and therapeutic intent.

A sympathetic, nonjudgmental, and sequential approach can lessen the worry and potential resistance of the patient when discussing the difficult topic of suicide. When a patient acknowledges active suicidal thoughts, resistance can be decreased by talking through the patient's history of suicidal thoughts and behavior before returning to the current situation. The clinician may say something like, *Before we look in detail into what's going on now, can you tell me about the first time you ever thought about killing yourself? Have you attempted suicide in the past?* Exploration of all past suicide attempts may require several encounters or interactions, and such an in-depth series of sessions may not be possible, depending on the clinical setting. Current risk, however, can be understood with good accuracy by exploring the first attempt and the most serious of past attempts (Joiner et al. 2003), with the patient identifying the most serious or "worst" attempt subjectively. Rudd (2006) has recommended the use of an "extended evaluation" for patients who may become suicidal repeatedly or chronically. A longer, more intensive evaluation may require three to five sessions before the clinician makes a collaborative decision with the patient about providing ongoing care and treatment.

It is not unusual for suicidal patients, particularly those with chronic suicidal behavior (Nock 2009), to also engage in repetitive self-harm. Although self-harm and suicidal behavior can co-occur, differentiating between the two is important for an accurate understanding of the present level of risk.

Consideration of contextual factors influencing suicidal intent in the current situation and in each past suicide attempt is essential to a rigorous assessment of suicide risk in the clinical interview. The PMOR mnemonic—short for Precipitant, Motivation, Outcome, Reaction—is helpful in this process (Table 4–1). Responses to the questions posed in Table 4–1 can help the clinician elicit and assess the subjective and objective indicators of intent. Although there is no exact or exactly accurate algorithm for evaluating the markers of objective intent, the patient's answers provide a way of examining differences and similarities across past suicidal crises. Recognizing the progression and trajectory of suicidal intent for a patient is vitally important. If there is a pattern of escalating lethality, it will be apparent across the past history and the course of the patient's life situation and health condition.

Time constraints are usually a big factor in initial psychiatric evaluations and may affect subsequent care in many systems. It is essential that the clinician take responsibility for pacing the discussion with the patient. When necessary, the clinician may have to defer detailed history taking regarding previous crises or suicide attempts to later sessions. Three to five sessions may be necessary in order to fully understand a patient's suicidal history. If the situation is too acute, or if the clinical setting does not permit a longitudinal evaluation and the patient will not be immediately hospitalized, the clinician should document the situation, deferring the historical review to the next clinician or the next encounter, clearly indicating that such an extensive review is needed and remains incomplete.

Once the patient's suicide history has been explored, as noted in Step 3 of the flowchart in Figure 4–1, the clinician should transition back to the current crisis. A sequence of questions can be advanced, bringing the patient from the past to the present. The clinician may ask, *Can you tell me about the first time you ever thought about suicide [or attempted suicide]? Has suicide crossed your mind in the past few months? Now let's talk in more detail about the suicidal thoughts [or attempt] that brought you here today.*

As the clinician brings the focus to the present, he or she needs to again determine how specific the patient's thinking and behavior are in relation to suicide. The clinician should ask about frequency, intensity, and duration of suicidal thoughts; about when and where the patient has thought about committing suicide; and about access to means. When asking about means of committing suicide, the clinician should not prompt the patient with options to choose from. One indicator of intent is the specificity of the patient's own thinking. Prompts can intrude and undermine an accurate assessment by depriving patients of the opportunity to state their thoughts in their own words and unique narrative voice. Prompts can also lead to an unbalanced exchange

TABLE 4–1.   Contextual factors of past attempts (PMOR mnemonic)

	Questions for the patient
Precipitant?	
What triggered the crisis, according to the patient?	*What triggered your thinking about attempting suicide? What was going on in your life at the time you made the suicide attempt?*
Motivation for the attempt?	
Did the patient want to die?	*What were your reasons for dying? Did you want to die when you [method]?*
What did the patient actually do?	*Please tell me exactly what you did.*
What was the patient's perception of lethality?	*Did you think [method] would kill you?*
Outcome?	
Was there any associated injury? If so, was medical care required? If required, did the patient follow through and get recommended medical care?	*Were you injured by the suicide attempt? Did you receive medical care? Why did you choose not to get medical care when it was recommended?*
How did the patient end up accessing care? Was care seeking initiated by the patient? Was it by random chance?	*How did you get to the hospital? Did you call someone?*
Did the patient take active steps to prevent discovery or rescue?	*Did you take steps to try to prevent discovery or rescue when you made the suicide attempt? Did you time the attempt or otherwise make it difficult for someone to find you?*
Reaction?	
What was the patient's emotional reaction to surviving the suicide attempt?	*How do you feel about surviving? Did you learn anything helpful about yourself [or others] from the previous attempt?*

Source.   Reprinted from Rudd MD: "The Clinical Risk Assessment Interview," in *The American Psychiatric Publishing Textbook of Suicide Assessment and Management,* 2nd Edition. Edited by Simon RI, Hales RE. Washington, DC, American Psychiatric Publishing, 2012, pp 57–74. Copyright 2012, American Psychiatric Publishing. Used with permission.

between the clinician and patient that can undermine the development of a sound and beneficial therapeutic relationship. Using the patient's own words (i.e., directly quoting speech about suicidal thoughts) conveys that you are, and will be, listening.

The clinician should be certain to explore whether the patient has been thinking about more than one method of suicide and about access to means for each method. The clinician must direct the interview to achieve saturation; the clinician should continue to ask the patient about possible methods and access until the patient says no other methods have been considered. Until questioned thoroughly, patients will sometimes withhold their most ready or accessible means. Asking about multiple methods communicates not only that the clinician cares about the patient but also that he or she is going to be thorough, specific, and detailed in the evaluation process. This process also communicates that the patient's thoughts are important to—but do not frighten or intimidate—the clinician, which in turn helps the therapeutic relationship to progress. An example of a sequence of questions that clinicians may ask about suicide, reinforcing the rubric of frequency, intensity, and duration along contextual dimensions, is provided below (Rudd 2012):

- How are you thinking about killing yourself?
- Do you have access to [method]?
- Have you made arrangements or planned to get access to [method]?
- Have you thought about any other way to kill yourself? [Ask this question until the patient says that no other methods have been considered.]
- How often do you think about killing yourself? Once a day, more than once a day, once a week, monthly?
- You said you think about suicide every day. How many times a day?
- When you have these thoughts, how long do they last? A few seconds, minutes, or longer?
- On average, how much time [every day, week, or month] do you spend thinking about suicide?
- What exactly do you think about [or do] for that [period of time]?
- When you have these thoughts, how intense or severe are they? Can you rate them on a scale of 1 to 10, with 1 being "not severe at all" and 10 being "so severe that I will act on them."
- Have you thought about when you would kill yourself?
- Have you thought about where you would kill yourself?
- Have you thought about taking steps or timing your attempt to prevent anyone from finding or stopping you?
- Have you shared your thoughts about suicide with others? Who? And when? And how often?
- If you were to commit suicide, what would happen to others in your life?
- Have you prepared for your death?
- Have you rehearsed or practiced your suicide?
- Do you have any intention of acting on your thoughts? Can you rate your intent on a scale of 1 to 10, with 1 being "no intent at all" and 10 being "certain that I'll act on them as quickly as I can"?

In the service of caring for patients longitudinally, the clinician's use of this degree of detail to assess suicidal thinking helps to estimate risk and to track patterns of suicidal thinking and behavior over time. A patient may improve and may evidence or experience little risk except morbid ruminations or infrequent thoughts of suicide. With chronic suicidality, simple comments or notes in the chart about the presence or absence of suicidal thoughts are insufficient. A patient may have been having suicidal thoughts for decades—the mere presence or absence of suicidal thinking is thus, in this case, not a particularly helpful indicator of escalating risk. Some patients may think about suicide intermittently but without intent. Other patients may think about suicide with sincere intent very often, yet not act on the cognition. Still other patients may continue to think about suicide daily even while making considerable progress, such as reduced amount of time focused on suicide or diminished intensity of the experience.

Evaluating Risk and Protective Factors

Evaluation of risk and protective factors is an essential feature of all 10 formalized clinical practice guidelines and of 6 out of 10 suicide prevention resource documents published in the United States (Bernert et al. 2014). Thus, a detailed assessment of suicidal thinking should be complemented by an assessment of additional risk and protective factors, integrated within a basic framework for shared and collaborative clinical decision making. It is expected that a complete and comprehensive intake history, diagnostic interview, mental status exam, and cultural formulation will also be conducted as a part of psychiatric and psychological evaluations.

There are a number of empirically supported domains essential to accurate assessment of suicide risk (Rudd et al. 2004), as detailed in Table 4–2. One of us (M.D.R.) has recommended that domains include identifiable precipitant(s), the patient's current symptomatic presentation, presence of hopelessness, nature of suicidal thinking, previous suicidal behavior, impulsivity and self-control, and protective factors. Beyond these particular domains, all clinicians should be keenly aware of the emerging evidence regarding suicide warning signs (Rudd et al. 2006), with acute symptoms of anxiety, sleep disturbance, and feelings of being a burden to others being of particular concern. The clinician may elect to include systematic measures (e.g., of hopelessness, of sleep disturbance) to complement the psychiatric interview.

One approach to assessing each of the domains in Table 4–2 involves moving in sequential fashion from the precipitating event to the patient's current situation and symptoms, to hopelessness, and then to active suicidal thinking and intent. As noted before, it is important to be empathic and nonjudgmental in the interview and to intervene with normalizing statements when resistance begins to play a role in the interaction. For instance, if a patient appears anxious or dysphoric, the clinician can say, *It's not unusual for someone who's been depressed and anxious to feel hopeless. Do you feel hopeless?* If hopelessness is endorsed, the clinician can transition to morbid thoughts and eventually to suicidal thinking, offering an opening for further discussion. The clinician can support the patient and destigmatize the patient's symptoms in the context of the identified disorder. This approach to the interview represents a strategic clinical intervention that serves to reduce anxiety about disclosing difficult material to the clinician. Figure 4–2 (from Rudd 2012) illustrates this approach to the overall interview.

Such hierarchical questioning may not be needed if suicidal thoughts and behaviors led to the clinical encounter. In routine clinical care, however, gentle and thorough inquiry is extremely useful, especially in caring for individuals who are in special populations, such as adolescents, elders, displaced persons, physically ill individuals, and members of underrepresented minority groups. A progressive approach to the interview reduces nervousness or anxiety and associated resistance and facilitates the therapeutic relationship, which will lead to a more accurate risk assessment. Evidence suggests that there is heightened risk among certain subpopulations (e.g., Native American adolescents, physically ill elders, transgender or gender-nonconforming individuals) and during certain sensitive time periods (e.g., first-episode psychosis, recent discharge from an inpatient psychiatric unit, divorce or widowhood). Individuals in these subpopulations or in these specific sensitive time periods may feel especially

---

TABLE 4–2.   **Eight additional domains of risk assessment**

---

1. **Predisposition to suicidal behavior**

   Past history of psychiatric diagnoses (increased risk with recurrent disorders, comorbidity, and chronicity), including major depressive disorder, bipolar disorder, schizophrenia, substance abuse, and personality disorders such as borderline personality disorder

   Past history of suicidal behavior (increased risk with previous attempts, high lethality, and chronic disturbance; those having made multiple attempts [i.e., two or more] are considered at chronic risk)

   Recent discharge from inpatient psychiatric treatment (increased risk within first year of release; risk is highest during the first month after discharge)

   Same-sex sexual orientation or nonconforming gender identity

   Male gender

   History of abuse (sexual, physical, or emotional)

   Family history of suicide

2. **Identifiable precipitants or stressors**

   Significant loss (e.g., financial loss, loss of interpersonal relationship[s], professional loss, loss of identity, rupture of sense of belonging)

   Chronic or acute health problems (loss of independence, autonomy, or function)

   Relationship instability (loss of meaningful relationships and related support and resources)

   Feelings of being a burden to others

3. **Symptomatic presentation (have patient rate severity on 1–10 scale)**

   Depressive symptoms (e.g., anhedonia, low self-esteem, sadness, dyssomnia, fatigue; increased risk when combined with anxiety and substance abuse)

   Bipolar disorder (increased risk early in disorder's course)

   Anxiety (increased risk with trait anxiety and acute agitation)

   Schizophrenia (increased risk following active phases)

   Borderline and antisocial personality features

   Sleep disorder or disruption

4. **Presence of hopelessness (have patient rate severity on 1–10 scale)**

   Severity of hopelessness

   Duration of hopelessness

5. **Nature of suicidal thinking**

   Current ideation frequency, intensity, and duration

   Presence of suicidal plan (increased risk with specificity)

   Availability of means (multiple methods)

   Lethality of means (including both medical and perceived lethality)

   Active suicidal behaviors

   Suicidal intent (subjective and objective markers)

6. **Previous suicidal behavior**

   Frequency and context of previous suicidal behaviors

   Perceived lethality and outcome

   Opportunity for rescue and help seeking

   Preparatory behaviors (including rehearsal)

   Presence and utility of a suicide crisis or coping card

TABLE 4–2.   **Eight additional domains of risk assessment** *(continued)*

---

7. **Impulsivity and self-control (have patient rate on 1–10 scale)**

    Subjective self-control

    Objective control (e.g., substance abuse, impulsive behaviors, aggression)

8. **Protective factors**

    Presence of social support (support needs to be both present and accessible—make sure that relationships are healthy)

    Problem-solving skills and history of coping skills

    Active participation in treatment

    Presence of hopefulness

    Children present in the home

    Pregnancy

    Religious commitment

    Cultural beliefs

    Life satisfaction (have the patient rate life satisfaction on a scale of 1–10; life satisfaction should correspond with the patient's stated reasons for living and dying)

    Intact reality testing

    Fear of social disapproval

    Fear of suicide or death (suggests that the patient has not yet habituated to the idea of death, a very good sign)

Source.   Reprinted from Rudd MD: "The Clinical Risk Assessment Interview," in *The American Psychiatric Publishing Textbook of Suicide Assessment and Management,* 2nd Edition. Edited by Simon RI, Hales RE. Washington, DC, American Psychiatric Publishing, 2012, pp 57–74. Copyright 2012, American Psychiatric Publishing. Used with permission.

isolated or untrusting of the health care system, and accurate risk assessments can be very difficult to attain.

Most identifiable precipitants and stressors can be understood as losses—that is, interpersonal loss, financial loss, identity loss, or loss of a sense of wholeness or safety (Berk and Adrian 2018; Rudd 2012). The clinician should suspend his or her own view of the precipitant or stressor and instead seek to evaluate the precipitant or stressor according to the mindset of the suicidal individual. The clinician needs to weigh acute and chronic health problems, along with acute family challenges associated with displacement, divorce, death of a loved one, or other disruptions. Medical illnesses have been associated with increased suicide risk. The risk is heightened when the medical illness occurs in the context of psychiatric disorder(s). Serious physical health conditions commonly lead to loss of independence, an experience that can give rise to feelings of frustration, fears of becoming a burden to others, and hopelessness.

Monitoring the patient's symptoms over time is critical. For patients who are experiencing psychotic symptoms and are thinking of killing themselves, the clinical response in most settings will be acute hospitalization and stabilization. For chronically suicidal individuals without psychosis, the immediate management approach is less straightforward. After clarifying the diagnosis, the clinician will need to evaluate symptoms and their severity.

Hopelessness has been found in clinical experience and through empirical evidence to have great salience for suicidal intent. Accordingly, as indicated in Table 4–2, hope-

Precipitant: *Is there anything in particular that happened that triggered thoughts about suicide?*

Symptomatic presentation: *Tell me about how you've been feeling lately. It sounds like you've been feeling depressed. Have you been feeling anxious, nervous, or panicky? Have you been down, low, or blue lately? Have you had trouble sleeping [additional symptoms of depression and anxiety]?*

Hopelessness: *It's not unusual for someone who's been feeling depressed to feel hopeless, like things won't change or get any better. Do you ever feel that way?*

Morbid ruminations: *It's not unusual when you're feeling depressed and hopeless to have thoughts about death and dying. Do you ever think about death or dying?*

Suicidal thinking: *It's not unusual when feeling depressed, hopeless, and having thoughts about death and dying to have thoughts about suicide. Have you ever thought about suicide?*

FIGURE 4–2. Hierarchical approach to the interview as a whole: an example.

Source. Reprinted from Rudd MD: "The Clinical Risk Assessment Interview," in *The American Psychiatric Publishing Textbook of Suicide Assessment and Management,* 2nd Edition. Edited by Simon RI, Hales RE. Washington, DC, American Psychiatric Publishing, 2012, pp 57–74. © 2012 American Psychiatric Publishing. Used with permission.

lessness is treated as a separate domain. It is not just the presence or absence of hopelessness that is important, but also the duration and severity of hopelessness. Hopelessness can be assessed with a few straightforward questions. As with the other symptoms, we would suggest the use of a simple scale to track the severity of reported hopelessness over time. For example: *Can you rate your hopelessness on a scale of 1 to 10, with 1 being very hopeful and optimistic about the future and 10 being so hopeless that you see suicide as the only option?* Patients who report enduring hopelessness are at greater risk for suicide, both acutely and chronically. Formal scales, such as the Beck Hopelessness Scale, may also be employed in assessing hopelessness and tracking symptoms over time.

Impulsivity is a difficult feature of suicidality, yet very critical. Assessment of impulsivity includes biological as well as psychological and social dimensions. An individual with a head injury or an individual struggling with substance dependence will commonly have particular difficulty with impulse control. To explore subjective aspects of impulsivity, the clinician can ask the patient, *Do you feel in control right now? Do others think you are an impulsive person? Do you ever feel out of control?* Based on the patient's response, the clinician must decide whether there is a disconnect between what the patient says about him- or herself and what the history or other reports suggest about the patient's impulsivity.

Resilience and the presence (or absence) of protective factors are increasingly recognized for their importance in suicidality and in the patient's ability to cope in life despite suicidal cognitions and behaviors. Evidence of resilience and the presence of protective factors can be assessed in a number of ways. Clinicians may ask a number of questions, such as, *Even though you've had a very difficult time, something has kept you going. What are your reasons for living? In the past, what has kept you going in hard times like this?* In considering suicide risk, social support represents an important protective factor. Signs of social support should not be vague or remote; social support needs to be both available and accessible. Simple questions like the following can help assess the availability of support: *Do you have family and friends whom you can talk to and who you know will be supportive? How easy is it to reach them? What usually happens when you ask for support [from family or friends]? Who can you turn to in times of crisis?* The presence of a strong therapeutic relationship can be an important protective factor for patients coping with suicidal thoughts and behaviors.

Patients with chronic or intermittent suicidal thoughts may carry a coping card with them in their backpack, purse, or wallet. The card can be very simple—an index card that states the name of the patient, his or her clinician, and the phone number of individuals who may be called upon for emotional support in a time of crisis. A safety plan developed in partnership with the patient should be outlined on the coping card. The card may also outline positive reasons for living and describe the emotional strengths of the struggling individual.

Role of Cultural Competence in Suicide Risk Assessment

A culture is defined by its unique constellation of values, attitudes, beliefs, behaviors, and rituals. *Cultural competence* relates to the ability to work in a world with many distinct cultures and many individuals who live within and across those cultures. Such work entails awareness, knowledge and skills, and a mindset of humility and acceptance of differences across cultures. Attitudes toward mental illness, suicide, death, and related topics are deeply culturally relevant, and data suggest that suicidal behavior varies greatly across cultures. For these reasons, cultural competence is vitally important in suicide risk assessment.

Many issues should be assessed in a culturally competent suicide assessment, including differences in degree of acculturation; differences in cultural attitudes toward suicide; variations in prevalence of risk factors such as unemployment, poverty, and substance use; differences in predominant religious beliefs; differences in care seeking and health disparities; differences across age groups; and differences in discerning and reporting suicide. Widely varying views of suicide are held across cultures and ethnic groups today and historically. Decriminalization of suicide, followed by legalization and extensive adoption of assisted suicide in many areas of Europe, represents one example of rapidly changing cultural perspectives. Assessment of patients will entail an exploration of their personal views about suicide as shaped by these culturally salient contextual influences. Cultural factors may also greatly affect a patient's willingness to engage in the therapeutic relationship with the clinician and accept recommended treatment.

Suicide is handled very differently in different countries throughout the world. The reasons for these difference relate to systems-based issues (are emergency services available?) as well as cultural value-based issues (how is mental illness understood?) and related issues (what is the role of the family in care and decision making?). The World Health Organization has emphasized the importance of approaching suicide as a profound contributor to world health and the need for additional research on suicide across diverse countries and across the age spectrum, on parasuicidal behaviors, and on different models of care (Ravindranath et al. 2012). Approaches to suicide assessment will evolve with more refined understanding of the considerations that may influence the individual experiencing suicidal thoughts.

Summing Up and Looking Ahead

Suicide represents a tremendous public health burden throughout the world. Assessment of suicide risk in the clinical interview is immensely challenging. A comprehensive assessment, including a full differential diagnosis, history, mental status examination, and cultural assessment, should be undertaken for every patient for whom suicidality is a concern. Clinicians should have a framework to guide their approach to the evaluation of suicide risk, and we have presented a six-step flowchart that helps to focus the clinical interview and to facilitate therapeutic engagement and future planning (see Figure 4–1). Suicidal thoughts, morbid rumination, and thoughts of self-harm are three domains of suicidal cognition that should be evaluated and tracked over time.

Suicidal intent is very difficult to discern, and specificity of the patient's suicidal thoughts, behaviors, and plans should be queried very carefully. Identified targeted domains, including precipitant(s), suicidal thinking and past behavior (to include an assessment of subjective and objective markers of intent), symptom presentation, hopelessness, impulsivity, self-control, protective factors, and cultural influences should always be covered in the assessment.

Documentation of the suicide risk assessment should include suicide risk factors and protective factors, including cultural dimensions of the situation that may contribute positively or negatively to the level of risk, along with an overall assessment rating, the progression and trajectory of suicidal intent, and treatment and management interventions and safety plans in alignment with these clinical observations and assessments.

Documentation in the electronic health record should reflect the care and thoroughness of the suicide risk assessment and should include detailed information about risk and protective factors, relevant aspects of the patient's past history of suicidal ideation and attempts, access to means, and key features of the assessment noted earlier. Inclusion of findings from rating scales may be valuable, but such findings do not alone suffice as a suicide assessment or its documentation. A description of possible safety tools such as a crisis or coping card may be included in the documentation—a coping card provides information on resources and steps to be taken by the patient when he or she feels suicidal. The safety plan and interventions should be documented carefully, as should the intended follow-up arrangements.

For those patients who do not have psychosis as the fundamental driver of their chronic and recurrent suicidality, Chiles et al. (2019) have suggested that the therapeutic goals and strategies for managing suicidality in ongoing care include the following, plus reduction of symptoms that may be associated with a mental disorder: 1) destigmatizing suicidal behavior; 2) reframing the patient's suicidal behavior as a solution to overwhelming pain; 3) addressing the likelihood of recurrent suicidal behavior; 4) activating more constructive coping and problem-solving behavior; 5) developing mindfulness and emotional acceptance skills; 6) developing personal goals and life direction; and 7) transitioning from therapy and establishing a future safety plan with appropriate follow-up, when necessary. For patients whose suicidality is governed by an underlying psychosis, the risk of suicide will in all likelihood continue to be quite high. In these patients, it is critical that the underlying mental disorder be treated intensively. In all cases, efforts to foster resilience and enrich the factors that protect against suicide are worthwhile and may bring enduring benefit.

On a broader level in society, clinicians who care for people with suicidal thoughts and behaviors may be in a unique position to lessen the stigma associated with suicidality. Supporting greater understanding of the contributors to suicide and the positive role of early recognition and warning signs may lessen suffering and help address one of the most significant health burdens throughout the world.

Key Clinical Points

- Suicide rates are increasing, and suicide is among the leading preventable causes of premature mortality among young people, elders, and other special populations. Suicide is the proximal cause of death of many mental and physical disorders.

- Suicide is difficult to predict accurately.

- Establishing a therapeutic alliance with the patient is an essential first step in strengthening the accuracy of a suicide assessment. Efforts to diminish the shame and emotional pain of the suicidal individual are important in the process of establishing this alliance.

- Suicidal thoughts should be differentiated from morbid ruminations and thoughts of self-harm. Suicidal thoughts may be a strategy for problem solving or emotional regulation and should not be interpreted in all cases as an authentic wish to die.

- Past suicide attempts should be assessed in relation to precipitants, motivation, outcomes, and reactions (PMOR).

- In assessing intent, the clinician should look for the following: 1) a combination of sources of preexisting distress, 2) an event or experience that led to a rupture in the patient's sense of place or belonging, and 3) access to means of committing suicide.

- Risk and protective factors are important to evaluate in a comprehensive suicide assessment.

- Documentation of the suicide risk assessment should include suicide risk factors and protective factors, including cultural dimensions of the situation that may contribute positively or negatively to the level of risk, along with an overall assessment rating, the progression and trajectory of suicidal intent, and treatment and management interventions and safety plans in alignment with these clinical observations and assessments.

References

Berk MS, Adrian M: The suicidal student, in Student Mental Health: A Guide for Psychiatrists, Psychologists, and Leaders Serving in Higher Education. Edited by Roberts LW. Washington, DC, American Psychiatric Association Publishing, 2018, pp 321–338

Bernert RA, Hom MA, Roberts LW: A review of multidisciplinary clinical practice guidelines in suicide prevention: toward an emerging standard in suicide risk assessment and management, training and practice. Acad Psychiatry 38(5):585–592, 2014 25142247

Bryan CJ, Rudd MD: Advances in the assessment of suicide risk. J Clin Psychol 62(2):185–200, 2006 16342288

Chiles JA, Strosahl KD, Roberts LW: Clinical Manual for Assessment and Treatment of Suicidal Patients, 2nd Edition. Washington, DC, American Psychiatric Association Publishing, 2019

Gould MS, Marrocco FA, Kleinman M, et al: Evaluating iatrogenic risk of youth suicide screening programs: a randomized controlled trial. JAMA 293(13):1635–1643, 2005 15811983

Jacobs DG, Baldessarini RJ, Conwell Y, et al: Practice Guideline for the Assessment and Treatment of Patients With Suicidal Behaviors. Arlington, VA, American Psychiatric Association, 2010. Available at: http://psychiatryonline.org/pb/assets/raw/sitewide/practice_guidelines/guidelines/suicide.pdf. Accessed July 16, 2018.

Joiner TE: Why People Die by Suicide. Cambridge, MA, Harvard University Press, 2005

Joiner TE Jr, Steer RA, Brown G, et al: Worst-point suicidal plans: a dimension of suicidality predictive of past suicide attempts and eventual death by suicide. Behav Res Ther 41(12):1469–1480, 2003 14583414

Joiner TE Jr, Van Orden KA, Witte TK, et al: Main predictions of the interpersonal-psychological theory of suicidal behavior: empirical tests in two samples of young adults. J Abnorm Psychol 118(3):634–646, 2009 19685959

Lane-McKinley K: Creating a culture of belonging, respect, and support on campus, in Student Mental Health: A Guide for Psychiatrists, Psychologists, and Leaders Serving in Higher Education. Edited by Roberts LW. Washington, DC, American Psychiatric Association Publishing, 2018, pp 17–32

Nock MK: Understanding Nonsuicidal Self-Injury: Origins, Assessment, and Treatment. Washington, DC, American Psychological Association, 2009

Ravindranath D, Deneke E, Riba M: Emergency services, in The American Psychiatric Publishing Textbook of Suicide Assessment and Management, 2nd Edition. Edited by Simon RI, Hales RE. Washington, DC, American Psychiatric Association Publishing, 2012, pp 283–303

Rudd MD: The Assessment and Management of Suicidality. Sarasota, FL, Professional Resource Exchange, 2006

Rudd MD: The clinical risk assessment interview, in The American Psychiatric Publishing Textbook of Suicide Assessment and Management, 2nd Edition. Edited by Simon RI, Hales RE. Washington, DC, American Psychiatric Association Publishing, 2012, pp 57–74

Rudd MD, Joiner TE, Rajab H: Treating Suicidal Behavior. New York, Guilford, 2004

Rudd MD, Berman AL, Joiner TE Jr, et al: Warning signs for suicide: theory, research, and clinical applications. Suicide Life Threat Behav 36(3):255–262, 2006 16805653

Simon RI: Suicide risk assessment: gateway to treatment and management, in The American Psychiatric Publishing Textbook of Suicide Assessment and Management, 2nd Edition. Edited by Simon RI, Hales RE. Washington, DC, American Psychiatric Association Publishing, 2012, pp 3–28

Stone DM, Simon TR, Fowler KA, et al: Vital signs: trends in state suicide rates—United States, 1999–2016 and circumstances contributing to suicide—27 states, 2015. MMWR Morb Mortal Wkly Rep 67(22):617–624, 2018 29879094

Wenzel A, Brown C, Beck AT: Cognitive Therapy for Suicidal Patients: Scientific and Clinical Applications. Washington, DC, American Psychological Association, 2008

Recommended Reading

Berk MS: Evidence-Based Treatment Approaches for Suicidal Adolescents: Translating Science Into Practice. Washington, DC, American Psychiatric Association Publishing, 2019

Bernert RA, Hom MA, Roberts LW: A review of multidisciplinary clinical practice guidelines in suicide prevention: toward an emerging standard in suicide risk assessment and management, training and practice. Acad Psychiatry 38(5):585–592, 2014

Chiles JA, Strosahl KD, Roberts LW: Clinical Manual for Assessment and Treatment of Suicidal Patients, 2nd Edition. Washington, DC, American Psychiatric Association Publishing, 2019

Michel K, Jobes DA (eds): Building a Therapeutic Relationship With the Suicidal Patient. Washington, DC, American Psychological Association, 2010

Russell ST, Joyner K: Adolescent sexual orientation and suicide risk: evidence from a national study. Am J Public Health 91(8):1276–1281, 2001

CHAPTER 5

Laboratory Testing and Neuroimaging Studies in Psychiatry

Sandra A. Jacobson, M.D.
Elisabeth A. Wilde, Ph.D.

General Approach to Laboratory Testing

Excellence in psychiatric care can be achieved only when all components of the patient evaluation—including the history, review of systems, functional assessment, physical and mental status examinations, and laboratory evaluation—are brought to bear on diagnosis and management. A good working knowledge of general medicine equips the clinician to make predictions as to the likelihood that particular laboratory tests will be helpful and thus to use these resources judiciously. These predictions take into account not only the patient's signs and symptoms but also other pertinent variables such as patient demographics and the setting in which the patient is seen. For example, a head computed tomography (CT) scan in an elderly patient with a suspected stroke seen in the emergency department would be useful whether positive or negative for blood, whereas the same test in a patient attending a clinic for mild neurocognitive disorders might not be as informative as an alternative such as a brain magnetic resonance imaging (MRI) scan.

Recommended test panels for psychiatric hospital admission and other indications have been published and have gained fairly wide acceptance. These panels are discussed in later sections (see "Suggested Psychiatric Screening Laboratory Evaluation" and "Diagnostic Testing in Specific Clinical Situations"). Some of the tests included are *screening* tests, for which the goal is to detect common disorders among a large subgroup of patients. These tests are mostly inexpensive and noninvasive. Others are *diagnostic* tests, which are performed to determine whether a hypothesized condition is present or to exclude such a condition. Diagnostic tests cover a very broad range of medical tests, including subspecialty tests, and many of these tests can be expensive and/or invasive. These are the tests for which informed predictions constitute best practice.

Cost of Laboratory Testing

With the exception of genetic testing and neuroimaging, laboratory testing generally does not contribute significantly to the cost of psychiatric care, although charges for tests vary considerably from one testing facility to another. Charges are generally highest at hospital and clinic laboratories and lowest at freestanding ("walk-in") laboratories. Information on laboratory charges is not readily available to either patients or clinicians, but an idea of what might be considered a fair price for individual lab tests can be obtained from the Healthcare Bluebook (www.healthcarebluebook.com). It is worth noting that the everyday workhorses of laboratory testing in clinical psychiatry—blood and urine labs—offer very good value. At the other end of the cost spectrum, specialized genetic testing can be expensive, and insurance company policies differ as to what tests are covered.

Reference Ranges

Reference ranges cited in this chapter and other published sources are only general guides. In all cases, reference intervals supplied by the testing laboratory take precedence, because ranges may not apply to testing methods in all laboratories.

The Clinical Laboratory as a Resource

When laboratory findings are unclear or introduce questions, laboratory staff can be an excellent resource for clinicians in interpreting test data and planning an approach to a diagnostic evaluation. Laboratory professionals can also answer questions about patient preparation for testing, optimal time of day for drawing samples, and interpretation of results. Similarly, when neuroimaging is requested, it is always good practice to review films in person with the radiologist, because the more clinical information provided to the radiologist, the more detailed and useful the interpretation of visual findings.

Clinical Laboratory Testing in Psychiatry

Clinical tests useful in psychiatric practice include blood, cerebrospinal fluid (CSF), stool, and urine tests as well as neuroimaging, neurophysiological tests, certain genetic tests, basic cardiopulmonary tests, and skin testing for tuberculosis. Table 5–1 lists individual tests, each discussed in the following section.

Blood Tests

Blood Alcohol Level

The blood alcohol level (BAL) is used to diagnose alcohol intoxication or withdrawal and to monitor drinking among individuals in treatment. When alcohol is ingested on an empty stomach, peak levels are reached within 1 hour. A small amount of the in-

TABLE 5–1.   **Clinically useful tests in psychiatric practice**

Blood tests	**Neuroimaging**
Blood alcohol level	Head computed tomography
Chemistries (metabolic panels)	Brain magnetic resonance imaging
Complete blood count	SPECT
Hemoglobin A_{1C} (HbA_{1C})	Positron emission tomography
HIV testing	
Lipid panel	**Neurophysiological tests**
Pregnancy testing (quantitative β-hCG)	Electroencephalogram (EEG)
Sexually transmitted infection testing	Quantitative EEG
Thyroid testing (TSH, free T_4)	Evoked potentials
Tuberculosis blood tests	MSLT/MWT
Vitamin levels (folate, thiamine, B_{12})	Electromyogram
	Polysomnogram
Cardiopulmonary studies	
Chest X ray	**Skin testing**
Electrocardiogram	Tuberculin skin test (Mantoux)
Cerebrospinal fluid studies	**Stool tests**
Cell count and differential	Fecal occult blood testing (guaiac test)
Protein	Fecal immunochemical testing
Glucose	
β-Amyloid (1–42)	**Urine tests**
Tau protein	Pregnancy (qualitative β-hCG)
	Urine dipstick testing
Genetic testing	Urinalysis
Apolipoprotein E genotyping	Urine drug screening
CYP genotyping	

Note.   CYP = cytochrome P450; hCG = human chorionic gonadotropin; MSLT/MWT = multiple sleep latency test/maintenance of wakefulness test; SPECT = single-photon emission computed tomography; T_4 = thyroxine; TSH = thyroid-stimulating hormone.

gested alcohol is excreted through the lungs and in urine, but most is metabolized in the liver to acetaldehyde and then to carbon dioxide and water. A normal liver can metabolize about 1 drink (12 oz of beer, 5 oz of wine, or 1.5 oz of 80-proof liquor) per hour. When more than 1 drink per hour is consumed, the alcohol level in the circulation rises.

A BAL of 0.08% or greater (>80 mg/dL; >17.4 mmol/L) is consistent with legal intoxication in all 50 states. Higher levels may be encountered clinically—for example, with reports of binge drinking in emergency department patients. A low BAL in the presence of symptoms of alcohol intoxication may predict serious impending withdrawal and should be treated accordingly.

Chemistries (Metabolic Panels)

Chemistries are indicated for hospital admission, mental status changes in a hospitalized patient, screening before starting a new psychotropic drug, monitoring for adverse effects of psychotropic drugs, and routine health assessment for patients with chronic mental illness for whom the psychiatrist serves in a primary care capacity. Although blood chemistries can be ordered individually, bundled test panels are a less costly alternative. Two panels in common use are the basic metabolic panel (BMP) and the comprehensive metabolic panel (CMP). Both panels provide a rapid assessment of the patient's acid–base status, kidney function, electrolytes, and glucose levels. The CMP, in addition, provides data on liver function and proteins. Table 5–2 lists individual tests included in the two panels.

Given that liver function is a critical variable in psychotropic metabolism and has a high probability of abnormality in certain psychiatric populations (e.g., those with alcohol use disorder), the CMP is often the preferred panel in psychiatric practice. The difference in cost between the two panels usually is negligible, as discussed a few paragraphs below.

One of the most important uses of the CMP is the identification of drug-induced hepatobiliary injury. A hepatotoxic drug reaction is suspected when the criteria for Hy's law are met:

- Aspartate aminotransferase (AST) or alanine aminotransferase (ALT) is three or more times the upper limit of normal.
- Bilirubin is two or more times the upper limit of normal.
- Alkaline phosphatase is two or less times the upper limit of normal.
- There is no other known reason for liver injury.

On the other hand, a cholestatic drug reaction is suspected when the following criteria are met:

- Alkaline phosphatase is more than three times the upper limit of normal.
- AST and ALT levels are normal or only minimally elevated.

The Healthcare Bluebook (www.healthcarebluebook.com) listed a fair price of $28 for the BMP and $34 for the CMP in greater metropolitan Phoenix, Arizona, on January 14, 2019, but prices vary considerably, both regionally and from one laboratory to another. The highest price listed on the same date for the same practice area was $171+ for the BMP and $146+ for the CMP.

In general, it is more expensive to have lab work performed at a hospital or clinic and less expensive to have it performed at an independent laboratory. All laboratories that handle human samples are required to meet the same regulatory standards. The so-called direct-access laboratories perform venipuncture and return metabolic panel results even without a doctor's order. In general, turnaround times are longer for these laboratories by 1–2 days.

Complete Blood Count

The complete blood count (CBC) is an automated count of blood cells that reports the following information: white blood cell (WBC), red blood cell (RBC), and platelet counts; platelet volume; hemoglobin content; hematocrit; and red cell indices (mean corpuscular volume, mean corpuscular hemoglobin, mean corpuscular hemoglobin concentration, and red cell distribution of width). The CBC can be ordered with platelets or with a WBC differential.

TABLE 5–2.   **Metabolic panels: basic (BMP) versus comprehensive (CMP) included tests**

Test	BMP	CMP
Glucose	X	X
Calcium	X	X
Albumin		X
Total protein		X
Sodium	X	X
Potassium	X	X
Carbon dioxide	X	X
Chloride	X	X
Blood urea nitrogen	X	X
Creatinine	X	X
Alanine transaminase (ALT)		X
Aspartate transaminase (AST)		X
Bilirubin		X
Alkaline phosphatase		X

Note.   BMP=basic metabolic panel; CMP=comprehensive metabolic panel.

The normal hematocrit is roughly 45%, which is about three times the hemoglobin value. The normal range for adult females is 36%–48%, whereas the normal range for adult males is 42%–52% (Fischbach and Dunning 2015). The lower limit of normal may be slightly lower for individuals of African or Afro-Caribbean ancestry. The normal platelet count in adults is $140–400 \times 10^3/mm^3$ (Fischbach and Dunning 2015). Critical values for hemoglobin, hematocrit, and platelets are shown in Table 5–3.

Hemoglobin A_{1C}

Glycosylated hemoglobin (HbA_{1C}) forms gradually over the 120-day life span of RBCs, with the amount formed corresponding to the average blood glucose concentration during that interval. The HbA_{1C} value is a better reflection of blood sugar control than fasting blood sugar but is not a replacement for fasting blood sugar, which is used to determine the need for immediate intervention. For comparison, HbA_{1C} values can be converted to estimated average glucose (eAG) values, which correspond more closely to fasting blood sugar or glucose meter values. The conversion can be made using published tables or can be calculated from the formula $28.7 \times A_{1C} - 46.7 = eAG$.

The HbA_{1C} reference interval is 4.0%–5.6%. HbA_{1C} values of 5.7%–6.4% represent an increased risk for developing diabetes. HbA_{1C} values of 6.5% or more are diagnostic of diabetes; in this case, the test is confirmed on a second sample (ARUP Laboratories 2018). In psychiatric practice, HbA_{1C} may be useful in the evaluation of patient adherence to diabetic treatment regimens and in patients with suspected metabolic syndrome. Pretest fasting is not necessary.

HIV Testing

The Centers for Disease Control and Prevention (CDC) recommends that everyone between the ages of 13 and 64 years be tested for HIV at least once as part of routine

TABLE 5–3.   **Complete blood count critical values**

Critical values	Potential consequences
Hemoglobin	
<5.0 g/dL	Multisystem organ failure; may be fatal
>20 g/dL	Denser concentration of hemoglobin, blood thickening, capillary clogging
Hematocrit	
<20%	Heart failure; may be fatal
>60%	Spontaneous clotting
Platelets	
$<20\times10^3/mm^3$	Spontaneous bleeding, bruising
$>1,000\times10^3/mm^3$	Bleeding from abnormal platelet function

Source. Fischbach and Dunning 2015.

health care and that any individual at risk be tested at least yearly. Several tests are in current use, both in the laboratory and for at-home screening. The currently recommended test is antigen/antibody testing, which is performed on a blood sample to detect the HIV p24 antigen and antibodies to HIV-1 and HIV-2. The inclusion of the p24 antigen facilitates slightly earlier detection of HIV (American Association for Clinical Chemistry 2018b).

The current CDC recommendations for HIV screening are as follows:

1. Screen for HIV using a combination antigen/antibody test.
2. If positive, perform a second HIV antibody test that distinguishes HIV-1 from HIV-2.
3. If the results from the first and second tests are not in agreement, perform an HIV-1 RNA test (nucleic acid test) (American Association for Clinical Chemistry 2018c).

Cost and insurance coverage of the nucleic acid test should be established before the test is ordered. It is important to note that patient counseling is mandatory with HIV testing (Centers for Disease Control and Prevention 2017, 2018).

Lipid Panel

Lipid screening is recommended at least every 4–6 years for adults age 20 years and older who have no risk factors for heart disease. More frequent testing is recommended for individuals who have risk factors such as smoking, obesity, hypertension, diabetes, unhealthy diet, sedentary lifestyle, older age, or personal/family history of heart disease or heart attack (American Association for Clinical Chemistry 2018d). For screening purposes, a lipid panel is performed, which includes total cholesterol, low-density lipoprotein cholesterol (LDL-C), high-density lipoprotein cholesterol (HDL-C), and triglycerides. In the standard panel, LDL-C is calculated, but that calculation is accurate only if the triglyceride content is less than 400 mg/dL. If the triglyceride content exceeds that limit, use of the extended panel is recommended, in which LDL-C is measured directly.

It is important that the patient fast for 9–12 hours before testing (American Association for Clinical Chemistry 2018d). If the test is nonfasting, only the total cholesterol and HDL-C will be usable. In this case, if the cholesterol is 200 mg/dL or greater or the HDL-C is less than 40 mg/dL, a follow-up fasting profile is required to determine LDL-C. The patient should abstain from alcohol use for 24 hours before the test. Drugs that affect cholesterol levels (e.g., statins) should be withheld for 24 hours before the test. Table 5–4 shows reference lipid values for adults.

Pregnancy Testing

Pregnancy tests are performed in women of reproductive age for whom treatment with potentially teratogenic medications or a procedure such as electroconvulsive therapy or transcranial magnetic stimulation is being considered. Testing is based on the detection of human chorionic gonadotropin (hCG), a hormone produced by the developing placenta that is elevated in pregnancy, with certain tumors, and at menopause. Of the two subunits of hCG (α and β), the β subunit is the more sensitive and specific for early pregnancy. β-hCG can be detected quantitatively in blood and qualitatively in urine. For routine pregnancy testing, a urine test can be used, as discussed in a later section (see "Pregnancy [Qualitative Beta–Human Chorionic Gonadotropin]" under "Urine Tests"). For nonroutine testing and for evaluation of conditions other than pregnancy, quantitative testing of β-hCG in blood is recommended. This test is the more sensitive and specific one to detect early pregnancy and estimate gestational age and to diagnose conditions such as ectopic pregnancy. The reference value for β-hCG in blood in nonpregnant women and men is less than 5.0 IU/L (Fischbach and Dunning 2015). In pregnant women, a range of β-hCG levels is seen, depending on the gestational age of the fetus. Factors that can interfere with the blood test include lipemia and specimen hemolysis.

Sexually Transmitted Infection/Disease Testing

Risk factors for sexually transmitted infection (STI) include being young (age <25 years), having a new or multiple sex partners, having a sex partner with an STI, using condoms inconsistently in a relationship that is not mutually monogamous, having a history of STI, and having a history of exchanging sex for money or drugs (U.S. Preventive Services Task Force 2014). Screening for STIs in individuals at risk may become the responsibility of the psychiatrist, particularly for patients with no identified primary care physician or clinic. STI screening guidelines published by the CDC in 2015 should be consulted (Centers for Disease Control and Prevention 2015).

Syphilis Testing

Testing for syphilis is indicated in patients with newly diagnosed HIV infection or other STIs such as gonorrhea, for patients who are pregnant, and for patients presenting with a skin rash, chancre, or other suggestive physical signs of syphilis (American Association for Clinical Chemistry 2018e). Although neurosyphilis is associated with dementia, behavioral changes, and mood disorders, syphilis testing is not universally performed in the course of a workup for major neurocognitive disorder unless there is a history of sexual risk behaviors.

For syphilis screening using blood, the rapid plasma reagin (RPR) test is used, with titers drawn if reactive. The Venereal Disease Research Laboratory (VDRL) test can be

TABLE 5–4.   Lipid values for adults (age 18 years and older): reference ranges

Total cholesterol		HDL cholesterol	
Desirable	<200 mg/dL	Desirable (females)	≥50 mg/dL
Borderline high	200–239 mg/dL	Desirable (males)	≥40 mg/dL
Triglycerides		**LDL cholesterol**	
Normal	<150 mg/dL	Desirable	<100 mg/dL
Borderline high	150–199 mg/dL	Above desirable	100–129 mg/dL
High	200–499 mg/dL	Borderline high	130–159 mg/dL
		High	160–189 mg/dL
		Very high	≥190 mg/dL

Note.   HDL= high-density lipoprotein; LDL= low-density lipoprotein.
Source.   National Lipid Association and National Cholesterol Education Program guidelines for lipids. Compiled from Test ID: LPSC (Lipid Panel, Fasting), in Mayo Medical Laboratories: Rochester 2018 Test Catalog, Laboratory Reference Edition (Sorted By Test Name; Current as of August 30, 2018). Available at: https://www.mayomedicallaboratories.com/test-catalog/Clinical+and+Interpretive/8053. Accessed September 3, 2018.

used as an alternative screen, with titers drawn if positive. RPR is preferred because the VDRL test has a higher rate of false-positive results (American Association for Clinical Chemistry 2018e). If either one of these tests is positive, treponemal testing should be performed (American Association for Clinical Chemistry 2018e), using one of the following tests:

- Fluorescent treponemal antibody absorption (FTA-Abs)
- Microhemagglutination tests for antibodies to *Treponema pallidum*
- Immunoglobulin M (IgM) antibody detection by enzyme-linked immunosorbent assay (ELISA)

If these tests are reactive (positive for antibodies), the diagnosis of syphilis is likely, and the disease should be staged and treated (American Association for Clinical Chemistry 2018e).

For suspected neurosyphilis, RPR is performed on serum, and VDRL is performed on CSF (American Association for Clinical Chemistry 2018e). If the serum RPR is negative but a suspicion for neurosyphilis remains, FTA-Abs should be performed on serum because some patients with late syphilis have a false-negative RPR test (American Association for Clinical Chemistry 2018e). In HIV patients, the affected site usually is the central nervous system (CNS). The organism *Treponema pallidum* cannot be cultured in vitro. If a skin lesion is present, a scraping from the lesion may be examined by dark-field microscopy to attempt to identify the bacterium.

False-positive RPR or VDRL results may be seen in the presence of HIV disease, herpes simplex virus infection, autoimmune disease, pregnancy, and many other conditions. False-positive FTA-Abs results may be seen in individuals of advanced age as well as persons with autoimmune disease, febrile illness, or other conditions (Fischbach and Dunning 2015).

Thyroid Function Testing

Thyroid-stimulating hormone (TSH) secreted by the anterior pituitary gland stimulates the thyroid gland to release stored triiodothyronine (T_3) and thyroxine (T_4), hormones responsible for the regulation of metabolism and other critical functions. TSH secretion is, in turn, regulated by thyrotropin-releasing hormone from the hypothalamus and by feedback inhibition from T_3 and T_4.

Functioning of the hypothalamic-pituitary-thyroid axis can be evaluated by measurement of hormones in the blood. In the past, a panel of thyroid tests was used, but with the introduction of more sensitive TSH testing, a simple TSH assay is now recommended. When a thyroid disorder is suspected or screening is indicated, a third-generation TSH is the best initial screening test (Kluesner et al. 2018). If the test is normal, no further testing is needed. If the TSH is not normal, free T_4 is checked. If pituitary hypothyroidism is suspected, free T_4 is checked initially with TSH. Reference values for TSH are shown in Table 5–5. If the normal range reported by the laboratory differs from that in the table, the laboratory range takes precedence. The reference range for free T_4 in adults is 0.7–2.0 ng/dL (Fischbach and Dunning 2015). For patients taking levothyroxine, the upper limit of normal is up to 5.0 ng/dL (Fischbach and Dunning 2015). A qualitative scheme for clinical interpretation of TSH and free T_4 levels is shown in Table 5–5.

Tuberculosis Blood Tests

Even in countries with a low prevalence of tuberculosis, the index of suspicion for tuberculosis exposure should be high in certain populations, including individuals who are homeless, who reside in nursing homes or correctional facilities, or who have traveled to or emigrated from countries with a high tuberculosis burden (U.S. Preventive Services Task Force 2016). Populations at particular risk for developing tuberculosis disease include the elderly, the very young, and individuals who are immunocompromised. For tuberculosis screening, either the Mantoux skin test or a blood test that measures interferon-γ release in response to the presence of the tuberculosis bacillus is used. These tests do not distinguish latent tuberculosis from active disease; a positive screen must be followed up with diagnostic tests such as sputum smear/culture, chest X ray, or CSF or other body fluid or tissue samples. Interferon-γ release assays are used for patients who have received the bacillus Calmette-Guérin (BCG) vaccine, in whom the skin test may be positive because of the vaccine. Interferon-γ release assays are known by various trade names, and each test has its own published standards for determining whether its results are positive or negative for tuberculosis (Franken et al. 2007; Piana et al. 2007).

Vitamin Levels

Folate (Vitamin B$_9$ or folic acid).   Folate is a water-soluble vitamin with a number of important molecular, cellular, and metabolic functions. Regular intake of folate is required and is critical during the first trimester of pregnancy to avoid neural tube defects in the developing fetus. Low folate levels have been shown to be associated with depression and poor response to antidepressants, but the literature is mixed as to whether folate augmentation of antidepressant medication is useful (Bedson et al.

TABLE 5–5.   **Thyroid testing**

TSH reference values

Normal	
Adults 21–54 years	0.4–4.2 µU/mL
Adults 55–87 years	0.5–8.9 µU/mL
Borderline hyperthyroidism	0.1–0.29 µU/mL
Probable hyperthyroidism	<0.1 µU/mL
Borderline hypothyroidism	5.1–7.0 µU/mL
Probable hypothyroidism	>7.0 µU/mL
Target level with T_4 replacement therapy	0.5–3.5 µU/mL
Critical value (thyrotoxicosis)	<0.1 µU/mL

Interpretation of basic thyroid function tests

TSH level	Free T_4 level	Condition
High	Low	Hypothyroidism
High	Normal	Subclinical hypothyroidism[a]
Low	High	Hyperthyroidism[b]
Low	Normal	Subclinical hyperthyroidism
Low	Low	Illness (nonthyroidal)

Note.   TSH=thyroid-stimulating hormone.
[a]If TSH is high and free T_4 is normal, thyroid antibodies are checked.
[b]If TSH is low and free T_4 is high, thyroid antibodies are checked (specifically, thyroid-stimulating immunoglobulin, thyroid peroxidase antibody, and TSH receptor antibody).
Source.   Col et al. 2004; Fischbach and Dunning 2015.

2014; Fava and Mischoulon 2009; Owen 2013). Low folate levels also are associated with dementia in certain patient populations, and folate is one of the lab tests routinely ordered in the workup for cognitive impairment. Newly admitted psychiatric patients with various diagnoses are more likely than the general population to have low folate levels (Lerner et al. 2006). In past years, RBC folate was the recommended test for folate deficiency, but on the basis of more recent studies, serum folate is now considered the test of choice by many specialists (De Bruyn et al. 2014; Farrell et al. 2013; Mayo Medical Laboratories 2018). In the presence of macrocytic anemia, when folate is checked, vitamin B_{12} is checked simultaneously; serum total homocysteine and methylmalonic acid levels can then help distinguish folate and vitamin B_{12} deficiencies. The patient should fast for 6–8 hours before testing, and the collected specimen must be protected from light exposure. Serum folate levels of 4.0 ng/mL or higher are considered normal (de Benoist 2008).

Thiamine (vitamin B_1).   This vitamin is a coenzyme in several important biochemical pathways and has a role in cognition, circulation, and numerous other functions. The body has a limited capacity to store thiamine, and severe deficiency can occur in as little as several weeks. Populations at risk for thiamine deficiency include adults with alcohol use disorder, eating disorders, or HIV, as well as individuals who have undergone gastric bypass surgery and elderly patients being treated with diuretic drugs. Thiamine requirements are directly correlated with carbohydrate intake. In any patient with suspected thiamine deficiency, thiamine must be replaced before glucose to prevent precipitation of Wernicke encephalopathy in a marginally deficient patient. Neuropsychiatric signs of thiamine deficiency include Wernicke-Korsakoff syndrome, sensorimotor dysfunction, ataxia, nystagmus, ophthalmoplegia, confusion, and coma. The severe deficiency syndrome can be fatal. Among individuals who do survive, residual memory and cognitive impairment may persist after treatment. The reference range for thiamine in whole blood is 2.5–7.5 µg/dL, and the reference range in serum or plasma is 0.2–0.4 µg/dL (Fischbach and Dunning 2015).

Cyanocobalamin (Vitamin B$_{12}$).   In addition to the classic presentation of subacute combined degeneration (with mental status changes in association with weakness, sensory deficits, and unsteady gait), symptoms of B$_{12}$ deficiency include delirium, psychosis, cognitive impairment, somnolence, irritability, and olfactory and visual changes (Langan and Goodbred 2017). Screening for B$_{12}$ deficiency may be advisable in adults older than 75 years, patients with alcohol use disorders, strict vegetarians, patients with inflammatory bowel disease or gastric/small bowel resection, and patients taking metformin, proton pump inhibitors, or H$_2$-blocking drugs (Langan and Goodbred 2017).

When B$_{12}$ deficiency is suspected, serum B$_{12}$ levels and a CBC should be obtained. A B$_{12}$ level of less than 150 pg/mL is consistent with deficiency; a workup for pernicious anemia may be indicated. A level of 400 pg/mL or higher is normal. For a level of 150–399 pg/mL or in the presence of deficiency symptoms, the methylmalonic acid (MMA) level is checked. If the MMA is low, B$_{12}$ deficiency is excluded. If the MMA level is high, B$_{12}$ deficiency is confirmed; a workup for pernicious anemia may be indicated (Langan and Goodbred 2017).

Cardiopulmonary Studies

Chest X Ray

A standard chest film can help diagnose a number of heart and lung conditions. A routine upright chest X ray has two views: posterior to anterior and left lateral. For bedridden patients, only an anterior-to-posterior film may be possible. Upright films are preferred because supine films do not show fluid levels. The procedure takes only a few minutes, and exposure to radiation is minimal unless the test is often repeated. According to updated guidelines, a chest X ray is appropriately performed for patients with suspected acute or unstable chronic cardiopulmonary disease and for elderly patients (age >70 years) who are unable to provide an accurate history or to undergo a reliable physical examination (Expert Panel on Thoracic Imaging et al. 2016).

Electrocardiogram

The electrocardiogram (ECG) records in real time the electrical activity of the heart and can be used to identify ischemia, infarction, cardiac hypertrophy, conduction delays, the source of abnormal rhythms, and tissue inflammation such as pericarditis. It can also be used to evaluate the function of implanted pacemakers and defibrillators. The ECG tracing may show the effects of electrolyte derangements, certain systemic diseases, and drugs that act on the heart.

The long-standing recommendation that an ECG be performed for all patients 40 years and older who are admitted to the hospital has been questioned because of low cost-benefit. However, given that certain patient populations reportedly have an elevated risk of sudden cardiac death, ECG should still be considered in selected cases. For example, among patients with schizophrenia, the adjusted risk ratio for sudden cardiac death was found to be 5.46 ($P<0.05$) in one study (Hou et al. 2015), and among patients with alcohol dependence, it was found to be 16.97 ($P<0.019$) (Wu et al. 2015). A study employing a decision analytic model found that ECG screening for prolonged QT interval for all patients on admission to psychiatric hospitals was cost-effective in reducing the rate of sudden cardiac death (Poncet et al. 2015). ECG screening is indicated prior to electroconvulsive therapy (Lafferty et al. 2001), particularly for patients older than 50 years or those with a prior abnormal ECG or known heart disease. ECG also is recommended for patients being considered for psychotropic drugs that affect cardiac conduction, such as antipsychotics, tricyclic antidepressants, and lithium (van Noord et al. 2009). ECG is, of course, also indicated for patients with chest pain or signs of myocardial infarction, syncope, or irregular pulse.

As shown in Figure 5–1, a normal heart cycle consists of a P wave, the QRS complex, and a T wave; a U wave also may be seen. This cycle is repeated at regular intervals. The P wave occurs with atrial depolarization, the QRS complex occurs with ventricular depolarization, and the T wave occurs with ventricular repolarization. The U wave represents nonspecific recovery afterpotentials.

The ECG is analyzed according to the following parameters: rate, rhythm, intervals, voltages, axis, and presence of abnormal waveforms. Table 5–6 lists rules that help identify the normal ECG, and Table 5–7 shows ECG results: normal, abnormal, and critical. Critical findings should prompt an immediate cardiology consultation.

Cerebrospinal Fluid Studies

In psychiatric practice, a lumbar puncture may be indicated for patients with delirium or a mental status change of unknown cause, a seizure of unknown cause, clinical suspicion of meningitis, another suspected CNS infection, or an unexplained fever in an immunocompromised patient (Irani 2009). CSF β-amyloid (1–42) and tau protein levels are used in specialty clinics and research settings in the evaluation of major neurocognitive disorder, as discussed later in this section (see "Cerebrospinal Fluid Beta-Amyloid (1–42)" and "Cerebrospinal Fluid Tau Protein" subsections). Ellenby et al. (2006) created an informative video detailing the method of performing a lumbar puncture (available via pay-per-view or subscription from the *New England Journal of Medicine* website).

Patient preparation is required before lumbar puncture. Anticoagulant therapy must be held (or the effects reversed) before the procedure so that the international normalized ratio is less than 1.2 (Irani 2009). In the presence of focal neurological signs, papilledema, new-onset seizures, or altered level of consciousness, a head CT or brain MRI should be performed before the procedure. The patient should be questioned about lumbar spine surgery or disease that might limit access to the subarachnoid space. Contraindications to lumbar puncture include a mass lesion in the posterior fossa, an intracranial lesion with mass effect seen on CT or MRI, a midline shift on CT or MRI, poor visualization of the fourth ventricle or quadrigeminal cistern on CT or

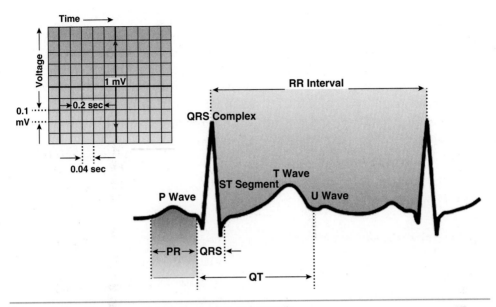

FIGURE 5–1. Electrocardiogram waves and intervals.

To view this figure in color, see Plate 1 in Color Gallery in middle of book.

The P wave represents atrial activation; the PR interval is the time from onset of atrial activation to onset of ventricular activation. The QRS complex represents ventricular activation; the QRS duration is the duration of ventricular activation. The ST–T wave represents ventricular repolarization. The QT interval is the duration of ventricular activation and recovery. The U wave probably represents "afterdepolarizations" in the ventricles.

Source. Reprinted from the ECG Learning Center (https://ecg.utah.edu/), a webpage created by the Spencer S. Eccles Health Sciences Library, University of Utah, and available under a Creative Commons CC-BY license. Content copyright ©1997, Frank G. Yanowitz, M.D., Professor of Medicine (Retired), University of Utah School of Medicine, Salt Lake City.

TABLE 5–6.   Ten rules for a normal electrocardiogram

1. The PR interval should be 120–200 milliseconds (ms) (three to five small squares).
2. The QRS complex should not be longer than 110 ms (fewer than three small squares).
3. The QRS complex should be mostly upright in leads I and II.
4. The QRS and T waves should have the same general polarity (up or down) in limb leads.
5. All waves in aVR are downgoing (negative).
6. The R wave should grow across precordial leads (V_1–V_6), at least to V_4.
7. The ST segment should start at baseline in all leads except V_1 and V_2, where it may start above the baseline.
8. P waves should be upright in leads I, II, and V_2–V_6.
9. Q waves should be absent, except for small Q waves of <0.04 second in leads I, II, and V_2–V_6.
10. The T wave must be upright in leads I, II, and V_2–V_6.

Note. A 12-lead ECG consists of three bipolar limb leads (I, II, and III), three unipolar limb leads (aVR, aVL, and aVF), and six unipolar chest leads, also called precordial or V leads (V_1, V_2, V_3, V_4, V_5, and V_6).
Source. Prepared by Professor Douglas Chamberlain, M.D., Honorary Professor of Resuscitation Medicine, Cardiff University; in public domain.

TABLE 5–7.   Results of electrocardiogram (ECG) testing

Normal ECG results

Heart rate (HR)	60–100 beats/minute
Rhythm	Normal sinus rhythm or sinus arrhythmia
PR interval	120–200 ms (0.12–0.20 second)
QRS interval	80–110 ms (0.08–0.11 second)
QT interval	350–430 ms[a]
P wave voltage	0.1–0.3 mV
T wave voltage	0.2–0.3 mV
Top of R wave to bottom of S wave	1 mV
Axis	+90° to −30° in adult

Abnormal ECG results

Bradycardia	HR <60 beats/minute
Tachycardia	HR >100 beats/minute
Atrial fibrillation	HR is rapid Rhythm is irregular Absence of P waves that usually precede QRS complexes
Atrial flutter	HR is rapid (ventricular rate about 150 beats/minute) QRS is narrow ECG baseline has a sawtooth appearance
First-degree heart block	PR interval >0.20 ms Each P wave is followed by QRS
Second-degree heart block	Some P waves have no following QRS
Third-degree (complete) heart block	Complete dissociation of P waves and QRS
QTc prolongation	QTc >450 ms for men QTc >470 ms for women
Premature ventricular contractions (PVCs) (also called ventricular premature depolarizations [VPDs])	A wide QRS that closely follows a normal QRS When a PVC occurs after every normal QRS, the pattern is called bigeminy When a PVC occurs after every other normal QRS, the pattern is called trigeminy When three or more PVCs occur in a row, the pattern is ventricular tachycardia
ST segment depression	The normal ST segment serves as the isoelectric line on the ECG tracing An ST segment below the baseline signifies ischemia
ST segment elevation	The normal ST segment serves as the isoelectric line on the ECG tracing An ST segment above the baseline signifies infarction

TABLE 5–7.	Results of electrocardiogram (ECG) testing *(continued)*
Critical ECG results	
Ventricular tachycardia	HR > 100 with three or more irregular heartbeats in a row
Ventricular fibrillation	Very rapid HR Uncoordinated Fatal unless treated immediately
Torsades de pointes	Bradycardia Prolonged QT QRS that rotates around the isoelectric baseline
Severe bradycardia	HR <40 Often symptomatic (dizziness, syncope, etc.)

[a]QT interval varies with heart rate, gender, time of day. Corrected QT (QTc)=QT / R-R interval.

MRI, an international normalized ratio greater than 1.5, a platelet count less than 50,000/mm^3, or a lumbar skin or tissue infection (Irani 2009).

CSF samples should be examined as soon as possible or frozen until examination. As a routine, the report returned from the laboratory will include cell counts (with a differential for WBCs if cell count is greater than 5), total protein, albumin, glucose, IgG, IgA, IgM, oligoclonal bands if present, specific antibodies if present (e.g., measles, rubella), lactate if requested, and the appearance of the CSF by visual inspection.

Cerebrospinal Fluid Cell Count and Differential

Normally, the CSF has few or no cells. In adults, a small number of lymphocytes and monocytes in a ratio of about 2 to 1 may be seen. RBCs are normally not present, except when the spinal tap has traumatized surrounding tissues. CSF cell counts include the number of RBCs, number of WBCs, and cell types. The total cell count is a sensitive indicator of acute inflammation or infection in the CNS. The reference range for WBCs in adults is 0–5 WBCs/mm^3 (40%–80% lymphocytes, 15%–45% monocytes, 0%–6% neutrophils) (Fischbach and Dunning 2015). The reference range for WBCs in children is 0–15 WBCs/mm^3 (Fischbach and Dunning 2015). In young children, a larger proportion of monocytes may be seen. Increased cell counts are seen in the presence of meningitis, encephalitis, metastatic tumors, and inflammatory reactions. The specific cell type that is increased helps guide further workup and treatment.

Cerebrospinal Fluid Total Protein

An elevation in the measured CSF protein level is a reliable indicator of CNS pathology. Table 5–8 shows normal protein levels by age group and levels representative of different pathological conditions. Special studies may be needed to determine the composition of protein or to identify pathological processes such as myelin breakdown. A false elevation of protein can result from a traumatic tap. In this case, the protein level is highest in tube 1 and falls progressively in tubes 2–4. This spurious elevation can be corrected if the same tube is used for protein and cell counts: subtract 1 mg/dL of protein for every 1,000 RBCs/mm^3. Generally, low CSF protein values have little clinical significance but can be seen in CNS trauma with CSF leakage, CSF volume removal, intracranial hypertension, or hyperthyroidism (Irani 2009).

TABLE 5–8.	Cerebrospinal fluid (CSF) protein levels (mg/dL)
Normal range	
15–45	10–40 years
20–50	40–50 years
20–55	50–60 years
30–60	>60 years
Critical values	
>60	Warrants a thorough investigation in the absence of diabetes or recent stroke
>1,000	Suggests subarachnoid obstruction of CSF flow; the lower the anatomic block, the higher the value
100–500	Consistent with increased permeability of the blood–CSF barrier
Mean values in various CNS diseases	
418	Bacterial meningitis
270	Cerebral hemorrhage
115	Brain tumor
77	Aseptic meningitis
69	Brain abscess
68	Neurosyphilis
43	Multiple sclerosis
32	Acute alcoholism
31	Epilepsy

Note. CNS=central nervous system.
Source. Fischbach and Dunning 2015; Irani 2009.

Cerebrospinal Fluid Glucose

The normal range of CSF glucose reflects the serum glucose level in the 1–4 hours before sampling. In adults, the normal range of CSF glucose is 45–80 mg/dL (about two-thirds of the serum glucose level) (Irani 2009). In children, the normal range is 35–75 mg/dL (Irani 2009). CSF glucose levels less than 40 mg/dL are always pathological in adults. Decreased CSF glucose levels are found in encephalitis, meningitis, CNS cancer, subarachnoid hemorrhage, hypoglycemia, and CNS inflammatory diseases such as sarcoidosis. Increased CSF glucose levels are found in traumatic brain injury, hyperglycemia, uremia, cerebral hemorrhage, and other conditions.

Cerebrospinal Fluid Beta-Amyloid (1–42)

CSF β-amyloid (1–42) is not a routine part of the CSF analysis and is performed only in designated laboratories. The assay is technically difficult, and the sample requires special collection and handling. The test is performed in conjunction with CSF tau protein (see next section) in the workup of cognitive impairment to provide evidence for or against the diagnosis of Alzheimer's disease. CSF β-amyloid (1–42) levels are lower in Alzheimer's disease patients compared with age-matched cognitively normal patients, but the mechanism underlying this difference is not entirely understood. At present, the test is used primarily in clinical research settings. Overlap of normal and pathological values of CSF β-amyloid (1–42) and poor correlation with cognitive measures render this test of limited value in individual patients, but work is ongoing to improve the sensitivity and specificity of the test (Dean and Shaw 2010; de Leon et al. 2004). One testing laboratory, Athena Diagnostics, calculates a β-amyloid (1–42) tau index (AT index) that differentiates Alzheimer's disease from normal aging, depression, alcohol-related dementia, and other dementing conditions. When the AT index is in the range consistent with Alzheimer's disease, tau protein (phosphorylated tau [P-Tau]) aids in distinguishing Alzheimer's from other forms of dementia with reasonable sensitivity and specificity. Laboratory reference values are returned with the report of test results. Recently, a more sensitive digital ELISA assay was developed that may be used on plasma rather than CSF samples to quantify β-amyloid (1–42) (Song et al. 2016).

Cerebrospinal Fluid Tau Protein

CSF tau is a special study available only through designated labs and is usually performed in tandem with CSF β-amyloid (1–42), as noted earlier. Tau protein is reported as total tau and P-Tau. As noted in the previous section, Athena Diagnostics has developed an AT index that is able to distinguish Alzheimer's disease from normal aging and other pathological conditions. When the AT index is in the range consistent with Alzheimer's disease, P-Tau helps to distinguish it from other forms of dementia with good sensitivity and specificity (Mitchell 2009). Laboratory reference values are returned with the report of test results.

Genetic Testing

Genetic tests in current clinical use that are covered in this section include genotyping of apolipoprotein E (apoE) alleles and cytochrome P450 (CYP) isoenzymes. Useful information about other genetic tests and associated diseases can be found at the Genetic Testing Registry (GTR) website (www.ncbi.nlm.nih.gov/gtr) (Rubinstein et al. 2013). In most settings, genetic tests are laboratory sendouts, and it is important to inquire directly with the testing laboratory about costs and specimen handling before sending samples. This type of testing can be expensive and may not be covered by medical insurance policies.

Apolipoprotein E Genotyping

Of the three *APOE* alleles—ε2, ε3, and ε4—the most common is ε3, which is present in more than 50% of the general population. The ε4 allele has a direct correlation with brain amyloid plaque burden, and its presence is the strongest genetic risk factor for the development of late-onset Alzheimer's disease (Liu et al. 2013). The ε2 allele appears to confer some degree of protection from this condition. The association between ε4 and Alzheimer's disease is strongest when the patient has a positive family history of dementia. The association is further strengthened when two copies of ε4 are present (Farrer et al. 1997). Although the ε4 allele has a worldwide frequency of 13.7%, the frequency among individuals with Alzheimer's disease is about 40% (Farrer et al. 1997).

Clinical apoE genotyping is characterized by low sensitivity and poor positive predictive value (Elias-Sonnenschein et al. 2011). It does not predict whether Alzheimer's disease will develop in an asymptomatic individual. It is not useful for screening or in the early stages of a dementia diagnostic evaluation. In fact, about 42% of patients with Alzheimer's disease do not have an ε4 allele. The specific context in which apoE testing may be useful is in a patient who meets clinical criteria for Alzheimer's disease. In this case, the finding of an ε4/ε4 genotype increases the probability that Alzheimer's disease is the correct diagnosis to about 97% (Elias-Sonnenschein et al. 2011; Petersen et al. 1996). ApoE genotyping is performed by a limited number of laboratories (accessible through the GTR website [www.ncbi.nlm.nih.gov/gtr]) (Rubinstein et al. 2013). When apoE genotyping is performed, patient counseling is required.

Cytochrome P450 Genotyping

CYP genotyping reveals genetically based variations in the activity of certain CYP isoenzymes, including CYP2D6 and CYP2C19, which are of particular interest in psychopharmacology. The testing is now widely available for clinical use, with indications that include poor antidepressant response, unexpected or severe adverse effects of antidepressants, poor antipsychotic response, and extrapyramidal effects of certain antipsychotics at low dosages (de Leon et al. 2006; Samer et al. 2013). Either saliva or whole blood is sampled.

Test results returned from CYP2D6 genotyping include the categorization of the patient's sample as reflecting ultrarapid, extensive, intermediate, or poor metabolizer status. Poor metabolizer status indicates an absence of enzyme activity, whereas ultrarapid metabolizer status indicates excessive enzyme activity. Extensive metabolizer status indicates normal enzyme activity, whereas intermediate status indicates slightly reduced enzyme activity. Poor metabolizers (and, to a lesser extent, intermediate metabolizers) may develop higher serum levels of a drug, with potential toxicity. It is recommended, for example, that pimozide dosages greater than 4 mg/day in adults should not be used without CYP2D6 genotyping (Rogers et al. 2012). Ultrarapid metabolizers may have drug levels too low to be clinically effective. In addition to pimozide, psychotropic drugs metabolized by CYP2D6 include aripiprazole, atomoxetine, duloxetine, haloperidol, risperidone, venlafaxine, vortioxetine, and zuclopenthixol. Recommendations regarding drug dosing in both poor metabolizers and ultrarapid metabolizers of CYP2D6 are regularly updated; package inserts should be consulted before prescribing one of these drugs or changing the dosage.

Test results returned from CYP2C19 genotyping also include the categorization of the patient's sample as reflecting ultrarapid, extensive, intermediate, or poor metabolizer status. Again, both ultrarapid and poor metabolizer status may indicate the need for a change of drug or a dosage adjustment as well as careful attention to therapeutic drug monitoring. Even with intermediate metabolizer status, drug–drug and drug–metabolite inhibition of enzyme activity must be considered. Psychotropic drugs metabolized by CYP2C19 include citalopram, escitalopram, sertraline, and tricyclic antidepressants.

In general, the findings on CYP genotyping published by the Evaluation of Genomic Applications in Practice and Prevention Working Group in 2007 still hold. CYP genotyping is more accurate and easier to interpret with more common polymorphisms than with rarer variants or gene duplications or deletions. In addition, the literature on clinical validity and utility is not robust. In spite of these limitations, however, a number of insurance companies have agreed to cover CYP2D6 and

CYP2C19 genotyping, recognizing the potential cost savings of avoiding hospitalization and serial drug trials in selected patients.

Neurophysiological Testing

Electroencephalography

The electroencephalogram (EEG) records electrical potential differences between electrode pairs on the scalp or between a scalp electrode and a reference electrode. These potentials reflect underlying electrical activity in the cerebral cortex and, indirectly, that in deeper structures. Frequencies of the electrical activity captured range from 0.5 Hz to approximately 35 Hz, and the range is divided into bands, shown in Figure 5–2.

For the EEG procedure, electrodes are attached to the scalp in standard positions, using an arrangement known as the 10–20 system (or an extended version of that system), and several different patterns of electrode pairings ("montages") are captured. Reference electrodes are placed on the ear or mastoid, or an averaged reference is created electronically. Ideally, recordings capture the fully awake, drowsy, and sleeping states. To achieve the sleep state, the patient may require sleep deprivation on the night before the test. Several stimulation procedures designed to elicit epileptiform patterns are performed during the test, including hyperventilation and photic stimulation. If the referring question relates to a specific provocation (e.g., seizures when listening to music), the provocation should be simulated during testing. To capture epileptiform or ictal activity arising from the temporal lobes (e.g., in partial seizures), anterior temporal and ear electrodes may be used; nasopharyngeal electrodes offer no advantage and are uncomfortable for the patient. If the referring question relates to encephalopathy, the patient may require specific alerting procedures; for example, the patient may be asked to count backward from 20, or the technician might provide a tapping stimulus to maintain wakefulness for a brief interval of recording. Figure 5–3 shows a normal EEG tracing (A) and an abnormal tracing obtained from a patient with delirium (B), described in the text below.

As a diagnostic tool, the routine EEG is inexpensive and noninvasive. Because it involves no ionizing radiation or contrast agents, the EEG can be repeated as often as needed. The patient should be reassured that the EEG only records electrical activity and does not deliver an electrical stimulus. Electrode application may require the use of collodion, an adhesive gel that requires vigorous cleansing for removal. The patient should avoid sedatives before testing. If a hypnotic is required to capture sleep during the recording, chloral hydrate is often used, but clonidine is used in children, and there is increasing interest in the use of dexmedetomidine; all three drugs have negligible effects on EEG activity. Sleep deprivation may be needed to ensure that an adequate sleep sample is obtained (e.g., in the case of suspected seizures). A commonly used sleep deprivation protocol involves awakening the patient at 4:00 A.M. and then keeping the patient awake without naps or stimulants until the time of testing.

The EEG is a useful adjunct to the clinical examination in confirming the diagnosis and monitoring the course of delirium. The EEG in delirium is characterized by generalized slow-wave activity in the delta and theta ranges, slowing of the posterior dominant frequency, disorganization of the background rhythm, and loss of reactivity to eye opening and closing (Jacobson and Jerrier 2000). Figure 5–3B shows an EEG

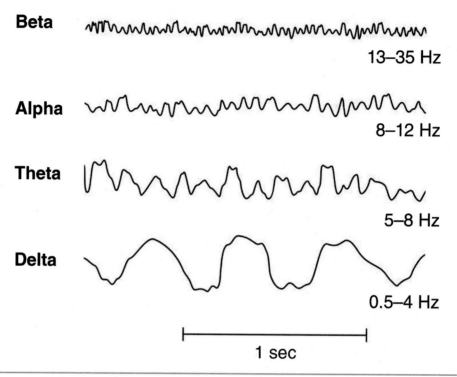

FIGURE 5–2.   Electroencephalographic frequency bands.

Note.   Figure shows the appearance of waveforms recorded in each of the four basic EEG frequency bands.

tracing obtained from a patient with clinical signs of delirium. The EEG can be used to distinguish delirium from primary psychosis, because it is usually normal in the latter condition. It can be used to detect the presence of delirium superimposed on dementia, in which case the amount of slow-wave activity may be greatly increased over the baseline tracing. Serial EEGs can be helpful in gauging response to the treatment of delirium, showing improvement in slowing and increase in alpha frequency (Jacobson et al. 1993). Other uses of the EEG in psychiatry are listed in Table 5–9.

The use of electroencephalography in the diagnosis of attention deficit/hyperactivity disorder (ADHD) has been controversial. A number of studies have identified increased brain theta activity (a higher theta/beta ratio) and reduced resting state 13- to 15-Hz activity over the sensorimotor cortex (sensorimotor rhythm) in ADHD, although these findings have not been consistent across studies (Lenartowicz and Loo 2014). When EEG neurofeedback is used to influence these variables, pre- and posttreatment differences may be negligible, even though symptoms of inattention and impulsivity are improved (Arns et al. 2014). It is likely that both the heterogeneity of the disorder and differences in recording conditions among studies have contributed to this inconsistency. In any event, both diagnostic testing and neurofeedback therapy are commercially available for this indication.

Quantitative Electroencephalography

Digital EEG data capture and computerized analysis have expanded the capabilities of electroencephalography and introduced a number of new variables such as abso-

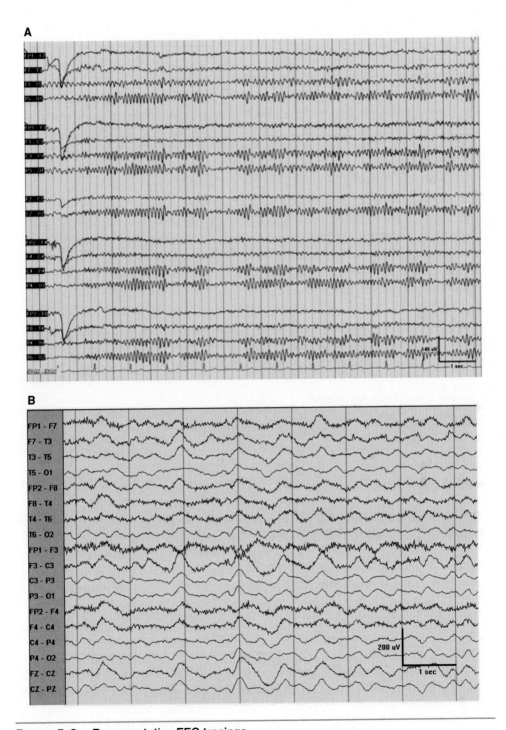

FIGURE 5–3. Representative EEG tracings.

(A) Tracing of a normal EEG from a longitudinal bipolar montage. Beta activity predominates frontally, and a clear alpha rhythm predominates posteriorly that emerges with eye closure *(large deflection at start of tracing)*. **(B)** EEG tracing of a patient with delirium, showing generalized slow-wave activity in the delta range and gross disorganization with no discernible posterior dominant (alpha) rhythm.

TABLE 5–9.   Selected examples of electroencephalogram (EEG) use in psychiatry

Attention-deficit/hyperactivity disorder

- Inconsistent findings of increased brain theta activity, increased theta/beta ratio, and reduced resting state 13- to 15-Hz activity over the sensorimotor cortex (sensorimotor rhythm) are noted.
- Neurofeedback may improve inattention and impulsivity without affecting these EEG measures.

Delirium

- Distinguish delirium from catatonia and primary psychosis.
- Diagnose delirium when superimposed on dementia.
- Monitor a course of treatment for delirium.

Nonconvulsive status epilepticus

- This presentation disproportionately affects elderly women.
- Patient presents with ongoing oneiric (dream-like) state or stupor.
- EEG shows sustained ictal activity.

Seizures

- Distinguish seizures from pseudoseizures if an ictal event is captured and neither spike nor spike-and-wave activity is seen.
- Caveats: Interictal EEG may be normal, some patients have both seizures and pseudoseizures, and deep epileptogenic foci may only be captured with depth recordings.

Sporadic Creutzfeldt-Jakob disease

- In early stages, the EEG is normal or shows a small amount of theta slowing.
- In late stages, periodic bursts of high-voltage polyphasic sharp waves are seen every 1–2 seconds in a burst–suppression pattern. These complexes are often symmetric but may be of higher voltage over one hemisphere.

Subacute sclerosing panencephalitis

- EEG shows periodic complexes consisting of 2–4 high-amplitude delta waves, usually bisynchronous and symmetrical, repeated every 5–7 seconds.
- The complexes correspond to the clinical occurrence of myoclonic jerks.
- Less commonly, frontal rhythmic delta activity or reduced EEG amplitude between complexes, bisynchronous spike-and-wave activity, random frontal spikes, or focal spike-and-slow-wave activity is seen.

Toxic effects of lithium

- EEG may show a disorganized rhythm, interspersed slow-wave activity, and/or triphasic waves.

lute and relative power in different frequency bands, spectral edge frequency, and signal coherence. The patient interface for quantitative EEG (qEEG) is the same as that for EEG, with an extended 10- to 20-electrode placement system used. Indications and patient preparation are the same as for conventional EEG. In the past, qEEG was used mostly in research settings, but most of the newer clinical EEG systems are now digital, with at least the theoretical potential to provide more complex analyses. Digital systems retain the ability to generate analog displays of EEG data in real time, so that visual examination ("reading") can still take place as a check on qEEG findings. Digital systems can also generate spatial displays of data, which are often superimposed on an outline of the brain ("brain maps").

Depending on the referring question, the qEEG may be analyzed and reported as numerical data, brain maps, or a real-time tracing that includes activation procedures (hyperventilation and photic stimulation). For conditions such as delirium, with persistent (nonperiodic) EEG correlates, it is possible to utilize only a few seconds of captured EEG for analysis, making qEEG a preferred modality in the case of a patient unable to cooperate fully. The use of an extended electrode array with digital analysis also facilitates three-dimensional dipole localization in seizure evaluation as well as other, more complex analyses.

Normal findings on qEEG include the following:

- Alpha power (absolute and relative) is highest over occipital areas and is symmetric.
- No appreciable slow-wave (delta or theta) power is observed in wakefulness.
- Other reference values are per laboratory report.

Examples of abnormal findings on qEEG include the following:

- Delta and theta power increased in a generalized distribution may be consistent with delirium or medication effects.
- Reduced alpha power in occipital areas may be consistent with dementia or medication effects.
- Increased beta activity may be consistent with anxiety or sedative-hypnotic use/ withdrawal.

The use of qEEG does not eliminate the need to have experienced neurophysiologists involved in data interpretation. Artifacts may be introduced that confound recordings, such as eye movements appearing as delta power in frontotemporal areas or muscle activity as beta power. In addition, EEG studies that do not explicitly produce and document alerting stimuli for patients with delirium or other conditions of reduced consciousness are considered incomplete. Many psychotropic drugs affect the EEG, usually increasing either slow-wave power (e.g., antipsychotics or mood stabilizers) or beta power (e.g., sedative-hypnotics or alcohol).

Evoked Potentials

Using a modification of the techniques used to capture EEG data, electrical potentials can be elicited in response to auditory, visual, somatosensory, or cognitive stimuli and can then be recorded. Each stimulus results in a small-magnitude electrical change in the brain. Stimuli are given repetitively, and the changes are averaged to yield the evoked potential. These methods have mostly been used to evaluate problems such as suspected optic nerve lesions in patients with multiple sclerosis or to assess brain stem function in comatose patients. However, because evoked potential testing provides clinically useful information about the processing of sensory stimuli, it could be helpful in distinguishing medical from psychogenic causes of certain symptoms. For example, visual evoked potentials could be useful in differentiating psychogenic blindness from true blindness.

Of potentially greater interest to psychiatrists are the evoked potential components that follow the initial evoked potentials, such as midlatency evoked responses and even later event-related potentials. One such event-related potential—the P300, named for the time of its appearance after the stimulus (between 250 and 500 ms)—has been found to be abnormal in individuals at risk of developing psychosis (Bodatsch et al. 2015) and in individuals with Alzheimer's disease (Frodl et al. 2002). The P300 is an endogenous potential believed to reflect processes involved in the brain's evaluation of a stimulus.

Multiple Sleep Latency Test

The multiple sleep latency test (MSLT) is indicated to confirm the clinical diagnosis of primary hypersomnia (narcolepsy) and to determine the effectiveness of treatment for this condition. It can also be used to evaluate daytime hypersomnolence in patients with other neuropsychiatric conditions, including those with Parkinson's disease, chronic fatigue syndrome, or major depressive disorder. The MSLT is often performed in a sleep laboratory on the day after an overnight polysomnography study (discussed later in this chapter in the subsection "Polysomnography"). The patient should be instructed to avoid caffeine until the MSLT is completed. The goal of the test is to quantify the patient's degree of daytime somnolence. The patient is given the opportunity to nap at least four times at 2-hour intervals throughout the day and is instructed not to resist the urge to fall asleep. EEG, electrooculogram, electromyogram (EMG), and ECG are monitored to determine times of sleep onset and offset, as well as rapid eye movement (REM) sleep, and to monitor heart rate and rhythm.

On the MSLT, the average time to sleep onset for patients without daytime hypersomnolence is 10–20 minutes (Rack et al. 2005). If the average time to sleep onset were less than 8 minutes, the test would be considered positive for hypersomnolence. Sleep-onset REM periods may also be seen in patients with narcolepsy. If more than two sleep-onset REM periods are observed, narcolepsy without cataplexy can be diagnosed (Rack et al. 2005).

The related maintenance of wakefulness test (MWT) provides an index of the patient's ability to stay awake during the daytime. In this test, the patient is instructed to resist the urge to fall asleep; otherwise, the protocol is much like the MSLT (Sullivan and Kushida 2008). As with the MSLT, the patient should be instructed to avoid caffeine after the polysomnogram until the MWT is completed.

Electromyography and Nerve Conduction Tests

Electromyography and nerve conduction tests (NCTs) evaluate the electrical activity of muscles (EMG) and nerves (NCT) as a means of assessing their function. In electromyography, needles are inserted into muscle tissue, and electrodes are attached to skin. Recordings are made at rest and with voluntary muscle contraction. In NCTs, electric current is applied to the nerve (sensory or motor) so that the velocity of nerve transmission can be measured. One important use of the EMG/NCT in psychiatric practice relates to the workup of somatoform disorders, in which normal test results aid in excluding muscle or nerve pathology as a cause of symptoms such as weakness or paralysis. In addition, conditions such as undiagnosed myasthenia gravis may come to the attention of psychiatrists because of symptoms such as weakness and fatigue, and in certain patients, an EMG/NCT would be indicated before a diagnosis of depression were considered. Both myositis associated with atypical antipsychotic use and peripheral neuropathy associated with alcoholism and vitamin deficiencies could also be indications for an EMG/NCT.

The EMG procedure takes 30–60 minutes. A normal EMG shows no electrical activity when the muscle is at rest. On NCTs, nerve conduction velocities vary with the nerve studied, but range from 40 to 70 meters/second (Chémali and Tsao 2005; Daube 1996). The patient should be instructed to bathe or shower before the test and to avoid application of cosmetics (including powders, deodorants, and lotions). In addition, the patient should avoid caffeine and tobacco prior to testing (Chémali and Tsao 2005; Daube 1996).

Polysomnography

Traditionally, polysomnography has required an overnight stay in a sleep laboratory while the patient undergoes monitoring of multiple parameters during sleep, including EEG, eye movements, ECG, EMG of chin muscle, EMG of anterior tibialis muscle, respiratory effort of chest and abdomen, oral/nasal airflow, and oxygen saturation. Video data are also captured. Home sleep study is now an option using ambulatory equipment. Regardless of where the study takes place, digital recording and computerized analysis have greatly simplified the detection of sleep-related events and the scoring of sleep stages and events (Flemons 2002).

Polysomnographic study can facilitate the diagnosis and characterization of a number of conditions commonly seen in psychiatric practice, including nocturnal panic attacks, sleep apnea with treatment-resistant depression, cognitive impairment associated with nocturnal oxygen desaturation, and various parasomnias (Fois et al. 2015). Table 5–10 lists common indications for polysomnography. The primary indication is to evaluate sleep-disordered breathing (sleep apnea) (Flemons 2002). For this purpose, apnea and hypopnea events are monitored. Apnea occurs when airflow stops for more than 10 seconds. Hypopnea occurs when airflow is reduced by 50% for more than 10 seconds. The apnea/hypopnea index (AHI) is the sum of apneas and hypopneas per hour of sleep. Results of polysomnographic studies related to the AHI can be helpful in reinforcing the need for weight loss in patients with obstructive sleep apnea, because the AHI can significantly improve with weight loss. Table 5–11 lists normal and abnormal findings in polysomnographic studies.

Skin Testing: Tuberculin Skin Test (Mantoux)

Psychiatric populations at particular risk of developing tuberculosis (TB) include recent immigrants, those who are homeless, those with alcoholism or intravenous drug use histories, and residents of congregate living facilities such as prisons, nursing homes, and residential facilities for adults with chronic mental illness. TB skin testing is used to determine whether an individual has been infected with TB For the tuberculosis skin test, a small amount of purified protein derivative is injected intradermally into the patient's forearm, and 48–72 hours later, the site is examined for induration (not erythema). The diameter of induration (measured perpendicular to the long axis of the arm) and the person's risk of being infected (and of progressing to disease if infected) are used to determine whether the test is positive. An induration of 5 mm or greater is considered a positive test result in a person with HIV infection, an organ

TABLE 5–10.   Indications for polysomnography

Evaluation of sleep-disordered breathing (including sleep apnea)
Confirmation of diagnosis of restless legs syndrome
Detection of periodic limb movements of sleep
Evaluation of rapid eye movement behavior disorder
Confirmation of suspected nocturnal seizures
Confirmation of suspected nocturnal panic attacks (and to exclude seizures)
Confirmation of other parasomnias such as sleepwalking

TABLE 5–11.   Polysomnogram report: normal and abnormal findings

Normal findings

Sleep variable

Sleep onset and offset times	Normal sleep time
Proportion of each sleep stage	Normal proportions of REM and non-REM sleep (sleep stages N1, N2, and N3)
Number of arousals during sleep	Normal
Periodic leg movements or jerks	Absent or negligible
Oxygen saturation	>90%
Oxygen desaturation index	Fewer than five events per hour of saturation <90%
Abnormal snoring	Absent
ECG rate and rhythm disturbances	Absent
Apnea/hypopnea index (AHI)	≤5 apneas/hypopneas per hour in a patient with OSA symptoms (<10 per hour after age 60 years)

Abnormal findings

AHI findings confirming a clinical diagnosis of OSA

Mild sleep apnea	AHI=5–14
Moderate sleep apnea	AHI=15–30
Severe sleep apnea	AHI >30

Other abnormal findings

Desaturation
Disrupted sleep architecture
Abnormal leg movements
Abnormal behaviors

Note.   ECG=electrocardiogram; OSA=obstructive sleep apnea; REM=rapid eye movement.

transplant recipient, a person with recent exposure to tuberculosis disease, or a patient immunosuppressed by prednisone or a tumor necrosis factor alpha (TNF-α) antagonist. An induration 10 mm or greater is considered a positive test result in recent immigrants from endemic countries or residents/employees of congregate living, and an induration of 15 mm or greater is a positive result in an individual with no risk factors (American Thoracic Society 2000).

False-positive results can occur among patients who have received the BCG vaccine, and such patients should be tested instead with tuberculosis blood testing (discussed in earlier section "Tuberculosis Blood Tests"). False-positive results also can be seen in patients with a nontuberculosis mycobacteria infection. False-negative results can occur among patients with cutaneous anergy, those with a viral illness such as chicken pox, or those who have recently been vaccinated with a live virus such as smallpox or measles (Centers for Disease Control and Prevention 2016).

Stool Tests: Fecal Occult Blood Test and Fecal Immunochemical Test

Patients treated with selective serotonin reuptake inhibitors (SSRIs) or serotonin-norepinephrine reuptake inhibitors may be at increased risk of bleeding from the gastrointestinal tract because of platelet effects of these drugs. The risk may be further increased among elderly people, individuals with a history of gastrointestinal bleeding from ulcers, and those coadministered aspirin or a nonsteroidal anti-inflammatory drug (NSAID). Screening for blood in stool is performed using either a high-sensitivity fecal occult blood test (FOBT; stool guaiac) or the fecal immunochemical test (FIT). A positive FOBT result indicates bleeding somewhere in the gastrointestinal tract, whereas a positive FIT result indicates bleeding in the lower gastrointestinal tract (American Association for Clinical Chemistry 2018a). A positive test result from either method is an indication for follow-up. False-negative results may be returned with either method in the case of intermittent bleeding.

At present, FOBT and FIT are considered to be equivalent in colorectal cancer screening but would not be expected to be equivalent for the detection of upper gastrointestinal bleeding. The FIT test is more acceptable to patients because stool is collected with a brush and sequestered in a liquid buffer–filled vial (Imperiale et al. 2004). In addition, no patient preparation is needed for FIT testing. For FOBT, the patient must be instructed to avoid aspirin, NSAIDs, dental procedures, vitamin C, and foods that can cause spurious results, such as red meat, broccoli, turnips, and horseradish. Even so, in an elderly SSRI-treated patient with anemia and a history of gastric or duodenal ulcer, the high-sensitivity FOBT may be the test of choice.

Urine Tests

Pregnancy (Qualitative Beta–Human Chorionic Gonadotropin)

Pregnancy tests are indicated for women who could become pregnant for whom potentially teratogenic medications are considered and before procedures such as electroconvulsive therapy. As discussed in an earlier section (see "Pregnancy Testing" under "Blood Tests"), β-hCG detected qualitatively in urine is the test of choice for routine pregnancy testing. The test yields a positive result shortly after the first missed menstrual period. Currently marketed home pregnancy tests are accurate when used according to package instructions. For nonroutine pregnancy testing or testing for any condition other than pregnancy, the blood test should be used.

For urine testing, the first morning urine specimen is used because it has the highest concentration of β-hCG. If a random specimen is used, it must not be dilute; specific gravity should be greater than 1.005 (Fischbach and Dunning 2015). Specimens containing clearly visible blood (i.e., with gross hematuria) should be discarded. The urine test returns a result of positive (pregnant) or negative (not pregnant). Certain factors can interfere with urine testing: false-positive results can be seen in the presence of proteinuria, hematuria, excess pituitary gonadotropin, and certain drugs (including phenothiazines and methadone) (Fischbach and Dunning 2015). False-negative results can be seen if the specimen is obtained too early in pregnancy or the urine is too dilute.

Urine Dipstick Testing

Using a commercially available test kit, it is possible to screen for infection and other abnormalities in the urine without involving the laboratory. Specific instructions included in each test kit must be followed. Dipstick results should be interpreted in the context of clinical signs and symptoms, because both false-negative and false-positive results can occur.

Urinalysis

Routine urinalysis (with urine sent to the laboratory) provides a quick and inexpensive screen for urinary tract infection, kidney and liver disease, and hyperglycemia. It is a standard component of a basic laboratory workup and a critical element of testing for elderly patients with mental status changes. If either leukocyte esterase or nitrite is positive on initial testing, the specimen is examined under the microscope for WBCs and bacteria. If both are positive, a urinary tract infection is likely, and a culture should be performed (Simerville et al. 2005). The persistence of anything more than trace proteinuria is a critical and early indicator of renal dysfunction (Fischbach and Dunning 2015). Significant or persistent hematuria (with intact RBCs) should raise the question of glomerular disease (Fischbach and Dunning 2015). The presence of myoglobin (occult blood with no intact RBCs) is seen in patients undergoing electroconvulsive therapy and in neuroleptic malignant syndrome.

The patient's first morning urine specimen should be used, with 10 mL constituting a sufficient sample. Failure to use the first morning specimen can result in a false-negative nitrite test. The patient should be instructed to void directly into a clean, dry container. It is no longer recommended that the patient use antibacterial wipes to clean the perineum before urinating. It is important that the urine specimen be examined within 1 hour of collection or refrigerated immediately and examined within 24 hours. Although catheterization for urinalysis is not routine, urine specimens obtained by any other means can be contaminated by feces, vaginal discharge, or menstrual blood.

Urine Drug Screen

Toxicology screening for drugs of abuse is often performed in the emergency department and is also used to monitor known substance abusers in treatment programs. For this purpose, a random urine sample is tested for a selected panel of drugs. Which drugs are included depends in part on abuse patterns in the community, although these patterns change over time, and some abused drugs are not routinely assayed. It may be necessary for the clinician to request specific drugs for inclusion. For certain drugs, such as γ-hydroxybutyrate (GHB), detection is difficult because of rapid clearance. Currently, most test panels include opioids, cocaine, amphetamines, barbiturates, benzodiazepines, phencyclidine, and cannabinoids (marijuana). Results that are returned as positive—above a predetermined cutoff level—can be followed up with more sensitive and specific testing that identifies the exact drug. As an alternative to the panel, tests can be ordered individually.

Different windows of detection apply to different drug classes (Moeller et al. 2008; Reisfield and Bertholf 2008). For amphetamines, cocaine, and opioids, urine screening detects drug use in the past 2–3 days. For chronic cannabinoid use (marijuana and its metabolites), urine screening detects drug use in the past several weeks. For barbiturates, urine detection depends on the specific drug; short-acting barbiturates are detected in urine up to 24 hours after use, and long-acting drugs are detected up to 3 weeks. For specific legal or employment purposes, samples other than urine may be used. Saliva samples can detect drugs used within the previous 24 hours. Hair samples can detect drug use within the past 2–3 months. Sweat samples can be collected over a period of days to weeks on an absorbent patch and can indicate drug use during that period. For alcohol screening, blood is most often used, as discussed in the earlier section "Blood Alcohol Level."

False-positive results can occur with urine drug screening by antibody-based immunoassay because of cross-reactivity (Keary et al. 2012). For example, drugs such as rifampin and fluoroquinolones and unwashed poppy seeds can cause false-positive results on opioid screening, and excessive use of a Vicks inhaler can cause false-positive results on amphetamine screening. Positive specimens can be further tested in the laboratory using gas chromatography–mass spectroscopy for specific drug identification so that false-positive results are not reported out. False-negative results can result from dilution of urine, although laboratories performing urine drug screening use urine specific gravity and creatinine to check for this possibility. In these cases, the report to the clinician may indicate that the sample was negative but diluted.

Neuroimaging Studies in Psychiatry

Current neuroimaging methods provide both structural and functional data about the brain. Structural imaging techniques such as CT and MRI provide a fixed image of the brain's anatomy. Functional neuroimaging techniques such as positron emission tomography (PET, PET-CT, and PET-MRI), single-photon emission computed tomography (SPECT), magnetic resonance spectroscopy (MRS), and arterial spin labeling provide information about brain metabolism, blood flow, presynaptic uptake of transmitter precursors, neurotransmitter transporter activity, and postsynaptic receptor activity. Functional scans should always be interpreted in the context of the underlying structural images. Through use of these techniques, one can identify abnormal functioning in a brain that appears to be structurally normal. Alternatively, abnormalities in brain structure can lead to altered functioning (e.g., a brain tumor).

Structural Neuroimaging Modalities

Computed Tomography

CT scanning involves a focused beam of X rays that passes through the brain at different angles, and the collected data are combined to provide a cross-sectional view of the brain. The X rays are attenuated as they pass through tissue, which absorbs their energy. The degree of energy absorption varies on the basis of the radiodensity of the tissue. This differential X ray attenuation is transformed into a two-dimensional grayscale map of the brain, with bone appearing most radiopaque (white) and air the least radiopaque (black). Brain tissue, CSF, and water have varying degrees of radiopacity.

In comparison with MRI, CT is more widely available, is less expensive, and requires shorter scanning time, and it is relatively more comfortable and convenient. Thus, CT is efficient in ruling out conditions that are life-threatening or that may require surgical intervention, such as a hemorrhage or brain tumor. CT also has limitations; it involves some radiation exposure, provides poor visualization of the posterior fossa (e.g., brain stem and cerebellum), and has limited capability to discriminate between gray and white matter due to their similar radiodensities.

Magnetic Resonance Imaging

MRI takes advantage of the fact that hydrogen nuclei in the body have paramagnetic properties, such that their spins align in a magnetic field. Magnetic pulses align the protons, and when the pulses are terminated, the protons relax toward their native positions and release energy at a detectable radio frequency. The energy released is nonionizing and considered to be safe. The collective magnetic behavior of the realigning hydrogen atoms within the magnetic field defines T1, or longitudinal relaxation, and T2, or transverse relaxation.

MRI can distinguish between hydrogen nuclei in free water and those in blood, fat, or muscle on the basis of differential relaxation rates in different tissues. The spatial resolution of the images produced is determined by the strength of the magnet. Most clinical MRI scanners use a magnet strength of 1.5 or 3.0 tesla.

As opposed to CT, where descriptors predominantly use the terms *density* (hypodense, isodense, hyperdense) and *attenuation* (hypoattenuation, hyperattenuation), MRI descriptors focus on *intensities* (hyperintense, isointense, hypointense).

MRI T2-weighted images are useful for visualizing lesions because they show edema as an increase in signal intensity. Hemorrhage and other blood-related lesions are also visible on T2-weighed imaging. T1-weighted images are useful for demonstrating structural anatomy. Gradient echo images can show past hemorrhages. Fluid-attenuated inversion recovery images are useful in identifying scarring (gliosis) of past infarcts, as well as the extent of past small-vessel ischemic change. Table 5–12 notes the characteristic appearance of tissue signals on T1-weighted, T2-weighted, and proton density–weighted MRI. Figure 5–4 shows the classic appearance of the brain on CT and different conventional MRI sequences that are commonly used.

Comparison of Computed Tomography and Magnetic Resonance Imaging

MRI has several advantages over CT. First, it allows superior visualization of brain tissue, providing enhanced gray and white matter discrimination and allowing quantitative or volumetric measurements. Deep brain structures such as the cerebellum and brain stem are better visualized with MRI. Furthermore, axial, coronal, and sagittal images may be acquired, allowing multiplanar visualization. Table 5–13 provides a summary comparison of CT and MRI scanning modalities. Figure 5–5 provides a comparison of images available with CT and MRI.

TABLE 5–12.   **Comparison of tissue signal on T1-weighted, T2-weighted, and PD-weighted MRI**

	T1	T2	PD
Gray matter	Intermediate (gray)	Intermediate to high (light gray)	Intermediate to high (light gray)
White matter	High (white)	Intermediate to low (dark gray)	Intermediate (gray)
Cerebrospinal fluid or water	Low (black)	High (white)	Intermediate to low (dark gray)
Fat	High (white)	Low (black)	Low (black)
Air	Low (black)	Low (black)	Low (black)
Edema	Intermediate (gray)	High (white)	High (white)
Demyelination or gliosis	Intermediate (gray)	High (white)	High (white)
Ferritin deposits (e.g., in basal ganglia)	Intermediate to low (dark gray)	Low (black)	Low (black)
Calcium bound to protein	High (white)	Intermediate to low (dark gray)	Intermediate to low (dark gray)
Proteinaceous fluid	High (white)	Variable	Variable

Note.   On fast spin echo sequences (a faster variant of the spin echo sequence), fat appears bright in T2- and PD-weighted images.
MRI=magnetic resonance imaging; PD=proton density.
Source.   Adapted from Wilde EA, Hunter JV, Bigler ED: "A Primer of Neuroimaging Analysis in Neurorehabilitation Outcome Research." *NeuroRehabilitation* 31:227–242, 2012.

Clinical Use of Computed Tomography and Magnetic Resonance Imaging in Psychiatry

Structural imaging (CT or MRI) is useful in identifying medical causes of psychiatric symptoms, such as stroke, brain tumor, traumatic injury, infection, or developmental abnormalities. Any patient presenting with focal neurological signs should undergo structural imaging. In addition, structural imaging is indicated in the initial workup for neurocognitive disorders, with MRI being the modality preferred for this indication. Although, in general, the threshold for obtaining structural imaging is lower in the geriatric population than in the general adult population, routine screening in the absence of focal neurological signs or deficits is discouraged on the basis of low yield.

Other Structural Imaging Techniques

Magnetic resonance spectroscopy.   MRS is based on the same principles as MRI, but rather than relying on the resonance of hydrogen protons, MRS detects other signals of interest, including protium (^{1}H), phosphorus 31 (^{31}P), lithium 7 (^{7}Li), fluorine 19 (^{19}F), sodium 23 (^{23}Na), and carbon 13 (^{13}C). MRS provides information about neuronal injury by measuring several markers of cellular integrity and function, including *N*-acetyl aspartate, creatine, choline, and myoinositol, as well as other markers of potential clinical relevance that can be detected at high and ultrahigh magnetic fields, such as brain glutathione, glycine, glutamine, glutamate, and γ-aminobutyric acid

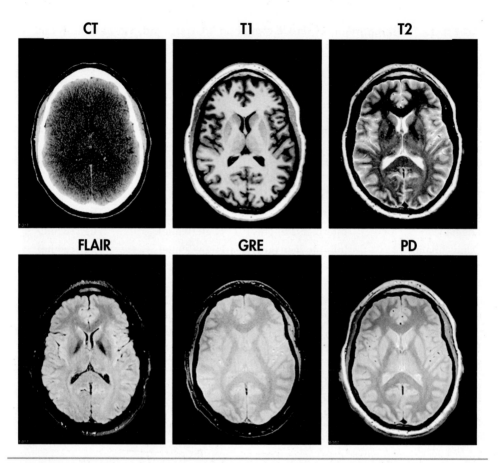

FIGURE 5–4.   Comparison of computed tomography (CT) and various magnetic resonance imaging (MRI) modalities.

The images are derived at the same level within the same individual and demonstrate the characteristic appearance of white matter, gray matter, and cerebrospinal fluid on CT and various conventional sequences in common use in clinical practice. FLAIR=fluid attenuated inversion recovery; GRE=gradient recalled echo; PD=proton density.

Source.   Images courtesy of Elisabeth A. Wilde, Ph.D., Department of Neurology, University of Utah, Salt Lake City, Utah; and Erin D. Bigler, Ph.D., Departments of Psychology and Neuroscience, Brigham Young University, Provo, Utah, and Department of Neurology, University of Utah, Salt Lake City, Utah.

(GABA; Godlewska et al. 2017). Each of these compounds produces a characteristic spectral peak, allowing quantification of the distribution of the compound within regions of the brain. MRS has been applied extensively to research psychiatric disorders, including major depressive disorder, bipolar disorder, psychosis, and schizophrenia. MRS has also been used to assess pharmacokinetics and pharmacodynamics of various psychotropic medications. Its clinical use is currently limited in primary psychiatric disorders.

Diffusion tensor imaging.   Diffusion tensor imaging (DTI) measures the diffusion of water in brain tissues, allowing quantification of orientation and structure via metrics such as fractional anisotropy and mean diffusivity, as well as qualitative aspects of white matter tracts via tractography. In DTI, diffusion-weighted pulse sequences that are sensitive to the random motion of water are used to quantify how water dif-

TABLE 5–13. **Comparison of CT and MRI**

	CT	MRI
Mechanism	X-ray attenuation	Proton magnetic resonance
Imaging planes	Axial (transverse) only	Axial, coronal, sagittal
Image acquisition time	Short (1–10 minutes)	Longer (30–45 minutes)
Slice thickness	2–5 mm	1–3 mm
Spatial resolution	1–2 mm	<1 mm
Cost	$300–$500+	$800–$1,000+
Advantages	Widely available Rapid acquisition Useful in evaluating for acute, life-threatening conditions such as hemorrhage or trauma Less expensive Fewer contraindications	No radiation exposure Gray–white contrast excellent Better resolution Excellent visualization of posterior fossa
Disadvantages	Radiation exposure Limited visualization of posterior fossa	Unable to use if metal or pacemakers are present Longer acquisition time

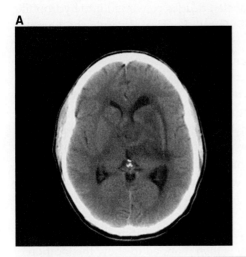
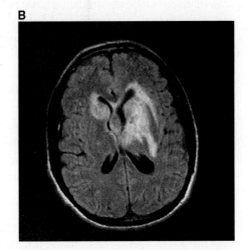

FIGURE 5–5. Side-by-side comparison of structural imaging modalities: computed tomography (CT) and magnetic resonance imaging (MRI).

The sensitivity of head CT versus MRI of the brain in the same patient is demonstrated here in a patient who presented with memory loss. **(A)** The head CT scan shows a large area of decreased density consistent with edema. It is difficult to ascertain whether there is an underlying mass or what its shape might be.

(B) The brain MRI (T2 image) also demonstrates an area of increased intensity of about the same shape as the CT abnormality. The patient was found to be HIV positive, and a subsequent brain biopsy revealed that the mass was a B-cell lymphoma.

Source. Images courtesy of Paul E. Schulz, M.D., Department of Neurology, University of Texas Health Science Center at Houston (UT Health), Houston, Texas.

fuses along axes. A matrix of water diffusion speed, the diffusion tensor, is calculated for every voxel in an image. The speed of water diffusion is generally constant in all directions. However, in white matter, water diffusion is faster parallel to axons rather than perpendicular to axons, ostensibly because myelin sheaths and white matter tracts constrain and direct water diffusion. Alterations in diffusion are used to identify damage to the structural integrity of white matter tracts, as seen in traumatic brain injury, stroke, and multiple sclerosis. This information can also be used to map white matter tracts that have been compromised by pathological processes or developmental anomalies. DTI and other advanced diffusion methods have been used in research studies of neurocognitive disorders, schizophrenia, mood and anxiety disorders, neurodevelopmental disorders, substance-related disorders, and brain injury. The clinical utility of DTI is currently limited, partially owing to the lack of normative data for comparison. Figure 5–6 illustrates white matter tracts that can be visualized with DTI.

Functional Neuroimaging Modalities

Single-Photon Emission Computed Tomography

SPECT provides images of cerebral blood flow and brain activity. The technique involves the injection of a radioactive tracer attached to a drug such as technetium-99m-hexamethylpropyleneamine oxime (HMPAO) or technetium-99m-ethyl cysteinate dimer (ECD), lipophilic drugs that are able to diffuse across the blood–brain barrier and into neurons. Once inside the cell, the radiolabeled drug is converted into hydrophilic compounds that are unable to diffuse out of the cell. Physical decay of the tracer attached to HMPAO or ECD leads to high-energy photon emissions that are measured by SPECT detectors. A computer creates visual images from the captured data, using various algorithms and filtering techniques to correct for background noise and motion.

Tracer uptake and cerebral blood flow are high in gray matter, where neuronal bodies and synapses reside, and low in white matter, which is composed of metabolically less active axons. Thus, the cortex and subcortical structures appear bright, or "hot," on SPECT, whereas white matter appears "cold," or dark. SPECT may be useful in the differential diagnosis of neurocognitive disorders, including those involving abnormalities of the dopamine transporter (e.g., dementia with Lewy bodies).

Positron Emission Tomography

In PET scanning, a radionuclide is coupled with a biologically active molecule or drug, and the concentration of radionuclide activity is then mapped to show the location of the coupled molecule or drug. If the coupled molecule is fluorodeoxyglucose (FDG), the scan gives information about tissue metabolic activity. In fact, a number of different isotopes are available for use with PET, including oxygen 15 (^{15}O), nitrogen 13 (^{13}N), and carbon 11 ^{11}C, but fluorine 18 (^{18}F) coupled with glucose (FDG) is most commonly employed in clinical PET scanning. ^{18}F has a long enough half-life that it is possible to produce the isotope at an off-site facility. In addition, it is less critical that the patient's mental state or activity be standardized with this isotope than with isotopes with very short half-lives, such as ^{15}O. When other molecules—such as florbetapir (^{18}F-AV-45), which binds to β-amyloid protein—are appended in place of a glucose analogue, brain amyloid deposits in patients with suspected Alzheimer's disease can be visualized in vivo. This compound has a long enough half-life that it can be express-shipped between

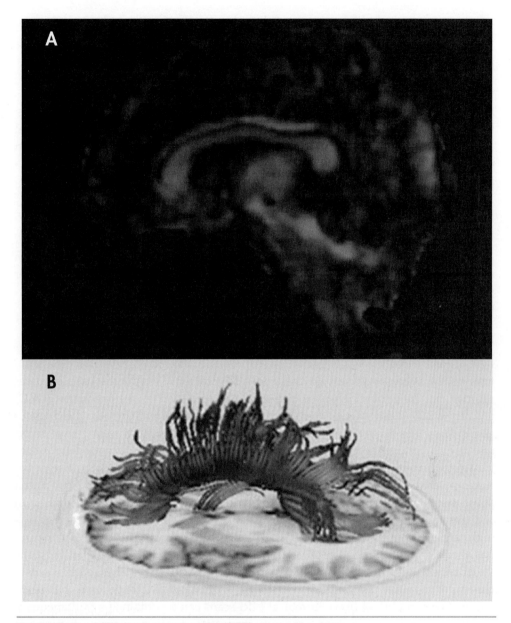

FIGURE 5–6. Diffusion tensor imaging (DTI).

To view this figure in color, see Plate 2 in Color Gallery in middle of book.

(A) Fractional anisotropy color map derived from DTI in the sagittal plane. *Red* indicates white matter fibers coursing in a right–left direction, *blue* indicates fibers running in a superior–inferior direction, and *green* reflects fibers oriented in an anterior–posterior direction. **(B)** Fiber tracking using DTI of the total corpus callosum overlaid on a T1-weighted inversion recovery image from the same brain.

Source. Images courtesy of Elisabeth A. Wilde, Ph.D., Department of Neurology, University of Utah, Salt Lake City, Utah.

states for use. As a rule, PET scanning in clinical and research settings also includes anatomic imaging with CT or MRI to coregister metabolic findings with anatomy.

Comparison of Single-Photon Emission Computed Tomography and Positron Emission Tomography

SPECT is more widely available compared with other functional imaging modalities, less expensive, and technically easier than PET imaging. PET offers superior spatial and temporal resolution. Both imaging modalities provide only limited visualization of anatomic structures. Table 5–14 presents a comparison of SPECT, PET, and functional MRI (fMRI) modalities.

Clinical Use of Positron Emission Tomography and Single-Photon Emission Computed Tomography in Psychiatry

Functional imaging using PET or SPECT combined with structural imaging is useful in the evaluation of neurocognitive disorders and traumatic brain injuries, among other neuropsychiatric conditions. Figure 5–7 shows a comparison of structural and functional neuroimaging modalities, and Figure 5–8 compares SPECT and PET images.

Functional Magnetic Resonance Imaging

fMRI measures the level of oxygenation in brain tissue to map the neuroanatomic activation that occurs with various challenges. Several fMRI techniques have been developed, but the most widely used is the blood oxygenation level–dependent (BOLD) technique. BOLD fMRI is based on the magnetic susceptibility of blood, whose hemoglobin fluctuates between a paramagnetic, deoxygenated state in resting-state blood and an isomagnetic, oxygenated state. Deoxyhemoglobin acts as an endogenous contrast agent. Increased neuronal activity in response to a sensorimotor, cognitive, or behavioral challenge results in an increase in regional cerebral blood flow and a subsequent decrease in regional deoxyhemoglobin concentration. Oxygen saturation changes in blood due to cognitive challenge or sensory stimuli result in a corresponding change in T2-weighted magnetic resonance signal intensity, thus allowing neuronal activation to be mapped neuroanatomically through the BOLD signal. fMRI scans are obtained when the subject is at rest and when the subject is engaged in a sensorimotor or cognitive task, and the two images are compared to determine changes in regional cerebral blood flow. Structural MRI scans can be obtained simultaneously, and these images can be coregistered with the fMRI scans to more precisely pinpoint neuroanatomic locations of regional activation.

fMRI has many advantages compared with other functional imaging techniques in that it provides superior spatial and temporal resolution in relation to PET and SPECT, is minimally invasive, and does not involve exposure to harmful ionizing radiation. It is being used extensively in research to study the neurocircuitry involved in psychotic disorders, mood and anxiety disorders, substance-related disorders, and neurocognitive and neurodevelopmental disorders. Furthermore, the effects of psychotropic medications are being studied via fMRI, with the hope of understanding the regional brain effects of acute and chronic treatment with these medications. Despite the insights into structure–function relations that fMRI has revealed, fMRI is not yet used as a diagnostic or treatment modality.

TABLE 5–14. Comparison of SPECT, PET, and fMRI

	SPECT	PET	fMRI
Measures	Cerebral perfusion	Cerebral glucose metabolism	Oxygen saturation of blood
Typical radiotracer half-life	^{99m}Tc T$_{\frac{1}{2}}$=6 h	^{18}F T$_{\frac{1}{2}}$=110 min ^{15}O T$_{\frac{1}{2}}$=2 min ^{13}N T$_{\frac{1}{2}}$=10 min ^{11}C T$_{\frac{1}{2}}$=20 min	N/A
Temporal resolution	Fair	Good	Great
Spatial resolution	6–9 mm	4–5 mm	3 mm
Scan time	30 min	10–30 min	30–60 min
Cost	$1,500	$2,000–$4,000	$800–$1,000
Advantages	Less expensive Technically easier method Relative stability of radiotracer	More precise and direct quantification of brain function Shorter radiation exposure time Markers for some receptors or enzymes of interest may be available Markers for some receptors or enzymes of interest may be available	No ionizing radiation exposure Ability to scan subject multiple times Superior temporal and spatial resolution
Disadvantages	Limited structural anatomic visualization Radiation exposure	Limited structural anatomic visualization Prohibitive cost Short half-life of many radiotracers Radiation exposure Problematic for diabetes patients because of glucose load from tracer (FDG-PET)	Limited clinical utility

Note. FDG = fluorodeoxyglucose; fMRI=functional magnetic resonance imaging; N/A=not applicable; PET=positron emission tomography; SPECT=single-photon emission computed tomography.

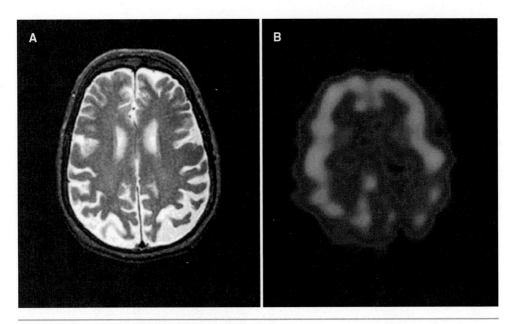

FIGURE 5–7. Side-by-side comparison of structural and functional neuroimaging: magnetic resonance imaging (MRI) and positron emission tomography (PET).

To view this figure in color, see Plate 3 in Color Gallery in middle of book.

(A) Axial view of brain MRI (fluid attenuated inversion recovery [FLAIR] sequence) and (B) corresponding PET scan of a patient with Alzheimer's disease. The MRI scan (A) shows prominent atrophic change in the posterior regions of the brain, consistent with the striking reduction of metabolic activity in the posterior parietal lobes on PET imaging (B).

Source. Image courtesy of Ziad Nahas, M.D., M.S.C.R., Department of Psychiatry, Medical College of South Carolina, Charleston, South Carolina.

More recently, the use of fMRI to study the brain at rest (often termed resting-state fMRI) has enabled researchers to investigate the functional architecture of the brain. Measures of resting-state functional connectivity have been shown to be reproducible and consistent across laboratories and to be sensitive to brain changes that occur in a number of conditions, including schizophrenia, bipolar disorder, major depressive disorder, anxiety disorders, posttraumatic stress disorder, drug addiction, and other psychiatric and neurological disorders.

Magnetoencephalography

Magnetoencephalography measures extracranial magnetic signals generated by the positive ionic flow of cortical pyramidal cells in the brain. It is noninvasive, does not entail exposure to ionizing radiation, and has excellent spatial and temporal resolution. It is currently being used to localize epileptiform activity by coregistration with structural MRI data and has been used to presurgically map auditory and somatosensory cortical areas to be avoided during neurosurgical procedures. Magnetoencephalography is also being used in research contexts to study possible cortical reorganization, cerebral lateralization, and auditory sensory memory abnormalities in patients with psychotic and other psychiatric and neurological disorders.

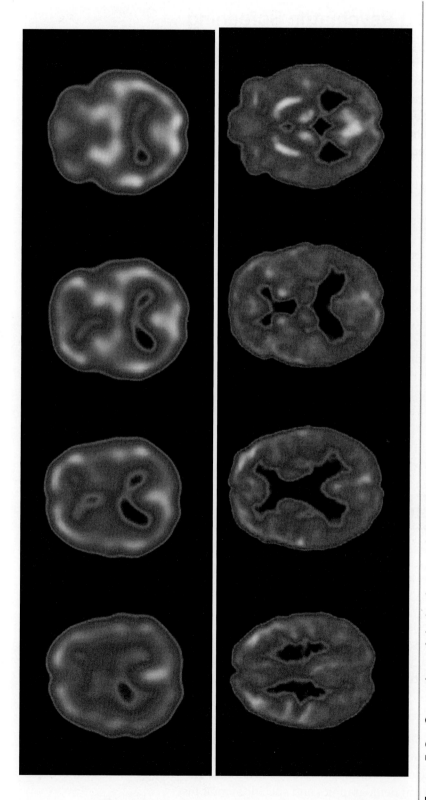

Figure 5–8. Comparison of single-photon emission computed tomography (SPECT) and positron emission tomography (PET).

To view this figure in color, see Plate 4 in Color Gallery in middle of book.

SPECT (*top row*) and PET (*bottom row*) images from two patients with clinically similar degrees of mild cognitive impairment. The PET scan shows parietal abnormalities, suggesting that this patient may be at risk of developing Alzheimer's disease. The PET scan also shows superior resolution compared with the SPECT scan.

Source. Images courtesy of Paul E. Schulz, M.D., Department of Neurology, University of Texas Health Science Center at Houston (UTHealth), Houston, Texas.

Suggested Psychiatric Screening Laboratory Evaluation

What tests should be included in standard laboratory screening for psychiatric patients in general is not well established. For certain populations—the elderly, the homeless, patients in alcohol and drug treatment programs, HIV-positive individuals, and patients hospitalized on medical and surgical units—medical issues often are found to underlie psychiatric symptoms. For other populations, including healthy adults in outpatient mental health care, medical issues are less likely to be a factor. Not surprisingly, then, clinical practice varies in terms of what laboratory tests are ordered and how often labs are checked. Whether a test is appropriate for a particular patient depends on the setting in which the patient is seen and the purpose of the testing. There does appear to be agreement that a laboratory evaluation is indicated for the following categories of patients: patients presenting for the first time with a major psychiatric syndrome (e.g., psychosis, a major mood disorder), patients with delirium or an initial presentation of a neurocognitive disorder, and patients with alcohol or drug use disorders.

On admission to an inpatient psychiatry service, patients may receive the basic screening laboratory evaluation shown in Table 5–15. For patients who are at risk of metabolic syndrome or are being started on a drug with potential to cause significant weight gain, a lipid panel and hemoglobin A1C may be added. For patients at risk of a cardiac complication such as QT prolongation, ECG is recommended. For women older than 50 years and for patients presenting with mood disorders or anxiety, TSH may appropriately be checked. Screening for sexually transmitted infections may be performed for patients with known risk behaviors. If there is a question of pregnancy, urine or serum pregnancy testing may be performed.

Diagnostic Testing in Specific Clinical Situations

Table 5–16 lists additional laboratory tests useful in the diagnosis of selected conditions, as discussed briefly in the following sections.

Delirium

Laboratory tests listed in Tables 5–15 and 5–16 are performed to determine the medical causes of delirium. If the diagnosis of the delirium syndrome itself is questioned, an EEG could help distinguish delirium from psychosis, catatonia, or dementia with behavioral disturbance, as discussed earlier (see section "Electroencephalography").

New-Onset Major Depressive Disorder

For a patient presenting with a first episode of major depressive disorder, especially if symptoms are atypical, laboratory tests listed in Tables 5–15 and 5–16 may be performed to exclude medical causes or contributors. The choice of tests will be determined by patient demographics and specific symptoms.

TABLE 5–15.   **Screening laboratory evaluation in psychiatry**

For psychiatric admission or general screening purposes
Complete blood count with platelets
Comprehensive metabolic panel
Urinalysis
Urine drug screen with alcohol
HIV testing (from which patients may opt out)

For patients at risk of metabolic syndrome or to be started on a drug associated with significant weight gain (e.g., an atypical antipsychotic)
Lipid panel
Hemoglobin A1C

For patients at risk of QT prolongation or other cardiac complications (see text)
Electrocardiogram

For women older than 50 years
Third-generation thyroid-stimulating hormone

Consider (depending on patient characteristics)
Pregnancy testing
Sexually transmitted infection screening

New-Onset Mania

For a patient presenting with a first episode of mania, particularly if the patient is older than 50 years or has physical signs potentially suggestive of secondary mania (e.g., exophthalmos or left hemiparesis), laboratory tests listed in Tables 5–15 and 5–16 may be performed to exclude medical causes or contributors.

New-Onset Psychosis

For a patient presenting with a first episode of psychosis, especially if symptoms are atypical or the patient is outside the normal age range of presentation for primary disease, laboratory tests listed in Tables 5–15 and 5–16 may be performed to exclude medical causes or contributors. The choice of tests will be determined by patient demographics and specific symptoms.

Major and Mild Neurocognitive Disorders

Standard practice in the evaluation of major neurocognitive disorder is to test for vitamin B_{12} deficiency and hypothyroidism and to obtain structural neuroimaging (noncontrast head CT scan or MRI). The same recommendations apply to the evaluation of mild neurocognitive disorder, because this condition represents a risk factor for progression to major neurocognitive disorder. Additional tests that may be useful in identifying the cause of major neurocognitive disorder include syphilis screening for patients with a history of risk behaviors; erythrocyte sedimentation rate or C-reactive protein to exclude vasculitis; methylmalonic acid for earlier detection of vitamin B_{12} deficiency; serum folate for folate deficiency; EEG to exclude conditions such as non-

TABLE 5–16.   Additional laboratory testing for selected conditions

Delirium

In elderly patients and in nonelderly patients with cardiopulmonary symptoms:

ECG	Chest X ray

If the cause(s) of delirium is/are still not identified, consider the following:

ESR or CRP	BAL
Serum ammonia level	Medication levels
Antinuclear antibody	Head CT or brain MRI
Vitamin B$_{12}$, folate levels	EEG if not done previously
RPR	

In the appropriate clinical setting, consider the following:

CSF analysis	Arterial blood gases
Urine porphyrins	Blood cultures

New-onset major depressive disorder

Folate level	Medication levels (e.g., TCAs or mood stabilizers)
Third-generation TSH	Urine pregnancy screening, if indicated
Antithyroid antibodies	EEG (to exclude epileptiform activity)
RPR	Brain MRI or head CT
BAL	

New-onset mania

Third-generation TSH	Urine pregnancy screening
RPR	EEG (to exclude epileptiform activity)
Urine toxicology	Brain MRI or head CT
BAL	

New-onset psychosis

Antinuclear antibody	Anti-NMDA receptor antibodies (CSF)
Antithyroid antibodies	Ceruloplasmin, free serum copper levels
Cortisol (blood and 24-hour urine)	Head CT with contrast or MRI with gadolinium
CSF analysis	MRI with gadolinium (if CT was done first)
ECG	Serum testosterone level
EEG	Spot urine for porphyrin precursors
ESR or CRP	Syphilis testing (RPR, VDRL, FTA-Abs)
CSF analysis	Third-generation TSH
Heavy-metal screening	Urine pregnancy screening
Levels of prescribed drugs	Vitamin B$_{12}$ level (and MMA if equivocal)
Rheumatoid factor	

Major neurocognitive disorder

Vitamin B$_{12}$ level	Third-generation TSH

Additional tests to consider:

Apolipoprotein E ε genotyping	CSF studies (routine; 14-3-3 protein)
ESR or CRP	Fasting lipids, triglycerides, and blood sugar
MMA or serum total homocysteine	Syphilis serology in patients at risk
EEG	

TABLE 5–16.   **Additional laboratory testing for selected conditions *(continued)***

Major neurocognitive disorder *(continued)*

In research settings:

Volumetric MRI	CSF assay of Aβ42 protein and tau proteins
FDG-PET imaging	Tau PET imaging
Amyloid PET imaging	DaT SPECT imaging (DaTscan)

Anxiety

The basic laboratory workup for anxiety includes only the following:

Third-generation TSH	Metabolic panel (BMP or CMP) to check calcium and glucose

Depending on the patient's history and examination, other elements of the workup might include one or more of the following:

Antithyroid antibodies	ECG, Holter monitor, cardiac stress testing, and/or echocardiogram
Plasma free metanephrines	
Urine porphyrin precursors	Chest X ray, pulmonary function tests, and/or arterial blood gas
Pulmonary CT scan	
EEG	Chest X ray, pulmonary function tests, and/or arterial blood gas

Note. Aβ42=β-amyloid (42); BAL=blood alcohol level; BMP=basic metabolic panel; CDT=carbohydrate-deficient transferrin; CMP=comprehensive metabolic panel; CRP=C-reactive protein; CSF=cerebrospinal fluid; CT=computed tomography; DaT=dopamine transporter; ECG=electrocardiogram; EEG=electroencephalogram; ESR=erythrocyte sedimentation rate; FDG=fluorodeoxyglucose; FTA-Abs=fluorescent treponemal antibody absorption; GGT=γ-glutamyltransferase; MMA=methylmalonic acid; MRI=magnetic resonance imaging; NMDA=*N*-methyl-D-aspartate; PET=positron emission tomography; RPR=rapid plasma reagin; SPECT=single-photon emission computed tomography; TCA=tricyclic antidepressant; TSH=thyroid-stimulating hormone; VDRL=Venereal Disease Research Laboratory.

convulsive status epilepticus and subacute sclerosing panencephalitis; and CSF studies to exclude CNS inflammation or infection. Assay of 14-3-3 protein in CSF may be used to confirm a clinical suspicion of Creutzfeldt-Jakob disease in a patient with a rapidly progressive neurocognitive disorder and neurological signs such as myoclonic jerks. ApoE ε genotyping may be used to improve the specificity of the diagnosis of Alzheimer's disease in a patient who meets clinical criteria; the presence of the ε4/ε4 genotype significantly increases the probability that Alzheimer's disease is the correct diagnosis. When a vascular etiology of major neurocognitive disorder is suspected, fasting lipids, triglycerides, and blood sugar may be checked. Testing recommendations for selected conditions are summarized in Table 5–16.

PET and SPECT imaging have been at the forefront of research on the diagnosis and pathogenesis of Alzheimer's disease and other major neurocognitive disorders. The Centers for Medicare and Medicaid Services (2004) has ruled that FDG-PET testing is reasonable and necessary for distinguishing Alzheimer's disease from frontotemporal dementia and for research purposes, provided that certain conditions are met. Other approved indications have been slow to emerge, in part because of the cost of testing. Amyloid PET scans can distinguish amyloid-based major neurocognitive disorders (e.g., Alzheimer's disease and major neurocognitive disorder with Lewy bodies) from non-amyloid-based major neurocognitive disorders. Tau PET imaging (^{18}F-AV-1451) has enabled researchers to perform disease staging—previously done only postmortem—for subjects across the spectrum of cognitively normal to mild neurocognitive disorder to major neurocognitive disorder (Schwarz et al. 2016). Dopamine transporter SPECT imaging (DaTscan; [^{123}I] ioflupane) can distinguish Parkinson's disease and related disorders from conditions with similar symptoms but without cognitive effects, such as essential tremor.

Anxiety Disorder

Anxiety disorder due to another medical disorder may be episodic or chronic and unremitting. Both presentations have numerous potential causes, including use of and withdrawal from prescribed drugs and substances of abuse. A suggested laboratory evaluation for anxiety is shown in Table 5–16.

Substance-Related Disorders

Alcohol Use Disorder

Laboratory findings listed in Table 5–17 can provide evidence for or against a diagnosis of alcohol use disorder suspected on clinical grounds. Recent drinking can be confirmed through use of breath analysis, saliva ethanol, BAL, or urine ethanol. A metabolite of ethanol, ethyl glucuronide, can also be measured in urine; this metabolite remains detectable for up to 5 days, longer than ethanol itself (Mayo Medical Laboratories 2018). In males, measurement of the liver enzyme γ-glutamyltransferase (GGT) and percentage carbohydrate-deficient transferrin (%CDT) together provides the most a reliable indicator of recent drinking; in females, measurement of GGT alone better correlates with recent drinking (Rinck et al. 2007). GGT and %CDT begin to normalize within days of cessation of drinking and return to normal levels within 2 weeks. In a patient with known alcohol use disorder, the BAL can be used to diagnose intoxication or withdrawal, the latter when BAL is zero in the presence of suggestive signs and symptoms.

Patients with alcohol use disorder often are found to have other blood lab abnormalities, including low magnesium, low phosphate, low blood sugar, anemia, low platelets, and abnormal blood clotting times (Magarian et al. 1992). In addition, in the presence of alcohol-related dementia, CT or MRI may show generalized atrophy. In the presence of motor findings suggestive of cerebellar degeneration, CT or MRI may show atrophy of the cerebellar cortex, most often in the anterior and superior segments of the vermis. Alcohol-related myopathy and polyneuropathy can be diagnosed with EMG/NCT.

Drug Use Disorders

Although urine, oral fluid, or blood can be used for drug testing, screening is normally performed on a random urine sample for a panel of drugs selected by that laboratory as relevant in view of community use patterns. The classes of drugs most often included in screening panels have been opioids, cocaine, amphetamines, barbiturates, benzodiazepines, phencyclidine (PCP), and cannabinoids (marijuana). Tests can be ordered individually as an alternative to the panel. Positive screening tests are confirmed by more sensitive and specific assays. False-negative results can be obtained from dilute urine or because of rapid drug elimination (e.g., with γ-hydroxybutyrate). Adulterants in street drugs are not assayed. Complicating the interpretation of opioid screening is the fact that some opioids are metabolized to other opioids, such that their presence may indicate metabolism rather than additional abuse. The American Society

---

TABLE 5–17.   **Positive laboratory findings in alcohol use disorder**

Gamma-glutamyltransferase (GGT)

Elevated: >47 U/L in men or >25 U/L in women, consistent with 4+ drinks daily for 4 weeks or more

Percentage carbohydrate-deficient transferrin (%CDT)

Elevated: >2.6%

Alanine transaminase/aspartate transaminase (AST/ALT) ratio

Elevated: >2:1

Mean corpuscular volume (erythrocytes) (MCV)

Elevated: >101 (age and gender dependent)

Uric acid

Elevated: ≥7 mg/dL (age and gender dependent)

Serum total homocysteine

Elevated: >15 μmol/L

Source.   Magarian et al. 1992; Rinck et al. 2007.

of Addiction Medicine issued useful guidelines in 2017 for the use of drug testing in clinical practice (Jarvis et al. 2017).

Psychotropic Medication Monitoring

Therapeutic drug monitoring, in which trough drug levels are routinely checked, is available for a subset of psychotropics with established therapeutic ranges. These include mainly mood stabilizers and tricyclic antidepressants. For other drugs, random levels can be measured to confirm either suspected toxicity or noncompliance, the latter with zero or low levels. Table 5–18 lists therapeutic and toxic ranges for selected psychotropics.

Other laboratory tests may be indicated for monitoring potential adverse effects of particular psychotropics and for screening to ensure that these medications can safely be initiated. These "safety labs" are beyond the scope of this chapter but are specified for medication classes and individual drugs in texts referenced in the "Recommended Readings" section at the end of the chapter (see Jacobson 2012, 2017).

Conclusion

What tests should be included in standard laboratory screening for psychiatric patients in general is not well established. In certain populations, however, medical issues often are found to underlie psychiatric presentations. A good working knowledge of general medicine equips the clinician to make predictions regarding the likelihood that particular diagnostic tests will be helpful and thus to use laboratory resources judiciously. Such predictions take into account not only the patient's signs and symptoms but also other pertinent variables such as patient demographics and the setting in which the patient is seen. A basic laboratory screening panel is suggested, along with additional tests to be considered for patients with selected psychiatric presentations.

TABLE 5–18.   Therapeutic and toxic drug levels

Drug	Therapeutic level (trough)	Toxic level (random)
Amitriptyline (+nortriptyline)	80–200 ng/mL	>500 ng/mL
Amoxapine (+8-hydroamoxapine)	200–400 ng/mL	Unknown[a]
Aripiprazole	109–585 ng/mL[b]	Unknown[a]
Carbamazepine, total	4–12 μg/mL	≥15 μg/mL
Carbamazepine, free	1–3 μg/mL	≥4 μg/mL
Clozapine	>350 ng/mL	>1,200 ng/mL
Clozapine+norclozapine	>450 ng/mL	—
Desipramine	100–300 ng/mL	>400 ng/mL
Doxepin (+nordoxepin)	50–150 ng/mL	>500 ng/mL
Haloperidol	5–16 ng/mL	Unknown[a]
Reduced haloperidol	10–80 ng/mL	—
Imipramine (+desipramine)	175–300 ng/mL	>400 ng/mL
Lamotrigine	2.5–15 μg/mL	>20 μg/mL
Levetiracetam	12–46 μg/mL	Unknown[a]
Lithium	0.5–1.2 mmol/L	>1.6 mmol/L
Nortriptyline	70–170 ng/mL	>500 ng/mL
Olanzapine	10–80 ng/mL[b]	Unknown[a]
Perphenazine	5–30 ng/mL (0.5–2.5 ng/mL for low-dose therapy)	Unknown[a]
Phenytoin, total	10–20 μg/mL	≥30 μg/mL
Phenytoin, free	1–2 μg/mL	≥2.5 μg/mL
Percentage free phenytoin	8%–14%	—
Quetiapine	100–1,000 ng/mL[b]	Unknown[a]
Risperidone (+9-OH-risperidone)	10–120 ng/mL	Unknown[a]
Thiothixene	10–30 ng/mL	Unknown[a]
Trazodone	800–1,600 ng/mL	Unknown[a]
Valproate, total	50 μg/mL (trough) to 125 μg/mL (peak)	≥151 μg/mL
Valproate, free	5–25 μg/mL	>30 μg/mL
Ziprasidone	Up to 220 ng/mL[b]	—

[a]Level unknown or not well established.
[b]Expected steady-state levels in patients receiving recommended dosages (not therapeutic ranges).
Source.   Data from Mayo Medical Laboratories: Rochester 2018 Test Catalog, Laboratory Reference Edition (sorted by test name; current as of August 30, 2018). Available at: https://www.mayomedicallaboratories.com/test-catalog/. Accessed September 3, 2018.

Key Clinical Points

- With several notable exceptions, laboratory testing generally does not contribute significantly to the cost of psychiatric care, although charges for tests vary considerably from one testing facility to another. Charges are generally highest at hospital and clinic laboratories and lowest at freestanding (walk-in) laboratories.

- When laboratory findings are unclear or introduce questions, laboratory staff can be an excellent resource for clinicians in the interpretation of test data and in planning an approach to a diagnostic evaluation.

- When neuroimaging is requested, it is always a good practice to review films in person with the radiologist, because the more clinical information provided to the radiologist, the more detailed and useful the interpretation of visual findings.

- Clinical tests useful in the current practice of psychiatry include blood, CSF, stool, and urine tests as well as neuroimaging, neurophysiological tests, certain genetic tests, basic cardiopulmonary tests, and skin testing for tuberculosis.

- Neuroimaging does not yet play a diagnostic role in any of the primary psychiatric disorders, but it is still an important part of the clinical workup for psychiatric patients with focal neurological signs and for patients with cognitive decline to rule out underlying medical causes of symptoms.

- Imaging may be helpful when atypical clinical features are present, such as an older age at onset of psychiatric illness.

- Structural imaging techniques such as CT and MRI provide a fixed image of the brain's anatomy. Functional neuroimaging techniques such as PET and SPECT provide information about brain metabolism, blood flow, presynaptic uptake of neurotransmitter precursors, neurotransmitter transporter activity, and postsynaptic receptor activity.

- Clinicians are advised to become familiar with the basic laboratory screening evaluation suggested in the text or to develop a panel appropriate to their own work setting.

- Psychiatric clinicians need to be aware that certain patient populations are at elevated risk of sudden cardiac death and should conduct regular ECG monitoring for evidence of QT prolongation.

- Less urgent but no less important, clinicians need to be aware of the potential toxic effects of psychotropic drugs on the liver and of how these effects can be detected through use of Hy's law.

References

American Association for Clinical Chemistry: Fecal Occult Blood Test and Fecal Immunochemical Test, in Lab Tests Online. 2018a. Available at: https://labtestsonline.org/tests/fecal-occult-blood-test-and-fecal-immunochemical-test. Accessed September 4, 2018.

American Association for Clinical Chemistry: HIV Antibody and HIV Antigen (p24), in Lab Tests Online. 2018b. Available at: https://labtestsonline.org/tests/hiv-antibody-and-hiv-antigen-p24. Accessed September 4, 2018.

American Association for Clinical Chemistry: HIV Viral Load, in Lab Tests Online. 2018c. Available at: https://labtestsonline.org/tests/hiv-viral-load. Accessed September 4, 2018.

American Association for Clinical Chemistry: Lipid Panel, in Lab Tests Online. 2018d. Available at: https://labtestsonline.org/tests/lipid-panel. Accessed September 4, 2018.

American Association for Clinical Chemistry: Syphilis Tests, in Lab Tests Online. 2018e. Available at: https://labtestsonline.org/tests/syphilis-tests. Accessed September 4, 2018.

American Thoracic Society: Targeted tuberculin testing and treatment of latent tuberculosis infection. MMWR Recomm Rep 49(RR-6):1–51, 200, 2000 10881762

Arns M, Heinrich H, Strehl U: Evaluation of neurofeedback in ADHD: the long and winding road. Biol Psychol 95:108–115, 2014 24321363

ARUP Laboratories: Hemoglobin A1c (0070426), in Laboratory Test Directory. May 21, 2018. Available at: http://ltd.aruplab.com/Tests/Pub/0070426. Accessed November 24, 2018.

Bedson E, Bell D, Carr D, et al: Folate Augmentation of Treatment–Evaluation for Depression (FolATED): randomised trial and economic evaluation. Health Technol Assess 18(48):vii–viii, 1–159, 2014 25052890

Bodatsch M, Brockhaus-Dumke A, Klosterkötter J, et al: Forecasting psychosis by event-related potentials—systematic review and specific meta-analysis. Biol Psychiatry 77(11):951–958, 2015 25636178

Centers for Disease Control and Prevention: STD 2015: 2015 Sexually Transmitted Diseases Treatment Guidelines. June 4, 2015. Available at: https://www.cdc.gov/std/tg2015/default.htm. Accessed November 18, 2018.

Centers for Disease Control and Prevention: Tuberculin Skin Testing (Fact Sheet). May 11, 2016. Available at: https://www.cdc.gov/tb/publications/factsheets/testing/skintesting.htm. Accessed November 18, 2018.

Centers for Disease Control and Prevention: HIV Infection: Detection, Counseling, and Referral. January 4, 2017. Available at: https://www.cdc.gov/std/tg2015/hiv.htm. Accessed November 18, 2018.

Centers for Disease Control and Prevention: HIV Screening and Testing: Guidelines and Recommendations. March 16, 2018. Available at: https://www.cdc.gov/hiv/guidelines/testing.html. Accessed November 18, 2018.

Centers for Medicare and Medicaid Services: Decision memo for positron emission tomography (FDG) and other neuroimaging devices for suspected dementia (CAG-00088R). September 15, 2004. Available at: https://www.cms.gov/medicare-coverage-database/details/nca-decision-memo.aspx?NCAId=104. Accessed January 21, 2019.

Chémali KR, Tsao B: Electrodiagnostic testing of nerves and muscles: when, why, and how to order. Cleve Clin J Med 72(1):37–48, 2005 15691056

Col NF, Surks MI, Daniels GH: Subclinical thyroid disease: clinical applications. JAMA 291(2):239–243, 2004 14722151

Daube JR: Clinical Neurophysiology. Philadelphia, PA, FA Davis, 1996

de Benoist B: Conclusions of a WHO Technical Consultation on folate and vitamin B12 deficiencies. Food Nutr Bull 29 (2 suppl):S238–S244, 2008 18709899

De Bruyn E, Gulbis B, Cotton F: Serum and red blood cell folate testing for folate deficiency: new features? Eur J Haematol 92(4):354–359, 2014 24351103

de Leon MJ, DeSanti S, Zinkowski R, et al: MRI and CSF studies in the early diagnosis of Alzheimer's disease. J Intern Med 256(3):205–223, 2004 15324364 de Leon J, Armstrong SC, Cozza KL: Clinical guidelines for psychiatrists for the use of pharmaco-genetic testing for CYP450 2D6 and CYP450 2C19. Psychosomatics 47(1):75–85, 2006 16384813

Dean RA, Shaw LM: Use of cerebrospinal fluid biomarkers for diagnosis of incipient Alzheimer disease in patients with mild cognitive impairment. Clin Chem 56(1):7–9, 2010 19926774

Elias-Sonnenschein LS, Viechtbauer W, Ramakers IH, et al: Predictive value of APOE-ε4 allele for progression from MCI to AD-type dementia: a meta-analysis. J Neurol Neurosurg Psychiatry 82(10):1149–1156, 2011 21493755

Ellenby MS, Tegtmeyer K, Lai S, Braner DA: Videos in clinical medicine. Lumbar puncture. N Engl J Med 355(13):e12, 2006 17005943

Evaluation of Genomic Applications in Practice and Prevention Working Group: Recommendations from the EGAPP Working Group: testing for cytochrome P450 polymorphisms in adults with nonpsychotic depression treated with selective serotonin reuptake inhibitors. Genet Med 9(12):819–825, 2007 18091431

Expert Panel on Thoracic Imaging, McComb BL, Chung JH, et al: ACR appropriateness criteria routine chest radiography. J Thorac Imaging 31(2):W13-5, 2016 26891074

Farrell CJ, Kirsch SH, Herrmann M: Red cell or serum folate: what to do in clinical practice? Clin Chem Lab Med 51(3):555–569, 2013 23449524

Farrer LA, Cupples LA, Haines JL, et al: Effects of age, sex, and ethnicity on the association between apolipoprotein E genotype and Alzheimer disease. A meta-analysis. JAMA 278(16):1349–1356, 1997 9343467

Fava M, Mischoulon D: Folate in depression: efficacy, safety, differences in formulations, and clinical issues. J Clin Psychiatry 70 (suppl 5):12–17, 2009 19909688

Fischbach F, Dunning MB: A Manual of Laboratory and Diagnostic Tests, 9th Edition. Philadelphia, PA, Wolters Kluwer Health/Lippincott Williams & Wilkins, 2015

Flemons WW: Clinical practice. Obstructive sleep apnea. N Engl J Med 347(7):498–504, 2002 12181405

Fois C, Wright MA, Sechi G, et al: The utility of polysomnography for the diagnosis of NREM parasomnias: an observational study over 4 years of clinical practice. J Neurol 262(2):385–393, 2015 25408370

Franken WP, Timmermans JF, Prins C, et al: Comparison of Mantoux and QuantiFERON TB Gold tests for diagnosis of latent tuberculosis infection in Army personnel. Clin Vaccine Immunol 14(4):477–480, 2007 17301213

Frodl T, Hampel H, Juckel G, et al: Value of event-related P300 subcomponents in the clinical diagnosis of mild cognitive impairment and Alzheimer's disease. Psychophysiology 39(2):175–181, 2002 12212666

Godlewska BR, Clare S, Cowen PJ, et al: Ultra-high-field magnetic resonance spectroscopy in psychiatry. Front Psychiatry 8:123, 2017 28744229

Hou PY, Hung GC, Jhong JR, et al: Risk factors for sudden cardiac death among patients with schizophrenia. Schizophr Res 168(1–2):395–401, 2015 26210551

Imperiale TF, Ransohoff DF, Itzkowitz SH, et al: Fecal DNA versus fecal occult blood for colorectal-cancer screening in an average-risk population. N Engl J Med 351(26):2704–2714, 2004 15616205

Irani DN: Cerebrospinal Fluid in Clinical Practice. Philadelphia, PA, Saunders Elsevier, 2009

Jacobson SA: Laboratory Medicine in Psychiatry and Behavioral Science. Washington, DC, American Psychiatric Publishing, 2012

Jacobson SA: Clinical Laboratory Medicine for Mental Health Professionals. Arlington, VA, American Psychiatric Association Publishing, 2017

Jacobson SA, Jerrier H: EEG in delirium. Semin Clin Neuropsychiatry 5(2):86–92, 2000 10837097

Jacobson SA, Leuchter AF, Walter DO, et al: Serial quantitative EEG among elderly subjects with delirium. Biol Psychiatry 34(3):135–140, 1993 8399804

Jarvis M, Williams J, Hurford M, et al: Appropriate use of drug testing in clinical addiction medicine. J Addict Med 11(3):163–173, 2017 28557958

Keary CJ, Wang Y, Moran JR, et al: Toxicologic testing for opiates: understanding false-positive and false-negative test results. Prim Care Companion CNS Disord 14(4), 2012 23251863

Kluesner JK, Beckman DJ, Tate JM, et al: Analysis of current thyroid function test ordering practices. J Eval Clin Pract 24(2):347–352, 2018 29105255

Lafferty JE, North CS, Spitznagel E, et al: Laboratory screening prior to ECT. J ECT 17(3):158–165, 2001 11528304

Langan RC, Goodbred AJ: Vitamin B12 deficiency: recognition and management. Am Fam Physician 96(6):384–389, 2017 28925645

Lenartowicz A, Loo SK: Use of EEG to diagnose ADHD. Curr Psychiatry Rep 16(11):498, 2014 25234074

Lerner V, Kanevsky M, Dwolatzky T, et al: Vitamin B12 and folate serum levels in newly admitted psychiatric patients. Clin Nutr 25(1):60–67, 2006 16216392

Liu CC, Liu CC, Kanekiyo T, et al: Apolipoprotein E and Alzheimer disease: risk, mechanisms and therapy. Nat Rev Neurol 9(2):106–118, 2013 23296339

Magarian GJ, Lucas LM, Kumar KL: Clinical significance in alcoholic patients of commonly encountered laboratory test results. West J Med 156(3):287–294, 1992 1595246

Mayo Medical Laboratories: Rochester 2018 Test Catalog, Laboratory Reference Edition (Sorted By Test Name; Current as of August 30, 2018). Available at: https://www.mayomedicallaboratories.com/test-catalog/. Accessed September 3, 2018.

Mitchell AJ: CSF phosphorylated tau in the diagnosis and prognosis of mild cognitive impairment and Alzheimer's disease: a meta-analysis of 51 studies. J Neurol Neurosurg Psychiatry 80(9):966–975, 2009 19465413

Moeller KE, Lee KC, Kissack JC: Urine drug screening: practical guide for clinicians. Mayo Clin Proc 83(1):66–76, 2008 18174009

Owen RT: Folate augmentation of antidepressant response. Drugs Today (Barc) 49(12):791–798, 2013 24524097

Petersen RC, Waring SC, Smith GE, et al: Predictive value of APOE genotyping in incipient Alzheimer's disease. Ann NY Acad Sci 802:58–69, 1996 8993485

Piana F, Ruffo Codecasa L, Baldan R, et al: Use of T-SPOT.TB in latent tuberculosis infection diagnosis in general and immunosuppressed populations. New Microbiol 30(3):286–290, 2007 17802911

Poncet A, Gencer B, Blondon M, et al: Electrocardiographic screening for prolonged QT interval to reduce sudden cardiac death in psychiatric patients: a cost-effectiveness analysis. PLoS One 10(6):e0127213, 2015 26070071

Rack M, Davis J, Roffwarg HP, et al: The multiple sleep latency test in the diagnosis of narcolepsy. Am J Psychiatry 162(11):2198–2199, author reply 2199, 2005 16263876

Reisfield GM, Bertholf RL: "Practical guide" to urine drug screening clarified. Mayo Clin Proc 83(7):848–849, author reply 849, 2008 18614000

Rinck D, Frieling H, Freitag A, et al: Combinations of carbohydrate-deficient transferrin, mean corpuscular erythrocyte volume, gamma-glutamyltransferase, homocysteine and folate increase the significance of biological markers in alcohol dependent patients. Drug Alcohol Depend 89(1):60–65, 2007 17234365

Rogers HL, Bhattaram A, Zineh I, et al: CYP2D6 genotype information to guide pimozide treatment in adult and pediatric patients: basis for the U.S. Food and Drug Administration's new dosing recommendations. J Clin Psychiatry 73(9):1187–1190, 2012 23059146

Rubinstein WS, Maglott DR, Lee JM, et al: The NIH genetic testing registry: a new, centralized database of genetic tests to enable access to comprehensive information and improve transparency. Nucleic Acids Res 41(Database issue):D925–D935, 2013 23193275

Samer CF, Lorenzini KI, Rollason V, et al: Applications of CYP450 testing in the clinical setting. Mol Diagn Ther 17(3):165–184, 2013 23588782

Schwarz AJ, Yu P, Miller BB, et al: Regional profiles of the candidate tau PET ligand 18F-AV-1451 recapitulate key features of Braak histopathological stages. Brain 139 (Pt 5):1539–1550, 2016 26936940

Simerville JA, Maxted WC, Pahira JJ: Urinalysis: a comprehensive review. Am Fam Physician 71(6):1153–1162, 2005 15791892

Song L, Lachno DR, Hanlon D, et al: A digital enzyme-linked immunosorbent assay for ultra-sensitive measurement of amyloid-β 1–42 peptide in human plasma with utility for studies of Alzheimer's disease therapeutics. Alzheimers Res Ther 8(1):58, 2016 27978855

Sullivan SS, Kushida CA: Multiple sleep latency test and maintenance of wakefulness test. Chest 134(4):854–861, 2008 18842919

U.S. Preventive Services Task Force: Summaries for patients. Screening for chlamydia and gonorrhea: U.S. Preventive Services Task Force Recommendation Statement. Ann Intern Med 161(12):1–30, 2014 25243662

U.S. Preventive Services Task Force, Bibbins-Domingo K, Grossman DC, et al: Screening for latent tuberculosis infection in adults: U.S. Preventive Services Task Force Recommendation Statement. JAMA 316(9):962–969, 2016 27599331

van Noord C, Straus SM, Sturkenboom MC, et al: Psychotropic drugs associated with corrected QT interval prolongation. J Clin Psychopharmacol 29(1):9–15, 2009 19142100

Wu SI, Tsai SY, Huang MC, et al: Risk factors for sudden cardiac death among patients with alcohol dependence: a nested case-control study. Alcohol Clin Exp Res 39(9):1797–1804, 2015 26207644

Recommended Readings

Fischbach F, Dunning MB: A Manual of Laboratory and Diagnostic Tests, 9th Edition. Philadelphia, PA, Wolters Kluwer Health/Lippincott Williams & Wilkins, 2015

Frey KA, Lodge MA, Meltzer CC, et al: ACR-ASNR practice parameter for brain PET/CT imaging dementia. Clin Nucl Med 41(2):118–125, 2016

Jacobson SA: Laboratory Medicine in Psychiatry and Behavioral Science. Washington, DC, American Psychiatric Publishing, 2012

Jacobson SA: Clinical Laboratory Medicine for Mental Health Professionals. Arlington, VA, American Psychiatric Association Publishing, 2017

Jarvis M, Williams J, Hurford M, et al: Appropriate use of drug testing in clinical addiction medicine. J Addict Med 11(3):163–173, 2017

Linden DE: The challenges and promise of neuroimaging in psychiatry. Neuron 12:8–22, 2012

Poncet A, Gencer B, Blondon M, et al: Electrocardiographic screening for prolonged QT interval to reduce sudden cardiac death in psychiatric patients: a cost-effectiveness analysis. PLoS One 10(6):e0127213, 2015

Simerville JA, Maxted WC, Pahira JJ: Urinalysis: a comprehensive review. Am Fam Physician 71(6):1153–1162, 2005

CHAPTER 6

The Social Determinants of Mental Health

Ruth S. Shim, M.D., M.P.H.

Michael T. Compton, M.D., M.P.H.

For the past 40 years or so, the biopsychosocial model has been an organizing framework for case formulation in clinical psychiatry. The basic sciences and neuro-imaging, interventional and effectiveness research, and epidemiology have advanced our understanding of the pathophysiology, treatment, and prevalence and comorbidity of psychiatric disorders; however, societal and environmental factors and their contributions to the development of mental illnesses and substance use disorders continue to warrant research and programmatic attention. *Social determinants of mental health* are defined as societal, environmental, and economic conditions that influence and affect mental health outcomes at the population level. In considering the current state of psychiatry as well as future directions for the field, the importance of social factors that contribute to mental health should not be underestimated. These factors are primarily responsible for disparities and inequities in mental health services access, treatment quality, and outcomes seen within and between population groups. In this chapter we discuss the importance of social determinants of mental health, present up-to-date evidence on specific social determinants, explain the relevance of these social determinants to clinical psychiatry, and consider action points that could help reduce mental health inequities, prevent mental illnesses and substance use disorders, and promote mental health at the population level.

Core Concepts

Several concepts are essential to understanding the relevance of social determinants of mental health not only to public health but also to clinical psychiatry (Table 6–1). The concept of *social determinants of health* is widely accepted and discussed in public health and global health circles and usually includes some limited reference to the contribution of adverse social circumstances and experiences to mental health problems or substance misuse. The effects of unfavorable social determinants of *mental* health, while not distinctly different from unfavorable social determinants of health overall, deserve special emphasis because of the significant morbidity, disability, and mortality associated with mental illnesses and substance use disorders and the extent to which disparities and inequities persist in mental health care.

Social justice, as defined by the philosopher David Miller (1999), refers to the distribution of good (advantages) and bad (disadvantages) in society, and, more specifically, how these things *should be* distributed in society. Social justice is concerned with the equitable allocation of resources to people by social institutions. Social justice can be considered to represent the moral foundation of public health, and health care and mental health care can be considered a resource, or a good, in society. For this reason, devising strategies to improve adverse social determinants of health is a means of advancing social justice.

Health disparities are differences in health status among distinct segments of the population, including differences that occur by gender, race or ethnicity, education or income, disability status, or geographic area. *Health inequities* are disparities in health that are a result of systemic, avoidable, and unjust social and economic policies and practices that create barriers to opportunity. In the United States, there is ongoing debate about the use of these definitions and their importance in setting priorities for allocation of resources to help reduce health status inequalities among different populations (Braveman et al. 2011b).

Risk factors are characteristics that predate a disorder or outcome that are statistically associated with the risk of developing that disorder or outcome. *Protective factors* are characteristics that predate a disorder or outcome that significantly reduce the risk of developing that disorder or outcome. Adverse social determinants of mental health can be considered to be precursors to risk factors; targeting interventions toward these adverse social determinants at the population level may help reduce risk factors and increase protective factors.

Whereas social determinants drive risk and protective factors, social norms and public policies can be thought of as the underlying drivers of the social determinants of mental health. *Social norms* are the values, attitudes, and biases that a society shares about people or populations, and *public policies* are the laws and codified rules that govern society. Some public policies and some social norms can lead to unequal distribution of opportunity, which in turn drives the social determinants of mental health. Public policies and social norms also interact with each other. Specifically, laws and policies can shape attitudes and perceptions, and social norms can lead to the creation of laws and policies.

Adverse Social Determinants of Mental Health

In the following subsections, we discuss 10 core social determinants that can contribute to mental health problems (summarized in Figure 6–1).

TABLE 6–1.   **Social determinants of mental health: definitions of important concepts**

Social determinants of mental health	Societal, environmental, and economic conditions that influence and affect mental health outcomes across various populations
Social justice	The distribution of good (advantages) and bad (disadvantages) in society—and, more specifically, how these things *should be* distributed in society
Health disparities	Differences in health status among distinct segments of the population, including differences that occur by gender, race or ethnicity, education or income, disability status, or geographic area
Health inequities	Disparities in health that are a result of systemic, avoidable, and unjust social and economic policies and practices that create barriers to opportunity
Risk factors	Characteristics that predate a disorder or outcome and are statistically associated with risk for developing that disorder or outcome
Protective factors	Characteristics that predate a disorder or outcome that significantly reduce the risk of developing that disorder or outcome
Social norms	The values, attitudes, and biases that a society shares about people and populations
Public policies	The laws and codified rules that govern society

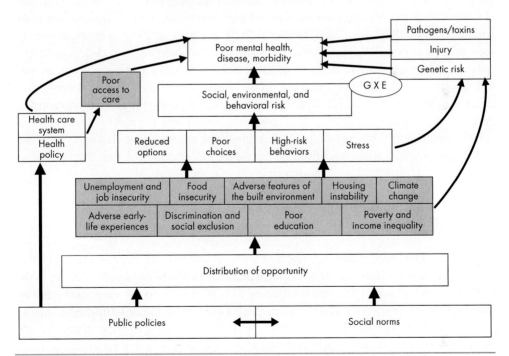

FIGURE 6–1.   Adverse social determinants of mental health: a conceptual model.

G×E=gene-by-environment interaction.

Source.   Adapted from Figure 1–1 (p. 15) from The Group for the Advancement of Psychiatry (GAP) Prevention Committee: "Overview of the Social Determinants of Mental Health," in *The Social Determinants of Mental Health*. Edited by Compton MT, Shim RS. Washington, DC, American Psychiatric Publishing, 2015. Copyright 2015, American Psychiatric Association. Used with permission.

Discrimination and Social Exclusion

Ample evidence supports a link between discrimination (or perceived discrimination) in its various forms (whether based on race/ethnicity, gender, religion, sexual orientation, social class, or other characteristics) and adverse mental health outcomes (Krieger 2014). Furthermore, the intersecting nature of the various forms of discrimination experienced by an individual or group of individuals is increasingly being recognized in regard to its effects on mental health. Several studies have found associations between discrimination and multiple adverse mental health outcomes, including substance use disorders, depression, and posttraumatic stress disorder (PTSD), in diverse population groups, including American Indians and Alaska Natives, African Americans, immigrants to the United States, and lesbian, gay, bisexual, and transgender (LGBT) populations (Newcomb and Mustanski 2010; Viruell-Fuentes et al. 2012; Walters et al. 2011).

Adverse Early-Life Experiences

Adverse early-life experiences are defined as inconsistent, threatening, hurtful, traumatic, or neglectful social interchanges experienced by infants, children, or adolescents. The original Adverse Childhood Experiences (ACE) Study, which involved more than 17,000 members of the Kaiser Permanente health maintenance organization in San Diego, California, found strong, graded relationships between the number of adverse childhood experiences and the risk of mood and anxiety disorders, cigarette smoking, and alcohol and illicit drug use (Dube et al. 2001; Felitti et al. 1998). Among marginalized or diverse populations, the many associations between adverse childhood experiences and poor mental health outcomes (including anxiety and depression, as well as tobacco, alcohol, and marijuana use, to name just a few) have been repeatedly documented (Mersky et al. 2013). In particular, there is a powerful graded relationship between the number of adverse childhood experiences and the risk of attempted suicide in adulthood (Dube et al. 2001). Independent associations also exist between childhood physical abuse and lifetime prevalence of attention-deficit/hyperactivity disorder (ADHD), PTSD, and bipolar disorder (Sugaya et al. 2012).

Poor Education

Many pathways link education to health outcomes (Braveman et al. 2011a). Life expectancy in the United States is correlated with educational attainment. Using relative risk estimates of mortality, a seminal study of death attributable to social factors in the United States estimated that approximately 245,000 deaths in the year 2000 were attributable to low educational attainment (Galea et al. 2011). Poor educational quality is closely linked to residential segregation, and students living in areas of high neighborhood-level poverty are much more likely to attend schools that are distressed and underresourced. Other studies have found an association between lower educational attainment and risk of developing late-life depression (Chang-Quan et al. 2010), among other mental health outcomes. Low educational attainment, poor quality of education, and educational inequality all have impacts on risk for, and outcomes of, diverse mental illnesses and substance use disorders.

Poverty and Income Inequality

Poverty is generally detrimental across a host of psychiatric outcomes. Childhood family poverty is independently associated with PTSD and major depressive disorder (Nikulina et al. 2011). Beyond associations between poverty and adverse mental health outcomes, income inequality and wealth inequality (or the differences in individuals' stock of valuable possessions) are also detrimental to mental health. At the population level, income inequality has been independently associated with depression (Pabayo et al. 2014), schizophrenia (Burns et al. 2014), and mental illness in general throughout the world (Pickett and Wilkinson 2010).

Unemployment and Job Insecurity

Insecurity in employment is associated with mental disorders, especially in industrialized countries (Moynihan 2012). Numerous studies document associations between employment and mental health. Research has revealed a link between the suicide rate and the unemployment rate in the United States (Reeves et al. 2012). Shutdowns of manufacturing plants and downturns of economies in various cities in the United States—and associated unemployment, underemployment, and job insecurity—have been related to adverse mental health and substance use outcomes; for example, there are higher rates of depression, anxiety, and alcohol use disorder among people living in those communities (Broman et al. 2012).

Food Insecurity

Food insecurity—a state of lacking reliable access to a sufficient quantity of affordable and nutritious food—is associated with many adverse mental health outcomes. Among adolescents, food insecurity has been associated with mood, anxiety, and substance use disorders, independent of other socioeconomic status measures (McLaughlin et al. 2012). In children, food insecurity increases the risk of depression, anxiety, and hyperactivity/inattention (Melchior et al. 2012). The adverse effects of food insecurity on mental health are particularly evident among young people but are clearly observable across the life span (Gundersen and Ziliak 2015).

Housing Instability

Housing instability is a major public health concern, one that signi0ficantly affects health outcomes among children and adults. Specifically, unstable living conditions and homelessness can lead to poor mental health outcomes. For children living in poverty, frequent moves are associated with attentional and behavioral problems (Ziol-Guest and McKenna 2014). In adults, residential instability—which includes frequent moves, often driven by lack of money to pay rent—is associated with higher rates of depression (Davey-Rothwell et al. 2008). Multiple studies have found additional associations between poor housing quality and housing instability and mental health.

Adverse Features of the Built Environment

The *built environment* is defined as all aspects of our surroundings that are built by human beings. All aspects of the built environment are dictated by public policy, and they can either promote mental health or increase risk for mental illnesses and substance use disorders. Features of the built environment include public works infrastructure, built green space, housing, and schools and workplaces. The effects of the built environment on mental health can be either direct (e.g., limited exposure to green space and associated risk of depression) or indirect (e.g., transportation systems designed in a way that limits social cohesion, physical activity, and/or access to health care). Unfavorable aspects of the built environment are associated with a range of adverse mental health and substance use disorder outcomes, particularly depression, anxiety, and alcohol use disorders (Diez Roux and Mair 2010).

Climate Change

Scientists have hypothesized that climate change affects the mental health of populations through exposure to climate-related catastrophic events such as floods, hurricanes, and bush fires and through the impact of such events on community well-being. The trauma of experiencing a life-threatening natural disaster can increase the likelihood of developing acute stress disorder, depression, PTSD, and anxiety disorders. Disruptions in community functioning and relationships, including loss of social cohesion, forced migration, and rises in violence and crime, are also potential correlates of climate change (Trombley et al. 2017).

Poor Access to Care

Lack of health insurance can lead to many negative health outcomes. In addition to not having proper access to necessary treatment when one needs health services, the uncertainty and added financial burden can increase the likelihood of mental health problems, including depression and anxiety. A natural experiment that compared individuals in Oregon with Medicaid coverage versus no health insurance found lower rates of depression in the Medicaid-insured population (Baicker et al. 2013). Research has also repeatedly demonstrated inequities in access to mental health care when comparing minority racial/ethnic populations in need of services with white populations (Wells et al. 2001). Lack of mental health parity in insurance coverage has also contributed to disparities and inequities in health outcomes for people with substance use disorders and mental illnesses.

Relevance of Social Determinants to Clinical Psychiatry Across the Life Span

References in the clinical literature to the social determinants of health have multiplied in the past two decades, and the social determinants are increasingly being integrated into measures of population health and mental health. For example, *Healthy People 2020,* a 10-year agenda of diverse goals set by the federal government with the purpose of improving the nation's health, includes social determinants of health as a set of outcomes to be measured (Centers for Disease Control and Prevention 2018). This recognition of and attention to social determinants is highly encouraging from a public health standpoint, but the implications for day-to-day clinical practice are not as clear. Nevertheless, there are ways that we can begin to incorporate an understanding of these social determinants into our interactions with patients as we develop tailored treatment plans and help our patients to work toward achieving recovery.

For children, adolescents, and young adults, early-childhood trauma, poor education, food insecurity, and other unfavorable circumstances are important social determinants of mental health that can set the stage for a host of adverse mental health outcomes, both in childhood and in adulthood. Screening for each of these issues is critical, as is tailoring interventions to address social factors that potentially contribute to adverse mental health outcomes. Potential measures may include screening all patients for adverse early-life experiences and implementing trauma-informed care as an overarching approach in clinical settings. Another example of a point of intervention would be the use of effective screening tools to evaluate children for food insecurity and to connect parents of food-insecure children to resources for nutritious food (e.g., federal/state food and nutrition assistance programs, local food banks).

For adults, issues related to income inequality, poverty, unemployment, and housing instability or poor housing quality are especially relevant. The I-HELP mnemonic—Income supports, Housing, Employment/education, Legal status, and Personal stability—can help identify target areas for screening and intervention (Kenyon et al. 2007). For adults who report difficulty in one or more of these areas, referrals to appropriate resources can help them begin to ameliorate some of the potential underlying causes of poor mental health.

For older adults, issues related to social isolation, access to health care, and the built environment may have particular relevance. Supports should be in place to provide older adults with help in accessing positive social relationships, feeling connected as contributing members of society, and navigating their physical environments free from physical or psychosocial challenges.

In the clinical assessment of all patients, special consideration should be given to adverse social determinants most relevant at certain points in the life span. Although universal screening focused on each of the key social determinants would be ideal, given the magnitude of their potential contribution to mental health and mental illness outcomes, competing priorities in clinical settings would make such screening difficult, if not impossible. However, mental health care practitioners should tailor specific screening assessments for use in patients whose presentations suggest that adverse social circumstances may underlie the complexity of their clinical symptoms. For example, although it would be optimal if all children undergoing a psychiatric assessment could be assessed for the presence of food insecurity, those children presenting with symptoms of anxiety or hyperactivity should consistently be screened, because food insecurity can contribute to or cause such symptoms. Similarly, screening measures for poverty should be considered in all patients, regardless of their physical appearance and independent of assumptions providers might have about their financial situation. All patients, regardless of their background or appearance, should be asked whether they have experienced any forms of discrimination or feelings of social exclusion or social isolation. If we can incorporate an awareness of the social determinants of mental health into our standardized assessments and ongoing treatment plans, we will form stronger connections with our patients and be better able to identify possible points of intervention to target the underlying factors that contribute to inequities and adverse mental health outcomes.

Case Examples of the Relevance of Social Determinants in Clinical Settings

The following case vignettes are presented to illustrate two scenarios in which a patient's adverse experiences related to social factors likely contribute significantly to that patient's presenting symptoms.

Case 1

A 26-year-old Navajo woman presents for evaluation of ongoing symptoms of anxiety and depression. She describes her childhood as having been difficult and traumatic; her father was not in the picture, and her mother had a serious alcohol use disorder. The woman reports that starting in early adolescence, she went back and forth between living with her mother on a reservation and staying with her grandparents, who lived in a nearby city. At age 17, she started an on-again/off-again relationship with her then-boyfriend. They were together for a total of 9 years and had two sons. During this time, her primary focus in life was on trying to maintain employment and housing to support her two children. She feels very strongly that her depression and anxiety symptoms are specifically and directly related to her housing status: "When I have a stable place to stay, I do fine. When I'm on the verge of being evicted or when we're bouncing around shelters, that's when my depression is really bad." She is requesting evaluation to start antidepressant medication.

Case 2

A 30-year-old Iranian woman presents for management of new-onset anxiety symptoms. She is in the third year of a family medicine residency and states that in recent months, more and more patients have made disparaging comments and offhand remarks about the hijab she wears. Some patients have asked if they could be seen by another doctor. She states that more than one patient has referred to her as a "terrorist doctor" and that she has felt unsafe in her interactions with certain patients. She has approached the medical director of the main clinic where she rotates regarding these feelings, and although he expressed sympathy for her situation, he also remarked that "from a customer service perspective, the patient is always right" and that the clinic would attempt to find an alternate provider for patients who had concerns. In recent weeks, she has begun to develop anxiety around evaluating new patients, because she is never sure whom she will encounter. She has noticed that she has had some difficulty remembering patients' histories and has had problems in synthesizing and organizing case presentations to her attending physician (supervisor). She has not been sleeping well and worries that she will not successfully complete her residency program.

Addressing the Social Determinants of Mental Health

Table 6–2 provides suggestions for how psychiatrists and other mental health care providers might begin to address adverse social determinants of mental health from a clinical perspective.

TABLE 6–2.	Examples of ways to help improve adverse social determinants of mental health in clinical settings
Discrimination and social exclusion	Use the DSM-5 Cultural Formulation Interview during all diagnostic evaluations
Adverse early-life experiences	Screen (using the ACE score calculator) for adverse early-life experiences
Poor education	Implement supported education in practice settings
Unemployment and job insecurity	Implement supported employment in your practice settings
Poverty and income inequality	Create a local resource list for your practice setting to help support individuals experiencing poverty or a financial crisis
Food insecurity	Use the 1- or 2-item food insecurity screen in all initial assessments
Housing instability	Screen patients with the I-HELP screening tool
Adverse features of the built environment	Educate your clinic/community about mental health impact assessments
Climate change	Work with clinicians, staff, and patients to develop and support ride-sharing programs to reduce pollutant emissions
Poor access to care	Consider expanding available appointments in your practice or clinic to outside of traditional work hours (evenings or weekends)

Note. ACE score calculator=Adverse Childhood Experiences score calculator (Felitti et al. 1998); DSM-5 Cultural Formulation Interview (American Psychiatric Association 2013, pp. 752–757); food insecurity screen (Hager et al. 2010; I-HELP screening tool=Income supports, Housing, Employment/education, Legal status, and Personal stability (Kenyon et al. 2007).

Just as psychiatrists and other mental health professionals consider countertransference that might impact clinical encounters and thus outcomes, they should also consider ways in which they may be contributing to or perpetuating structural factors that interfere with rapport and impact outcomes. Most important, unconscious (or implicit) bias can play a detrimental role in daily interactions with patients. There have been many documented examples of how unconscious bias results in poor delivery of health care to marginalized population groups, but less is known about specific ways that unconscious bias leads to disparities and inequities in mental health care (Santry and Wren 2012). Given the more subjective nature of psychiatry relative to other fields of medicine, and coupled with the significance of the therapeutic alliance in shaping mental health recovery, the impact of unconscious bias may be even more crucial in psychiatry and may contribute to mental health disparities and inequities.

While clinical interventions can be invaluable for beginning to address the social determinants of mental health on an individual basis, lasting impact requires a population-based approach. Distribution of opportunity is the main driver of the social determinants of mental health and is influenced by the social norms and public policies that shape how opportunity is distributed in a society.

Social Norms

Social norms are deeply held beliefs that are ingrained in the fabric of our society. Some are suppressed, and others are reinforced by charismatic leaders who set tone and precedent for what is appropriate in our shared culture. In addition, social norms can be affected by laws and policies that serve to move public perceptions in a particular direction and change our understanding of fairness or what is right and wrong. Attitudes and values around social exclusion, discrimination, and acceptance are some of the most powerful social norms that govern our societal behavior. Furthermore, social norms help to form the unconscious bias that individuals (and health care providers) hold toward others in society.

Therefore, to impact the social norms that drive opportunity and thus impact the social determinants of mental health, psychiatrists and other mental health providers have a responsibility to help create and uphold social norms of tolerance, inclusion, acceptance, respect, and dignity for all. It is incumbent on psychiatrists and other mental health professionals, as experts in human behavior, to be aware of the role and impact of conscious and unconscious bias, and to better understand how structural forces have historically collided to create mental health inequities and social determinants that affect mental health outcomes today. Psychiatrists and other mental health professionals should not shy away from addressing uncomfortable topics related to issues of social exclusion and should be vocal about confronting any observed violations of health-promoting social norms of tolerance and inclusion.

Public Policies

Many laws, policies, and programs exist to prevent detrimental effects of the social determinants. Antidiscrimination laws that have shifted social norms and helped to improve social determinants of mental health include several amendments of the U.S. Constitution, the Civil Rights Act of 1964, the Voting Rights Act of 1965, the Fair Housing Act, the Equal Opportunity Act, the Americans with Disabilities Act, the Lilly Ledbetter Fair Pay Act of 2009, the Matthew Shepard and James Byrd Jr. Hate Crimes Prevention Act, and the Fair Sentencing Act of 2010, to name a few (Krieger 2014). Yet many laws and policies worsen the social determinants of mental health. Psychiatrists and mental health providers have a responsibility to advocate for laws and policies—at local, state, and federal levels—that promote, rather than harm, mental health and improve mental health outcomes for all.

Future Directions

Although it is increasingly clear that social disadvantage and unfavorable life circumstances contribute to adverse mental health outcomes and inequities, there are still important research questions to be answered, and greater innovation is needed to bring about meaningful change. Individual determinants do not exert their effects in a vacuum, and research must focus on understanding the complex ways that many social determinants of mental health interact with each other to influence mental health outcomes. Future research directions include acquiring a better understanding of how social and environmental factors interact with genetics (e.g., gene-by-environment interactions and epigenetic modification), deciphering the biological mechanisms or mediators through which social and environmental factors change the body and brain, and quantifying the impact of diverse and interacting social determinants on specific disease outcomes.

Innovation is needed to invigorate this area of psychiatry, as it has done for neuroimaging and other aspects of the field. Innovative screening and assessment strategies are necessary. Clinical and policy approaches to improving the social determinants of mental health would benefit from innovation, perhaps best accomplished through collaboration with other diverse professional groups (e.g., behavioral economists, urban planners, educators, public health experts). Policies and programs that have demonstrated effectiveness in altering the social determinants of mental health must be better disseminated and implemented, just as biomedical technological advances have been. Finally, innovative methods of teaching health care professionals, as well as trainees from undergraduate students to postdoctoral fellows and junior faculty, need to be tested and shared.

Key Clinical Points

- The social determinants of mental health are societal, environmental, and economic conditions that influence and affect mental health outcomes across various populations.

- Taking action to change adverse social determinants of mental health holds promise for reducing mental health disparities and inequities and improving outcomes among individuals with mental illnesses and substance use disorders.

- Key social contributors to mental illness include discrimination and social exclusion, adverse early-life experiences, poor education, poverty and income inequality, unemployment and job insecurity, food insecurity, housing instability, adverse features of the built environment, climate change, and poor access to health care.

- Adverse social influences on mental health are largely underpinned by an unequal and unfair distribution of opportunity, which in turn is founded upon certain social norms (i.e., opinions, attitudes, biases) and public policies (i.e., laws and codified rules).

- Psychiatrists and other mental health professionals can play diverse roles in addressing the social determinants of mental health, and thus potentially improving population mental health; these roles include developing clinical programs and advocacy focused on specific social determinants as well as working collaboratively to change social norms and public policies so that they promote, rather than undermine, mental health.

References

American Psychiatric Association: Diagnostic and Statistical Manual of Mental Disorders, 5th Edition. Arlington, VA, American Psychiatric Association, 2013

Baicker K, Taubman SL, Allen HL, et al: The Oregon experiment—effects of Medicaid on clinical outcomes. N Engl J Med 368(18):1713–1722, 2013 23635051

Braveman P, Egerter S, Williams DR: The social determinants of health: coming of age. Annu Rev Public Health 32:381–398, 2011a 21091195

Braveman PA, Kumanyika S, Fielding J, et al: Health disparities and health equity: the issue is justice. Am J Public Health 101 (suppl 1):S149–S155, 2011b 21551385

Broman CL, Hamilton VL, Hoffman WS: Stress and Distress Among the Unemployed: Hard Times and Vulnerable People. New York, Springer, 2012

Burns JK, Tomita A, Kapadia AS: Income inequality and schizophrenia: increased schizophrenia incidence in countries with high levels of income inequality. Int J Soc Psychiatry 60(2):185–196, 2014 23594564

Centers for Disease Control and Prevention: Social Determinants of Health. Last updated December 9, 2018. Available at: https://www.healthypeople.gov/2020/topics-objectives/topic/social-determinants-of-health. Accessed December 9, 2018.

Chang-Quan H, Zheng-Rong W, Yong-Hong L, et al: Education and risk for late life depression: a meta-analysis of published literature. Int J Psychiatry Med 40(1):109–124, 2010 20565049

Davey-Rothwell MA, German D, Latkin CA: Residential transience and depression: does the relationship exist for men and women? J Urban Health 85(5):707–716, 2008 18581237

Diez Roux AV, Mair C: Neighborhoods and health. Ann N Y Acad Sci 1186:125–145, 2010 20201871

Dube SR, Anda RF, Felitti VJ, et al: Childhood abuse, household dysfunction, and the risk of attempted suicide throughout the life span: findings from the Adverse Childhood Experiences Study. JAMA 286(24):3089–3096, 2001 11754674

Felitti VJ, Anda RF, Nordenberg D, et al: Relationship of childhood abuse and household dysfunction to many of the leading causes of death in adults. The Adverse Childhood Experiences (ACE) Study. Am J Prev Med 14(4):245–258, 1998 9635069

Galea S, Tracy M, Hoggatt KJ, et al: Estimated deaths attributable to social factors in the United States. Am J Public Health 101(8):1456–1465, 2011 21680937

Gundersen C, Ziliak JP: Food insecurity and health outcomes. Health Aff (Millwood) 34(11):1830–1839, 2015 26526240

Hager ER, Quigg AM, Black MM, et al: Development and validity of a 2-item screen to identify families at risk for food insecurity. Pediatrics 126(1):e26–e32, 2010 20595453

Kenyon C, Sandel M, Silverstein M, et al: Revisiting the social history for child health. Pediatrics 120(3):e734–e738, 2007 17766513

Krieger N: Discrimination and health inequities. Int J Health Serv 44(4):643–710, 2014 25626224

McLaughlin KA, Green JG, Alegría M, et al: Food insecurity and mental disorders in a national sample of U.S. adolescents. J Am Acad Child Adolesc Psychiatry 51(12):1293–1303, 2012 23200286

Melchior M, Chastang JF, Falissard B, et al: Food insecurity and children's mental health: a prospective birth cohort study. PLoS One 7(12):e52615, 2012 23300723

Mersky JP, Topitzes J, Reynolds AJ: Impacts of adverse childhood experiences on health, mental health, and substance use in early adulthood: a cohort study of an urban, minority sample in the U.S. Child Abuse Negl 37(11):917–925, 2013 23978575

Miller D: Principles of Social Justice. Cambridge, MA, Harvard University Press, 1999

Moynihan R: Job insecurity contributes to poor health. BMJ 345:e5183, 2012 22859778

Newcomb ME, Mustanski B: Internalized homophobia and internalizing mental health problems: a meta-analytic review. Clin Psychol Rev 30(8):1019–1029, 2010 20708315

Nikulina V, Widom CS, Czaja S: The role of childhood neglect and childhood poverty in predicting mental health, academic achievement and crime in adulthood. Am J Community Psychol 48(3–4):309–321, 2011 21116706

Pabayo R, Kawachi I, Gilman SE: Income inequality among American states and the incidence of major depression. J Epidemiol Community Health 68(2):110–115, 2014 24064745

Pickett KE, Wilkinson RG: Inequality: an underacknowledged source of mental illness and distress. Br J Psychiatry 197(6):426–428, 2010 21119145

Reeves A, Stuckler D, McKee M, et al: Increase in state suicide rates in the USA during economic recession. Lancet 380(9856):1813–1814, 2012 23141814

Santry HP, Wren SM: The role of unconscious bias in surgical safety and outcomes. Surg Clin North Am 92(1):137–151, 2012 22269267

Sugaya L, Hasin DS, Olfson M, et al: Child physical abuse and adult mental health: a national study. J Trauma Stress 25(4):384–392, 2012 22806701

Trombley J, Chalupka S, Anderko L: Climate change and mental health. Am J Nurs 117(4):44–52, 2017 28333743

Viruell-Fuentes EA, Miranda PY, Abdulrahim S: More than culture: structural racism, intersectionality theory, and immigrant health. Soc Sci Med 75(12):2099–2106, 2012 22386617

Walters KL, Mohammed SA, Evans-Campbell T, et al: Bodies don't just tell stories, they tell histories: embodiment of historical trauma among American Indians and Alaska Natives. Du Bois Review: Social Science Research on Race 8:179–189, 2011

Wells K, Klap R, Koike A, et al: Ethnic disparities in unmet need for alcoholism, drug abuse, and mental health care. Am J Psychiatry 158(12):2027–2032, 2001 11729020

Ziol-Guest KM, McKenna CC: Early childhood housing instability and school readiness. Child Dev 85(1):103–113, 2014 23534607

Recommended Readings

Blas E, Kurup AS (eds): Equity, social determinants and public health programmes. Geneva, Switzerland, World Health Organization, 2010

Compton MT, Shim RS (eds): The Social Determinants of Mental Health. Washington, DC, American Psychiatric Publishing, 2015

Compton MT, Shim RS: The social determinants of mental health. Focus 13:419–425, 2015

Marmot M, Wilkinson R (eds): Social Determinants of Health. Oxford, UK, Oxford University Press, 2005

Marmot M, Friel S, Bell R, Houweling TA, et al: Closing the gap in a generation: health equity through action on the social determinants of health. Lancet 372(9650):1661–1669, 2008

Wilkinson RG, Marmot MG (eds): The Solid Facts: Social Determinants of Health, 2nd Edition. Geneva, Switzerland, World Health Organization, 2003

Wilkinson RG, Pickett K: The Spirit Level: Why Equality Is Better for Everyone. New York, Penguin Books, 2010

World Health Organization, Calouste Gulbenkian Foundation: Social Determinants of Mental Health. Geneva, Switzerland, World Health Organization, 2014

CHAPTER 7

Ethical Considerations in Psychiatry

Laura Weiss Roberts, M.D., M.A.

Laura B. Dunn, M.D.

Ethics is an endeavor. It refers to ways of understanding what is good and right in human experience. It is about discernment, knowledge, and self-reflection, and it is sustained through seeking, clarifying, and translating. It is the concrete expression of moral ideals in everyday life. Ethics is about meaning, and it is about action.

Roberts 2002a

Psychiatrists understand the hardships and heroism of their patients, people who have been affected by illnesses or conditions that are often misunderstood and cause great suffering, significant disability, and even, at times, loss of life. Psychiatrists learn about the most sensitive aspects of their patients' lives and witness the strengths of their patients as they bear the burdens of disease and its repercussions. Patients with mental illness trust that psychiatrists will value and respect them as human beings. To be worthy of that trust, psychiatrists must develop and work to maintain a deep capacity for self-reflection and sensitivity to the ethical nuances of their work (Roberts 2016; Roberts and Dyer 2004).

The high value of ethics to psychiatry stems from the unique place of psychiatry within medicine. As specialist physicians trained in human behavior, psychiatrists are asked to bring expertise to complex situations that require an understanding of ethics, medicine, and psychology, as well as an understanding of the often complex psychosocial dimensions of patients' lives. Psychiatrists are often called upon to help clarify and resolve ethical dilemmas that arise in the care of medical patients, to join ethics committees, and to reflect publicly on ethical questions confronted by health care institutions and society.

Ethical behavior is fundamental to medical professionalism, which in turn is grounded in service to others in society. The "litmus test" of professionalism is the willing acceptance by the professional of the ethical obligation to place the interests of the patient and society before his or her own (Roberts 2016). The capacity to appreciate the ethical aspects of everyday practice, to apply ethical principles and enact ethical behaviors, and to reflect on the ethical impact of decisions is fundamental to professionalism in medicine. Moreover, it is important to understand that professional "codes" of conduct promulgated by organizations (e.g., the American Medical Association or the American Psychiatric Association [APA]) should not be viewed as sufficient stand-alone or immutable guides to ethical behavior, as these codes are incomplete, subject to changing social norms, and unable to address emerging ethical and legal issues in a rapidly evolving biomedical landscape.

Essential Ethical Skills of Psychiatrists

Psychiatrists whose work embodies the highest ethical standards tend to rely on a set of core "ethics skills" that are learned during or before medical training and are continually practiced and refined during their career (Table 7–1) (Roberts 2016; Roberts and Dyer 2004). Acquiring these skills in support of professional conduct in psychiatry is itself a developmental process, with certain predictable issues and milestones that occur in relation to the nature of psychiatrists' work and the roles with which they are entrusted (Jain et al. 2011).

The first of these core skills is the ability to identify ethical issues as they arise. For some, this identification will be an intuitive insight (e.g., an internal sense that "something is not right"). For others, it will be derived more logically (e.g., awareness that involuntary treatment or the care of "VIP" patients can pose specific ethical problems). The ability to recognize ethical issues requires some familiarity with key ethics concepts and the interdisciplinary field of bioethics (Table 7–2). As a corollary, this ability presupposes the psychiatrist's capacity to observe and translate complex phenomena into patterns, using the common language of the profession (e.g., conflicts between autonomy and beneficence, as might arise when a depressed older adult, whose somatic delusions caused her to stop eating and thus to lose a significant amount of her body mass, is deemed incapable of refusing medical treatment and is hospitalized involuntarily).

The second skill is the ability to understand how one's personal values, beliefs, and sense of self may affect one's care of patients. For instance, a psychiatrist who is emotionally invested in his or her ability to "do good" as a healer should recognize that this emotional investment may subtly influence his or her judgment when evaluating the decisional capacity of a patient who refuses medically necessary treatments. A psychiatrist with a strong commitment to personal self-care (e.g., healthy eating and daily exercise) may have difficulty working effectively with a patient who engages voluntarily in unhealthy or risky behaviors. The ability to appreciate this aspect of the doctor–patient relationship is important for safeguarding the ethical decision making of the professional who seeks to help serve the well-being and aims of the patient.

TABLE 7–1.	**Essential ethics skills in clinical practice**

1. The ability to identify and describe ethical features of a patient's care and to outline various relevant dimensions of ethical dilemmas
2. The ability to see how one's own life experiences, attitudes, and knowledge may influence one's care of a patient (e.g., awareness of one's biases and countertransference)
3. The ability to identify one's areas of clinical expertise (i.e., scope of clinical competence) and to work within those boundaries
4. The ability to anticipate ethically risky or problematic situations (e.g., boundary crossings)
5. The ability to gather additional information and to seek consultation and additional expertise in order to clarify and, ideally, resolve ethical conflicts
6. The ability to build additional ethical safeguards into the patient care situation

TABLE 7–2.	**Glossary of ethics terms**
Term	**Definition**
Altruism	The virtue of acting for the good of another person rather than for oneself
Autonomy	The principle honoring the individual's capacity to make decisions for him- or herself and to act on the basis of such decisions
Beneficence	The principle of engaging in actions to bring about good for others
Compassion	The virtue of recognizing the experience of another person and acting with kindness and regard for his or her welfare
Confidentiality	The professional obligation of physicians not to disclose information or observations related to patients without their permission
Fidelity	The virtue of promise keeping
Honesty	The virtue of truthfulness
Integrity	The virtue of coherence, and of adherence to professionalism, in intention and action
Justice	The principle of fairness in the distribution of benefits and burdens
Nonmaleficence	The principle of avoiding harm toward others
Respect	The virtue of fully regarding and according intrinsic value to someone or something

Source. Adapted from Roberts (2016).

The third key ethics skill is an awareness of the limits of one's medical knowledge and expertise and a willingness to practice within those limits. Providing competent care within the scope of one's expertise fulfills both the positive ethical duty of doing good and the obligation to "do no harm." In some real-world situations, however, psychiatrists may at times feel compelled to perform services outside their areas of expertise. Such situations may occur with increasing frequency as the number of psychiatrists available to provide needed care to a growing population appears to be shrinking (National Council Medical Director Institute 2017). In some regions (e.g., rural, isolated, economically disadvantaged, war-torn, or disaster areas), psychiatrist shortages are so severe that psychiatrists face the ethical dilemma of either providing care for which they lack adequate training or being unable to treat the many patients who need help (Roberts 2016). In such settings, clinicians may feel ethically justified in choosing to do their best in the clinical situation while simultaneously trying to resolve the underlying problem. A rural psychiatrist may expand his or her areas of competence, for instance, by obtaining consultation by telephone from an expert in another region (Roberts 2004).

The fourth skill is the ability to recognize high-risk situations in which ethical problems are likely to arise. Ethically high-risk situations may be obvious, such as in circumstances in which a psychiatrist must step out of the usual treatment relationship to protect the patient or others from harm. These situations include involuntary treatment and hospitalization, reporting child or elder abuse, or informing a third party of a patient's intention to inflict harm. Other ethically high-risk situations may be harder to recognize—for example, providing clinical care to people with whom one has other relationships (e.g., relatives or friends)—but may create vulnerability for poor decision making and ethical mistakes.

The fifth skill is the willingness to seek information and consultation when faced with an ethically or clinically difficult situation and the ability to make use of offered guidance. Just as psychiatrists should tackle clinically difficult cases by reviewing the psychiatric literature and consulting with more experienced colleagues, psychiatrists should clarify and solve ethically difficult situations by referring to ethics codes and guidelines and consulting with colleagues and ethics committees.

The final essential ethics skill is the ability to build appropriate ethical safeguards into one's work. For example, a psychiatrist who treats children and adolescents would be wise to routinely inform new patients and their parents, at the onset of treatment, about the limits of confidentiality and the physician's legal mandate to report child abuse. The early-career psychiatrist who arranges to continue routine mentoring sessions as he gets his practice established and the later-career psychiatrist who joins a peer-supervision group to improve her ability to care for a new patient population are further illustrations of this skill. As psychiatric practice increasingly involves collaborative work with other clinicians (e.g., primary care providers), documentation in the electronic health record (EHR) of large organizations, use of cloud-based and other digital technologies, and other changes to the traditional, independent model of psychiatric practice, other needs and opportunities for ethical safeguards will arise (Shenoy and Appel 2017).

Practical Ethical Problem Solving

Many clinicians use an eclectic approach to ethical problem solving that intuitively makes use of both inductive and deductive reasoning. Such an approach does not typically yield one "right" answer but rather an array of possible and ethically justifiable approaches that may be acceptable in the current situation. In the clinical setting, a widely used approach to ethical problem solving is the "four-topics method" described by Jonsen et al. (2006). This method entails gathering and evaluating information about 1) clinical indications, 2) patient preferences, 3) patient quality of life, and 4) contextual or external influences on the ethical decision-making process.

Many ethical dilemmas in clinical care involve a conflict between the first two topics of the four-topics method: clinical indications and patient preferences. Examples of such dilemmas include a depressed cancer patient who refuses life-prolonging che-motherapy and a young person undergoing a "first psychotic break" who is brought to a hospital for treatment against his or her will. In each of these situations, the pref-erences of the patient are at odds with what is medically beneficial, creating a conflict for the physician between the duties of beneficence and respecting patient autonomy. To work through such dilemmas, it is critical to clarify what is clinically necessary and to fully and thoughtfully explore the patient's preferences. Why does the patient re-fuse treatment? Does the patient have the cognitive and emotional capacity to make this decision at this time? What is the full range of medically beneficial options? How urgent is the clinical situation, and is time available for discussion, collaboration, and perhaps compromise? If the patient does not have decision-making capacity, the di-lemma is at least temporarily resolved by identifying an appropriate alternative deci-sion maker. If the patient does have the ability to provide informed consent—involv-ing capacity for decision making and for voluntarism—then, under most foreseeable circumstances, his or her preferences must be followed. Engaging the patient in a con-versation in which the physician describes the full range of treatment options and demonstrates sensitivity to the reasons for the patient's refusal may help the physi-cian craft a solution that the patient can willingly accept and that the physician can justify as medically beneficial.

Physician Well-Being as an Ethical Imperative

Caring for patients is a great privilege and a source of fulfillment for health profession-als, yet it is increasingly recognized that the sustained, intensive work effort and per-sonal sacrifice involved in being a physician or physician-in-training can take their toll on physician well-being over time (Gengoux and Roberts 2018). Negative conse-quences of diminished well-being are serious and have been well documented. Con-sequences may include emotional exhaustion; greater likelihood of medical mistakes and boundary violations; lack of empathy and engagement; lessened overall resil-ience; substance use; greater vulnerability to mental health issues and relationship is-sues; occupational, functional, or social impairment; the emergence of suicidality; and decisions to drop out of medical training or depart early from the profession of medi-cine (Brown et al. 2009; Shanafelt et al. 2010). More positively, it is increasingly recog-nized that physicians who proactively take care of their own health are more likely to support the preventive health practices of their patients, to experience joy in their work, to deliver high-quality care, and to see improved health or service outcomes (Schrijver et al. 2016). Because physicians are entrusted with the health of large numbers of pa-tients over their careers, and because of the tremendous need to preserve the health care workforce, many stakeholders have converged to support physician well-being as an ethical imperative of the medical profession (Baker and Sen 2016; Smith 2017).

Over the past three decades, the physician well-being literature has examined work-related stress in medicine and has documented the phenomenon of physician "burnout" (Brady et al. 2018). *Burnout* is a syndrome that is defined by emotional ex-haustion, depersonalization, and a decreased sense of personal accomplishment (Maslach and Jackson 1981). High workload, lack of alignment with organizational values, lack of autonomy, and other factors contribute to this syndrome (Dyrbye and

Shanafelt 2016). More than half of all physicians report having experienced burnout (Shanafelt et al. 2015), and burnout has been identified in physicians at each stage of career development (Dyrbye et al. 2014; Raj 2016). Studies suggest that nearly half of medical students and nearly three-quarters of residents endorse all or some features of the syndrome (Ishak et al. 2009). Women (McMurray et al. 2000) and physicians working in fast-paced, high-stakes fields of medicine are at greatest risk for burnout (Shanafelt et al. 2012). Moreover, compared with other working adults, physicians are more likely to be dissatisfied with their work–life balance (Shanafelt et al. 2012). Importantly, early empirical findings suggest that the burden of caring for patients has not been the single greatest concern among physicians; the time-intensity and isolation associated with the increasingly heavy burden of the EHR have been identified as the biggest threats to physician well-being (Robertson et al. 2017).

Such evidence suggests, as does a proliferation of physicians' blogs and posts online, that loss of control over practice parameters, increasing demands for productivity, and mounting administrative burdens contribute to burnout. Although psychiatrists tend to rank lower than other specialties in terms of the proportion reporting symptoms of burnout in survey studies (Parks 2017), there is a need to understand what factors are protective and what factors are damaging. For instance, as more and more psychiatrists begin to work in large health care systems, and as the shortage of psychiatrists becomes more apparent (Weiner 2018), clinicians will increasingly face "unfunded mandates" to provide care for greater numbers of patients while using the same or fewer resources. This imbalance may increase burnout and should be addressed urgently.

The effort–reward imbalance model (Siegrist 1996), which has three main components—efforts, rewards, and overcommitment—has been utilized to examine physician burnout in a number of studies (Rasmussen et al. 2016). Both extrinsic rewards (e.g., respect from colleagues, financial rewards, security) and intrinsic rewards (e.g., meaningful work, career and personal development) are important to physicians. When efforts (the pressure, demands, and duties of being a physician) are out of balance with rewards, stress and burnout are likely. Moreover, overcommitment (exerting high efforts despite low rewards) heightens vulnerability to burnout. Therefore, in addition to the urgent need for systems-wide changes to address the increasing burdens on physicians, it is also important that physicians develop self-awareness of their own vulnerabilities (e.g., a tendency to overcommitment) in order to redress effort–reward imbalance.

Self-awareness and strong self-care practices have long been appreciated for their importance in psychiatry. The sibling profession of psychology similarly has emphasized how well-being and professional competence are tightly linked (Rupert et al. 2015). The evolving domains of positive psychiatry, positive psychology, and physician health suggest that well-being can be intentionally nurtured and reinforced (Lyubomirsky et al. 2005; Seligman et al. 2005). The experiences of high professional accomplishment and of personal meaning and belonging allow physicians to respond to the challenges of their work with resilience and greater emotional engagement (MacKinnon and Murray 2018).

Psychiatrists, as experts in mental health, play an important role in helping colleagues engage in well-being practices and in intervening when colleagues may be at risk for impairment. Psychiatrists can also lead and foster institutional or systemic efforts to strengthen physician well-being, such as leadership development, collaborative practice improvements, and well-being activities, which are valued by stakeholders and have a growing evidence base for their effectiveness in staving off professional burnout (Schrijver et al. 2016). Psychiatrists will play an increasingly important role as leaders in medicine in the future and can help to emphasize the links among physician well-being, clinical competence, improved patient care practices, and population health while stressing the importance of well-being as an ethical imperative of the health professions (Roberts 2016).

Key Ethical Issues in Psychiatry

Ethical decision making can be extremely challenging in the field of psychiatry, given the complexities of the doctor–patient relationship and the need for careful attention to ethical safeguards when working with people with disorders and with treatments that affect mental processes. Maintaining treatment boundaries is important for all clinicians but is especially important in the intimacy of the psychotherapeutic relationship. The concept of doctor–patient confidentiality, similarly, is an important safeguard in all of medicine but is particularly relevant for patients with stigmatized illnesses, for whom treatment may involve revealing deeply private information. Additionally, the process of informed consent for treatment may require more careful efforts in psychiatry because patients with severe and persistent mental illness may have episodic, fluctuating, and/or progressive impairments of decisional capacity (Baruth and Lapid 2017). Finally, all physicians have an obligation to use their power ethically, but psychiatrists must routinely and appropriately use legal power to impose involuntary treatment and hospitalization. These and other key ethical issues in psychiatry are discussed in more detail in the following sections.

Maintaining Therapeutic Boundaries

Professional therapeutic boundaries, which have been defined as "the edge or limit of appropriate behavior by the psychiatrist in the clinical setting" (Gabbard 2009a), are essential for all physicians but have been most thoroughly defined in the context of psychoanalysis and psychodynamic therapy (Gabbard 2009a). Maintenance of therapeutic boundaries ensures that the psychiatrist does not exploit or take advantage of the patient. While some behaviors are clearly "boundary violations" regardless of context (e.g., sexual behavior with a patient), other behaviors—referred to as "boundary crossings"—must be evaluated in the context of the treating relationship, the type of therapy, and other factors, such as cultural customs (e.g., accepting a small gift from a patient). In supportive psychotherapy, for instance, self-disclosure may be used as an intentional technique to establish rapport and relatedness with the patient (see Chapter 34, "Supportive Psychotherapy"). In long-term psychodynamic psychotherapy, the same act of self-disclosure could have a paradoxically negative impact, rendering the relationship more fragile. Professional judgment is therefore important in evaluating actions that touch upon boundaries.

Boundary violations are actions by the psychiatrist that are outside normal professional limits and have the potential to harm patients. The most widely studied boundary violation is sexual contact. Although sexual and romantic entanglements between psychiatrists and patients were not uncommon in the early days of psychiatry, the damage caused by such relationships eventually became evident (Epstein 1994). Sexual contact between patients and physicians has been prohibited by the APA since 1973 (American Psychiatric Association 2001). A review of qualitative and quantitative studies of therapists who had sexual relations with their patients suggests that risk factors for such behavior include inadequate training, isolation from colleagues, and narcissistic pathology (Epstein 1994). Sexual contact with former patients is also understood as being inherently exploitative because feelings of transference do not disappear when treatment ends (American Psychiatric Association 2001). In addition, sexual or romantic involvement with key third parties, such as the parent or spouse of a patient, threatens the therapeutic relationship and presents a conflict of interest that should be avoided (American Psychiatric Association 2017).

Nonsexual boundary violations have been less well studied. These transgressions include seeing patients outside normal office hours and in nonclinical locations, engaging in social or business relationships with patients, accepting gifts from patients, and engaging in nonsexual physical contact with patients (Epstein 1994; Gabbard 2009a). All of these violations carry the potential to exploit the patient or harm the treatment relationship and therefore should be avoided.

The term "boundary crossing" has been used to describe a subtle, nonsexual transgression that is helpful to the patient because it advances the treatment (Gutheil and Gabbard 1998). As an example of a boundary crossing, Gabbard (2009a) described the situation of a guarded, paranoid patient who offered her psychiatrist a cookie. By accepting this token gift graciously, the psychiatrist helped the patient feel more relaxed in the treatment setting and more willing to discuss her symptoms. Boundary crossings of this type are common and not unethical, but differentiating boundary crossings from boundary violations may be difficult in the course of treatment. In general, even though the patient is encouraged to share intimate feelings, thoughts, and memories in psychotherapy and in much of clinical care, the physician avoids such deeply personal disclosures, adopting instead a posture of neutrality that helps to ensure that the patient feels safe and that the interaction remains focused on patient well-being.

Confidentiality

Respect for the privacy of patients' personal information has been an established ethical duty of physicians for millennia. Hippocrates (2012) stated the ethical duty of confidentiality as follows: "What I may see or hear in the course of treatment…In regard to the life of men…I will keep to myself, holding such things to be shameful to be spoken about." Effective treatment—and, in particular, effective psychotherapy—would not be possible if patients did not feel free to disclose intensely personal information under the assumption of confidentiality.

From the standpoint of U.S. law, doctor–patient confidentiality is a legal privilege granted to patients. The privilege requires physicians to keep patient information private unless the physician is legally compelled to make a disclosure or the patient waives the privilege. Although this seems straightforward in theory, there are many gray areas in which a physician's legal and ethical duties may conflict in practice. In remote rural settings where clinicians and patients are neighbors, friends, and relatives, confidentiality poses extraordinary challenges.

Specific protections for personal health information, including a higher level of protection for psychotherapy notes, were enacted with the Health Insurance Portability and Accountability Act of 1996. Differentiating between "medical care" and "psychotherapy" can be difficult, however. As psychotherapy notes are granted a higher level of privacy protection under the law, the APA recommends keeping the following types of information in psychotherapy notes separate from medical notes: "intimate personal content or facts; details of fantasies and dreams; process interactions; sensitive information about other individuals in the patient's life; the therapist's formulations, hypotheses, or speculations; topics/themes discussed in therapy sessions" (American Psychiatric Association Council on Psychiatry and the Law 2002, p. 1).

Several limits on confidentiality are recognized. Patients should be informed of limits to confidentiality when entering treatment (although there is disagreement about how best to enact this duty). Patients should not be asked to sign a blanket waiver of general consent to disclosure, because many patients would not want all of their personal mental health information disclosed to a third-party payer, for example. When patients consent to specific, limited disclosures of their information (e.g., for third-party payment or for a court proceeding), disclosure may occur. In these instances, the minimum amount of information necessary for the situation should be revealed—that is, a rigorously upheld "need to know" approach should be taken.

A nonconsenting patient may have the privilege of confidentiality suspended based on the physician's overriding duties to others. These situations typically involve child or elder abuse or threatened violence. The legal case of *Tarasoff v. Regents of the University of California* demonstrated the notion that psychiatrists have a "duty to protect" members of the public from the violent intentions of their patients.

In general, patients should reasonably be able to expect that the information they tell their psychiatrist or other mental health professional will be kept confidential and that disclosure will not occur without their consent. Unfortunately, several studies have shown that many patients are not informed about specific safeguards for their confidentiality and do not seek treatment out of fear about lack of confidentiality (Roberts and Dyer 2004).

In an era of EHRs, digitized medical information, passive data collection through digital applications, an "open notes" movement (in which patients increasingly have ready access to their entire medical record), and a push toward national health identifiers (Torous and Roberts 2017), it remains unclear whether, how, and to what degree special privacy protections for mental health treatment will continue to be guarded. A number of hospitals, clinics, and organizations have developed approaches for handling sensitive information in the medical record. For example, "lockbox" or "break the glass" approaches require special access for personnel viewing mental health records. Marking an electronic progress note as "sensitive," in most cases, will nevertheless allow numerous providers to access that record. Moreover, patients now have unprecedented access to their own medical charts, test results, and diagnoses as documented by providers through EHR systems. Providers who document in such systems should strive to understand who will have access to the patient's mental health records and to include only medically necessary information while strictly limiting content that is not relevant to the overall medical care of the patient. Ensuring privacy of genetic and genomic data stored electronically is another evolving issue that promises to raise new challenges related to confidentiality in psychiatric care (Hoge and Appelbaum 2012).

Informed Consent and Decision-Making Capacity

Informed consent is the process by which individuals make free, knowledgeable decisions about whether to accept a proposed plan for assessment and/or treatment. Informed consent is a cornerstone of ethical practice. The philosophical basis for informed consent is found in our societal and cultural respect for individual persons and affirmation of individuals' freedom of self-determination. An adequate process of informed consent therefore reflects and promotes the ethical principle of autonomy. Promoting autonomy alone without incorporating other ethical principles, however, fails to create an environment for true informed consent that enhances a patient's meaningful decision making. The principle of beneficence is also crucial. The clinician must thoroughly appraise to what degree the consent process meets the patient's need for information. The clinician must also appraise whether the patient has the opportunity to make a choice consistent with his or her authentic preferences and values (Roberts 2002b).

Informed consent is not just a legal requirement. Informed consent is part of an overall therapeutic relationship and an opportunity for respectful dialogue that may enhance the relationship and patient care. The informed consent process should consist of repeated opportunities, over time, to gather relevant clinical information and discuss and clarify patients' (and, when appropriate, families' or caregivers') values, preferences, informational needs, decisional abilities, and decision-making processes.

The phrase *decision-making capacity* differs from the term *competency* in that competency to perform a specific function or competency in a particular life domain is a legal determination made through a judicial or other legal process. Legal jurisdictions have differing standards for establishing competency (Appelbaum and Grisso 1995). *Decisional capacity* refers to a determination made by a clinical professional. Psychiatrists are often called upon to make determinations of the decisional capacity of nonpsychiatric patients. A detailed understanding of the concept of decisional capacity is therefore important for all psychiatrists and is especially crucial for those who perform consultation-liaison work and for those involved in the care of patients with disorders characterized by cognitive impairment (Bourgeois et al. 2017). Moreover, being able to explain and teach standards and strategies for assessing capacity to nonpsychiatric colleagues is a critical skill, as many clinicians have not been adequately trained to do even basic screening for capacity (Armontrout et al. 2016).

The use of surrogate consent, as well as the use of involuntary or court-mandated treatment, is predicated, in part, on the absence of intact decision-making capacity. Careful assessment of these component abilities is key in evaluating the appropriateness of seeking involuntary treatment for any patient. A patient who refuses treatment but whose understanding, appreciation, reasoning, and indication of a choice are adequate has the right to refuse treatment. An ill individual may thoroughly understand the medical facts presented by the clinicians but erroneously believe that those facts do not apply to his or her situation, thereby showing a lack of appreciation. For example, a man with a gangrenous foot may fully understand the facts about gangrene and its treatment, but he may refuse treatment because he believes that his foot is completely healthy.

It is important to remember that even patients who accept recommended treatment may do so while lacking adequate capacity for their decisions. Thus, although most consultation requests involve patient refusal of recommended treatment, there may be good reasons to carefully assess and document incapacity (or fluctuating capacity, as is frequently seen in hospitalized patients who develop delirium), and to seek consent from a surrogate decision maker, even in cases where a patient is accepting treatment (Owen et al. 2013). Although there is no clear index for deciding how stringent the standard for consent should be, a general rule of thumb is to use a "sliding scale" approach (Appelbaum 2007). Decisions involving higher risks or greater risk–benefit ratios generally require a more stringent standard for decisional capacity, whereas more routine, lower-risk decisions generally require a less rigorous standard for decisional capacity. For example, the standard for understanding the procedure, risks, benefits, and alternatives related to an invasive treatment (such as deep brain stimulation) should be substantially higher than the standard for a relatively low-risk treatment (such as selective serotonin reuptake inhibitor treatment).

Crucially, a judgment of capacity is independent of the patient's diagnosis and the severity of the illness. This is a key point to reemphasize to nonpsychiatric colleagues, who may assume that patients with psychiatric disorders lack capacity de facto. Patients with schizophrenia, bipolar disorder, mania, severe depression, or any other mental illness may possess or lack decisional capacity to accept or refuse a variety of procedures and treatments, from pharmacotherapy to electroconvulsive treatment. Although disease process, age, and cognitive functioning may substantially impair patients' abilities to make a fully informed, meaningful choice about treatment, empirical evidence suggests that many people with severe mental illness commonly have adequate ability to make treatment decisions (Okai et al. 2007). The physician must determine each patient's capacity to make a specific decision at the time of assessment. There is often a need to reassess capacity, which is best viewed not as a static trait but as a trait that fluctuates over time.

When an individual is deemed to lack decisional ability, a surrogate or alternative decision maker is asked to make choices on behalf of that person. Psychiatric advance directives may be useful for persons with mental illnesses that cause fluctuating or progressive impairment. For example, a patient with a history of recurrent psychosis may create an advance directive requesting hospitalization and involuntary medication treatment if he or she becomes incapable of making decisions during a future relapse. Psychiatric advance directives potentially allow patients with severe and relapsing mental illnesses to maintain control over their treatment during periods of incapacity. Advance directives are used only when patients lack decisional capacity, however, and patients can change their advance directives at any time.

Working Therapeutically in the Ethical Use of Power

The psychiatrist holds a position of power. This power not only stems from the psychiatrist's professional education and consequent privileges, but also from special powers granted to the psychiatrist by the state, which include the ability to involuntarily hospitalize patients and the ability to act as a gatekeeper to health care services, such as prescribed medication. By contrast, most patients enter psychiatric treatment at a time of great personal vulnerability. Additionally, psychiatric disorders may impair patients' abilities to reason, feel, and behave in an effective manner. The highly unequal power relationship between the psychiatrist and the patient can leave the weaker party, the patient, less able to identify and advocate for his or her interests and thus more vulnerable to exploitation.

The most egregious ethical violations in the history of psychiatry have been blatant abuses of power. Some abuses of power have involved individual sociopathic practitioners who exploited their patients for financial gain, sexual gratification, or sadistic pleasure. Other abuses of power have involved entire communities of psychiatrists who have allowed their skills and legal powers to be misused to harm patients. In Nazi Germany, psychiatrists killed thousands of patients in mental hospitals in the name of eugenic goals. Psychiatrists in the Soviet Union in the previous century diagnosed political dissidents with dubious "mental disorders" and subjected them to unnecessary treatments, including long-term involuntary hospitalization. Recently, similar allegations have been made against psychiatrists in several European countries (e.g., Belgium, the Netherlands), where a new unethical practice of euthanasia and assisted suicide for treatable psychiatric disorders is emerging (e.g., Kim et al. 2016; Thienpont et al. 2015).

Psychiatrists, like other physicians, are entrusted with the responsibility of judging when involuntary treatment may be necessary to protect the health and safety of a person affected by mental illness. Many important ethical issues surround this use of power, for example, via involuntary hospitalization, outpatient commitment, or involuntary medication treatment for patients whose mental illness makes them a danger to themselves or others. Involuntary treatment is a clear example of conflicting ethical principles: the obligation to respect patient autonomy and the obligation of beneficence (see Table 7–2). Choosing not to override a patient's refusal of treatment would demonstrate respect for patient autonomy, but blind adherence to a patient's wishes may not be ethically justifiable and may, in fact, cause harm. For the suicidal patient who refuses hospitalization, the patient who expresses homicidal ideas, or the patient whose mental illness seriously jeopardizes his or her safety, for example, involuntary treatment may be necessary and justifiable.

Wise practitioners will reflect on the following sequence in ethically high-risk situations.

- Understand treatment refusal as a possible expression of distress.
- Ascertain the reasons for refusal.
- Allow the patient to discuss his or her preferences and fears.
- Explain the reason for the intervention in simple language.
- Offer options for the disposition of treatment.
- Appropriately enlist the assistance of family and friends.
- Request support from nursing and support staff.
- Assess decisional capacity and, if necessary, have recourse to the courts.
- Attend to side effects—both long and short term, serious and bothersome.
- Employ emergency treatment options where available.
- Work to preserve the therapeutic alliance.
- Utilize treatment guardians (i.e., legally appointed alternate decision makers, sometimes called guardians or conservators) where appropriate.

Patient Abandonment

According to accepted ethical standards in medicine, physicians are "free to choose whom to serve" (American Psychiatric Association 2013). Once an ongoing doctor–patient relationship has been established, however, the physician may not ethically abandon the patient. As a practical matter, nonabandonment means that the psychiatrist must arrange for clinical coverage when he or she is on vacation and must give adequate notice to patients when closing his or her practice (American Psychiatric Association 2017). It is not considered patient abandonment to transfer a patient's care to another physician if the treating psychiatrist is not able to provide necessary care and if the situation is not an emergency. A transfer of care may occur because the treating physician is not trained in the therapeutic modality that the patient needs or because, despite diligent work, it has not been possible to form or repair a therapeutic alliance. Nevertheless, psychiatrists must be aware that a covert, even unconscious form of patient abandonment may occur when countertransference issues or burnout causes a psychiatrist to subtly encourage a difficult patient to leave treatment. Self-reflective clinicians who recognize this pattern can support their patients by seeking consultation or supervision (Roberts and Dyer 2004).

Managing Overlapping Roles and Potential Conflicts of Interest

In addition to their roles as clinicians, psychiatrists take on a variety of roles in the medical community and in society (e.g., as educators of medical students and residents, administrators of academic programs and health care systems, clinical researchers and basic scientists, and consultants to industry). Because the ethical duties required by one role may not align precisely with the ethical duties of another role, psychiatrists in multiple roles often face ethical binds. Conflicts of interest that arise are not necessarily unethical but must be managed in a way that allows the psychiatrist to fulfill expectations of professionalism and maintain a fiduciary relationship with patients.

There are many strategies for helping to ensure that conflicts between roles do not distort the judgment of professionals. Strategies include disclosure and documentation; focused, more intensive supervision and oversight committees; retrospective review; financial disclosure; role recusal; and other safeguards (Roberts 2016).

Financial conflicts of interest pertaining to patient care represent a significant threat to the integrity of the profession of medicine. The most obviously unacceptable conflicts of interest include those in which physicians have a clear-cut financial arrangement that could adversely influence the treatment of patients. For example, fee-splitting arrangements in which a psychiatrist is paid to refer patients to a consultant are unethical because the payment may compromise the psychiatrist's judgment about the clinical merits of the referral. Similarly, accepting bonuses from hospitals for referring patients may co-opt the physician's professional judgment. Physicians who work for managed care or accountable care organizations may also face conflicts of interest, for example, when plans or organizations provide incentives that encourage physicians to order less expensive treatments and tests or that constrain the number or types of treatments that can be offered. Guidelines for ethical practice in organized care settings established by the APA in 1997 require that managed-care psychiatrists disclose such incentives to patients (American Psychiatric Association 2001).

Currently, organizations within medicine differ in their approaches and guidelines for dealing with relationships with the pharmaceutical industry (Institute of Medicine 2009). At a minimum, psychiatrists should learn and work within the guidelines specified by their own organizations and work environments. Academic departments of psychiatry and psychiatric residency training programs increasingly play an important role in educating physicians about the ethical issues involved in relationships with the pharmaceutical industry.

Another type of conflict of interest, sometimes referred to as a "dual agency" situation, arises for psychiatrists who have additional professional duties that may not be fully congruent with their role as a physician. An extreme example is the forensic psychiatrist asked to evaluate an inmate on death row to determine whether the inmate is "sane enough" to be executed. In this instance, the forensic psychiatrist's first duty is to veracity—telling the truth—in the service of society above all other interests, including the interests of the individual being evaluated. In such a situation, it is essential that the forensic psychiatrist disclose the ethical obligations and limits of his or her role in relation to the interests of the individual being evaluated.

Ethical binds occur with many types of dual roles. Research psychiatrists who provide clinical care for their study volunteers may struggle to maintain the integrity of the doctor–patient relationship in the face of the demands of the research protocol. Similarly, medical trainees, supervisors, and administrative psychiatrists may find that their roles as students, teachers, and managers challenge their ability to put the needs of patients first (Roberts 2016). In public health settings, psychiatrists may find it challenging to balance fidelity to individual patients with the legitimate need to be good stewards of social resources and distribute them fairly. Managing these multiple roles requires physicians to recognize the potential for ethical binds, institute safeguards when possible, and fully inform patients (Roberts 2016).

Ethical Interactions With Colleagues and Trainees

As members of a profession, psychiatrists are expected to behave ethically toward their colleagues, both individually and collectively. The APA's *Principles of Medical Ethics* explicitly states that physicians should "respect the rights" of colleagues and "strive to report physicians deficient in character or competence, or engaging in fraud or deception, to appropriate entities" (American Psychiatric Association 2013). Although the first statement encourages collegial behavior, the second suggests the importance of self-governance in the medical professions and the need to report colleague misconduct and impairment.

Intervening in and reporting colleague misconduct or impairment are some of the most difficult ethical imperatives of the conscientious psychiatrist. When psychiatrists bring legitimate cases of physician misconduct to light, they fulfill the ideals of beneficence and nonmaleficence by protecting the physician's current and future patients. Nevertheless, a number of psychological barriers to reporting colleague impairment have been identified, including overidentification with the impaired physician, collusion with the colleague's denial and minimization, and a tendency to overvalue confidentiality and protect the colleague's reputation and career at the expense of safety (Roberts and Miller 2004).

To help psychiatrists overcome their reluctance to report problem behavior, Overstreet (2001) suggested a useful four-step procedure for working through the issue. First, the psychiatrist should become informed about the reporting requirements of his or her state. In some localities, physicians may experience legal penalties if they fail to report physician impairment. Second, the psychiatrist should seek to more fully understand the situation, including how his or her own feelings may complicate the ability both to observe the colleague's behavior objectively and to report it. Third, all of the options that fulfill the duty to "strive to expose" the misconduct should be considered. Just as there is a range of physician misbehaviors, there can be a range of appropriate responses. These may include speaking privately with the colleague, informing the colleague's supervisor or administrative chief, filing an ethics complaint with the district APA branch, and/or notifying the state licensing board. Finally, the psychiatrist should choose the most appropriate option or options as a first step, knowing that other options are available should the situation persist (Overstreet 2001).

It is important to note that the reporting physician is not expected to make a definitive judgment about whether or not a colleague is practicing competently. Worrisome professional behavior should be investigated by appropriate professional bodies such as the APA (American Psychiatric Association 2013) and state licensing boards. Furthermore, as a practical matter, an impaired physician may be greatly helped by the impetus to accept treatment. To that end, many states have enacted laws regarding physician impairment based on model legislation proposed by the American Medical Association Council on Mental Health. These statutes are designed to encourage appropriate treatment and rehabilitation rather than approaches that may be seen as merely punitive (Roberts 2016; Roberts and Dyer 2004).

The ethical obligations of psychiatric faculty toward trainees involve many of the same requirements as with colleagues, but with the added obligations of a "fiduciary-like" relationship (Mohamed et al. 2005). The relationship between an attending physician and a resident or medical student is similar to the doctor–patient relationship. In both relationships there is a power differential, the possibility of transference feelings, and, in some cases, the potential for the weaker party to be exploited. The propriety of sexual relationships between supervising physicians and trainees has therefore become increasingly controversial due to the potential negative impact on the trainee, on the patients whose care is being supervised, and on the training program as a whole.

Specific ethical issues arise in medical school and residency training because of the need for trainees to provide care that is beyond their current level of expertise. The third-year medical student who performs a lumbar puncture for the first time, the new intern responsible for evaluating the suicide risk of a patient in an emergency department, and the inexperienced resident with a severely regressed therapy patient, for example, must all provide medical care outside of their current zone of competence in order to learn skills that will benefit future patients. This process requires treating patients as a means to an end, a violation of the principle of respect for persons. Yet the thorough training of psychiatrists is clearly beneficent from a public health standpoint. Handling this ethical dilemma requires the informed consent of patients as willing participants in the educational setting as well as safeguards to ensure that trainees practice only marginally beyond their current capabilities and with adequate supervision (Roberts 2016).

Emerging Ethical Issues in Psychiatry

Genetic Testing and Other Biomarker Testing

While genetic testing and testing of other biomarkers (e.g., neuroimaging, electroencephalographic testing) have not become routine in clinical psychiatric practice, these emerging modalities are likely to raise ethical issues for psychiatrists in the near future. These issues will be related to autonomy (Does the patient fully comprehend and voluntarily agree to the testing?), beneficence (Would testing have clear benefits for the patient?), nonmaleficence (Are there any foreseeable harms to the patient from undergoing testing?), and justice (Is access to testing fair and nonexploitative of vulnerable populations?).

Psychiatric genetic testing may have a number of possible goals, including predictive testing, diagnostic testing, testing that may aid treatment decision making (e.g., pharmacogenomics testing), or testing to aid in reproductive decision making (Hoge and Appelbaum 2012). A 2011 review of studies that examined the perspectives of patients, family members, and psychiatrists regarding psychiatric genetic testing found strong interest in diagnostic and predictive testing among patients and family members, as well as substantial interest in predictive testing for offspring. Concerns about the possibility of discrimination based on genetic testing were also found, however (Lawrence and Appelbaum 2011).

Genetic testing may raise patients' and/or family members' expectations regarding diagnostic or predictive accuracy; thus, a robust informed consent process that highlights the limits of prediction of these tests is important. As genetic testing and other biomarker testing move from the bench to the clinic, and to direct-to-consumer platforms, psychiatrists will need to be versed in both the potential benefits and the potential negative impacts of these modalities. In general, psychiatrists do not view themselves as adequately prepared to review genetic test results with patients (Hoop et al. 2008b). Moreover, despite recommendations that patients and/or families who undergo genetic testing receive genetic counseling, psychiatrists appear to be less likely than other physicians to have access to referrals to genetic counseling for their patients (Costain et al. 2014).

In a small 2008 survey of psychiatrists regarding the probable impact of genetic testing on psychiatry, psychiatrists were generally optimistic about the clinical benefits of genetic testing for pharmacogenetics as well as diagnostic and susceptibility testing (Hoop et al. 2008a). These psychiatrists also strongly endorsed the importance of legal and ethical safeguards surrounding such testing, including informed consent, confidentiality, and pre- and posttest counseling. Interestingly, while psychiatrists strongly support laws aimed at preventing genetic discrimination (e.g., the Genetic Information Nondiscrimination Act, or GINA), it is unclear how well psychiatrists (either in practice or in training) understand the scope and the limitations of these laws. For example, GINA is aimed at preventing discrimination in terms of employment and health insurance but does not protect against discrimination for purposes of obtaining life insurance or long-term care insurance. As direct-to-consumer genetic testing becomes more available, psychiatrists should be aware of the limits on both confidentiality and legal protections when patients ask questions or bring in results for interpretation.

Social Media, Electronic Footprints, and Digital Health

Another emerging area of ethical significance for psychiatrists (and all medical professionals) is the maintenance of ethics and professionalism in the digital age. The Internet, e-mail, blogs, social networking, and other online media pose a number of new ethical challenges (Mostaghimi and Crotty 2011; Torous and Roberts 2017).

All psychiatrists need to make conscientious and informed choices about whether, how, what, and how much to interact and disclose online. Given that the majority of psychiatry trainees, and an increasing number of physicians, have social media accounts, outright avoidance or rejection of social media has become impractical. Moreover, these sites now play integral and positive roles for many physicians as facilitators of social interaction. Furthermore, if psychiatrists act carefully and proactively, they can maintain appropriate boundaries, ethics, and professionalism online. Suggested guidelines center on basic issues of trust, privacy, professional standards of conduct, and awareness of the potential implications of all digital content and interactions (Gabbard et al. 2011). Simply put, online expression should be viewed as "the new millennium's elevator," where psychiatrists have little control over who hears what they say (Mostaghimi and Crotty 2011, p. 561).

Additional ethical issues are emerging as digital medicine and digital health tools rapidly proliferate. For example, there are now apps to help patients self-monitor their symptoms, digital technologies for medication adherence tracking, and predictive analytics relevant to mental health. A recent study used machine-learning methods to build a model that predicted suicidal behavior from longitudinal EHRs (Barak-Corren et al. 2017). The ethical implications of such "big data" approaches in psychiatry have been minimally explored. While there may be numerous benefits of such approaches for population-level and individual health, other concerns (e.g., patient privacy and informed consent for EHR data mining) must be weighed alongside potential benefits.

From an ethical perspective, novel digital health tools ideally will be used as an adjuvant strategy in support of the goals of the therapeutic relationship (Torous and Roberts 2017). Modern psychiatric practitioners should become knowledgeable about the digital apps used and digital activities engaged in by their patients and discuss these tools with them, including potential value and potential liability. For instance, a patient may use a daily diary app that tracks symptoms and behaviors. This diary may be positively incorporated into the therapeutic process with the clinician. A patient may be uncertain or unaware, however, of how passive data collection through devices, apps, and programs may be encroaching upon his or her privacy; this topic may be important to consider because of its implications for the patient's security and well-being.

Future Directions

For the past several decades, major topics of ethical reflection in psychiatry have included traditional topics such as boundary issues in psychotherapy, informed consent, confidentiality, role conflicts, and involuntary treatment. More recently, several new avenues for ethical inquiry have opened as new diagnostic and therapeutic modalities have been invented. First, technological advances continue to create new and unforeseen ethical challenges. For example, scientific advances in genomics and genetics, neuroscience, neuroimaging, biomarker testing, digital health tools, and data analytics, to name a few, are bringing new technologies for diagnosing predisposition to neuropsychiatric conditions, evaluating current levels of symptoms, and even predicting future behavior and risk of disease. Both the risks and the benefits of such advances could be substantial, and empirical and conceptual ethics research is needed to guide proper usage.

Second, the severe shortage of psychiatrists, the shortage of psychiatric inpatient and outpatient services, and the numerous pressures on psychiatrists to meet greater needs with fewer resources represent a trend with important ethical implications and both financial and political roots. From 1998 to 2013, the United States experienced a 35% decrease in the number of psychiatric beds (i.e., from 34 to 22 beds per 100,000 population). Meanwhile, the suicide rate increased 24% between 1999 and 2014 (Bastiampillai et al. 2016). Furthermore, despite parity laws, in community settings in the United States, low Medicare and Medicaid reimbursement rates for psychiatric procedures coupled with reductions in funding for the uninsured have placed extreme pressures on psychiatrists to provide ethical, clinically appropriate care to large inpatient caseloads within relatively brief outpatient appointments (Gabbard 2009b).

Clinical psychiatry, in sum, is ethically laden and ethically rich work. In the professional life of a psychiatrist, ethics helps to inform and shape day-to-day choices, including not only the decisions surrounding clearly problematic situations such as involuntary treatment but also the routine decisions of clinical practice. In this work, serving the well-being and interests of patients must take precedence over other concerns, and adherence to ethical standards of the field is essential; these are the requirements of professionalism. Through each of these actions, and through our ongoing attempts to become more discerning, more self-aware, and more respectful, we embody ethics for our patients and as an expression of our profession.

Key Clinical Points

- Cultivating an understanding of ethics is vital to providing competent clinical care as well as fulfilling the varied duties and roles of a psychiatrist.

- Ethical conduct is an expression of professionalism that is grounded in service to others in society.

- Central ethics skills include the ability to identify ethical issues as they arise; the ability to understand how one's personal values, beliefs, and sense of self may affect clinical care practices; an awareness of the limits of one's medical knowledge and expertise and a willingness to practice within those limits; the ability to recognize high-risk situations; the willingness to seek information and consultation appropriately and make use of obtained guidance; and the foresight to build safeguards into one's clinical work.

- Physician well-being is an ethical imperative in medicine. Failure to attend to personal well-being can lead to many adverse consequences for patients and health professionals. Positive self-care by physicians is linked with improved patient care practices and greater professional fulfillment.

- Maintenance of therapeutic boundaries is an ethical as well as a clinical responsibility in the care of patients.

- Boundary violations are actions by the psychiatrist that are outside usual professional limits and that may harm patients. Sexual relationships with patients are boundary violations and are not permissible, as noted in the APA ethics guidelines.

- Informed consent is an ethically and legally fundamental aspect of psychiatric practice and essential to psychiatrists' obligation to respect patient autonomy to make unconstrained, knowledgeable decisions about their own care whenever possible.

- Involuntary treatment is an example of an ethically complex area in which the obligations of respecting patient autonomy and of seeking to do good and avoid harm are often in conflict.

- Confidentiality is a patient privilege that requires physicians to keep patient information private unless the patient waives the privilege or the physician is compelled by law to disclose information; confidentiality in the electronic era is extraordinarily challenging.

- Conflicting roles and interests are encountered by physicians throughout medicine and may undermine public trust in the profession.

- The reporting of suspected misconduct or impairment is an ethical duty of members of a profession.

- Remaining mindful of ethical obligations toward trainees is an important ethical responsibility of supervising psychiatrists.

- Newly emerging diagnostic and therapeutic modalities in psychiatry will pose many ethical challenges in the future; attentiveness to these issues and commitment to the well-being and interests of patients and others in society will help ensure that psychiatrists will address the dilemmas of the future in accordance with the aims of the profession.

References

American Psychiatric Association: Ethics Primer of the American Psychiatric Association. Washington, DC, American Psychiatric Association, 2001

American Psychiatric Association: The Principles of Medical Ethics With Annotations Applicable to Psychiatry, 2013 Edition. Washington, DC, American Psychiatric Association, 2013. Available at: https://www.psychiatry.org/File%20Library/Psychiatrists/Practice/Ethics/principles-medical-ethics.pdf. Accessed March 7, 2018.

American Psychiatric Association: Opinions of the Ethics Committee on The Principles of Medical Ethics. Washington, DC, American Psychiatric Association, 2017. Available at: https://www.psychiatry.org/File%20Library/Psychiatrists/Practice/Ethics/Opinions-of-the-Ethics-Committee.pdf. Accessed March 7, 2018.

American Psychiatric Association Council on Psychiatry and the Law: Resource Document on Psychotherapy Notes Provision of the Health Insurance Portability and Accountability Act (HIPAA) Privacy Rule. APA Official Actions. Washington, DC, American Psychiatric Association, 2002

Appelbaum PS: Clinical practice. Assessment of patients' competence to consent to treatment. N Engl J Med 357(18):1834–1840, 2007 17978292

Appelbaum PS, Grisso T: The MacArthur Competence Study, III: abilities of patients to consent to psychiatric and medical treatments. Law Hum Behav 19(2):149–174, 1995 11660292

Armontrout J, Gitlin D, Gutheil T: Do consultation psychiatrists, forensic psychiatrists, psychiatry trainees, and health care lawyers differ in opinion on gray area decision-making capacity cases? A vignette-based survey. Psychosomatics 57(5):472–479, 2016 27400660

Baker K, Sen S: Healing medicine's future: prioritizing physician trainee mental health. AMA J Ethics 18(6):604–613, 2016 27322994

Barak-Corren Y, Castro VM, Javitt S, et al: Predicting suicidal behavior from longitudinal electronic health records. Am J Psychiatry 174(2):154–162, 2017 27609239

Baruth JM, Lapid MI: Influence of psychiatric symptoms on decisional capacity in treatment refusal. AMA J Ethics 19(5):416–425, 2017 28553898

Bastiampillai T, Sharfstein SS, Allison S: Increase in US suicide rates and the critical decline in psychiatric beds. JAMA 316(24):2591–2592, 2016 27812693

Bourgeois JA, Cohen MA, Erickson JM, et al: Decisional and dispositional capacity determinations: neuropsychiatric illness and an integrated clinical paradigm. Psychosomatics 58(6):565–573, 2017 28734555

Brady KJS, Trockel MT, Khan CT, et al: What do we mean by physician wellness? A systematic review of its definition and measurement. Acad Psychiatry 42(1):94–108, 2018 28913621

Brown SD, Goske MJ, Johnson CM: Beyond substance abuse: stress, burnout, and depression as causes of physician impairment and disruptive behavior. J Am Coll Radiol 6(7):479–485, 2009 19560063

Costain G, Esplen MJ, Toner B, et al: Evaluating genetic counseling for individuals with schizophrenia in the molecular age. Schizophr Bull 40(1):78–87, 2014 23236078

Dyrbye L, Shanafelt T: A narrative review on burnout experienced by medical students and residents. Med Educ 50(1):132–149, 2016 26695473

Dyrbye LN, West CP, Satele D, et al: Burnout among U.S. medical students, residents, and early career physicians relative to the general U.S. population. Acad Med 89(3):443–451, 2014 24448053

Epstein RS: Psychological characteristics of therapists who commit serious boundary violations, in Keeping Boundaries: Maintaining Safety and Integrity in the Psychotherapeutic Process. Washington, DC, American Psychiatric Press, 1994, pp 239–254

Gabbard GO: Boundary violations, in Psychiatric Ethics, 4th Edition. Edited by Bloch S, Green SA. New York, Oxford University Press, 2009a, pp 251–270

Gabbard GO: Deconstructing the "med check." Psychiatric Times 26(9), 2009b. Available at: http://www.psychiatrictimes.com/articles/deconstructing-"med-check". Accessed March 7, 2018.

Gabbard GO, Kassaw KA, Perez-Garcia G: Professional boundaries in the era of the internet. Acad Psychiatry 35(3):168–174, 2011 21602438

Gengoux GW, Roberts LW: Enhancing wellness and engagement among healthcare professionals. Acad Psychiatry 42(1):1–4, 2018 29297148

Gutheil TG, Gabbard GO: Misuses and misunderstandings of boundary theory in clinical and regulatory settings. Am J Psychiatry 155(3):409–414, 1998 9501754

Hippocrates: The oath, in Internet Encyclopedia of Philosophy: Hippocrates (c. 450–c. 380 B.C.E.), 2012. Available at: http://www.iep.utm.edu/hippocra/#SH2a. Accessed March 7, 2018.

Hoge SK, Appelbaum PS: Ethics and neuropsychiatric genetics: a review of major issues. Int J Neuropsychopharmacol 15(10):1547–1557, 2012 22272758

Hoop JG, Roberts LW, Green Hammond KA, et al: Psychiatrists' attitudes regarding genetic testing and patient safeguards: a preliminary study. Genet Test 12(2):245–252, 2008a 18452395

Hoop JG, Roberts LW, Hammond KA, Cox NJ: Psychiatrists' attitudes, knowledge, and experience regarding genetics: a preliminary study. Genet Med 10(6):439–449, 2008b 18496226

Institute of Medicine: Conflict of Interest in Medical Research, Education, and Practice. Washington, DC, National Academies Press, 2009. Available at: https://www.nap.edu/catalog/12598/conflict-of-interest-in-medical-research-education-and-practice. Accessed March 7, 2018.

Ishak WW, Lederer S, Mandili C, et al: Burnout during residency training: a literature review. J Grad Med Educ 1(2):236–242, 2009 21975985

Jain S, Dunn LB, Warner CH, et al: Results of a multisite survey of U.S. psychiatry residents on education in professionalism and ethics. Acad Psychiatry 35(3):175–183, 2011 21602439

Jonsen AR, Siegler M, Winslade WJ: Clinical Ethics, 6th Edition. New York, McGraw-Hill, 2006

Kim SYH, De Vries RG, Peteet JR: Euthanasia and assisted suicide of patients with psychiatric disorders in the Netherlands 2011 to 2014. JAMA Psychiatry 73(4):362–368, 2016 26864709

Lawrence RE, Appelbaum PS: Genetic testing in psychiatry: a review of attitudes and beliefs. Psychiatry 74(4):315–331, 2011 22168293

Lyubomirsky S, Sheldon KM, Schkade D: Pursuing happiness: the architecture of sustainable change. Review of General Psychology 9(2):111–131, 2005

MacKinnon M, Murray S: Reframing physician burnout as an organizational problem: a novel pragmatic approach to physician burnout. Acad Psychiatry 42(1):123–128, 2018 28247366

Maslach C, Jackson SE: The measurement of experienced burnout. Journal of Organizational Behavior 2(2):99–113, 1981

McMurray JE, Linzer M, Konrad TR, et al: The work lives of women physicians results from the physician work life study. J Gen Intern Med 15(6):372–380, 2000 10886471

Mohamed M, Punwani M, Clay M, et al: Protecting the residency training environment: a resident's perspective on the ethical boundaries in the faculty-resident relationship. Acad Psychiatry 29(4):368–373, 2005 16223900

Mostaghimi A, Crotty BH: Professionalism in the digital age. Ann Intern Med 154(8):560–562, 2011 21502653

National Council Medical Director Institute: The Psychiatric Shortage: Causes and Solutions. March 28, 2017. Available at: https://www.thenationalcouncil.org/wp-content/uploads/2017/03/Psychiatric-Shortage_National-Council-.pdf. Accessed February 14, 2018.

Okai D, Owen G, McGuire H, et al: Mental capacity in psychiatric patients: Systematic review. Br J Psychiatry 191(4):291–297, 2007 17906238

Overstreet MM: Duty to report colleagues who engage in fraud of deception, in Ethics Primer of the American Psychiatric Association. Washington, DC, American Psychiatric Association, 2001, pp 51–56

Owen GS, Szmukler G, Richardson G, et al: Decision-making capacity for treatment in psychiatric and medical in-patients: cross-sectional, comparative study. Br J Psychiatry 203(6):461–467, 2013 23969482

Parks T: Report reveals severity of burnout by specialty. AMA Wire, January 31, 2017. Available at: https://wire.ama-assn.org/life-career/report-reveals-severity-burnout-specialty. Accessed February 14, 2018.

Raj KS: Well-being in residency: a systematic review. J Grad Med Educ 8(5):674–684, 2016 28018531

Rasmussen V, Turnell A, Butow P, et al: Burnout among psychosocial oncologists: an application and extension of the effort-reward imbalance model. Psychooncology 25(2):194–202, 2016 26239424

Roberts LW: Ethics as endeavor in psychiatry: principles, skills, and evidence. Psychiatric Times 19(12):33–34, 36, 2002a

Roberts LW: Informed consent and the capacity for voluntarism. Am J Psychiatry 159(5):705–712, 2002b 11986120

Roberts LW: Caring for people in small communities, in Concise Guide to Ethics in Mental Health Care. Edited by Roberts LW, Dyer AR. Washington, DC, American Psychiatric Publishing, 2004, pp 167–184

Roberts LW: A Clinical Guide to Psychiatric Ethics. Arlington, VA, American Psychiatric Publishing, 2016

Roberts LW, Dyer AR: Concise Guide to Ethics in Mental Health Care. Washington, DC, American Psychiatric Publishing, 2004

Roberts LW, Miller MN: Ethical issues in clinician health, in Concise Guide to Ethics in Mental Health Care. Edited by Roberts LW, Dyer AR. Washington, DC, American Psychiatric Publishing, 2004, pp 233–242

Robertson SL, Robinson MD, Reid A: Electronic health record effects on work-life balance and burnout within the I^3 population collaborative. J Grad Med Educ 9(4):479–484, 2017 28824762

Rupert PA, Miller AO, Dorociak KE: Preventing burnout: what does the research tell us? Professional Psychology: Research and Practice 46(3):168–174, 2015

Schrijver I, Brady KJ, Trockel M: An exploration of key issues and potential solutions that impact physician wellbeing and professional fulfillment at an academic center. PeerJ 4:e1783, 2016 26989621

Seligman MEP, Steen TA, Park N, et al: Positive psychology progress: empirical validation of interventions. Am Psychol 60(5):410–421, 2005 16045394

Shanafelt TD, Balch CM, Bechamps G, et al: Burnout and medical errors among American surgeons. Ann Surg 251(6):995–1000, 2010 19934755

Shanafelt TD, Boone S, Tan L, et al: Burnout and satisfaction with work-life balance among US physicians relative to the general US population. Arch Intern Med 172(18):1377–1385, 2012 22911330

Shanafelt TD, Hasan O, Dyrbye LN, et al: Changes in burnout and satisfaction with work-life balance in physicians and the general US working population between 2011 and 2014. Mayo Clin Proc 90(12):1600–1613, 2015 26653297

Shenoy A, Appel JM: Safeguarding confidentiality in electronic health records. Camb Q Healthc Ethics 26(2):337–341, 2017 28361730

Siegrist J: Adverse health effects of high-effort/low-reward conditions. J Occup Health Psychol 1(1):27–41, 1996 9547031

Smith TM: Ethics of physician wellbeing: what the AMA code says. AMA Wire, April 12, 2017. Available at: https://wire.ama-assn.org/life-career/ethics-physician-wellbeing-what-ama-code-says. Accessed February 14, 2018.

Thienpont L, Verhofstadt M, Van Loon T, et al: Euthanasia requests, procedures and outcomes for 100 Belgian patients suffering from psychiatric disorders: a retrospective, descriptive study. BMJ Open 5(7):e007454, 2015 26216150

Torous J, Roberts LW: The ethical use of mobile health technology in clinical psychiatry. J Nerv Ment Dis 205(1):4–8, 2017 28005647

Weiner S: Addressing the escalating psychiatrist shortage. AAMC News, February 13, 2018. Available at: https://news.aamc.org/patient-care/article/addressing-escalating-psychiatrist-shortage/. Accessed February 28, 2018.

Recommended Readings

American Psychiatric Association: Ethics Primer of the American Psychiatric Association. Washington, DC, American Psychiatric Association, 2001

American Psychiatric Association: Opinions of the Ethics Committee on The Principles of Medical Ethics. Washington, DC, American Psychiatric Association, 2009

American Psychiatric Association: The Principles of Medical Ethics With Annotations Applicable to Psychiatry, 2013 Edition. Washington, DC, American Psychiatric Association, 2013

Appelbaum PS, Grisso T: Assessing patients' capacities to consent to treatment. N Engl J Med 319:1635–1638, 1988

Beauchamp TL, Childress JF: Principles of Biomedical Ethics, 6th Edition. New York, Oxford University Press, 2008

Emanuel EJ, Wendler D, Grady C: What makes clinical research ethical? JAMA 283:2701–2711, 2000

Grisso T, Appelbaum PS, Hill-Fotouhi C: The MACCAT-T: a clinical tool to assess patients' capacities to make treatment decisions. Psychiatr Serv 48:1415–1419, 1997

Jonsen AR, Siegler M, Winslade WJ: Clinical Ethics, 6th Edition. New York, McGraw-Hill, 2006

Roberts LW, Dyer AR: Concise Guide to Ethics in Mental Health Care. Washington, DC, American Psychiatric Publishing, 2004

Roberts LW, Mines J, Voss C, et al: Assessing medical students' competence in obtaining informed consent. Am J Surg 178:351–355, 1999

Roberts LW, Geppert CM, Bailey R: Ethics in psychiatric practice: essential ethics skills, informed consent, the therapeutic relationship, and confidentiality. J Psychiatr Pract 8:290–305, 2002

Roberts LW: A Clinical Guide to Psychiatric Ethics. Washington, DC, American Psychiatric Association Publishing, 2016

Roberts LW, Reicherter D: Professionalism and Ethics in Medicine: A Study Guide for Physicians and Physicians-in-Training. New York, Springer, 2015

Roberts LW, Hoop JG: Professionalism and Ethics: Q & A Self-Study Guide for Mental Health Professionals. Washington, DC, American Psychiatric Association Publishing, 2008

Rubenstein L, Pross C, Davidoff F, et al: Coercive US interrogation policies: a challenge to medical ethics. JAMA 294:1544–1549, 2005

Schouten R: Impaired physicians: is there a duty to report to state licensing boards? Harv Rev Psychiatry 8:26–39, 2000

Online Resources

American Medical Association Principles of Medical Ethics: https://www.ama-assn.org/delivering-care/ama-principles-medical-ethics

American Medical Association Virtual Mentor, Ethics Education Resources: http://virtualmentor.ama-assn.org/

APA Ethics Resources and Standards: http://www.psychiatry.org/practice/ethics/resources-standards

CHAPTER 8

Legal Considerations in Psychiatry

Michael Kelly, M.D.

Anne McBride, M.D.

John Hearn, M.D.

The codification of legal concepts is almost as old as civilization itself. Distinctions between civil and criminal law can be traced back to ancient Mesopotamia, where the Code of Ur-Nammu (~2100 B.C.) and Code of Hammurabi (~1800 B.C.) addressed issues as disparate as capital punishment (e.g., "an eye for an eye, a tooth for a tooth"), theft, fair wages, and divorce. In the United States today, the law is broadly divided into two categories. Whereas the civil code aims to settle disagreements between private parties (e.g., disputed business deals, financial compensation for personal injury), the criminal code serves to hold people accountable for actions deemed unlawful through a system of punishment. The juvenile justice system is built on a foundation of rehabilitation for minors who break the law. Several levels of court systems (e.g., superior courts, appellate courts, state supreme courts) make up the U.S. legal system at the federal and state level. The application of the law, standards of evidence, and potential damages and punishments vary depending on jurisdiction (e.g., federal vs. state) and whether a case involves civil or criminal matters.

Psychiatry and the U.S. Legal System

The U.S. legal system is largely rooted in British common law, developed in the eleventh century as a means to apply the "king's justice" across different territories. Seventeenth-century British common law is also where the Western notion of criminal intent, or *mens rea*, took root. The concept of *mens rea* had a profound impact on criminal proceedings in that the unlawful act itself, the *actus reus*, could be mitigated, and in some cases voided entirely, on the basis of a defendant's apparent degree of *mens rea* or lack thereof. (A Glossary of Legal Terms is provided in the Appendix to this chapter.)

The U.S. legal system intersects with the field of psychiatry in a multitude of ways. American psychiatrist Isaac Ray was one of the first to consider the moral and legal implications of a defendant's mental state at the time of a crime. In his landmark work, *Treatise on the Medical Jurisprudence of Insanity,* Ray (1838) characterized the ways in which a defendant's ability to distinguish right from wrong might be influenced by underlying mental illness. In a famous instance of cross-pollination between American ideas and British common law, Dr. Ray's work was quoted extensively in the 1843 trial of Daniel M'Naghten.

Daniel M'Naghten, a Scotsman from Glasgow, was by all accounts a highly competent and successful woodturner. Mr. M'Naghten sold his business in 1840 and eventually moved to London. Around this time, he began to report that he was being persecuted by members of the conservative Tory Party. Mr. M'Naghten's mental state eventually devolved into a delusional belief system centered on the notion that he was being persecuted by then–British prime minister Robert Peel. Mr. M'Naghten ultimately attempted to shoot Prime Minister Peel and in the process killed Peel's personal secretary, Edward Drummond. Mr. M'Naghten's attorneys, with the aid of Dr. Isaac Ray's writings, successfully argued that Mr. M'Naghten was "not guilty on the ground of insanity." Mr. M'Naghten was subsequently committed to the State Lunatic Asylum at Bethlem Royal Hospital, where he lived out the rest of his days. Widespread public backlash over this ruling led Queen Victoria to charge lawmakers with creating a set of standards by which an individual could be found legally insane. They eventually settled on the following criteria: "To establish a defence on the ground of insanity, it must be clearly proved that at the time of the committing of the act, the party accused was labouring under such a defect of reason, from disease of the mind, as not to know the nature and quality of the act he was doing; or, if he did know it, that he did not know he was doing what was wrong" (*M'Naghten's Case* 1843).

The "M'Naghten standard," as it is often called, established enduring legal principles that form the basis of many state sanity statutes today. Under this standard, a mentally ill defendant may demonstrate his insanity by meeting at least one of two criteria. First, a person may be unable to know the nature and quality of the act (e.g., someone is so disorganized that they are unaware of their actions). Alternately, a mentally ill defendant may argue that because of a mental illness, he was unable to distinguish right from wrong (e.g., killing someone on the basis of a delusional belief that the defendant was saving the world from destruction). Although the M'Naghten standard is by no means a common clinical concern for most psychiatrists, it has had a substantial impact on the U.S. criminal justice system and how mental health professionals are used by the courts.

Clinical Practice and the Law

Every practicing psychiatrist should understand the law as it relates to negligence, confidentiality and privilege, mandated reporting, informed consent, the duty to protect, and medicolegal aspects of institutionalized care, among others. What follows is a brief overview of these topics and the landmark legal cases that serve to guide practicing psychiatrists. For a brief summary of these important clinical concepts, please refer to Table 8–1.

TABLE 8–1.   **Clinical pearls and associated case law**

Term	Definition
Confidentiality and privilege	*Confidentiality* refers to a patient's right and the physician's duty to keep all information obtained during the course of treatment private. *Privilege* describes a patient's right to prevent his or her treatment provider from being compelled to disclose information provided in confidence to a court or some other entity. Thus, privilege falls within the patient's dominion and may be waived at his or her discretion. However, there are some notable exceptions to both confidentiality and privilege.
Mandated reporting	Standards vary across jurisdictions, but most require that a psychiatrist demonstrate a reasonable suspicion that a vulnerable person (e.g., child, elderly individual, or developmentally disabled adult) has been abused and/or neglected.
Informed consent	American courts have ruled that competent patients are entitled to make voluntary, knowing (i.e., based on relevant information), and intelligent (competent) health care decisions. In practical terms, patients or their substitute decision makers should be told about potential risks, benefits, prognosis (*with and without treatment*), and alternative treatments (*risks and benefits*) to make informed decisions.
Duty to protect	After a series of lengthy legal battles, the California Supreme Court ruled in *Tarasoff v. Regents of the University of California* (1976) that a therapist has a duty to protect a potential victim from foreseeable danger. Justice Mathew O. Tobriner succinctly summed up the court's opinion by writing, "The protective privilege ends where the public peril begins."
Civil commitment	Involuntary civil commitment is generally reserved only for those individuals at risk of self-harm or harm to others or those who are gravely disabled.
Right to treatment	The rulings in *Wyatt v. Stickney* (1971) and *Youngberg v. Romeo* (1982) outlined the minimally adequate standards of care afforded to civilly committed persons while acknowledging the states' interests in running mental health facilities.
Right to refuse treatment	The contrasting models outlined in *Rennie v. Klein* (1983) and *Rogers v. Commissioner of Department of Mental Health* (1983) have shaped the process by which jurisdictions across the United States handle treatment refusal in locked settings. Unlike the decision in *Rennie v. Klein*, which largely deferred to medical decision makers, *Rogers* gave judges great discretion in determining patients' wishes.
Expert versus fact witness	Given the potential conflicts of interest, clinicians who take on an expert witness role for one of their patients run the risk of presenting actual or potential bias as a result of their dual role.
Suicidal patients	Courts do not expect that psychiatrists will be able to predict whether a patient will complete or attempt suicide; however, standard of care necessitates that psychiatrists perform and document a competent suicide risk assessment.
Violence risk	Although there is no expectation that a psychiatrist will accurately predict whether a patient will become violent toward others, standard of care dictates that a psychiatrist perform competent violence risk assessments.
Subpoenas	In general, the first step a clinician should take after receiving a subpoena is to seek advice from his or her institutional or personal legal counsel.

TABLE 8–1.	Clinical pearls and associated case law *(continued)*
Term	**Definition**
Sexual misconduct	Psychiatrists who engage in sexual misconduct or other forms of grossly unprofessional behavior are at risk for civil liability, professional disciplinary actions, and criminal prosecution.
Dual agency	Ethical guidelines strongly discourage psychiatrists from taking the role of treatment provider and court expert with the same patient.

Negligence

In professional malpractice cases, negligence is associated with the "four D's." The four D's are duty of care (e.g., the doctor–patient relationship), dereliction of duty (e.g., failing to meet an accepted standard of care), direct cause (e.g., the injury to patient occurred as a direct result of the physician's actions), and damages (e.g., personal injury, psychic harm, or death). Put another way, negligence requires a "dereliction of duty directly causing damages" (Sadoff 1975). Professional negligence is commonly referred to as *malpractice.* Malpractice cases are tried in civil rather than criminal court. For a psychiatrist to be deemed negligent, plaintiffs must demonstrate that each aspect of the four D's was committed by a preponderance of evidence (i.e., more likely than not).

A study in the *New England Journal of Medicine* (Jena et al. 2011, p. 629) reviewed malpractice claims from 1991 through 2005 for "all physicians who were covered by a large professional liability insurer with a nationwide client base" and found that psychiatrists were the least likely medical specialty to be sued (i.e., 2.6% annually). A more recent study in *JAMA Internal Medicine* (Schaffer et al. 2017) revealed a rate of only 4.3 successful malpractice claims involving psychiatrists per 1,000 physicians from 1992 to 2014. Of note, the same study showed that more than half of the paid malpractice claims involving psychiatrists between 2004 and 2014 involved patient death. In fact, the leading cause of malpractice claims against psychiatrists is patient suicide (Scott and Resnick 2006).

Confidentiality and Privilege

Physicians are well acquainted with the concept of confidentiality. Simply put, *confidentiality* refers to a patient's right and the physician's duty to keep all information obtained during the course of treatment private. *Privilege* describes a patient's right to prevent his or her treatment provider (e.g., psychiatrist, primary care physician, psychologist) from being compelled to disclose information provided in confidence to a court or some other entity. Thus, privilege falls within the patient's dominion and may be waived at his or her discretion. However, there are some notable exceptions. Table 8–2 outlines some situations in which physicians may share a patient's personal health information without obtaining consent.

A number of landmark cases help to illustrate the ways in which patient information may be appropriately shared by psychiatrists. For example, the case of *In re Lifschutz* (1970) illustrates the distinction between confidentiality and privilege. In 1968, a San Francisco Bay Area high school physics teacher named Joseph Housek filed a lawsuit against one of his students at Burlingame High School. Mr. Housek claimed

---

TABLE 8–2.   Common exceptions to confidentiality and privilege

---

Mandatory reporting (e.g., cases of suspected child abuse and/or neglect, elder abuse)

Civil commitment of persons presenting a danger to themselves or others

A therapist's duty to protect a third party from a dangerous patient threatening harm

Criminal and civil proceedings where mental health issues have been raised by the defendant

Waiver

    A patient who signs a release of information has *explicitly* waived his or her right to privacy.

    A patient who asks to bring a significant other to a therapy session has *implicitly* waived his or her right to privilege.

    A patient has waived privilege when he or she is the plaintiff in a lawsuit that makes mental health the focus of litigation (e.g., files a lawsuit claiming psychological injury).

---

physical injuries, pain and suffering, and severe emotional distress after being hit in the jaw by the student. When the student's attorney learned that Mr. Housek had spent 6 months under the care of a psychiatrist (Dr. Joseph Lifschutz) 10 years prior to the incident in question, he subpoenaed Dr. Lifschutz and requested all of Mr. Housek's prior treatment records.

At the subsequent deposition, Dr. Lifschutz refused to acknowledge whether he had treated Mr. Housek and declined to turn over any previous treatment records. As a result, Dr. Lifschutz was held in contempt of court and subsequently spent a few days in the San Mateo County Jail. Dr. Lifschutz and his attorney (incidentally, the great-grandnephew of Dr. Sigmund Freud) claimed that psychotherapists held "absolute privilege," similar to that between a member of the clergy and a penitent. The Supreme Court of California took up the matter and concluded that "no constitutional right enables the psychotherapist to assert an absolute privilege concerning all psychotherapeutic communications." Dr. Lifschutz's stand, although unsuccessful, was pioneering in that it helped courts define the scope of confidentiality and privilege inherent to the therapist–patient relationship (Roberts 2017).

The case of *Doe v. Roe* (1977) played a major role in protecting patient confidentiality. A woman ("Ms. Doe") brought a lawsuit in the New York Supreme Court, New York County, because her previous psychiatrist ("Dr. Roe") published a book, without her consent, that included many details from their sessions. According to the case briefs, Dr. Roe's book "reported verbatim and extensively the patient's thoughts, feelings, emotions, fantasies, and biographies." Ms. Doe filed suit in the hopes of halting publication of the book and sought to receive compensation in the form of damages.

Adding insult to injury, Dr. Roe and her husband, a psychologist, claimed that their right to publication was protected under the First Amendment. Drs. Roe also declared that the publication's scientific merit transcended Ms. Doe's right to privacy. Fortunately for Ms. Doe and mental health professionals everywhere, the trial court sided with Ms. Doe, noting that "patients could only reveal their most intimate and socially unacceptable instincts and urges, immature wishes, and perverse sexual thoughts in an atmosphere of unusual trust." The court ordered that publication of the book should cease and awarded Ms. Doe $20,000 in compensatory damages. The court did not award Ms. Doe punitive damages because Dr. Roe and her husband's "acts were not willful, malicious or wanton—they were merely stupid."

In the case of *Jaffee v. Redmond* (1996), the U.S. Supreme Court was tasked to decide whether federal courts should uphold psychotherapist–patient privilege. During the summer of 1991, a police officer in suburban Chicago, Mary Lu Redmond, was first to respond to a disturbance at an apartment complex. Bystanders told Officer Redmond that a stabbing had occurred, prompting her to call for an ambulance. Moments later, several men emerged from the apartment, one of them brandishing a pipe. Another, Mr. Ricky Allan, brandished a butcher knife. Officer Redmond drew her service revolver and told Mr. Allan to put down the knife. He did not comply. Officer Redmond ultimately shot and killed Mr. Allan on the basis of her belief that he was about to stab another person.

In the aftermath of the shooting, Officer Redmond attended 50 therapy sessions with a licensed clinical social worker. The executor of Mr. Allan's estate filed a lawsuit in federal court claiming that Officer Redmond used excessive force during the incident in question. When Officer Redmond and her therapist refused to disclose her treatment records, citing psychotherapist–patient privilege, the trial judge ruled that Officer Redmond had no legal justification for withholding her records. The judge further explained to the jury that they were free to assume that the contents of the records would have portrayed Officer Redmond in an unfavorable light. The jury ultimately sided with Mr. Allan's executor and awarded his family $545,000.

The case was appealed and eventually reached the U.S. Supreme Court, which held that federal rules protected information disclosed to psychiatrists, psychologists, and licensed clinical social workers during the course of psychotherapy. Relying on amicus briefs from the American Psychiatric Association and the American Psychological Association, the court reasoned that effective psychotherapy is contingent on

> an atmosphere of confidence and trust in which the patient is willing to make a frank and complete disclosure of facts, emotions, memories, and fears. Because of the sensitive nature of the problems for which individuals consult psychotherapists, disclosure of confidential communications made during counseling sessions may cause embarrassment or disgrace. For this reason, the mere possibility of disclosure may impede development of the confidential relationship necessary for successful treatment.

Jaffee had a major impact on the creation of special protections afforded to psychotherapy notes under the *Health Insurance Portability and Accountability Act of 1996* (HIPAA; P.L. 104–191), requiring that they remain private.

HIPAA was implemented in 1996. With few exceptions, psychotherapy notes under HIPAA cannot be released without explicit authorization from the patient. Furthermore, insurers are prohibited from making treatment and/or payment contingent on whether psychotherapy notes are disclosed. Despite the appearance of added privacy afforded to psychotherapy notes by HIPAA, there is a fair amount of fine print worth mentioning (Appelbaum 2002; Brendel and Bryan 2004; Corley 2013). For instance, psychotherapy notes must be stored separately from the rest of a patient's medical records to qualify for added protections.

Corley's (2012) paper "Protection for Psychotherapy Notes Under the HIPAA Privacy Rule: As Private as a Hospital Gown" pointed out that "the definition of psychotherapy notes does not include a summary of diagnosis, symptoms, functional status, treatment plan, prognosis and progress, as well as type of treatment, frequency of treatment, counseling session start and stop times, clinical tests, and medication"

(p. 492). Thus, psychotherapy notes may not be as "protected" as many mental health providers believe. Although an in-depth discussion on the merits of HIPAA is beyond the scope of this chapter, it behooves psychiatrists to be aware of these limitations and consider their implications.

Mandated Reporting

All states have statutes pertaining to the mandatory reporting of suspected child abuse. In addition, most jurisdictions mandate the reporting of maltreatment involving other vulnerable populations, including the elderly and adults with developmental disabilities. Many states also have laws requiring the reporting of intimate partner violence and nonaccidental injury. Standards vary across jurisdictions, but most require that a psychiatrist demonstrate a reasonable suspicion that a vulnerable person (e.g., child, elderly individual, or developmentally disabled adult) has been abused and/or neglected. In jurisdictions with laws that address intimate partner violence, psychiatrists are expected to report all adults with suspicious injuries, not just those in vulnerable populations. Readers interested in learning more about reporting requirements in their jurisdictions are encouraged to visit the U.S. Department of Health and Human Services website (www.hhs.gov) or to download the "Compendium of State and U.S. Territory Statutes and Policies on Domestic Violence and Health Care," available online from Futures Without Violence (2013).

Informed Consent

Informed consent is based on three elements: information sharing, decisional capacity, and voluntarism. In common usage, the terms *competence* and *capacity* are frequently used interchangeably in both the legal and psychiatric literatures (Appelbaum 2007). However, these terms have quite different meanings in a medicolegal context. Determinations of "competence" or "incompetence" are made by a judge, whereas decisions related to "capacity" or "decisional capacity" are based on clinical appraisals of an individual's ability to function in regard to a specific demand or situation (Mishkin 1989).

Psychiatrists routinely evaluate decisional capacity in clinical contexts. In 2007, Paul Appelbaum succinctly described the basic components of decisional capacity as follows: "Legal standards for decision-making capacity for consent to treatment vary somewhat across jurisdictions, but generally they embody the abilities to communicate a choice, to understand the relevant information, to appreciate the medical consequences of the situation, and to reason about treatment choices" (Appelbaum 2007, p. 1835). From a legal standpoint, only "competent" persons can provide informed consent for treatment. A person who has been deemed "incompetent" in the eyes of the law requires a substitute decision maker to provide informed consent to initiate treatment. Historically, determinations of legal competence were based largely on a person's cognitive abilities. However, the Massachusetts Supreme Judicial Court ruled in *In the Guardianship of John Roe* (1992) that a man with schizophrenia was incompetent to make decisions about his treatment *not* because of any cognitive limitations but because of his persistent denial that he had an actual illness. This ruling expanded the circumstances under which an individual could be deemed incompetent and served to illustrate the complex ways in which mental illness may alter one's ability to make medical decisions.

The case of Mary Schloendorff highlights further parameters involving informed consent. Following the Great San Francisco Earthquake of 1906, Ms. Schloendorff, an elocutionist and guitar teacher from San Francisco, moved to New York City. In 1908, Ms. Schloendorff presented to New York Hospital with stomach pains and eventually agreed to an "ether exam" of her pelvis (i.e., a pelvic examination under anesthesia). Prior to losing consciousness, Ms. Schloendorff made it clear to her doctors that she did not wish to receive an operation. However, doctors subsequently located a fibroid tumor and removed it against Ms. Schloendorff's previously stated wishes. Unfortunately, Ms. Schloendorff developed gangrene as a complication of surgery, which necessitated that multiple fingers on her left hand later be amputated. Ms. Schloendorff filed a lawsuit against the hospital, and in 1914 the New York State Court of Appeals ruled that she was the victim of medical battery, given that "every human being of adult years and sound mind has a right to determine what shall be done with his own body; and a surgeon who performs an operation without his patient's consent commits an assault for which he is liable in damages. This is true except in cases of emergency where the patient is unconscious and where it is necessary to operate before consent can be obtained" (*Schloendorff v. Society of New York Hospital* 1914).

American notions of informed consent have evolved substantially since 1914. For instance, in the case of *Natanson v. Kline* (1960), the Kansas Supreme Court ruled that informed consent was a hallmark feature of nonnegligent appropriate medical care. The court also held that the adequacy of informed consent should be judged on the basis of what a "reasonable medical practitioner" would have disclosed to a patient under similar circumstances. The reasonable medical practitioner standard is still used in some jurisdictions around the United States.

A subsequent case in the U.S. Court of Appeals for the District of Columbia Circuit, *Canterbury v. Spence* (1972), ruled that a physician is required to provide a level of detail about medical care that a "reasonable person" would want to know before deciding whether to undergo treatment. The court added that such disclosure should include a discussion of serious associated risks (e.g., major injury, death), even when there is a low likelihood of such complications. Many jurisdictions around the United States began shifting toward the "reasonable person" standard following the *Canterbury v. Spence* ruling. Overall, there are significant legal precedents dictating that physicians obtain informed consent from patients. Failing to do so can be grounds for negligence.

More recently, in the case of *Long v. Jaszczak* (2004), the Supreme Court of North Dakota ruled that the obligation to obtain informed consent from a patient prior to initiating treatment lies squarely on the treating physician and not the institution he or she works for. In this case, a woman who presented with recurrent urinary tract infections was ordered to undergo an intravenous pyelogram. Unfortunately, the patient experienced an allergic reaction and died from anaphylactic shock. The woman's grieving husband later sued the hospital and the treating physicians because she was not informed about the potential for death associated with the procedure. The court ruled in favor of the husband, stating that a "reasonable person" would have considered the possibility of death associated with the procedure a significant factor when voluntarily making an informed and intelligent decision to pursue or decline a procedure.

More specific to the practice of psychiatry, the case of *Clites v. State of Iowa* (1982) involved a developmentally disabled man who was prescribed antipsychotics in an institutional setting for a number of years without proper monitoring. He eventually developed tardive dyskinesia, and his father sued the institution for negligence. The Iowa Court of Appeals ultimately ruled that prescribing antipsychotics without informing patients and/or guardians about the nature of treatment and possible side effects can constitute grounds for malpractice.

In *Zinermon v. Burch* (1990), a disoriented and psychotic gentleman, Mr. Darrell Burch, was found walking along a Tallahassee, Florida, highway in 1981. Mr. Burch was admitted to a private psychiatric hospital, where he received treatment with an antipsychotic medication for 3 days. Still psychotic, Mr. Burch was later transferred to a Florida state mental hospital, where he signed voluntary admission forms, despite Florida's requirement that adults seeking voluntary treatment at state hospitals do so by "making application by express and informed consent."

Mr. Burch later sued the state of Florida, claiming that he had been incompetent to voluntarily consent to admission and thereby unfairly deprived of his civil liberties. The U.S. Supreme Court ruled that Mr. Burch had a valid claim in that the state of Florida violated his procedural due process rights provided under the Fourteenth Amendment. This decision highlights the importance of ensuring that persons are able to consent to voluntary psychiatric admission as a means of preserving their civil liberties.

Common Exceptions to Informed Consent: Emergencies, Waiver, Therapeutic Privilege, Incompetence

There are some situations in which medical professionals are not required to obtain informed consent. These exceptions include emergency situations, patient waivers of informed consent, therapeutic privilege, and the treatment of legally incompetent patients.

Emergencies

Informed consent is not necessary when a patient requires treatment to save his or her life or to prevent serious harm. In these situations, it is sometimes impossible to obtain informed consent from the patient or legal guardian who may consent on the patient's behalf. It is important to note, however, that an emergency does not give physicians carte blanche, as exemplified by the tragic case of *Shine v. Vega* (1999).

In 1990, a 29-year-old woman named Catherine Shine presented to a Boston emergency room in the midst of an asthma attack. Ms. Shine was treated with oxygen and medication and then decided to leave the hospital. Ms. Shine's treating physician, Dr. Vega, determined that it would be unsafe for Ms. Shine to leave the hospital in her condition, despite her objections, on the basis of the results of a recent blood gas test. Ms. Shine eventually made a break for the door only to be apprehended by security.

Ms. Shine was then placed in four-point restraints and intubated against her will. Two years later, Ms. Shine experienced a severe asthma attack and refused to go to the emergency room because of her fears of being intubated again. Unfortunately, Ms. Shine passed away as the result of this untreated asthma attack. Ms. Shine's family later sued Dr. Vega, claiming that his behavior 2 years prior was the direct cause of

Ms. Shine's refusal to seek help and, ultimately, her death. Dr. Vega claimed that he was compelled to treat Ms. Shine over her objections because she was in emergent danger; however, the Massachusetts Supreme Judicial Court did not share this opinion. The court ruled that a "competent patient's refusal to consent to medical treatment cannot be overridden whenever the patient faces a life-threatening situation."

Cruzan v. Director of Missouri Department of Health (1990) involved a family's request to remove their daughter from life support after she had been in a persistent vegetative state for some time. The hospital refused to remove life support without a formal court order. Over the next couple of years, the case would rise to the level of the U.S. Supreme Court. The Supreme Court ruled that Missouri's requirement that "clear and convincing evidence" be shown in order to terminate life support in cases involving incompetent patients was constitutional. The ruling also set forth several key precedents, including the following:

1. The so-called right to die is not constitutionally protected.
2. In the absence of a living will, advanced directives, or clear and convincing evidence of a patient's previous wishes, the state must err on the side of preserving life.
3. States may create their own right-to-die standards, as opposed to the court mandating a national standard.

Thus, some key points for psychiatrists to consider regarding informed consent in emergency situations include the following: 1) Informed consent is not required when a patient requires treatment to save his or her life or to prevent serious danger when it is impossible to obtain informed consent. 2) Treatment may continue only until the patient is out of immediate danger. 3) A competent person who has the capacity to make decisions about treatment can always refuse treatment. 4) A competent patient's previously stated preferences cannot be rescinded just because of an emergency (Brendel and Schouten 2007).

Waiver

Competent patients can knowingly and voluntarily "waive" their rights to informed consent and may defer to their physician's judgment regarding treatment decisions. For example, a patient may decide that he does not want to be informed about possible side effects of a particular medication. In these cases, psychiatrists should thoroughly document that a patient has the capacity to waive the right to informed consent in the manner described.

Therapeutic Privilege

A particularly risky and rarely invoked exception to informed consent in some jurisdictions relates to the concept of therapeutic privilege. Therapeutic privilege involves the withholding of information from patients if the treating physician determines that the information would lead to physical and/or emotional harm. For example, in *Canterbury v. Spence* (1972) the U.S. Court of Appeals for the District of Columbia Circuit expressed the following:

> It is recognized that patients occasionally become so ill or emotionally distraught on disclosure as to foreclose a rational decision, or complicate or hinder the treatment, or perhaps even pose psychological damage to the patient. Where that is so, the cases have

generally held that the physician is armed with a privilege to keep the information from the patient, and we think it clear that portents of that type may justify the physician in action he deems medically warranted.

The concept of therapeutic privilege is not without criticism. For instance, some have argued that withholding information from competent patients is unethical or, at the very least, a slippery slope with a potential for abuse (Abigail 2011; Cox and Fritz 2016; Edwin 2008; Johnston and Holt 2006). According to the American Medical Association's *AMA Code of Medical Ethics,* "Withholding pertinent medical information from patients in the belief that disclosure is medically contraindicated creates a conflict between the physician's obligations to promote patient welfare and to respect patient autonomy" (American Medical Association Council on Ethical and Judicial Affairs 2016, Opinion 2.1.3). The *AMA Code of Medical Ethics* also says the following: "The obligation to communicate truthfully about the patient's medical condition does not mean that the physician must communicate information to the patient immediately or all at once. Information may be conveyed over time in keeping with the patient's preferences and ability to comprehend the information" (Opinion 2.1.3).

Thus, although jurisdictions may allow a physician to invoke therapeutic privilege, the physician who does so may have a difficult time providing an adequate justification for doing so in court.

Incompetence

The interchangeability of the terms *competence* and *capacity* in legal and medical literature can be confusing. In general, patients who are deemed incompetent for the purposes of medical decision making are not able to provide informed consent; however, the incompetent patient's legal guardian (or designated health care proxy) may provide informed consent on his or her behalf.

The examples here highlight some of the important principles of which psychiatrists should be mindful in their clinical practices. Most notably, a competent patient has a right to decide what happens to his or her body, and standard of care necessitates that informed consent must be obtained. The degree of disclosure required when obtaining informed consent varies across jurisdictions but generally involves physicians disclosing what a reasonable medical practitioner would disclose or what a reasonable person would need to know in order to make informed health care decisions.

American courts have ruled that competent patients are entitled to make voluntary, knowing (i.e., based on relevant information), and intelligent (competent) health care decisions. In practical terms, patients or their substitute decision makers should be told about potential risks, benefits, prognosis (*with and without treatment*), and alternative treatments (*risks and benefits*) in order to make informed decisions.

Duty to Protect

Courts have weighed in on therapists' duty to protect third parties from dangerous patients in a variety of well-known cases. Perhaps the most famous example is the case of *Tarasoff v. Regents of the University of California* (1976). Mr. Prosenjit Poddar was a graduate student at the University of California (UC), Berkeley, where he was studying naval architecture. Mr. Poddar met a fellow student, Ms. Tatiana Tarasoff, at a folk dancing class in 1968. By all accounts, Mr. Poddar and Ms. Tarasoff started off as friendly acquaintances and shared a New Year's Eve kiss. Unfortunately, Mr. Poddar became obsessed with Ms. Tarasoff and stalked her.

Mr. Poddar began seeing a therapist at the student mental health clinic, Dr. Lawrence Moore. Mr. Poddar eventually told Dr. Moore that he planned to kill Ms. Tarasoff. Dr. Moore notified campus police and recommended that Mr. Poddar be civilly committed; however, Dr. Moore's supervisor disagreed. Mr. Poddar was not committed, and Ms. Tarasoff was never provided a warning about Mr. Poddar's stated plans. Mr. Poddar eventually tracked down Ms. Tarasoff at her parents' home and stabbed her to death.

Ms. Tarasoff's parents sued UC Berkeley and Mr. Poddar's therapist, Dr. Moore. After a series of lengthy legal battles, the California Supreme Court ruled that a therapist has a duty to protect a potential victim from foreseeable danger. Justice Mathew O. Tobriner succinctly summed up the court's opinion by writing, "The protective privilege ends where the where the public peril begins."

In the 40-plus years since the *Tarasoff* decision, psychiatrists' duty to protect has expanded on the basis of court rulings from a number of jurisdictions. For example, in the case of *Lipari v. Sears, Roebuck and Company* (1980), a Nebraska court expanded on the language of *Tarasoff* by ruling that potential victims of violence did not need to be readily identifiable, so long as it could be "reasonably foreseen" that a "class of persons" was in harm's way. In *Naidu v. Laird* (1988), the Supreme Court of Delaware found that a psychiatrist who discharged a patient during a voluntary state hospital admission 5 months prior was liable for a man's death in a motor vehicle accident caused by the former patient. According to the court, the psychiatrist did not properly review the patient's extensive history of psychiatric hospitalizations and medication noncompliance prior to discharge, and this negligence was the "proximate cause" of the motor vehicle accident victim's death.

Medicolegal Aspects of Institutionalized Care

Civil Commitment

All states have statutes addressing the involuntary commitment of persons who are deemed to be a "danger to self" or "danger to others." Most states also include a third criterion for mentally ill persons who are unable to meet their basic needs (e.g., adequate food, clothing, shelter), sometimes referred to as "grave disability." Although all psychiatrists are well acquainted with these terms, it is important for psychiatrists to understand the case law underpinning these concepts.

Attitudes toward the mentally ill became more humanitarian in the European and American era of postenlightenment. In the mid-nineteenth century, elaborate state hospitals were constructed in the United States with a focus on aesthetic beauty, which was believed to promote healing. However, the standards for civil commitment at this time in history were vague, low, and indeterminate. Commitment standards were also largely based on an arguably paternalistic notion that involuntary hospitalization was preferable to living on the streets (Arrigo 1992–1993). As a result of these standards, American state hospitals became overcrowded, underfunded, and inhumane.

The changing social climate of the 1960s led jurisdictions across the United States to place greater value on patient autonomy in matters related to involuntary psychiatric care. States began moving away from a paternalistic "need for treatment" model to that of a "dangerousness model" (Testa and West 2010). The sweeping changes in public values and perception of civil commitment are reflected in a case decided by the U.S. Supreme Court in 1975, *O'Connor v. Donaldson*.

In 1956, Mr. Kenneth Donaldson left his home in Philadelphia to visit his parents in Florida. During his stay, Mr. Donaldson told his father that be believed a neighbor back home was poisoning him. Concerned, Mr. Donaldson's father filed a petition for a sanity hearing that led to his son being diagnosed with paranoid schizophrenia. Kenneth Donaldson was civilly committed to a state hospital in Chattahoochee, Florida. There, he refused to take antipsychotic medication, in part on the basis of his religious beliefs as a Christian Scientist. Mr. Donaldson would spend the next 15 years of his life receiving "milieu therapy" in the state hospital, sometimes going years without having a single progress note written. Despite Mr. Donaldson not exhibiting dangerous or violent behavior during his stay, the hospital's superintendent, Dr. J.B. O'Connor, ignored multiple offers from Mr. Donaldson's friends to provide a safe haven for him if released. Mr. Donaldson remained in the hospital until Dr. O'Connor retired. He was released a few months later with the help of hospital staff who sympathized with his plight. Mr. Donaldson then sued Dr. O'Connor, claiming that he had been deprived of his constitutional right to liberty. A jury agreed with Mr. Donaldson, as did the U.S. Court of Appeals for the Fifth Circuit and the U.S. Supreme Court, which reasoned that "a State cannot constitutionally confine, without more, a nondangerous individual who is capable of surviving safely in freedom by himself or with the help of willing and responsible family members or friends." In pointing out the injustice Mr. Donaldson endured, the Supreme Court added the following: "May the State fence in the harmless mentally ill solely to save its citizens from exposure to those whose ways are different? One might as well ask if the State, to avoid public unease, could incarcerate all who are physically unattractive or socially eccentric."

The U.S. Supreme Court's decision in *O'Connor v. Donaldson* (1975) has shaped civil commitment standards in jurisdictions throughout the country. The decision led to a shift from a relatively paternalistic treatment model to one that prioritized patient autonomy. On the basis of the court's ruling, involuntary civil commitment would be reserved only for those individuals at risk of self-harm or harm to others or those who were gravely disabled.

The Right to Treatment

The case of *Wyatt v. Stickney* (1971) was the first case to address the minimally adequate conditions for persons committed involuntarily to psychiatric facilities (Perlin 2005). The case continued for more than three decades and was the longest-running mental health lawsuit in the history of the United States. Mr. Wyatt was a 15-year-old Tuscaloosa native who was admitted to Bryce State Hospital because of misbehavior at a local group home. Despite having been previously labeled a juvenile delinquent, Mr. Wyatt did not have a formal psychiatric diagnosis (Wilson Carr 2004). Mr. Wyatt would later become part of a class action lawsuit that alleged inhumane conditions at Bryce Hospital. The federal district court in Alabama ruled that patient conditions were indeed deficient, adding that involuntarily confined patients "unquestionably have a constitutional right to receive such individual treatment as will give each of them a realistic opportunity to be cured or to improve his or her mental condition." The court specifically outlined three minimum standards that all psychiatric hospitals must meet:

1. A humane psychological and physical environment
2. Qualified staff in numbers sufficient to administer adequate treatment
3. Individualized treatment plans

The U.S. Supreme Court case of *Youngberg v. Romeo* (1982) addressed the rights of developmentally disabled institutionalized persons under the Fourteenth Amendment. Nicholas Romeo was a 33-year-old developmentally disabled man who reportedly functioned around the level of a 1.5-year-old child. Mr. Romeo's mother had Nicholas committed to Pennhurst State School and Hospital in Pennsylvania following the death of her husband.

Mr. Romeo sustained multiple injuries during his first 3 years at Pennhurst, which prompted his mother to file a lawsuit against the hospital's superintendent. The case was appealed to the U.S. Supreme Court, which ruled in favor of Mr. Romeo and his mother. In particular, the court ruled that state facilities must provide freedom from bodily restraint, safe conditions, and care by staff skilled in techniques aimed at minimizing the need for involuntary restraint. Despite this ruling, the court's opinion included language that recognized the state's authority in managing mental health facilities. The ruling sought to balance patient autonomy with the state's interests and advised that courts "should not second-guess the expert administrators on matters on which they are better informed." The court added that a professional's decision should be "presumptively valid" unless it is determined that the decision was "such a substantial departure from accepted professional judgment…as to demonstrate that the person responsible actually did not base the decision on such a judgment."

The court chose its words carefully in the *Romeo* opinion by asserting that mental health professionals' treatment decisions were to be considered "presumptively valid" unless it could be proven that these decisions were a "substantial departure from accepted professional judgment." In wording its opinion this way, the U.S. Supreme Court made it easier for federal courts to steer clear of making decisions that might affect the day-to-day operations of state institutions. This language also indicates that involuntarily committed persons must prove that their providers were more than merely negligent, as is the case with most medical or psychiatric malpractice cases, to successfully claim that their rights to freedom from unnecessary restraint were violated (Bersoff 1993). In summary, the rulings in *Wyatt* and *Romeo* outlined the minimally adequate standards of care afforded to civilly committed persons while acknowledging the states' interests in running these mental health facilities.

The Right to Refuse Treatment

The process by which a patient may refuse treatment is controversial and varies across jurisdictions. A classic paper by Appelbaum and Gutheil (1979) discussed the implications of courts relying on theoretical ideas rather than practical experience in deciding whether civilly committed persons may refuse psychiatric care. The authors expressed concern that overreliance on high-minded ideals, as opposed to more practical clinical knowledge, might leave some civilly committed patients vulnerable to "rotting with their rights on." In other words, the authors questioned whether mentally ill patients are best served by refusing treatment, however technically or legally appropriate these refusals might be. Two landmark legal cases have addressed the rights of civilly committed persons to refuse treatment. The contrasting models outlined in *Rennie v. Klein* (1983) and *Rogers v. Commissioner of Department of Mental Health* (1983) have shaped the process by which jurisdictions across the United States handle treatment refusal in locked settings.

John Rennie was a former pilot and flight instructor who developed severe and persistent mental illness during his early thirties. He had been hospitalized numerous times and frequently refused to take antipsychotic medication on discharge. Mr. Rennie filed a lawsuit during his twelfth hospitalization at Ancora State Psychiatric Hospital in New Jersey, claiming that he had a constitutional right to refuse antipsychotic medication in nonemergent situations, despite his being involuntarily hospitalized.

The U.S. Court of Appeals for the Third Circuit agreed with Mr. Rennie yet also concluded that a patient's right to refuse treatment with antipsychotics could be overridden "whenever, in the exercise of professional judgment, such an action is deemed necessary to prevent the patient from endangering himself or others." The court also ruled that treatment providers who wish to administer antipsychotic medications to an unwilling patient in a nonemergent setting must provide a rationale to additional professional staff for their review and approval.

The court's decision in *Rennie* was influenced by the professional judgment standard referenced earlier in the case of *Youngberg v. Romeo* (1982). Jurisdictions that defer to the judgment of psychiatrists as described in *Rennie* are said to follow a treatment-driven model. Legal and patient advocacy groups are typically not in favor of treatment-driven models because of the implied loss of patient autonomy and increased vulnerability to unscrupulous providers and/or errors in provider judgment.

In the case of *Rogers v. Commissioner of Department of Mental Health* (1983), seven patients at Boston State Hospital, including Ms. Rubie Rogers, filed a lawsuit against the Department of Mental Health on behalf of "all present and future voluntary and involuntary patients at the May and Austin Units of the Boston State Hospital who have been secluded or medicated without their consent." The Supreme Judicial Court of Massachusetts ruled that committed persons are to be considered competent unless a judge finds them incompetent through an adversarial hearing. Notably, the court also ruled that if a patient is deemed incompetent, "a judge, using a substituted-judgment standard, shall decide whether the patient would have consented to the administration of antipsychotic drugs."

Substituted judgment, as defined by the *Rogers* court, was based on the following six factors:

1. The patient's previously "expressed preferences regarding treatment"
2. The strength of the incompetent patient's religious convictions, to the extent that they may contribute to refusal of treatment
3. The impact on the patient's family from the patient's viewpoint
4. The probability of adverse side effects
5. The patient's prognosis with treatment
6. The patient's prognosis without treatment

Unlike the decision in *Rennie v. Klein* (1983), which largely deferred to medical decision makers, *Rogers* gave judges great discretion in determining patients' wishes. Jurisdictions that invoke such processes are said to follow a rights-driven model. Critics of this model claim that the process is expensive, inefficient, impractical, and akin to allowing patients to "rot with their rights on."

The courts have also addressed the right to refuse treatment by persons involved in the criminal justice system. For instance, in the case of *Sell v. United States* (2003), the U.S. Supreme Court outlined the standards by which the government may medicate a pretrial detainee back to trial competence against his or her wishes. The U.S. Supreme Court's decision in *Sell* was heavily influenced by its rulings in *Washington v. Harper* (1990) and *Riggins v. Nevada* (1992). In the case of *Washington v. Harper*, the court ruled that the decision to medicate dangerous prisoners against their will may be made via an administrative, rather than judicial, hearing. In *Riggins v. Nevada*, the court held that a person who is standing trial cannot be forced to take antipsychotic medication without first determining whether such treatment is medically necessary and the least intrusive option.

Additional Forensic Issues in Clinical Practice

There are many other situations in which clinicians may interact with the legal system. In this section, we summarize some of the key legal concepts with which all mental health providers should be familiar.

Testifying as a Fact Witness

A *fact witness* is someone with knowledge about a case who testifies about personal observations and related facts. In short, fact witnesses report facts, not their opinions. Clinicians are sometimes called to testify as fact witnesses in cases in which defendants' mental status is a consideration. By contrast, expert witnesses rely on their knowledge, skill, training, and expertise to provide opinions that help the court come to a conclusion. Definitions for what constitutes an expert witness may vary across jurisdictions. Given the potential conflicts of interest, clinicians who take on an expert witness role for one of their patients run the risk of presenting actual or potential bias as a result of their dual role.

Suicidal Patients

Patient suicides are the most common reason for which psychiatrists are sued (Baerger 2001; Packman et al. 2004). Given that suicides are rare and difficult to predict, a patient's attempted or completed suicide does not automatically imply negligent psychiatric care. For instance, a tragic case from New York in 2001 involved a woman who was hospitalized for attempting suicide by jumping from a moving car in the setting of postpartum depression. The woman later denied having attempted suicide throughout her hospitalization; however, 1 week into her admission she took her own life after being granted a 12-hour pass to return home. The court in this case ruled that even if a psychiatrist fails "to predict that a patient will harm himself or herself if released, the psychiatrist cannot be held liable for a mere error in professional judgment."

Courts do not expect that psychiatrists will be able to predict whether a patient will complete or attempt suicide; however, standard of care necessitates that psychiatrists perform and document a competent suicide risk assessment (Simon 2002). Furthermore, the psychiatrist's safety plan should be commensurate with the patient's estimated level of suicide risk. It is also worth noting that the use of no-harm contracts for patients who are thinking about suicide has no empirical basis and offers no protection in malpractice litigation (Garvey et al. 2009; Lewis 2007).

Violence Risk Assessment

Assessing violence risk is both a challenging and everyday aspect of a psychiatrist's job. Psychiatrists typically assess for the presence or absence of violent fantasies or thoughts in a variety of clinical settings. Although there is no expectation that a psychiatrist will accurately predict whether a patient will become violent toward others, standard of care dictates that a psychiatrist perform competent violence risk assessments. An important consideration in a clinical violence risk assessment is an understanding of the subtype of violence a patient is displaying and/or is prone to engage in. The literature often refers to such subtypes as *reactive* (i.e., "hot") versus *predatory* (i.e., "cold") aggression. Hot aggression tends to occur in the heat of the moment in response to an identifiable trigger and subsides over time. By contrast, cold aggression can be more challenging to identify because a person who calmly plans to execute violence on another is not likely to broadcast his or her intentions.

Additional considerations when performing violence risk assessments include dynamic and static risk factors. Dynamic risk factors are subject to change. Examples of dynamic risk factors include substance intoxication, access to firearms, medication noncompliance, and absence of a stable living situation. Static risk factors, on the other hand, are not subject to change and are largely demographic or historical in nature. A history of previous violence, male gender, and early childhood trauma history are all examples of static variables that can influence violence risk.

The Epidemiologic Catchment Area Surveys study (Swanson et al. 1990) illustrates the interaction between historical and dynamic risk factors. This study found that persons with a history of severe mental illness were at a slightly increased risk of becoming violent in the community. However, the combination of untreated severe mental illness and active substance use problems markedly increased the risk of violence.

Disability

Despite the frequency with which psychiatrists are asked to comment on their patient's disability status, there are data to suggest that psychiatrists receive little training in residency related to psychiatric disability (Christopher et al. 2010). Common types of disability evaluations include workers' compensation, fitness for duty, social security, and those related to the Americans with Disabilities Act. The term *disability* is not a clinical term but rather a legal one with specific criteria based on the government agency involved and/or type of evaluation that is being performed. Clinicians interested in a cogent summary of disability evaluations are encouraged to review the American Academy of Psychiatry and the Law practice guideline for the forensic evaluation of psychiatric disability (Gold et al. 2008).

Subpoenas

A subpoena is a writ (i.e., formal order issued by the court) requiring testimony and/ or the turning over of evidence (e.g., treatment records) in court or at a deposition. Subpoenas are often a cause for anxiety among psychiatrists. In general, the first step a clinician should take after receiving a subpoena is to seek advice from his or her institutional or personal legal counsel. Clinicians should also seek to clarify their patients' wishes regarding the potential of waiving psychotherapist–patient privilege. Last, clinicians should never attempt to alter or destroy records after receiving a subpoena.

Sexual Misconduct

Romantic and sexual relationships with patients are never appropriate for obvious reasons. These issues were addressed in the state of New York in the landmark case *Roy v. Hartogs* (1976). Here, Ms. Julie Roy sought treatment from a psychiatrist, Dr. Renatus Hartogs, who prescribed sexual intercourse as part of her "therapy." The sexual relationship went on for approximately 13 months before it was terminated by Dr. Hartogs. Ms. Roy filed a lawsuit claiming that she sustained emotional and mental injuries because of Dr. Hartogs's unprofessional behavior. The court found in favor of Ms. Roy, who was ultimately awarded $25,000 in compensatory damages.

Psychiatrists who engage in sexual misconduct or other forms of grossly unprofessional behavior are at risk for civil liability, professional disciplinary actions, and criminal prosecution. Malpractice claims related to sexual misconduct require proof by a preponderance of the evidence (i.e., more likely than not) that the exploitation occurred and caused harm (e.g., worsening psychiatric condition). Professional disciplinary actions often include temporary or permanent loss of professional licensure. Approximately half of states have statutes criminalizing sexual conduct with current patients, and some have extended this prohibition to former patients (Morgan 2013).

Dual Agency

A key ethical consideration at the intersection of clinical and forensic psychiatry is dual agency. The term *dual agency* refers to clinicians who attempt to fulfill both clinical and forensic roles within the same case. The ethical guidelines of the American Psychiatric Association and the American Academy of Psychiatry and the Law strongly discourage psychiatrists from taking the role of treatment provider and court expert for the same patient.

Conclusion

Psychiatrists should have a basic understanding of the laws that guide clinical practice. Understanding concepts such as negligence, confidentiality and privilege, mandated reporting, informed consent, the duty to protect, and medicolegal aspects of institutionalized care, among others, provides a foundation for psychiatrists to maintain an ethical and proficient practice. Knowledge of case law on topics involving the overlap of psychiatry and the law can provide relevant context for the practitioner.

Key Clinical Points

- With some exceptions such as emergencies, psychiatrists are required to obtain informed consent (intelligent, knowing, and voluntary) from all competent persons prior to initiating treatment.

- Psychiatrists have a duty to maintain patient confidentiality unless authorized to disclose personal health information by the patient, on court order, or when mandated by law (e.g., reporting suspected child abuse).

- Clinicians should take into consideration both static (e.g., age, psychiatric history, violence history) and dynamic (e.g., treatment compliance, access to weapons, intoxication) risk factors when performing a violence risk assessment.

- Practitioners typically have a duty to protect a reasonably identifiable victim from foreseeable imminent harm.

- Clinicians are advised to speak with their personal or institutional legal counsel prior to responding to a subpoena.

- Ethical standards dictate that psychiatrists avoid conflicts of interest inherent to acting both as treatment provider and forensic expert whenever possible.

References

Abigail S: The obstacle of therapeutic privilege in healthcare mediation. American Journal of Mediation, Vol. 5, 2011. Available at: http://www.americanjournalofmediation.com/docs/The%20Obstacle%20of%20Therapeutic%20Privilege%20in%20Healthcare%20Mediation(1).pdf. Accessed September 10, 2017.

American Medical Association Council on Ethical and Judicial Affairs: AMA Code of Medical Ethics. Chicago, IL, American Medical Association, 2016

Appelbaum PS: Privacy in psychiatric treatment: threats and responses. Am J Psychiatry 159(11):1809–1818, 2002 12411211

Appelbaum PS: Clinical practice. Assessment of patients' competence to consent to treatment. N Engl J Med 357(18):1834–1840, 2007 17978292

Appelbaum PS, Gutheil TG: "Rotting with their rights on": constitutional theory and clinical reality in drug refusal by psychiatric patients. Bull Am Acad Psychiatry Law 7(3):306–315, 1979 549703

Arrigo BA: Paternalism, civil commitment and illness politics: assessing the current debate and outlining a future direction. J Law Health 7(2):131–168, 1992–1993 11652819

Baerger DR: Risk management with the suicidal patient: lessons from case law. Professional Psychology: Research and Practice 32(4):359–366, 2001

Bersoff DN: Judicial deference to nonlegal decisionmakers: imposing simplistic solutions on problems of cognitive complexity in mental disability law. Southern Methodist University Law Review 46:329–372, 1993

Brendel RW, Bryan E: HIPAA for psychiatrists. Harv Rev Psychiatry 12(3):177–183, 2004 15371073

Brendel RW, Schouten R: Legal concerns in psychosomatic medicine. Psychiatr Clin North Am 30(4):663–676, 2007 17938039

Christopher PP, Boland RJ, Recupero PR, et al: Psychiatric residents' experience conducting disability evaluations. Acad Psychiatry 34(3):211–215, 2010 20431102

Corley SO: Protection for psychotherapy notes under the HIPAA Privacy Rule: as private as a hospital gown. 22 Health Matrix: The Journal of Law–Medicine 22(2):489–534, 2013. Available at: http://scholarlycommons.law.case.edu/healthmatrix/vol22/iss2/8. Accessed September 10, 2017.

Cox CL, Fritz Z: Should non-disclosures be considered as morally equivalent to lies within the doctor-patient relationship? J Med Ethics 42(10):632–635, 2016 27451425

Edwin A: Don't lie but don't tell the whole truth: the therapeutic privilege—is it ever justified? Ghana Med J 42(4):156–161, 2008 19452024

Futures Without Violence: Compendium of State and U.S. Territory Statutes and Policies on Domestic Violence and Health Care. Futures Without Violence, 2013. Available at: https://www.futureswithoutviolence.org/userfiles/file/HealthCare/Compendium%20Final%202013.pdf. Accessed July 20, 2018.

Garvey KA, Penn JV, Campbell AL, et al: Contracting for safety with patients: clinical practice and forensic implications. J Am Acad Psychiatry Law 37(3):363–370, 2009 19767501

Gold LH, Anfang SA, Drukteinis AM, et al: AAPL practice guideline for the forensic evaluation of psychiatric disability. J Am Acad Psychiatry Law 36 (4 suppl):S3–S50, 2008 19092058

Jena AB, Seabury S, Lakdawalla D, et al: Malpractice risk according to physician specialty. N Engl J Med 365(7):629–636, 2011 21848463

Johnston C, Holt G: The legal and ethical implications of therapeutic privilege—is it ever justified to withhold treatment information from a competent patient? Clinical Ethics 1(3):146–151, 2006

Lewis LM: No-harm contracts: a review of what we know. Suicide Life Threat Behav 37(1):50–57, 2007 17397279

Mishkin B: Determining the capacity for making health care decisions, in Issues in Geriatric Psychiatry (Advances in Psychosomatic Medicine, Vol 19). Edited by Billig N, Rabins PV. Basel, Switzerland, Karger, 1989, pp 151–166

Morgan S: Criminalization of Psychotherapist Sexual Misconduct. Washington, DC, National Association of Social Workers, May 2013. Available at: http://c.ymcdn.com/sites/www.naswca.org/resource/resmgr/imported/7_13_legal_issue.pdf. Accessed July 20, 2018.

Packman WL, Pennuto TO, Bongar B, et al: Legal issues of professional negligence in suicide cases. Behav Sci Law 22(5):697–713, 2004 15378596

Perlin ML: "May you stay forever young": Robert Sadoff and the history of mental disability law. J Am Acad Psychiatry Law 33(2):236–244, 2005 15985668

Ray I: A Treatise on the Medical Jurisprudence of Insanity. Boston, MA, Little, Brown, 1838

Roberts S: Dr. Joseph Lifschutz, 92, dies; asserted confidentiality right for therapists. New York Times, April 28, 2017. Available at: www.nytimes.com/2017/04/28/science/joseph-lifschutz-dead-confidentiality-psychiatry.html. Accessed July 20, 2018.

Sadoff RL: Forensic Psychiatry: A Practical Guide for Lawyers and Psychiatrists. Springfield, IL, Thomas, 1975

Schaffer AC, Jena AB, Seabury SA, et al: Rates and characteristics of paid malpractice claims among US physicians by specialty, 1992–2014. JAMA Intern Med 177(5):710–718, 2017 28346582

Scott CL, Resnick PJ: Patient suicide and litigation, in Textbook of Suicide Assessment and Management. Edited by Simon RI, Hales RE. Washington, DC, American Psychiatric Publishing, 2006, pp 530–531

Simon RI: Suicide risk assessment: what is the standard of care? J Am Acad Psychiatry Law 30(3):340–344, 2002 12380411

Swanson JW, Holzer CE III, Ganju VK, et al: Violence and psychiatric disorder in the community: evidence from the Epidemiologic Catchment Area surveys. Hosp Community Psychiatry 41(7):761–770, 1990 2142118

Testa M, West SG: Civil commitment in the United States. Psychiatry (Edgmont) 7(10):30–40, 2010 22778709

Wilson Carr L: Wyatt vs. Stickney. Alabama Disability Advocacy Program, July 2004. Available at: http://adap.ua.edu/ricky-wyatt.html. Accessed July 20, 2018.

Legal Citations

Canterbury v Spence, 464 F2d 772 (DC Cir 1972), cert denied, Spence v Canterbury, 409 US 1064 (1972)

Clites v State of Iowa, 322 NW2d 917 (Iowa Ct App 1982)

Cruzan v Director of Missouri Department of Health, 497 US 261, 110 S Ct 2841, 111 L Ed2d 224 (1990)

Doe v Roe, 93 Misc 2d 201, 400 NYS2d 668, 400 NYS 2 (Sup Ct 1977)

Health Insurance Portability and Accountability Act of 1996, Pub L No 104–191, 110 Stat 1936

In the Guardianship of John Roe, 411 Mass 666 (1992)

In re Lifschutz, 2 Cal 3d 415 (1970)

Jaffee v Redmond, 518 US 1 (1996)

Lipari v Sears, Roebuck and Company, 497 F Supp 185 (D Neb 1980)

Long v Jaszczak, 688 NW2d 173 (ND 2004)

M'Naghten's Case, 10 CL & F. 200, 8 Eng. Rep. 718 (1843)

Naidu v Laird, 539 A2d 1064 (Del 1988)

Natanson v Kline, 186 Kan 393, 350 P2d 1093 (1960)

O'Connor v Donaldson, 422 US 563, 95 S Ct 2486, 45 L Ed2d 396 (1975)

Rennie v Klein, 462 F Supp 1131 (D NJ 1978), remanded, 476 F Supp 1294 (D NJ 1979), aff'd in part, modified in part and remanded, 653 F2d 836 (3d Cir 1980), vacated and remanded, 458 US 1119 (1982), 720 F2d 266 (3rd Cir. 1983)

Riggins v Nevada, 504 US 127 (1992)

Rogers v Commissioner of Department of Mental Health, 390 Mass 489, 458 NE2d 308 (Mass 1983)

Roy v Hartogs, 85 Misc2d 891, 381 NYS2d 587, 381 NYS 587 (App Term 1976)

Schloendorff v Society of New York Hospital, 211 NY 125, 105 NE 92 (1914)

Sell v United States, 539 US 166 (2003)

Shine v Vega, 429 Mass 456, 709 NE2d 58 (1999)

Tarasoff v Regents of the University of California, 17 Cal 3d 425, 551 P2d 334; 131 Cal Rptr 14 (1976)

Washington v Harper, 494 US 210 (1990)

Wyatt v Stickney, 325 F Supp 781 (MD Ala 1971)

Youngberg v Romeo, 457 US 307 (1982); on remand, Romeo v Youngberg, 687 F2d 33 (3rd Cir 1982)

Zinermon v Burch, 494 US 113, 110 S Ct 975, 108 L Ed2d 100 (1990)

Recommended Readings

Benedek EP, Ash P, Scott CL (eds): Principles and Practice of Child and Adolescent Forensic Mental Health. Washington, DC, American Psychiatric Publishing, 2009

Gold LH: Clinical Guide to Mental Disability Evaluations. Edited by Vanderpool DL. Berlin, Germany, Springer, 2013

Gold LH, Anfang SA, Drukteinis AM, et al: AAPL practice guideline for the forensic evaluation of psychiatric disability. J Am Acad Psychiatry Law 36 (4 suppl):S3–S50, 2008

Schouten R (ed): Mental Health Practice and the Law. New York, Oxford University Press, 2017

Scott C (ed): DSM-5 and the Law: Changes and Challenges. New York, Oxford University Press, 2015

Appendix: Glossary of Legal Terms

Actus reus   Literally translated from Latin as "guilty act"; the physical act of a crime.

Appellate   Related to an appeal; appellate courts review, and may overturn, the decisions of lower courts.

Burden of proof   The duty of proving one's case; in criminal cases the state has the burden of proof to demonstrate a defendant's guilt; in civil cases, this burden falls on the plaintiff.

Case law   Previous court rulings by which legal precedents are set.

Damages   Money that is awarded to plaintiffs in civil cases; can be compensatory or punitive (to punish the defendant).

Defendant   A person facing criminal or civil charges.

Discovery   Information related to a legal matter; compiled and disclosed to both sides prior to a hearing or trial.

Felony   A relatively serious criminal act; generally involves sentences greater than 1 year.

Jurisdiction   A court's authority to hear a particular type of case; may also indicate the geographical area over which a court may try cases.

Mens rea   Literally translated from Latin as "guilty mind"; the intention of wrongdoing related to the commission of an illegal act.

Misdemeanor   Less serious criminal acts; punishment limited to 1 year of imprisonment.

Plaintiff   A person or entity who files a complaint with the court.

Plea   In criminal cases, a defendant's statement of guilt, innocence, or insanity prior to a trial.

Pro se   Refers to situations in which defendants choose to represent themselves in court.

Standard of proof   The degree to which a prosecutor or plaintiff must prove a defendant's guilt.

Subpoena   A court order that compels an individual to appear and provide testimony.

Voir dire   A process by which the court determines an expert witness's expertise and qualifications prior to testimony.

PART II

Psychiatric Disorders

CHAPTER 9

Neurodevelopmental Disorders

David S. Hong, M.D.
Lawrence K. Fung, M.D., Ph.D.
Antonio Hardan, M.D.

In this chapter, we consider the DSM-5 diagnostic class of neurodevelopmental disorders (American Psychiatric Association 2013). As the name implies, disorders within this class represent impairments in a broad range of cognitive, motor, or sensory functions that typically change dynamically across developmental stages. These conditions are characterized by symptoms that are acquired or inherited and that demonstrate divergence from an expected trajectory of skill acquisition over time. Etiologies for disorders within this class are highly heterogeneous. Indeed, the nature of these developmental effects is such that definitions of pathology may encompass individuals falling in the lower tail of population-wide dimensional traits, as well as individuals affected by more specific pathophysiological processes. Regardless of cause, it is important to approach disorders in this category with a comprehensive evaluation of a number of cognitive functions; careful consideration of genetic, familial, and environmental risk factors; and contextualization within a developmental framework. As with other diagnostic classes, impairments in this group of disorders must demonstrate significant impact on adaptive functioning, generally manifesting in learning or work environments.

Development can follow a number of patterned trajectories, as illustrated in Figure 9–1.

Intellectual Disabilities

The DSM-5 intellectual disabilities category encompasses conditions characterized by delayed development of general mental abilities, which is associated with significant

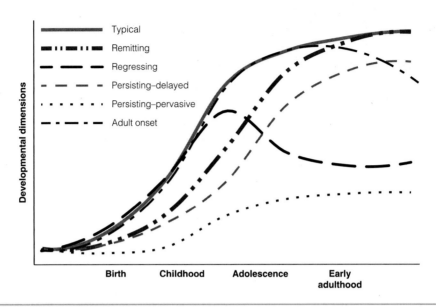

FIGURE 9–1. Developmental trajectories.

Potential trajectories of development include the following: **Typical:** development that is steady, relatively linear, and rapid throughout childhood and adolescence, and to a lesser degree in adulthood; **Remitting:** development characterized by a pattern of delayed maturation throughout childhood and adolescence that ultimately converges with the trajectory of chronological-age peers in adulthood; **Regressing:** development that appears relatively typical in early stages, only to diverge or regress from the trajectory of chronological-age peers at a later stage; **Persisting–delayed:** development that is steady but persistently slower over time; **Persisting–pervasive:** development that appears to halt at a specific developmental stage; and **Adult onset:** development that diverges from the trajectory of chronological-age peers in late adolescence or adulthood.

deficits in daily adaptive functioning. Diagnoses in this group include intellectual disability, global developmental delay, and unspecified intellectual disability, depending on criteria met.

Clinical Features

While prior versions of DSM defined intellectual disability primarily by intelligence quotient (IQ) scores, the current DSM-5 schema incorporates both intellectual abilities and level of adaptive functioning as determinants for diagnostic criteria (American Psychiatric Association 2013). In concert, the term *intellectual disability* has replaced the earlier term *mental retardation,* a change reflecting current practices both within the clinical domain and across other related educational and professional fields. These changes represent an increasing conceptualization of intelligence as a construct representing both psychometrically defined intellectual function and the interaction of cognitive abilities with the ability to navigate one's environment.

The definition of intellectual disability is agnostic of etiology, a stance reflected in the fact that there are no exclusion criteria for the disorder. As a result, the clinical features of intellectual disability can be quite varied as long as evidence for deficits in intellectual and adaptive functioning is present. However, a unifying theme in these conditions is evidence for impairments in well-established cognitive faculties: verbal comprehension, working memory, perceptual reasoning, quantitative reasoning, abstract thought, and cognitive efficacy. While these dimensions are typically psychometrically defined or measured, clinical manifestations of intellectual disability will often take the form of global delays in achieving cognitive, academic, or social milestones. While there is a degree of interindividual heterogeneity in the extent to which different cognitive domains are affected, as a general guideline, there should be evidence that most domains are affected in order to meet criteria for this diagnosis. In cases where specific cognitive functions appear substantially more affected than others, diagnoses associated with those particular cognitive faculties may be appropriate (e.g., specific learning disorders, communication disorders, autism spectrum disorder). Broader impairments in intellectual ability may manifest as difficulties with reasoning and practical understanding throughout stages of development, but may also manifest as impaired communication abilities, gullibility, or poor management of emotions or behavior. In certain instances, behavioral correlates of cognitive deficits may appear more uniform, as is commonly the case in syndromic disorders with a well-defined genetic basis. Conditions such as trisomy 21 (Down syndrome), fragile X syndrome, and Rett syndrome, among others, may commonly present with specific cognitive profiles or patterns of cognitive ability that are shared among individuals affected with these conditions. These "behavioral phenotypes" in neurogenetic conditions offer further insight into the biological processes underlying intellectual function, as well as providing important leads for clinicians to pursue in the treatment of these disorders.

An important innovation in DSM-5 is the increased emphasis on adaptive functioning (as opposed to intellectual capacity alone) as a foundational criterion for the diagnosis. In accordance with this heightened emphasis, behavioral manifestations of the condition are required to include evidence for difficulties in meeting standards for personal independence and social responsibility within the appropriate sociocultural and developmental context. Specifiers of severity of intellectual disability have similarly shifted to an emphasis on adaptive functioning rather than on psychometric scores, highlighting the importance of this domain in defining psychopathology. The adaptive functioning components considered in DSM-5 encompass competence in *conceptual, social,* and *practical* domains. Related behaviors in these domains include academic function, problem solving and judgment, interpersonal abilities, and self-management of activities of daily living, among others. These features are similarly affected by physical and psychiatric comorbidities, and impairments in these domains may be complex and multifactorial. It is important to use careful clinical judgment in assessing impairments in these domains within an appropriate sociocultural context.

Prevalence and Epidemiology

Prevalence estimates for intellectual disability in the general population are varied, with meta-analyses indicating that rates are approximately between 0.5% and 1.5%, with commonly accepted figures estimating 1% prevalence (Maenner et al. 2016; Maulik et al. 2011). These estimates have remained relatively stable in recent years. Intellectual disability has been identified in all races and cultures, as reflected in international data. However, significant differences have been reported based on disparities in socioeconomic status, sex, and age. These reports include findings that intellectual disability is less prevalent in younger than in older children, and less prevalent in adults than in youth. Sex differences in prevalence have also been identified, with higher prevalence rates in males relative to females (i.e., a male-to-female ratio of 1.6 to 1) (Maenner et al. 2016). However, these findings appear to be moderated by severity, with greater sex disparities in mild to moderate severity cases and greater sex equivalence in severe cases. Findings for differences in prevalence based on race have been mixed.

Development and Course

By definition, intellectual disability is identified earlier in development (age <18 years) either by clinical history or by presentation at time of diagnosis. This earlier detection may be related to the fact that most etiologies underlying intellectual disability are likely inborn or acquired during early development. Differences may present in timing of diagnosis, with more severe intellectual disabilities being associated with earlier manifestation of deficits—and, by corollary, earlier identification of disorder. In contrast, milder forms of intellectual disability may escape detection until individuals are placed in settings with higher cognitive demands, such as academic or other learning environments. Acquired forms of intellectual disability will correlate with the timing of the insult, such as postinfectious sequelae, head trauma, or (more rarely) neurodegenerative conditions with onset during the developmental period.

Regarding course, intellectual disabilities generally tend to follow a fairly stable trajectory over development, particularly after stabilization in early childhood (age <7 years). The underlying inference is that causal insults resulting in intellectual disability generally tend to be time-limited and nonprogressive, and it is possible for future gains in cognitive and adaptive functioning to occur relative to an individual's baseline cognitive function. Developmental course in these instances is likely influenced by multiple factors, including efficacy and timing of interventions, as well as the inherent nature of the underlying etiology. Relatedly, due to the heterogeneity of causes underlying intellectual disability, there will also be subsets of individuals with intellectual disability that may not achieve age-related gains in cognitive or adaptive functioning; or that may demonstrate progressive declines in function relative to age norms, or even show patterns of regression from previously acquired cognitive or adaptive skills. In these specific instances, a diagnosis of neurocognitive disorder may also be considered.

Etiology and Risk/Prognostic Factors

In keeping with the complex biological processes underlying neurodevelopment and related cognitive functions, there are numerous channels through which cognitive development may be disrupted. These span both inborn and acquired mechanisms and reflect both genetic and environmental factors. While the majority of cases of intellectual disability are of unknown etiology, rapidly expanding knowledge of genetic mechanisms underlying cognition suggests that up to 55%–70% of moderate-to-severe cases of intellectual disability may be related to genetic causes, with more than 700 genes associated with intellectual disability already identified (Vissers et al. 2016). Genetic etiologies include single-gene disorders, copy number variants, and chromosomal abnormalities. Intellectual disability has also been linked to environmental causes, including pre- or perinatal exposure to infectious agents or teratogens, congenital or hypoxic conditions, malnutrition, severe psychological neglect and deprivation, and head trauma, among others.

Diagnostic Evaluation

Whereas establishment of onset of symptoms in the developmental period (DSM-5 Criterion C) is often straightforward, diagnostic evaluation for other criteria in intellectual disability may be challenging, particularly when considering chronological age at the time of assessment, developmental ability, or severity of the symptoms. However, there are numerous useful approaches for establishing that diagnostic criteria are met, including collateral history from informants and utilization of standardized instruments. In the instance that individuals are presenting for assessment early in development (age <5 years), determination of clinical severity of intellectual deficits may not be reliable. For individuals in this age range who demonstrate delays in meeting developmental milestones, a diagnosis of global developmental delay would be appropriate.

Assessment for deficits in intellectual functions (DSM-5 Criterion A) involves clinical assessment and standardized intelligence testing. Diagnostic testing in this dimension will therefore include psychometric measures of intelligence; commonly used tests include the Wechsler intelligence scales and the Differential Abilities Scale. These assessments typically incorporate age- and sex-based norms for a representative population-based sample. Intellectual disability for Criterion A is then defined as scores approximately two standard deviations below the expected population mean. On assessments with a full-scale IQ population mean of 100 with a standard deviation of 15, scores below 70 (±5 points for measurement error) would be considered evidence of cognitive impairment. Psychometric properties of assessments have been extensively documented in the literature and should be carefully considered, including practice effects; score validity in the face of discrepant subtest scores; accuracy of the measurement in reflecting innate intellectual ability as related to confounding factors of motivation or attention; and other communication, sensory, language, or cultural biases that may affect testing performance.

The potential limitations of intelligence testing in accurately classifying disability underscore the importance of DSM-5 Criterion B, which requires evidence for impaired adaptive functioning in everyday life across academic/intellectual, social, and practical domains. Diagnostic evaluation of this dimension often encompasses clinical evaluation and collateral information from other reliable informants, or standardized testing instruments specifically geared toward assessment of adaptive behavior, such as the Vineland Adaptive Behavior Scales. Importantly, severity of intellectual disability is classified in DSM-5 on the basis of adaptive functioning deficits rather than intelligence scores through use of the specifiers *mild, moderate, severe,* and *profound.* As with assessment of cognitive function, careful clinical judgment is warranted in determination of adaptive functioning, with appropriate context for social norms for the patient to be considered when making a diagnosis.

Given the high prevalence of syndromic causes associated with intellectual disability, diagnostic evaluations should necessarily include comprehensive clinical evaluation of developmental, medical, and family histories to assist in establishing a specific etiology whenever possible. Careful physical examination with particular sensitivity to neurological signs or dysmorphic features is also needed. Referral for further genetic evaluation or workup with chromosomal microarray and fragile X testing is also routine in newly diagnosed cases of intellectual disability. In rare instances where assessment of clearly evident intellectual deficits is difficult due to associated sensory or physical impairment or disruptive behaviors that impede the process, a DSM-5 diagnosis of *unspecified intellectual disability* may be considered.

Comorbid Psychiatric Disorders

Intellectual disability is highly comorbid with other psychiatric disorders, particularly in view of the fact that there are no exclusion criteria for the disorder. A number of disorders can affect cognitive function, likely increasing the rates of concurrent diagnoses. From an alternative perspective, conditions such as attention-deficit/hyperactivity disorder (ADHD), autism spectrum disorder (ASD), mood and anxiety disorders, and disruptive behavior disorders have a much higher prevalence in individuals with intellectual disability.

Treatment

Treatment planning for intellectual disability often requires interdisciplinary collaboration across clinical, educational, and community domains. While there is sparse evidence for disease-modifying interventions for deficits in global cognitive function, behavioral and educational strategies may significantly improve adaptive functioning over the developmental period. Similarly, comprehensive management of comorbid symptoms, including therapy and medication management, may significantly affect long-term clinical outcomes. For individuals with a higher burden of symptoms, clinical treatment tends to be interdisciplinary in nature and requires substantial case management support to coordinate care across different environments.

Communication Disorders

Human language represents the capacity to convey information between individuals and comprises a set of developmentally emergent skills that support this important social function. Abilities within this domain include generating units of communication (whether in the form of signed or spoken language), developing a semiotic system to assign meanings to these signs, and learning to place these signs within a context to effectively relay information to others. Disorders in communication may disrupt any of these functions, potentially influencing an individual's ability to effectively navigate the social or academic environment. Based on this general framework, communication disorders are categorized in DSM-5 under the domains of language, speech, and communication, which respectively encompass the various aspects of facility in understanding and using a symbolic system; effectively producing sound; and functional implementation of verbal and nonverbal actions to interact with others. This group of conditions are often underrecognized in psychiatric settings despite their high prevalence in the population and often require collaboration with providers outside of psychiatric practice, such as speech and language pathologists, occupational and physical therapists, and educators. Further complicating this category, consensus diagnoses around communication disorders continue to be a subject of debate, reflecting the complex and interdisciplinary nature of these conditions.

Language Disorder

Clinical Features

As the name implies, language disorder represents a category of deficits in the acquisition and use of language. Whereas previous DSM editions defined expressive and mixed receptive–expressive subtypes, DSM-5 more broadly defines impairments in the capacity to effectively produce, receive, or comprehend language signals within this diagnostic category, while still recognizing that deficits may be more pronounced in either the receptive or the expressive domain. There has been considerable evolution in the definition of *language disorder* in recent years even outside of DSM, with other terms such as "developmental language disorder" and "specific language impairment" causing some confusion, although interdisciplinary efforts are ongoing to achieve consensus around these terms.

The relatively broad array of skills supporting language means that deficits may manifest in numerous ways. Clinical presentations may include difficulties with grammar; i.e., individuals may demonstrate errors in the morphemes, or form of language, spanning appropriate use of tenses or plurals, verbs and nouns, comprehension of complex syntax, and so on. Alternatively, deficits may manifest as impoverished language repertoires and vocabulary or difficulty in effectively using these forms in discourse. In contrast to other aspects of speech or communication, individuals with language disorders may still have intact articulation or communication skills, such as relatively facile use of nonverbal gestures.

Prevalence and Epidemiology

Language deficits are common in childhood, with prevalence estimates ranging from approximately 3% to 9% (Norbury et al. 2016), and are even more likely to be overrepresented in individuals referred to child and adolescent psychiatry.

Development and Course

Much like other cognitive domains, there is a clear developmental trajectory evident in the acquisition of language, with most individuals achieving adult levels of language ability by adolescence. However, there is substantial interindividual variation in the rate and consistency of language development in early childhood. This heterogeneity limits the sensitivity and specificity of assessment of impairments in the early developmental period, particularly in children younger than 3 years. However, the presence of language deficits by 4 years of age appears to be predictive of later language problems, with increased prevalence of deficits in later developmental stages (Weindrich et al. 2000).

Etiology and Risk/Prognostic Factors

Language disorders appear to be highly heritable, indicating a strong contribution of genetic factors. Clear genetic etiologies have yet to be identified but likely represent a complex multigenic process. However, a number of single-gene candidates have been implicated in language disorders, including *FOXP2* and *CNTNAP2*, among others (Newbury et al. 2010). It is likewise clear that language development is sensitive to environmental factors, including associations with social advantage, early exposure to language, and environmental insults occurring both in utero and during later development. It is also important to note that the ambient language environment to which individuals are exposed during language acquisition substantially influences development and may manifest as many nonpathological variations in language structure and grammar. Similarly, individual factors such as cognitive strategies for information processing and motivation to attend to language acquisition may further affect developmental trajectories in this domain.

Diagnostic Evaluation

Language evaluation should be considered within the larger context of environment, exposure to language throughout development, and other sociocultural contexts, such as primary languages and dialects used in the home. As part of routine screening, or when suspicion for language deficits arises, a thorough evaluation for underlying sensory and structural neurological issues, such as hearing impairment or global intellectual disability, should be considered. Based on DSM-5 criteria, language deficits arising from a specific identified structural etiology would exclude a language disorder diagnosis as currently defined; however, acquired language deficits secondary to neurological disorders such as epilepsy would potentially meet criteria for the disorder. In addition to a thorough clinical evaluation to rule out other psychopathology, diagnostic evaluation should include standardized assessments to assess global intellectual ability and language ability, as well as evaluation of sensorimotor functions to rule out other structural etiologies. Evaluations will synthesize information from multiple informants and will typically be conducted in collaboration with neuropsychology and speech/language pathology services. As yet, imaging-based tools for diagnostic evaluation remain elusive, despite an increased understanding of the neural circuitry underlying language and comprehension functions.

Comorbid Psychiatric Disorders

Language disorder is frequently identified with other neurodevelopmental disorders, including specific learning disorder, ADHD, and motor and coordination disorders.

Treatment

Current treatment paradigms are centered on language development and target instruction of specific language skills. Given the relatively varied domains within language that may be primarily affected, intervention plans should rely heavily on individualized assessment and related treatment goals and are typically administered in coordination with speech and language pathologists. Treatment is tailored to the developmental age of the individual and may focus on phonology, morphology, syntax, vocabulary environment, and pragmatics. Multiple approaches to language instruction have been developed, spanning developmental stages and encompassing early intervention with family and individuals, structured academic intervention in an individual or group context within school or clinical settings, modification of the environmental milieu to enhance language, and structured behavioral treatment to increase specific communication behaviors. Technology is increasingly being incorporated into treatment plans, particularly for individuals with severe deficits, which may entail picture communication symbols or other augmentative and alternative communication devices. There is little evidence supporting use of pharmacological agents in language disorder.

Speech Sound Disorder

Clinical Features

Speech sound disorder encompasses deficits in the articulation or phonology of spoken language. Individuals with this condition may have difficulty using phonemes, the basic units of spoken language, to produce intelligible speech. This function entails both phonological awareness of speech sounds and the ability to translate that awareness into speech through motor coordination of orofacial musculature and management of airstream production. Symptoms in this domain may manifest clinically as differences in speech patterns, including substitutions of one phonetic sound for another, additions or deletions of sounds/syllables in a word, and distorting sounds in a word independent of local dialect or accents.

Prevalence and Epidemiology

Speech sound disorders are fairly common, with prevalence estimates as high as 2%–4% (L. Law et al. 2000; Shriberg et al. 1999).

Development and Course

Similar to language disorder, early development of speech is fairly variable in typical development. However, typically, most children will use intelligible speech by 4 years of age and will have mastered phonemes by 8 years of age. Developmental timing of specific phonemes may vary, which may relate to their inherent complexity. However, evidence of persistent misarticulation of sounds beyond developmental norms may indicate a potential speech sound disorder. Longer-term outcomes for speech sound disorder indicate an ongoing developmental pattern, with most children affected by this condition improving over time.

Etiology and Risk/Prognostic Factors

The etiology of a developmental speech sound disorder as defined in DSM-5 is still unknown. Similarly, the functions supporting speech encompass a broad range of cognitive (phonological) and motor coordination skills, indicating that underlying etiologies are also likely heterogeneous. Furthermore, a number of related conditions may affect speech production, including neurological disorders and sensory or hearing problems.

Diagnostic Evaluation

Similar to other communication disorders, speech sound disorder evaluation typically comprises a comprehensive assessment of speech and language ability through clinical interview, standardized measures assessing language, and thorough assessment for medical and physical factors. Diagnostic evaluation should carefully screen for other conditions with a clear functional neurological basis that may affect speech production, including audiological examination and orofacial abnormalities. Global intellectual disability and contextualization of speech relative to the child's cultural and linguistic environment needs to be carefully assessed. Further screening to rule out other psychopathology impeding speech production in specific contexts, such as social anxiety or selective mutism, should also be considered.

Comorbid Psychiatric Disorders

As with other communication disorders, speech sound disorder is commonly diagnosed with other neurodevelopmental conditions. Language disorder may be comorbid with this diagnosis, particularly when expressive deficits have been identified. If articulation is primarily involved, other motor coordination issues may be present, with a diagnosis of developmental coordination disorder as an additional comorbidity.

Treatment

Careful screening and assessment may lead to interventions for speech/language pathology, educational intervention, and other psychiatric and medical interventions as required. Treatment is focused on increasing speech intelligibility, with emphasis on the production of whole words rather than individual phonemes. As is the case with other language disorders, treatment is often coordinated by speech and language pathologists and the educational system and may focus on behavioral approaches to enhance coordination of oral motor function to improve speech production. In more severe cases, augmentative and alternative communication devices are used. Although the evidence base for long-term efficacy of these interventions is limited, evidence supports improved outcomes relative to individuals who do not receive intervention.

Childhood-Onset Fluency Disorder (Stuttering)

Clinical Features

Childhood-onset fluency disorder, or stuttering, affects a specific aspect of speech—that of oral fluency, which pertains to the rate and continuity of speech production. Clinical evidence of dysfluency may take the form of repetitions of sounds or syllables ("s-s-s-orry") or blocking and prolongations of sounds. Symptoms may also manifest as word substitutions to avoid problematic words or excessive physical tension to produce words. Symptoms may demonstrate substantial variability, both from day to day and over a period of years. Severity of symptoms may be dependent on context or perceived pressure in situations where speech occurs. It is not uncommon for clinical manifestations to be detected by compensatory strategies adopted by individuals who stutter, including avoidance behaviors.

Prevalence and Epidemiology

Similar to other communication disorders, stuttering is relatively common, with prevalence estimates ranging from 1% to 5% in the general population (Yairi and Ambrose 2013). As with other neurodevelopmental disorders, there appears to be a sex difference, with slightly increased male predominance. The association of dysfluency with race or ethnicity is unclear.

Development and Course

As opposed to many other communication disorders, where atypical patterns emerge nearer to school age, the vast majority of childhood-onset fluency issues will be evident prior to 5 years of age. There appears to be an age-related effect, with children more likely to be affected relative to adolescents or adults. One interpretation of these findings is that a cohort of youth will experience remission in symptoms over the course of development. Similar to tic disorders, periods of dysfluency may occur in early development that do not demonstrate a pervasive pattern throughout development. Dysfluency that emerges after adolescence is identified as an adult-onset dysfluency and is typically associated with a specific neurological or medical condition. As such, it would not meet criteria for childhood-onset fluency disorder as defined in DSM-5.

Etiology and Risk/Prognostic Factors

A specific etiology has yet to be identified for childhood-onset fluency disorder; however, twin studies indicate a higher concordance among monozygotic relative to dizygotic twins, demonstrating a degree of heritability.

Diagnostic Evaluation

Clinical evaluation for dysfluencies incorporates a broad assessment of function and sampling of language abilities, including standardized measures of speech production and fluency such as the Stuttering Severity Instrument. Cultural and language contexts for the individual should always be considered. A thorough evaluation of avoidance and anxiety behaviors and other psychopathology, as well as a review of academic, medical, and family history, should be undertaken within the context that they may represent accessory behaviors to underlying dysfluency or independent comorbidity. When evidence of dysfluency is present, evaluation and treatment should be carried out in coordination with speech and language pathologists. Alternative or co-occurring diagnoses should be considered, including other language or learning disorders, other forms of dysfluency, and neurological conditions affecting fluency, as well as cultural and environmental factors.

Comorbidity

Childhood-onset fluency disorder may co-occur with other language-based disorders, tic or motor disorders, and ADHD. It is also more commonly identified in certain syndromic conditions, such as ASD and Down syndrome.

Treatment

Treatment for speech dysfluency is typically provided by speech and language pathologists and incorporates multiple strategies that address speech patterns directly, as well as secondary behaviors that influence the individual's functioning. Given the evidence of age effects on symptom course, the individual's developmental stage is typically considered in determining the need for intervention as well as the intensity and goals of treatment. Meta-analyses suggest that although most studies of treatment efficacy in stuttering are at risk for bias, there is indication for positive effects (Herder et al. 2006); however, there is also a high degree of interindividual variability in course. When indicated, intervention may focus on speech modification and efficiency, and may include working with individuals and families to reduce negative perceptions of dysfluency and accessory behaviors. Educational accommodations and coordination of care with school systems are frequently incorporated in the treatment plan to improve adaptive functioning.

Social (Pragmatic) Communication Disorder

Clinical Features

Social (pragmatic) communication disorder (SPCD) is a new category in DSM-5 that relates to deficits in the pragmatic aspects of language. The disorder is characterized by impairments in communicating for social purposes, adjusting communication to match the context of the conversation, observing rules of typical conversation, and understanding implicit meanings. Per DSM-5, symptoms must have their onset at an early age, and the symptoms must not be attributable to another psychiatric, neurological, or medical disorder. Unlike individuals with ASD, individuals with SPCD do not have restricted and repetitive behaviors.

Prevalence and Epidemiology

The prevalence of SPCD is not available at this time. A recent study found that SPCD is not qualitatively distinct from ASD and that patients diagnosed with SPCD have ASD traits that are insufficiently severe for an ASD diagnosis (Mandy et al. 2017).

Etiology and Risk/Prognostic Factors

Currently it is not clear whether SCPD represents a mild subtype or variant of ASD. Therefore, strong scientific evidence is lacking to support any specific etiologies for SPCD. Diagnostic evaluation is based on clinical interview and DSM-5 criteria.

Treatment

Given the relatively recent emergence of this diagnostic category, no evidence-based treatments have been developed for SPCD to date. However, it is reasonable to assume that the interventions used to treat social communication deficits in ASD (e.g., social skills training) may also be applicable for patients with SPCD.

Autism Spectrum Disorder

Clinical Features

ASD is a neurodevelopmental disorder characterized by impairments in social communication and social interaction, repetitive and stereotyped behaviors, and/or sensory aberrations. ASD is a highly heterogeneous condition with a wide spectrum of presentations, which can range from nonverbal individuals with severe core and comorbid symptomatology (as first described by Leo Kanner) to individuals with high intellectual capacity but enough core symptoms to impact their daily living. Per DSM-5, the diagnosis of ASD requires the presence of all three social communication criteria and at least two of the four additional criteria, with onset of symptoms in the early developmental period. The three social communication criteria are 1) deficits in social-emotional reciprocity, 2) deficits in nonverbal communicative behaviors used for social interaction, and 3) deficits in developing, maintaining, and understanding relationships. The four additional criteria for ASD are as follows: 1) stereotyped or repetitive motor movements; 2) cognitive inflexibility or ritualized patterns of verbal or nonverbal behavior; 3) highly restricted, fixated interests that are abnormal in intensity or focus; and 4) hyperreactivity or hyporeactivity to sensory input or unusual interest in sensory aspects of the environment. To further describe interindividual differences, specifiers for the DSM-5 ASD diagnosis are provided to denote the following: severity (level of support required); absence or presence of accompanying intellectual impairment; absence or presence of accompanying language impairment; association with a known medical or genetic condition or environmental factor; association with another neurodevelopmental, mental, or behavioral disorder; and presence of catatonia.

Prevalence and Epidemiology

When autism was initially described, it was considered a rare condition. In the mid-1970s, the U.S. prevalence was estimated at 5 cases per 10,000 children. Reported prevalence has increased substantially since that time, with the most recent estimated prevalence being 1 in 68 children at age 8 years, and with pronounced sex differences (i.e., a male-to-female ratio of 4 to 1) (Christensen et al. 2016). The prevalence of ASD in adults has been less investigated; however, the largest epidemiological study in adults with ASD identified a prevalence of 1 in 102 and a male-to-female ratio of 9 to 1 in the United Kingdom (Brugha et al. 2011). In all countries in which multiple studies have been conducted, there is a pattern of increasing prevalence over time. Clearly, some of the increase is attributable to improved detection, increased awareness, and use of broader diagnostic criteria. However, these factors do not appear to fully explain the dramatic rise in ASD. This phenomenon appears to apply to all socioeconomic levels, races, and ethnicities.

Development and Course

The developmental trajectories of core and comorbid symptoms of ASD are dependent on multiple factors, including IQ, age at initiation of intervention, and type and duration of intervention. Later functional and adaptive outcomes are highly related to overall cognitive ability. Educational, vocational, economic, community, and family supports play an important role in promoting positive adaptation. In addition, the availability of high-quality intensive early intervention for an increasing number of young children may alter long-term clinical outcomes for ASD.

In a recent study involving 203 children ages 1–4 years with ASD, participants were assessed over a 3-year period (Visser et al. 2017). During this early developmental period, five different trajectories were identified:

- A mild–stable group (48% of cohort; mean baseline nonverbal IQ [NV-IQ)] of 93). Children in this group maintained their NV-IQs throughout the assessment period. They also had the highest scores on ADHD-related traits.
- A moderate–stable group (22% of cohort; mean baseline NV-IQ of 72). Over the assessment period, these children showed a slight increase in NV-IQs.
- A severe–stable group (20% of cohort; mean baseline NV-IQ of 45). Children in this group showed no language improvement, persistently low NV-IQs, and marked increases in attention problems over time.
- A severe-to-moderate change group (5% of cohort; mean baseline NV-IQ of 61). In addition to improvement on ASD scores, these children improved on language, NV-IQ, and ADHD-related traits.

- A moderate-to-mild/nonspectrum change group (5% of cohort (mean baseline NV-IQ of 83). Together with improvement on ASD scores, these children showed improvements on language, NV-IQ, and ADHD-related traits.

Existing literature suggests that the vast majority of children diagnosed with ASD will retain the diagnosis into adulthood. Although ASD is a lifelong condition, symptoms usually improve with age, with periods of waxing or waning of specific symptoms, in some cases to the extent that individuals may no longer meet criteria for an ASD diagnosis as they age.

Etiology and Risk/Prognostic Factors

ASD has multiple putative etiologies; according to AutDB (a curated database for autism research; www.mindspec.org/autdb.html), more than 800 genes have been associated with ASD to date, with more than 70 risk loci strongly associated with the disorder (Sanders et al. 2015). Genetic factors play a strong role, although few specific genes accounting for any substantial percentage of cases have been discovered. ASD is highly heritable, with most recent studies estimating the proportion of risk attributable to genetic factors at 40% to 50% (Hallmayer et al. 2011; Sandin et al. 2014). A large population-based study involving more than 2 million Swedish children and 2.6 million siblings found a relative recurrence risk of 10.3 for full siblings, 3.3 for maternal half-siblings, and 2.9 for paternal half-siblings (Sandin et al. 2014). Genetic causes, such as chromosomal abnormalities and de novo copy number variations (Iossifov et al. 2014), are implicated in about 10%–20% of individuals with ASD. Genetic causes of ASD may be classified into syndromic and nonsyndromic. Many genetic syndromes are highly associated with ASD, including fragile X syndrome, which is the most common monogenetic cause of ASD. Approximately 28% of males and 11% of females with fragile X syndrome met DSM-5 criteria for ASD (Wheeler et al. 2015). Other genetic syndromes with a high prevalence of ASD include Rett syndrome (61%), Cohen syndrome (54%), Cornelia de Lange syndrome (43%), tuberous sclerosis complex (36%), Angelman syndrome (34%), and neurofibromatosis type 1 (18%) (Richards et al. 2015). Among individuals with nonsyndromic ASD, no single genetic etiology accounts for more than 0.2% of cases based on large gene-sequencing studies (Vorstman et al. 2017).

Risk of ASD has been found to be associated with environmental factors, such as older paternal age and birth complications. Other environmental influences include prenatal exposure to thalidomide or valproic acid. Although a subject of much debate, immunization has been confirmed in definitive studies not to have a causal role in ASD (DeStefano et al. 2013; Madsen et al. 2002; Parker et al. 2004). However, evidence of immune dysregulation in individuals with ASD has been gradually accumulating (Estes and McAllister 2015).

Diagnostic Evaluation

Guidelines for the assessment of ASD have been published by various professional organizations, including a practice parameter published by the American Academy of Child and Adolescent Psychiatry (Volkmar et al. 2014). In general, there are two levels of evaluation: Level 1 screening involves routine developmental surveillance by primary care physicians for young children, and Level 2 evaluation involves a more thorough diagnostic assessment by experienced clinicians (e.g., child and adolescent psychiatrists, pediatric neurologists, developmental and behavioral pediatricians, child psychologists, speech and language pathologists) for children in whom screening identifies significant ASD symptomatology. The Level 2 assessment typically involves a review of presenting symptoms; a psychiatric review of systems; a psychiatric and behavioral history; a detailed developmental, school, medical, and social history obtained from parents and care providers; a review of available records (e.g., school reports, neuropsychological testing); and direct observation of and interaction with the child.

Although standardized instruments are not required to establish a diagnosis of ASD, many clinics use such instruments in routine assessments for ASD. Currently, the gold standard diagnostic tool for direct assessment of symptoms is the Autism Diagnostic Observation Schedule, a 40-minute semistructured interaction formatted into multiple modules that are developmentally appropriate from infancy through adulthood and across the range of functioning levels. In some clinical and most research settings, the Autism Diagnostic Interview—Revised (ADI-R) is used to establish the developmental history required for ASD diagnosis. The ADI-R is a semistructured comprehensive interview for parents or caregivers of children and adults being assessed for ASD.

A critical part of the process of case formulation is differential diagnosis to determine whether presenting symptoms are due to ASD, an independent condition, or the presence of co-occurring disorders. For example, poor eye contact and low social initiative are common manifestations in children and adults with ASD, but these symptoms are also frequently found in children with depression or anxiety and in individuals with schizoid personality disorder or avoidant personality disorder. However, whereas individuals with ASD often have abnormal psychomotor function and inattention, these symptoms are typically absent in schizoid and avoidant personality disorders. Another condition commonly included in the differential diagnosis of ASD is obsessive-compulsive disorder (OCD). However, whereas rituals and compulsions can be part of both ASD and OCD symptomatology, they tend to be ego-syntonic in ASD but ego-dystonic in OCD. Furthermore, the compulsions in ASD are typically related to sensory-seeking behaviors or restricted interests, whereas the compulsions in OCD are related to contamination fears, superstitions, and repeated doubts.

Comorbid Psychiatric Disorders

Psychiatric comorbidity is generally considered the rule rather than the exception in individuals with ASD. The prevalence of specific comorbid psychiatric conditions is dependent on age and intellectual functioning. Among children between the ages of 10 and 14 years, the most common comorbid diagnoses were found to be social anxiety disorder (prevalence of 29%), ADHD (28%), and oppositional defiant disorder (28%) (Simonoff et al. 2008). In adults with ASD, depression and anxiety were the most common comorbidities, and in ASD populations with comorbid intellectual disability, anxiety and OCD were found to be the most common psychiatric comorbidities (Buck et al. 2014).

Comorbid Medical Conditions

Medical comorbidities in multiple body systems (e.g., gastrointestinal, neurological, immunological) occur in children and adolescents with ASD. In a retrospective prevalence study involving more than 14,000 individuals with ASD younger than 35 years of age, the most common medical comorbidities were epilepsy (19%) and bowel disorders (12%) (Kohane et al. 2012). Another study found that food allergies and sensitivities were more common in children with ASD than in typically developing controls and that these issues appeared to correlate with behavioral problems (Lyall et al. 2015).

Treatment

Behavioral interventions are the most effective and widely used treatments for core symptoms of ASD. It is therefore imperative that initial diagnosis be followed by provision of validated behavioral treatments as soon as possible. Systematic reviews of early intensive interventions indicate that the Early Intensive Behavioral Intervention (EIBI) and the Early Start Denver Model (ESDM) have the strongest evidence for improving language and cognitive skills in children with ASD (Warren et al. 2011). The EIBI approach is based on principles of operant conditioning (reinforcement and negative consequences) and applied behavior analysis. EIBI involves several years of one-to-one intervention for 35–40 hours per week, carried out in the home (and occasionally in community settings). The ESDM approach incorporates similar behavioral principles but is more developmentally based, focusing on dyadic interactions, joint play, and activity routines between adult and child in which teaching opportunities are embedded in the play. Outcome studies for both approaches demonstrate large and significant gains in IQ and language compared with control conditions (Warren et al. 2011).

Pharmacological interventions are used primarily to treat comorbid symptoms rather than the core symptoms of ASD. Studies have provided support for use of risperidone or aripiprazole to treat irritability and associated aggressive behaviors (Fung et al. 2016), although these agents have significant adverse effects, including extrapyramidal side effects, somnolence, and weight gain. Stimulants have been shown to be effective in treating comorbid ADHD symptoms in individuals with ASD. The use of serotonin reuptake inhibitors lacks sufficient strength of evidence to evaluate benefit–risk profiles, although these medications are used clinically to manage repetitive behaviors and anxiety.

Attention-Deficit/Hyperactivity Disorder

Clinical Features

ADHD involves persistent impairments along core axes of inattention or hyperactivity–impulsivity. Broadly, clinical manifestations of *inattention* may be seen in behaviors such as frequent distraction, carelessness due to difficulty sustaining focus, and disorganization in management of materials or time. Behavioral aspects of *hyperactivity* are seen in excessive motor activity or restlessness in inappropriate contexts, fidgeting, or talkativeness. In the related domain of *impulsivity,* clinical features may be identified in social intrusiveness or action without accompanying self-monitoring. These features are reflected in DSM-5 schema, where a unified ADHD symptom structure is defined and is then further specified by *presentations* as predominantly inattentive, hyperactive/impulsive, or a combination of the two. An important aspect of the symptoms is that they are not context-dependent, but instead manifest in multiple settings (e.g., home and school). Indeed, ADHD features will often manifest with substantial impairments in academic or interpersonal environments, often resulting in learning difficulties, social rejection by peers and family, or elevated interpersonal conflict. Also, as with other disorders in this category, symptoms must first appear during the developmental period; in the case of ADHD, this period is defined as prior to age 12 years, which is expanded from prior definitions (e.g., before age 7 years in DSM-IV [American Psychiatric Association 1994]).

Prevalence and Epidemiology

ADHD is now the most common pediatric behavioral disorder, with epidemiological studies indicating prevalence rates between 5% and 10% in the general population (Danielson et al. 2018; Thomas et al. 2015). Meta-analyses indicate that prevalence rates are fairly consistent across countries, and differences identified appear to be strongly influenced by methodological variations in assessment of childhood behavior (Polanczyk et al. 2014). There do appear to be disparities in ADHD prevalence based on age and sex. Rates of ADHD are lower in adulthood relative to childhood, with most estimates for adulthood ADHD ranging between 2.5% and 5.0% (Kessler et al. 2006). Similarly, there appear to be sex differences in prevalence, with male:female ratios ranging from 2:1 to 4:1; however, there is some debate regarding the potential influence of referral bias, in that girls may be less likely to be referred for evaluation of ADHD, as well as evidence indicating that girls with ADHD are more likely than boys to be diagnosed with the inattentive presentation (Quinn and Madhoo 2014). Some studies that specifically focused on girls with ADHD suggest that whereas there may be a protective effect in terms of global prevalence of the disorder relative to boys, affected girls may also carry an increased disease burden, particularly during the adolescent period, when they are more likely to have issues associated with self-harm or emotional dyscontrol (Hinshaw et al. 2012).

Development and Course

As required by DSM-5 Criterion B, ADHD symptoms must be present by the early stages of development (age <12 years). Indeed, many individuals with ADHD will be identified by school age due to the emergence of impairments in home and learning environments. However, it is also not uncommon for ADHD to be diagnosed in adolescence or adulthood, at which point clinicians must rely on retrospective recollections of symptom onset, as well as confirmation through collateral information. There is concern for heterogeneity in ADHD symptomatology, particularly given the fairly significant symptom variation over time and context. It is not yet clear whether this variation represents the evolving nature of the disorder, differences in underlying biological mechanisms, or biases in the application of diagnostic criteria. Indeed, among children receiving a diagnosis of ADHD prior to 7 years of age, approximately 10% will not meet criteria for any psychiatric disorder after a follow-up period of 5–10 years, while another 20%–25% will later meet criteria for a psychiatric condition other than ADHD (E.C. Law et al. 2014). However, after the age of 7 years, the diagnosis appears to be relatively stable, although the stability of the initial presentation (or subtype, as defined in DSM-IV-TR [American Psychiatric Association 2000]) may vary across developmental stages, particularly when initial symptoms are in the hyperactive–impulsive domain (Lahey et al. 2005; E.C. Law et al. 2014).

A fundamental issue in the current conceptualization of ADHD is its definition as a disorder of childhood. Longitudinal data indicate that individuals with ADHD may be separated into cohorts with diverging trajectories of disease burden, including "remitters" and "persisters" with varying degrees of severity. This disparity in developmental course is reflected in lower rates of ADHD in adulthood, with prevalence roughly half that in children, and likely represents the etiological heterogeneity of ADHD. One consideration is that a subset of children with ADHD represent delayed maturational processes relative to chronological age in prefrontal cortices, while other cohorts indicate disruptions in more specific circuitry underlying attentional and inhibitory processes. However, a common feature in the developmental course is the finding that symptoms associated with the hyperactivity domain generally decrease over time in most individuals with the diagnosis. Finally, there is also newer evidence suggesting the existence of a cohort of individuals with adult-onset ADHD who do not meet historical criteria for childhood ADHD (Moffitt et al. 2015); however, this group would not meet criteria for ADHD as defined by DSM-5.

Etiology and Risk/Prognostic Factors

Behavioral and cognitive domains implicated in ADHD represent sophisticated and effortful higher-order cognitive functions. Given the extensive infrastructure supporting these multidimensional executive and control processes, there are numerous processes that are vulnerable to disruption during neurodevelopment. These include genetic causes, as is supported by findings of high degrees of heritability in twin and family-based studies (>80%). Recent consortia of genetic data have identified several candidate genes implicated in ADHD, although the limited odds ratios associated with these single-gene polymorphisms support the multifactorial nature of genetic processes underlying ADHD symptomatology, but also provide important pathways that underlie attentional processes (Faraone and Larsson 2018). Similarly, multiple physiological and environmental risk factors for ADHD have been identified, including low birth weight; infant malnutrition; unhealthy maternal diet; maternal smoking during pregnancy; child abuse; exposure to teratogens or environmental toxins; and sensory, sleep, and metabolic impairments, among many other potential causes.

Diagnostic Evaluation

Evaluation of ADHD may be challenging, given the heterogeneous clinical nature of these symptoms, which are often temporally and contextually variable. Similarly, attentional and inhibitory deficits in childhood often overlap with a number of other psychiatric conditions that commonly present during this developmental stage, necessitating rigorous screening and assessment practices to ensure accurate application of diagnoses. Diagnoses will typically be based on a thorough clinical assessment, entailing history of deficits in both inattentive and hyperactive–impulsive domains. History taking will focus on determining the age at onset of symptom presentation and placing symptoms within the context of a developmental and sociocultural framework. Family and medical histories are needed to identify potential etiologies and to rule out other potential diagnostic classifications. Collateral information is critical, often due to varying levels of perception of symptom burden based on reporter source and diagnostic criterion requiring presence of symptoms in multiple settings. Therefore, observer reports from family members, teachers, coworkers, or roommates are essential. Despite variability in symptom scale reports based on reporter source, standardized assessments are also important sources of information. Historical records from school settings and parental observations are particularly useful in establishing a diagnosis in adults presenting for evaluation. Neuropsychological testing may be helpful but is not required for a diagnosis of ADHD. In fact, despite strong evidence that neuropsychological domains are disproportionately affected in ADHD relative to typical development, the specific cognitive domains affected are heterogeneous, and identification of clear neuropsychological phenotypes has remained elusive, although there continues to be progress in this area.

To account for a stable core diagnostic structure in ADHD, which may vary over time in phenomenology, DSM-5 provides three classes of specifiers to characterize 1) the symptom presentation in the previous 6 months, defined as predominantly inattentive, hyperactive/impulsive, or combined; 2) the degree of severity as mild, moderate, or severe based on level of functional impairment; and 3) whether symptoms that had previously met full criteria are in partial remission at the time of evaluation.

In cases in which full criteria for ADHD are not met, DSM-5 allows assignment of the diagnostic category *other specified attention-deficit/hyperactivity disorder* to indicate the presence of symptoms characteristic of ADHD causing clinically significant distress or impairment that do not meet the full criteria for ADHD or another neurodevelopmental disorder. Therefore, a diagnosis of "other specified attention-deficit/hyperactivity disorder," followed by "with insufficient symptoms" in the relevant domain (e.g., inattention, hyperactivity/impulsivity), may be assigned. In presentations where criteria are not met but significant impairment related to ADHD is present, a diagnosis of *unspecified attention-deficit/hyperactivity disorder* may be assigned without identifying the domain with insufficient symptoms.

Comorbid Psychiatric Disorders

ADHD is a condition where comorbidity is the norm rather than the exception, with more than 60% of individuals identified with a comorbid diagnosis (Larson et al. 2011). Frequently diagnosed conditions include oppositional defiant disorder, specific learning disorder, and motor disorders, as well as mood and anxiety disorders. Core symptomatology associated with attentional, hyperactive–impulsive, or executive functions may interact with or cumulatively affect functioning in academic, social/interpersonal, or self-concept domains, resulting in the emergence of secondary psychiatric comorbidities.

Treatment

There are a number of effective interventions for ADHD that have a high degree of efficacy, with estimates that up to 75% of children receiving treatment will receive benefit (Pliszka 2007). In contrast to many other psychiatric conditions with onset in the developmental period, pharmacological treatments are often provided as first-line treatment rather than psychosocial intervention. Pharmacological treatment approaches such as the Texas Children's Medication Algorithm Project outline empirically based practices (Pliszka et al. 2000), including first-line treatment with stimulants, encompassing the methylphenidate and mixed amphetamine salt classes as well as atomoxetine. Other evidence-based approaches include alpha-agonists, bupropion, and tricyclic agents. While pharmacological intervention is effective and generally well tolerated, adverse side effects are frequently reported and require close monitoring and supervision.

Also, despite earlier findings discounting the efficacy of behavioral interventions relative to medication response, a number of therapies may positively influence outcomes in ADHD. Therapy modalities include organizational skills training and cognitive-behavioral therapy. Additionally, coordination with educational or work environments to provide appropriate accommodations to support learning and attentional functions may result in significant improvements. Close monitoring and management of comorbid psychiatric and physical conditions affecting sleep, mood, and disruptive behavior are also indicated with appropriate empirically based therapies. Nutritional supplementation with fatty acids has shown a small effect size in prior studies, as have cognitive training and neurofeedback paradigms; however, recent meta-analyses have not demonstrated consistent evidence for the efficacy of nonpharmacological interventions, at least in the short term (Goode et al. 2018).

Specific Learning Disorder

Clinical Description

Specific learning disorder encompasses impairments in academic skills and learning. From a nosological perspective, specific learning disorder impairments are differentiated from communication disorders in that they represent difficulties in the acquisition or application not of language abilities, but rather of specific core academic skills, which is also in line with a broader sociological inference that historically this diagnosis would not have been relevant in preliterate societies. However, within a biological framework, learning disorders likely arise from deficits in functional neural circuits and have substantial impacts on adaptive functioning over development, similar to other neurodevelopmental disorders. Furthermore, specific learning disorder is distinguished from global intellectual disability in that specific learning functions are affected, which in DMS-5 are separated into reading, written expression, and mathematics domains. These areas of learning may be affected singly or together; however, multiple diagnoses should exceed what would be expected if intellectual disability were present. Clinical symptoms will reflect challenges in these domains, typically emerging in academic settings. Persistent difficulties in core academic skills are the hallmark of this disorder, although a number of biological and environmental factors must be carefully considered, given the multifactorial nature of successful learning. Signs may include evidence of difficulties or impairments in reading accuracy, fluency, or comprehension; in recognition and manipulation of phonemes; in sequencing of numbers and letters; or in arithmetic, number sense, and mastery of math facts. Other indications may include errors in spelling or grammar; difficulty with recall and comprehension; and impaired clarity or organization of written expression. As always with neurodevelopmental disorders, expected standards for developmental age should be considered, as well as environmental, cultural, and socioeconomic impacts on symptom presentation.

Prevalence and Epidemiology

Epidemiological evidence indicates that specific learning disorder is highly prevalent, with rates as high as 10% across all domains (Altarac and Saroha 2007). While sex differences have been identified, these differences have also recently been the subject of some debate, although generally a male-predominant pattern has been consistently reported, with male-to-female ratios ranging from 1.5:1 to 3:1. Specific learning disorder is seen across cultures but may vary in its manifestations relative to spoken and written language systems. Effects of socioeconomic factors on learning are also broadly studied in education and demonstrate a substantial impact.

Development and Course

In line with societal and developmental expectations, evidence of specific learning disorder will typically emerge during formal schooling in elementary school, where the primary focus is acquisition of reading, writing, and arithmetic skills. There is also likely intraindividual variation based on early cognitive development, development and efficacy of compensatory strategies, and degree of environmental scaffolding. While deficits typically will be evident at school age, for a subset of individuals, functional impairments may not emerge until adolescence, when academic and cognitive loads increase.

Etiology and Risk/Prognostic Factors

A clear etiology for learning disorders has yet to be identified; however, advances have been made in understanding the neuroanatomical processes supporting reading, writing, and mathematics functions. There is evidence for genetic contributions to learning issues, with higher incidence rates in first-degree relatives. Similarly, environmental factors such as prenatal exposure to nicotine, prematurity, and low birth weight have been associated with the condition. Learning processes are closely tied to attentional function, and co-occurring attentional disorders negatively influence long-term learning outcomes. Specific learning disorder has a lifelong trajectory; however, environmental demands and individual compensation for academic skills may vary substantially between years spent in formal schooling and in adulthood.

Diagnostic Evaluation

Diagnosis of specific learning disorder requires thorough assessment of academic skills and intellectual ability. A broad array of standardized measurements have been developed to assess these domains. Importantly, the diagnosis of specific learning disorder has evolved from prior conceptualizations based on a discrepancy model between academic performance and intellectual ability and/or variability between academic domains, toward a developmentally informed framework assessing for the presence of academic difficulties that persist despite targeted intervention addressing potential impairments. Evaluations are interdisciplinary in nature and typically occur in either clinical or educational settings; they encompass thorough medical, family, and psychiatric assessment, as well as neuropsychological testing and behavioral observation.

Comorbid Psychiatric Conditions

Unsurprisingly, specific learning disorder is highly comorbid with other neurodevelopmental conditions—in particular, communication disorders, ADHD, and motor disorders. Over time, difficulties in learning may negatively influence self-concepts and lead to anxiety or mood disorders.

Treatment

A number of programs have been developed to address these issues; these programs primarily focus on development of phonological awareness and decoding skills for dyslexia and explicit instruction in numeracy and arithmetic skills for difficulties in the mathematics domain. Studies of interventions to date have been relatively small in scale; however, they indicate moderate to large effect sizes, with improvement in target domains (Swanson 1999; Swanson and Sachse-Lee 2000). These programs will typically be implemented through special education within the educational system or through independent work with educational specialists in the community. Accommodations embedded in learning environments may also improve overall functioning and reduce associated comorbidity. In contrast, there is limited evidence indicating utility of pharmacological interventions for specific learning disorder.

Motor Disorders

Developmental Coordination Disorder

Clinical Description

Developmental coordination disorder (DCD) is characterized by delays in development of coordinated motor skills, often manifesting as clumsiness and slowness, as well as inaccuracy of performance of gross and/or fine motor skills. These deficits are not better explained by other neurological disorders (e.g., cerebral palsy) or psychiatric conditions (e.g. intellectual disability).

Prevalence and Epidemiology

DCD is estimated to affect about 5%–6% of school-aged children.

Etiology and Risk/Prognostic Factors

The symptoms exhibited in DCD are hypothesized to associate with basic processes of motor learning, anticipatory control of movement, and cognitive control. Structural magnetic resonance imaging (MRI) studies have shown reduced cortical thickness in the right medial orbitofrontal cortex of children with DCD compared with typically developing control subjects (Wilson et al. 2017). Diffusion-weighted imaging studies suggest altered structural connectivity across the entire brain network in children with DCD, as well as reduced white matter integrity in sensorimotor structures (Wilson et al. 2017). In a meta-analysis of seven functional MRI studies involving 86 children with

DCD and 84 typically developing control subjects, children with DCD showed greater activation relative to controls in parts of the thalamus, but reduced activation in the cerebellum, middle frontal gyrus, superior frontal gyrus, supramarginal gyrus, and inferior parietal lobule, during a manual dexterity task (Fuelscher et al. 2018).

Diagnostic Evaluation

DCD should be diagnosed by a multidisciplinary team of professionals qualified to examine the specific DSM-5 criteria for the disorder. Ideally, the team should include a physician and an occupational therapist or physical therapist. Diagnostic tools such as the Movement Assessment Battery for Children, second edition (Movement ABC-2), the Bruininks–Oseretsky Test of Motor Proficiency, second edition, and the Developmental Coordination Disorder Questionnaire (DCDQ) are commonly used to assess coordinated motor skills (Harris et al. 2015). The differential diagnosis for DCD includes motor impairments due to another medical condition, intellectual disability, ADHD, ASD, and joint hypermobility syndrome.

Treatment

A systematic review and meta-analysis of motor-based interventions in DCD involving 30 studies revealed positive benefits for activity-oriented approaches, body function–oriented approaches combined with activities, active video games, and small group programs (Smits-Engelsman et al. 2018). In another meta-analysis with 2,585 participants (2,250 children with DCD and 335 typically developing children), motor skills interventions were found to be effective in improving short-term cognitive, emotional, and other psychological aspects of motor competence and performance in children with DCD (Yu et al. 2018).

Stereotypic Movement Disorder

Clinical Description

Stereotypic movement disorder (SMD) is broadly characterized by involuntary, coordinated, repetitive, seemingly driven but apparently purposeless motor behaviors, such as hand flapping, opening and closing of hands, head banging, and self-biting, that cannot be attributed to other medical conditions or psychiatric disorders. The stereotypies usually begin in early childhood (before 3 years of age).

Prevalence and Epidemiology

Simple stereotypic movements such as rocking are common in young typically developing children. SMD usually involves more complex stereotypic movements. The prevalence of SMD is approximately 3%–4%. The prevalence of SMD-like behaviors is higher (4%–16%) in individuals with intellectual disability (Arron et al. 2011; Harris 2010).

Etiology and Risk/Prognostic Factors

Stereotypic behaviors are associated with lower cognitive functioning. Many neuro-genetic disorders, such as Rett syndrome, Lesch-Nyhan syndrome, and Smith-Magenis syndrome, are characterized by stereotypic and self-injurious behaviors. According to DSM-5, SMD can be diagnosed only if the repetitive motor behaviors are not attributable to neurological, neurodevelopmental, or mental disorders. Therefore, by definition, SMD is always idiopathic.

Diagnostic Evaluation

SMD is a diagnosis of exclusion. Diagnostic tools for SMD include rating scales such as the Stereotypy Severity Scale, the Repetitive Behavior Scale—Revised, and the Behavior Problems Inventory. The differential diagnosis of SMD includes neurological conditions such as complex motor tics, benign hereditary chorea, and bobble-head doll syndrome; psychiatric disorders such as intellectual disability, ASD, trichotillomania, excoriation (skin-picking) disorder, and OCD; and other neurogenetic disorders such as fragile X syndrome, Cornelia de Lange syndrome, neuroacanthocytosis, Rett syndrome, Lesch-Nyhan syndrome, and Smith-Magenis syndrome.

Treatment

Evidence-based treatments for SMD are lacking. Behavior modification techniques, including habit reversal and differential reinforcement of other behaviors, have been employed. The combination of these techniques showed significant reduction in stereotyped motor movements in a small group of children and adolescents with SMD (Miller et al. 2006).

Tic Disorders

Clinical Description

A tic is a sudden, rapid, recurrent, nonrhythmic motor movement or vocalization. Examples of simple motor tics include eye blinking, shoulder shrugging, eye rolling, nose twitching, mouth pouting, head jerking, muscle tensing, and finger flexing; examples of simple phonic tics include throat clearing, coughing, gulping, snorting, sniffing, grunting, barking, belching, and hiccuping. Common complex motor tics include touching, flexing of abdomen, kissing, squatting, jumping, copropraxia, and echopraxia; examples of common complex phonic tics are coprolalia, echolalia, and palilalia. Classification of tic disorders depends on the presence and/or absence of motor and vocal tics and the duration of symptoms. The DSM-5 diagnostic criteria for Tourette's disorder require a history of multiple motor tics and at least one vocal tic, lasting for more than 1 year since first tic onset (which must have occurred before age 18 years); the symptoms must not be attributable to another medical condition or the physiological effects of a substance. The diagnostic criteria for persistent motor or vocal tic disorder are the same as those for Tourette's disorder, except that the tics must involve either the motor or the vocal domain (but not both). Provisional tic disorder can involve symptoms consistent with either Tourette's disorder or persistent tic disorders; however, the diagnosis is reserved for cases in which the duration of symptoms since first tic onset is less than 1 year. In cases in which tics are present but do not meet full criteria for a defined disorder, a DSM-5 diagnosis of *other specified tic disorder* or *unspecified tic disorder* may be considered. As with other neurodevelopmental conditions, DSM-5 diagnostic criteria require the presence of significant distress or impairment in social, occupational, or other important areas of functioning.

Prevalence and Epidemiology

Among the tic disorders, Tourette's disorder has been the most studied. According to a systematic review and meta-analysis (Scharf et al. 2015), the population prevalence of Tourette's disorder is between 0.3% and 0.9%. There is also evidence of sex differences, with a male to female predominance of 4:1. Based on twin studies, the concordance rate for Tourette's disorder was found to be 53%–56% in monozygotic twins and 8% in dizygotic twins (Price et al. 1985). When the diagnostic criteria were broadened from Tourette's disorder to any tic disorder, the concordance rates increased to 77%–94% for monozygotic twins and 23% for dizygotic twins (Price et al. 1985).

Etiology and Risk/Prognostic Factors

The genetics of Tourette's disorder was summarized in a 2012 review of the literature (Deng et al. 2012). Various candidate genes have been proposed to be associated with Tourette's disorder, including genes involved in dopaminergic neurotransmission (dopamine receptor genes [*DRD1–DRD5*] and dopamine β-hydroxylase [*DBH*]), γ-aminobutyric acid (GABA)-ergic neurotransmission (*GABRB3*), serotonin neurotransmission (*HTR1A, HTR1DA,* and *TDO2*), and adrenergic and noradrenergic neurotransmission (*COMT, MAOA ADRA2A, ADRA2C, PNMT*). Other candidate genes include *IMMP2L*, which encodes inner mitochondrial membrane peptidase 2; *CNTNAP2*, which encodes a membrane protein located at the nodes of Ranvier of myelinated axons; and *SLITRK1*, which is thought to be involved in neurite outgrowth, synapse formation, and neuronal survival. Some candidate genes for Tourette's disorder are also implicated in other disorders, including OCD (*CNTNAP2*), ASD (*NLGN4X, CNTNAP2*), and ADHD (*DRD2, SLITRK1*). Studies of alternative splicing (Tian et al. 2011) offer new insights into genetic mechanisms of a number of neurodevelopmental disorders, suggesting, for example, atypical exon expression in Tourette's disorder.

In addition to genetic studies, effects of environmental factors on Tourette's disorder have been investigated. Proposed risk factors for Tourette's disorder include stress and infection during pregnancy. Immune response to pathogens such as group A streptococcus (GAS) has been associated with tic disorders in a large population of children (Kurlan 1998). In particular, antistreptolysin O (ASO) titers were found to be significantly higher in children with a history of tics than those without such a history (Cardona and Orefici 2001). Various studies that have investigated the role of cytokines, immunoglobulins, specific immune cell subpopulations, and gene expression profiling of peripheral lymphocytes have collectively supported the presence of elevated systemic immune response in individuals with Tourette's disorder (Martino et al. 2015).

Development and Course

Tics manifest similarly across the life span. In patients with Tourette's disorder, onset of tic symptoms is typically between the ages of 4 and 6 years. The severity of symptoms is often at its peak between the ages of 10 and 12 years, with a decline in severity during adolescence. Many adults with Tourette's disorder experience less significant symptoms. However, a small percentage of individuals with Tourette's disorder will have persistently severe or worsening symptoms in adulthood.

Diagnostic Evaluation

As previously described, diagnosis of tics disorders is based on the clinical history. The specific diagnosis depends on the duration of symptoms and whether both motor and vocal tics are manifested. Physical examination is usually not needed, but a careful neurological examination can be helpful to exclude other causes. The differential diagnosis for Tourette's disorder includes stereotypic movement disorder, substance-induced and paroxysmal dyskinesias, myoclonus, obsessive-compulsive and related disorders, and medical conditions associated with motor stereotypies, such as chorea and dystonia.

Comorbid Psychiatric Conditions

Neuropsychiatric comorbidities such as OCD, ADHD, depression, rage attacks, sleep issues, and migraine are common in patients with Tourette's disorder. OCD is the most common comorbidity in patients with Tourette's disorder (Hirschtritt et al. 2015). The prevalence of OCD in male and female patients with Tourette's disorder was estimated to be 64% and 71%, respectively (Hirschtritt et al. 2015). Comorbid ADHD also has a higher prevalence in male than in female patients with Tourette's disorder (59% vs. 42.3%). In contrast, comorbid mood disorders (27% vs. 39%) and anxiety disorders (32% vs. 48%) have a lower prevalence in male than in female patients with Tourette's disorder (Hirschtritt et al. 2015).

Treatment

Interventions for Tourette's disorder can be categorized under pharmacological, behavioral, physical, and dietary treatments. In a systematic review of 40 trials, α_2-adrenergic receptor agonists (clonidine and guanfacine) showed strong evidence for effective treatment of Tourette's disorder (Whittington et al. 2016). Trials of both atypical antipsychotics (aripiprazole, risperidone, ziprasidone) and typical antipsychotics (haloperidol, pimozide) demonstrated their efficacy in treating tic symptoms; however, these agents carry the risk of more side effects than the α_2-adrenergic receptor agonists. When combined with pharmacological treatment, habit reversal training (delivered alone or as part of a treatment package such as Comprehensive Behavioral Intervention for Tics) was found to be effective (Dutta and Cavanna 2013); nevertheless, evidence of efficacy of behavioral therapies when administered alone is still limited.

Although medication and behavioral treatments are effective for many patients with Tourette's disorder, a significant proportion of patients with the disorder fail to respond to these treatments. Some will continue to experience debilitating symptoms through adulthood. In these cases, deep brain stimulation (DBS) appears to be a potential treatment option. Based on a systematic review and meta-analysis of DBS involving 156 cases of Tourette's disorder, DBS resulted in significant improvement in 53% of cases, as measured by the Yale Global Tic Severity Scale (YGTSS) (Baldermann et al. 2016). It is unclear which neuroanatomic regions represent the most promising target. The optimal surgical approach remains unknown. Although optimization of DBS protocols is still evolving, DBS is a potentially viable approach for a subset of severely affected patients who do not respond to conventional pharmacological and behavioral treatments.

Conclusion

Neurodevelopmental disorders represent a category of disorders emerging in childhood, representing a broad range of cognitive, motor, and academic skills that diverge from expected levels of function at any particular point in development. When considered within a larger developmental framework, cross-sectional observations identify specific manifestations of a longitudinal profile that may follow a number of different trajectories. The heterogeneity of these paths reflects the complex etiologies underlying these presentations, their interplay with environmental factors, and the potential influence of interventions on long-term adaptive outcomes. Within this context, while disease-modifying treatments largely remain elusive, interventions targeting symptom modification may substantially improve adaptive functioning for affected individuals. Clinicians working in this domain should be particularly sensitive to the need for comprehensive evaluation of this set of disorders and the high degree of comorbidity and frequent involvement of multiple domains of function. Interventions for neurodevelopmental disorders encompass numerous methodologies and—perhaps more than many other DSM-5 disorder categories—require extensive coordination of care across multiple disciplines.

Key Clinical Points

- Typical development of cognitive, language, motor, and academic skills follows a global time-dependent course on a macroscopic scale.

- There is significant individual variability in the exact timing of acquisition of these skills.

- Persistent divergence from these trajectories across developmental stages may be indicative of delays, underlying pathology, or maladaptive environmental factors.

- Etiologies are often heterogeneous; however, emergence of neurodevelopmental deficits requires thorough and comprehensive evaluation with particular sensitivity to screen for syndromic features.

- Early detection and intervention may be particularly important in this group of disorders.

- Assessment and management of symptoms are often interdisciplinary and require coordination across multiple providers and environments.

- Treatment plans should be tailored based on a developmental framework.

- Interventions often rely heavily on behavioral modalities to enhance skill acquisition over time to support the highest level of function possible for each developmental stage.

- While pharmacological interventions are often limited, they may be useful in symptom management.

- Neurodevelopmental disorders may be limited to early developmental stages, but many individuals will be affected, sometimes severely, across the life span. For this reason, establishment of long-term systems of care is often necessary.

- Much future work is needed to develop disease-modifying treatments and interventions.

References

Altarac M, Saroha E: Lifetime prevalence of learning disability among US children. Pediatrics 119 (suppl 1):S77–S83, 2007 17272589

American Psychiatric Association: Diagnostic and Statistical Manual of Mental Disorders, 4th Edition. Washington, DC, American Psychiatric Association, 1994

American Psychiatric Association: Diagnostic and Statistical Manual of Mental Disorders, 4th Edition, Text Revision. Washington, DC, American Psychiatric Association, 2000

American Psychiatric Association: Diagnostic and Statistical Manual of Mental Disorders, 5th Edition. Arlington, VA, American Psychiatric Association, 2013

Arron K, Oliver C, Moss J, et al: The prevalence and phenomenology of self-injurious and aggressive behaviour in genetic syndromes. J Intellect Disabil Res 55(2):109–120, 2011 20977515

Baldermann JC, Schüller T, Huys D, et al: Deep brain stimulation for Tourette syndrome: a systematic review and meta-analysis. Brain Stimulat 9(2):296–304, 2016 26827109

Brugha TS, McManus S, Bankart J, et al: Epidemiology of autism spectrum disorders in adults in the community in England. Arch Gen Psychiatry 68(5):459–465, 2011 21536975

Buck TR, Viskochil J, Farley M, et al: Psychiatric comorbidity and medication use in adults with autism spectrum disorder. J Autism Dev Disord 44(12):3063–3071, 2014 24958436

Cardona F, Orefici G: Group A streptococcal infections and tic disorders in an Italian pediatric population. J Pediatr 138(1):71–75, 2001 11148515

Christensen DL, Baio J, Van Naarden Braun K, et al; Centers for Disease Control and Prevention (CDC): Prevalence and characteristics of autism spectrum disorder among children aged 8 years: Autism and Developmental Disabilities Monitoring Network, 11 sites, United States, 2012. MMWR Surveill Summ 65(3):1–23, 2016 27031587

Danielson ML, Bitsko RH, Ghandour RM, et al: Prevalence of parent-reported ADHD diagnosis and associated treatment among U.S. children and adolescents, 2016. J Clin Child Adolesc Psychol 47(2):199–212, 2018 29363986

Deng H, Gao K, Jankovic J: The genetics of Tourette syndrome. Nat Rev Neurol 8(4):203–213, 2012 22410579

DeStefano F, Price CS, Weintraub ES: Increasing exposure to antibody-stimulating proteins and polysaccharides in vaccines is not associated with risk of autism. J Pediatr 163(2):561–567, 2013 23545349

Dutta N, Cavanna AE: The effectiveness of habit reversal therapy in the treatment of Tourette syndrome and other chronic tic disorders: a systematic review. Funct Neurol 28(1):7–12, 2013 23731910

Estes ML, McAllister AK: Immune mediators in the brain and peripheral tissues in autism spectrum disorder. Nat Rev Neurosci 16(8):469–486, 2015 26189694

Faraone SV, Larsson H: Genetics of attention deficit hyperactivity disorder. Mol Psychiatry June 11, 2018 (Epub ahead of print) 29892054

Fuelscher I, Caeyenberghs K, Enticott PG, et al: Differential activation of brain areas in children with developmental coordination disorder during tasks of manual dexterity: an ALE meta-analysis. Neurosci Biobehav Rev 86:77–84, 2018 29339004

Fung LK, Mahajan R, Nozzolillo A, et al: Pharmacologic treatment of severe irritability and problem behaviors in autism: a systematic review and meta-analysis. Pediatrics 137 (suppl 2):S124–S135, 2016 26908468

Goode AP, Coeytaux RR, Maslow GR, et al: Nonpharmacologic treatments for attention-deficit/hyperactivity disorder: a systematic review. Pediatrics 141(6):e20180094, 2018 29848556

Hallmayer J, Cleveland S, Torres A, et al: Genetic heritability and shared environmental factors among twin pairs with autism. Arch Gen Psychiatry 68(11):1095–1102, 2011 21727249

Harris JC: Advances in understanding behavioral phenotypes in neurogenetic syndromes. Am J Med Genet C Semin Med Genet 154C(4):389–399, 2010 20981768

Harris SR, Mickelson EC, Zwicker JG: Diagnosis and management of developmental coordination disorder. CMAJ 187(9):659–665, 2015 26009588

Herder C, Hinshaw SP, Owens EB, Zalecki C: Effectiveness of behavioral stuttering treatment: a systematic review and meta-analysis. Contemporary Issues in Communication Science and Disorders 33:61–73, 2006

Hinshaw SP, Owens EB, Zalecki C, et al: Prospective follow-up of girls with attention-deficit/hyperactivity disorder into early adulthood: continuing impairment includes elevated risk for suicide attempts and self-injury. J Consult Clin Psychol 80(6):1041–1051, 2012 22889337

Hirschtritt ME, Lee PC, Pauls DL, et al; Tourette Syndrome Association International Consortium for Genetics: Lifetime prevalence, age of risk, and genetic relationships of comorbid psychiatric disorders in Tourette syndrome. JAMA Psychiatry 72(4):325–333, 2015 25671412

Iossifov I, O'Roak BJ, Sanders SJ, et al: The contribution of de novo coding mutations to autism spectrum disorder. Nature 515(7526):216–221, 2014 25363768

Kessler RC, Adler L, Barkley R, et al: The prevalence and correlates of adult ADHD in the United States: results from the National Comorbidity Survey Replication. Am J Psychiatry 163(4):716–723, 2006 16585449

Kohane IS, McMurry A, Weber G, et al: The co-morbidity burden of children and young adults with autism spectrum disorders. PLoS One 7(4):e33224, 2012 22511918

Kurlan R: Tourette's syndrome and "PANDAS": will the relation bear out? Pediatric autoimmune neuropsychiatric disorders associated with streptococcal infection. Neurology 50(6):1530–1534, 1998 9633690

Lahey BB, Pelham WE, Loney J, et al: Instability of the DSM-IV subtypes of ADHD from preschool through elementary school. Arch Gen Psychiatry 62(8):896–902, 2005 16061767

Larson K, Russ SA, Kahn RS, Halfon N: Patterns of comorbidity, functioning, and service use for US children with ADHD, 2007. Pediatrics 127(3):462–470, 2011 21300675

Law EC, Sideridis GD, Prock LA, Sheridan MA: Attention-deficit/hyperactivity disorder in young children: predictors of diagnostic stability. Pediatrics 133(4):659–667, 2014 24639272

Law J, Boyle J, Harris F, et al: Prevalence and natural history of primary speech and language delay: findings from a systematic review of the literature. Int J Lang Commun Disord 35(2):165–188, 2000 10912250

Lyall K, Van de Water J, Ashwood P, Hertz-Picciotto I: Asthma and allergies in children with autism spectrum disorders: results from the CHARGE Study. Autism Res 8(5):567–574, 2015 25722050

Madsen KM, Hviid A, Vestergaard M, et al: A population-based study of measles, mumps, and rubella vaccination and autism. N Engl J Med 347(19):1477–1482, 2002 12421889

Maenner MJ, Blumberg SJ, Kogan MD, et al: Prevalence of cerebral palsy and intellectual disability among children identified in two U.S. National Surveys, 2011–2013. Ann Epidemiol 26(3):222–226, 2016 26851824

Mandy W, Wang A, Lee I, Skuse D: Evaluating social (pragmatic) communication disorder. J Child Psychol Psychiatry 58(10):1166–1175, 2017 28741680

Martino D, Zis P, Buttiglione M: The role of immune mechanisms in Tourette syndrome. Brain Res 1617:126–143, 2015 24845720

Maulik PK, Mascarenhas MN, Mathers CD, et al: Prevalence of intellectual disability: a meta-analysis of population-based studies. Res Dev Disabil 32(2):419–436, 2011 21236634

Miller JM, Singer HS, Bridges DD, Waranch HR: Behavioral therapy for treatment of stereotypic movements in nonautistic children. J Child Neurol 21(2):119–125, 2006 16566875

Moffitt TE, Houts R, Asherson P, et al: Is adult ADHD a childhood-onset neurodevelopmental disorder? Evidence from a four-decade longitudinal cohort study. Am J Psychiatry 172(10):967–977, 2015 25998281

Newbury DF, Fisher SE, Monaco AP: Recent advances in the genetics of language impairment. Genome Med 2(1):6, 2010 20193051

Norbury CF, Gooch D, Wray C, et al: The impact of nonverbal ability on prevalence and clinical presentation of language disorder: evidence from a population study. J Child Psychol Psychiatry 57(11):1247–1257, 2016 27184709

Parker SK, Schwartz B, Todd J, Pickering LK: Thimerosal-containing vaccines and autistic spectrum disorder: a critical review of published original data. Pediatrics 114(3):793–804, 2004 15342856

Pliszka SR: Pharmacologic treatment of attention-deficit/hyperactivity disorder: efficacy, safety and mechanisms of action. Neuropsychol Rev 17(1):61–72, 2007 17242993

Pliszka SR, Greenhill LL, Crismon ML, et al: The Texas Children's Medication Algorithm Project: report of the Texas Consensus Conference Panel on Medication Treatment of Childhood Attention-Deficit/Hyperactivity Disorder, I: attention-deficit/hyperactivity disorder. J Am Acad Child Adolesc Psychiatry 39(7):908–919, 2000 10892234

Polanczyk GV, Willcutt EG, Salum GA, et al: ADHD prevalence estimates across three decades: an updated systematic review and meta-regression analysis. Int J Epidemiol 43(2):434–442, 2014 24464188

Price RA, Kidd KK, Cohen DJ, et al: A twin study of Tourette syndrome. Arch Gen Psychiatry 42(8):815–820, 1985 3860194

Quinn PO, Madhoo M: A review of attention-deficit/hyperactivity disorder in women and girls: uncovering this hidden diagnosis. Prim Care Companion CNS Disord 16(3), 2014 25317366

Richards C, Jones C, Groves L, et al: Prevalence of autism spectrum disorder phenomenology in genetic disorders: a systematic review and meta-analysis. Lancet Psychiatry 2(10):909–916, 2015 26341300

Sanders SJ, He X, Willsey AJ, et al; Autism Sequencing Consortium: Insights into autism spectrum disorder genomic architecture and biology from 71 risk loci. Neuron 87(6):1215–1233, 2015 26402605

Sandin S, Lichtenstein P, Kuja-Halkola R, et al: The familial risk of autism. JAMA 311(17):1770–1777, 2014 24794370

Scharf JM, Miller LL, Gauvin CA, et al: Population prevalence of Tourette syndrome: a systematic review and meta-analysis. Mov Disord 30(2):221–228, 2015 25487709

Shriberg LD, Tomblin JB, McSweeny JL: Prevalence of speech delay in 6-year-old children and comorbidity with language impairment. J Speech Lang Hear Res 42(6):1461–1481, 1999 10599627

Simonoff E, Pickles A, Charman T, et al: Psychiatric disorders in children with autism spectrum disorders: prevalence, comorbidity, and associated factors in a population-derived sample. J Am Acad Child Adolesc Psychiatry 47(8):921–929, 2008 18645422

Smits-Engelsman B, Vinçon S, Blank R, et al: Evaluating the evidence for motor-based interventions in developmental coordination disorder: a systematic review and meta-analysis. Res Dev Disabil 74:72–102, 2018 29413431

Swanson HL: Reading research for students with LD: a meta-analysis of intervention outcomes. J Learn Disabil 32(6):504–532, 1999 15510440

Swanson HL, Sachse-Lee C: A meta-analysis of single-subject-design intervention research for students with LD. J Learn Disabil 33(2):114–136, 2000 15505942

Thomas R, Sanders S, Doust J, et al: Prevalence of attention-deficit/hyperactivity disorder: a systematic review and meta-analysis. Pediatrics 135(4):e994–e1001, 2015 25733754

Tian Y, Liao IH, Zhan X, et al: Exon expression and alternatively spliced genes in Tourette syndrome. Am J Med Genet B Neuropsychiatr Genet 156B(1):72–78, 2011 21184586

Visser JC, Rommelse NNJ, Lappenschaar M, et al: Variation in the early trajectories of autism symptoms is related to the development of language, cognition, and behavior problems. J Am Acad Child Adolesc Psychiatry 56(8):659–668, 2017 28735695

Vissers LELM, Gilissen C, Veltman JA: Genetic studies in intellectual disability and related disorders. Nat Rev Genet 17(1):9–18, 2016 26503795

Volkmar F, Siegel M, Woodbury-Smith M, et al; American Academy of Child and Adolescent Psychiatry (AACAP) Committee on Quality Issues (CQI): Practice parameter for the assessment and treatment of children and adolescents with autism spectrum disorder. J Am Acad Child Adolesc Psychiatry 53(2):237–257, 2014 24472258

Vorstman JAS, Parr JR, Moreno-De-Luca D, et al: Autism genetics: opportunities and challenges for clinical translation. Nat Rev Genet 18(6):362–376, 2017 28260791

Warren Z, McPheeters ML, Sathe N, et al: A systematic review of early intensive intervention for autism spectrum disorders. Pediatrics 127(5):e1303–e1311, 2011 21464190

Weindrich D, Jennen-Steinmetz C, Laucht M, et al: Epidemiology and prognosis of specific disorders of language and scholastic skills. Eur Child Adolesc Psychiatry 9(3):186–194, 2000 11095041

Wheeler AC, Mussey J, Villagomez A, et al: DSM-5 changes and the prevalence of parent-reported autism spectrum symptoms in Fragile X syndrome. J Autism Dev Disord 45(3):816–829, 2015 25234484

Whittington C, Pennant M, Kendall T, et al: Practitioner Review: Treatments for Tourette syndrome in children and young people: a systematic review. J Child Psychol Psychiatry 57(9):988–1004, 2016 27132945

Wilson PH, Smits-Engelsman B, Caeyenberghs K, et al: Cognitive and neuroimaging findings in developmental coordination disorder: new insights from a systematic review of recent research. Dev Med Child Neurol 59(11):1117–1129, 2017 28872667

Yairi E, Ambrose N: Epidemiology of stuttering: 21st century advances. J Fluency Disord 38(2):66–87, 2013 23773662

Yu JJ, Burnett AF, Sit CH: Motor skill interventions in children with developmental coordination disorder: a systematic review and meta-analysis. Arch Phys Med Rehabil 99(10):2076–2099, 2018 29329670

Recommended Readings

Barkley RA: Attention-Deficit Hyperactivity Disorder: A Handbook for Diagnosis and Treatment, 3rd Edition. New York, Guilford Press, 2005

Harris JC: Intellectual Disability: A Guide for Families and Professionals. New York, Oxford University Press, 2010

The Individuals with Disabilities Education Act (IDEA). Available at: https://sites.ed.gov/idea/. Accessed on February 4, 2019.

Ji N, Findling RL: An update on pharmacotherapy for autism spectrum disorder in children and adolescents. Curr Opin Psychiatry 28(2):91–101, 2015 25602248

Mueller A, Hong DS, Shepard S, Moore T: Linking ADHD to the neural circuitry of attention. Trends Cogn Sci 21(6):474–488, 2017 28483638

O'Hare A, Bremner L: Management of developmental speech and language disorders, part 1. Arch Dis Child 101(3):272–277, 2016 26208514

Peterson RL, Pennington BF: Developmental dyslexia. Annu Rev Clin Psychol 11:283–307, 2015 25594880

CHAPTER 10

Schizophrenia Spectrum and Other Psychotic Disorders

Ryan E. Lawrence, M.D.

T. Scott Stroup, M.D., M.P.H.

Jeffrey A. Lieberman, M.D.

Schizophrenia is a brain disorder that manifests its symptoms in adolescence and young adulthood and is characterized by positive symptoms (hallucinations and delusions), negative symptoms (social withdrawal and decreased engagement in activities), disorganization (illogical thought processes or behaviors), and cognitive impairment. The disease course is variable, but the consequences can include hospitalization, relapses, disability, unemployment, homelessness, violence, suicide, and medical complications.

Disease Burden

Although estimates of the prevalence of schizophrenia vary across studies, a systematic review reported that the median lifetime prevalence of schizophrenia is 0.48%. Expanding the inclusion criteria to include schizophreniform and schizoaffective disorders increased prevalence estimates by 18%–90% (Simeone et al. 2015).

The economic burden of schizophrenia in the United States was estimated to be $155.7 billion for 2013. The largest components were excess costs associated with unemployment, productivity loss due to caregiving, and direct health care costs. Estimates include excess direct health care costs of $37.7 billion, direct non–health care costs of $9.3 billion, and indirect costs of $117.3 billion compared with costs of individuals without schizophrenia (Cloutier et al. 2016).

Clinical Presentation

Core Symptoms

Core features of schizophrenia include positive symptoms, thought disorganization, negative symptoms, and cognitive impairment (Table 10–1).

Positive Symptoms

Positive symptoms can take many forms, including hallucinations, hyperactivity and hypervigilance, mood lability, grandiosity, suspiciousness, and hostility. Psychological studies trace positive symptoms to errors in cognitive processing. Altered perceptions, misattribution of environmental cues, attentional deficits, bias toward threatening information, and a tendency to jump to conclusions on the basis of limited information have all been implicated.

Disorganization

Disorganization encompasses conceptual disorganization, disorientation, posturing and mannerisms, bizarre behavior, stereotyped thinking, poor attention, and inappropriate affect (Ventura et al. 2010). Disorganization is more socially impairing than hallucinations or delusions and is associated with a worse prognosis. Although individuals may learn to ignore hallucinations or to avoid talking about or acting on delusions, disorganization is harder to mask. Disorganization also correlates with deficits in attention/vigilance, reasoning, problem solving, processing speed, and performance on IQ tests (Ventura et al. 2010).

Negative Symptoms

Lists of negative symptoms have varied over time, but the National Institute of Mental Health Measurement and Treatment Research to Improve Cognition in Schizophrenia (NIMH MATRICS) studies focused on affective flattening, alogia, avolition, asociality, and anhedonia as the central symptoms (Foussias et al. 2014). More severe negative symptoms are associated with worse functional outcomes, including impairments in occupational functioning, household integration, social functioning, engagement in recreational activities, and quality of life (Foussias et al. 2014).

Cognitive Impairment

Schizophrenia is associated with significant cognitive impairment. Cognitive deficits can include impairments in processing speed, working memory, verbal learning, executive function, and social cognition. Performance on IQ tests tends to be lower than that of healthy control subjects: eight points lower in the premorbid phase, then declining several more points after illness onset (Meier et al. 2014).

Complications

Suicide

Individuals with schizophrenia are at increased risk of suicide. The lifetime suicide mortality rate in schizophrenia is 4%–6%, and between 2% and 12% of all suicides are attributable to schizophrenia (Popovic et al. 2014).

TABLE 10–1.   Common schizophrenia symptoms

Positive symptoms	Negative symptoms	Disorganization	Cognitive impairment
Hallucinations Hyperactivity Hypervigilance Mood lability Grandiosity Suspiciousness Hostility	Flat affect Reduced speech and activity Reduced social engagement Anhedonia	Disorientation Bizarre posturing Illogical behavior Poor attention Inappropriate affect	Slow processing speed Memory and learning deficits Poor executive function Poor social cognition Difficulties with abstract thinking

Note.   Symptoms must be present for at least 6 months for an individual to receive a diagnosis of schizophrenia.

Among both inpatients and outpatients with schizophrenia, suicide risk factors include depression, a prior suicide attempt (risk remains high for 2 years following an attempt), and multiple psychiatric admissions. Among outpatients with schizophrenia, several additional risk factors have been identified: hopelessness (even without comorbid depression), younger age, closer proximity to illness onset (especially in the first few years), older age at illness onset, male sex, recent hospital admission (during or immediately after discharge; risk remains elevated for the following year), and substance misuse or dependence (Popovic et al. 2014).

Clozapine has been shown to reduce suicide risk. It is not known whether clozapine produces this effect by reducing psychotic symptoms, by ameliorating depressive symptoms, or by increasing the frequency of clinical contacts as patients see clinicians for weekly blood draws. Other antipsychotics may be helpful but do not have consistent evidence of protecting against suicide.

Substance Abuse

Half of individuals with schizophrenia meet criteria for a comorbid substance use disorder at some point in their lifetime. The most commonly abused substances (aside from tobacco and caffeine) are alcohol, marijuana, and cocaine. A number of risk factors for substance use disorders have been found: male sex, younger age at schizophrenia onset, more extrapyramidal side effects, more depressive symptoms, and a preponderance of positive symptoms over negative symptoms. Comorbid substance use disorders are associated with lower quality-of-life scores, a higher incidence of violent behaviors, a greater likelihood of homelessness, a greater likelihood of unemployment, and worse treatment adherence. Substance use disorders make schizophrenia treatment more difficult and increase treatment costs (Thoma and Daum 2013).

Nicotine use is far more common among persons with schizophrenia than among the general population. Most patients with schizophrenia who smoke began smoking before illness onset, suggesting that smoking is not solely a response to schizophrenia symptoms or to antipsychotic medication (smoking increases the metabolism of many antipsychotic drugs and may reduce blood levels and side effects). Individuals with schizophrenia report that smoking helps to alleviate symptoms and to improve concentration. Experimental evidence supports patients' claims that nicotine helps them to concentrate. Administering nicotine to patients with schizophrenia restored P50 sensory gating (an electroencephalographic finding common in schizophrenia). Acute nicotine administration has been shown to improve sustained attention, recognition memory, and working memory. Although evidence is mixed, there are some indications that nicotine attenuates negative symptoms, positive symptoms, anxiety, and depression. Future schizophrenia treatments might exploit these nicotine receptors (Featherstone and Siegel 2015).

Treating comorbid substance abuse may improve outcomes. Among antipsychotics, clozapine has been associated with decreased cocaine craving, decreased smoking rates, decreased alcohol use, decreased overall substance use, and increased abstinence. Naltrexone can help patients with alcohol problems. Disulfiram has been used with some success but carries concerns about worsening psychotic symptoms. Acamprosate and topiramate are not well studied in schizophrenia.

Depression

Approximately 25% of patients with schizophrenia have comorbid depression. It is associated with more impaired functioning, more personal suffering, higher relapse rates, more hospitalizations, and suicide.

Comorbid depression can be difficult to diagnose because its symptoms overlap with the negative symptoms of schizophrenia, especially anhedonia, anergia, and blunted affect. However, true depression is marked by the subjective experience of sad mood or guilty thoughts. Recognizing depression is challenging when patients have impaired communication skills. However, distinguishing between depression and negative symptoms is important, because depression is a risk factor for suicide.

Before depression can be diagnosed, alternative etiologies must be ruled out (e.g., thyroid dysfunction, anemia, substance abuse, medication side effects). Akinesia caused by antipsychotic drugs can resemble depression. Reducing the antipsychotic dosage or adding an anticholinergic agent to treat parkinsonism can sometimes improve depressive symptoms. In some cases, depressive symptoms emerge prior to a psychotic relapse, but these typically last only a few days or weeks before they are surpassed by more prominent and definitive psychotic symptoms.

The literature on treatment of comorbid depression in schizophrenia is limited but does support use of antidepressants. Newer antipsychotics, especially those with serotonergic activity, are often preferred. Electroconvulsive therapy may also have a role, although the evidence is limited.

Violence

Most patients with schizophrenia are not violent, and most episodes of violence do not result in any significant injury. However, schizophrenia, especially untreated psychosis, is a risk factor for violence. A review of violence during first episodes of psychosis found that one-third of persons experiencing a first episode of psychosis commit an act of violence before entering treatment. One in six patients experiencing a first psychotic episode commits an act of serious violence (i.e., assault causing any degree of injury, sexual assault, or assault with a weapon). Fewer than 1% of first-episode patients commit an act of severe violence resulting in severe or permanent injury (Nielssen et al. 2012).

In the Clinical Antipsychotic Trials of Intervention Effectiveness (CATIE) study, 19% of patients had exhibited violent behavior at some point prior to the study (Swanson et al. 2008). Predictors of violence were childhood conduct problems, substance misuse, a history of victimization, economic deprivation, and living with other people (rather than living alone). Patients with a history of violence were more likely to discontinue their medication and to leave the study compared with those with no baseline history of violence. A history of violence was a predictor of violence in the next 6 months. Higher levels of negative symptoms were associated with a significantly lower risk of violence (Swanson et al. 2008).

Antipsychotic medications reduce the incidence of violent behaviors. However, longitudinal studies indicate that persons with a history of violence continue to be at risk of further violence (Nielssen et al. 2012). In the CATIE study, all antipsychotics tested (perphenazine, quetiapine, risperidone, ziprasidone, olanzapine) reduced the incidence of violence (Swanson et al. 2008). Clozapine has also been shown to reduce violence and is the treatment of choice for persistently violent individuals on inpatient units.

Medical Comorbidity

Mortality rates in patients with schizophrenia are two to four times higher than those in the general population, and the average life span in these patients is up to 25 years shorter than that in the general population. Although some of this variation is attributable to the increased suicide rate and higher rate of traumatic injuries associated with the illness, medical comorbidities also play a major role. Cardiovascular disease accounts for a large share of this premature mortality. In comparison with control populations, patients with schizophrenia have higher rates of cardiovascular disease, deaths from cardiovascular disease, and sudden deaths. Risk factors for cardiovascular disease that are common among individuals with schizophrenia include smoking, obesity, diabetes, dyslipidemia, lack of exercise, and the cardiac side effects of antipsychotic drugs.

Related to cardiovascular disease is the constellation of risk factors labeled *metabolic syndrome* (weight gain, insulin resistance, hypertension, elevated triglycerides, and decreased high-density lipoprotein cholesterol levels). A meta-analysis estimated a point prevalence of 32.5% for metabolic syndrome in adults with schizophrenia (Mitchell et al. 2013). Some antipsychotic medications—in particular, olanzapine and clozapine—are associated with high levels of weight gain and metabolic problems. When risk factors are considered individually, half of patients with schizophrenia are overweight, one in five has hyperglycemia, and two in five have lipid abnormalities (Mitchell et al. 2013).

Of the infectious diseases, HIV and hepatitis are more common among patients with schizophrenia than in the general population. Increased rates of osteoporosis have been noted among patients with schizophrenia, possibly related to elevated prolactin levels from antipsychotic medication, sedentary lifestyle and lack of exercise, smoking, other substance use, dietary and vitamin deficiencies, decreased sun exposure, and polydipsia-induced electrolyte imbalances.

Polydipsia is a poorly understood complication of schizophrenia that can cause (potentially fatal) hyponatremia. Risk factors include younger age at schizophrenia onset, male sex, white race, heavy smoking, poor antipsychotic response, and tardive dyskinesia.

Other medical complications have been described. High prolactin levels can cause galactorrhea, amenorrhea, sexual dysfunction, and urinary incontinence. Pregnancies among women with schizophrenia have higher rates of complications compared with those among control subjects, possibly due to cigarette smoking, illicit drugs, or alcohol use.

Much medical comorbidity among psychiatric patients goes unrecognized by both patients and caregivers. Some evidence suggests that patients with schizophrenia have a higher pain tolerance or that antipsychotic medications may reduce pain sensitivity, resulting in fewer complaints to the physician. Additionally, patients with known somatic delusions may not be fully evaluated for their complaints. Current efforts to create medical or behavioral health homes are intended to improve the integration of medical and psychiatric care and have the potential to improve the recognition of medical illnesses and thus improve outcomes.

Case Examples

The following case examples illustrate two potential presentations and illness trajectories in schizophrenia.

Case 1

A 19-year-old man with no psychiatric history leaves home to attend a university. Early in his first semester, he stops attending class and instead spends all of his time in the library collecting newspaper articles about international espionage. In his second semester, he is brought to the emergency department after campus safety officers find him breaking into the biology building. On psychiatric interview he insists that researchers in the university laboratory are inventing viruses and deliberately poisoning the campus water supply, as evidenced by the fact that the plant in his dorm room is dying. The patient begins taking an antipsychotic medication and has a good response, showing reduced preoccupation with his delusions. He returns home to live with his parents, remains stable on his medication, and is able to complete his undergraduate degree at the local university. On graduation, he obtains a full-time job in a small business owned by a family friend. He continues to have periods of symptom exacerbation, requiring temporary increases in his medication and an occasional hospitalization, but each time he is able to return to work afterward.

Case 2

A 27-year-old woman is brought to the emergency department by her parents. For the past year, she has been increasingly socially withdrawn. She was fired from her job for missing work without calling. She stopped socializing with friends and currently spends all of her time in her bedroom. She leaves her room only to get food from the kitchen. On presentation, she is malodorous, disheveled, and wearing wrinkled and stained clothing. During the interview, she gives only brief answers to questions and often appears distracted, frequently looking over her shoulder, even though nobody else is in the room. She admits occasionally hearing voices of two people saying she is a bad person. She begins taking an antipsychotic, which reduces the auditory hallucinations. However, she continues to live with her parents, does not return to work, and spends most of her time watching television.

Initial Assessment

As with any change in mental status, a presentation consistent with schizophrenia warrants a medical evaluation to look for alternative diagnoses and reversible causes. A diagnosis of a psychotic disorder is based predominantly on history, observed behavior, and subjective reports obtained from the mental status evaluation. The history and physical examination should pay special attention to any family history of neurological disease, mental illness, personal exposure to drugs or chemicals, and exposure to infectious agents. Routine laboratory testing, especially for newly diagnosed patients, should include a complete blood count, serum electrolytes (including calcium), blood urea nitrogen and creatinine, liver function tests, thyroid function tests, vitamin B_{12} level, HIV and syphilis tests, and drug screening. Other diagnostic tests, including neuroimaging, electroencephalography, and genotypic and serological assessments, are not usually performed for patients presenting with a first episode of psychosis unless there is suspicion of an underlying medical condition such as a neurodegenerative disease or substance-induced psychosis. If clinically indicated, ceruloplasmin testing, chest radiography, or lumbar puncture may be performed.

Differential Diagnosis

Table 10–2 lists medical conditions that can result in psychotic symptoms and that should be considered in the differential diagnosis of schizophrenia.

When medical etiologies have been ruled out and the symptoms are attributed to a primary psychiatric disorder, careful attention must be paid to the timing of symptoms (taking into account age of patient, the sequence of symptoms, time correlation with other symptoms, duration of symptoms), the nature of the symptoms, and any associated features before arriving at a diagnosis. Table 10–3 summarizes important differences among the psychotic disorders.

In brief psychotic disorder, delusions, hallucinations, or disorganized speech lasts for more than 1 day but resolves within 1 month. Classically, people experiencing a brief psychotic disorder will change from a nonpsychotic state to a psychotic state suddenly (e.g., within 2 weeks), without a prodrome.

The core symptoms of schizophreniform disorder are similar to those of schizophrenia, but the disturbance lasts from 1 to 6 months. Unlike schizophrenia, schizophreniform disorder does not have impaired social and occupational functioning as a diagnostic criterion.

Delusional disorder is characterized by one or more delusions that are present for longer than 1 month. The type of delusion is variable, and delusions might involve erotomanic, grandiose, jealous, persecutory, or somatic themes or a mixture of them. Functioning is not markedly impaired, and behavior is not obviously odd (apart from the impact of the delusions). Individuals with delusional disorder tend to behave appropriately when their delusions are not being discussed or acted on. However, social, marital, work, or legal problems can result from delusional beliefs or actions taken in response to delusions.

TABLE 10–2.   **Medical differential diagnosis: conditions that can result in psychosis**

Medical condition	Considerations
Neoplasms	Mental status changes are common in primary and metastatic brain tumors.
Neurovascular events	Hemineglect and seizures can resemble delusions.
Seizures	Temporal lobe seizures can be associated with olfactory hallucinations and religious delusions.
Neurodegenerative disorders	Dementia, Huntington's disease, and Creutzfeldt-Jakob disease are all associated with psychosis.
White matter diseases	Metachromatic leukodystrophy, X-linked adrenoleukodystrophy, Pelizaeus-Merzbacher disease, cerebrotendinous xanthomatosis, adult-onset Niemann-Pick type C, and multiple sclerosis may be associated with symptoms of psychosis.
Systemic lupus erythematosus	Psychosis occurs in 5%–15% of patients.
Delirium	Electrolyte disturbances and poor oxygenation associated with many illnesses may cause psychosis. Steroids, opiates, benzodiazepines, and polypharmacy can cause delirium.
Endocrine disorders	Hypo- and hyperthyroidism, hypo- and hyperparathyroidism, Addison's disease, and Cushing's disease may cause psychosis.
Intoxication	Amphetamines, cocaine, phencyclidine (PCP, angel dust), methylenedioxypyrovalerone (bath salts), hallucinogens (e.g., lysergic acid diethylamide [LSD], mescaline, psilocybin), dextromethorphan at high doses, and cannabis can trigger psychotic symptoms.
HIV, AIDS	HIV-associated psychosis can occur directly from the viral infection and typically involves a sudden onset (no prodrome), delusions (87% of patients), hallucinations (61% of patients), and mood symptoms (81% of patients).
Other infections	Patients with syphilis, tuberculosis, or other central nervous system infections may develop psychotic symptoms.
Limbic encephalitis	Limbic encephalitis is subacute and involves short-term memory loss, psychosis, behavior changes, and seizures involving the medial temporal lobes and the amygdalae.
Mitochondrial disorders	Mitochondrial disorders usually involve multiple organ systems, so a past medical history of multiple medical problems affecting several organs is often suggestive.

Debate exists over whether delusional disorder exists on a continuum with schizophrenia or is a distinct entity. Although there are clear similarities, differences also exist, with delusional disorder characterized by better premorbid adjustment, better overall functioning, higher rates of being married, older age at onset, fewer hospital-

TABLE 10–3. **Brief comparison of psychotic disorders**

Disorder	Characteristics suggestive of the diagnosis	Symptom onset and duration
Schizophrenia	Prodromal phase with nonspecific symptoms is followed by enduring symptoms in multiple domains (positive, negative, disorganization, or cognitive).	Symptoms last more than 6 months.
Schizoaffective disorder	Symptoms resemble schizophrenia, but affected persons may not have impaired social or occupational functioning.	Psychotic symptoms are continuously present for more than 6 months, and depression or bipolar mood symptoms are present more than half of the time.
Schizophreniform disorder	Persons may not have impaired social or occupational functioning.	Symptoms last from 1 to 6 months.
Brief psychotic disorder	The onset is sudden, with no prodromal phase.	Symptoms last more than 1 day but resolve within 1 month.
Delusional disorder	Functioning is not impaired, and behavior is not odd, aside from the impact of the delusion.	Symptoms last more than 1 month.
Bipolar mania or depression with psychotic features	Content can vary but may be mood congruent.	Psychosis occurs only during the mood episode.

izations, fewer delusions (average of two), and better psychosocial functioning (personal care, social functioning, paid work) after 1 year. However, delusional disorder is also characterized by a more chronic course, more severe delusions, higher levels of delusional conviction, and poorer response to antipsychotic medications. Cognitive-behavioral therapy can help delusion-related affective states, but there is currently no effective treatment to improve insight and to reduce delusional conviction (Peralta and Cuesta 2016).

Psychosis can also occur during the manic phase of bipolar I disorder or during a major depressive episode with psychotic features. If delusions or other psychotic symptoms occur exclusively during manic or depressive episodes, then the diagnosis would be bipolar disorder or major depressive disorder with psychotic features.

Schizoaffective disorder is diagnosed when the core symptom criteria for schizophrenia co-occur with a manic or major depressive episode but are preceded or followed by at least 2 weeks of delusions or hallucinations without a major mood episode. To meet DSM-5 (American Psychiatric Association 2013) criteria for schizoaffective disorder, a major mood episode must be present for half (or more) of the total duration of the illness. Impaired social or occupational functioning is not a diagnostic criterion, reflecting a belief that schizoaffective disorder has a somewhat better prognosis than schizophrenia.

The categories *other specified schizophrenia spectrum and other psychotic disorder* and *unspecified schizophrenia spectrum and other psychotic disorder* are used when a patient's presentation does not fit any of the categories previously described. The "other specified" designation is used when the clinician wishes to indicate the reasons that full criteria for a specific psychotic disorder are not met. Examples of presentations that could qualify for this designation include attenuated psychosis syndrome and persistent auditory hallucinations without other psychotic features.

Natural History of Schizophrenia

The natural history of schizophrenia involves four stages of illness: premorbid, prodromal, progressive, and chronic–residual.

Premorbid Stage

In the premorbid stage of illness, individuals who will eventually develop schizophrenia do not yet exhibit significant signs or symptoms of the illness. A number of studies have identified subtle differences between individuals who later develop schizophrenia and those who do not, including physical abnormalities, motor abnormalities, and deficits in intellectual and social functioning. However, these differences are not sufficiently sensitive or specific to predict which individuals will develop schizophrenia, and premorbid deficits are usually not severe enough to draw the attention of mental health practitioners. Premorbid abnormalities tend not to progress until the prodromal stage is reached.

Prodromal Stage

The prodromal stage is characterized by signs and symptoms that suggest impending psychosis. These may include attenuated psychotic symptoms (e.g., exaggerated thoughts with partially preserved insight), transient psychotic symptoms (e.g., brief in duration, spontaneously remitting), or a significant decrease in functioning in conjunction with a genetic risk for schizophrenia or in conjunction with a schizophrenia spectrum personality disorder. Symptoms might include impairments in thought, language, perception, motor function, bodily sensations, stress tolerance, emotion, affect, or socialization. Among young adults who are identified as possibly being in a prodromal state (also called clinical high-risk or ultrahigh-risk individuals), approximately one-third convert to a full psychotic illness over 3-year follow-up. Currently, there is no way to determine which clinically high-risk individuals will convert to psychosis, and there is no known treatment that prevents conversion to a psychotic illness.

In acknowledgment of the importance of identifying individuals who are at high risk of developing schizophrenia and of devising treatments to delay or prevent conversion to psychosis, criteria for an attenuated psychosis syndrome were developed and placed under "Conditions for Further Study" in DSM-5 Section III. Key elements of this syndrome include at least one psychotic symptom (delusion, hallucination, or disorganized speech), with relatively intact reality testing, that is intermittently present (at least once per week for the past month) and is sufficiently severe to warrant clinical attention.

Progressive Stage

The progressive stage of schizophrenia begins when overt psychotic symptoms appear (positive symptoms, negative symptoms, or disorganization) and cause significant social and occupational dysfunction. The progressive stage often lasts 5–10 years and is characterized by progressive deterioration in functioning, progressive worsening of symptoms, and worsening of structural brain abnormalities. Accumulating evidence indicates that repeated or extended psychotic episodes have deleterious effects on the illness course and that antipsychotic medications can slow or arrest progression of structural changes in the brain.

Typically, patients who are treated relatively early in the course of their illness experience a substantial reduction in symptoms. Positive symptoms respond best, and in some cases fully, whereas cognitive and negative symptoms tend to be less prominent at the onset of psychosis, are less treatment responsive, and persist in at least a large subset of individuals. After psychotic symptom response, partial or complete, the majority of patients will not continue medication (either because they stop on their own or because their doctors agree to taper and discontinue their medication after a period of stability). However, most of these patients will subsequently experience relapse of psychotic symptoms. In the context of repeated relapses, patients often achieve remissions that are less complete than what previously occurred. Clinical deterioration is common during this cycle of relapses and remissions and is characteristic of the progressive stage of illness. Notably, the progressive phase of illness is the period of highest suicide risk.

Several structural brain changes have been observed during the progressive phase. In multiple studies, gray matter volumes have been shown to decrease in a progressive manner when comparisons are made between prodromal patients and first-episode patients. Thinning of the cortex, particularly the frontal, temporal, and parietal cortex, has been a frequently reported finding. Progressive reductions of white matter integrity in the frontal cortex have also been reported as patients make the transition from the prodromal stage to psychosis. Additionally, lateral ventricular enlargement, which may be present at the start of illness, has also been shown to progress.

Chronic–Residual Stage

Five to 10 years after entering the progressive stage of schizophrenia, patients typically enter what may be called the chronic–residual stage, which is characterized by persistent residual symptoms and disability that may remain stable and without progression. Outcomes are highly variable. Chronic illness and poor functioning are extremely common, but a minority of patients show near-remission or full remission between exacerbations. Worse outcomes are often associated with more severe symptoms, treatment-resistant symptoms, and earlier age at onset.

In many cases, once the chronic-residual state is reached, cognitive deficits and negative symptoms remain relatively stable, whereas positive symptoms continue to fluctuate. Treatment resistance is more common in this stage than in earlier stages.

Even when symptoms persist, many patients still achieve a meaningful recovery in which illness is not the dominant part of their lives. Overall mortality remains increased because of suicide and medical comorbidity.

Interventions and Clinical Management

Treatment Goals

Between exacerbations, the treatment goals include helping the patient to attain his or her best possible level of functioning, minimizing psychotic symptoms, preventing exacerbations, and minimizing adverse medication effects. When exacerbations occur, extra attention is given to maintaining safety and controlling psychotic symptoms, which might necessitate higher medication dosages, more frequent appointments, or hospitalization. Optimal treatment includes both pharmacological and psychosocial interventions.

Antipsychotic Drugs

Since the first antipsychotic, chlorpromazine, was introduced in the early 1950s, more than 60 similar antipsychotic medications have been developed, all of which modulate the effects of dopamine and block postsynaptic dopamine type 2 (D_2) receptors to varying degrees. Antagonism of dopamine in the mesolimbic and mesocortical pathways is thought to account for the drugs' antipsychotic effect. Antipsychotics also interact with other neurotransmitter systems, a fact that contributes to their side-effect profiles and may influence their therapeutic effects. Antipsychotics have a robust effect on positive symptoms and disorganization but have little effect on negative symptoms. Continuous treatment with antipsychotic medication is recommended for most patients because antipsychotic discontinuation is associated with higher relapse rates.

For most patients, the onset of antipsychotic drug action appears within a few days of starting treatment, and the effect often builds over several weeks. The full effect may take several months to develop. However, not all antipsychotic medications work for all patients. A response during the first 2–4 weeks of treatment is highly predictive of long-term response. Patients experiencing a first episode of psychosis often respond well to lower dosages of antipsychotics and may be more sensitive to side effects if higher dosages are used. Other patients (e.g., those who have experienced multiple episodes or long-term illness) may take longer to respond and may require higher dosages. Not all individuals diagnosed with schizophrenia have a robust response to antipsychotic medications. Those who continue to have significant psychotic symptoms and substantial disability despite multiple trials of antipsychotics are said to have treatment-resistant schizophrenia. Clozapine is the only antipsychotic that is proven to work better than other drugs for treatment-resistant schizophrenia.

Adverse Effects of Antipsychotics

Antipsychotics can have numerous adverse effects (Table 10–4). The side-effect profile is a primary consideration when selecting an antipsychotic medication. Some of the most prominent adverse effects are rigidity, bradykinesia, and tremor resembling Parkinson's disease; severe restlessness known as akathisia; and abnormal involuntary movements known as tardive dyskinesia. These neurological effects, known as extrapyramidal side effects (EPS), were extremely problematic in the early decades of antipsychotic use, but they have been mitigated by the use of lower dosages and by the introduction of newer antipsychotics with lower tendencies to cause EPS.

TABLE 10–4.   Side effects of selected antipsychotic drugs in common use

Drug	Recommended dosage range (mg/day)	Half-life (hours)	Weight/metabolic side effects	EPS/TD	Prolactin elevation	Sedation	Anticholinergic side effects	Hypotension
			Side effects[a]					
Aripiprazole	10–30	75	–	+	–	+	–	–
Amisulpride	50–1,200	12	–/+	+	+++	–/+	–	–/+
Asenapine	10–20	24	+	+	+	++	–	+
Chlorpromazine	300–1,000	6	+++	+	++	+++	+++	+++
Clozapine	150–600	12	+++	–	–	+++	+++	+++
Fluphenazine	5–20	33	+	+++	+++	+	–	–
Haloperidol	5–20	21	+	+++	+++	++	–	–
Iloperidone	12–24	14	++	–	+	+	+	+++
Loxapine	30–100	4	++	++	++	++	+	+
Lurasidone	40–120	18	+	++	–	++	–	–
Olanzapine	10–30	33	+++	+	+	++	++	+
Paliperidone	6–12	23	++	++	+++	+	–	+
Perphenazine	12–48	10	++	++	++	++	–	–
Quetiapine	300–750	6	++	–	–	++	–	++
Risperidone	2–8	20	++	++	+++	+	–	++
Thioridazine	300–800	24	+++	+	++	+++	+++	+++
Thiothixene	15–50	34	++	+++	++	+	–	–
Trifluoperazine	15–50	24	++	+++	++	+	–	+
Ziprasidone	120–160	7	–	+	+	+	–	+

Note.   EPS/TD=extrapyramidal side effects/tardive dyskinesia.

[a] Magnitude of risk indicated as follows: –=minimal risk; +=low risk; ++=moderate risk; +++=high risk.

Source.   Adapted from Stroup TS, Lieberman JA, Marder SA: "Pharmacotherapies," in *Essentials of Schizophrenia*. Edited by Lieberman JA, Stroup TS, Perkins DO. Washington, DC, American Psychiatric Publishing, 2011, pp. 173–206. Copyright 2011, American Psychiatric Publishing. Used with permission.

Many antipsychotics have cardiovascular effects. Some effects (e.g., tachycardia, orthostatic hypotension) are relatively benign, although orthostatic hypotension can be problematic early in treatment and with elderly patients at risk of falling. Other effects (e.g., QT prolongation, myocarditis) are more severe and potentially life-threatening. QT prolongation (defined as a QT interval longer than 450 ms) can precipitate torsades de pointes arrhythmia, so electrocardiographic monitoring is important. Although the absolute risk of torsades de pointes is very low, even when QT prolongation occurs, the antipsychotic should still be changed to an alternative if possible. Myocarditis and agranulocytosis can occur with any antipsychotic but are most closely associated with clozapine.

One of the most dangerous antipsychotic adverse effects is neuroleptic malignant syndrome. Signs and symptoms include dystonia, rigidity, fever, autonomic instability, delirium, myoglobinuria, elevated creatine kinase, elevated leukocytes, and elevated hepatic enzymes. The prevalence is low (<1% of patients taking antipsychotics), but the condition can be fatal. Risk factors for neuroleptic malignant syndrome include acute agitation, young age, male gender, preexisting neurological disability, physical illness, dehydration, rapid dosage escalation, use of high-potency antipsychotics, and use of intramuscular formulations. Treatment usually involves intravenous fluids, supportive care, and transfer to an intensive care unit.

Weight gain, diabetes, hyperlipidemia, and hypercholesterolemia are common adverse effects of antipsychotics. Clozapine, olanzapine, quetiapine, and risperidone are especially likely to have these effects; however, all patients taking any antipsychotic should receive regular monitoring of body weight, blood pressure, serum lipids, and glucose, especially when a new antipsychotic medicine is started or when the dosage is changed. When patients develop metabolic side effects, physicians should consider changing to another antipsychotic medication with less significant weight and metabolic side effects or should help the patient to manage these side effects by using adjunctive agents (e.g., metformin, topiramate, amantadine) and lifestyle modification (e.g., diet, exercise).

Choosing an Antipsychotic

There is no single best antipsychotic drug or dosage for all patients. Drug selection is a process that requires consideration of the patient's current symptoms, past medication response (or nonresponse), comorbid conditions, concurrent treatments, and patient preference. Medication management after a new antipsychotic drug is started requires careful monitoring of the patient's response and adverse effects, ongoing risk–benefit assessment, and judicious switching or management of side effects when necessary.

The optimal antipsychotic medication choice is influenced by the stage of the patient's illness. For first-episode patients, avoiding unnecessary side effects that may have adverse health consequences or may taint an individual's opinion about medications is a key consideration. Prudent first-line choices are those with low or moderate risk of EPS, weight gain, and metabolic problems.

Relapses are often triggered by medication nonadherence, substance use, and stressful life events. When a patient has a relapse, the antipsychotic should be chosen on the basis of the patient's response history, the patient's comorbid conditions, the drug's adverse-effect profile, and the patient's preference. Rapid dosage escalation, high loading doses, and dosages above the recommended range are not advised; these tactics typically increase the rate of side effects without improving efficacy.

Although many patients diagnosed with schizophrenia benefit greatly from antipsychotic medications, at least 30% of patients have only a partial response, and another 10%–20% have little or no response. The first step for patients with a poor medication response is to ensure that there has been an adequate antipsychotic drug trial, with adequate dosing, duration (at least 2–4 weeks), and adherence. Additionally, clinicians should assess whether comorbid substance use, concurrent use of other prescribed medicines, pharmacokinetic and pharmacodynamic interactions, physical illness, and/or poor social environment and support might have contributed to the nonresponse. For patients who show any response to the initial antipsychotic, that agent should be continued for another 4–10 weeks. For patients who show any response to a second antipsychotic, that agent should be continued for 5–11 weeks. If, after 2–4 weeks of treatment, the patient has shown little or no response to an antipsychotic, the medication should be changed, preferably to an antipsychotic that is pharmacologically dissimilar. Clozapine is indicated when a patient has not benefited sufficiently from two adequate trials of different antipsychotics (Hasan et al. 2012).

Changing an Antipsychotic

There is no definitive method on how best to change from one antipsychotic to another. Preferred methods are to cross-taper (i.e., gradually decreasing the dosage of the first medicine while gradually increasing the dosage of the second) or to overlap and taper (i.e., continue the first medicine at the full dosage while gradually increasing the dosage of the second medicine to its target dosage, and then tapering off the first medicine) (Hasan et al. 2012).

Other Biological Interventions

Benzodiazepines

Benzodiazepines are often prescribed for patients diagnosed with schizophrenia. They are not effective for psychotic symptoms but may have a short-term role for treating anxiety, insomnia, or agitation. Caution is necessary, because benzodiazepines combined with antipsychotics can increase the mortality risk in patients with schizophrenia (Tiihonen et al. 2012).

Lithium and Anticonvulsants

Neither lithium nor anticonvulsant medication (valproic acid, carbamazepine) is effective as monotherapy for schizophrenia. However, these medications are often used in conjunction with antipsychotic medications. Evidence supporting this combination is sparse, and the benefits may be limited to helping control associated symptoms (e.g., affective symptoms, impulsivity, aggression), rather than treating the core symptoms of schizophrenia.

Antidepressants

Antidepressants (combined with antipsychotics) play an important role in treating comorbid depressive symptoms among patients with schizophrenia. There is not strong evidence that antidepressants improve negative symptoms or other core symptoms of schizophrenia.

Other Somatic Treatments

Guidelines suggest that electroconvulsive therapy may be useful as an add-on to antipsychotic treatment, especially for patients with treatment-resistant symptoms that have not responded to clozapine or for patients who cannot tolerate clozapine. Catatonic patients seem most responsive to electroconvulsive therapy (Hasan et al. 2012).

Repetitive transcranial magnetic stimulation has not consistently shown benefit in double-blind, randomized controlled trials.

Psychological Interventions

Cognitive-behavioral therapy has a strong evidence base supporting its use among patients with schizophrenia. It is especially valuable for treating psychotic symptoms that have not responded to medications. In this treatment, the patient chooses symptoms and problem areas, and the therapist supportively guides the patient to implement coping methods and to develop more rational cognitive perspectives about the symptoms. The therapist does not directly challenge the patient's beliefs as irrational, but rather elicits the patient's beliefs about the symptoms and draws on the natural coping mechanisms the patient has developed to deal with the symptoms. Specific techniques include belief modification (gently challenging delusional beliefs, starting with loosely held delusions first), behavioral experiments (examining evidence for and against distressing beliefs), focusing/reattribution (helping patients to reattribute auditory hallucinations to an internal source), normalizing psychotic experiences (helping patients to view symptoms as responses to life stresses, making the symptoms seem more normal), and thought challenging (identifying "mistakes" in thinking).

Family psychoeducation is useful for individuals with schizophrenia who are in regular contact with family members or significant others. Family psychoeducation includes family support, education, crisis intervention, problem-solving skills training, and coping skills training.

Personal therapy is a long-term therapy (sometimes lasting for years) that focuses on affect regulation and promotes adaptive responses to emotional stress. It incorporates illness education workshops, social skills training, and behavioral exercises that build awareness of oneself and others.

Social Interventions

Two social interventions that may be especially helpful to patients with schizophrenia are assertive community treatment (ACT) and supported employment. ACT is often reserved for frequently hospitalized patients and those with treatment nonadherence in the community. ACT teams are multidisciplinary and may include a psychiatrist, a nurse, a substance abuse counselor, and a case manager. ACT team members share a caseload that is intended to be small enough to allow frequent contact with the patient. ACT team members can see patients at a clinic or out in the community.

Supported employment starts with the principle that any person with schizophrenia who wants to work should be helped to obtain and maintain employment. The supported employment model uses individually tailored job development (emphasizing patient preference and choice), a rapid job search (rather than prolonged preemployment preparation), ongoing job supports, and integration of vocational and mental health services.

Etiology and Pathophysiology

Environmental Factors

A variety of environmental factors are associated with higher rates of schizophrenia: advanced paternal age, increased maternal parity, obstetric complications (including low birth weight for gestational age), being born in the winter or spring, marijuana use, psychostimulant use, prior *Toxoplasma gondii* infection, living in an urban setting, and migration. Some of these associations have plausible explanations (advanced paternal age may increase the possibility of de novo mutations, infection might trigger neuroinflammation), but many others have yet to be explained (Kotlar et al. 2015).

Genetic Factors

For decades it has been known that schizophrenia has a genetic component. Adoption studies found that schizophrenia rates are higher when a biological parent had schizophrenia than when an adoptive parent had schizophrenia. Data from monozygotic and dizygotic twin studies suggest that genetic factors account for more than half of the total variance in phenotype. Identifying the genes responsible for schizophrenia has proven to be difficult, leading many to believe that the genetic factors underlying schizophrenia are heterogeneous. Nevertheless, a number of genetic risk factors and candidate genes have been identified (Kotlar et al. 2015).

Genome-wide association studies have identified many (>100) common single nucleotide polymorphisms that seem to confer small increases in the risk of developing schizophrenia. Some of these single nucleotide polymorphisms implicate genes involved with G protein–coupled receptor functioning (*DRD2, GRM3*), glutamatergic neurotransmission (*GRIN2A, SRR, CLCN3, GRIA1*), neuronal calcium signaling (*CACNA1C, CACNAII, CACNB2, RIMSI*), and broader synaptic functioning (*KCTD13, CNTN4, PAK6*). Genes encoding the major histocompatibility complex have also been implicated; C4 in the major histocompatibility complex plays an important role in shaping synaptic structures on neurons. Additionally, transforming growth factor–beta (TGF-β) signaling and B or T cell activation have been implicated in schizophrenia. Despite these many discoveries, these common risk loci collectively explain less than 5% of the disease variance (Foley et al. 2017).

Several copy number variants—rare chromosomal rearrangements involving deletion, duplication, inversion, or translocation of DNA—have been found to greatly increase the risk of developing schizophrenia and other neurodevelopmental disorders. Many of the important copy number variants that have been discovered so far affect N-methyl-D-aspartate (NMDA) receptors and neuronal activity-regulated cytoskeleton-associated postsynaptic signaling complexes. Examples of copy number variants that are associated with schizophrenia include 1q21.1, 2p16.3 (*NRXN1*), 3q29, 7q11.2,

15q13.3, distal 16p11.2, proximal 16p11.2, and 22q11.2. Although some of these genes confer a high risk for developing schizophrenia, only a small number of patients (<2.5%) carry known or probable risk loci (Foley et al. 2017).

So far, these genetic findings apply to a small minority of patients with schizophrenia. However, they point toward important molecular mechanisms that may generate a fuller understanding of the biology underlying schizophrenia, which may lead to a greater variety of treatments and to more targeted treatments.

Neurodevelopment and Neurodegeneration

Neurodevelopmental theories have proposed that abnormal brain development, perhaps starting as early as the prenatal period, makes persons more susceptible to developing schizophrenia later in life. A number of observations point to a neurodevelopmental component in schizophrenia. Prenatal insults such as maternal infection (e.g., influenza, toxoplasmosis, poliovirus, herpes simplex virus, rubella), malnutrition or starvation, and maternal smoking are associated with increased rates of schizophrenia among offspring. Perinatal obstetric complications and childhood viral infections are sometimes associated with schizophrenia. Individuals with schizophrenia are also more likely to have shown delays in attaining motor and speech milestones. Children who later develop schizophrenia may show deficits in verbal and visual knowledge, processing speed, working memory, and IQ scores. Consistent with this neurodevelopmental hypothesis, postmortem brain transcriptome-profiling studies by microarray and next-generation RNA sequencing have found that rare coding variants associated with schizophrenia risk are enriched in genes that are preferentially expressed during fetal development. Epigenetic mechanisms during early brain development have also been implicated, with patients showing different patterns of DNA methylation in comparison with control subjects (Birnbaum and Weinberger 2017).

There is also evidence for neurodegeneration in schizophrenia, beginning with the observation that many patients with schizophrenia show progressive deterioration over time. Patients show a general decrease of brain mass from the onset of the disorder, loss of cortical gray matter, and reduced volume of the amygdala, hippocampus, and frontal and temporal lobes. Decreases of specific cell types have been reported in schizophrenia (e.g., striatal cholinergic interneurons, cortical parvalbumin-containing and calbindin-containing γ-aminobutyric acid–ergic [GABAergic] cells, nonpyramidal neurons in hippocampal sector CA2, cortical nicotinamide adenine dinucleotide phosphate [NADPH]-diaphorase positive neurons, and hypothalamic nitric oxide synthase-containing neurons). Most studies do not show gliosis patterns that might be expected when there is cell injury and death, suggesting that apoptotic processes are involved. There is also evidence for reduced white matter integrity at the onset of schizophrenia and accelerated decline in the chronic stages of the illness (Kochunov and Hong 2014).

Neurotransmitters

Because antipsychotic medications all seem to act by antagonizing dopamine D_2 receptors, dopamine has been central to discussions about the etiology of schizophrenia. The dopamine hypothesis posits that patients with schizophrenia have increased dopaminergic activity, especially in the mesolimbic dopamine pathway. Consistent with this hypothesis, positron emission tomography studies have shown that patients with schizophrenia have increased dopamine activity in the striatum and midbrain origins of neurons. Antipsychotics cause varying degrees of blockade at the dopamine D_2 receptor in the mesolimbic pathway, which effectively treats the positive symptoms of schizophrenia. Notably, antipsychotic medications do little for cognitive symptoms and negative symptoms, suggesting that other neurotransmitters are also involved in schizophrenia (Yang and Tsai 2017).

Glutamate has been hypothesized to play a role in schizophrenia. Glutamate is the most abundant neurotransmitter in the brain. It is mediated by NMDA receptors, and its pathways involve the cortex, limbic system, and thalamus—regions that are implicated in schizophrenia. Glutamate levels have been found to be lower in the cerebrospinal fluid of patients with schizophrenia. NMDA receptor antagonists such as phencyclidine and ketamine can trigger psychotic symptoms. Anti-NMDA receptor encephalitis can result in psychotic symptoms that resemble schizophrenia (Yang and Tsai 2017).

A role for serotonin has been suggested by the observation that lysergic acid diethylamide (LSD) causes hallucinations. However, there is currently no direct evidence for serotonergic dysfunction in the pathogenesis of schizophrenia (Yang and Tsai 2017).

The high rates of smoking among patients with schizophrenia and patients' reports that smoking helps with sedation, reduces negative symptoms, and counteracts medication side effects have led to proposals that schizophrenia involves a defect in nicotinic cholinergic receptors and that acetylcholine might play an important role in schizophrenia (Yang and Tsai 2017).

Alterations in the GABA neurotransmitter system have been reported in clinical and basic neuroscience schizophrenia studies and in animal models. GABA is the primary inhibitory neurotransmitter in the central nervous system. GABA abnormalities may contribute to problems with neural synchrony, γ oscillations, and working memory impairments (synchrony of neural oscillations is important for memory, perception, and consciousness) (Yang and Tsai 2017).

Neural Network Abnormalities

Functional neuroimaging studies have allowed visualization of brain activity during the performance of tasks. Early literature focused on brain regions that showed increased or decreased activity, giving rise to regional interpretations of altered activity in schizophrenia such as "hypofrontality." However, accumulating evidence suggests that regions with underactivation and overactivation in schizophrenia are widely distributed across the brain. This finding is consistent with the global nature of brain dysfunction in schizophrenia and suggests that it is unlikely that schizophrenia can be fully understood in terms of an anatomically localized abnormality of brain function (Crossley et al. 2016).

More recently, focus has shifted toward interpreting abnormal activation patterns in terms of disrupted interactions between regions or disruptions of brain connectivity. Diffusion tensor magnetic resonance imaging studies have shown numerous disruptions of white matter tracts among preclinical, first-episode drug-naive, and chronic stages of schizophrenia. For example, positive symptoms have been linked to white matter alterations (increased fractional anisotropy or decreased mean diffusivity) in the inferior fronto-occipital fasciculus, inferior longitudinal fasciculus, and superior longitudinal fasciculus, and negative symptoms have been linked to disruption of interhemispheric fibers and long association tracts passing through the temporal lobe (Canu et al. 2015).

Network analysis of the human brain (prominent in efforts to construct a connectome) has highlighted the important role of brain hubs: regions that enable efficient neuronal signaling, communication, and integration of distributed neural information. Because brain hubs perform higher-level integrative functions, they are points of vulnerability where disconnection or dysfunction can have wide-reaching consequences. Neuroimaging data from multiple sources have implicated hub dysfunction in schizophrenia: topological analysis of differential activation in schizophrenia showed that underactivations were concentrated in hubs, structural abnormalities in brain disorders (including schizophrenia) are preferentially located in hubs, and network analyses of resting-state functional MRI scans have shown a reduced probability of identifying high-degree hubs in patients with schizophrenia (Crossley et al. 2016).

Conclusion

Schizophrenia is a complex mental disorder that imposes a costly burden on patients, families, and society. Scientific research has made important progress expanding knowledge of its etiology, pathophysiology, phenomenology, and natural history, but much remains to be discovered. Fortunately, pharmacological and psychosocial treatments have been developed that suppress symptoms, enhance functioning, and improve the quality of life for many individuals with schizophrenia. With the application of existing information and the prospect of new knowledge through scientific research, clinicians have reason for optimism about the future of schizophrenia prevention and treatment.

Key Clinical Points

- Schizophrenia has a variable course; some people recover and function at a high level, whereas others are severely disabled.

- Longer periods of untreated psychosis are associated with poorer outcomes; early intervention has the potential to reduce disability.

- Antipsychotic medications are the cornerstone of treatment, but optimal treatment also includes psychosocial interventions such as assertive community treatment, family psychoeducation, and supported employment.

- Continuous long-term treatment with antipsychotics is recommended; relapse is far more likely when medications are stopped.

- Clozapine is the only antipsychotic proven to be more effective than other antipsychotics in treatment-resistant schizophrenia; its underuse is a barrier to improved outcomes.

References

American Psychiatric Association: Diagnostic and Statistical Manual of Mental Disorders, 5th Edition. Arlington, VA, American Psychiatric Association, 2013

Birnbaum R, Weinberger DR: Genetic insights into the neurodevelopmental origins of schizophrenia. Nat Rev Neurosci 18(12):727–740, 2017 29070826

Canu E, Agosta F, Filippi M: A selective review of structural connectivity abnormalities of schizophrenic patients at different stages of the disease. Schizophr Res 161(1):19–28, 2015 24893909

Cloutier M, Aigbogun MS, Guerin A, et al: The economic burden of schizophrenia in the United States in 2013. J Clin Psychiatry 77(6):764–771, 2016 27135986

Crossley NA, Mechelli A, Ginestet C, et al: Altered hub functioning and compensatory activations in the connectome: a meta-analysis of functional neuroimaging studies in schizophrenia. Schizophr Bull 42(2):434–442, 2016 26472684

Featherstone RE, Siegel SJ: The role of nicotine in schizophrenia. Int Rev Neurobiol 124:23–78, 2015 26472525

Foley C, Corvin A, Nakagome S: Genetics of schizophrenia: ready to translate? Curr Psychiatry Rep 19(9):61, 2017 28741255

Foussias G, Agid O, Fervaha G, et al: Negative symptoms of schizophrenia: clinical features, relevance to real world functioning and specificity versus other CNS disorders. Eur Neuropsychopharmacol 24(5):693–709, 2014 24275699

Hasan A, Falkai P, Wobrock T, et al: World Federation of Societies of Biological Psychiatry (WFSBP) guidelines for biological treatment of schizophrenia, part 1: update 2012 on the acute treatment of schizophrenia and the management of treatment resistance. World J Biol Psychiatry 13(5):318–378, 2012 22834451

Kochunov P, Hong LE: Neurodevelopmental and neurodegenerative models of schizophrenia: white matter at the center stage. Schizophr Bull 40(4):721–728, 2014 24870447

Kotlar AV, Mercer KB, Zwick ME, et al: New discoveries in schizophrenia genetics reveal neurobiological pathways: a review of recent findings. Eur J Med Genet 58(12):704–714, 2015 26493318

Meier MH, Caspi A, Reichenberg A, et al: Neuropsychological decline in schizophrenia from the premorbid to the postonset period: evidence from a population-representative longitudinal study. Am J Psychiatry 171(1):91–101, 2014 24030246

Mitchell AJ, Vancampfort D, Sweers K, et al: Prevalence of metabolic syndrome and metabolic abnormalities in schizophrenia and related disorders—a systematic review and meta-analysis. Schizophr Bull 39(2):306–318, 2013 22207632

Nielssen OB, Malhi GS, McGorry PD, et al: Overview of violence to self and others during the first episode of psychosis. J Clin Psychiatry 73(5):e580–e587, 2012 22697204

Peralta V, Cuesta MJ: Delusional disorder and schizophrenia: a comparative study across multiple domains. Psychol Med 46(13):2829–2839, 2016 27468631

Popovic D, Benabarre A, Crespo JM, et al: Risk factors for suicide in schizophrenia: systematic review and clinical recommendations. Acta Psychiatr Scand 130(6):418–426, 2014 25230813

Simeone JC, Ward AJ, Rotella P, et al: An evaluation of variation in published estimates of schizophrenia prevalence from 1990–2013: a systematic literature review. BMC Psychiatry 15:193, 2015 26263900

Swanson JW, Swartz MS, Van Dorn RA, et al: Comparison of antipsychotic medication effects on reducing violence in people with schizophrenia. Br J Psychiatry 193(1):37–43, 2008 18700216

Thoma P, Daum I: Comorbid substance use disorder in schizophrenia: a selective overview of neurobiological and cognitive underpinnings. Psychiatry Clin Neurosci 67(6):367–383, 2013 23890122

Tiihonen J, Suokas JT, Suvisaari JM, et al: Polypharmacy with antipsychotics, antidepressants, or benzodiazepines and mortality in schizophrenia. Arch Gen Psychiatry 69(5):476–483, 2012 22566579

Ventura J, Thames AD, Wood RC, et al: Disorganization and reality distortion in schizophrenia: a meta-analysis of the relationship between positive symptoms and neurocognitive deficits. Schizophr Res 121(1–3):1–14, 2010 20579855

Yang AC, Tsai SJ: New targets for schizophrenia treatment beyond the dopamine hypothesis. Int J Mol Sci 18(8):1689, 2017 28771182

Recommended Readings

Lieberman JA, Stroup TS, Perkins D (eds): Essentials of Schizophrenia. Washington, DC, American Psychiatric Publishing, 2012

Saks ER: The Center Cannot Hold: My Journey Through Madness. New York, Hyperion, 2007

Stroup TS, Lieberman JA: Clinical Antipsychotic Trials of Intervention Effectiveness: The CATIE Project. Cambridge, UK, Cambridge University Press, 2010

Torrey EF: Surviving Schizophrenia: A Manual for Families, Patients, and Providers, 5th Edition. New York, Harper Perennial, 2006

Yung A, Phillips L, McGorry PD (eds): Treating Schizophrenia in the Prodromal Phase: Back to the Future. London, Taylor & Francis, 2004

Online Resources

National Alliance on Mental Illness: Schizophrenia. www.nami.org/Learn-More/Mental-Health-Conditions/Schizophrenia

National Institute of Mental Health: Schizophrenia. www.nimh.nih.gov/health/topics/schizophrenia/index.shtml

Schizophrenia Research Forum: www.schizophreniaforum.org

CHAPTER 11

Bipolar and Related Disorders

Shefali Miller, M.D.

Michael Ostacher, M.D.

Trisha Suppes, M.D., Ph.D.

Bipolar disorder is a chronic, severe mental illness involving instability of mood and energy, manifested by fluctuations between depressive and hypomanic or manic episodes. In this chapter, we provide an overview of the phenomenology, epidemiology, and pathogenesis of bipolar and related disorders and summarize current treatment strategies.

Phenomenology of Bipolar and Related Disorders

Historical Concepts: Manic-Depressive Illness

Observations of melancholia and mania were recorded as early as ancient Greece in the writings of Hippocrates and Aristotle. Their descriptions indicated an emerging understanding of mood disturbance as biologically based, potentially emanating from excesses of black and yellow bile (Goodwin and Jamison 2007). The idea that mania and depression may represent opposite poles of a single illness gained increasing acceptance in the nineteenth century and was eventually solidified by Emil Kraepelin, who developed a coherent disease model of manic-depressive illness in the early twentieth century. Kraepelin differentiated manic-depressive illness from dementia praecox (schizophrenia), a distinction that aligns with modern nosology. However, contrary to current diagnostic classifications, he conceptualized all recurrent mood disorders (both unipolar and bipolar) as falling under a unitary disease model of manic-depressive illness (Goodwin and Jamison 2007).

Current Concepts: Bipolar and Related Disorders

In contrast to Kraepelin's unitary model of mood disorders, DSM-5 (American Psychiatric Association 2013) dedicates a separate chapter to bipolar and related disorders, which is located between the chapters for schizophrenia and depressive disorders (Table 11–1). This chapter structure intentionally positions bipolar disorders as intermediate on a spectrum between psychotic disorders, on the one hand, and unipolar recurrent mood disorders, on the other hand, reflecting the substantive genetic, neurobiological, and phenomenological overlap across these disease categories. With this new chapter order, DSM-5 acknowledges dimensional conceptualizations of psychiatric illness (Insel et al. 2010) while simultaneously reinforcing categorical distinctions that maintain bipolar disorders as clinically and biologically separate from schizophrenia and unipolar depressive disorders.

Mood Episodes

As outlined in DSM-5, individuals with bipolar disorder may experience episodes of depression, hypomania, and/or mania. In alignment with the previous edition, DSM-IV (American Psychiatric Association 1994), DSM-5 requires a history of mania or hypomania for a bipolar I or II disorder diagnosis, respectively. Notably, DSM-5 departs from DSM-IV by eliminating the mixed episode as a specific episode type and replacing it with the mixed features specifier, which can be applied to major depressive, hypomanic, or manic episodes (see Table 11–1). It is important to understand mood disorder diagnosis as essentially unidirectional. For instance, if a patient has met criteria for unipolar major depressive disorder and then goes on to develop a full spontaneous manic episode, the diagnosis will move to bipolar I disorder. Even if the majority of the patient's subsequent course continues to be depressed, the diagnosis of bipolar I disorder will be retained, and past history will need to be considered with respect to treatment recommendations.

Major Depressive Episode

The DSM-5 diagnostic criteria for a major depressive episode (Table 11–2) are essentially unchanged from the DSM-IV criteria. The diagnosis requires the presence of depressed mood and/or loss of interest or pleasure most of the day, nearly every day, for at least 2 weeks. Additional symptoms must be present during the same 2-week period, yielding a total of five or more symptoms, including significant change in weight or appetite, insomnia or hypersomnia, psychomotor agitation or retardation, fatigue, feelings of worthlessness or excessive or inappropriate guilt, impaired concentration or indecisiveness, and recurrent thoughts of death. The symptoms must be of sufficient severity to cause significant distress and/or functional impairment and must not be attributable to the direct physiological effects of a substance or medical condition.

As noted, DSM-5 introduced the "with mixed features" specifier that can be applied to major depressive episodes in either bipolar or unipolar depression (see Table 11–1). The specifier is applied when full criteria are met for a major depressive episode and at least three nonoverlapping mood elevation symptoms (i.e., elevated or expansive mood, inflated self-esteem, overtalkativeness, flight of ideas or racing thoughts, increased energy or goal-directed activity, impulsivity/high-risk behavior, and decreased need for sleep) are present during most days of the episode. Overlapping

TABLE 11–1. Bipolar and related disorders: summary of major changes from DSM-IV to DSM-5

DSM-IV	DSM-5
Bipolar disorders and unipolar depressive disorders are placed together in the "Mood Disorders" chapter	"Bipolar and Related Disorders" is a separate chapter placed between "Schizophrenia Spectrum and Other Psychotic Disorders" and "Depressive Disorders"
Criterion A for manic/hypomanic episode requires "a distinct period of abnormally and persistently elevated, expansive, or irritable mood"	Criterion A for manic/hypomanic episode requires "a distinct period of abnormally and persistently elevated, expansive, or irritable mood *and abnormally and persistently increased activity or energy*"
"Mixed episode" subtype Separate episode type Requires presence of full syndromal criteria for mania and depression during the same week Applies only to bipolar disorder	"With mixed features" specifier Can be applied to a major depressive, hypomanic, or manic episode Subthreshold (three or more) nonoverlapping opposite-pole symptoms qualify for use of the specifier Can apply to either bipolar disorder or major depressive disorder
An antidepressant-induced manic/hypomanic episode is diagnosed as a substance-induced manic/hypomanic episode.	An antidepressant-induced manic/hypomanic episode can be diagnosed as a manic/hypomanic episode if full syndromal criteria persist beyond the expected physiological effects of the antidepressant
Presentations that do not meet full criteria for a specific disorder diagnosis may be designated as "bipolar disorder not therwise specified"	Presentations that do not meet full criteria for a specific disorder diagnosis may be designated as either "other specified bipolar and related disorder" or "unspecified bipolar and related disorder"
Anxiety is not included within diagnostic criteria for bipolar disorder mood episodes	Specifier "with anxious distress": Applies to major depressive, hypomanic, or manic episodes Requires presence of two or more anxiety-related symptoms during most days of episode

TABLE 11–2.   **Essential features of DSM-5 major depressive episode**

Minimum duration	2 weeks
Minimum number of symptoms	Five Criterion A symptoms (at least one of which must be depressed mood or loss of interest or pleasure) present nearly every day of the episode
Other features	Symptoms cause distress or functional impairment Primary substance or medical etiologies have been ruled out Consider presence of specifiers (e.g., anxious distress, mixed features, psychosis, rapid cycling)

Note.   For the complete diagnostic criteria, please refer to pp. 125–126 in DSM-5 (American Psychiatric Association 2013).

mood elevation symptoms (i.e., those that may occur during either depressive or mood elevation episodes), including irritability, distractibility, and psychomotor agitation, are not counted toward the mixed features specifier for major depressive episodes. DSM-5 indicates that if full criteria are simultaneously met for both a major depressive episode and a manic episode, the diagnosis of manic episode with mixed features would apply, given the high degree of clinical severity and functional impairment associated with mania. In contrast, DSM-5 does not provide diagnostic guidelines for scenarios in which full criteria are simultaneously met for both major depressive and hypomanic episodes, although it might be expected that this presentation would be coded as depression with mixed features.

Manic Episode and Hypomanic Episode

The DSM-5 criteria for manic and hypomanic episodes (Table 11–3) are largely identical to those in DSM-IV but added to Criterion A the requirement that "abnormally and persistently elevated, expansive, or irritable mood" be accompanied by "abnormally and persistently increased activity or energy" (see Table 11–1). Three of the following additional mood elevation symptoms (four if mood is only irritable) must be present and must represent an observable change from the individual's usual behavior: inflated self-esteem, decreased need for sleep, overtalkativeness, flight of ideas or racing thoughts, distractibility, increased goal-directed activity, or impulsivity/high-risk behavior. Manic episodes are distinguished from hypomanic episodes by their minimum duration (7 days [fewer if hospitalization is necessary] for manic vs. 4 days for hypomanic) and severity (manic requires that psychosis, psychiatric hospitalization, and/or severe functional impairment be present during the episode, whereas hypomanic requires that none of these be present). It is important to note that in contrast to DSM-IV, DSM-5 changes the concept of antidepressant-induced mania by allowing the diagnosis of an autonomous manic or hypomanic episode in situations where symptoms meeting a fully syndromal mood episode emerged during antidepressant treatment but persisted beyond the expected physiological effect of the antidepressant treatment (see Table 11–1). Thus, these patients are now diagnosed with manic or hypomanic episodes and would qualify for having a lifetime diagnosis of bipolar I or II disorder rather than a diagnosis of substance-induced mood disorder (as would have been the case in DSM-IV).

TABLE 11–3.   **Essential features of DSM-5 manic or hypomanic episode**

Minimum duration	Mania: 1 week (or less if hospitalization is necessary) Hypomania: 4 days
Minimum number of symptoms	Criterion A (elevated, expansive, or irritable mood and increased activity or energy) *plus* three Criterion B symptoms (four if mood is only irritable) present nearly every day of the episode
Other features	Marked functional impairment, psychosis, or need for psychiatric hospitalization must be *present* for mania and *absent* for hypomania Primary substance or medical etiologies have been ruled out Consider presence of specifiers (e.g., anxious distress, mixed features, psychosis, rapid cycling)

Note.   For the complete diagnostic criteria, please refer to pp. 124–125 in DSM-5 (American Psychiatric Association 2013).

As noted earlier, DSM-5 introduced a "with mixed features" episode specifier that could be met during a manic or hypomanic episode (see Table 11–1). The specifier is applied when full criteria are met for either a manic or hypomanic episode, concurrent with at least three nonoverlapping symptoms of depression, that is, depressed mood, loss of interest or pleasure, psychomotor retardation, fatigue, feelings of worthlessness or excessive/inappropriate guilt, or recurrent thoughts of death. Overlapping depressive symptoms (i.e., those that may occur during either depressive or mood elevation episodes), including weight/appetite change, sleep disturbance, impaired concentration, and psychomotor agitation, are not counted toward the mixed features specifier for manic or hypomanic episodes. The importance of this specifier is that it more accurately reflects actual clinical practice; previously, full criteria for mania (and not hypomania) needed to be met concurrently with a major depressive episode for 1 week for a mixed episode to be diagnosed, with the array of clinical presentations in which prominent depressive symptoms (not necessarily meeting full episode criteria for depression) occurred during mania having no place in the diagnostic schema and depressive symptoms during hypomania being overlooked completely.

Bipolar and Related Disorders Diagnoses

Bipolar I Disorder and Bipolar II Disorder

As in DSM-IV, DSM-5 requires a history of at least one manic episode for the diagnosis of bipolar I disorder, whereas a history of a major depressive episode is not required. Nevertheless, most patients with bipolar I disorder experience problems with depression as well as mania, and as many as half initially present with a major depressive episode (Goodwin and Jamison 2007), thus calling attention to the need for careful history taking when initiating treatment for a mood episode. About 5% of individuals with bipolar I disorder might be expected to experience unipolar mania, although some will develop depressive episodes later in life (American Psychiatric Association 2013). A diagnosis of bipolar II disorder requires a history of at least one hypomanic episode, at least one major depressive episode, and no manic episodes. Although by definition bipolar II disorder is characterized by less severe mood elevation episodes compared with bipolar I disorder, longitudinal data suggest that both bipolar subtypes are associated with equally severe courses and outcomes, particularly with respect to time spent with depressive symptoms (Kupka et al. 2007).

Cyclothymic Disorder

Cyclothymic disorder can be diagnosed in individuals presenting with chronic (≥2 years in adults, ≥1 year in children and adolescents) symptoms of depression and mood elevation without any history of major depressive, manic, or hypomanic episodes. If an individual who meets criteria for cyclothymic disorder subsequently (i.e., after the initial 2 years in adults or 1 year in children and adolescents) experiences a major depressive, manic, or hypomanic episode, the diagnosis would become major depressive disorder, bipolar I disorder, or other specified bipolar and related disorder (i.e., hypomanic episode without prior major depressive episode), and the cyclothymic disorder diagnosis would be dropped.

Substance/Medication-Induced Bipolar and Related Disorder

The diagnosis of substance/medication-induced bipolar and related disorder should be applied to periods of significant and persistent mood disturbance involving elevated, expansive, or irritable mood, possibly (but not necessarily) in combination with depressed mood or anhedonia, emerging in the context of substance intoxication or withdrawal or medication exposure. Symptoms that predated the onset of the substance/medication use or withdrawal or persisted for a significant duration (e.g., about 1 month) after the substance/medication exposure or acute withdrawal period ended are better classified as primary (i.e., not substance/medication-induced) bipolar and related disorders. Substances commonly associated with mood disturbance include alcohol, phencyclidine, hallucinogens, amphetamines, cocaine, and opioids. Psychotropic medications that may contribute to secondary mood disorders include antidepressants, sedative-hypnotic/anxiolytic agents (e.g., barbiturates, benzodiazepines), stimulants (e.g., methylphenidate), and other depression treatments (e.g., electroconvulsive therapy [ECT], light therapy). Certain medications have also been associated with mood disturbance, such as analgesics (e.g., opiates), anti-infectives (e.g., interferon, isoniazid), steroids, hormonal contraceptives, and neurological agents (e.g., anticholinergics, baclofen, levodopa).

Bipolar and Related Disorder Due to Another Medical Condition

The diagnosis of bipolar and related disorder due to another medical condition is applied when persistently elevated, expansive, or irritable mood and persistently increased activity or energy develop in the context of another medical condition and, on the basis of available evidence, are believed to be a direct pathophysiological consequence of that medical condition. Some medical conditions that have been associated with manic syndromes include traumatic brain injury, epilepsy, cerebral malignancies, paraneoplastic syndromes, multiple sclerosis, dementia, stroke, hypercortisolemia, thyroid dysfunction, HIV/AIDS, and neurosyphilis.

Other Specified or Unspecified Bipolar and Related Disorder

Another change from DSM-IV to DSM-5 was the elimination of the diagnostic classification "bipolar disorder not otherwise specified," which was replaced with two new classifications, "other specified bipolar and related disorder" and "unspecified bipolar and related disorder." These diagnostic categories are intended to capture scenarios in which individuals exhibit significant mood elevation and depressive symptoms yet fail to meet full diagnostic criteria for any of the aforementioned bipolar or related disorder diagnoses. The diagnosis of other specified bipolar and related disorder should be accompanied by a description indicating why the individual did not meet criteria for a specific bipolar and related disorder (e.g., short-duration hypomanic episodes and major depressive episodes, hypomanic episodes with insufficient symptoms and major depressive episodes, hypomanic episode without prior major depressive episode, or short-duration cyclothymia), whereas the diagnosis of unspecified bipolar and related disorder should be made if the clinician chooses not to specify such a reason and/or insufficient data are available to make a specific diagnosis (e.g., in an emergency department setting).

Ongoing Considerations in Bipolar Disorder Nosology

As our understanding of bipolar disorder phenomenology continues to evolve with ongoing research, the diagnostic boundaries laid out in DSM-5 are likely to be further debated and revised. For example, recent analyses involving observational data sets have raised questions regarding the "with mixed features" specifier criteria, particularly the requirements that three opposite-pole symptoms be present (which may be overly stringent) (Miller et al. 2016) and that such symptoms be nonoverlapping (which may exclude clinically significant mixed symptomatology) (Kim et al. 2016). Another analysis suggested that the DSM-5 requirement for increased energy/activity during mood elevation episodes reduced the prevalence of manic and hypomanic episodes without significantly affecting the clinical validity of these constructs (Machado-Vieira et al. 2017), although a different analysis observed no notable changes (Gordon-Smith et al. 2017). Also warranting additional investigation are depressive episodes with short-duration hypomania (2–3 days), designated in DSM-5 as a condition for further study (Section III), given data suggesting that this phenotype may be more clinically and biologically similar to bipolar disorder than to major depressive disorder (American Psychiatric Association 2013).

Finally, as alluded to earlier, the nosology outlined in DSM-5 retained a largely categorical structure for mood disorder diagnosis, distinguishing bipolar disorder from unipolar depressive disorder as well as from psychotic spectrum illnesses (e.g., schizoaffective disorder) and from personality disorders (e.g., borderline personality disorder), conditions that share considerable clinical and/or biological overlap with bipolar disorder. The categorical approach of DSM-5 may continue to have clinical and research utility—for example, by providing greater clarity to patients and families desiring a definitive diagnosis or by permitting clinical trials to be organized around categorical diagnoses so as to increase the likelihood of enrolling clinically homogeneous participants. Nevertheless, there is growing interest in a dimensional approach that would highlight continuity and overlap across psychiatric presentations and potentially reorganize diagnostic groupings around shared biological, environmental, and psychological indicators (Insel et al. 2010). Future DSM revisions may increasingly incorporate such perspectives as research in these areas continues to accumulate.

Differential Diagnosis of Bipolar and Related Disorders

About half of patients with bipolar disorder will experience depression as their first mood episode, leading to challenges in making an initial bipolar diagnosis. Indeed, bipolar disorder patients will commonly be misdiagnosed initially with unipolar major depressive disorder (Bobo 2017), leading to unfortunate delays in appropriate treatment and the potential for exacerbation of the illness by exposure to antidepressants without concurrent antimanic agents. Early age at onset (i.e., younger than 25 years) of the first major depressive episode, a first-degree family history of bipolar disorder, and the presence of psychotic features associated with depression are key risk factors that may lead a clinician to suspect a possible bipolar diagnosis in a patient initially presenting with depression (Bobo 2017). In presentations involving manic symptoms with concurrent psychotic features, the differential diagnosis may include bipolar I disorder, schizoaffective disorder, or possibly even schizophrenia. The subsequent time course (episodic vs. chronic) of the illness and relative preponderance of mood versus psychotic symptoms will ultimately help to clarify the diagnosis in such situations. Borderline personality disorder is another psychiatric condition with considerable symptomatic overlap with bipolar disorder, especially in terms of the prominence of affective instability, irritability, functional difficulties, and impulsivity in both illnesses. A long-standing, pervasive pattern of poor emotional and interpersonal functioning, a history of trauma at a young age, and the persistence of marked emotional lability and environmental reactivity even outside the context of significant mood episodes or symptoms might suggest a diagnosis of borderline personality disorder. Finally, a detailed history should be obtained to rule out substance-related and/or general medical etiologies contributing to bipolar mood symptoms. However, as noted previously, fully syndromal manic or hypomanic episodes that persist beyond the expected physiological duration of a substance exposure are considered by DSM-5 to qualify as primary mood elevation episodes.

Comorbidity in Bipolar and Related Disorders

Findings from the World Health Organization World Mental Health Survey Initiative showed that three-quarters of individuals with bipolar disorder (type I, type II, or subthreshold) met criteria for at least one comorbid psychiatric disorder (Merikangas et al. 2011). Of these, more than half had at least three comorbidities, the most common of which were anxiety disorders in 62.9%, behavior disorders (e.g., attention-deficit/hyperactivity disorder [ADHD], oppositional defiant disorder) in 44.8%, and substance use disorders in 36.6% (Merikangas et al. 2011). Bipolar disorder is commonly associated not only with psychiatric comorbidity but also with increased risk of medical comorbidity and mortality compared with rates found in the general population (Bobo 2017). The metabolic adverse effects of many medications used to treat bipolar disorder can compound these problems.

Suicide and Bipolar and Related Disorders

The estimated annual rates of attempted and completed suicide among bipolar disorder patients are 3.9% and 1.4%, respectively, which are considerably higher than the corresponding rates among the general population (0.5% and 0.02%, respectively)

(Baldessarini et al. 2006). Moreover, patients with bipolar disorder are more likely than individuals in the general population to complete suicide attempts, as demonstrated by the higher ratio of completed to attempted suicide in individuals with bipolar disorder (approximately 1:3) compared with that in the general population (1:20 to 1:40) (Baldessarini et al. 2006). Bipolar disorder patients in depressive or mixed mood states may be at particularly heightened risk for suicide (Baldessarini et al. 2006).

Cognitive and Psychosocial Functioning in Bipolar and Related Disorders

Cognitive impairment has been consistently demonstrated in bipolar disorder patients compared with healthy individuals during both euthymic periods and acute mood episodes (Wingo et al. 2009). As with cognitive impairment, poor psychosocial functioning has been demonstrated in bipolar disorder across both euthymic periods and acute mood episodes and appears to correlate with neurocognitive impairment (Wingo et al. 2009). Functional impairment is worsened during acute episodes, and functional recovery tends to lag behind symptomatic recovery (Wingo et al. 2009). Quality of life, a measure reflecting subjective well-being across multiple life domains, is consistently lower in bipolar disorder patients than in the general population, with reductions in quality of life correlating more strongly with depressive than with manic/hypomanic symptoms (Amini and Sharifi 2012).

Phenomenology of Bipolar and Related Disorders in Women and Special Age Groups

Women

Some data suggest that women are more likely than men to experience bipolar II disorder and less likely to experience bipolar I disorder (Baldassano et al. 2005; Merikangas et al. 2011). The National Comorbidity Survey Replication, however, found no effect of sex on the prevalence of bipolar disorder across bipolar subtypes (Merikangas et al. 2007). Female gender has been associated with increased rates of rapid cycling and depressive or mixed symptoms in some studies (Altshuler et al. 2010; Miller et al. 2016; Suppes et al. 2005) but not in others (Baldassano et al. 2005). In comparison with bipolar men, women with bipolar disorder may also have higher rates of lifetime suicide attempts as well as anxiety and eating disorder comorbidities but lower rates of comorbid alcohol dependence (Altshuler et al. 2010; Baldassano et al. 2005), although women with bipolar disorder have been shown to be at greater risk of alcoholism in comparison with women in the general population (Frye et al. 2003). The postpartum and perimenopausal periods may be especially high-risk times for mood episode recurrence in women with bipolar disorder (Perich et al. 2017).

Children and Adolescents

Although DSM-5 diagnostic criteria require the occurrence of discrete major depressive, hypomanic, and/or manic episodes to render a bipolar diagnosis, many children and adolescents with bipolar disorder will present with more chronic, subsyndromal, and often mixed mood symptoms (Leibenluft 2011), creating diagnostic challenges.

Moreover, symptomatic overlap between bipolar disorder and other pediatric conditions (e.g., oppositional defiant disorder, ADHD, disruptive mood dysregulation disorder) can lead to misdiagnosis and delays in appropriate treatment (Leibenluft 2011). A first-degree family history of bipolar disorder in a young patient with emerging mood and/or behavioral symptoms should raise significant concern for a possible bipolar diagnosis and warrants careful consideration of the risks and benefits of treatment before exposure to antidepressants and stimulants, each of which should be avoided as monotherapy in patients with bipolar disorder. Certain prodromal features may be particularly salient for the diagnosis of bipolar disorder in at-risk youth. A prospective longitudinal study involving 359 offspring (ages 6–18 years) of parents with bipolar disorder identified the presence of anxiety/depression, affective lability, and subsyndromal manic symptoms as being highly predictive of subsequent progression to bipolar spectrum illness, with as many as 49% of individuals with all three risk factors eventually receiving a bipolar disorder diagnosis (Hafeman et al. 2016).

Older Adults

Approximately 25% of individuals with bipolar disorder are older than 50–60 years (Sajatovic et al. 2015) and warrant special consideration in light of the higher prevalence of medical comorbidities, sensitivity to treatment-related adverse effects, and complex psychosocial challenges that may be associated with this age group. Although many older adults living with bipolar disorder first develop the illness earlier in life, a small subset (5%–10% of all bipolar disorder patients) experience their first manic or hypomanic episode after age 50 years, with such late-onset cases more likely to be secondary to general medical, primarily cerebrovascular/neurological, conditions (Sajatovic et al. 2015). The few studies to date that have specifically examined clinical phenomenology in older compared with younger adults with bipolar disorder have found largely similar illness characteristics, with the exceptions of potentially decreased rates of suicide attempts and psychiatric hospitalizations and increased rates of cognitive dysfunction in older adults (Sajatovic et al. 2015).

Epidemiology of Bipolar and Related Disorders

The lifetime prevalence of bipolar disorder in the United States is approximately 4.5%, according to the National Comorbidity Survey Replication (1.0% for bipolar I disorder, 1.1% for bipolar II disorder, and 2.4% for subthreshold bipolar disorder) (Merikangas et al. 2007), although a subsequent worldwide population study reported a lower prevalence, of 2.4% (0.6% for bipolar I disorder, 0.4% for bipolar II disorder, and 1.4% for subthreshold bipolar disorder) (Merikangas et al. 2011). Although less common than major depressive disorder, bipolar disorder yields substantial societal burden and represents the twelfth leading cause of disability worldwide across age groups (World Health Organization 2008). Bipolar disorder tends to emerge in the late teens to early twenties, with a mean onset age ranging from 18 years for bipolar I disorder to 22 years for subthreshold bipolar disorder (Merikangas et al. 2011). Although a global report suggested women are overrepresented among bipolar II disorder samples (Merikangas et al. 2011), a United States–based population report found comparable rates of male and female patients across bipolar subtypes (Merikangas et al. 2007). Sociodemographic correlates of bipolar disorder include lower educational levels and higher rates of unemployment/disability, but bipolar disorder prevalence does not appear to be related to race/ethnicity or family income (Merikangas et al. 2007). A first-degree family history of bipolar disorder and onset of first depressive episode prior to age 25 years are important risk factors for the development of bipolar disorder (Bobo 2017).

Pathogenesis of Bipolar and Related Disorders

A strong genetic component to the pathogenesis of bipolar disorder has long been supported by family, twin, and adoption studies, with estimates of heritability (i.e., the proportion of phenotypic variability that can be attributed to genetic rather than environmental factors) ranging from 73% to 93% (Bobo 2017). More recent large-scale genome-wide association studies (GWASs) have suggested that bipolar disorder is a polygenic disease, with hereditary risk likely due to cumulative effects of multiple small-effect genes. Possible biological pathways of bipolar disorder pathogenesis supported by GWAS data include disruptions in calcium channels, second-messenger systems, hormonal regulation, and glutamate receptor signaling (Sigitova et al. 2017). Of note, recent GWAS data have identified genetic heterogeneity between bipolar I and bipolar II disorder and genetic overlap with schizophrenia that appears greater for bipolar I disorder than for bipolar II disorder (Charney et al. 2017), lending molecular support to the phenotypic separation of the two bipolar subtypes.

Putative mechanisms of action of many pharmacological treatments for bipolar disorder suggest a likely role for monoamines (norepinephrine, serotonin, dopamine) and other neurotransmitters (γ-aminobutyric acid [GABA], glutamate) in the pathophysiology of bipolar disorder (Sigitova et al. 2017). Such theories are further supported by findings such as abnormal neurotransmitter levels in the plasma and cerebrospinal fluid and abnormal neurotransmitter receptor expression in the postmortem brains of bipolar disorder patients (Sigitova et al. 2017). Additional lines of evidence posit mechanisms such as hormonal pathway (e.g., hypothalamic-pituitary-adrenal axis) dysfunction (Belvederi Murri et al. 2016), inflammatory dysregulation (Rosenblat and McIntyre 2016), and abnormal cellular signaling (Sigitova et al. 2017) in the pathogenesis of bipolar disorder.

Structural and functional neuroimaging studies have also contributed importantly to our understanding of the neurobiological substrates of bipolar disorder. Structural imaging studies in bipolar disorder patients have demonstrated decreased gray matter volumes in prefrontal and subcortical regions, findings that appear to correlate with illness progression and may normalize with lithium treatment (Phillips and Swartz 2014). Functional neuroimaging studies examining prefrontal, limbic, and striatal neurocircuitry, pathways that have been implicated in diverse emotional, cognitive, and reward-processing functions, have identified numerous abnormalities in the functioning of these circuits in bipolar disorder patients compared with healthy individuals (Phillips and Swartz 2014).

In summary, although much remains to be understood with respect to bipolar disorder pathogenesis, multiple areas of investigation, including genetics, neurochemistry, and neuroimaging, hold promise to elucidate potential contributors to the development of this complex and disabling condition.

Treatment of Bipolar and Related Disorders

Evidence-based strategies for the treatment of bipolar and related disorders are organized around the three main phases of the illness: acute mania, acute bipolar depression, and longer-term maintenance treatment. U.S. Food and Drug Administration (FDA) approvals for bipolar disorder treatments are granted for specific indications (e.g., acute bipolar depression) on the basis of the demonstration of superior efficacy and adequate safety of the medication compared with placebo for that particular phase of illness in large randomized, double-blind clinical trials. It is important to note that almost all FDA indications were granted specifically for bipolar I disorder because patients with other bipolar subtypes were typically excluded from large registration studies. For this reason, there are very limited systematic data to support evidence-based treatment strategies for bipolar II disorder, which tend to be extrapolated from data on bipolar I disorder treatment. FDA-approved medications for bipolar I disorder encompass mood stabilizers (lithium, valproate, carbamazepine, and lamotrigine), second-generation antipsychotics (SGAs; olanzapine, risperidone, quetiapine, ziprasidone, aripiprazole, asenapine, lurasidone, and cariprazine), and one SGA–antidepressant combination therapy (olanzapine plus fluoxetine). The off-label use of medications for the treatment of bipolar disorder is also common, with clinicians often utilizing agents such as antidepressants, anxiolytics/hypnotics, and other anticonvulsants in situations where inefficacy, intolerability, and/or excessive cost may limit the utility of FDA-approved medications. A summary of FDA-approved medications for bipolar I disorder is provided in Table 11–4.

Treatment of Acute Manic Episodes

As of the fall of 2018, there were 11 FDA-approved medications for acute mania, including three mood stabilizers (lithium, divalproex, and carbamazepine), one first-generation antipsychotic (chlorpromazine, not discussed in detail), and seven SGAs (olanzapine, risperidone, quetiapine, ziprasidone, aripiprazole, asenapine, and cariprazine). All of these agents, with the exception of lithium, are also approved for the treatment of DSM-IV mixed episodes. (Lithium has not been studied systematically for mixed episodes; given the removal of mixed episodes from DSM-5, it is not clear that it is less effective for mania in patients with the mixed features specifier.) Most of the SGAs are approved as both monotherapy and adjunctive therapy (added to lithium or divalproex/valproate), with the exceptions of ziprasidone and cariprazine, which are approved only as monotherapy.

Mood Stabilizers

Lithium.   In 1970, lithium became the first medication to receive FDA approval for the treatment of bipolar I disorder, specifically for acute mania. Lithium treatment has also been associated with decreased risk of suicidality (Baldessarini et al. 2006). Certain clinical features may predict a greater likelihood of response to lithium, such as classic euphoric mania, fewer prior episodes, and family history of lithium response. In contrast, individuals presenting with mixed states or rapid cycling (i.e., four or more mood episodes within 1 year) may be less likely to respond to lithium (Bobo 2017).

TABLE 11–4.   FDA-approved medications for bipolar I disorder

	Acute mania	Acute bipolar depression	Longer-term maintenance	Children and adolescents
Lithium	X		X	X (mania, maintenance)
Divalproex	X			
Carbamazepine	X			
Lamotrigine			X	
Chlorpromazine	X			
Olanzapine	X[a]		X	X (mania)
OFC		X		X (depression)
Risperidone	X[a]		X[b]	X (mania)
Quetiapine	X[a]	X[c]	X[d]	X (mania)
Ziprasidone	X		X[d]	
Aripiprazole	X[a]		X[e]	X (mania,[a] maintenance)
Asenapine	X[a]			
Lurasidone		X[a]		
Cariprazine	X			

Note.   FDA=U.S. Food and Drug Administration; OFC=olanzapine–fluoxetine combination.
[a]Monotherapy and adjunctive (added to lithium or divalproex/valproate) therapy.
[b]Long-acting injectable formulation only.
[c]Approved for acute depressive episodes in both bipolar I disorder and bipolar II disorder.
[d]Adjunctive (added to lithium or divalproex/valproate) therapy only.
[e]Both oral and long-acting injectable formulations approved for monotherapy; oral formulation also approved for adjunctive (added to lithium or valproate) therapy.

The history of lithium, the first medication specifically targeting bipolar disorder, is an interesting one. In the United States, the arrival of lithium in the 1970s led to a better diagnostic approach for separating schizophrenia and bipolar disorder. Prior to lithium use, much was made of the specific nature of psychotic symptoms as denoting schizophrenia, but studies done in the 1970s both overseas and in the United States made it clear that one could not distinguish diagnoses on the basis of psychotic symptom details (Pope and Lipinski 1978). Additionally, as recently as the late 1980s there was debate about the need for ongoing treatment in patients with bipolar I disorder, and even lithium holidays were recommended. A meta-analysis published in 1991 provided definitive evidence that patients with bipolar I disorder needed lifelong treatment to avoid relapse, and also that medication changes should be gradual in bipolar I disorder so as not to destabilize the patient (Suppes et al. 1991).

The FDA has issued a black box warning for lithium toxicity, which can entail vomiting, diarrhea, ataxia, and confusion and may occur at dosages close to the therapeutic level. Because lithium is reabsorbed in the proximal tubule, serum levels are sensitive to fluctuations in hydration status, such that maintaining adequate hydration (particularly in contexts involving significant fluid loss, such as vomiting and diarrhea) is important for preventing toxicity. More common adverse effects of lithium include tremor, gastrointestinal side effects (nausea, vomiting, diarrhea), sedation, weight gain, polyuria, and polydipsia. Lithium use has also been associated with renal and thyroid toxicity, thus requiring routine monitoring of kidney and thyroid function. For treatment of acute mania, lithium can be initiated at 600–900 mg/day, with controlled-release formulations likely to yield better tolerability and permit less frequent dosing (twice daily or even once at bedtime). The lithium dosage should be increased as tolerated to a likely target range of 1,200–1,800 mg/day to achieve a 12-hour serum trough level of 0.8–1.2 mEq/L, with greater clinical benefit for acute mania likely to be achieved in the 1.0–1.2 mEq/L window.

Divalproex.   Divalproex received FDA approval for monotherapy treatment of acute mania in 1994. Divalproex treatment may be beneficial in clinical presentations associated with poor lithium response, such as mixed states and rapid cycling (Bobo 2017).

Divalproex has FDA black box warnings for hepatotoxicity, teratogenicity (neural tube defects, major fetal malformations, and decreased IQ), and pancreatitis. Because of concerns regarding teratogenicity and polycystic ovary syndrome, divalproex may not be a treatment of choice for young women of reproductive potential. Divalproex also carries a class warning for increased risk of suicidality in individuals prescribed anticonvulsants. More common adverse effects associated with divalproex include gastrointestinal side effects (nausea, diarrhea, dyspepsia), weight gain, sedation, alopecia, and elevated transaminases (thus warranting routine monitoring of hepatic function tests in patients taking divalproex). Divalproex can be initiated at 750 mg/day, although initial loading of divalproex at a dosage of 20 mg/kg can be useful and adequately tolerated in acute mania. Divalproex dosage can subsequently be increased in 250-mg/day increments every 1–2 days to achieve a 12-hour serum trough level of 50–125 µg/mL, with greater clinical benefit for acute mania likely to be achieved in the 85–125 µg/mL window.

Carbamazepine.   Carbamazepine received FDA approval for acute mania in 2004. Nevertheless, complex drug interactions and adverse effects have limited the utility of carbamazepine such that it is largely considered a second-line treatment for acute mania. Notably, carbamazepine is an inducer of cytochrome P450 3A4 (CYP3A4), of which many psychotropic medications (including carbamazepine) are substrates. Thus, carbamazepine treatment may result in heightened metabolism and hence decreased efficacy of concomitant medications. Indeed, autoinduction of carbamazepine metabolism via CYP3A4 induction may result in a drop in carbamazepine serum levels several weeks into therapy.

Carbamazepine has black box warnings for serious dermatological reactions (e.g., toxic epidermal necrolysis and Stevens-Johnson syndrome) as well as aplastic anemia and agranulocytosis. Patients of Asian descent may be at particularly increased risk for dermatological complications; genetic screening of such individuals for the HLA-B*1502 allele (the presence of which would warrant avoidance of carbamazepine exposure) may mitigate this risk. The FDA has also issued a class warning for increased risk of suicidality in individuals with epilepsy or psychiatric disorders prescribed anticonvulsants. Common adverse effects reported with carbamazepine treatment include dizziness, somnolence, blurred vision, nausea, vomiting, and ataxia. Carbamazepine is associated with congenital malformations, including spina bifida, and therefore should not be administered during pregnancy. For acute mania, carbamazepine extended-release capsules can be initiated at 200 mg twice daily and increased by 200 mg every day to reach a dosage of 600–1,600 mg/day, targeting a serum level of 6–12 µg/mL.

Second-Generation Antipsychotics

Although lithium was the mainstay of treatment for bipolar disorder for many decades, the early 2000s witnessed a dramatic increase in the number of FDA-approved medications for bipolar disorder, primarily for treatment of acute manic and mixed episodes. SGAs compose the majority of these recently approved agents. Results from large controlled studies generally support use of SGAs as primary mood stabilizers, regardless of whether psychotic symptoms are present. Although the efficacy of SGAs for acute mania has been demonstrated in randomized, double-blind, placebo-controlled multicenter trials, the utility of these agents may be limited by tolerability concerns, particularly with respect to sedation and metabolic adverse effects (weight gain, diabetes, and hyperlipidemia). The American Diabetes Association has recommended that patients taking SGAs should be monitored regularly for changes in weight, with consideration for a medication switch if the patient gains 5% or more of their baseline weight (American Diabetes Association et al. 2004). In addition, fasting blood glucose, lipids, and blood pressure should be assessed at baseline, 3 months after initiating the SGA, and annually (glucose and blood pressure) or every 5 years (lipids) thereafter (American Diabetes Association et al. 2004). Of note, the FDA has issued a class-level box warning for all first- and second-generation antipsychotics, alerting clinicians to increased mortality risk associated with the use of antipsychotics for dementia-related psychosis in elderly patients. In addition, certain SGAs (namely, aripiprazole, quetiapine, olanzapine–fluoxetine combination, lurasidone, and brexpiprazole) carry an antidepressant class warning for increased risk of suicidality in individuals ages 24 years or younger.

Olanzapine. In 2000, olanzapine became the first SGA to receive FDA approval for treatment of bipolar disorder, particularly for management of acute manic and mixed episodes. An adjunctive (added to lithium or valproate) indication for acute manic and mixed episodes was obtained in 2003. Olanzapine treatment has been associated with potentially problematic somnolence and metabolic adverse effects (weight gain, diabetes, and hyperlipidemia), with as many of 30%–40% of individuals receiving olanzapine in clinical trials experiencing clinically significant weight gain (7% or more of baseline weight) (Nashed et al. 2011). Indeed, olanzapine is associated with greater risk of weight gain and other metabolic abnormalities than most other SGAs (American Diabetes Association et al. 2004). In acutely manic patients, olanzapine can be initiated at 10–15 mg/day and increased in 5-mg/day increments up to a maximum recommended dosage of 20 mg/day.

Risperidone. Risperidone was FDA approved for treatment of acute manic and mixed episodes in 2003 as both monotherapy and adjunctive (added to lithium or valproate) therapy. Common adverse effects associated with risperidone include extrapyramidal symptoms and weight gain. Compared with other SGAs, risperidone is considered to carry intermediate risk for metabolic adverse effects (American Diabetes Association et al. 2004). For treatment of acute mania, risperidone can be initiated at 2–3 mg/day and increased in 1-mg/day increments up to a maximum recommended dosage of 6 mg/day.

Quetiapine. In 2004, quetiapine received FDA approval for monotherapy and adjunctive (added to lithium or divalproex) treatment of acute manic and mixed episodes. In 2008, an extended-release formulation of quetiapine received FDA approval for the same indications. Sedation and weight gain are the most common adverse effects associated with quetiapine. Similar to risperidone, quetiapine is considered to carry intermediate risk for metabolic adverse effects (American Diabetes Association et al. 2004). As noted earlier, quetiapine carries an antidepressant class warning for increased risk of suicidality in patients younger than 25 years. The immediate-release formulation of quetiapine can be initiated at 100 mg/day for treatment of acute mania, increasing in 100-mg increments daily up to 400 mg/day, then in 200-mg increments daily up to a maximum recommended dosage of 800 mg/day. The extended-release formulation of quetiapine can be initiated at 300 mg/day for treatment of acute mania, increased up to 600 mg/day on day 2, and adjusted as tolerated and indicated to a target dosage of 400–800 mg/day on day 3.

Ziprasidone. In 2004, the FDA approved ziprasidone as monotherapy for the treatment of acute manic and mixed episodes. Extrapyramidal symptoms, sedation, and akathisia are common adverse effects associated with ziprasidone. Compared with other SGAs, ziprasidone carries relatively low risk for metabolic adverse effects (American Diabetes Association et al. 2004) and, indeed, may yield weight loss in certain patients (Wang et al. 2011). Ziprasidone should be administered with food; although the prescribing information suggests dosing ziprasidone twice daily with meals, sedating effects can be mitigated by dosing ziprasidone once daily at dinner or at bedtime with a snack. For acute mania, ziprasidone can be initiated at 80 mg/day, increased on day 2 to 120–160 mg/day, and adjusted on the basis of efficacy and tolerability to a maximum recommended dosage of 160 mg/day.

Aripiprazole. Aripiprazole is FDA approved for monotherapy (since 2004) and adjunctive (added to lithium or valproate; since 2008) treatment of acute manic and mixed episodes. Akathisia is the most common—and potentially the most problematic—adverse effect associated with aripiprazole. Other potential adverse effects include sedation and extrapyramidal symptoms. Similar to ziprasidone, aripiprazole is considered to have relatively low risk for metabolic adverse effects (American Diabetes Association et al. 2004). Aripiprazole carries an antidepressant class warning for increased risk of suicidality in patients younger than 25 years. In acutely manic patients, aripiprazole can be initiated at a dosage as high as 15 mg/day for monotherapy treatment or 10–15 mg/day when administered in combination with lithium or valproate. A dosage of 15 mg/day may prove adequate for treatment of acute mania, although aripiprazole may be increased as necessary and tolerated to a maximum recommended dosage of 30 mg/day.

Asenapine. Asenapine is FDA approved for monotherapy (since 2009) and adjunctive (added to lithium or valproate; since 2010) treatment of acute manic and mixed episodes. Asenapine must be administered sublingually and thus may contribute to problems with oral hypoesthesia/paresthesia and bitter taste. Other common adverse effects associated with asenapine include somnolence and dizziness. In acute mania studies, 5.8% of patients receiving asenapine showed clinically significant weight gain (7% or more of baseline body weight), compared with 0.5% of patients receiving placebo. For monotherapy treatment of acute mania, asenapine can be initiated at 10 mg twice daily, which is also the maximum recommended dosage, and decreased to 5 mg twice daily if necessary on the basis of tolerability concerns. For adjunctive treatment of acute mania, asenapine can be initiated at 5 mg twice daily and increased as needed and tolerated to 10 mg twice daily.

Cariprazine. In 2015, cariprazine became the most recently FDA approved monotherapy treatment for acute manic and mixed episodes. As with aripiprazole, akathisia may be the most problematic potential adverse effect associated with cariprazine. In placebo-controlled acute mania studies, 20%–21% of patients receiving cariprazine reported akathisia, compared with only 5% of patients receiving placebo. The proportions of patients experiencing shifts from baseline to endpoint in fasting glucose or lipids or in weight (gains of 7% or greater) were similar in those receiving cariprazine and those receiving placebo. Cariprazine can be administered in one daily dose, starting at 1.5 mg/day for acutely manic patients and increasing to 3 mg/day on day 2. Thereafter, the dosage of cariprazine can be increased as needed and tolerated in 1.5- to 3-mg/day increments up to a maximum daily dosage of 6 mg/day.

Treatment of Acute Bipolar Depression

As of the fall of 2018, only three medications were FDA approved for the treatment of acute bipolar depression: olanzapine–fluoxetine combination therapy, quetiapine, and lurasidone. Of these, olanzapine–fluoxetine combination and lurasidone are approved for depressive episodes associated with only bipolar I disorder, whereas quetiapine is approved for both bipolar I and bipolar II depression, making quetiapine the only FDA-approved treatment for bipolar II disorder. In addition, two positive trials of cariprazine for bipolar I depression have been reported, and the drug is under review by the FDA for this indication (Gedeon Richter 2017). The small number of FDA-approved treatments for bipolar depression stands in stark contrast to the predominance of depression over the longitudinal course of bipolar disorder, with one prospective study finding that bipolar disorder patients spent three times more days depressed than manic/hypomanic (Kupka et al. 2007). Thus, treatment of bipolar depression represents a substantial unmet need in available pharmacological interventions. Notably, the three currently approved bipolar depression treatments all involve SGAs, thus raising the tolerability concerns discussed earlier with respect to sedation, metabolic adverse effects, increased mortality risk (in elderly patients for dementia-related psychosis), and suicidality (in individuals younger than 25 years). For this reason, clinicians commonly use off-label treatments for acute bipolar depression, including antidepressants, lamotrigine, and other agents such as modafinil and armodafinil, given their tolerability advantages over SGAs despite less robust evidence of efficacy. The three FDA-approved medications for acute bipolar depression are discussed in detail here.

Olanzapine–Fluoxetine Combination

In 2003, olanzapine–fluoxetine combination became the first medication to receive FDA approval for the treatment of depressive episodes associated with bipolar I disorder, having demonstrated superior efficacy compared with both olanzapine monotherapy and placebo for treatment of acute bipolar depression. Nevertheless, problematic (≥7%) weight gain and sedation were common adverse effects associated with olanzapine–fluoxetine combination therapy (experienced by 19.5% and 20.9% of exposed patients, respectively), thus potentially limiting the utility of this treatment for many patients with acute bipolar depression. As previously noted for other SGAs, olanza-pine–fluoxetine combination carries FDA black box warnings for increased mortality risk in elderly individuals with dementia-related psychosis and increased risk of sui-cidal thinking and behavior in individuals younger than 25 years. For treatment of acute bipolar depression, olanzapine–fluoxetine combination can be initiated at 6 mg/25 mg, administered once daily at bedtime, and increased as necessary and tolerated to a dosage range of 6–12 mg/day for olanzapine and 25–50 mg/day for fluoxetine.

Quetiapine

Quetiapine received FDA approval in 2006 for the monotherapy treatment of acute de-pressive episodes in bipolar I disorder and bipolar II disorder patients. The extended-release formulation of quetiapine received FDA approval for a similar indication in 2008. As previously noted, sedation and weight gain are the most common adverse effects associated with quetiapine, with sedation likely to be the primary limiting fac-tor in achieving a therapeutic dose. Quetiapine also has FDA black box warnings for increased mortality risk in elderly patients with dementia-related psychosis and in-creased risk of suicidal thinking and behavior in individuals younger than 25 years. In acutely depressed bipolar disorder patients, quetiapine (either immediate or extended release) should be dosed once daily at bedtime, starting at 50 mg on day 1 and increas-ing to 100, 200, and 300 mg on days 2–4, respectively. Tolerability limitations (primarily related to sedation) may require more gradual dosing in 25- to 50-mg/day increments, particularly in bipolar II disorder patients, who may be more sensitive to the sedating side effects of quetiapine (Suppes et al. 2008).

Lurasidone

In 2013, lurasidone became the most recent medication to obtain FDA approval for the treatment of depressive episodes associated with bipolar I disorder as both mono-therapy and adjunctive (added to lithium or valproate) therapy. Notably, lurasidone lacks an indication for acute mania because large randomized, placebo-controlled studies were not conducted to evaluate its efficacy in the treatment of acute mania. Lurasidone treatment may commonly be associated with adverse effects of akathisia, nausea, and sedation. However, compared with other SGAs, lurasidone appears to have a favorable tolerability profile with respect to metabolic adverse effects, with only 2.4%–3.1% of individuals receiving lurasidone in controlled studies for bipolar depression experiencing clinically significant weight gain (7% or more of baseline weight), compared with 0.3%–0.7% of placebo-treated patients. Similar to olanza-pine–fluoxetine combination and quetiapine, lurasidone has black box warnings for increased mortality risk in elderly patients with dementia-related psychosis and in-creased suicidality risk in individuals younger than 25 years. Lurasidone should be administered once daily with food. For treatment of acute bipolar I depression, lurasi-done can be initiated as either monotherapy or adjunctive (added to lithium or val-proate) therapy at 20 mg/day and increased as necessary and tolerated to a final dosage range of 20–120 mg/day.

Longer-Term Maintenance Treatment of Bipolar and Related Disorders

Whereas the acute treatment phase begins with the onset of a new mood episode, with the goal of reducing symptoms and achieving remission from the episode, the longer-term maintenance phase begins after resolution of the acute episode, with the goal of preventing future mood episode recurrence. As of the fall of 2018, seven medications have received FDA approval for use in longer-term maintenance treatment of bipolar I disorder: lithium, lamotrigine, olanzapine, risperidone, quetiapine, ziprasidone, and aripiprazole.

Often, clinicians are advised to treat patients in the maintenance phase with the same medication(s) to which they responded during the acute phase. Nevertheless, some medications (i.e., divalproex, carbamazepine, asenapine, lurasidone, and cariprazine) have acute indications but lack maintenance indications, whereas one medication (lamotrigine) has a maintenance indication but lacks an acute indication. As a result, as patients transition from acute to maintenance treatment, clinicians may at times need to decide whether to continue treating with medications that are off-label for the maintenance phase of illness or to switch to or add a different agent with a maintenance indication. Another important aspect of longer-term maintenance treatment is the need to optimize tolerability, which in fact may supersede efficacy as the primary goal of treatment during this phase. Thus, clinicians will often adjust medication dosages downward during the maintenance phase, finding that dosages and/or serum levels that were necessary during acute mood episodes are no longer adequately tolerated for longer-term treatment. However, it is recommended that such dosage adjustments be pursued only very cautiously, with slow and gradual reductions, while carefully monitoring patients for signs of clinical worsening barring the need for a faster discontinuation due to medical necessity.

Mood Stabilizers

Lithium.   The efficacy of lithium for bipolar disorder preventive treatment is well established (Bobo 2017). The targeted serum lithium concentration for maintenance is 0.6–0.8 mEq/L, commonly corresponding to dosages ranging from 900 to 1,200 mg/day. Unlike acute mania treatment, which may necessitate dosing at the higher end of the therapeutic range, longer-term preventive efficacy may be attainable at lower serum concentrations (i.e., in the 0.6–0.8 mEq/L range), thus ensuring enhanced tolerability. Indeed, even lower lithium levels (0.4–0.6 mEq/L) may be considered in certain contexts, such as adjunctive treatment for bipolar I disorder patients or monotherapy treatment for bipolar II disorder patients (Goodwin and Jamison 2007). Certainly, lower levels are associated with lower rates of renal and thyroid abnormalities and have fewer side effects, although overall, lower levels are also associated with a greater relapse risk.

Lamotrigine.   Lamotrigine received FDA approval in 2003 for the longer-term maintenance treatment of bipolar I disorder. Although lamotrigine yielded benefit compared with placebo for both mania and depression prevention, the depression prevention benefit was more robust. Notably, lamotrigine does not have an acute bipolar depression indication because of its failure to separate from placebo in five large-scale bipolar depression studies, although pooled meta-analytic data support its potential benefit in alleviating acute depressive symptoms in bipolar I disorder patients (Geddes et al. 2009). Thus, lamotrigine is commonly used in the acute depressive and longer-term maintenance phases of bipolar disorder. In contrast, lamotrigine is generally considered to lack acute antimanic efficacy.

Compared with other mood stabilizers and SGAs, lamotrigine is generally better tolerated, with less propensity to cause sedation or metabolic adverse effects. However, lamotrigine use has been associated with rare but life-threatening rashes, including Stevens-Johnson syndrome, resulting in lamotrigine carrying a black box warning for serious rash. Most cases of serious rash have emerged during the first 1–2 months of treatment with lamotrigine, thus warranting very slow and cautious initial dosage titration. In addition, patients missing more than four consecutive doses of lamotrigine are advised to reinitiate the dosage titration from the beginning to lower the risk of rash associated with abrupt reexposure to a full dose. As with carbamazepine, the risk for dermatological complications may be increased in patients of Asian descent, and genetic screening of such individuals for the *HLA-B*1502* allele (the presence of which would warrant avoidance of lamotrigine exposure) may mitigate this risk. Lamotrigine also carries a class warning for increased risk of suicidality in individuals prescribed anticonvulsants.

Lamotrigine can be initiated at 25 mg/day for 2 weeks, followed by 50 mg/day for 2 weeks, then 100 mg/day for 1 week, and finally increasing to the target maintenance dosage of 200 mg/day. Because drug interactions affect lamotrigine serum concentrations, the dosage titration should be halved when lamotrigine is prescribed concurrently with valproate (i.e., start at 12.5 mg/day or, alternatively, 25 mg every other day for 2 weeks, then increase to 25 mg/day for 2 weeks, then increase to 50 mg/day for 1 week, then finally increase to a target dosage of 100 mg/day) or doubled when lamotrigine is prescribed concurrently with carbamazepine (i.e., start at 50 mg/day for 2 weeks, then increase to 100 mg/day for 2 weeks, then increase to 200 mg/day for 1 week, then increase to 300 mg/day for 1 week, then finally increase to a target dosage of 400 mg/day). Hormonal contraceptives can also reduce the serum concentration of lamotrigine by up to half, thus potentially necessitating higher maintenance dosages in patients taking lamotrigine concurrently with hormonal contraceptives.

Second-Generation Antipsychotics

Five SGAs have been FDA approved for the longer-term maintenance treatment of bipolar disorder, yet their indications vary with respect to monotherapy versus adjunctive (added to lithium or divalproex/valproate) treatment and oral versus long-acting injectable formulations. Thus, as of the fall of 2018, the following SGAs carried bipolar maintenance indications: olanzapine (monotherapy only), risperidone long-acting injectable (both as monotherapy and as an adjunct to lithium or valproate), quetiapine (both immediate- and extended-release; adjunctive to lithium or divalproex only), ziprasidone (adjunctive to lithium or valproate only), and aripiprazole (both as monotherapy [oral tablets or long-acting injectable Abilify Maintena] and as an adjunct to lithium or valproate [oral tablets only]). The adverse-effect profiles and monitoring parameters for these SGAs were previously discussed. The SGA bipolar maintenance studies were completed in enriched samples; that is, only subjects who were stable in treatment for a long period on the treatment in question were randomly assigned to maintenance treatment compared with placebo, so the generalizability of these study findings is difficult to extrapolate from the small proportion of initial subjects who were ultimately started on the SGA. However, in some sense this study design follows clinical practice, in which patients generally are maintained on the medication(s) that successfully helped them to stabilize.

Although the prescribing information for these agents generally recommends continuing the medication at the same dosage on which the patient was stabilized during acute treatment, clinicians may find it necessary to reduce dosages during maintenance treatment because of tolerability challenges. The recommended maintenance dosage ranges for olanzapine (5–20 mg/day), quetiapine immediate or extended release (400–800 mg/day), ziprasidone (80–160 mg/day), and oral aripiprazole (15–30 mg/day) are comparable to the dosage recommendations for acute mania. For risperidone long-acting injectable, the recommended dosage for both monotherapy and adjunctive (added to lithium or valproate) therapy is 25 mg administered intramuscularly every 2 weeks, although some patients may benefit from dosages up to 37.5–50 mg every 2 weeks. Prior to initiating risperidone long-acting injectable, a brief trial of oral risperidone should be initiated to ensure adequate tolerability, and oral risperidone should be continued for 3 weeks following administration of the first intramuscular dose. For aripiprazole long-acting injectable (Abilify Maintena), the recommended starting and maintenance dosage is 400 mg administered intramuscularly monthly, although if tolerability concerns are encountered, a dosage reduction to 300 mg monthly may be appropriate. Prior to initiating aripiprazole long-acting injectable, a trial of oral aripiprazole for up to 2 weeks is recommended to establish tolerability; oral aripiprazole 10–20 mg/day should be continued for 14 days following the first intramuscular dose.

Antidepressants

The use of antidepressants in individuals with bipolar and related disorders is a topic of considerable controversy. Although antidepressants are considered the first-line treatments for unipolar major depressive disorder, controlled data suggest that they lack efficacy for the acute or prophylactic treatment of bipolar depression (although it should be noted that most controlled studies enrolled primarily bipolar I disorder patients) (Sidor and Macqueen 2011). Of additional concern is the potential risk of a treatment-emergent affective switch in bipolar disorder patients exposed to antidepressants. Although some meta-analytic data suggest that this risk may be lower than previously thought (Sidor and Macqueen 2011), particularly in patients with bipolar II disorder (Altshuler et al. 2017), others have suggested that clinical trial data underestimate actual switch rates, which tend to be higher in naturalistic/observational studies (Goodwin and Jamison 2007). Nevertheless, risk of an antidepressant-induced affective switch may be mitigated through concurrent treatment with antimanic mood-stabilizing agents (Bobo 2017).

Despite concerns regarding inefficacy and destabilizing effects on mood, antidepressants are among the most widely used pharmacotherapies for individuals with bipolar disorder, being prescribed in as many as 50% of patients (Baldessarini et al. 2007), likely in part because of the scarcity of adequately tolerated alternative agents for bipolar depression. Indeed, some data have indicated that for those bipolar disorder patients who do initially respond to antidepressant treatment, longer-term continuation of antidepressant therapy is likely to be beneficial for prevention of depressive recurrence (Pacchiarotti et al. 2013). In addition, emerging data suggest differential antidepressant response rates in patients with bipolar II compared with bipolar I depression, with the former group potentially receiving greater benefit (Liu et al. 2017), although more research in this area is needed.

In an effort to synthesize these often-conflicting data, the International Society for Bipolar Disorders Task Force issued a consensus statement in 2013 providing clinical recommendations for antidepressant use in bipolar disorder (Pacchiarotti et al. 2013). Their primary recommendations were as follows:

1. Adjunctive antidepressants may be used for acutely depressed bipolar I or II disorder patients who previously had a positive response to antidepressants.
2. Adjunctive antidepressants should be avoided in acutely depressed bipolar I or II disorder patients experiencing two or more concurrent core manic symptoms in the presence of psychomotor agitation or rapid cycling.
3. Adjunctive antidepressants may be continued for longer-term maintenance treatment if the depressive symptoms recur following antidepressant discontinuation.
4. Antidepressant monotherapy should be avoided in patients with bipolar I disorder as well as in patients with bipolar II disorder who are experiencing two or more concurrent core manic/hypomanic symptoms.

In addition, the Task Force recommended that antidepressants be discontinued if treatment-emergent manic symptoms develop and that antidepressants be avoided in patients with rapid cycling, current mixed features, or a history of treatment-emergent mood elevation.

Other Interventions

Patients with bipolar disorder who fail to respond to or tolerate evidence-based pharmacotherapies may be candidates for alternative interventions such as ECT, repetitive transcranial magnetic stimulation (rTMS), and ketamine infusion. In clinical practice, ECT has long been considered a highly effective intervention for treatment-refractory bipolar depression or mania and may be particularly useful for populations in which pharmacological exposure is contraindicated (e.g., pregnant women). Nevertheless, few controlled studies have investigated the efficacy of ECT for treatment of bipolar disorder. One systematic review identified only three controlled studies of ECT for acute mania, all of which had small sample sizes, and no controlled studies of ECT for acute bipolar depression (Versiani et al. 2011). However, several noncontrolled studies comparing unipolar and bipolar depressed samples demonstrated similar response to ECT in both populations. The authors were cautious about drawing conclusions regarding the efficacy of ECT in bipolar disorder, given the lack of methodologically rigorous data, but noted that most clinical trials involving bipolar disorder patients demonstrated high response rates with ECT (Versiani et al. 2011). ECT is reserved for emergency life-saving care and treatment-resistant illness because it carries a risk of cognitive side effects, although these effects typically are limited to short-term memory deficits that usually reverse following termination of treatment. Nevertheless, the potential for irreversible memory loss limits the utility of ECT as a longer-term maintenance treatment. Additional adverse effects may include headaches and nausea or vomiting.

A growing evidence base supports the use of rTMS, which involves daily electromagnetic stimulation of the left prefrontal cortex, for treatment-resistant unipolar depression. In contrast, there are very limited controlled data investigating the use of rTMS for bipolar depression (Nahas et al. 2003), and its benefits for this indication remain unclear. Nevertheless, if it is shown to be effective for bipolar disorder, rTMS offers certain advantages over ECT with respect to convenience (because rTMS can be conducted on an outpatient basis), noninvasiveness (general anesthesia is not required for rTMS), and limited side effects and therefore may prove to be an appropriate intervention for individuals with treatment-refractory bipolar depression. The efficacy of rTMS for acute mania has not been established.

Ketamine is another novel treatment that has demonstrated rapid, albeit transient, antidepressant effects in bipolar disorder patients (Parsaik et al. 2015). In three randomized controlled trials, a single intravenous infusion of ketamine was shown to reduce overall depression scores, with particular benefits for reducing anhedonia and suicidal thoughts, with effects lasting up to 14 days (Parsaik et al. 2015). Ketamine was fairly well tolerated in these trials, although some participants did experience dissociative symptoms (Parsaik et al. 2015), a known potential adverse effect of ketamine. Thus, ketamine may prove to be a future treatment option for bipolar disorder patients requiring short-term stabilization of acute, severe depressive symptoms, although its potential utility as a longer-term treatment remains to be established.

Psychotherapeutic Treatment

Although pharmacological interventions are the mainstay of bipolar disorder management, adjunctive psychotherapy is an important component of a comprehensive treatment plan. Psychosocial interventions, when added to medications, can improve outcomes for bipolar disorder patients by alleviating subsyndromal mood symptoms, enabling early detection of emerging mood episodes, increasing medication adherence, enhancing interpersonal functioning, and potentially targeting comorbid conditions such as anxiety and personality disorders. Four evidence-based psychosocial interventions for bipolar disorder have been evaluated in randomized controlled trials: group psychoeducation, family-focused therapy, cognitive-behavioral therapy, and interpersonal and social rhythm therapy (Reiser et al. 2017).

Psychoeducational psychotherapy aims to enhance the individual's understanding of the disorder and improve treatment adherence. Family-focused therapy involves a psychoeducational component in addition to family therapy sessions and training in communication and problem-solving skills. Cognitive-behavioral therapy is a manualized psychosocial intervention that aims to identify and change maladaptive patterns of cognition and behavior. Interpersonal and social rhythm therapy, in contrast, emphasizes the need to stabilize daily routines and circadian rhythms on the basis of the notion that abnormalities in circadian rhythms and sleep–wake cycles underlie mood episode recurrence. The controlled studies for these varied psychotherapeutic interventions have primarily demonstrated their benefit in preventing mood episode recurrence in euthymic patients, whereas their efficacy in treating acute mood episodes may prove less robust (Reiser et al. 2017).

Treatment Considerations in Women and Special Age Groups

Women

The treatment of women with bipolar and related disorders can be complicated by factors such as interactions between reproductive hormones and psychotropic medications; mood instability resulting from hormonal changes during the perimenstrual, postpartum, and perimenopausal periods; and the potential for teratogenic and other adverse effects of medications during pregnancy and breastfeeding. In women with bipolar disorder, exposure to psychotropic medications has been associated with increased rates of menstrual irregularities and polycystic ovary syndrome. Certain SGAs may cause hyperprolactinemia, which can lead to complications such as galactorrhea or amenorrhea. Treatment with valproate may be contraindicated in women of reproductive potential, given its association with polycystic ovary syndrome and teratogenicity. Carbamazepine should also be avoided during pregnancy because of its association with congenital malformations. Lamotrigine dosages greater than 200 mg/day during pregnancy have been associated with increased risk for cleft lip and palate. As noted earlier, drug interactions between hormonal contraceptives and lamotrigine may necessitate higher than typical dosages of lamotrigine to achieve adequate therapeutic benefit. However, treatment with hormonal contraceptives may prove beneficial for perimenstrual exacerbation of mood symptoms; alternatively, luteal-phase dosing of mood-stabilizing medications (i.e., increasing the dosage during the week prior to menses, then reducing again at menses onset) can yield benefit in such instances.

Children and Adolescents

Few medications are FDA approved specifically for the treatment of children and adolescents with bipolar disorder (see Table 11–4). Children and adolescents with bipolar disorder may be more sensitive than adults to the adverse effects of psychiatric medications, particularly with respect to metabolic adverse effects and weight gain. Thus, pharmacological treatment of pediatric patients with bipolar disorder requires careful monitoring of tolerability concerns while limiting exposure to the minimum necessary dosage of the minimum necessary number of medications. Management of bipolar and related disorders in pediatric populations may be further complicated by ambiguous initial presentations, potentially leading to misdiagnosis and exposure to antidepressants that may destabilize mood. Comorbid ADHD is also common among bipolar youth and often leads to treatment with stimulant medications, which may increase vulnerability to mixed symptoms or manic episodes, particularly if these agents are administered without concurrent mood stabilizers.

Older Adults

There are limited data to inform definitive treatment guidelines for older adults with bipolar and related disorders because such patients tend to be excluded from large randomized controlled studies. Treatment of older populations may be complicated by comorbid medical conditions and complex medication regimens leading to higher rates of drug interactions as well as increased vulnerability to adverse effects (particularly with respect to central nervous system effects). Most guidelines recommend treating older patients with lower dosages and using more stringent monitoring parameters to compensate for age-related changes in renal clearance, as well as to avoid drug interactions with concomitant medications (Dols et al. 2016). Older adults may receive adequate benefit from mood stabilizers such as lithium at the lower end of the therapeutic serum level range, although systematic data evaluating this proposition are lacking (Dols et al. 2016).

Conclusion

In summary, bipolar disorder is a chronic mental illness characterized by episodes of depression as well as mania and/or hypomania. Accurate diagnosis of bipolar disorder requires careful consideration of current and past clinical features, family history, and the potential influences of medication/substance exposures and/or general medical conditions. Treatment strategies for bipolar disorder may vary according to the phase of illness (i.e., acute mania, acute depression, or longer-term maintenance) but commonly involve mood stabilizers and/or second-generation antipsychotics, in combination with psychosocial interventions.

Key Clinical Points

- Bipolar and related disorders affect as many as 4% of people and are characterized by fluctuating episodes of depression and mania/hypomania.

- Current diagnostic classifications conceptualize bipolar and related disorders as biologically and phenomenologically intermediate between psychotic disorders and unipolar depressive disorders.

- The pathogenesis of bipolar and related disorders entails a strong genetic component, with heritability estimates ranging from 70% to 80%, yet genome-wide association studies suggest contributions of many small-effect rather than few large-effect genes.

- Pharmacological treatment of bipolar and related disorders is guided by illness phase, with varying agents being FDA approved for acute manic episodes, acute bipolar depressive episodes, and longer-term maintenance treatment of bipolar I disorder.

- There are very limited data to guide treatment of bipolar II disorder, with quetiapine being the only FDA-approved bipolar II disorder treatment (for acute depression) and some data suggesting potential efficacy of antidepressants for this patient population.

- FDA-approved medications have the most robust evidence for efficacy and therefore should generally be considered first-line agents; nevertheless, tolerability or efficacy limitations may lead to the use of off-label medications, including standard antidepressants and other adjunctive treatments, and neuromodulatory approaches such as electroconvulsive therapy and repetitive transcranial magnetic stimulation.

- Certain psychotherapies have some evidence base for their use in bipolar disorder and should be offered concurrently with medication management.

References

Altshuler LL, Kupka RW, Hellemann G, et al: Gender and depressive symptoms in 711 patients with bipolar disorder evaluated prospectively in the Stanley Foundation bipolar treatment outcome network. Am J Psychiatry 167(6):708–715, 2010 20231325

Altshuler LL, Sugar CA, McElroy SL, et al: Switch rates during acute treatment for bipolar II depression with lithium, sertraline, or the two combined: a randomized, double-blind comparison. Am J Psychiatry 174(3):266–276, 2017 28135846

American Diabetes Association, American Psychiatric Association, American Association of Clinical Endocrinologists, et al: Consensus development conference on antipsychotic drugs and obesity and diabetes. Diabetes Care 27(2):596–601, 2004 14747245

American Psychiatric Association: Diagnostic and Statistical Manual of Mental Disorders, 4th Edition. Washington, DC, American Psychiatric Association, 1994

American Psychiatric Association: Diagnostic and Statistical Manual of Mental Disorders, 5th Edition. Arlington, VA, American Psychiatric Association, 2013

Amini H, Sharifi V: Quality of life in bipolar type I disorder in a one-year followup. Depress Res Treat 2012:860745, 2012 23326652

Baldassano CF, Marangell LB, Gyulai L, et al: Gender differences in bipolar disorder: retrospective data from the first 500 STEP-BD participants. Bipolar Disord 7(5):465–470, 2005 16176440

Baldessarini RJ, Pompili M, Tondo L: Suicide in bipolar disorder: risks and management. CNS Spectr 11(6):465–471, 2006 16816785

Baldessarini RJ, Leahy L, Arcona S, et al: Patterns of psychotropic drug prescription for U.S. patients with diagnoses of bipolar disorders. Psychiatr Serv 58(1):85–91, 2007 17215417

Belvederi Murri M, Prestia D, Mondelli V, et al: The HPA axis in bipolar disorder: systematic review and meta-analysis. Psychoneuroendocrinology 63:327–342, 2016 26547798

Bobo WV: The diagnosis and management of bipolar I and II disorders: clinical practice update. Mayo Clin Proc 92(10):1532–1551, 2017 28888714

Charney AW, Ruderfer DM, Stahl EA, et al: Evidence for genetic heterogeneity between clinical subtypes of bipolar disorder. Transl Psychiatry 7(1):e993, 2017 28072414

Dols A, Kessing LV, Strejilevich SA, et al: Do current national and international guidelines have specific recommendations for older adults with bipolar disorder? A brief report. Int J Geriatr Psychiatry 31(12):1295–1300, 2016 27442023

Frye MA, Altshuler LL, McElroy SL, et al: Gender differences in prevalence, risk, and clinical correlates of alcoholism comorbidity in bipolar disorder. Am J Psychiatry 160(5):883–889, 2003 12727691

Geddes JR, Calabrese JR, Goodwin GM: Lamotrigine for treatment of bipolar depression: independent meta-analysis and meta-regression of individual patient data from five randomised trials. Br J Psychiatry 194(1):4–9, 2009 19118318

Gedeon Richter: Allergan and Richter announce positive topline results from phase III study of cariprazine for the treatment of bipolar I depression. December 18, 2017. Available at: https://www.richter.hu/en-US/investors/announcements/Pages/extraord171218.aspx. Accessed February 16, 2018.

Goodwin FR, Jamison K: Manic-Depressive Illness: Bipolar Disorders and Recurrent Depression, 2nd Edition. New York, Oxford University Press, 2007

Gordon-Smith K, Jones LA, Forty L, et al: Changes to the diagnostic criteria for bipolar disorder in DSM-5 make little difference to lifetime diagnosis: findings from the U.K. Bipolar Disorder Research Network (BDRN) study. Am J Psychiatry 174(8):803, 2017 28760020

Hafeman DM, Merranko J, Axelson D, et al: Toward the definition of a bipolar prodrome: dimensional predictors of bipolar spectrum disorders in at-risk youths. Am J Psychiatry 173(7):695–704, 2016 26892940

Insel T, Cuthbert B, Garvey M, et al: Research Domain Criteria (RDoC): toward a new classification framework for research on mental disorders. Am J Psychiatry 167(7):748–751, 2010 20595427

Kim H, Kim W, Citrome L, et al: More inclusive bipolar mixed depression definition by permitting overlapping and non-overlapping mood elevation symptoms. Acta Psychiatr Scand 134(3):199–206, 2016 27137894

Kupka RW, Altshuler LL, Nolen WA, et al: Three times more days depressed than manic or hypomanic in both bipolar I and bipolar II disorder. Bipolar Disord 9(5):531–535, 2007 17680925

Leibenluft E: Severe mood dysregulation, irritability, and the diagnostic boundaries of bipolar disorder in youths. Am J Psychiatry 168(2):129–142, 2011 21123313

Liu B, Zhang Y, Fang H, et al: Efficacy and safety of long-term antidepressant treatment for bipolar disorders—a meta-analysis of randomized controlled trials. J Affect Disord 223:41–48, 2017 28715727

Machado-Vieira R, Luckenbaugh DA, Ballard ED, et al: Increased activity or energy as a primary criterion for the diagnosis of bipolar mania in DSM-5: findings from the STEP-BD study. Am J Psychiatry 174(1):70–76, 2017 27523498

Merikangas KR, Akiskal HS, Angst J, et al: Lifetime and 12-month prevalence of bipolar spectrum disorder in the National Comorbidity Survey replication. Arch Gen Psychiatry 64(5):543–552, 2007 17485606

Merikangas KR, Jin R, He JP, et al: Prevalence and correlates of bipolar spectrum disorder in the world mental health survey initiative. Arch Gen Psychiatry 68(3):241–251, 2011 21383262

Miller S, Suppes T, Mintz J, et al: Mixed depression in bipolar disorder: prevalence rate and clinical correlates during naturalistic follow-up in the Stanley Bipolar Network. Am J Psychiatry 173(10):1015–1023, 2016 27079133

Nahas Z, Kozel FA, Li X, et al: Left prefrontal transcranial magnetic stimulation (TMS) treatment of depression in bipolar affective disorder: a pilot study of acute safety and efficacy. Bipolar Disord 5(1):40–47, 2003 12656937

Nashed MG, Restivo MR, Taylor VH: Olanzapine-induced weight gain in patients with bipolar I disorder: a meta-analysis. Prim Care Companion CNS Disord 13(6), 2011 22454806

Pacchiarotti I, Bond DJ, Baldessarini RJ, et al: The International Society for Bipolar Disorders (ISBD) task force report on antidepressant use in bipolar disorders. Am J Psychiatry 170(11):1249–1262, 2013 24030475

Parsaik AK, Singh B, Khosh-Chashm D, et al: Efficacy of ketamine in bipolar depression: systematic review and meta-analysis. J Psychiatr Pract 21(6):427–435, 2015 26554325

Perich TA, Roberts G, Frankland A, et al: Clinical characteristics of women with reproductive cycle-associated bipolar disorder symptoms. Aust NZ J Psychiatry 51(2):161–167, 2017 27687774

Phillips ML, Swartz HA: A critical appraisal of neuroimaging studies of bipolar disorder: toward a new conceptualization of underlying neural circuitry and a road map for future research. Am J Psychiatry 171(8):829–843, 2014 24626773

Pope HG Jr, Lipinski JF Jr: Diagnosis in schizophrenia and manic-depressive illness: a reassessment of the specificity of "schizophrenic" symptoms in the light of current research. Arch Gen Psychiatry 35(7):811–828, 1978 354552

Reiser RP, Thompson LW, Johnson SL, et al: Bipolar Disorder. Boston, MA, Hogrefe, 2017

Rosenblat JD, McIntyre RS: Bipolar disorder and inflammation. Psychiatr Clin North Am 39(1):125–137, 2016 26876323

Sajatovic M, Strejilevich SA, Gildengers AG, et al: A report on older-age bipolar disorder from the International Society for Bipolar Disorders Task Force. Bipolar Disord 17(7):689–704, 2015 26384588

Sidor MM, Macqueen GM: Antidepressants for the acute treatment of bipolar depression: a systematic review and meta-analysis. J Clin Psychiatry 72(2):156–167, 2011 21034686

Sigitova E, Fišar Z, Hroudová J, et al: Biological hypotheses and biomarkers of bipolar disorder. Psychiatry Clin Neurosci 71(2):77–103, 2017 27800654

Suppes T, Baldessarini RJ, Faedda GL, et al: Risk of recurrence following discontinuation of lithium treatment in bipolar disorder. Arch Gen Psychiatry 48(12):1082–1088, 1991 1845226

Suppes T, Mintz J, McElroy SL, et al: Mixed hypomania in 908 patients with bipolar disorder evaluated prospectively in the Stanley Foundation Bipolar Treatment Network: a sex-specific phenomenon. Arch Gen Psychiatry 62(10):1089–1096, 2005 16203954

Suppes T, Hirschfeld RM, Vieta E, et al: Quetiapine for the treatment of bipolar II depression: analysis of data from two randomized, double-blind, placebo-controlled studies. World J Biol Psychiatry 9(3):198–211, 2008 17853277

Versiani M, Cheniaux E, Landeira-Fernandez J: Efficacy and safety of electroconvulsive therapy in the treatment of bipolar disorder: a systematic review. J ECT 27(2):153–164, 2011 20562714

Wang PW, Hill SJ, Childers ME, et al: Open adjunctive ziprasidone associated with weight loss in obese and overweight bipolar disorder patients. J Psychiatr Res 45(8):1128–1132, 2011 21371718

Wingo AP, Harvey PD, Baldessarini RJ: Neurocognitive impairment in bipolar disorder patients: functional implications. Bipolar Disord 11(2):113–125, 2009 19267694

World Health Organization: The Global Burden of Disease: 2004 Update. Geneva, World Health Organization, 2008. Available at: http://www.who.int/healthinfo/global_burden_disease/GBD_report_2004update_full.pdf. Accessed August 31, 2015.

Recommended Readings

Altshuler LL, Sugar CA, McElroy SL, et al: Switch rates during acute treatment for bipolar II depression with lithium, sertraline, or the two combined: a randomized double-blind comparison. Am J Psychiatry 174(3):266–276, 2017

Goodwin FR, Jamison K: Manic-Depressive Illness: Bipolar Disorders and Recurrent Depression, 2nd Edition. New York, Oxford University Press, 2007

Ketter TA: Handbook of Diagnosis and Treatment of Bipolar Disorder. Washington, DC, American Psychiatric Publishing, 2010

Kupka RW, Altshuler LL, Nolen WA, et al: Three times more days depressed than manic or hypomanic in both bipolar I and bipolar II disorder. Bipolar Disord 9(5):531–535, 2007

Merikangas KR, Akiskal HS, Angst J, et al: Lifetime and 12-month prevalence of bipolar spectrum disorder in the National Comorbidity Survey replication. Arch Gen Psychiatry 64(5):543–552, 2007

CHAPTER 12

Depressive Disorders

Sagar V. Parikh, M.D.

Michelle B. Riba, M.D., M.S.

John F. Greden, M.D.

It has been 6 years since DSM-5 (American Psychiatric Association 2013) was unveiled with significant changes from DSM-IV-TR (American Psychiatric Association 2000), and, in particular, with some important modifications in the "Depressive Disorders." DSM-5 depressive disorders include the categories listed in Table 12–1.

The list of modifications has clinical and research implications. The "Mood Disorders" chapter of DSM-IV-TR was split into two separate chapters in DSM-5, "Bipolar and Related Disorders" and "Depressive Disorders," and the number of categories in each of these chapters has increased (see Table 12–1). The separation sought to reflect that bipolar disorders have a similar degree of phenomenological and genetic overlap with schizophrenia and with depression (Hopper 2018). Clinicians must remain cognizant of the fact that most cases of bipolar disorder first present as depression, but long-term treatment implications may differ dramatically; thus, the switch from major depressive disorder (MDD) to bipolar disorder is one of the most common and important diagnostic transitions in psychiatry (Uher et al. 2014). New to the depressive disorders diagnostic class are disruptive mood dysregulation disorder (DMDD) and premenstrual dysphoric disorder (PMDD). "Specifiers" are additional descriptors of severity, course, or comorbid clinical features and are available for improved objective clinical documentation. Risk of self-harm may be assessed and characterized within the DSM-5 Level 1 Cross-Cutting Symptom Measure for the purpose of communicating risk and prevention planning integral to the clinical evaluation based on DSM-5 criteria. Minor differences in the wording of the criteria for major depressive episode are seen from DSM-III (American Psychiatric Association 1980) to the current DSM-5; in more than 35 years of research, a core uniform definition of major depressive episode has essentially been used. Finally, bereavement is no longer considered an exclusion to a depressive disorder diagnosis within the first 2 months of the loss.

TABLE 12–1.   **DSM-5 depressive disorders**

Disruptive mood dysregulation disorder
Major depressive disorder, single or recurrent episodes
Persistent depressive disorder (dysthymia)
Premenstrual dysphoric disorder
Substance/medication-induced depressive disorder
Depressive disorder due to another medical condition
Other specified depressive disorder
Unspecified depressive disorder

The rationale, although complex, is fundamentally simple. DSM-5 emphasizes specifiers aimed toward helping to further subcategorize and manage disease patterns (Table 12–2 lists the DSM-5 specifiers for depressive disorders). The coexistence of at least three manic/hypomanic symptoms (insufficient for a manic episode) within a major depressive episode is indicated in DSM-5 by the specifier "with mixed features." There is no clear evidence that individuals with this symptom profile will develop bipolar disorder; however, the clinical manifestation of mixed features may have treatment and etiological relevance. Episode severity may now be coded independently of presence of psychotic features. Psychosis is specified according to mood congruency; mood-congruent psychotic features are consistent with underlying mood (e.g., psychotic guilt), whereas mood-incongruent psychotic features are generally bizarre and unexplained by mood symptoms. The presence of psychosis is often, but not always, associated with greater severity.

New diagnostic categories were placed in the depressive disorders class after careful scientific review of the evidence. PMDD has been moved from DSM-IV-TR Appendix B, "Criteria Sets and Axes Provided for Further Study" (American Psychiatric Association 2000), to become a stand-alone diagnosis. DMDD refers to the presentation of children with severe, recurrent temper outbursts. Although initial clinical impressions suggested that these phenomena may be related to childhood bipolar disorder, long-term outcome studies found that children with this presentation developed MDD.

The "Depressive Disorders" chapter in DSM-5 Section II coupled with the "Assessment Measures" chapter in DSM-5 Section III reflects refinements aimed at improving the recognition and treatment of these disorders by encouraging the clinician to record and consider important dimensional measures that are not conveyed by the categorical diagnoses themselves in arriving at a treatment plan for a specific patient. The Level 1 Cross-Cutting Symptom Measure is highlighted within DSM-5 to improve characterization and rate the severity of comorbid symptoms (e.g., anxiety, substance abuse) that have been shown to have a significant effect on clinical outcome of treatment as well as on risk of self-harm in individuals with mood disorders.

Disruptive Mood Dysregulation Disorder

DMDD is a new disorder in DSM-5 whose core phenomenology is characterized by frequent and severe verbal and/or behavioral outbursts (in response to common

TABLE 12–2.   **DSM-5 specifiers for depressive disorders**

With anxious distress (specify current severity)

With mixed features

With melancholic features

With atypical features

With psychotic features

With catatonia

With peripartum onset

With seasonal pattern (specify current severity)

Note.   For the complete text of these specifiers, please refer to DSM-5 pp. 184–188.

stressors) that are pervasive, are outside the developmental stage, and occur in the background of a chronic negative mood. The onset is between ages 6 and 10 years. The diagnosis emerges from research on severe mood dysregulation and irritability and observations on the overlapping phenomenology of bipolar disorder and specific mood symptoms of irritability (Leibenluft 2011). It is placed in the depressive disorders diagnostic class because longitudinal follow-up evidence predicted emergence of depressive disorders (and not bipolar disorder) both in a short-term follow-up of 2 years (Stringaris et al. 2010) and in a long-term follow-up 20 years later (Stringaris et al. 2009). Children previously considered to be within the bipolar spectrum are anticipated to be included in this new diagnostic category.

Phenomenology and Diagnostic Features

The key phenomenological feature of DMDD is irritability that is both acutely reactive and persistently chronic. Reactive agitated temper outbursts, profound and beyond what would be expected in the developmental stage, occur at least three times weekly in response to daily frustrations. The verbal component of irritability includes shouting and screaming, with wanton disregard for the feelings of others; the physical and behavioral aspect may include reckless aggression toward people, animals, or property. The nature and extent of the outbursts must be assessed in three settings and documented (e.g., home, school, and social settings with peers) and must be considered to be severe in one setting (requiring the supervising adult to suspend the current activity to focus on the management of the child). The agitated outbursts must be frequent, occurring on average three times weekly over the course of 1 year and on the background of a chronic irritable, upset, or angry mood present nearly every day. The chronic irritable mood will characteristically be described by the parent or caretaker as being the child's temperament.

Epidemiology

Prevalence

Because minimal epidemiological data are available, estimates of irritability in youth that use criteria very similar to those for DSM-5 DMDD suggest that the overall prevalence of the disorder ranges from around 0.8% to 3.3% (Copeland et al. 2013).

Course and Development

The chronic irritability and random temper outbursts of youths with DMDD in response to mundane provocations showed several distinctive features in comparison with those of youths with classic episodic bipolar disorder (Leibenluft 2011). Individuals with DMDD are less likely to have a parent with bipolar disorder and are more likely to develop MDD (Stringaris et al. 2009, 2010), and the specific symptoms (irritable outbursts) of DMDD become less common with the transition to adulthood (Leibenluft et al. 2006). The lack of association of childhood dysregulation of mood with later bipolar disorder was also found in a longitudinal study of Dutch children followed to adulthood (Althoff et al. 2010). The current research and understanding of the clinical course of childhood irritability and dysregulated moods clearly place DMDD in the DSM-5 class of depressive disorders rather than among bipolar and related disorders.

Etiological Factors

Risk and protective etiological factors of DMDD are not known. Children with DMDD frequently present with a complex psychiatric and temperamental history with an extensive pattern of irritability and other comorbidities that manifest before the full criteria of the syndrome are met. The family history is generally noncontributory. Children with a dysregulated mood profile on the Child Behavior Checklist have been found to have a substantial background of psychosocial adversity, which may be either a cause or an effect of the syndrome (Jucksch et al. 2011).

Differential Diagnosis

Individuals with pediatric bipolar disorder exhibit discrete episodic periods of mood disturbance with sustained volitional and cognitive changes. The phenomenology, including duration, is similar to that of bipolar disorder in the young adult population. In contrast, DMDD is a disorder with acute temperamental outbursts on a background of chronic irritability. Distinct periods of euphoria, grandiosity, racing thoughts, and lack of need for sleep in a sustained energized state characterize bipolar disorder rather than DMDD. An explosive, chronically cranky, sensitive, and unhappy child will more likely have DMDD.

Oppositional defiant disorder will be frequently, if not invariably, found in children with DMDD. Oppositional defiant disorder may be diagnosed before age 6 years, after which there may be debate as to which diagnostic category is most applicable to the clinical course. The primary phenomenology of explosive irritability on a background of a chronic state of anger and irritability warrants application of DMDD as a primary diagnosis. The absence of the chronic unhappy irritability criteria (including time duration) would support oppositional defiant disorder as the sole diagnosis.

Attention-deficit/hyperactivity disorder (ADHD) may frequently coexist with DMDD, and the diagnosis is made according to the criteria of ADHD. The chronic irritability of DMDD may contribute to the appearance of boredom and difficulty maintaining focus that are part of ADHD. The impulsivity of ADHD is unlikely to be confused with the profound outbursts of temper in DMDD.

MDD and persistent depressive disorder (dysthymia) often have irritability as a prominent clinical symptom. The lack of irritable outbursts and temper tantrums would call for a diagnosis of persistent depressive disorder in a chronically irritable and upset child. Should the *average* weekly number of outbursts over the course of a year be estimated to be three or more by the parent or caregiver, the DMDD diagnosis should be considered. There may be variable numbers of symptoms of depression in the context of DMDD, and there is evidence that DMDD frequently evolves into MDD. Once the criteria for MDD are met, MDD becomes the preferred diagnostic category. Future investigations are needed to clarify treatment implications.

Intermittent explosive disorder is an exclusion diagnostic category for a child with frequent outbursts of temper (similar to a child with DMDD) but with no evidence of persistent mood disruption between outbursts. A child with chronic and persistent annoyed, sensitive, and irritable mood with temper outbursts would receive a diagnosis of DMDD; a child with "normal" mood between temper outbursts would receive a diagnosis of intermittent explosive disorder.

Substance use disorders should not be overlooked despite a person's young age because young individuals may be exposed to a variety of substances in their environment. On occasion, these exposures may have developed from prescription medications. Comorbidities should always be considered.

Comorbid Diagnoses

It is anticipated that DMDD will have many comorbid diagnoses. Three diagnostic categories—bipolar disorder, intermittent explosive disorder, and oppositional defiant disorder—are exclusionary. The presence of symptoms from mood, anxiety, and developmental disorders is expected, and the formulation of the patient's clinical problems provides for prioritization of such problems and emphasis of the preferred diagnostic category. As a clinical axiom, diagnostic co-occurrences are best considered a norm, not an exception.

Management

The formulation of DMDD within the class of depressive disorders rather than within the bipolar and related disorders class has implications for therapeutic management. The current approach to management is symptomatic and problem focused. Optimal treatment for individuals with DMDD is not clear, and several individual and combined treatments are under consideration; however, there is no currently validated treatment for this disorder. Clinical trials involving antidepressants and other medication classes are predicated on the inclusion of DMDD within the class of depressive disorders. Aggressive outbursts are prominent features of the disorder. Effect sizes of between 0.43 and 0.5 were found in a trial of risperidone plus concurrent stimulant medication and parent training for treatment of serious aggression in the context of childhood ADHD (Aman et al. 2014). Irritability has been shown to be responsive to selective serotonin reuptake inhibitors (SSRIs) in the context of a nonbipolar illness. If a manic episode occurs in the context of antidepressant therapy, the clinician should reconsider the overall diagnosis, with bipolar disorder a strong possibility. A small placebo-controlled study of lithium treatment of DMDD was negative, whereas results of trials of divalproex and risperidone have provided some support for use of these agents in management of the irritability (Leibenluft 2011). Although no formal psychotherapy trials have been reported, anecdotal reports indicate that irritability and aggression have improved with behavioral management strategies.

Prognosis

In a longitudinal study (Brotman et al. 2006), subjects were monitored for more than 15 years in four distinct assessment "waves" for the evidence for DMDD (called "severe mood dysregulation" in the study). The fact that DMDD was found in only one wave for 80% of the participants implies that the diagnosis may be time limited (i.e., DMDD was not diagnosed at each assessment time point). The risk of developing MDD in early adulthood was predicted by the mood dysregulation diagnosis in only one of the assessment waves. Other functional outcomes have not been published and await further research (Leibenluft 2011).

Major Depressive Disorder

MDD is a unique diagnostic category in the current descriptive understanding of the illness. This diagnosis represents the clinical manifestation of heterogeneous illnesses likely to have complex biopsychosocial brain-change etiologies with symptom patterns that may change in quality and severity over the lifetime of the individual. Neuroscience, medical, and psychological texts, as well as literature and art in most cultures, provide articulate descriptions and interpretations of the perceived underlying pathophysiology of depression. Central to the definition is a disordered affect. *Affect* is defined as the objective and behavioral expression of internal mood states with concomitant observable motor components in the form of expressive features of facial and other bodily movements. Diminished volitional and cognitive expressions are generally, but not always, aligned with the degree of disordered and depressed mood.

The term *depression* is complicated because, in addition to referring to the heterogeneous manifestation of the medical disorders that are captured by the concept of major depression, with single or recurrent episodes, it is used in daily language with its own culturally determined meanings. DSM-5 represents the current approach to the clinical understanding of MDD, putting a framework around the observations and providing a clinical base for the etiological and translational research that is ongoing and will ultimately lead to further clarification of understandings of specific etiologies, pathways, and treatments.

Phenomenology and Diagnostic Features

The core feature of MDD is the major depressive episode, represented by Criteria A–C of the DSM-5 diagnostic criteria for MDD.

Criterion A in DSM-5 requires the individual to have experienced at least five of nine listed symptoms simultaneously during a 2-week period and to have undergone a change from previous functioning. Either depressed mood or anhedonia (loss of interest or pleasure) must be one of the symptoms. The depressed mood of MDD goes beyond transient mood changes experienced in response to the vicissitudes of everyday life, which may lead to temporary demoralization but can usually be relieved by situational remediation. The depressed mood of a major depressive episode is objective and sustained and preoccupies most (>50%) of the time nearly every day. The patient often describes the mood as a profound sense of hopelessness or internal emptiness. In less mature individuals (e.g., children, people with intellectual disabilities), the expression of depressed mood may be irritability with a cranky, easily annoyed disposition that is sustained.

Anhedonia is the second anchor criterion of depression. Its insidious onset in the absence of depressed mood may be associated with diminished capacity to recognize the presence of a depressive episode. Key to the assessment is the qualitative change and reference points that include timelines and activities. People who know the patient well (e.g., family members) may be immeasurably helpful in providing necessary clinical data to establish these criteria.

Several vegetative signs and symptoms are included in the criteria for a depressive episode. Appetite change and unintended weight loss reflect the physical and metabolic symptoms related to depression; the desire to eat, the pleasure of a favorite food, and the volitional drive of self-care are diminished. Patterns of sleep disturbances within a depressive episode vary across individuals, and an individual may experience episode variability and evolution of the depressive sleep pattern over time. Characteristically, the individual feels that he or she is not getting enough sleep and experiences fatigue or exhaustion during waking hours. The patterns of insomnia include initial insomnia (difficulty falling asleep), middle insomnia (waking during the night), and terminal insomnia (early-morning awakening and difficulty falling back asleep). A subgroup of individuals show "reverse vegetative" symptoms, wherein the eating and sleeping patterns are reversed from the typical pattern; these individuals experience increased appetite and carbohydrate craving, and their sleep patterns, compared with baseline, are characterized by oversleeping, often more than 10 hours per day.

Altered psychomotor activity is expressed in agitation or retardation. Psychomotor agitation is an inner irritability with an objective motor component, such as the hand wringing of a depressed elderly person or the gesticulated pacing of a fretting despondent individual. Psychomotor retardation refers to the notable slowing of all objective body activity, including walking, eating, talking, and gestures. Fatigue and loss of energy may be subjective, objective, or both.

Thoughts and cognitive processes are disrupted. The content of thought is often disrupted, and individuals with MDD may have unfavorable thoughts toward themselves and their own actions that are not consistent with the rational assessment of an observer. An individual with MDD may have feelings of unworthiness or excessive or inappropriate guilt that are delusional (e.g., unfounded blaming of self for a major catastrophe). The individual's thinking may be disrupted by the diminished ability to think or concentrate or by indecisiveness. The capacity to perform at previously documented levels is impaired (e.g., a professor will have difficulty reading and critiquing research papers, a carpenter will have difficulty organizing and executing tasks of the day that were previously done with ease, pleasure, and a sense of self-fulfillment).

Recurrent thoughts of death and suicide are a common feature of the depressive episode. Immediate risk is indicated if an individual has a plan to kill himself or herself or has prepared and planned for his or her own demise (e.g., has recently prepared a will and planned for disposition of property). Direct questions such as "Do you have thoughts of killing yourself?" are helpful. The depressed patient is more likely than not to have contemplations of death that may be magnified by the current depressive episode, and delineation of the extent and frequency of these thoughts should guide treatment.

The Level 1 Cross-Cutting Symptom Measure provided in the "Assessment Measures" chapter of DSM-5 Section III is a very pragmatic self-rated instrument to assess symptoms and severity; it is highly recommended that clinicians use this or a similar clinical measure in their evaluations. Baseline assessment instruments ideally are suitable for ongoing measurement-based care, perhaps one of the most neglected components of psychiatric treatment delivery. The DSM-5 "Assessment Measures" chapter also refers to the Patient-Reported Outcomes Measurement Information System (PROMIS) instruments (www.nihpromis.org), which have been used extensively in clinical outcomes research (www.nihpromis.org/science/PublicationsYears). In addition, the 9-item depression module from the Patient Health Questionnaire (PHQ-9) (Kroenke et al. 2001), a validated tool for assessment of DSM-5 depressive symptom severity, is useful because it combines categorical and dimensional assessments of the symptoms. The Level 1 Cross-Cutting Symptom Measure, the PROMIS instruments, and the PHQ-9 are relatively easy to use, time efficient, and internally consistent measures of mood symptoms (based on self-report). It is anticipated that use of such measures will be expected by insurers and administrative oversight entities. The Columbia-Suicide Severity Rating Scale has gained widespread adoption for suicide assessments (Posner et al. 2011).

Epidemiology

Prevalence

Estimates of the lifetime prevalence of MDD (all using DSM-IV [American Psychiatric Association 1994] criteria) are variable and range from over 17% in the United States to approximately 10% for many developed countries, with lower rates in Asia (World Health Organization 2017). The 2015 National Survey on Drug Use and Health (NSDUH) reported a 12-month prevalence of 6.7% for MDD in the United States, with the majority of respondents reporting severe disability in at least one of four major roles (home management, work, close relationships with others, and social life) (National Institute of Mental Health 2017). In almost all countries, women are approximately twice as likely as men to experience depression. In the United States, young adults (ages 18–25 years) have the highest rates of depression of all age groups (Center for Behavioral Health Statistics and Quality 2016), whereas globally, depression prevalence is highest in the 50- to 64-year age group. Overall, depression is the largest cause of disability worldwide (World Health Organization 2017).

Course of Illness: Recurrent Versus Single Episode

DSM-5 differentiates a single episode from recurrent episodes of MDD. For episodes to be considered recurrent, they must have been preceded by a period of at least 2 months during which criteria for MDD were not met. The signs and symptoms of recurrent and single episodes of MDD are identical; it is the course of the illness that categorizes the disorder. Clearly, the illness begins with a single episode; however, in many cases, the episodes are destined to become recurrent, with higher recurrence in those who do not achieve full remission in the index episode or those who discontinued treatments that had achieved response/remission. At least half of individuals with a single episode will experience a recurrence in their lifetime, with higher rates for those who have experienced at least two episodes (Forte et al. 2015).

The purported length of depressive episodes is in the range of 5–6 months, with approximately 20% of episodes becoming chronic (i.e., lasting beyond 2 years), but this pattern becomes quite different for those individuals who develop chronicity or treatment-resistant depression, found to be about 30% of those treated (Greden 2003; Greden et al. 2011). The course of symptoms throughout an episode varies according to the success of targeted treatment of symptoms. Because volition and energy may pick up early in treatment relative to mood and emotional symptoms, a patient may feel distressed that others comment that he or she appears somewhat better even though he or she still feels emotionally lousy, sad, and overwhelmed. The improvement in volition and energy is generally a good sign of initial response to treatment; however, the lag in improvement in mood relative to volition may result in despondency and suicidal behavior.

Risk and Prognostic Factors

Environmental factors. Adverse childhood experiences, particularly when there are multiple experiences of diverse types, comprise a set of potent risk factors for MDD and are often associated with poor response to treatment. Major current research focuses on the epigenetic factors as a mechanism of neurobiological translation of stress into depression (Nestler 2014). Stressful life events are well recognized as precipitants of major depressive episodes, but the presence or absence of adverse life events near the onset of episodes does not appear to provide a useful guide to prognosis or treatment selection.

Genetic and physiological factors. First-degree family members of individuals with MDD have a risk for MDD that is two to four times higher than that in the general population. Relative risks appear to be higher for early-onset and recurrent forms. Heritability has been estimated at 40% in the general population and 67% in populations at high risk for MDD (Guffanti et al. 2016). Major efforts are under way to use new approaches to psychiatric genetics to identify biological pathways that suggest or identify biomarkers and open the door to new treatment development. Progress is being made (CONVERGE Consortium 2015; Hyde et al. 2016; Hyman 2017; Power et al. 2017).

Course modifiers. Features associated with lower recovery rates, other than current episode duration, include psychosis, prominent anxiety, personality disorders, and severe symptomatology. The risk of recurrence falls slowly as time in remission increases and is higher when the preceding episode was severe, especially in younger individuals and in those who have already experienced multiple episodes (Kanai et al. 2003). The persistence of even mild depressive symptoms during remission is a powerful predictor of recurrence. An increasing number of prior episodes also predicts higher risk of recurrences (Greden 2003; Greden et al. 2011). Essentially, all major non-mood-related disorders increase the risk of an individual developing depression (Kessler et al. 1997). Major depressive episodes that develop in the context of another disorder often follow a more refractory course. Substance use, anxiety, and borderline personality disorders are among the most common of these, and the presenting depressive symptoms may obscure and delay their recognition (Kessler et al. 2005). However, sustained clinical improvement in depressive symptoms may depend on the appropriate treatment of underlying illnesses. Chronic or disabling medical conditions also increase risks for major depressive episodes. Such prevalent illnesses as diabetes, morbid obesity, and cardiovascular disease are often complicated by depressive episodes, which are more likely to become chronic than are depressive episodes in medically healthy individuals (McIntyre et al. 2012). Recent investigations suggest that co-occurring depressive and cardiovascular or cancer illnesses may share common inflammatory mechanisms that alter interleukin and cytokine abnormalities, concomitantly altering both brain and other organ functions (Miller and Raison 2016).

Suicidal Ideation

The possibility of suicidal behavior exists at all times during major depressive episodes. Sadly, suicide rates have increased during the past decade (Caine 2017). Although the most consistently described risk factor is a past history of suicide attempts or threats, most completed suicides are *not* preceded by unsuccessful attempts. Other features associated with an increased risk for completed suicide include male sex, being a member of a sexual minority group, being single or living alone, and having prominent feelings of hopelessness (Turecki and Brent 2016). Transgender struggles have recently been identified as a variable in suicide risk (Marshall et al. 2016). Recent investigations also suggest that alterations in inflammatory mechanisms may increase acute risk of suicide (Brundin et al. 2016), and opioid use most recently has become linked with an increasing risk of death by suicide (Ashrafioun et al. 2017). The presence of borderline personality disorder markedly increases risks for future suicide attempts.

Clinical Expression Related to Gender and Age

Despite consistent differences between genders in prevalence rates for depressive disorders and in suicide rates, there appear to be no clear differences by gender in phenomenology, course, or treatment response. The higher prevalence in females is the most reproducible finding in the epidemiology of MDD. Risks for suicide attempts are higher in women; however, risks for death from suicides in women are lower, largely attributable to greater use of more lethal means among men. There are no consistent differences between genders in symptoms, course, treatment response, or functional consequences.

Similarly, there are no clear effects of current age on the course or treatment response of MDD. Some symptom differences exist, however, such that reverse vegetative symptoms are more likely in younger individuals, and melancholic symptoms, particularly psychomotor slowing, are more common in older individuals. The likelihood of suicide attempts lessens in middle and late life, although the risk of death by suicide does not. Differentiating unipolar depression from bipolar disorder is vital; in MDD, there may be a later age at onset, fewer total lifetime episodes, and longer episodes, but these differences are small enough to probably not be useful in diagnostic formulations (Kessler et al. 2012).

There are inadequate data about specific effects of aging on long-term course of untreated MDD, but available data consistently suggest that untreated or inadequately treated individuals with MDD appear to experience more recurrences as years pass; they are also aging, of course. Additionally, with each episode, they experience longer episodes that occur closer together, and these episodes appear to become more difficult to treat with each ensuing episode (Greden 2003; Greden et al. 2011; Kupfer et al. 1992).

Etiological Factors

Although MDD is characterized as a syndrome that ostensibly represents a single disease, it is widely understood that there are many different types of MDD phenotypes and that the etiologies of each of these types may differ (Fried and Nesse 2015; Otte et al. 2016; Robinson and Jorge 2016; van Loo et al. 2012). To elaborate, the phenotypes or symptoms considered characteristic of a depressive syndrome may be similar for different underlying causes, such as serotonergic versus glutamatergic neurotransmitter disturbances, sleep apnea, inflammatory dysregulation, head trauma, cocaine abuse, and others. As a result, the search for etiological factors in "major depression" invariably leads to significant findings only in distinct subsets of individuals experiencing clinical MDD, suggesting and perhaps even mandating a consideration of the term *depressions* rather than simply major depression. Early attempts to clarify the different subtypes of MDD were based on constellations of symptoms, which ultimately did not prove reliable and did not lead to discrete etiological factors associated with different depression subtypes (Arnow et al. 2015; van Loo et al. 2012). A broader, more integrative view of mental health and mental disease allows for an appreciation of the scope of etiological factors for the constellation of specific forms of depression that all are identified by the clinical syndrome "major depression." As a clinical result, because of this heterogeneity, one treatment size never fits all.

One of the most helpful early discussions seeking to aid understanding of the complex etiologies behind a heterogeneous disorder such as MDD was presented in *The Perspectives of Psychiatry* by McHugh and Slavney (1998), which postulated that there are (at least) four perspectives to approaching and understanding these illnesses and phenomena. The *biological* perspective considers the increased genetic risk in affected family members, as well as biochemical and immunological factors such as inflammatory molecules and stress-related markers in the endocrine system. The *behavioral* perspective takes into account the role of motivated behaviors contributing to the clinical picture, including unhealthy lifestyle choices and related behaviors; smoking, drinking, unhealthy eating habits leading to obesity, and gambling are examples of behaviors that compromise moods and contribute to the etiology of MDD. Personality features and temperament contributing to mood disorders are captured in the *dimensional* perspective. Finally, the *life story* perspective describes the influences that life events and environmental influences may have on the development of the disorder (in 2019 terminology, these might be referred to as epigenetic modifiers of gene expression). A number of recent reviews identify specific research findings that implicate social and environmental influences (Bustamante et al. 2016; Wittenborn et al. 2016), brain–body interactions (McEwen 2017; Miller and Raison 2016), and the specific neurobiology of depression characterized by genetics, epigenetic factors, inflammatory markers, neuroendocrine alterations, and neuroimaging changes both structural and functional (Brakowski et al. 2017; Drysdale et al. 2017; Fabbri et al. 2017; Kraus et al. 2017; Lin and Turecki 2017; Yohn et al. 2017; Zhang et al. 2016). More promising, utilizing these frameworks allows for identification of biomarkers that may predict risk for depressions and, in particular, may aid treatment selection (Fonseka et al. 2018; Gadad et al. 2018; Lam et al. 2016a; Strawbridge et al. 2017).

Differential Diagnosis

The list of medical diseases that may have depressive symptoms as a concomitant feature is extensive. It includes diseases of most organ systems of the body. A newly diagnosed patient with depression clearly warrants a comprehensive medical examination that includes standard hematological and biochemistry screens as well as other screens indicated by the physical examination. Neither neuroimaging nor electroencephalographic investigations are routinely indicated. Given the potential interaction between many psychiatric medications and cardiac function, as well as the higher rate of cardiovascular disease in mood disorders, it is often helpful to get an electrocardiogram as part of the initial workup. The diagnostic formulation of the symptoms of a major depressive episode is especially difficult when they occur in an individual who also has a general medical condition (e.g., cancer, stroke, myocardial infarction, congestive heart failure, diabetes, pregnancy). Some of the criterion signs and symptoms of a major depressive episode are identical to those of general medical conditions (e.g., weight loss with untreated diabetes, fatigue with cancer, hypersomnia early in pregnancy, insomnia later in pregnancy or during the postpartum period). Such symptoms may appear to be linked with a major depressive diagnosis, but not when they are clearly and fully attributable to a general medical condition. Nonvegetative symptoms of dysphoria, anhedonia, feelings of guilt or worthlessness, sleep disturbances, impaired concentration or indecision, and suicidal thoughts should be assessed with particular care in such cases. Definitions of major depressive episodes that have been modified to include only these nonvegetative symptoms appear to perform in a fashion nearly identical to the complete DSM-5 definition.

A thorough psychiatric examination will consider and weigh the evidence for psychotic illness, such as schizophrenia, although there may be mood-congruent or mood-incongruent psychotic features within MDD that manifest with expressions of guilt. The more systematized and bizarre the psychotic features are, the greater the likelihood that a schizophrenia-phenotypic-spectrum illness is present. Bipolar disorder commonly begins with an episode of MDD, but a thorough review of the patient's history, including input from family members, may reveal concerns about bipolar disorder. At the moment, however, the diagnosis is based on the current phenomenology, not the concerns of the future or the symptoms of the family member. Anxiety and substance use disorders may be considered comorbid to depression—and commonly are—or may, in fact, be the primary disorder. An axiom by some is that for individuals with co-occurring depressive symptoms, anxiety, and panic, all should be treated concomitantly, with less regard for which was the primary presenting problem. The rationale is that anxiety is routinely a symptom itself and is extremely common during a depressive episode, and panic attacks occurring only during a depressive episode do not merit a separate diagnosis of panic disorder.

DSM-5 allows for specification of the current clinical status and severity (mild, moderate, or severe). Assessment tools that measure symptom severity in depression without psychotic features include the PHQ-9 (Kroenke et al. 2001) and the Quick Inventory of Depressive Symptomatology (Trivedi et al. 2004). A PHQ-9 score of 20 or greater indicates a severe classification, 15–19 is rated moderate, and 10–14 is considered mild severity. Assignment of a measure of severity is recommended to provide a dimensional measure for use in ongoing monitoring of disease. When measurement-based care, which ideally should always be employed, is then used, the effectiveness of treatments can then be objectively assessed and adjusted as needed. Disorder-specific severity measures and additional dimensional assessments can be found online at www.psychiatry.org/practice/dsm/dsm5/online-assessment-measures.

Management

Management of MDD is a balance between understanding principles based on research evidence typically done on groups of individuals and tailoring treatment to a specific individual. Major treatment guidelines have been published by many different groups, each with nuances of how to evaluate evidence, how to weigh side effects, and how to consider specific treatments in the context of all available interventions, costs, and patient preference. American Psychiatric Association treatment guidelines for MDD were last published in 2010 (American Psychiatric Association 2010) and thus are less useful than more recent ones. The National Institute for Health and Care Excellence (in press) in the United Kingdom has produced depression treatment guidelines that are useful for their consideration of the health economic impact of decisions and also for their stepwise approach to treatment based on number of symptoms and extent of disability. Guidelines published in Australia in 2015 were notable for the integration of MDD and bipolar disorder in the single document and for their careful attention to integrating multiple stakeholders into the feedback process for guideline creation (Malhi et al. 2015). In 2015, the British Association for Psychopharmacology produced guidelines for treating depressive disorders with antidepressants, with clear stepwise recommendations for acute management as a well as advice on how to deal with inadequate treatment response to an antidepressant (Cleare et al. 2015). The American College of Physicians published two key articles in 2016 regarding management of depression, with one article comparing the benefits and harms of second-generation antidepressants versus other treatments (Gartlehner et al. 2016) and the second article contrasting pharmacological versus nonpharmacological treatments (Qaseem et al. 2016). Although each of the preceding guidelines offers evidence-based and well-reasoned approaches to the management of depression, by far the most widely cited treatment guidelines for MDD are those produced by the Canadian Network for Mood and Anxiety Treatments (CANMAT). The five articles constituting the 2009 adult depression guidelines from CANMAT have been cited more than 800 times and are extensively used worldwide (Kennedy et al. 2009; Lam et al. 2009; Parikh et al. 2009; Ravindran et al. 2009). More recently, CANMAT 2016 guidelines for MDD treatment in adults offer current advice with an emphasis on both evidence and clinical utility and serve as the main guide for the following management principles (Kennedy et al. 2016; Lam et al. 2016a; MacQueen et al. 2016; Milev et al. 2016; Parikh et al. 2016; Ravindran et al. 2016).

Management of MDD in adults begins with a comprehensive biopsychosocial assessment, with particular attention to using either clinician or (preferably) patient self-report scales to capture both depression symptoms and disability. The two most widely used self-report scales include the PHQ-9 for depression symptoms and the Sheehan Disability Scale for assessing disability across domains, including work/school, social life, and family life/home responsibilities. After assessing symptoms and suicidality, key family, work, and physical health information should be obtained and used to formulate a diagnosis and differential.

Once the diagnosis is established as MDD, it is essential to provide psychoeducation to ensure that the patient understands the nature of depression and its treatment as well as the critical role of self-monitoring and self-management. Essential in this treatment initiation stage is the establishment of a collaborative tone with the patient, along with careful elicitation of patient preferences for testing and treatment. With this background, the systematic application of evidence-based treatments may commence. Regular use of monitoring scales such as the PHQ-9 is also essential to ongoing treatment. Family members may be vital allies for such monitoring and treatment adherence.

Initiation of a specific treatment is a balance between patient preference, evidence, and the severity of the illness. For mild to moderate depression, especially when precipitated by stresses or traumas, and when the illness is not a clear-cut repeat episode of MDD, several types of psychotherapy and antidepressant medication have the most evidence and should be considered for initiation as a monotherapy. For moderate to severe depression, pharmacotherapy usually produces a more rapid clinical response and may be particularly indicated as severity increases. In situations of extreme severity, hospitalization as well as electroconvulsive therapy (ECT) may be necessary. For situations where MDD is accompanied by psychotic symptoms, it is essential to use an antipsychotic medication as well as an antidepressant. The presence of significant suicidal ideation or intent automatically makes any episode of depression one of extreme severity and necessitates additional management.

In the situation of mild depression where the patient has an insistence on avoiding medications, in addition to psychotherapy there may be a role for complementary and alternative treatments. Examples would include vigorous exercise for 45 minutes at least three times a week, light therapy, and, although evidence is certainly not as robust, use of certain natural health products such as St. John's wort and omega-3 fatty acids. A number of other complementary and alternative treatments such as yoga and S-adenosyl-L-methionine (SAM-e) have some role as adjunctive treatments to formal evidence-based treatments like cognitive-behavioral therapy (CBT) and antidepressants.

Key psychological treatments that are first line for the acute management of MDD are CBT, interpersonal therapy, and behavioral activation. Most of the evidence for these treatments is for sessions given face-to-face either individually or in a group format, usually for 12–16 sessions provided over approximately 4 months. In addition to face-to-face therapy, CBT in particular has been adopted for use in specific self-help books, Internet sites, and a few smartphone apps, all of which have limited efficacy as stand-alone interventions but are quite useful as an adjunctive to face-to-face therapy or as adjunctive to antidepressants.

Key medication treatments that are first line for the acute management of MDD include all licensed antidepressants. Given that there are more than 40 antidepressants available on the market, there are important nuances involving efficacy, side-effect profile, and safety in overdose to guide which antidepressants should be considered first. From an efficacy perspective, an initial network meta-analysis in 2009 by Cipriani and colleagues identified that four antidepressants were slightly stronger than the rest, specifically escitalopram, mirtazapine, sertraline, and venlafaxine (Cipriani et al. 2009). In that same meta-analysis, escitalopram and sertraline were found to have lower dropout rates and hence were recommended as potential first choices. The same research group has just published (Cipriani et al. 2018) a new meta-analysis examining 21 antidepressants in 522 trials with 116,477 participants. In this study, although 8 of the 21 antidepressants showed evidence of slight superior efficacy, after using dropout rates as a proxy for side-effect burden, 6 antidepressants emerged as having slightly superior efficacy with good tolerability: agomelatine, escitalopram, mirtazapine, paroxetine, sertraline, and vortioxetine. On the basis of research evidence, it would be reasonable to consider initiation of antidepressant treatment with one of the six preceding antidepressants. However, such research evidence would have to be balanced against patient preference based on prior favorable outcome with specific medications, specific side-effect concerns of the individual patient, the physical health of the patient, and drug interaction potential.

Once an antidepressant is initiated, regular monitoring at 1- to 3-week intervals is recommended to evaluate clinical response, monitor suicidality, manage side effects, and ensure treatment adherence. Regular use of a depression scale such as the PHQ-9 can provide a more reliable indication of patient progress. Additional psychoeducation around depression and its treatment is particularly recommended after 4–6 weeks in treatment, as that is another peak time for treatment discontinuation by the patient.

Regardless of the treatment modality, patient improvement at 4 weeks after treatment initiation should be formally assessed. If there has been a less than 25% improvement in symptoms based on a rating scale, a discussion for treatment adjustment should be initiated with the patient. For psychological treatments alone, the individual should be invited to comment on whether he or she feels that any change in frequency of or approach to the psychotherapy could be beneficial. For antidepressant treatments, poor or no response after 4 weeks at a therapeutic dosage is highly predictive of eventual nonresponse. Therefore, poor or no response at 4 weeks should prompt a dosage increase, a change in antidepressants, or the addition of another treatment such as an additional medication or psychotherapy. It also may be a propitious moment to consider a pharmacogenomic assessment to determine whether the poor response may be attributable to the individual's pharmacokinetic (metabolism) phenotype, such as being an ultrarapid metabolizer and requiring higher dosages or being a poor or nonmetabolizer and experiencing adverse events. The results of such a pharmacogenomic assessment (Greden 2018) should be used to seek adjustment to a medication that is congruent with test results.

At the 4-week assessment, if there has been significant improvement, the existing treatment may continue. An adequate trial of an antidepressant would be 8 weeks in duration at a dosage at least in the midtherapeutic dosage range for that particular medication. After 8 weeks of antidepressant monotherapy at appropriate dosages, if response is poor, then it would be strongly recommended to conduct a pharmacogenomic assessment and, depending on results, either change the antidepressant, add an adjunctive medication to the antidepressant, or add psychotherapy if that has not been used. Patient preference, side-effect burden, availability of alternative treatments, and cost of treatment will all factor into the decision about next-step treatment. Numerous studies have attempted to assess whether switching medications or adding medications is superior; data are inadequate to indicate that precision medicine choices can be made; each of these changes may offer similar chances of success. Factors favoring switching antidepressants include the following: it was the first antidepressant trial that had been initiated, the side effects were particularly strong, or the response to the treatment was particularly modest. Alternatively, adjunctive medication should be considered when the initial antidepressant is well tolerated and is showing a greater than 25% response in terms of improvement on a depression rating scale. First-line treatments for adjunctive therapy to an antidepressant in the situation of partial response include low dosages of aripiprazole, quetiapine, or risperidone. Additional adjunctive medication choices that are second line but that may be particularly familiar or well tolerated include brexpiprazole, lamotrigine, lithium, bupropion, and the thyroid hormone T_3. CANMAT treatment guidelines should be consulted for specific details on dosing and sequencing of various medications and psychotherapy.

In addition to psychotherapy and medication, brain stimulation techniques, including ECT and repetitive transcranial magnetic stimulation, have first-line evidence for efficacy in adult MDD. In general, ECT will be reserved for severe depression or for situations of extreme clinical need, such as a highly suicidal patient, a patient with prominent psychotic symptoms, or a medically vulnerable patient with other health concerns, including pregnancy or medical conditions that interfere with use of antidepressant medications. Currently, transcranial magnetic stimulation is recommended only after failure of at least one antidepressant.

The acute phase of depression treatment involves 6–9 months of treatment. Depending on the patient's prior history of depression and other risk factors for recurrence, ongoing treatment recommendations will need to be tailored to the specific patient, with special consideration for prior history of recurrences. In terms of psychological treatments, CBT and mindfulness-based cognitive therapy have strong evidence for relapse prevention during the maintenance phase of depression. Significant evidence also exists for interpersonal therapy, the cognitive-behavioral analysis system of psychotherapy, and behavioral activation in the maintenance treatment for prevention of depression relapse. With respect to antidepressant treatment, once treatment response has been established and maintained for a number of months, maintenance of the same medication at the same dosage is recommended. If the person has had more than two previous major depressive episodes, long-term use of medication is recommended. Furthermore, should there be a prior history of doing well, remaining in remission, then discontinuing medications with a taper and relapsing, patient, clinician, and family would be advised to consider indefinite maintenance treatment to maintain wellness.

Current trial-and-error prescribing of antidepressants for MDD produces limited treatment success. Combinatorial pharmacogenomics may improve outcomes by identifying medications that will be less effective for genetic reasons. The use of pharmacokinetic and pharmacodynamic markers is being evaluated to aid early identification of medications that may not be adequately metabolized or may interact undesirably with other medications. Studies to date are limited by small sample sizes, limited randomization, no blinding, and short durations, but several large, long-term, double-blind, randomized trials now indicate that combinatorial pharmacogenomic testing improves both response and remission rates with statistical significance (Greden 2018).

Prognosis

Although precision-medicine-like pursuits for biomarkers and precision treatments continue, currently, there are no consistent predictors of optimal treatments (Lam et al. 2016b). Large-sample, controlled, long-term studies are sorely needed. The prognosis for MDD is influenced by vulnerability factors (untoward life events and stressful environmental influences) and protective factors (supportive relationships and nurturing environment). The chronicity of the disorder is exemplified in the 85% lifetime recurrence rate and the 1-year remission rate of around 40%. The prognosis is positively influenced by a long-term strategy for medical and psychological management that focuses on the patient as well as his or her family and environment and maximizes the protective factors and minimizes the vulnerabilities.

Persistent Depressive Disorder (Dysthymia)

Dysthymia (literally "bad mood") has long been recognized as a phenomenon in the context of a temperamental predisposition to depression, with overlapping symptoms and a chronicity that weighs heavily on the individual and family. Persistent depressive disorder is defined as a chronic low-grade depression characterized and defined by the presence of a depressed mood for at least 2 years (or 1 year in children and adolescents) and at least two of six designated symptoms of depression that are present most (>50%) of the time and that result in clinically significant distress or impairment. Persistent depressive disorder is not diagnosed in the context of a chronic psychotic disorder or when it is caused by a substance or another medical condition. Although often common, burdensome, and costly, persistent depressive disorder has not been a dedicated focus of research over the years. Much of what is known has been described by Akiskal (2016). Some mood disorder specialists view this diagnosis with suspicion, as possibly reflecting an inadequately or incompletely treated MDD, an underlying undiagnosed medical disorder, or the early, still-mild stages of an MDD.

Unlike the DSM-IV-TR criteria for dysthymic disorder, the DSM-5 criteria for persistent depressive disorder do not require the absence of a major depressive episode during the first 2 years of the mood disturbance or stipulate that criteria for cyclothymic disorder must never have been met. These requirements were dropped in DSM-5 because such information is unlikely to be reliably remembered in sufficient detail to provide clarity.

Phenomenology and Diagnostic Features

The core phenomenological feature of persistent depressive disorder is a long-standing subthreshold depression with vicissitudes of mood and temperament. Symptoms may change daily or weekly. The individual often has a sullen disposition with low energy and drive, preoccupation with guilt and failure, and a tendency to ruminate. Complaints and symptoms tend to outweigh the physical signs. Common subjective symptoms include sadness, diminished concentration or indecisiveness, a pervasive sense of hopelessness, and low self-worth or self-esteem and a generally "unhappy" aura; objective clinical signs include appetite and sleep disturbances (increased or decreased) and notable changes in energy levels. It is important to determine that these are not associated with pharmacological interventions. The illness is chronic, and the individual reports having "always been this way." This sense of chronicity is especially distressing for many. Should an individual alternate between mood states that sometimes reach criteria for major mood disorders, clinical approaches should consider whether periodic nonadherence is a variable or whether mood stabilizers such as lamotrigine might be beneficial. Clinicians should also be cautious about labeling mood fluctuations as "cyclothymic" and should make sure to give adequate consideration to the possibility of bipolar illness, because treatments will be different.

Epidemiology

Major epidemiological studies in the United States estimate that dysthymia has a population prevalence ranging from 1.5% to 3.3% (Vandeleur et al. 2017). The disorder is more commonly diagnosed among women and appears to be more commonly diagnosed among primary care populations. Up to 50% of those with the disorder, however, are undiagnosed and seek medical care for perceived physical reasons.

Differential Diagnosis

The presence of dysthymic or low-grade depressive symptoms should always prompt the clinician to inquire about confounding variables. First, have there been changes in physical health, especially in individuals who are older and have no previous psychiatric history? Many medical disorders may have dysthymic symptoms among the presenting clinical picture. A comprehensive medical examination at initial presentation is indicated before making this diagnosis. Second, have any new medications been introduced, and might they be producing symptoms suggestive of persistent depressive disorder? Benzodiazepines have the potential to be special offenders, notably when used by elderly patients. When prescribed for mild anxiety or sleep disturbances and then used chronically, they may induce the low energy or fatigue, poor concentration, and difficulty making decisions that are criteria for making this diagnosis.

From a psychiatric perspective, the differential diagnosis of persistent depressive disorder includes most major psychiatric illnesses. The first disorder to consider is MDD; the relationship between these two disorders is complex, with the two disorders perhaps being different degrees of severity for the same disorder, perhaps overlapping, with episodes fading in and out of each other and then resulting in the so-called and arguably inappropriate "double depression," which some consider a major depressive episode on top of a dysthymic disorder but others consider a waxing and waning of MDD. A rational diagnostic formulation is based on a medical history and mental status examination that encompass the four perspectives of psychiatric practice, as outlined by McHugh and Slavney (2012; see "Etiological Factors" subsection earlier in chapter), and the diagnostic criteria of DSM-5.

Specifiers for persistent depressive disorder have been formulated to aid the clinician's global view of the patient, allowing the rationale to be advanced that the individual is primarily someone with persistent depressive disorder but with specific clinical (e.g., melancholic, anxious, atypical, psychotic) features that might guide treatment selection or with episodes of MDD interspersed within the persistent depressive disorder. Persistent depressive disorder that begins before age 21 years is arbitrarily referred to as early onset, and illness that begins after age 21 years as late onset. Severity may be specified as mild, moderate, or severe on the basis of clinical impressions but preferably using objective assessment measures (see "Assessment Measures" chapter in DSM-5 Section III).

Management

The care and psychiatric management of a patient with persistent depressive disorder may be challenging because of chronicity and paucity of controlled trials. A meta-analytic review of 16 randomized trials (Cuijpers et al. 2010) concluded that psychotherapy had a small but significant effect but that it was less effective than pharmacotherapy in direct comparisons, especially SSRIs, and that combined pharmacotherapy and psychotherapy treatment was more effective than either alone. This pattern is comparable to that found with MDD. In clinical practice, concomitant anxiety occurs frequently and tends to result in many patients being treated concomitantly with SSRIs and an anxiolytic, usually a benzodiazepine. As already conveyed, the use of combined interventions, although most effective in many studies, makes it difficult to appreciate which are providing the most relief and which may even be a contributor to the perpetuation of some symptoms. Starting with one intervention for an adequate period, monitoring progress, and augmenting if needed with one treatment at a time may aid in determining the intervention or interventions that will be most effective. Symptom severity scales and functional outcome measures are essential for objectively monitoring progress. Should progress be made with the development of biomarkers, this diagnosis predictably—perhaps hopefully—may be absorbed into other categorizations.

Prognosis

Persistent depressive disorder is frequently a chronic illness that persists despite persistent, long-term, or seemingly aggressive treatment. Symptom severity may wax and wane, particularly if there is a reactive component in the temperament of the person with the disorder. The individual may experience long-term variability in symptoms, which can change in a gradual manner over time. Environmental conditions (e.g., bad relationships or enduring stressful emotional conditions) clearly influence clinical course. There is a risk for suicide, with risk variables being comparable to those for MDD and all known suicidal risk factors. Hopelessness often emerges because of the chronic nature of the disorder. Although at first glance the symptoms may appear less severe than those of MDD, their effects on vocational, personal, and social functioning may be devastating at the individual level, resulting in substantive loss of status, relationships, and occupational stability.

Premenstrual Dysphoric Disorder

On the basis of clinical features, PMDD was initially categorized as late luteal phase dysphoric disorder in DSM-III-R (American Psychiatric Association 1987) and was renamed PMDD in DSM-IV (American Psychiatric Association 1994). In several general community and clinical samples of women, PMDD has been shown to be a clinically significant psychiatric disorder with discriminate biological markers and to be amenable to a variety of pharmacological, hormonal, and psychotherapeutic treatments (Epperson et al. 2012). PMDD involves changes specific to the menstrual cycle, which include emotional lability as well as adverse changes in volition, energy, concentration ability, and self-perception. Many women experience headaches, abdominal pain, bloating, and growing discomfort prior to the onset of menstrual periods. Physiological disruptions in sleep and appetite are common (but are not necessary for the diagnosis), as are somatoform discomforts and sensations, including breast tenderness for some. Symptom severity usually peaks immediately prior to the onset of menstruation and then wanes quickly thereafter. Typically, 1 week after the onset of menstruation, there are minimal symptoms. The symptoms must have occurred in most (>50%) menstrual cycles during the past year and must have an adverse effect on work or social functioning.

Phenomenology and Diagnostic Features

PMDD may occur anytime after menarche and often changes as an individual grows older. Differentiation from "premenstrual syndrome" is sometimes perplexing for those who struggle and their families and friends. Such differentiation generally is perceived by patients and clinicians as simply a matter of severity and degree of disruption in work and relationships. It is important to obtain a good assessment, initially by history, of symptoms related to cognitive, emotional, and physical distress associated with functional impairment or avoidance. A clinician may be able to provide a provisional diagnosis of PMDD on the basis of history, but using rating scales of PMDD symptoms in a provisional manner for at least two symptomatic cycles is advised to confirm the diagnosis. The Premenstrual Tension Syndrome Rating Scales (Steiner et al. 2011) capture the clinical features in an objective self-rated manner.

At least one of the essential PMDD phenomenological features—mood lability, irritability, depressed mood, and anxiety (tension or feeling "keyed up")—must be present. Additional symptoms often present are listed in Criterion C; five symptoms from Criteria B and C must have been met for most (>50%) menstrual cycles in the past year. Typically, an anxious tension builds to a crescendo with irritability and apparent interpersonal conflict. Physical symptoms, which include bloating and general joint or soft tissue (including breast) discomfort, magnify daily and create a sense of being overwhelmed. Examples of disturbed functioning in home, work, and social life include conflict or challenges in performing roles.

The critical diagnostic feature is the timing of the onset and dissipation of symptoms surrounding the menstrual cycle. Symptoms and signs wax with the impending menses and wane following the onset of menstruation. The symptoms are minimal or absent in the week following cessation of menses.

Epidemiology

Prevalence

The 12-month prevalence of PMDD is between 1.8% and 5.8% (Gehlert et al. 2009; Wittchen et al. 2002). PMDD is not a culture-bound syndrome and has been observed in women in the United States, India, Europe, and Asia.

Course and Development

Although symptoms of PMDD often emerge in early adulthood, women often do not seek professional treatment until they are older than age 30. Women often try oral birth control pills to modify hormonal variability; modify their diets; seek improvements through exercise routines; change their work, school, or social routines and commitments to align with their menstrual cycles; and let their friends, family, and partners know when to expect mood lability and emotional lability. PMDD symptoms are often mitigated as a result of ovulatory changes, such as during pregnancy and after menopause.

Etiological Factors

The specific etiology for PMDD is not known, but reproductive hormones, genetics, serotonin, and endogenous opiates have been hypothesized as being involved. Proposed causes of PMDD include declining levels of ovarian steroid hormones in the late luteal phase of the menstrual cycle and a hormonal ratio imbalance related to high estrogen levels compared with progesterone levels. Lines of active inquiry include the roles of serotonergic and related transmitters, γ-aminobutyric acid (GABA), and growth factors such as brain-derived neurotrophic factor. Other endocrine equilibria, inflammatory factors, and genetic vulnerabilities may influence the expression of PMDD. Finally, psychological and social factors that destabilize the individual may contribute to the condition. A review of etiological factors provides additional discussion (Matsumoto et al. 2013). Psychological factors may also play an important role for some women regarding feelings of dyscontrol, poor coping, and feelings of anger and depression.

Differential Diagnosis

Colloquially, premenstrual syndrome (PMS) and PMDD are often used as interchangeable terms. PMS conventionally refers to subthreshold PMDD. The majority of menstruating women have symptoms of PMS but are not (by definition) impaired by this condition. Subthreshold criteria should be examined carefully to determine whether the individual has a specific mood, anxiety, or behavioral disorder. Symptoms of MDD and anxiety may become exacerbated during the menstrual period; any psychopathology may become more problematic during menses. If MDD symptoms predominate and are not connected to the menstrual cycle, MDD should be the primary diagnosis. The key determining features of PMDD are the progressive increase in severity of symptoms up to the onset of menses and the rapid waning of symptoms in the week following onset of menses. PMS will exacerbate existing illness, such as MDD; the menstrual period amplifies the experience of mood symptoms, and there is no rapid relief of symptoms within a week of menstruation onset. In PMDD, significant mood swings or changes within this time period is primary and required for diagnosis.

Management

The management of PMDD includes a discussion of environmental and medical interventions. Lifestyle modifications that are encouraged and recommended include reductions in use of caffeine, salt, alcohol, and tobacco. In addition, regular physical activity, relaxation, and psychotherapy are integrated (Zukov et al. 2010).

An impressive pharmacological observation is the rapid response of PMDD to SSRIs. An SSRI antidepressant may be used in the 7–10 days prior to the onset of menses or be taken on a regular basis. The relief of symptoms is usually immediate (within 24 hours). Long-term efficacy has not been adequately documented. Additional considerations include contraception medication, diuretics, nutritional supplements, and pain-relieving medications (Yonkers et al. 2008).

Cognitive-behavioral treatments have been found to benefit PMDD symptoms, especially when cognitive, emotional, or physical changes occur on a predictable basis related to the menses (Yonkers and Simoni 2018). Treating co-occurring psychiatric and other medical conditions may improve the severity of the PMDD symptoms.

Prognosis

Because of the long-term nature of PMDD, it is important to stress a multidisciplinary approach to care (psychiatry, obstetrics-gynecology, endocrinology), lifestyle changes (diet, exercise) that may be necessary, and the need to monitor daily and monthly symptoms over a period of time. Patients who respond to SSRIs may develop their own approach to determining when to start and stop the medication during their menstrual cycles. Systematic evaluation of therapeutic interventions with self-ratings of symptoms and response will guide the clinician and patient to an effective treatment strategy.

Substance/Medication-Induced Depressive Disorder

Substance/medication-induced depressive disorder (SMIDD) remained relatively unchanged from DSM-IV to DSM-5, and traditional consistencies persist. One major, important new consideration for clinicians is the development of an opioid epidemic in the United States. This prospect has become so significant that it requires high vigilance by clinicians (Volkow and Collins 2017). When combined with MDD or bipolar illness, use of opioids is likely to be shown to be a major risk variable for an increasing rate of suicide.

Although the criteria for SMIDD are straightforward, the underlying relationship between the effects of psychotropic substances and depressions is complex, is intertwined, and stems from the long-standing awareness that depressed individuals often use substances and individuals with addiction problems often become depressed. Most traditional substances of abuse can cause depressive disorder symptoms (Criterion A). SMIDD is essentially a clinical assessment that guides the clinician to determine that the MDD likely was caused by the physiological effects of a chemical substance with psychotropic properties. In SMIDD, the symptoms begin following use of a substance capable of inducing depression, as established by clinical (historical) or laboratory evidence of the substance use or dependence. Alternatively, SMIDD may begin in the context of substance withdrawal. Time durations may vary, but close associations, such as weeks or months, between initiation of substance use and onset of depression symptoms make the causal association more likely and the diagnosis more accurate.

A primary condition may exist. For example, a depressed patient who drinks to alleviate symptoms would be clearly excluded on the basis of the criteria. However, an alcohol-dependent person who becomes demoralized and overwhelmed by the effects of drinking may meet criteria for MDD for a significant portion of a 2-week period and might therefore be considered to have SMIDD. If the alcohol-dependent person is successfully withdrawn from alcohol and maintains sobriety for more than 1 month but continues to have signs and symptoms of depression, the diagnosis would be MDD and not SMIDD.

Phenomenology

The phenomenology and diagnostic features of the depression in SMIDD are identical to those of a depressive episode (see DSM-5 diagnostic criteria for MDD), and there are psychological and physical stigmata of substance abuse or dependence.

Epidemiology

A key concept in considering this diagnosis is that co-occurring substance abuse and depression are most often comorbid rather than causal (Blanco et al. 2012). Rates of psychiatric disorder, including depression, are generally high in the population of substance abusers who are seeking treatment. Results from the National Epidemiologic Survey on Alcohol and Related Conditions suggested that the lifetime prevalence of SMIDD is 0.26%–7% (American Psychiatric Association 2013).

Etiological Factors

The etiology of SMIDD must be linked to the taking of a chemical substance or the withdrawal from the same substance, with an ensuing major depressive episode. Depression has been clearly associated with the use of various substances. Examples include interferon or reserpine, which is widely quoted as a cause but is rarely seen clinically; β-blockers, common and typically prescribed to treat high blood pressure; corticosteroids, used to treat inflammatory conditions; benzodiazepine hypnotics, commonly used and often overused; hormone-altering medications, such as estrogen (Premarin); stimulants, such as methylphenidate (Ritalin); and anticholinergic agents, such as those used to treat bowel disorders. Some commonly used medications must also be considered, such as statins for hyperlipidemia and proton pump inhibitors to treat gastroesophageal reflux. Withdrawal from some of the same medication classes also can be causal for some (e.g., chemicals in the stimulant class).

A preliminary principle for the clinician evaluating a depressed patient motivated or known to be using non–medically prescribed substances is to carefully consider the possibility that the depression may be caused by the substance. DSM-5 stipulates that there must be evidence that the substance or its withdrawal is *capable* of producing a depressive disorder.

A potentially confounding issue is that the presence of depressive episodes prior to the use of substances may indicate an independent depressive disorder, with the disorder being exacerbated by the substance use. If the depressed mood remains after 1 month of abstinence, it should be considered independent of the substance.

Other clinically prescribed and common medications that may destabilize mood include steroids, interferon, β-blockers, and cytotoxic agents. A clear temporal association of depression with the initiation of medical therapy is the most informative historical evidence in the etiological link between the agent and the depressive episode. For that reason, interferon has been perceived as an ideal model for the study of SMIDD because of the relatively high frequency, predictable onset, and course of SMIDD in individuals taking the agent.

The recently developing opioid crisis has complex interactions and etiologies, and clinicians who manage patients with chronic pain and depression are critical in early detection, intervention, and prevention. It has long been known (Kroenke and Price 1993) that the more pain and physical symptoms an individual experiences, the more likely there is coexisting depression. It is well established that lengthy opioid use produces a depressive phenotype. The longer the use is and the higher the opioid doses are, the more likely it is that depression may ensue, often accompanied by higher risk for suicide. Habituation and addiction soon follow if use is sustained. Opioid overdoses are surging, increasing by several hundred percent since 2000, with more than 50,000 deaths estimated annually from overdose. Clinicians face obligations to inquire carefully about opiates among all depressed patients with pain, all those who recently have undergone surgical or dental procedures, and those at high risk because of prior substance misuse. Clinicians also face obligations to seek alternatives to opioids for pain alleviation and to limit the size of prescriptions if they are to be used. Such steps may be lifesaving.

Differential Diagnosis

SMIDD is a broad category, and the causal substance driving the depressive episode is less critical than the observation of an association between the substance and the depression. DSM-5 stipulates that the substance must be known to be capable of producing a depressive disorder. Although novel substances of abuse cannot yet be known to be capable of inducing SMIDD, their membership in the class of substances of abuse provides a compelling rationale for the possibility. An empirical test would be a month of abstinence from the suspected substance, and if the depression resolves, it is likely to have been caused by or associated with SMIDD. The depression is considered to be independent of the substance abuse if depression clearly occurred prior to the onset of abuse or continues once abstinence is reliably achieved for at least 1 month. Alternatively, the withdrawal of substances may precipitate a depression; in particular, stimulant substances are notorious for contributing to a depressive crash after a period of heavy use and bingeing. In these situations, the temporal relationship between use (starting and stopping) and the emergence of depression is the key. For some of the longer-acting benzodiazepines, however, the withdrawal syndrome may last beyond this time frame. Finally, as already emphasized, MDD and substance abuse may be comorbid conditions, occurring together, with one exacerbating the other in what often appears to be a self-perpetuating cycle of deteriorating mood and substance abuse. Indeed, that may be the most common situation.

The substance or substances associated with the SMIDD are indicated by coding accordingly. The DSM-5 criteria for SMIDD provide codes for the following: alcohol; phencyclidine; other hallucinogen; inhalant; opioid; sedative, hypnotic, or anxiolytic; cocaine; and other (or unknown) substance.

Management

The care of a patient with clear-cut SMIDD must address the primary clinical problem of the substance abuse as indicated by the severity and nature of the condition and co-morbid features. Debate over the years has centered on whether the depression should be treated concomitantly if a substance is clearly inducing the depression. By DSM-5 definition, depressive episodes will remit with the removal of the substance. However, recent neuroscience developments counteract a simplistic approach. Chronic cocaine use, for example, depletes dopaminergic brain stores, and simple cessation may not lead to disappearance of depressive symptoms. Depending on the nature of symptoms associated with the depression, the causes, and the temporal associations, concomitant treatment of both may be clinically warranted and, when uncertainty prevails, may be the wisest choice. Intensive interventions are clearly indicated when life-threatening conditions, suicidality, or inability to care for self are present.

Individuals taking clinically indicated medications (e.g., interferon, steroids) that are focused on a specific medical treatment and known to cause depression should be monitored closely for emerging depression. As symptoms and signs of depression emerge and the clinician anticipates the need for ongoing treatment, aggressive treatment should be implemented and continued for at least 1 month following discontinuation of the causal substance and longer if indicated by symptom persistence or recurrence.

Prognosis

The prognosis for SMIDD that is due to clinically indicated medications is generally good. Most patients taking interferon or steroids recover from an associated depression once the causal agent is no longer present. The prognosis (and diagnosis) is less clear when the purported causal substance has not been widely associated with SMIDD; for some substances, there may have been case reports in the world literature but no supportive systematic study showing significant effects that is replicated. An example of a medication widely associated with depression is propranolol, a β-blocker. Concerns raised following a letter to the editor in the *American Journal of Psychiatry* (Kalayam and Shamoian 1982) triggered several case reports and established the "link" between propranolol and depression, yet subsequent meta-analyses have not supported this link (Ko et al. 2002). The average psychiatrist, however, is still likely to associate propranolol with depression. Because of their widespread use, β-blocker medications require additional study.

The outcome and prognosis for SMIDD that is related to recreational substance abuse are dependent on a variety of variables: the duration of the abuse; the social, occupational, economic, and marital consequences of long-standing abuse; adherence to treatment interventions; rates of relapse; pending legal threats; and the success of the substance abuse interventions.

Too few studies support clear-cut prognostic determinations. In the 2001–2002 National Epidemiologic Survey on Alcohol and Related Conditions, SMIDD was associated with elevated severity measures and low rates of treatment (Blanco et al. 2012). Successful management of the abuse or addiction is a life-changing experience, and there is every expectation that the SMIDD will remit as well. However, depending on the substance, abuse over a lifetime may result in neurological damage and associated clinical phenomena (e.g., alcoholic dementia) that will adversely affect the prognosis according to the nature and severity of these phenomena.

Depressive Disorder Due to Another Medical Condition

A depressive disorder attributable to another medical condition is generally considered in the context of the medical disorder and its manifestations. The mere presence of chronic or debilitating physical illness is associated with an increased but variable risk of depression. The approach to this category of depression will be influenced by whether the clinician is approaching a patient with known medical disease (cancer, cardiovascular disease, diabetes, or neurological disease) and evaluating whether MDD is present or whether the patient is presenting with depressive symptoms and is in need of a comprehensive medical workup. All patients presenting with a new lifetime onset of depressive symptoms should be evaluated medically for physical illness, and a physical and laboratory assessment should be guided by the patient's primary care physician. For this reason, it behooves health personnel of various disciplines to make every effort to collaborate, work closely, and share data when evaluating and treating such patients.

In individuals with certain medical conditions, clinical symptoms of depression and emotional instability develop in a relatively predictable manner. These conditions include neurological disorders such as Huntington's disease, Parkinson's disease, and stroke. Cancer and rheumatological, endocrine, and inflammatory disorders commonly cause considerable demoralization and depression. Cardiovascular disorders such as myocardial infarction frequently result in significant depressive symptoms following infarction. DSM-5 stipulates that the episode of depression must be the direct physiological effect of another medical condition.

In the patient who has received a diagnosis of MDD in the past, it is unlikely that the current medical condition is the sole direct physiological cause of the depression, and the diagnosis of depressive disorder due to another medical condition would be unwarranted. A new lifetime onset of an episode, however, in the context of a recent cancer or rheumatological, inflammatory, or endocrine disorder can be arguably attributed to the underlying medical condition.

The phenomenology of the depressive episodes is essentially that of classic episodes. Depressions caused by general medical conditions have no distinctive mood features. It is critical to identify and treat these and all depressions, because management of the underlying medical conditions is negatively affected by the presence of depression. The treatment of the depression involves management of the underlying medical disorder as well as the depression. The underlying medical condition, particularly a neurological disorder, may impede and slow the rate of improvement of the depression. Many endocrine disorders (e.g., thyroid, parathyroid, or adrenal disease) must be primarily managed before the psychiatric and mood instability can be adequately addressed.

The prognosis of depression due to another medical condition is related to the prognosis of that other medical condition. Chronic medical conditions will continue to stress the physiology and impede the depression treatment; terminal cancers likewise will compromise medical and psychological systems. Successful management of medical conditions will affect the outcome of depression favorably, especially when the medical disorder and depression are treated concurrently. The role of inflammation is becoming progressively recognized as a potential variable in these comorbid/co-occurring conditions, and many more studies are indicated.

Other Specified or Unspecified Depressive Disorder

The diagnoses of other specified depressive disorder and unspecified depressive disorder are intended to be used for individuals who have symptoms of mood pathology but do not meet diagnostic criteria for a specific depressive disorder. In addition, the other specified or unspecified depressive disorder symptoms may not be attributable to the direct physiological effects of a substance or another medical condition. To avoid overuse of these diagnoses, the clinician should be critical and use these categories only for individuals whose symptoms cause significant distress or impairment that requires clinical care. Frequent reevaluation also is recommended whenever this diagnosis is employed, because temporal changes may clarify the clinical picture.

In DSM-IV-TR, the other specified and unspecified depressive disorders were in the category named "depressive disorder not otherwise specified (NOS)." PMDD was included in this category, but PMDD has been moved into its own disorder category in DSM-5. Likewise, minor depressive disorder (which has a lower threshold than MDD) was a NOS entity in DSM-IV-TR but now falls within the "other specified depressive disorder" DSM-5 category and is termed short-duration depressive episode (4–13 days).

Frequently, individuals with such presentations are evaluated in a busy emergency department or primary care office, where clinicians are pressed for time. These individuals clearly need monitoring for emerging psychopathology, and the symptom measures and assessment schedules in DSM-5 Section III are an excellent approach to beginning the ongoing evaluation process.

Lacking biomarkers and clear neuroscience measures, prior strategies for improving diagnoses, treatments, maintenance of wellness, and prevention for patients with psychiatric illnesses traditionally have relied on deep phenotyping. Current strategies have begun to rely progressively more on simple, inexpensive phenotyping, very large samples, and longitudinal monitoring. This suggests that using the label of "unspecified" should be discouraged.

Conclusion

In 2017, the World Health Organization determined that depressions were the most disabling of all illnesses being monitored (World Health Organization 2017). These illnesses clearly must be important foci for improving health care. Most scientific advances in knowledge are incremental, and such was the case for DSM-5 and the category and subcategories of depressive disorders. For example, the scientific observations of Leibenluft (2011) and others led to a significant shift in our understanding of dysregulated moods in youth and their outcomes, with greater frequency of MDD in early adulthood, and suggested that the clinical diagnostic category disruptive mood dysregulation disorder is *currently best placed* within the depressive disorders. The inclusion of PMDD within depressive disorders recognized the clinical research that emphasizes the dysphoric and depressive nature of the phenomenology that responds to antidepressant medication, especially when aided by other comprehensive interventions. The criteria for MDD itself have changed little from the criteria set forth in DSM-III because the *current understanding* of the disorder remains relatively constant and there has been no compelling scientific evidence to amend the criteria or the category.

The philosophy of DSM-5 was to be adaptive, integrative, and informative—incorporating the science that aids the understanding of psychiatric disease, integrating the understandings into a rational approach to categorizing disorders, and informing the community such that DSM-5 and its derivatives represent the *current clinical currency* for exchanging and mediating ideas. Depressive disorders represent a category that will surely experience dynamic shifts in understanding and organization, rapidly expanding in concert with emerging brain research and evolving editions of the *Diagnostic and Statistical Manual of Mental Disorders.*

Key Clinical Points

- Depressive disorders are a complex class of affective disturbances involving genetic, medical, volitional, stress, emotional, cognitive, brain, and psychological functioning. Assessment includes the dimensions of social, environmental, and biological elements.

- Major depressive disorder (MDD) is a common, treatable, characteristically recurrent and chronic disorder that is often associated with other medical and psychiatric illnesses. Untreated, its episodic course tends to worsen with each episode. MDD is the largest single underlying variable in deaths by suicide.

- Disruptive mood dysregulation disorder (DMDD) is an illness of childhood with irritability and aggressive outbursts outside of the expected range of behavior for the developmental stage. It is associated with development of depressive disorders in later years.

- Premenstrual dysphoric disorder (PMDD) shows many of the features of depression in the 7–10 days prior to menses and dissipates within a week following menstruation onset. This disorder responds quickly to selective serotonin reuptake inhibitors (SSRIs).

- Management of MDD optimally requires the integration of medical, psychological, social, exercise, sleep, and nutritional treatments. Currently, medical management usually begins with an SSRI or a serotonin–norepinephrine reuptake inhibitor, but major efforts are under way to develop biomarkers that will guide selection of precision treatments. Use of pharmacokinetic and pharmacodynamic (combinatorial pharmacogenomic) biomarkers is being evaluated to aid early identification of medications that may not be adequately metabolized or that may interact undesirably with other medications. If the patient lacks a minimal response within 3–5 weeks, the prudent course is to change or augment the current treatment plan aided by such emerging biomarker tools, as well as to reevaluate target diagnoses.

- For MDD and many of the depressive subtypes, combinations of antidepressant and psychotherapy routinely produce the most optimal outcomes. Combination treatment requires close coordination between the clinicians providing each component.

- New treatment interventions, such as glutamatergic (ketamine) administration, are generating an appropriate sense of excitement because of their apparently beneficial effects in individuals with treatment-resistant symptoms or with suicidal ideation. However, well-controlled, standardized research investigations and long-term maintenance strategies for these treatments are sorely needed.

- Comorbid medical and psychiatric disorders should be managed concurrently, rather than treating one disorder and waiting to see whether that leads to clinical improvement in the other.

References

Akiskal HS: Mood disturbances, in The Medical Basis of Psychiatry. Edited by Fatemi SH, Clayton PJ. New York, Springer, 2016, pp 459–475

Althoff RR, Verhulst FC, Rettew DC, et al: Adult outcomes of childhood dysregulation: a 14-year follow-up study. J Am Acad Child Adolesc Psychiatry 49(11):1105–1116, 2010 20970698

Aman MG, Bukstein OG, Gadow KD, et al: What does risperidone add to parent training and stimulant for severe aggression in child attention-deficit/hyperactivity disorder? J Am Acad Child Adolesc Psychiatry 53(1):47–60.e1, 2014 24342385

American Psychiatric Association: Diagnostic and Statistical Manual of Mental Disorders, 3rd Edition. Washington, DC, American Psychiatric Association, 1980

American Psychiatric Association: Diagnostic and Statistical Manual of Mental Disorders, 3rd Edition, Revised. Washington, DC, American Psychiatric Association, 1987

American Psychiatric Association: Diagnostic and Statistical Manual of Mental Disorders, 4th Edition. Washington, DC, American Psychiatric Association, 1994

American Psychiatric Association: Diagnostic and Statistical Manual of Mental Disorders, 4th Edition, Text Revision. Washington, DC, American Psychiatric Association, 2000

American Psychiatric Association: Practice Guideline for the Treatment of Patients With Major Depressive Disorder, 3rd Edition. Washington, DC, American Psychiatric Association, 2010

American Psychiatric Association: Diagnostic and Statistical Manual of Mental Disorders, 5th Edition. Arlington, VA, American Psychiatric Association, 2013

Arnow BA, Blasey C, Williams LM, et al: Depression subtypes in predicting antidepressant response: a report from the iSPOT-D trial. Am J Psychiatry 172(8):743–750, 2015 25815419

Ashrafioun L, Bishop TM, Conner KR, et al: Frequency of prescription opioid misuse and suicidal ideation, planning, and attempts. J Psychiatr Res 92:1–7, 2017 28364579

Blanco C, Alegría AA, Liu SM, et al: Differences among major depressive disorder with and without co-occurring substance use disorders and substance-induced depressive disorder: results from the National Epidemiologic Survey on Alcohol and Related Conditions. J Clin Psychiatry 73(6):865–873, 2012 22480900

Brakowski J, Spinelli S, Dörig N, et al: Resting state brain network function in major depression—depression symptomatology, antidepressant treatment effects, future research. J Psychiatr Res 92:147–159, 2017 28458140

Brotman MA, Schmajuk M, Rich BA, et al: Prevalence, clinical correlates, and longitudinal course of severe mood dysregulation in children. Biol Psychiatry 60(9):991–997, 2006 17056393

Brundin L, Sellgren CM, Lim CK, et al: An enzyme in the kynurenine pathway that governs vulnerability to suicidal behavior by regulating excitotoxicity and neuroinflammation. Transl Psychiatry 6(8):e865, 2016 27483383

Bustamante AC, Aiello AE, Galea S, et al: Glucocorticoid receptor DNA methylation, childhood maltreatment and major depression. J Affect Disord 206:181–188, 2016 27475889

Caine ED: Suicide and attempted suicide in the United States during the 21st century. JAMA Psychiatry 74(11):1087–1088, 2017 28903162

Center for Behavioral Health Statistics and Quality: 2015 National Survey on Drug Use and Health: Methodological summary and definitions. Rockville, MD, Substance Abuse and Mental Health Services Administration, September 2016. Available at: https://www.samhsa.gov/data/sites/default/files/NSDUH-MethodSummDefsHTML-2015/NSDUH-MethodSummDefsHTML-2015/NSDUH-MethodSummDefs-2015.htm. Accessed September 20, 2018.

Cipriani A, Furukawa TA, Salanti G, et al: Comparative efficacy and acceptability of 12 new-generation antidepressants: a multiple-treatments meta-analysis. Lancet 373(9665):746–758, 2009 19185342

Cipriani A, Furukawa TA, Salanti G, et al: Comparative efficacy and acceptability of 21 antidepressant drugs for the acute treatment of adults with major depressive disorder: a systematic review and network meta-analysis. Lancet 391(10128):1357–1366, 2018 29477251

Cleare A, Pariante CM, Young AH, et al: Evidence-based guidelines for treating depressive disorders with antidepressants: a revision of the 2008 British Association for Psychopharmacology guidelines. J Psychopharmacol 29(5):459–525, 2015 25969470

Cochran AL, Schultz A, McInnis MG, et al: A comparison of mathematical models of mood in bipolar disorder, in Computational Neurology and Psychiatry. Edited by Érdi P, Sen Bhattacharya B, Cochran AL. Cham, Switzerland, Springer, 2017, pp 315–341

CONVERGE Consortium: Sparse whole-genome sequencing identifies two loci for major depressive disorder. Nature 523(7562):588–591, 2015 26176920

Copeland WE, Angold A, Costello EJ, et al: Prevalence, comorbidity, and correlates of DSM-5 proposed disruptive mood dysregulation disorder. Am J Psychiatry 170(2):173–179, 2013 23377638

Cuijpers P, van Straten A, Schuurmans J, et al: Psychotherapy for chronic major depression and dysthymia: a meta-analysis. Clin Psychol Rev 30(1):51–62, 2010 19781837

Drysdale AT, Grosenick L, Downar J, et al: Resting-state connectivity biomarkers define neurophysiological subtypes of depression. Nat Med 23(1):28–38, 2017 27918562

Epperson CN, Steiner M, Hartlage SA, et al: Premenstrual dysphoric disorder: evidence for a new category for DSM-5. Am J Psychiatry 169(5):465–475, 2012 22764360

Fabbri C, Hosak L, Mössner R, et al: Consensus paper of the WFSBP Task Force on Genetics: genetics, epigenetics and gene expression markers of major depressive disorder and antidepressant response. World J Biol Psychiatry 18(1):5–28, 2017 27603714

Fonseka TM, MacQueen GM, Kennedy SH: Neuroimaging biomarkers as predictors of treatment outcome in major depressive disorder. J Affect Disord 233:21–35, 2018 29150145

Forte A, Baldessarini RJ, Tondo L, et al: Long-term morbidity in bipolar-I, bipolar-II, and unipolar major depressive disorders. J Affect Disord 178:71–78, 2015 25797049

Fried EI, Nesse RM: Depression is not a consistent syndrome: an investigation of unique symptom patterns in the STAR*D study. J Affect Disord 172:96–102, 2015 25451401

Gadad BS, Jha MK, Czysz A, et al: Peripheral biomarkers of major depression and antidepressant treatment response: current knowledge and future outlooks. J Affect Disord 233:3–14, 2018 28709695

Gartlehner G, Gaynes BN, Amick HR, et al: Comparative benefits and harms of antidepressant, psychological, complementary, and exercise treatments for major depression: an evidence report for a clinical practice guideline from the American College of Physicians. Ann Intern Med 164(5):331–341, 2016 26857743

Gehlert S, Song IH, Chang CH, et al: The prevalence of premenstrual dysphoric disorder in a randomly selected group of urban and rural women. Psychol Med 39(1):129–136, 2009 18366818

Greden JF: Physical symptoms of depression: unmet needs. J Clin Psychiatry 64 (suppl 7):5–11, 2003 12755646

Greden JF: Combinatorial pharmacogenomics significantly improves response and remission for major depressive disorder: a double-blind, randomized control trial. Abstract presented at the American Psychiatric Association Annual Meeting, New York, NY, May 7, 2018.

Greden JF, Riba MB, McInnis MG: Treatment Resistant Depression: A Roadmap for Effective Care. Washington, DC, American Psychiatric Publishing, 2011

Guffanti G, Gameroff MJ, Warner V, et al: Heritability of major depressive and comorbid anxiety disorders in multi-generational families at high risk for depression. Am J Med Genet B Neuropsychiatr Genet 171(8):1072–1079, 2016 27452917

Hopper L: Autism, schizophrenia, bipolar disorder share molecular traits, study finds. ScienceDaily, February 8, 2018. Available at: http://newsroom.ucla.edu/releases/autism-schizophrenia-bipolar-disorder-share-molecular-traits-study-finds. Accessed April 12, 2018.

Hyde CL, Nagle MW, Tian C, et al: Identification of 15 genetic loci associated with risk of major depression in individuals of European descent. Nat Genet 48(9):1031–1036, 2016 27479909

Hyman SE: A new hope for biological insights into depression. Biol Psychiatry 81(4):280–281, 2017 28089024

Insel TR: Join the disruptors of health science. Nature 551(7678):23–26, 2017 29094713

Jucksch V, Salbach-Andrae H, Lenz K, et al: Severe affective and behavioural dysregulation is associated with significant psychosocial adversity and impairment. J Child Psychol Psychiatry 52(6):686–695, 2011 21039485

Kalayam B, Shamoian CA: Propranolol, psychoneuroendocrine changes, and depression. Am J Psychiatry 139(10):1374–1375, 1982 7125003

Kanai T, Takeuchi H, Furukawa TA, et al: Time to recurrence after recovery from major depressive episodes and its predictors. Psychol Med 33(5):839–845, 2003 12877398

Kennedy SH, Milev R, Giacobbe P, et al: Canadian Network for Mood and Anxiety Treatments (CANMAT) clinical guidelines for the management of major depressive disorder in adults, IV: neurostimulation therapies. J Affect Disord 117 (suppl 1):S44–S53, 2009 19656575

Kennedy SH, Lam RW, McIntyre RS, et al: Canadian Network for Mood and Anxiety Treatments (CANMAT) 2016 clinical guidelines for the management of adults with major depressive disorder, section 3: pharmacological treatments. Can J Psychiatry 61(9):540–560, 2016 27486148

Kessler RC, Zhao S, Blazer DG, Swartz M: Prevalence, correlates, and course of minor depression and major depression in the National Comorbidity Survey. J Affect Disord 45(1–2):19–30, 1997 9268772

Kessler RC, Chiu WT, Demler O, et al: Prevalence, severity, and comorbidity of 12-month DSM-IV disorders in the National Comorbidity Survey Replication. Arch Gen Psychiatry 62(6):617–627, 2005 15939839

Kessler RC, Petukhova M, Sampson NA, et al: Twelve-month and lifetime prevalence and lifetime morbid risk of anxiety and mood disorders in the United States. Int J Methods Psychiatr Res 21(3):169–184, 2012 22865617

Ko DT, Hebert PR, Coffey CS, et al: Beta-blocker therapy and symptoms of depression, fatigue, and sexual dysfunction. JAMA 288(3):351–357, 2002 12117400

Kraus C, Castrén E, Kasper S, et al: Serotonin and neuroplasticity—links between molecular, functional and structural pathophysiology in depression. Neurosci Biobehav Rev 77:317–326, 2017 28342763

Kroenke K, Price RK: Symptoms in the community. Prevalence, classification, and psychiatric comorbidity. Arch Intern Med 153(21):2474–2480, 1993 8215752

Kroenke K, Spitzer RL, Williams JB: The PHQ-9: validity of a brief depression severity measure. J Gen Intern Med 16(9):606–613, 2001 11556941

Kupfer DJ, Frank E, Perel JM, et al: Five-year outcome for maintenance therapies in recurrent depression. Arch Gen Psychiatry 49(10):769–773, 1992 1417428

Lam RW, Kennedy SH, Grigoriadis S, et al; Canadian Network for Mood and Anxiety Treatments (CANMAT): Canadian Network for Mood and Anxiety Treatments (CANMAT) clinical guidelines for the management of major depressive disorder in adults, III: pharmacotherapy. J Affect Disord 117 (suppl 1):S26–S43, 2009 19674794

Lam RW, McIntosh D, Wang J, et al: Canadian Network for Mood and Anxiety Treatments (CANMAT) 2016 clinical guidelines for the management of adults with major depressive disorder, I: disease burden and principles of care. Can J Psychiatry 61(9):510–523, 2016a 27486151

Lam RW, Milev R, Rotzinger S, et al: Discovering biomarkers for antidepressant response: protocol from the Canadian biomarker integration network in depression (CAN-BIND) and clinical characteristics of the first patient cohort. BMC Psychiatry 16:105, 2016b 27084692

Leibenluft E: Severe mood dysregulation, irritability, and the diagnostic boundaries of bipolar disorder in youths. Am J Psychiatry 168(2):129–142, 2011 21123313

Leibenluft E, Cohen P, Gorrindo T, et al: Chronic versus episodic irritability in youth: a community-based, longitudinal study of clinical and diagnostic associations. J Child Adolesc Psychopharmacol 16(4):456–466, 2006 16958570

Lin R, Turecki G: Noncoding RNAs in depression. Adv Exp Med Biol 978:197–210, 2017 28523548

Machado-Vieira R, Gold PW, Luckenbaugh DA, et al: The role of adipokines in the rapid antidepressant effects of ketamine. Mol Psychiatry 22(1):127–133, 2017 27046644

MacQueen GM, Frey BN, Ismail Z, et al: Canadian Network for Mood and Anxiety Treatments (CANMAT) 2016 clinical guidelines for the management of adults with major depressive disorder, section 6: special populations: youth, women, and the elderly. Can J Psychiatry 61(9):588–603, 2016 27486149

Malhi GS, Bassett D, Boyce P, et al: Royal Australian and New Zealand College of Psychiatrists clinical practice guidelines for mood disorders. Aust N Z J Psychiatry 49(12):1087–1206, 2015 26643054

Marshall E, Claes L, Bouman WP, et al: Non-suicidal self-injury and suicidality in trans people: a systematic review of the literature. Int Rev Psychiatry 28(1):58–69, 2016 26329283

Matsumoto T, Asakura H, Hayashi T: Biopsychosocial aspects of premenstrual syndrome and premenstrual dysphoric disorder. Gynecol Endocrinol 29(1):67–73, 2013 22809066

McEwen BS: Integrative medicine: breaking down silos of knowledge and practice an epigenetic approach. Metabolism 69S:S21–S29, 2017 28118933

McHugh PR, Slavney PR: The Perspectives of Psychiatry. Baltimore, MD, Johns Hopkins University Press, 1998

McHugh PR, Slavney PR: Mental illness—comprehensive evaluation or checklist? N Engl J Med 366(20):1853–1855, 2012 22591291

McIntyre RS, Rosenbluth M, Ramasubbu R, et al: Managing medical and psychiatric comorbidity in individuals with major depressive disorder and bipolar disorder. Ann Clin Psychiatry 24(2):163–169, 2012 22563572

Milev RV, Giacobbe P, Kennedy SH, et al: Canadian Network for Mood and Anxiety Treatments (CANMAT) 2016 clinical guidelines for the management of adults with major depressive disorder, section 4: neurostimulation treatments. Can J Psychiatry 61(9):561–575, 2016 27486154

Miller AH, Raison CL: The role of inflammation in depression: from evolutionary imperative to modern treatment target. Nat Rev Immunol 16(1):22–34, 2016 26711676

National Collaborating Centre for Mental Health: Depression: The Treatment and Management of Depression in Adults. London, National Institute for Health and Care Excellence, 2009

National Institute for Health and Care Excellence: Depression in Adults: Treatment and Management Guidelines. London, National Institute for Health and Care Excellence (in press). Available at: www.nice.org.uk/guidance/indevelopment/gid-cgwave0725. Accessed December 17, 2018.

National Institute of Mental Health: Major Depression. Bethesda, MD, U.S. Department of Health and Human Services, 2017. Available at: www.nimh.nih.gov/health/statistics/prevalence/major-depression-among-adults.shtml. Accessed December 17, 2018.

Nestler EJ: Epigenetic mechanisms of depression. JAMA Psychiatry 71(4):454–456, 2014 24499927

Otte C, Gold SM, Penninx BW, et al: Major depressive disorder. Nat Rev Dis Primers 2:16065, 2016 27629598

Parikh SV, Segal ZV, Grigoriadis S, et al: Canadian Network for Mood and Anxiety Treatments (CANMAT) clinical guidelines for the management of major depressive disorder in adults, II: psychotherapy alone or in combination with antidepressant medication. J Affect Disord 117 (suppl 1):S15–S25, 2009 19682749

Parikh SV, Quilty LC, Ravitz P, et al: Canadian Network for Mood and Anxiety Treatments (CANMAT) 2016 clinical guidelines for the management of adults with major depressive disorder, II: psychological treatments. Can J Psychiatry 61(9):524–539, 2016 27486150

Posner K, Brown GK, Stanley B, et al: The Columbia-Suicide Severity Rating Scale: initial validity and internal consistency findings from three multisite studies with adolescents and adults. Am J Psychiatry 168(12):1266–1277, 2011 22193671

Power RA, Tansey KE, Buttenschøn HN, et al: Genome-wide association for major depression through age at onset stratification: Major Depressive Disorder Working Group of the Psychiatric Genomics Consortium. Biol Psychiatry 81(4):325–335, 2017 27519822

Qaseem A, Barry MJ, Kansagara D, et al: Nonpharmacologic versus pharmacologic treatment of adult patients with major depressive disorder: a clinical practice guideline from the American College of Physicians. Ann Intern Med 164(5):350–359, 2016 26857948

Ravindran AV, Lam RW, Filteau MJ, et al: Canadian Network for Mood and Anxiety Treatments (CANMAT) clinical guidelines for the management of major depressive disorder in adults, V: complementary and alternative medicine treatments. J Affect Disord 117 (suppl 1):S54–S64, 2009 19666194

Ravindran AV, Balneaves LG, Faulkner G, et al: Canadian Network for Mood and Anxiety Treatments (CANMAT) 2016 clinical guidelines for the management of adults with major depressive disorder, section 5: complementary and alternative medicine treatments. Can J Psychiatry 61(9):576–587, 2016 27486153

Robinson RG, Jorge RE: Post-stroke depression: a review. Am J Psychiatry 173(3):221–231, 2016 26684921

Steiner M, Peer M, Macdougall M, et al: The premenstrual tension syndrome rating scales: an updated version. J Affect Disord 135(1–3):82–88, 2011 21802738

Strawbridge R, Young AH, Cleare AJ: Biomarkers for depression: recent insights, current challenges and future prospects. Neuropsychiatr Dis Treat 13:1245–1262, 2017 28546750

Stringaris A, Cohen P, Pine DS, et al: Adult outcomes of youth irritability: a 20-year prospective community-based study. Am J Psychiatry 166(9):1048–1054, 2009 19570932

Stringaris A, Baroni A, Haimm C, et al: Pediatric bipolar disorder versus severe mood dysregulation: risk for manic episodes on follow-up. J Am Acad Child Adolesc Psychiatry 49(4):397–405, 2010 20410732

Trivedi MH, Rush AJ, Ibrahim HM, et al: The Inventory of Depressive Symptomatology, Clinician Rating (IDS-C) and Self-Report (IDS-SR), and the Quick Inventory of Depressive Symptomatology, Clinician Rating (QIDS-C) and Self-Report (QIDS-SR) in public sector patients with mood disorders: a psychometric evaluation. Psychol Med 34(1):73–82, 2004 14971628

Turecki G, Brent DA: Suicide and suicidal behaviour. Lancet 387(10024):1227–1239, 2016 26385066

Uher R, Payne JL, Pavlova B, et al: Major depressive disorder in DSM-5: implications for clinical practice and research of changes from DSM-IV. Depress Anxiety 31(6):459–471, 2014 24272961

van Loo HM, de Jonge P, Romeijn JW, et al: Data-driven subtypes of major depressive disorder: a systematic review. BMC Med 10:156, 2012 23210727

Vandeleur CL, Fassassi S, Castelao E, et al: Prevalence and correlates of DSM-5 major depressive and related disorders in the community. Psychiatry Res 250:50–58, 2017 28142066

Volkow ND, Collins FS: The role of science in addressing the opioid crisis. N Engl J Med 377(4):391–394, 2017 28564549

Wittchen HU, Becker E, Lieb R, et al: Prevalence, incidence and stability of premenstrual dysphoric disorder in the community. Psychol Med 32(1):119–132, 2002 11883723

Wittenborn AK, Rahmandad H, Rick J, et al: Depression as a systemic syndrome: mapping the feedback loops of major depressive disorder. Psychol Med 46(3):551–562, 2016 26621339

World Health Organization: Depression and Other Common Mental Disorders Global Health Estimates. Geneva, World Health Organization Press, 2017

Yatham LN, Kennedy SH, Parikh SV, et al: Canadian Network for Mood and Anxiety Treatments (CANMAT) and International Society for Bipolar Disorders (ISBD) 2018 guidelines for the management of patients with bipolar disorder. Bipolar Disord 20(2):97–170, 2018 29536616

Yohn CN, Gergues MM, Samuels BA: The role of 5-HT receptors in depression. Mol Brain 10(1):28, 2017 28646910

Yonkers KA, Simoni MK: Premenstrual disorders. Am J Obstet Gynecol 218(1):68–74, 2018 28571724

Yonkers KA, O'Brien PM, Eriksson E: Premenstrual syndrome. Lancet 371(9619):1200–1210, 2008 18395582

Zhang K, Zhu Y, Zhu Y, et al: Molecular, functional, and structural imaging of major depressive disorder. Neurosci Bull 32(3):273–285, 2016 27142698

Zukov I, Ptácek R, Raboch J, et al: Premenstrual dysphoric disorder—review of actual findings about mental disorders related to menstrual cycle and possibilities of their therapy. Prague Med Rep 111(1):12–24, 2010 20359434

Recommended Reading

Styron W: Darkness Visible: A Memoir of Madness. New York, Random House, 1990

Online Resources

American Psychiatric Association: DSM-5 Online Assessment Instruments: www.psychiatry.org/practice/dsm/dsm5/online-assessment-measures

Depression and Bipolar Support Alliance: www.dbsalliance.org

National Institute of Mental Health: Depression: www.nimh.nih.gov/health/topics/depression/index.shtml

National Network of Depression Centers: http://nndc.org

CHAPTER 13

Anxiety Disorders

Murray B. Stein, M.D., M.P.H., F.R.C.P.C.
Jitender Sareen, M.D., F.R.C.P.C.

Fear is a response to external threat. Fear or fearlike behaviors are seen in most mammals and are often used as animal models for anxiety. *Anxiety*, a common human emotion, is an affect; it is an internal state, focused very much on anticipation of danger. It resembles fear but occurs in the absence of an identifiable external threat, or it occurs in response to an internal threatening stimulus. Anxiety that is disabling or that results in extreme distress is considered to be "normal" only when it occurs under tremendous stress and is short-lived. In such instances, a diagnosis of an adjustment disorder (with anxiety) may be appropriate. When anxiety occurs in the absence of substantial stress or when it fails to dissipate when the stressor abates, an anxiety disorder is likely.

Anxiety disorders are commonly encountered in clinical practice. In most studies of primary care settings (e.g., Kroenke et al. 2007), anxiety disorders (10%–15% of patients) are more common than depressive disorders (7%–10% of patients). In a general psychiatric outpatient practice, anxiety disorders will comprise up to 40% of new referrals.

Much of the treatment of anxiety disorders can be successfully carried out by the primary care treatment provider (e.g., family doctor or internist) (Stein and Craske 2017). The psychiatrist usually plays a consultative role or manages the patients who are most difficult to treat.

In this chapter we briefly review the epidemiology of anxiety disorders, risk factors for these disorders, and comorbidity. This review is followed by a detailed discussion of specific anxiety disorders and their treatment.

The authors are grateful to Sarah Marie Raposo and Cara Katz for their assistance in the preparation of an earlier version of this chapter.

Epidemiology

Among mental disorders, anxiety disorders are the most prevalent conditions in any age category (Stein et al. 2017). They are associated with substantial cost to society due to disability and loss of work productivity. Anxiety disorders are also associated with increased risk of suicidal behavior (Thibodeau et al. 2013). Table 13–1 summarizes the prevalence rates, median ages at onset, and gender ratios of anxiety disorders in the U.S. general population (Kessler et al. 2012). Among anxiety disorders, phobias, particularly specific phobia and social anxiety disorder, are the most common conditions, with lifetime prevalence rates greater than 10%. Panic disorder, generalized anxiety disorder (GAD), agoraphobia, and separation anxiety disorder have lifetime prevalence rates between 2% and 7%. Social anxiety disorder and specific phobia have a lower median age at onset than the other anxiety disorders. On the basis of a systematic review of prevalence studies across 44 countries, it is estimated that between 10% and 15% of persons worldwide have an anxiety disorder (Baxter et al. 2013).

Risk Factors

Studies have shown a constellation of risk factors that, for the most part, are common to all of the anxiety disorders (Kessler et al. 2010). Female sex, younger age, single or divorced marital status, low socioeconomic status, poor social supports, and low education are associated with an increased likelihood of anxiety disorders. White individuals are more likely than individuals from ethnic minority groups to have anxiety disorders. Stressful life events and childhood maltreatment (Fonzo et al. 2016) are also strong risk factors for anxiety disorders. Among genetic and family factors, there is increasing evidence for the familial transmission of anxiety disorders through both genetic transmission and modeling (Craske et al. 2017; Eley et al. 2015).

Comorbidity

Anxiety disorders are highly comorbid with other mental disorders, personality disorders, and physical health conditions, with more than 90% of persons with an anxiety disorder having lifetime comorbidity with one or more of these disorders (El-Gabalawy et al. 2013). Comorbidity of anxiety disorders with other conditions often leads to poorer outcomes and affects treatment. The most common comorbidity is the presence of another anxiety disorder. Mood and substance use (including nicotine and alcohol) disorders also commonly co-occur with anxiety disorders. Because anxiety disorders often precede the onset of mood disorders and substance use, early interventions to treat anxiety disorders may prevent mood and substance use disorders. Anxiety disorders are also commonly comorbid with personality disorders, such as borderline, antisocial, and avoidant personality disorders (El-Gabalawy et al. 2013).

Physical health conditions are also common among patients with anxiety disorders (Craske and Stein 2016). Among the comorbid physical health conditions, the most prevalent are cardiovascular disease (Tully et al. 2016), respiratory illness (e.g.,

TABLE 13–1. Approximate lifetime and 12-month prevalence, gender ratio, and median age at onset for anxiety disorders in the U.S. general population

Disorder	Lifetime prevalence (%)	12-month prevalence (%)	Gender ratio, female:male	Median age at onset (years)
Panic disorder[a]	3.8	2.4	1.8:1	23
Agoraphobia[b]	2.5	1.7	1.8:1	18
Social anxiety disorder	10.7	7.4	1.4:1	15
Generalized anxiety disorder	4.3	2.0	1.8:1	30
Specific phobia	15.6	12.1	1.5:1	15
Separation anxiety disorder	6.7	1.2	1.6:1	16

[a]Regardless of presence or absence of agoraphobia.
[b]Regardless of presence or absence of panic disorder.
Source. Adapted from Kessler et al. 2012.

asthma), arthritis, and migraines. The onset of a serious physical illness might trigger the onset of an anxiety disorder, or conversely, anxiety and avoidance might lead to physical health problems.

Specific Anxiety Disorders

Separation Anxiety Disorder

Case Example

A 21-year-old single woman comes to her psychiatric appointment accompanied by her mother. The young woman has never had a driver's license, and she states that her mother drives her everywhere. She has come in because of recurrent physical complaints (including abdominal pain and headaches) that have baffled her primary care physician and so far defied diagnosis. Diagnostic interview reveals a long-standing history of dependence on the parents, which has worsened since the father's death by cancer several years prior. Childhood history is noteworthy for a lifelong history of fear and discomfort when separated from her parents. She never attended day camp or sleepaway camp as a child, and the parents never traveled without their daughter. Elementary school was marked by numerous absences due to a combination of physical complaints and outright school refusal.

Beginning with DSM-III (American Psychiatric Association 1980), separation anxiety disorder was included as a diagnosis in the chapter "Disorders Usually First Diagnosed in Infancy, Childhood, or Adolescence." In DSM-5 (American Psychiatric Association 2013), the decision was made to move some disorders with typical childhood onset into the respective adult chapters; hence the move of separation anxiety disorder into the "Anxiety Disorders" chapter. Interestingly, it was possible to diagnose separation anxiety in adults even prior to DSM-5—nothing in the criteria prohibited it—but its placement in the "Disorders Usually First Diagnosed in Infancy, Childhood, or Adolescence" chapter may have left the impression that the disorder was a "childhood-only" disorder. The new diagnostic criteria implicitly permit the diagnosis of separation anxiety disorder to be made even if the onset is in adulthood, which apparently is the case in a substantial minority (~40%) of individuals with the disorder (Silove et al. 2015).

Separation anxiety disorder should be diagnosed when there is evidence of developmentally inappropriate and excessive anxiety occurring on separation (or threat of separation) from significant attachment figures (Table 13–2). In children, this extreme anxiety is usually manifested by excessive crying, tantrums, physical complaints, and other manifestations of fear and avoidance of separation. Young children may have difficulty expressing the reason for their discomfort, but older children can usually explain their fearfulness that something bad will happen to these significant figures—typically the parents—if they are separated. In adults, the concerns about separation from significant others and the worry about harm befalling them are usually much more readily expressed, although the pattern of behavior can be so long-standing and ingrained, extending longitudinally since childhood, that both the patient and the significant other may rationalize the behaviors. Separation anxiety disorder is the appropriate diagnosis in many cases of "school phobia"; the other common explanatory diagnosis is social anxiety disorder.

Diagnosis and Clinical Evaluation

Prior to DSM-5, the diagnosis of separation anxiety disorder was not widely considered in the differential diagnosis of anxiety in adults, and therefore it is difficult to determine what kinds of diagnostic dilemmas might arise. Agoraphobia is a likely source of diagnostic confusion, because both separation anxiety and agoraphobia may include pervasive situational anxiety and avoidance, and both may be associated with excessive dependence and concerns about inability to function in certain situations if left alone. What differentiates them is the content of the cognitions, with separation anxiety disorder patients emphasizing the separation worries. Panic disorder will also enter the differential diagnosis, and in fact, patients with separation anxiety may have panic attacks when faced with an unwanted separation from a significant attachment figure. What distinguishes panic disorder from separation anxiety disorder is the unexpected nature of the panic attacks. Symptomatic overlap with GAD, wherein individuals have multiple worries that often involve the health and welfare of significant others, is expected to be substantial, but in separation anxiety, the worries should be limited to separation from significant others and the feared consequences thereof.

Etiology

Very little is known about the etiology of separation anxiety disorder (Strawn and Dobson 2017). It is believed to share a genetic basis, through traits such as neuroticism, with many of the other anxiety disorders. Genetic links with panic disorder are believed to be especially strong (Roberson-Nay et al. 2012).

Selective Mutism

Case Example

A 6-year-old boy is brought to the mental health clinic by his mother. He has been referred by his pediatrician because he will not speak in situations outside of the home.

TABLE 13–2.	Essential features of DSM-5 separation anxiety disorder

Anxiety is focused on separation from key attachment figures (usually parent[s], although the figure may be a significant other in the case of adults).

Patient may express concerns that when separated, the attachment figure(s) may leave the patient or get hurt or die.

Somatic symptoms (e.g., headaches, stomachaches) are frequently observed.

Note. For the complete diagnostic criteria, please refer to pp. 190–191 in DSM-5 (American Psychiatric Association 2013).

> Extensive speech and hearing assessment and psychoeducational testing prior to referral have failed to indicate any evidence of a communication or other developmental disorder. The boy performs above grade level on tests of comprehension and, according to parental report, language expression. Yet he had entered first grade 3 months prior to the referral and had not spoken to any teacher or teacher's aide or, as far as anyone could tell, any of the other children in the class. On evaluation by the psychiatrist, the boy smiles appropriately when greeted but looks downward or at his mother during most of the assessment. He occasionally nods or shakes his head in response to questions that require yes or no answers but sometimes does not respond at all. When pressed (gently) to respond verbally, he eventually whimpers and begins to cry, at which point the interview is terminated by the examiner. The mother indicates that her son speaks well—and frequently—when at home but that no one has ever witnessed him speaking to anyone other than her or his father. The boy does have play dates with other children his age, and he plays board games, participates in some sports (swimming), and enjoys watching television. He recently started passing short written notes to teachers and other children in his class in lieu of speaking.

Selective mutism was present in DSM-IV (American Psychiatric Association 1994) and its precursors (where it was referred to as "elective mutism") but resided in the "Disorders Usually First Diagnosed in Infancy, Childhood, or Adolescence" chapter. In DSM-5 the decision was made to move some disorders with typical childhood onset into the respective adult chapters, and after some deliberation about where to put selective mutism, it was decided that it belonged in the "Anxiety Disorders" chapter even though it had not previously been classified as an anxiety disorder.

Selective mutism is characterized by the failure of the individual (almost invariably a child) to speak in nearly all social situations, despite apparently normal language development and abilities, as evidenced by speech with familiar people (typically the parents) (Table 13–3). Onset is in early childhood; however, precise age-at-onset data are not available, nor are good epidemiological data on the prevalence of selective mutism (although it is considered to be relatively uncommon, affecting approximately 1 in 1,000 children according to some estimates) (Muris and Ollendick 2015).

Diagnosis and Clinical Evaluation

For children with selective mutism, the failure to speak is not limited to the presence of adults or other unfamiliar people; these children do not speak even when with their peers. The failure to speak is also consistent in that it occurs reliably across social situations and across time (Table 13–3). DSM-5 specifically reminds clinicians not to diagnose selective mutism until after the first month of the school year has passed, to ensure that the mutism is not merely a transient phenomenon related to initial dis-

TABLE 13–3.   **Essential features of DSM-5 selective mutism**

A child known to be capable of speaking (because she or he does it at home) fails to speak when in school or in other situations with unfamiliar people.

Child shows clear evidence of understanding and may communicate nonverbally (e.g., head nodding, following instructions, writing notes).

When old enough, most children acknowledge social fears underlying their avoidance.

Note.   For the complete diagnostic criteria, please refer to p. 195 in DSM-5 (American Psychiatric Association 2013).

comfort with starting school. Selective mutism is commonly diagnosed either in kindergarten or in first grade, and parents may be surprised by reports from the teacher that their child, who speaks well and often at home, has not said a word to anyone. The mutism must also be seen (usually in the eyes of the parents and/or teachers) to interfere with either academic or social aspects of school or other activities.

DSM-5 notes that the disorder should not be diagnosed if the failure to speak is due to a lack of knowledge of or comfort with the spoken language required in the social situation. Application of this criterion in clinical practice can require a nuanced interpretation of the criteria: Compared with other immigrants from that culture, is the failure to speak clearly aberrant? If so, a diagnosis of selective mutism could be applied. A similar rule of thumb may be applied to selective mutism in bilingual families.

Children with selective mutism may not be entirely mute in situations where they would be expected to speak. Sometimes a child with selective mutism will have one peer with whom speech is engaged, although often in a whisper or another shorthand form of verbal communication. The passing of notes (or, increasingly, electronic texts) is common among slightly older children who are able to write or text.

An area of difficulty in differential diagnosis pertains to the criterion that the mutism not be better accounted for by a communication disorder or a neurodevelopmental disorder. Whereas extreme stuttering, for example, would contraindicate the application of a selective mutism diagnosis, studies show that children with selective mutism are, as a group, more likely than children without selective mutism to have various language and speech problems. In such instances, the diagnosis of selective mutism may be applied, but attention to potentially remediable communication or other neurodevelopmental disorders should not be neglected in treatment planning.

Most children with selective mutism are socially anxious and, in fact, meet diagnostic criteria for social anxiety disorder, a finding that should not confound diagnosis but rather be a frequently expected comorbid finding. Some experts believe that most cases of selective mutism can be considered an early-onset severe subtype of social anxiety disorder, but further research is needed to test this hypothesis.

Etiology

Little is known about the etiology of selective mutism. As noted, the vast majority of children with selective mutism also meet criteria for a social anxiety disorder diagnosis, suggesting a possible shared etiology. A single yet-to-be-replicated study found an association between selective mutism and variation in the gene *CNTNAP2* (Stein et al. 2011); however, the implications of this finding are as yet unknown.

Specific Phobia

Case Example

A 25-year-old woman presents with a fear of needles. She describes repeated avoidance of medically recommended blood tests because of the fear of fainting. She understands that her fear is "irrational," but she is unable to overcome it. She has avoided getting blood tests recommended by her doctor, and she has had dental procedures without anesthetics because of her fear of needles. She reports a 10-year history of this fear. At age 15 years, she received an immunization in school and fainted as soon as she got up after getting the shot. She would like to start a family, and her doctor has recommended that she get some psychological help for her fears.

A key feature of specific phobia is that the fear or anxiety is limited to the phobic stimulus, which is a specific situation or object. DSM-5 has codes for specifying the various types of situations or objects that may be involved: animal, natural environment, blood-injection-injury, situational, and other (Table 13–4).

To differentiate specific phobias from normal fears that are very common in the general population, specific phobias must be persistent (although this characteristic, of course, depends on the opportunity for exposure to the situation or object), the fear or anxiety must be intense or severe (sometimes taking the form of a panic attack), and the individual must either be routinely taking steps to actively avoid the situation or object or be intensely distressed in its presence. As is the case for all phobias, the fear and/or avoidance in specific phobias must be disproportionate to the actual danger posed by the situation or object (Craske and Stein 2016).

Diagnosis and Clinical Evaluation

Specific phobias are most common in childhood, although they are also surprisingly prevalent among older adults. It is common for individuals with specific phobia, especially children, to have multiple specific phobias. Whereas individuals with situational, natural environment, and animal-specific phobias are likely to describe a typical fear response with autonomic hyperarousal (heart racing, tremor, shortness of breath) in the presence or the anticipation of the phobic stimulus, individuals with blood-injection-injury specific phobia often experience a vasovagal fainting or near-fainting response; this is one of those rare instances where patients with anxiety disorders can actually pass out rather than just worry about passing out. On first occurrence, a thorough neurological and cardiac evaluation is recommended to rule out another explanation for the loss of consciousness.

Differentiating specific phobia from agoraphobia can also be challenging. When the symptoms involve the typical agoraphobic cluster with concerns about being incapacitated in the situation, that diagnosis should be applied. Public speaking anxiety is another area where confusion with specific phobia can occur. By definition, public speaking anxiety is considered to be a form of social anxiety disorder, and in fact, it is mentioned as a specific example of the "performance only" specifier in DSM-5. What unites public speaking anxiety, which otherwise would fit the criteria for specific phobia, with social anxiety disorder is the content of the cognitions: people with public speaking anxiety, like other people with social anxiety, are uncomfortable and/or avoid situations involving scrutiny by others, fearing that they will do or say some-

TABLE 13–4.   **Essential features of DSM-5 specific phobia**

The individual has a focal fear related to a situation or object, such as heights, particular animals, insects, or blood.

The individual may have panic attacks when exposed to the feared situation or object.

Specific phobias are common in children; most outgrow them.

When fears are multifocal, agoraphobia should be considered in the differential diagnosis.

Public speaking fears are considered in the domain of social anxiety disorder (social phobia) rather than specific phobia.

Note.   For the complete diagnostic criteria, please refer to pp. 197–198 in DSM-5 (American Psychiatric Association 2013).

thing to embarrass themselves, look stupid, or otherwise be negatively evaluated, all core concerns in social anxiety disorder.

Etiology

Some specific phobias develop after a traumatic event (e.g., being bitten by a dog), but most patients with specific phobia do not recall any experiential precursor (e.g., most individuals with a snake phobia have never been bitten by a snake, and most with a flying phobia have never been in a plane crash). Temperamental characteristics that are risk factors for specific phobia, such as neuroticism or behavioral inhibition, are shared with other anxiety disorders (Craske et al. 2017). Although much is known about the brain circuitry and genes involved in fear (Craske et al. 2017), little is known about the specific function of these biological systems in specific phobia.

Social Anxiety Disorder

Case Example

A 36-year-old man was referred to a psychiatrist by his primary care physician after antidepressant treatment with sertraline up to 100 mg/day had failed to improve his depression. The patient reported having had depressive symptoms on and off since adolescence but had never sought treatment previously. The current episode was precipitated by a job layoff and the subsequent protracted search for a new job, which was ongoing. In addition to a history consistent with current major depressive disorder without suicidal ideation, the patient reported a history of past alcohol dependence and a recent increase in alcohol use. He also reported, on systematic questioning, having a lifelong history of discomfort in social situations, marked by fear of saying something foolish or being judged as stupid. He further reported that he had been having tremendous difficulty making phone calls as part of his job search and that he had been avoiding setting up job interviews and other networking appointments.

Social anxiety disorder, also known as social phobia, is characterized by a marked fear of social and performance situations that often results in avoidance. The concern in such situations is that the individual will say or do something that will result in embarrassment or humiliation. The core fear in social anxiety disorder is fear of negative evaluation, that is, the belief that when in situations where evaluation is possible, the individual will not measure up and will be judged negatively.

The median time of onset is in the late teens, but there are really two modes of onset of social anxiety disorder: onset in the teenage years and onset very early in life. Social anxiety disorder is frequently comorbid with major depressive disorder (MDD) and, in fact, seems to be an antecedent risk factor for its onset among young adults. The course of social anxiety disorder is typically continuous and lifelong. Despite the extent of suffering and impairment associated with social anxiety disorder, few individuals with the disorder seek treatment, and then only after decades of suffering.

DSM-5 uses the term *social anxiety disorder* as the preferred diagnostic moniker (rather than *social phobia*) to emphasize that the illness is, for the majority of patients, more than just a circumscribed phobia. In DSM-IV, the disorder name began with *social phobia* but emphasized the existence of a substantial subgroup of patients with pervasive social fears and avoidance, which was termed "generalized" social phobia. Framers of the DSM-5 criteria elected to delete the "generalized" subtype, instead noting the existence of a newly defined "performance only" specifier (Table 13–5). The effect of this change is (implicitly, if not explicitly) to acknowledge that many patients with social anxiety disorder have extensive social fears spanning multiple social situations that are *not* limited to performance situations and to identify a subtype ("performance only") in which the fears are much more circumscribed in this regard.

Diagnosis and Clinical Evaluation

Social anxiety disorder is not especially difficult to diagnose in a clinical context once an index of suspicion is high enough and appropriate queries are made. A patient who reports fear and avoidance of social situations because of concerns about embarrassment or humiliation and who experiences functional impairment and/or considerable distress in relation to these concerns almost certainly meets diagnostic criteria and may well benefit from treatment. Still, there are several areas in which the differential diagnosis can be somewhat more challenging.

Shyness (i.e., social reticence) spans a range from normative to extreme and is not in and of itself an indicator of psychopathology. Many persons with social anxiety disorder do consider themselves to be shy, and many report that their condition evolved from a background of childhood shyness. When shyness causes extreme distress or is associated with functional disability, then it is likely that appropriate questioning will lead to a diagnosis of social anxiety disorder.

Panic attacks are not unique to panic disorder; they can and do occur in individuals with social anxiety disorder when facing situations in which they feel scrutinized, or even when anticipating such situations. Directly asking about the cognitions the individual experiences during or in anticipation of the anxiety symptoms (e.g., "What were you thinking about when you felt anxious and uncomfortable?") is essential in differential diagnosis. Patients with social anxiety disorder attribute their anxiety symptoms to the evaluative situation, whereas patients with panic disorder experience their anxiety symptoms as unexpected or inexplicable.

Social anxiety disorder is frequently comorbid with MDD but should not be diagnosed separately if social avoidance is confined to depressive episodes. Social fears and discomfort are often part of the schizophrenia syndrome and at times, especially in the prodromal stages, can be difficult to distinguish from social anxiety disorder, but other evidence of psychotic symptoms will eventually surface. Eating disorders or obsessive-compulsive disorder may be associated with social evaluative anxiety

TABLE 13–5.   **Essential features of DSM-5 social anxiety disorder (social phobia)**

The individual has intense fear or anxiety about social situations involving possible scrutiny by others.

Anxiety and worry may occur well in advance, in anticipation of social situations, and the individual often avoids such situations.

Cognitions pertain to fears that the individual will do or say things to embarrass him- or herself or look foolish.

Individuals whose fears are restricted to public speaking and other formal performance situations would qualify for the "performance only" specifier.

Note.   For the complete diagnostic criteria, please refer to pp. 202–203 in DSM-5 (American Psychiatric Association 2013).

(e.g., persons are concerned that others will observe and judge them on the basis of their abnormal eating or checking behaviors), but a diagnosis of social anxiety disorder should be made only if independent social anxiety symptoms occur in situations unrelated to eating or compulsive behaviors, respectively.

Body dysmorphic disorder, which in DSM-5 is classified with the obsessive-compulsive and related disorders, is interesting in that it commonly involves concerns about how the individual will be judged by others. In the case of body dysmorphic disorder, however, the concern is that others will negatively evaluate perceived defects or flaws in the individual's physical appearance, whereas in social anxiety disorder the concern is that others will negatively evaluate the individual's internal self (e.g., personality, intelligence). Not surprisingly, there is considerable comorbidity between social anxiety disorder and body dysmorphic disorder.

Avoidant personality disorder will be diagnosable as a comorbid disorder in many patients with social anxiety disorder, particularly those with diagnoses that do *not* include the "performance only" specifier (i.e., diagnoses that would have been considered "generalized" in DSM-IV). Therefore, avoidant personality disorder would not be considered an alternative diagnosis but rather an additional diagnosis that may represent a marker of increased social anxiety disorder severity.

Etiology

The etiology of social anxiety disorder is not well understood, but an increasing understanding of the disorder as being multifactorially influenced by a variety of biopsychosocial risk factors is emerging. Social anxiety disorder shares with the other anxiety disorders the common risk factors of childhood maltreatment and familial risk. Studies of children who are behaviorally inhibited, meaning that they are hesitant to interact with and approach strangers in a variety of laboratory-based experimental paradigms, are at increased risk of developing social anxiety disorder by adolescence (Craske et al. 2017). Observational laboratory studies suggest that parent-to-child transmission of social fears and avoidance can occur as a result of parental modeling, although interactions with innate temperament also are in evidence. Twin studies comparing risk of social anxiety disorder in monozygotic versus dizygotic twin pairs demonstrate modest heritability, as do more recent heritability estimates of social anxiety as a trait from genome-wide association studies (Stein et al. 2017). Genetic studies are still in their infancy, with no well-replicated genes yet identified (Stein et al. 2017).

Social anxiety disorder seems to involve abnormal response in anxiety circuitry (involving the amygdala and insular cortex), findings that are shared with several other anxiety and trauma-related disorders. There is also some evidence from positron emission tomography studies that social anxiety disorder may involve pathology in the brain's serotonergic systems (Stein and Andrews 2015). Adults with social anxiety disorder demonstrate a variety of attentional, interpretative, and other cognitive biases (Craske et al. 2017), the origins of which are poorly understood.

Panic Disorder

Case Example

A 35-year-old woman was referred to a psychiatrist for assessment of anxiety and avoidance. At the assessment she described an incident 2 years prior to the referral when she woke up one night with chest pains and thought that she was having a heart attack. Accompanying symptoms were shortness of breath, racing heart, sweating, and dizziness. Her family took her to the emergency department, where she received a thorough medical workup. There was no evidence of any cardiac problems. After that day, she stopped driving because of the fear of having chest pains. She was unable to attend her children's sports events, go on buses, or go to church because of her fear. Although the patient was unable to define a specific stressor prior to the onset, a number of stressful life events had occurred before the incident 2 years earlier when she woke up with chest pains; these events included the death of a close friend from cancer and the loss of her husband's job. There was no prior history of emotional problems. There was a past history of asthma. When the patient was 12 years old, her father had died suddenly of a heart attack.

Although panic disorder as a diagnostic entity emerged only in 1980 with the publication of DSM-III, accounts of a clinically similar syndrome appeared much earlier (e.g., soldier's heart, neurocirculatory asthenia) (Wheeler et al. 1950). Along with paroxysmal autonomic nervous system arousal and catastrophic cognitions, these descriptions highlighted symptoms of profound fatigue, which are not part of current diagnostic criteria (although patients with panic disorder often report extreme fatigue after experiencing an attack). The military contexts in which these syndromes developed suggested a prominent association with stress and trauma, indicating a possible area of etiological overlap with posttraumatic stress disorder (PTSD), another disorder that often features panic attacks.

Diagnosis and Clinical Evaluation

Descriptions of panic disorder have changed only slightly between DSM-III and DSM-5, with the essential elements of the syndrome remaining unchanged. The DSM-5 diagnosis of panic disorder (Table 13–6) requires the presence of recurrent panic attacks along with either 1) worry about the possibility of future attacks or 2) development of phobic avoidance—staying away from places or situations the individual fears may elicit a panic attack or where escape or obtaining help in the event of an attack would be unlikely or difficult (e.g., driving on a bridge or sitting in a crowded movie theater)—or other change in behavior due to the attacks (e.g., frequent visits to the doctor because of concerns about undiagnosed medical illness). Panic attacks are sudden, sometimes unexpected episodes of severe anxiety (although they may become more context specific and less unexpected over time), accompanied by an array of physical (e.g., cardiorespiratory, otoneurological, gastrointestinal, and/or auto-

TABLE 13–6.	Essential features of DSM-5 panic disorder

The individual experiences recurrent unexpected panic attacks.

In response to the threat of these attacks, the individual exhibits changes in behavior (usually avoidance, which, if extensive enough, may warrant an additional diagnosis of agoraphobia) and/or excessive worry about the attacks and their implications.

Attacks may become less unexpected with time, but if they have always been predictably associated with certain situations or stimuli, other diagnoses, such as specific phobia, social anxiety disorder, or posttraumatic stress disorder, should be considered.

Note. For the complete diagnostic criteria, please refer to pp. 208–209 in DSM-5 (American Psychiatric Association 2013).

nomic) symptoms (Table 13–7). These attacks are extremely frightening, particularly because they seem to occur out of the blue and without explanation. The attacks are so aversive that the individual may avoid places or situations where prior attacks occurred (e.g., a shopping mall or supermarket) or where escape would be difficult (e.g., driving a car on a freeway) or embarrassing (e.g., sitting in a movie) in the event of an attack. At times, the individual may fear that a panic attack is a heart attack and may make recurrent visits to the emergency department seeking medical care. The individual may also become especially focused on his or her own physiology, being alert to changes in heart or respiratory rate that he or she believes—from experience in prior attacks—might herald a panic attack and avoiding activities (e.g., exercise) that might reproduce these feelings.

Over time—ranging from days to months to years—the experience of recurrent panic attacks in multiple situations may lead the individual to curtail many activities in an effort to prevent panic attacks from occurring in such situations. It is this pervasive phobic avoidance—which carries the diagnostic label *agoraphobia* (discussed in more detail later in this chapter)—that often leads to the extensive disability seen with panic disorder. Interestingly, however, the extent of phobic avoidance can vary widely among individuals, and the factors that influence this variation are largely unclear.

Whereas in DSM-IV the co-occurrence of panic disorder and agoraphobia was given a single diagnosis (i.e., panic disorder with agoraphobia), DSM-5 has diagnostically decoupled the two entities (i.e., there are separate diagnoses for panic disorder and for agoraphobia). Although it is to be expected that panic disorder and agoraphobia will frequently co-occur (about two-thirds of the time), the diagnoses were decoupled to draw attention to the fact that it is not unusual for agoraphobia to occur in the absence of a history of panic disorder.

Not all panic attacks, even when recurrent, are indicative of panic disorder. Panic attacks can occur in individuals with specific phobias when exposed to the feared object (common examples are heights, snakes, and spiders) or in individuals with social anxiety disorder when faced with (or in anticipation of) situations where they may be scrutinized. The difference in such situations is that the individual is keenly aware of the source of the fearful sensations, whereas in panic disorder these same types of sensations are experienced as unprovoked, unexplained, and often occurring "out of the blue." Panic attacks can also occur in individuals with PTSD, in whom exposure to reminders of a traumatic event can trigger such attacks and can be especially difficult to discern as such, unless a careful history of prior traumatic experiences is taken.

TABLE 13–7. **Essential features of DSM-5 panic attack specifier**

DSM-5 Note: Symptoms are presented for the purpose of identifying a panic attack; however, panic attack is not a mental disorder and cannot be coded. Panic attacks can occur in the context of any anxiety disorder as well as other mental disorders. When the presence of a panic attack is identified, it should be noted as a specifier (e.g., "posttraumatic stress disorder with panic attacks"). For panic disorder, the presence of panic attack is contained within the criteria for the disorder and panic attack is not used as a specifier. (American Psychiatric Association 2013, p. 214)

The individual experiences a sudden onset of extreme anxiety and associated physical symptoms (including but not limited to palpitations, sweating, dizziness) and cognitive symptoms (including but not limited to fear of dying or fear of losing control or losing one's mind).

Symptoms peak rapidly (usually within a few minutes) but may wax and wane for some time before dissipating.

Note. For the complete diagnostic criteria, please refer to p. 214 in DSM-5 (American Psychiatric Association 2013).

Because panic disorder mimics numerous medical conditions, patients often become high utilizers of health care, including physician visits, procedures, and laboratory tests. The DSM-5 diagnostic entity of illness anxiety disorder, which retains elements of its predecessor, hypochondriasis, in DSM-IV, applies to individuals who are preoccupied with having or acquiring a serious illness. Persons with panic disorder commonly believe that their intense somatic symptoms are indicative of a serious physical illness (e.g., cardiac, neurological). This belief may be particularly strong early in the course of the illness and in situations where these individuals fail to receive good care that includes appropriate diagnosis and education about their condition. In illness anxiety disorder, however, there is the belief that an illness is present *without the experience of strong somatic symptoms.*

Comorbid medical problems—such as mitral valve prolapse, asthma, Meniere's disease, migraine, and sleep apnea—can accentuate panic symptoms or be accentuated by them, but these co-occurring conditions would rarely, if ever, be considered the cause of an individual's panic attacks (Craske and Stein 2016). In contrast, panic attacks (and, when recurrent, panic disorder) can occur as a direct result of common conditions such as hyperthyroidism and caffeine and other stimulant (e.g., cocaine, methamphetamine) use/abuse and, more rarely, with disorders such as pheochromocytoma or complex partial seizures. In most instances, a thorough medical history, physical examination, routine electrocardiogram, thyroid-stimulating hormone blood level, and urine or blood drug screening are sufficient as a first-pass "rule out" for such conditions. Yet, when dictated by the patient's history, additional tests may be indicated (e.g., frequent palpitations indicating the need for a Holter monitor, echocardiogram, and/or cardiology consultation; profound confusion during or after attacks indicating the need for an electroencephalogram and/or neurology consultation). Importantly, although a diagnosis of panic disorder can be considered definitive without needing to rule out every rare medical condition with which it can be confused or comorbid, it is incumbent on the physician to revisit the medical differential diagnosis if the course of illness changes, if symptoms become atypical, or, critically, if the patient does not respond well to standard treatments.

Clinicians should be aware that patients with panic disorder may be at heightened risk of suicide. Panic attacks are now so well recognized in certain medical settings, such as the emergency department, that it is common practice to identify them appropriately as such, provide reassurance, and send the patient home. It is incumbent on clinicians in these settings to inquire about comorbid depression in general, and about suicidal ideation and plans in particular. It is the "anxious depressed" patient who is at especially high risk of suicide, rather than the depressed patient who is melancholic and exhibits psychomotor retardation, and patients with panic disorder should not be overlooked in this regard.

Without treatment, panic disorder tends to follow a relapsing and remitting course. Only a minority of patients experience symptom remission without subsequent relapse within a few years, although many experience notable improvement (albeit with a waxing and waning course).

Etiology

The etiology of panic disorder is not well understood. Research over the past several decades has continued to inform our understanding of the biological and psychological contributors to the development and maintenance of panic disorder. A substantial body of epidemiological evidence has accumulated on risk factors for panic disorder. As in most psychiatric disorders, a stress–diathesis model is commonly used to explain the genesis and maintenance of panic disorder. Studies have suggested that early-life trauma or maltreatment is an important risk factor, although this risk is not unique to panic disorder, but instead extends to other anxiety and depressive disorders (Craske and Stein 2016) as well as to dissociative disorders and certain personality disorders. Stressful life events likely contribute to the timing of onset as well as the maintenance of the disorder. Studies have also implicated cigarette smoking and nicotine dependence as a risk factor for later onset of panic disorder (reviewed in Craske et al. 2017).

Genetics.   Twin studies suggest that panic and other anxiety disorders are moderately heritable, and although several candidate genes (e.g., a common variant [rs4606] in the catechol-*O*-methyltransferase gene [*COMT*]) have been shown in meta-analyses to be associated with panic disorder, future studies with larger sample sizes and genome-wide approaches are needed to fully appreciate the multiple genes likely contributing to risk for panic disorder and its subtypes (Otowa et al. 2016).

Neurobiology.   Beginning in 1967 with Pitt's observation that hyperosmolar sodium lactate provoked panic attacks in patients with panic disorder but not in control subjects (Pitts and McClure 1967), a series of studies showed that agents with disparate mechanisms of action such as caffeine, isoproterenol, yohimbine, carbon dioxide, and cholecystokinin (CCK) had similar abilities to provoke panic in patients with panic disorder but not in control subjects. The studies of these challenge agents were originally proposed to indicate specific biochemical abnormalities in panic disorder. However, many investigators now agree that most of the effects elicited by these compounds can be explained on the basis of learning theories of panic disorder (see the next section, "Psychology"), which emphasize that patients with panic disorder misinterpret and are frightened by perceived perturbations in their physiological state.

In other words, patients' *beliefs* about their physiological state, rather than their physiology per se, seem to be at fault in patients with panic disorder.

Alterations in the functioning of fear circuitry are generally posited across many of the anxiety disorders, with dysfunction in the amygdala and its connections believed to play an important etiological role in the pathophysiology of an array of fear-based disorders, including panic disorder, social phobia, and PTSD (Etkin and Wager 2007; Figure 13–1). Functional neuroimaging data suggest that a particular brain structure, the insula, is involved in the intense awareness of somatic sensations experienced by patients with panic disorder and related disorders (Paulus and Stein 2010). The emergence of these data heralds much closer ties between psychological and biological theories of panic disorder in the years to come.

Psychology. Psychodynamic theories of panic disorder, which tend to emphasize underlying issues with anger and conflict, continue to hold some sway but have been relatively little studied empirically (Busch and Milrod 2009). Learning theory postulates that factors that increase the salience of bodily sensations are central to the onset and maintenance of panic disorder. One such factor is *anxiety sensitivity*, the belief that anxiety-related sensations are harmful. Individuals who score high on anxiety sensitivity are at increased risk of experiencing panic attacks and of developing panic disorder.

Heightened anxiety sensitivity is probably multifactorial, with studies suggesting that it may be acquired from recurrent aversive direct experiences (e.g., childhood maltreatment, physical illness such as asthma), vicarious observations (e.g., significant illnesses or deaths among family members), or parental reinforcement or modeling of distressed reactions to bodily sensations. These factors may contribute to a heightened state of *interoceptive attention* (attention to internal sensations) that primes the individual to experience panic attacks and to be intensely frightened by them when they occur. "Fear of fear" develops after the initial panic attacks and is believed to be the result of *interoceptive conditioning* (conditioned fear of internal cues such as pounding heart) and the subsequent misappraisal of these internal cues as indicating something threatening or dangerous (e.g., loss of control; heart attack or stroke).

Figure 13–2 illustrates the cycle of cognitive distortions and behavioral changes seen in panic disorder. It is this theoretical model that underlies the application of cognitive-behavioral therapy (CBT) to this disorder (Meuret et al. 2012).

Agoraphobia

Case Example

A 34-year-old man reports a 5-year history of avoidance of malls and movie theaters. He describes an episode in which he became physically ill, with vomiting and dizziness, at a restaurant. He was quite embarrassed, and since then, he has become anxious in many situations. He avoids crowds, buses, movie theaters, and malls. Because of anxiety, he will go shopping only with a family member present. He cannot attend his son's sports activities because of his anxiety. His wife and his children are quite frustrated with him.

Agoraphobia literally, in Greek, means "fear of the marketplace." Whereas large shopping venues certainly can be among the situations avoided by persons with agoraphobia, Criterion A of the DSM-5 diagnostic criteria for agoraphobia (Table 13–8) refers to marked fear or anxiety regarding two or more of the following five situa-

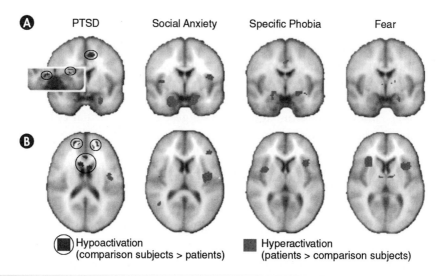

FIGURE 13–1. Clusters in which significant hyperactivation or hypoactivation was found in patients with posttraumatic stress disorder (PTSD), social anxiety disorder, or specific phobia relative to comparison subjects and in healthy subjects undergoing fear conditioning.

Results are shown for (A) amygdalae and (B) insular cortices. Note that within the left amygdala there were two distinct clusters for PTSD, a ventral anterior hyperactivation cluster and a dorsal posterior hypoactivation cluster. The right side of the image corresponds to the right side of the brain.

To view this figure in color, see Plate 5 in Color Gallery in middle of book.

Source. Reprinted from Etkin A, Wager TD: "Functional Neuroimaging of Anxiety: A Meta-analysis of Emotional Processing in PTSD, Social Anxiety Disorder, and Specific Phobia." *American Journal of Psychiatry* 164(10):1476–1488, 2007. Copyright 2007, American Psychiatric Association. Used with permission.

tions: 1) using public transportation, 2) being in open spaces, 3) being in enclosed places, 4) standing in line or being in a crowd, or 5) being outside of the home alone. What ties these types of situations together under the syndrome of agoraphobia is the person's fear of being incapacitated or unable to escape or obtain help in the event that certain symptoms (e.g., dizziness, heart racing, trouble concentrating) occur in these situations. The agoraphobic situations are actively avoided, require the presence of a companion, or are endured with intense fear or anxiety.

As noted earlier in the "Panic Disorder" section, agoraphobia is a common consequence of panic disorder. Yet agoraphobia can also occur without panic disorder, and although this has long been known to be the case, the decision to decouple agoraphobia from panic disorder in DSM-5 reflects, in part, the recognition that this scenario is not uncommon (e.g., the 12-month prevalence of agoraphobia without panic disorder in the National Comorbidity Survey Replication was 0.8% [Kessler et al. 2012]). Furthermore, the presumed causal evolution from panic disorder to agoraphobia—inherent in the DSM-IV conceptualization of the two disorders—has not been upheld.

Agoraphobia can be among the most disabling of the anxiety disorders. It can range in severity from avoidance of driving on busy freeways during rush hour to requiring a companion when venturing outside the home to being completely homebound. Dependence on others (e.g., to chauffeur children, to shop, to travel to and from work) frequently results. The extent of these phobic limitations may fluctuate over time. Whereas agoraphobia can begin at any age, it typically has its onset many

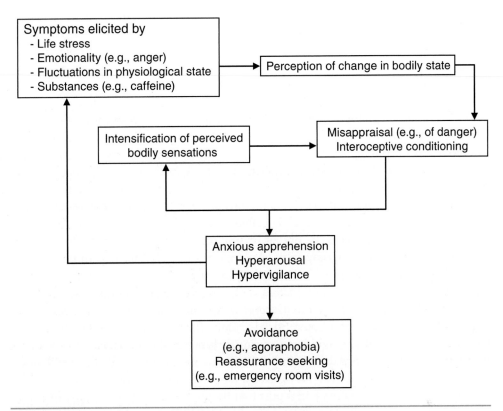

FIGURE 13–2. Cognitive and behavioral factors in panic disorder.

Source. Adapted from Roy-Byrne PP, Craske MG, Stein MB: "Panic Disorder." *Lancet* 368(9540):1023–1032, 2006. Copyright 2006, Elsevier.

TABLE 13–8. **Essential features of DSM-5 agoraphobia**

Fears relate to a characteristic set of situations, such as driving a car, flying in a plane, being in either very large or enclosed places, or being away from home.

Cognitions pertain to being trapped or incapacitated in these situations.

If fears are confined to just one of these situations (e.g., driving a car or going over bridges), then other diagnoses (e.g., specific phobia) should be considered.

Panic attacks are often, but not always, associated with (and may have preceded) the phobic avoidance seen in agoraphobia.

DSM-5 Note: Agoraphobia is diagnosed irrespective of the presence of panic disorder. If an individual's presentation meets criteria for panic disorder and agoraphobia, both diagnoses should be assigned. (American Psychiatric Association 2013, p. 218)

Note. For the complete diagnostic criteria, please refer to pp. 217–218 in DSM-5 (American Psychiatric Association 2013).

---

years later than other phobias and, unlike most other anxiety disorders, can surface in the elderly. In cases involving onset in late adulthood, agoraphobia can often be understood as an anxiety-based complication of physical limitations. For example, an individual who has experienced several episodes of vertigo might develop a fear of driving or walking without assistance, even when the vertiginous bouts subside. When fear and avoidance exceed the actual dangers posed to an individual in performing certain activities, even if the fears have (or had) a basis in genuine physical limitations, a diagnosis of agoraphobia may be applicable.

Diagnosis and Clinical Evaluation

Differentiating agoraphobia from specific phobia is not always easy. Individually, each of the situations within the typical agoraphobic clusters (see Table 13–8) could be considered a specific phobia if it were truly specific (i.e., isolated to that particular situation). What ties these situations together under agoraphobia is the fact that the individual will have *several* fears from these clusters of situations, accompanied by the aforementioned prototypical fears of being incapacitated, unable to escape, or unable to obtain help if symptoms emerge. So-called driving phobia will often, on more systematic questioning, prove to be one of several other transportation-related phobias that reveal a diagnosis of agoraphobia. Another disorder that may be difficult to differentiate from agoraphobia is PTSD, in which an individual may have multiple feared situations from the agoraphobia clusters, including leaving home; however, in PTSD, the fears and avoidance are tied to *memories* of specific traumatic experiences, which are typically absent in agoraphobia. Social anxiety disorder and agoraphobia can both be associated with fear and avoidance of similar types of situations (e.g., crowds), but the nature of the cognitions differs. Individuals with social anxiety disorder will report that they avoid situations because of fear of embarrassment or humiliation, whereas individuals with agoraphobia will report that they avoid situations because of fear of incapacitation or difficulty in escaping should help not be available.

Etiology

The etiology of agoraphobia, particularly as distinct from panic disorder, is not well understood. As already noted, many cases of agoraphobia are considered to be a complication of panic disorder, wherein repeated panic attacks—which are highly aversive—lead to fear and avoidance of situations in which the attacks have occurred or are considered likely to occur. There are also many cases of agoraphobia where no antecedent history of spontaneous panic attacks can be elicited. Although some of these cases may stem from a history of physical illness (e.g., vertigo) or other physical limitations (e.g., postural instability in Parkinson's disease) that serve to render the individuals fearful and concerned about their own ability to function in certain situations, such a history is absent in many—especially younger—individuals with agoraphobia.

Generalized Anxiety Disorder

Case Example

A 34-year-old woman who works as a sous chef at a restaurant is referred to a psychiatrist by her family physician for treatment of depression. When seen, she reports being chronically tense, nervous, and readily upset by a variety of life stressors. She worries that she will lose her job because of her inability to perform to the expected standard of her boss (although he has never expressed to her that he is dissatisfied with her work) and that she will spiral into penury and homelessness. She becomes tearful when describing these fears. On further questioning, she admits to having many worries beyond her work and her finances, including her own health and that of her dog, as well as more general concerns (e.g., about the state of the world economy). She also reports a long history of initial insomnia, describing how she lies in bed and rehashes the day's events and the next day's anticipated tribulations. Although her mood has been worse in the past 3–4 months than it was previously, the nervousness, worries, and insomnia have gone on "for years."

GAD is characterized by nervousness, somatic symptoms of anxiety, and worry. The name of the disorder has drawn criticism for its propensity to be referred to by some practitioners as "general anxiety disorder," leading to the assumption that all forms of anxiety fall under the diagnostic label *generalized anxiety disorder* (Table 13–9). Whereas nervousness, physical symptoms, and focal worries are indeed seen in virtually all of the anxiety disorders, what distinguishes GAD is the multifocal and pervasive nature of the worries. Individuals with GAD have multiple domains of worry, which can include finances, health (their own and that of their loved ones), safety, and many others.

GAD is encountered much more frequently by primary care physicians and other medical practitioners than by psychiatrists (Kroenke et al. 2007), likely because GAD typically occurs with somatic symptoms (e.g., headache, back pain and other muscle aches, gastrointestinal distress) for which patients seek help in the primary care setting. Insomnia is another common complaint in GAD for which patients may seek help in primary care, and it is one of the symptoms that can first lead practitioners to apply a diagnosis of MDD. Whereas initial insomnia is somewhat more typical of GAD and later insomnia with early-morning awakening is more typical of MDD, either type of insomnia can occur with either disorder, and in fact, GAD and MDD themselves very commonly co-occur. GAD has a later modal onset age than the other anxiety disorders and is fairly unique among the anxiety disorders in its relatively higher incidence in late life.

Diagnosis and Clinical Evaluation

The diagnosis of GAD is made when an individual reports characteristic *chronic* symptoms of nervousness, somatic symptoms, and worry that persist for 6 months or longer. Although GAD is not solely a diagnosis of exclusion, it is important to rule out other conditions that may have GAD-like symptoms. Foremost among these is MDD, which is often associated with nervousness, physical symptoms, and ruminative worries (although the worries tend to be more self-blaming in MDD than in GAD). GAD and MDD can co-occur, but both diagnoses should generally be made only when there is fairly clear evidence of independent evolution of symptoms. For example, an individual who has experienced typical GAD symptoms for several years may subsequently develop marked worsening of mood, loss of interest, and thoughts of suicide, a presentation that would warrant the dual diagnoses of GAD and MDD. In contrast, the onset of worry, nervousness, tearfulness, and suicidal ideation in a previously healthy individual would usually be best explained by the single diagnosis of MDD (although the presence of prominent anxiety symptoms might be noted by applying the "with anxious distress" specifier).

GAD may also co-occur with alcohol and other substance use disorders. When the chronology of symptom onset in relation to substance use is unclear, sometimes only a protracted course of abstinence can separate GAD from the effects of the substance use itself. GAD worries can usually be distinguished from obsessive ruminations that are part of obsessive-compulsive disorder by the more ego-dystonic and, at times, unusual concerns seen in the latter disorder. Health worries in GAD may completely

TABLE 13–9.	Essential features of DSM-5 generalized anxiety disorder

Chronic worry is the most characteristic feature.

Worries span multiple domains, such as home, family, and work/school.

Physical symptoms such as headache or gastrointestinal distress are common.

Note. For the complete diagnostic criteria, please refer to p. 222 in DSM-5 (American Psychiatric Association 2013).

overlap with those that can be attributed to illness anxiety disorder, but the latter should be diagnosed only if the concerns are solely health related. If health-related concerns are only one of multiple domains of worry, the diagnosis of GAD should be applied. As in panic disorder, GAD-like symptoms can be caused by certain physical ailments (e.g., hyperthyroidism) and substances (e.g., excessive caffeine use, stimulants); these possibilities should be considered in the differential diagnosis.

Etiology

Twin studies suggest that genetic factors influencing the risk of GAD show substantial overlap with genetic factors influencing the personality trait neuroticism. In addition, the high comorbidity between MDD and GAD is believed to be attributable, at least in part, to similar genetic but different environmental risk factors in the two disorders. No specific genes have been reliably associated with GAD to date, although further study of genes associated with the "worry" dimension of neuroticism (Nagel et al. 2018) may prove fruitful.

There have been relatively few functional neuroimaging studies in GAD, but there is some evidence that failure of anterior cingulate activation and connectivity with the amygdala during implicit regulation of emotional processing may play a role in the etiology of GAD (reviewed in Craske et al. 2017).

Other Anxiety Disorder Categories

Four additional anxiety disorder diagnostic categories are provided in DSM-5.

Substance/medication-induced anxiety disorder is characterized by prominent symptoms of panic or anxiety that are presumed to be due to the effects of a substance (e.g., a drug of abuse, a medication, a toxin) (American Psychiatric Association 2013).

Anxiety disorder due to another medical condition is characterized by clinically significant anxiety that is judged—on the basis of evidence from the history, physical examination, and/or laboratory findings—to be best explained as the direct pathophysiological consequence of another medical condition, such as thyroid disease or temporal lobe epilepsy (American Psychiatric Association 2013).

Finally, the categories other specified anxiety disorder and unspecified anxiety disorder may be applied to presentations in which symptoms characteristic of an anxiety disorder are present and cause clinically significant distress or impairment but do not meet full criteria for any specific anxiety disorder. For an "other specified" diagnosis, the clinician provides the specific reason that full criteria are not met; for an "unspecified" diagnosis, no reason need be given by the clinician.

Treatment of Anxiety Disorders

General Approach

Treatment of anxiety disorders can be extremely rewarding for clinicians because anxiety disorders tend to respond well to psychological and pharmacological treatments. Most patients with anxiety disorders can be well managed in the primary care setting (Rollman et al. 2017; Roy-Byrne et al. 2010; Stein and Craske 2017), with only the more difficult-to-treat cases necessitating care in the mental health specialty setting. Figure 13–3 illustrates a general approach to the treatment and management of anxiety disorders. A careful comprehensive assessment of anxiety symptoms, disability, presence of any comorbid mental and physical conditions, patient preferences for treatment, and access to evidence-based psychotherapies is important. Detailed assessment of the troubling anxiety symptoms, the key catastrophic cognitions, and the avoidance strategies used by the patient is critical to comprehensive treatment planning. Documentation of symptoms through panic diaries, worry diaries, or the use of self-report standardized scales (e.g., Overall Anxiety Severity and Impairment Scale [Campbell-Sills et al. 2009], GAD-7 [Kroenke et al. 2007]) can help both the patient and the therapist to track the course and severity of the anxiety problems, and these rating scales are indispensable aids to treatment.

The presence of current comorbidity with other mental disorders such as mood, substance use, and personality disorders (e.g., borderline) also affects the management of anxiety disorders. If the individual is severely depressed, it is important to prioritize treatment of the depression, usually with a combination of medications and therapy, at the same time as attending to the anxiety symptoms. If bipolar disorder is comorbid with an anxiety disorder, it may affect the type of medications used (e.g., possible need for mood stabilizers) for the treatment of the anxiety disorder. Alcohol and substance use disorders are frequently comorbid with anxiety disorders, and self-medication with alcohol and drugs to reduce tension and anxiety is common among people with anxiety disorders. Understanding the vicious cycle of anxiety symptoms, in which self-medication with alcohol and drugs leads to a rebound of anxiety, is important for both the patient and the clinician. Whereas in the past, recommendations specified that clinicians should insist on abstinence before treating comorbid anxiety and substance use disorders, current thinking favors concurrent treatment of both disorders whenever feasible.

Most patients prefer treatment of anxiety with psychotherapy, either alone or in combination with medications (Roy-Byrne et al. 2010). However, evidence-based psychotherapies administered by therapists well trained and experienced in those psychotherapies may not be readily accessible by all patients in all settings. Thus, medication treatment, which is more often available and covered by insurance, frequently becomes the de facto treatment for anxiety disorders. Even in such circumstances, however, it should be possible to optimize the care of patients receiving pharmacotherapy through use of appropriate educational, motivational, and behavioral information and resources (see the section "Pharmacotherapy" later in this chapter).

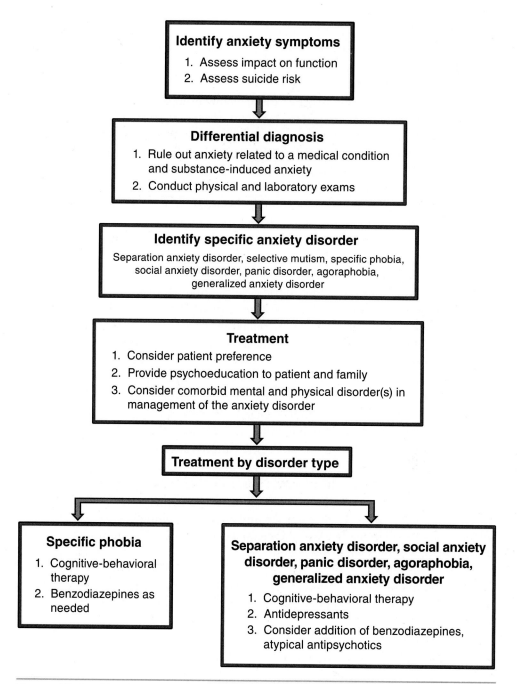

FIGURE 13–3.　Algorithm for the treatment and management of anxiety disorders.

Cognitive-Behavioral Therapy

Among the psychosocial interventions for anxiety disorders, CBT has the most robust evidence for efficacy and can be delivered in a variety of formats (e.g., individual, group, bibliotherapy, telephone based, computerized, Internet). CBT strategies for the various anxiety disorders differ somewhat in their focus and content, but despite this disorder-specific tailoring, they are similar in their underlying principles and approaches (Craske et al. 2011). All CBTs include the following core components: psychoeducation, relaxation training, cognitive restructuring, and exposure therapy.

Psychoeducation involves having the patient read material about the normal and abnormal nature of anxiety that enhances their understanding of the sources and meanings of anxiety. The cognitive model of anxiety disorders proposes that people with these disorders overestimate the danger in a particular situation and underestimate their own capacity to handle the situation. People with anxiety disorders often have catastrophic automatic thoughts in triggering situations. Patients are taught to become aware of these thoughts that precede or co-occur with their anxiety symptoms, and they learn to challenge these thoughts and change them (i.e., cognitive restructuring). The behavioral model of anxiety disorders posits that individuals respond to external and internal cues that elicit a sense of imminent danger. This sense of danger triggers a fight-or-flight response, leading the individual to avoid the triggering situation. Behavioral treatments of anxiety disorders aim to expose the individual to the anxiety-provoking situation and prevent the response of avoidance. Through systematic desensitization, patients gradually but in increasingly more challenging situations face the phobic stimuli that make them feel anxious. Another technique used in CBT is relaxation training through deep-muscle relaxation and/or breathing management.

As an illustration of the use of CBT strategies, consider the case of a woman with panic disorder who avoids malls. The patient would first be taught about the panic model (see Figure 13–3). The therapist would ask the patient to keep a diary of her panic attacks and to record details of each panic attack: where the attack occurred, what symptoms she experienced during the attack, and what she did to manage her anxiety. In treatment sessions, the patient would learn how to identify the "hot" thoughts that increase the anxiety. For example, if her panic attacks in shopping malls begin with chest pains, she might have the anxiety-provoking thought that "I could be having a heart attack." The patient would learn methods to challenge this thinking by looking at evidence for and against the fear that she is having a heart attack. Exposure therapy would also be used with this patient; exposure therapy for panic disorder often involves exercises that recreate the panic symptoms (i.e, interoceptive exposure). The technique most often used to recreate such symptoms is hyperventilation, because this phenomenon is common in panic attacks. When hyperventilation is used as a technique in exposure therapy, the patient and the therapist hyperventilate together for brief periods and the patient is taught that the physiological symptoms will resolve on their own. Next, the patient would be asked to make a hierarchical list of situations that she avoids because of anxiety. Over the course of the therapy, the patient would gradually face these anxiety-provoking situations and learn that her anxiety will resolve if she stays in the situation long enough.

CBT for adult anxiety disorders is efficacious and generally well accepted, and there is growing evidence that Internet-delivered CBT may be as efficacious as face-to-face CBT (Carlbring et al. 2018), particularly when therapist support is available online or by telephone. Internet-delivered CBT is extremely cost-effective, particularly when one considers that a relatively short-term (e.g., 10- to 20-week) investment in patient and therapist time and effort usually results in long-lasting (e.g., months, years, or decades) therapeutic effects. Group CBT for anxiety is also commonly employed, in part to lower costs but also to enable in-group access to in vivo exposure opportunities. There is some evidence that group CBT somewhat dilutes this modality's efficacy, but group CBT nonetheless remains popular for practical reasons. Most patients will accrue some, if not maximal, benefit from group CBT; if there is insufficient improvement, a follow-on course of more focused individual CBT could be considered.

Other Forms of Psychotherapy

Although less established than CBT for anxiety disorders, several other forms of psychotherapy can be considered currently or might be considered in the future if additional research confirms their effectiveness. Psychodynamic psychotherapy, although little studied in randomized controlled trials, may be a reasonable treatment option for patients with panic disorder (Busch and Milrod 2009). So-called third-wave psychotherapies such as acceptance and commitment therapy, mindfulness-based stress reduction, and various other therapies that target emotion regulation need to be further studied but may well be options in the future. Although interventions aimed at remediating particular cognitive (attentional or interpretative) biases in patients with anxiety disorders had showed promise in randomized controlled trials, meta-analyses of these trials have called into question the utility of these interventions (Cristea et al. 2016). It is still too early to wholeheartedly recommend any of these novel (or, in the case of psychodynamic psychotherapy, not new but possibly improved) therapies as a first-line treatment for anxiety disorders; however, this may well change in the coming years. Even though acceptability of and response to CBTs for anxiety disorders are high, there is ample room for new treatments that will meet the needs and preferences of patients who do not respond to standard therapies.

Pharmacotherapy

Pharmacotherapy is a good option for many patients with anxiety disorders, either in combination with CBT or as a stand-alone treatment (Stein and Craske 2017). However, in the latter instance, pharmacotherapy should never be prescribed without also prescribing the reading of educational materials, many of which can be accessed for low cost or no cost through the Internet. Unbiased high-quality information is available from the National Institutes of Health (www.nih.gov), the Anxiety and Depression Association of America (www.adaa.org), and UpToDate (www.uptodate.com; provides free access to medical information in materials written expressly for consumers), among others. Patients with anxiety disorders often come to treatment with the belief that they are alone in their symptoms and suffering (although such isolation is less and less common nowadays, with the advent of widespread access to information via the Internet). Providing patients with informational material that describes their symptoms, discusses at an appropriate level of depth and sophistication the theoretical underpinnings of their disorder(s), and outlines the treatment options available can be the most important therapeutic intervention a clinician makes. In some instances, the increased understanding and reassurance that come from this type of psychoeducation may be enough to curtail certain frightening symptoms (e.g., spontaneous panic attacks) and costly, disabling behaviors (e.g., frequent trips to the emergency department). Although such improvement from psychoeducation is not the norm, and most patients continue to have a need for specific therapeutic interventions, the provision of educational materials at least ensures that when patients seek professional treatment, they will do so as better-informed, more empowered consumers.

Another critical element in the provision of pharmacotherapy to patients with anxiety disorders is the prescription of exposure. Exposure instructions and practice are a critical component of CBT, but they can be readily incorporated into everyday pharmacotherapy of anxiety disorders. Patients should be instructed that whereas their antianxiety medications are intended to reduce their spontaneous and anticipatory anxiety, it is also important that they begin to face situations that have made them fearful in the past in order to learn that these situations can be successfully negotiated. Some patients take this advice and carry out their own exposure practice, whereas others can benefit from more explicit instructions and advice.

Several classes of medications are approved by the U.S. Food and Drug Administration (FDA) and similar regulatory agencies in other nations for use in the treatment of specific anxiety disorders. Although adherence to FDA-approved indications offers confidence that a certain level of evidence exists to support the drug's use for those conditions, any practitioner licensed and authorized to prescribe medications can choose to do so off-label. Given that pharmaceutical companies make decisions about which drugs to submit for the necessary (and costly) clinical trials required to obtain a specific indication based in large part on economics, it is the case that some efficacious antianxiety medications never obtain FDA approval. In such instances, the informed clinician can consider using any marketed medication that has a solid, peer-reviewed published evidence base of efficacy and safety.

The medication classes with the best evidence of efficacy and (when used properly) safety for the anxiety disorders (except for specific phobia, discussed in the "Benzodiazepines" subsection later in this section) are the antidepressants and the benzodiazepine anxiolytics. The antidepressants include selective serotonin reuptake inhibitors (SSRIs), serotonin–norepinephrine reuptake inhibitors (SNRIs), tricyclic antidepressants (TCAs), and monoamine oxidase inhibitors (MAOIs). There is also a role for several nonbenzodiazepine anxiolytics (e.g., buspirone, pregabalin) and possibly the atypical antipsychotics (for refractory anxiety). Although these pharmacotherapeutic agents are discussed in more detail in Chapter 29 in this volume, "Psychopharmacology," an overview of their utility is included here.

Selective Serotonin Reuptake Inhibitors and Serotonin–Norepinephrine Reuptake Inhibitors

Currently, six different SSRIs are available for clinical use in the United States: fluoxetine, sertraline, paroxetine (immediate- and controlled-release formulations), fluvoxamine, citalopram, and escitalopram. Although individual SSRIs have different FDA indications for particular anxiety disorders, clinicians tend to treat all SSRIs as having equal efficacy across the class, and there is no evidence to the contrary. As a class, the SSRIs are considered the first-line pharmacotherapy for each of the anxiety disorders because of their overall levels of efficacy, safety, and tolerability.

Currently, four SNRIs are available for clinical use in the United States: venlafaxine ER (extended-release), desvenlafaxine, duloxetine, and milnacipran. Nearly all research investigating SNRIs for anxiety disorders is based on venlafaxine ER or duloxetine, and either of these can be considered as a first- or second-line treatment for anxiety disorders, although some experts would relegate them to second-line status, given their more limited study in anxiety disorders.

Experts usually recommend an initial trial of an SSRI, beginning with the lowest available dosage, given that patients with anxiety disorders—particularly those with panic disorder, who attend to and fear physiological sensations—tend to be sensitive to medication side effects. The dosage is then increased gradually, in weekly or biweekly increments, until therapeutic dosages are reached. Time course of response is similar to that in MDD—that is, taking 4–6 weeks to see a clinically meaningful response (although this may occur sooner) and as long as 12–16 weeks to achieve an optimal response. There is a misconception that anxiety disorders respond to lower dosages of antidepressants than are needed to treat depression. This is not the case; in fact, average dosages for treating anxiety disorders are as high as—or higher than—those used to treat depression. Of course, it is also the case that many patients presenting with anxiety also have MDD, necessitating that full antidepressant dosages be used. However, clinicians may take an extra week or two to reach those dosages in patients with anxiety disorders, comorbid or otherwise.

There is no evidence that patients with anxiety disorders who fail to respond to an SSRI will respond to an SNRI. Thus, the next step would be either to try a different SSRI or to switch to an SNRI. For patients who experience a partial response to an SSRI or SNRI, adjunctive treatment with a benzodiazepine or other antianxiety agent may be considered. There is insufficient evidence of the utility of some of the newer antidepressants (e.g., vortioxetine, vilazodone) to recommend their use in the treatment of anxiety disorders (Schneier et al. 2017; Stein and Sareen 2015).

Tricyclic Antidepressants and Monoamine Oxidase Inhibitors

TCAs were widely used to treat anxiety disorders prior to the advent of the SSRIs. Because they tend to be less well tolerated than the SSRIs or SNRIs, TCAs are rarely used today for treating anxiety disorders. The same can be said of the MAOIs, whose side-effect profile and requirement for a special diet limit their utility. However, some experts feel that MAOIs may be efficacious for patients whose symptoms do not respond to other treatments and that they may be especially effective in the treatment of social anxiety disorder.

Benzodiazepines

Benzodiazepines are among the best-tolerated of the antianxiety agents and are highly efficacious. They have broad-spectrum efficacy across the anxiety disorders, including specific phobia. Benzodiazepines can be used as first-line agents for treating anxiety but may be best utilized as adjuncts or alternatives to ineffective antidepressant therapy (e.g., Pollack et al. 2014). Nonetheless, benzodiazepines also have some abuse liability and thus need to be prescribed with caution and probably not at all (or only with great care and a high level of supervision) to patients with a prior history of alcohol or any other substance abuse.

Benzodiazepines are the best-established pharmacotherapy for treating anxiety that is predictable and limited to particular situations (e.g., specific phobia such as flying phobia; social phobia such as public speaking or other performance anxiety), for which they can be prescribed on an as-needed basis. Prescription of benzodiazepines on an as-needed basis for unpredictable anxiety (e.g., panic disorder) is not recommended, because it is impossible for patients to anticipate when they will need to use them. Apart from as-needed use for occasionally recurring, predictable specific phobias, benzodiazepines should generally be prescribed for anxiety on a regular schedule—that is, anywhere from one to four times daily, depending on the pharmacokinetics of the particular benzodiazepine.

Nonbenzodiazepine Anxiolytics

Buspirone is a nonbenzodiazepine anxiolytic with efficacy limited to the treatment of GAD (Stein and Sareen 2015). Gabapentin and pregabalin have somewhat limited evidence for efficacy in treating anxiety disorders, although they are sometimes used as an alternative to benzodiazepines, often as an adjunct to antidepressants.

Atypical Antipsychotics

There is some (at present very limited) evidence that atypical antipsychotics (e.g., quetiapine, risperidone) may be efficacious as monotherapy or as an adjunct to antidepressants for treatment-resistant anxiety disorders (Craske and Stein 2016).

Combining Cognitive-Behavioral Therapy and Pharmacotherapy

Although the evidence is limited, several studies suggest that combining CBT and pharmacotherapy for anxiety disorders is superior to using either alone, particularly in children (Wang et al. 2017). Yet the efficacy of either pharmacotherapy or CBT is sufficiently high that clinicians may begin by choosing one or the other, primarily on the basis of patient preference. In patients who fail to respond sufficiently to an adequate therapeutic trial, the other modality can be added later.

Conclusion

Anxiety disorders are highly prevalent, frequently disabling conditions that often begin in childhood and persist into adulthood. They are generally very responsive to pharmacological and/or cognitive-behavioral treatments.

Key Clinical Points

- Anxiety disorders are extremely common.
- Anxiety disorders are frequently comorbid with major depressive disorder, particularly in clinical settings.

- Anxiety disorders are associated with increased risk for suicide; clinicians must therefore not neglect to ask about suicidality in patients assessed for anxiety disorders.

- Antidepressants are the pharmacological treatment of choice for most anxiety disorders. Benzodiazepines play a secondary role, and although they are usually safe and beneficial, their risks must be considered on a case-by-case basis.

- Efficacious cognitive-behavioral therapies (CBTs) exist for each of the anxiety disorders, and there are also some newer forms of CBT that can be used for multiple anxiety disorders.

References

American Psychiatric Association: Diagnostic and Statistical Manual of Mental Disorders, 3rd Edition. Washington, DC, American Psychiatric Association, 1980

American Psychiatric Association: Diagnostic and Statistical Manual of Mental Disorders, 4th Edition. Washington, DC, American Psychiatric Association, 1994

American Psychiatric Association: Diagnostic and Statistical Manual of Mental Disorders, 5th Edition. Arlington, VA, American Psychiatric Association, 2013

Baxter AJ, Scott KM, Vos T, et al: Global prevalence of anxiety disorders: a systematic review and meta-regression. Psychol Med 43(5):897–910, 2013 22781489

Busch FN, Milrod B: Psychodynamic treatment of panic disorder: clinical and research assessment, in Handbook of Evidence-Based Psychodynamic Psychotherapy. Edited by Levy RA, Ablon JS. New York, Humana Press, 2009, pp 29–44

Campbell-Sills L, Norman SB, Craske MG, et al: Validation of a brief measure of anxiety-related severity and impairment: the Overall Anxiety Severity and Impairment Scale (OASIS). J Affect Disord 112(1–3):92–101, 2009 18486238

Carlbring P, Andersson G, Cuijpers P, et al: Internet-based vs. face-to-face cognitive behavior therapy for psychiatric and somatic disorders: an updated systematic review and meta-analysis. Cogn Behav Ther 47(1):1–18, 2018 29215315

Craske MG, Stein MB: Anxiety. Lancet 388(10063):3048–3059, 2016 27349358

Craske MG, Stein MB, Sullivan G, et al: Disorder-specific impact of coordinated anxiety learning and management treatment for anxiety disorders in primary care. Arch Gen Psychiatry 68(4):378–388, 2011 21464362

Craske MG, Stein MB, Eley TC, et al: Anxiety disorders. Nat Rev Dis Primers 3:17024, 2017 28470168

Cristea IA, Kok RN, Cuijpers P: The effectiveness of cognitive bias modification interventions for substance addictions: a meta-analysis. PLoS One 11(9):e0162226, 2016 27611692

El-Gabalawy R, Tsai J, Harpaz-Rotem I, et al: Predominant typologies of psychopathology in the United States: a latent class analysis. J Psychiatr Res 47(11):1649–1657, 2013 23978394

Eley TC, McAdams TA, Rijsdijk FV, et al: The intergenerational transmission of anxiety: a children-of-twins study. Am J Psychiatry 172(7):630–637, 2015 25906669

Etkin A, Wager TD: Functional neuroimaging of anxiety: a meta-analysis of emotional processing in PTSD, social anxiety disorder, and specific phobia. Am J Psychiatry 164(10):1476–1488, 2007 17898336

Fonzo GA, Ramsawh HJ, Flagan TM, et al: Early life stress and the anxious brain: evidence for a neural mechanism linking childhood emotional maltreatment to anxiety in adulthood. Psychol Med 46(5):1037–1054, 2016 26670947

Kessler RC, Ruscio AM, Shear K, et al: Epidemiology of anxiety disorders. Curr Top Behav Neurosci 2:21–35, 2010 21309104

Kessler RC, Petukhova M, Sampson NA, et al: Twelve-month and lifetime prevalence and lifetime morbid risk of anxiety and mood disorders in the United States. Int J Methods Psychiatr Res 21(3):169–184, 2012 22865617

Kroenke K, Spitzer RL, Williams JB, et al: Anxiety disorders in primary care: prevalence, impairment, comorbidity, and detection. Ann Intern Med 146(5):317–325, 2007 17339617

Meuret AE, Wolitzky-Taylor KB, Twohig MP, et al: Coping skills and exposure therapy in panic disorder and agoraphobia: latest advances and future directions. Behav Ther 43(2):271–284, 2012 22440065

Muris P, Ollendick TH: Children who are anxious in silence: a review on selective mutism, the new anxiety disorder in DSM-5. Clin Child Fam Psychol Rev 18(2):151–169, 2015 25724675

Nagel M, Jansen PR, Stringer S, et al: Meta-analysis of genome-wide association studies for neuroticism in 449,484 individuals identifies novel genetic loci and pathways. Nat Genet 50(7):920–927, 2018 29942085

Otowa T, Hek K, Lee M, et al: Meta-analysis of genome-wide association studies of anxiety disorders. Mol Psychiatry 21(10):1391–1399, 2016 [Erratum in: Mol Psychiatry 21(10):1485] 26754954

Paulus MP, Stein MB: Interoception in anxiety and depression. Brain Struct Funct 214(5–6):451–463, 2010 20490545

Pitts FN Jr, McClure JN Jr: Lactate metabolism in anxiety neurosis. N Engl J Med 277(25):1329–1336, 1967 6081131

Pollack MH, Van Ameringen M, Simon NM, et al: A double-blind randomized controlled trial of augmentation and switch strategies for refractory social anxiety disorder. Am J Psychiatry 171(1):44–53, 2014 24399428

Roberson-Nay R, Eaves LJ, Hettema JM, et al: Childhood separation anxiety disorder and adult onset panic attacks share a common genetic diathesis. Depress Anxiety 29(4):320–327, 2012 22461084

Rollman BL, Belnap BH, Mazumdar S, et al: Telephone-delivered stepped collaborative care for treating anxiety in primary care: a randomized controlled trial. J Gen Intern Med 32(3):245–255, 2017 27714649

Roy-Byrne P, Craske MG, Sullivan G, et al: Delivery of evidence-based treatment for multiple anxiety disorders in primary care: a randomized controlled trial. JAMA 303(19):1921–1928, 2010 20483968

Schneier FR, Moskow DM, Choo TH, et al: A randomized controlled pilot trial of vilazodone for adult separation anxiety disorder. Depress Anxiety 34(12):1085–1095, 2017 29071764

Silove D, Alonso J, Bromet E, et al: Pediatric-onset and adult-onset separation anxiety disorder across countries in the World Mental Health Survey. Am J Psychiatry 172(7):647–656, 2015 26046337

Stein MB, Andrews AM: Serotonin states and social anxiety. JAMA Psychiatry 72(8):845–847, 2015 26083085

Stein MB, Craske MG: Treating anxiety in 2017: optimizing care to improve outcomes. JAMA 318(3):235–236, 2017 28679009

Stein MB, Sareen J: CLINICAL PRACTICE. Generalized anxiety disorder. N Engl J Med 373(21):2059–2068, 2015 26580998

Stein MB, Yang BZ, Chavira DA, et al: A common genetic variant in the neurexin superfamily member CNTNAP2 is associated with increased risk for selective mutism and social anxiety-related traits. Biol Psychiatry 69(9):825–831, 2011 21193173

Stein MB, Chen CY, Jain S, et al: Genetic risk variants for social anxiety. Am J Med Genet B Neuropsychiatr Genet 174(4):470–482, 2017 28512750

Strawn JR, Dobson ET: Individuation for a DSM-5 disorder: adult separation anxiety. Depress Anxiety 34(12):1082–1084, 2017 29211944

Thibodeau MA, Welch PG, Sareen J, et al: Anxiety disorders are independently associated with suicide ideation and attempts: propensity score matching in two epidemiological samples. Depress Anxiety 30(10):947–954, 2013 24108489

Tully PJ, Harrison NJ, Cheung P, et al: Anxiety and cardiovascular disease risk: a review. Curr Cardiol Rep 18(12):120, 2016 27796859

Wang Z, Whiteside SPH, Sim L, et al: Comparative effectiveness and safety of cognitive behavioral therapy and pharmacotherapy for childhood anxiety disorders: a systematic review and meta-analysis. JAMA Pediatr 171(11):1049–1056, 2017 28859190

Wheeler EO, White PD, Reed EW, Cohen ME: Neurocirculatory asthenia, anxiety neurosis, effort syndrome, neurasthenia: a 20 year follow-up study of 173 patients. JAMA 142(12):878–889, 1950 15410387

Recommended Readings

Craske MG, Stein MB: Anxiety. Lancet 388:3048–3059, 2016
Craske MG, Stein MB, Eley TC, et al: Anxiety disorders. Nat Rev Dis Primers 3:17024, 2017
Stein MB, Craske MG: Treating anxiety in 2017: optimizing care to improve outcomes. JAMA 318(3):235–236, 2017

Online Resources

Anxiety and Depression Association of America: https://adaa.org/
National Institute of Mental Health: www.nimh.nih.gov/index.shtml
UpToDate: www.uptodate.com/home (available by individual or institutional subscription to providers; grants free access to medical information in materials written expressly for consumers)

CHAPTER 14

Obsessive-Compulsive and Related Disorders

Darin D. Dougherty, M.D., M.M.Sc.

Sabine Wilhelm, Ph.D.

Michael A. Jenike, M.D.

In DSM-IV (American Psychiatric Association 1994) and DSM-IV-TR (American Psychiatric Association 2000), obsessive-compulsive disorder (OCD) was characterized as an anxiety disorder. In DSM-5 (American Psychiatric Association 2013), OCD was moved to a new chapter, titled "Obsessive-Compulsive and Related Disorders," together with associated disorders that were previously classified in other chapters (e.g., Somatoform Disorders; Impulse-Control Disorders Not Elsewhere Classified). Additionally, new disorders were added to the "Obsessive-Compulsive and Related Disorders" chapter, which now includes OCD, body dysmorphic disorder, hoarding disorder, trichotillomania (hair-pulling disorder), excoriation (skin-picking) disorder, substance/medication-induced obsessive-compulsive and related disorder, and obsessive-compulsive and related disorder due to another medical condition. The goal of this chapter is to review the "Obsessive-Compulsive and Related Disorders" chapter of DSM-5 and each of the disorders contained within this categorization.

Obsessive-Compulsive Disorder

Diagnosis

As its name suggests, OCD is characterized by the presence of obsessions and/or compulsions. *Obsessions* are unwanted, repetitive thoughts that usually involve themes of harm and danger. Early work in the field of OCD suggested that common obsession content included fear of contamination, pathological doubt, violent and/or sexual intrusive thoughts, symmetry concerns, and religious scrupulosity (Table 14–1). In con-

TABLE 14–1.   Frequency of common obsessions and compulsions in a clinic sample of 560 patients with obsessive-compulsive disorder

Obsessions	%	Compulsions	%
Contamination	50	Checking	61
Pathological doubt	42	Washing	50
Somatic	33	Counting	36
Need for symmetry	32	Need to ask or confess	34
Aggressive	31	Symmetry and precision	28
Sexual	24	Hoarding	18
Multiple obsessions	72	Multiple compulsions	58

Source.   Adapted from Rasmussen SA, Eisen JL: "Clinical and Epidemiologic Findings of Significance to Neuropharmacologic Trials of OCD." *Psychopharmacology Bulletin* 24:466–470, 1988.

trast, *compulsions* have been recognized as the repetitive behaviors that the sufferer performs in response to the distress associated with the content of the obsessions. Common compulsive behaviors have been noted to include excessive cleaning (e.g., hand washing), checking, ordering, rearranging, counting, repeating, and mental rituals (see Table 14–1). DSM-5 requires that individuals meet criteria either for obsessive thoughts or for compulsive behaviors (Criterion A) in order to receive a diagnosis of OCD. However, most patients with OCD have both obsessions and compulsions. In order to meet criteria for an OCD diagnosis, the obsessions or compulsions must be time-consuming (e.g., take more than 1 hour per day) or cause clinically significant distress or impairment in social, occupational, or other important areas of functioning (Criterion B). Additionally, the OCD symptoms cannot be attributable to the physiological effects of a substance or another medical condition (Criterion C) and may not be better explained by the symptoms of another DSM disorder (Criterion D). DSM-5 includes specifiers as to insight (good or fair, poor, or absent/delusional beliefs) and as to whether the OCD is tic related (i.e., whether the individual has a lifetime history of a chronic tic disorder).

Differential Diagnosis

The diagnosis of OCD is determined by the presence of obsessions and/or compulsions. Although this may seem straightforward, the differential diagnosis includes the ruminations of depression, the delusions of psychosis, anxiety symptoms associated with other anxiety disorders, and severe obsessive-compulsive personality disorder (OCPD). OCPD is defined as a rigid, perfectionistic personality type. A general rule of thumb is that whereas the behavioral patterns of OCPD tend to be experienced as ego-syntonic, the obsessions and compulsions of OCD are experienced as ego-dystonic. Despite the similarity of their names, OCPD is clearly a separate disorder from OCD and does not respond to the treatments used for OCD.

Psychiatric comorbidity is common in OCD; the Epidemiologic Catchment Area (ECA) study found that two-thirds of patients with OCD met criteria for at least one other psychiatric illness during their lifetime (Karno et al. 1988). The most common comorbid psychiatric diagnosis is major depressive disorder. Approximately one-third of individuals with OCD are currently experiencing a major depressive episode, and two-thirds will experience a major depressive episode during their lifetime. Other psychiatric illnesses commonly comorbid with OCD are anxiety disorders, eating disorders, and substance use disorders.

Clinical Course

The average age at onset of OCD is 21 years, with average onset age varying by gender (19 years for men, 22 years for women; Rasmussen and Eisen 1992). However, earlier onset is not rare; 21% of patients experience symptoms before puberty. Although onset may occur during other periods of life, late-onset OCD is relatively rare; thus, OCD-like symptoms appearing for the first time in an older individual may warrant a medical workup for a possible neurological cause.

    The clinical course of OCD is typically lifelong, with waxing and waning symptomatology. A minority of patients with OCD may experience a phasic or episodic course with periods of complete or partial remission. Women are at particular risk of symptom exacerbation or new-onset symptoms during pregnancy and the postpartum period. One study found that 57% of women experiencing postpartum depression also experienced obsessional thoughts (Wisner et al. 1999).

Epidemiology

Although OCD was once considered a rare disorder, data from a large sample of U.S. households in the ECA study suggested a lifetime prevalence of OCD of between 1.9% and 3.3% (Goodman 1999). Epidemiological studies from other countries throughout the world have generally found comparable lifetime prevalence rates of OCD. The disability associated with OCD is severe enough that the World Health Organization has listed OCD among the 10 medical illnesses most likely to cause disability (Murray and Lopez 1996).

Etiology

Psychodynamic Theory

Freud (1973) postulated that obsessions were defensive reactions to unconscious impulses, especially sexual and aggressive impulses. Obsessions served as a way to mask these impulses and/or control them. Unfortunately, although psychodynamic therapy may help to reveal the origins of obsessions, there is little evidence that doing so changes OCD symptoms.

Genetics

A review of twin studies found that there is a strong heritable component to OCD, including concordance rates of between 80% and 87% in monozygotic twins and between 47% and 50% in dizygotic twins (van Grootheest et al. 2005). OCD also tends to run in families, with a recent study of 1,209 first-degree relatives of OCD probands finding an increased risk of OCD among relatives of probands (8.2%) compared with control subjects (2.0%) (Hettema et al. 2001). Candidate gene studies have found a number of genes that may be associated with OCD, including many associated with serotonin, dopamine, and glutamate (Pauls et al. 2014). Larger-scale studies are needed to confirm these initial findings.

Neuroanatomy

While a thorough review of all that has been learned from neuroimaging studies is beyond the scope of this chapter, a general description of the neurocircuitry involved in the pathophysiology of OCD is presented. Parallel cortico-striato-thalamo-cortical (CSTC) circuits in the brain each subserve different functions ranging from oculomotor movement to cognition and affective functions. One of these CSTC circuits, termed the *ventral cognitive loop,* includes the orbitofrontal cortex, the caudate nucleus, and the dorsomedial thalamus. Numerous functional neuroimaging studies in OCD have found functional abnormalities in all nodes of this circuit—specifically, these brain regions are hyperactive at rest in patients with OCD compared with healthy volunteers, with the hyperactivity amplified during OCD symptom provocation and attenuated with successful treatment (Dougherty et al. 2010).

Treatment

Cognitive-Behavioral Therapy

A specific type of behavioral therapy, exposure and response prevention (ERP), has been used and refined since the 1960s for the treatment of OCD. As the name suggests, patients are first exposed to stimuli that trigger their specific OCD symptoms. For patients with contamination fears, this may involve touching a doorknob or a faucet handle that they perceive as being contaminated. Patients then prevent themselves from responding to the stimuli as they usually would (e.g., a patient who now feels contaminated will avoid washing his hands after touching the contaminated stimulus). Initially patients experience marked anxiety, and it can take a significant amount of time for the anxiety to decrease. As patients repeat their ERP exercises, both the amplitude of the anxiety and the time required for it to diminish will gradually decrease until patients become habituated to the stimuli.

ERP is a highly effective treatment for OCD and is considered to be the first-line intervention for the disorder. While many clinical trials of ERP in the treatment of OCD have been published, meta-analytic reviews provide the best general estimate of the response rates associated with ERP. Foa and Kozak (1996), defining "response" as a 30% or greater improvement in OCD symptoms, found that the response rate across more than a dozen studies was 76%–83%. Although pharmacotherapy of OCD is reviewed later in this chapter, it is noteworthy that the few studies that have compared ERP with pharmacotherapy (e.g., Foa et al. 2005) have found that ERP was superior. Additionally, some studies have suggested that combining ERP and pharmacotherapy results in lower relapse rates in patients with OCD when they discontinue pharmacotherapy.

Cognitive therapy (CT) is a form of psychotherapy that seeks to identify and modify maladaptive beliefs (Wilhelm et al. 2009). Meta-analyses of psychotherapies in OCD (Öst et al. 2015; Rosa-Alcázar et al. 2008) found similar effect size estimates for CT and ERP. In clinical practice, cognitive and behavioral treatments are often combined, and a meta-analysis by Öst et al. (2015) found that cognitive-behavioral therapy (CBT) performed well relative to a wait-list condition, placebo, and antidepressant medication.

Pharmacotherapy

The serotonin reuptake inhibitors (SRIs) represent the first-line pharmacotherapy intervention for OCD (Bandelow et al. 2008). The SRIs include all of the selective serotonin reuptake inhibitors (SSRIs) as well as clomipramine. Meta-analyses have generally found that 40%–60% of patients with OCD achieve response (defined as at least a 25%–35% decrease in OCD symptoms) when treated with SRIs (Greist et al. 1995). These meta-analyses, as well as a small number of head-to-head studies, have failed to demonstrate superior efficacy of any SRI over the others. When SRIs are used for treating OCD, it is important that high dosages be used (clomipramine up to 250 mg/day, fluoxetine up to 80 mg/day, paroxetine up to 60 mg/day, fluvoxamine up to 300 mg/day, sertraline up to 200 mg/day, citalopram up to 40 mg/day, and escitalopram up to 30 mg/day), because response rates are higher with high-dosage treatment compared with low-dosage treatment. Additionally, it is important for both the clinician and the patient to realize that response may not be achieved until after 8–12 weeks of treatment.

Other potential monotherapy approaches to the treatment of OCD generally involve other classes of antidepressants that affect the serotonergic system. Although data are much more limited for these classes, there is some support for the use of serotonin–norepinephrine reuptake inhibitors (SNRIs) and, possibly, monoamine oxidase inhibitors (MAOIs) (Dell'Osso et al. 2006). There is no evidence supporting the use of dopaminergic antidepressants (e.g., bupropion) in the treatment of OCD, and there is strong evidence from clinical trials that tricyclic antidepressants (TCAs) other than clomipramine are not effective in the treatment of OCD.

There have long been data supporting the use of dopaminergic antagonists to augment the effects of SRIs in the treatment of OCD. Although initial studies, by necessity, included only conventional antipsychotics, studies since the advent of the atypical antipsychotics also support their use as augmenting agents with the SRIs. Because of the lower extrapyramidal side-effect burden, most clinicians now use the atypical antipsychotics to augment SRIs for the treatment of OCD. However, the gains of lower extrapyramidal side-effect burden with the atypical antipsychotics are somewhat mitigated by the higher rates of metabolic syndrome with the atypical antipsychotics, so clinicians should use these agents with caution and an understanding of the risks and benefits. At this juncture, strong evidence exists only for risperidone and aripiprazole, although other atypical antipsychotics are commonly used as well (Veale et al. 2014b). Dosages are usually in the low to moderate range (e.g., risperidone 1–4 mg/day), and response after augmentation is typically seen within 1–4 weeks.

Another pharmacological approach to treatment of OCD involves agents that affect the glutamatergic system. Studies involving memantine, riluzole, and N-acetylcysteine have been promising (Pittenger et al. 2011), although further research is needed.

Neurosurgical Approaches

Although beyond the scope of this chapter, neurosurgical approaches may be efficacious for patients with intractable OCD that has not improved despite treatment with available conventional therapies. These approaches include ablative limbic system procedures such as anterior cingulotomy, anterior capsulotomy, subcaudate tractotomy, and limbic leucotomy, as well as deep brain stimulation (DBS) with electrodes placed at various brain targets (see also Chapter 30 in this volume, "Brain Stimulation

Therapies"). In 2009, the U.S. Food and Drug Administration (FDA) approved the use of DBS targeted at the ventral capsule/ventral striatum for treatment-refractory OCD (Keen et al. 2017).

Prognosis

Rates of full remission over different time periods (although all are over years, not months) reported in various studies have ranged from 6% to 43%; rates of partial remission reported in these same studies have ranged from 17% to 75% (Eisen et al. 2010). The longest follow-up study ever conducted (mean follow-up period of 47 years) found that almost half (48%) of patients reported clinical recovery (defined as no clinically relevant symptoms for at least 5 years). However, only 20% experienced full remission (i.e., complete absence of symptoms for at least 5 years) (Skoog and Skoog 1999).

Body Dysmorphic Disorder

Diagnosis

According to DSM-5 criteria, body dysmorphic disorder (BDD) is characterized by a preoccupation with one or more perceived defects or flaws in physical appearance that are not observable by or appear very mild to others (Criterion A). For an individual to be diagnosed with BDD, DSM-5 also requires that at some point during the course of the disorder, the individual has performed repetitive behaviors (e.g., mirror checking, excessive grooming, skin picking, reassurance seeking) or mental acts (e.g., comparing one's appearance with that of others) in response to his or her appearance concerns (Criterion B). Although there is no minimum threshold of daily time occupied by the preoccupation required to meet diagnostic criteria for BDD, the preoccupation must cause clinically significant distress or impairment in social, occupational, or other important areas of functioning (Criterion C). Finally, the appearance preoccupations must not be restricted to concerns with body fat or weight in an eating disorder (Criterion D). DSM-5 includes specification as to insight (good or fair, poor, absent/delusional beliefs) and as to presence of muscle dysmorphia (i.e., the belief that one's body build is too small or insufficiently muscular).

The diagnosis of BDD requires the preoccupation with perceived appearance defects as described. Patients believe that they look ugly, unattractive, abnormal, or deformed. The perceived defects can involve any area of the body. Behaviors such as comparing oneself with others and mirror checking are common. Many, if not most, patients with BDD attempt to hide or camouflage their perceived defects using clothing, hair growth, cosmetics, and so forth. Many will seek care from dermatologists and/or cosmetic surgeons. As opposed to the generally good insight seen in patients with OCD, most patients with BDD have poor insight into their illness. They tend to firmly believe that the perceived defect is present and not imagined. BDD patients often suffer from delusions of reference and believe that others are laughing at them or mocking them because of the perceived appearance flaw.

Muscle dysmorphia, a form of BDD appearing almost exclusively in males, consists of preoccupation with the idea that one's body is too small or not muscular enough (Phillips et al. 2010). These individuals actually look normal or even muscular. Most diet, exercise excessively, and lift weights. These individuals are at higher risk for anabolic steroid abuse. BDD by proxy is a form of BDD in which individuals are preoccupied with perceived defects in another person's appearance.

Differential Diagnosis

Perhaps the most important factor to consider in the differential diagnosis of BDD is the possibility of normal appearance concerns or actual clearly noticeable physical defects. Concerns with bodily defects that are clearly noticeable (i.e., not slight) are not diagnosed as BDD. Weight concerns occurring in the context of an eating disorder preclude the diagnosis of BDD. Finally, the feelings of low self-worth associated with major depressive disorder may manifest physically, and delusions associated with psychosis may focus on physical appearance.

Psychiatric comorbidity is common in BDD; major depressive disorder, with a lifetime prevalence of 75%, is the most common comorbid diagnosis. Approximately one-third of patients with BDD experience comorbid OCD during their lifetime, and almost 40% have comorbid social anxiety disorder at some point. Comorbid substance use disorders are also common.

Clinical Course

BDD symptoms typically emerge during early adolescence; the female-to-male gender ratio ranges from 1:1 to 3:2 (Phillips 2011). The course is usually chronic, with waxing and waning symptoms. The clinical features are generally similar for men and women, although some gender differences have been reported (Perugi et al. 1997; Phillips and Diaz 1997; Phillips et al. 2006a).

Epidemiology

The point prevalence of BDD in epidemiological studies ranges from 0.7% to 2%–4% (Phillips 2011). BDD is more common in patients with other psychiatric disorders, with a frequency of 8%–37% in patients with OCD, 11%–13% in patients with social phobia, 26% in patients with trichotillomania, and 39% in patients with anorexia nervosa (Phillips 2011). Individuals with BDD are more likely than individuals without BDD to report suicidal ideation and suicide attempts related to concerns about appearance (Buhlmann et al. 2010; Rief et al. 2006). Finally, as many as 55% of individuals with BDD are unmarried (Koran et al. 2008; Rief et al. 2006), and more than 20% are unemployed (Rief et al. 2006).

Etiology

Although BDD was classified as a somatoform disorder in DSM-IV and DSM-IV-TR, it has long been considered to be an OCD spectrum disorder. There are similarities between OCD and BDD in phenomenology, onset age, gender ratio, and treatment response to SRIs. However, because very few neuroimaging studies have been conducted in subjects with BDD, comparisons between the two disorders are not yet possible. Interestingly, and perhaps unique to the pathophysiology of BDD, functional magnetic resonance imaging studies have demonstrated abnormalities in brain regions associated with visual processing, with individuals with BDD showing a bias for processing details of visual images rather than focusing on the visual image as a whole (Feusner et al. 2010, 2011).

Treatment

Before we review CBT and pharmacotherapy for BDD, it is important to note that whereas many patients with BDD seek surgical and cosmetic treatment for their perceived appearance defects, patients with BDD are rarely satisfied with the results of these treatments. Therefore, surgical and cosmetic treatments should not be encouraged in patients with BDD.

Cognitive-Behavioral Therapy

As is the case with OCD, ERP appears to be a first-line treatment for BDD. For BDD, the exposures and response prevention are tailored to the individual's BDD symptoms. For example, exposures may involve going into social settings with the response prevention being resistance to mirror checking or excessive grooming. CBT for BDD also often involves cognitive restructuring in which inaccurate beliefs are identified and targeted. Unlike the treatment of OCD, BDD treatment often includes mirror retraining to address the distorted perception of appearance characteristic of BDD (Wilhelm et al. 2013). Although there are fewer studies of CBT for BDD than for OCD, existing studies (e.g., Veale et al. 2014a; Wilhelm et al. 2014) strongly support the efficacy of CBT in the treatment of BDD.

Pharmacotherapy

There are no FDA-approved medications for BDD. The SRIs have received the most study for the treatment of BDD, but the number of studies is still relatively small. There have been two controlled trials (one of clomipramine and one of fluoxetine) and four open-label trials (involving fluvoxamine, citalopram, and escitalopram) of SRI treatment in BDD. Intent-to-treat analyses of these data suggest that 63%–83% of patients with BDD will respond to treatment with SRIs (Phillips 2011). As is the case with OCD, higher dosages of the SRIs are generally required, and time until response may be as long as 12–16 weeks. Finally, although antipsychotic augmentation of SRIs is commonly used in clinical practice, only one controlled study of antipsychotic augmentation of SRI treatment for BDD has been reported (Phillips 2005). This trial found that pimozide augmentation was not more effective than placebo.

Prognosis

The largest (N=161) follow-up study of patients with BDD found that over 1 year, the probability of full remission was 9% and the probability of partial remission was 21%, even though 84.2% of participants were receiving mental health treatment during the 1-year period (Phillips et al. 2006b). However, 4-year remission rates as high as 60% have been reported following treatment with pharmacotherapy and/or psychotherapy (Phillips et al. 2005). Finally, in terms of disability, individuals with BDD have been found to be more disabled than individuals with depression, diabetes, or a recent myocardial infarction (Phillips 2000).

Hoarding Disorder

Diagnosis

Until the inclusion of hoarding disorder as a discrete illness in DSM-5, hoarding was considered to be a subtype of OCD. Evidence regarding pathophysiology and treatment response of hoarding symptoms (Mataix-Cols et al. 2010) strongly suggested that hoarding warranted its own diagnostic category separate from OCD. In DSM-5, hoarding is defined as a persistent difficulty in discarding or parting with possessions, regardless of their actual value (Criterion A). This difficulty is due to strong urges to save items and/or distress associated with discarding (Criterion B). This difficulty with discarding results in the accumulation of such a large amount of possessions in living areas or the workplace that the intended use of these areas is no longer possible (Criterion C). DSM-5 does allow for exceptions for Criterion C if areas are uncluttered because of the interventions of others. Although no specific quantities of time or items are required for diagnosis, the hoarding must cause clinically significant distress or impairment in social, occupational, or other important areas of functioning (Criterion D). Finally, the hoarding symptoms may not be attributable to another medical condition (Criterion E) or better explained by the symptoms of another mental disorder (Criterion F). DSM-5 includes specifiers to indicate the level of insight (good or fair, poor, or absent/delusional beliefs) and the presence of "excessive acquisition." The diagnosis of hoarding disorder is relatively straightforward, because the diagnosis relies on hoarding symptoms that result in impairment and/or distress.

Individuals with hoarding disorder often hoard items that they perceive as having utility or sentimental value (including, at times, animals). It has been noted that affected individuals may also report a fear of losing important information. If faced with the prospect of discarding items, individuals with hoarding disorder frequently experience significant distress. The volume of accumulated items is often staggering. Individuals may fill an entire home with hoarded items, sometimes to the detriment of their safety.

Differential Diagnosis

Some patients who have experienced brain trauma may exhibit hoarding behavior (e.g., damage to the ventromedial prefrontal and anterior cingulate cortices has been associated with hoarding symptoms). In these cases, the hoarding behavior would not begin until after the brain injury. Neurodevelopmental disorders such as autism spectrum disorder and Prader-Willi syndrome are sometimes associated with hoarding behavior. If the hoarding symptoms are directly due to obsessions or compulsions associated with OCD (fear of contamination or harm), then the diagnosis of hoarding disorder should not be considered. Additionally, individuals who exhibit hoarding behavior usually find the hoarding distressing. Finally, some patients with psychiatric diagnoses other than hoarding disorder may appear to be exhibiting hoarding behavior when, in fact, their debilitated state may prevent them from appropriately discarding items.

Approximately 75% of individuals with hoarding disorder have a comorbid mood or anxiety disorder (Frost et al. 2011). Additionally, 20% of individuals with hoarding disorder have comorbid OCD (Frost et al. 2011).

Clinical Course

Although onset age is not as well characterized for hoarding disorder as it is for OCD and BDD, some studies suggest that hoarding symptoms begin at around 11–15 years of age and gradually worsen until they interfere with the individual's life (Tolin et al. 2010). One study of hoarders found that symptom onset occurred by age 12 for 60% of participants and by age 18 for 80% (Grisham et al. 2006). As opposed to OCD, hoarding symptoms, while also chronic, are rarely associated with a waxing and waning course and instead show relatively little change over time (Tolin et al. 2010).

Epidemiology

Although no national epidemiology data are available regarding the prevalence of hoarding symptoms, community surveys estimate the point prevalence of clinically significant hoarding symptoms as approximately 2%–6% (e.g., Samuels et al. 2008). Two studies (Iervolino et al. 2009; Samuels et al. 2008) found higher prevalence in men than in women, whereas one study (Mueller et al. 2009) found no difference in prevalence between genders.

Etiology

Until DSM-5, hoarding had been considered to be a subtype of OCD. However, when the different OCD symptom factors were examined, hoarding was clearly distinct from the others (Bloch et al. 2008; Mataix-Cols et al. 2010). Additionally, multiple neuroimaging studies had revealed differences in the pathophysiology of OCD and hoarding (Mataix-Cols et al. 2004; Saxena et al. 2001; Tolin et al. 2009). There does appear to be a genetic component to the illness. Approximately 50% of hoarders report a first-degree relative who hoards, and twin studies suggest that approximately 50% of the variability in hoarding is attributable to genetic factors.

Treatment

One of the most difficult aspects of treating individuals with hoarding disorder is persuading them to accept treatment. Although their hoarding behavior often causes great distress to those around them, individuals with hoarding disorder may not themselves find these behaviors distressing. The first-line treatment of hoarding disorder is behavioral therapy that focuses on removing hoarded items from the environment (increasing outflow) and providing skills to decrease future hoarding (decreasing inflow) (Frost and Tolin 2008). Some data suggest that CBT (e.g., with the addition of motivational interviewing) may be a more effective approach to treating hoarding behavior (Steketee et al. 2010). There are few to no data regarding pharmacotherapy specifically for hoarding disorder, because it has only recently been considered a disorder separate from OCD. Overall, in pharmacological trials for OCD, hoarding appears to exhibit a lesser response to SRIs than do other OCD spectrum disorders (e.g., Bloch et al. 2014; Mataix-Cols et al. 1999).

Prognosis

Most studies have found hoarding symptoms to be chronic and unchanging. Individuals with hoarding disorder who participate in behavioral therapy show lower response rates than do individuals with OCD (Abramowitz et al. 2003; Mataix-Cols et al. 2002). This lower response may be partly due to poor motivation to engage in treatment and higher dropout rates. Some data suggest that CBT may be more effective than behavioral therapy alone for hoarding symptoms. Because hoarding had been considered a subtype of OCD rather than a distinct disorder until DSM-5, there is little prognostic data regarding pharmacotherapy for hoarding behavior.

Trichotillomania (Hair-Pulling Disorder)

Diagnosis

In DSM-IV and DSM-IV-TR, hair-pulling disorder was referred to as *trichotillomania*. Although the term *trichotillomania* was retained in DSM-5, the descriptor *hair-pulling disorder* was added parenthetically to the disorder name. Additionally, the diagnostic requirement in DSM-IV and DSM-IV-TR of a buildup of tension before hair pulling followed by a sense of gratification after hair pulling was removed in DSM-5 because it became clear that a large number of individuals do not experience these emotional states in association with their hair pulling. In DSM-5, the core diagnostic criterion of hair-pulling disorder is "recurrent pulling out of one's hair, resulting in hair loss" (Criterion A). In addition, the individual must have made repeated attempts to decrease or stop the hair pulling (Criterion B). There are no specified lower limits regarding time spent hair pulling or degree of hair loss, but the hair pulling must cause clinically significant distress or impairment in social, occupational, or other important areas of functioning (Criterion C). Finally, the hair pulling or hair loss may not be due to another medical condition (Criterion D) or better explained by the symptoms of another mental disorder (Criterion E).

Individuals with hair-pulling disorder may be drawn to pull hairs that have particular characteristics (e.g., "coarse" or "kinky"). They may pull hair from any part of the body, including scalp, eyebrows, eyelashes, arms, legs, and the pubic area (Table 14–2; Christenson et al. 1991a). Most individuals with hair-pulling disorder pull from multiple sites (see Table 14–2). Whereas some patients report pulling hair when distressed, others report hair pulling during states of relaxation; most report pulling during both conditions. Many patients report mirror-checking behaviors, although they may or may not pull in front of a mirror. Some will use implements (e.g., tweezers) instead of or in addition to their fingers for hair pulling. Some patients with hair-pulling disorder will eat their hair after pulling, resulting in a risk for trichobezoars, which can require surgical intervention. There is significant shame associated with both the hair loss and the inability to stop the hair pulling. As a result, many individuals with hair-pulling disorder hide their hair loss with hats, scarves, and long clothing.

Differential Diagnosis

It is of paramount importance to avoid misattributing hair loss caused by a medical condition to hair pulling. It is also possible that OCD or BDD may manifest symptoms consistent with hair-pulling disorder. For example, patients may pull their hair because they feel it is contaminated (OCD) or because they perceive it as a physical defect (BDD). If this is the case, hair-pulling disorder should not be considered as a

TABLE 14–2. **Phenomenology of hair pulling in a sample of 60 patients with chronic trichotillomania**

	Percentage of patients
Hair pulling at specific sites	
Scalp	75
Eyelashes	53
Eyebrows	42
Pubic area	17
Beard and face	10
Arms	10
Legs	7
Total number of pulling sites	
One	38
Two or more	62
Three or more	33
Four or more	10

Source.   Adapted from Christenson et al. 1991a.

diagnosis. In these instances, it may be difficult to ascertain whether patients have hair-pulling disorder instead of or in addition to OCD or BDD. Finally, individuals with psychotic disorders may remove hair as a result of a delusion or hallucination. The diagnosis of hair-pulling disorder would not apply in this case.

The most common psychiatric comorbidities associated with hair-pulling disorder are major depressive disorder and skin-picking disorder (Stein et al. 2008; Woods et al. 2006a).

Clinical Course

Onset of hair pulling frequently occurs around the onset of puberty, although it may begin before or after puberty as well (Mansueto et al. 1997). Some studies have found that when the behavior begins in early childhood, the hair pulling may be of brief duration and not require treatment. However, if the hair-pulling symptoms are of longer duration, the usual course is chronic with some waxing and waning of symptoms (Keuthen et al. 2001). Finally, females sometimes report worsening of symptoms before or during menstruation, a feature that might help explain the high female prevalence of the disorder.

Epidemiology

A 12-month prevalence rate of 0.6% for hair-pulling disorder has been reported in both community-based and college student samples (Christenson et al. 1991b; Duke et al. 2009). Most studies have found that females are much more commonly affected than males, with some studies estimating that 93% of individuals with hair-pulling disorder are female (Christenson et al. 1991a).

Etiology

Hair pulling is more common in persons with OCD and their first-degree relatives (Bienvenu et al. 2000, 2012), and genetic studies have shown a genetic vulnerability to hair-pulling disorder (Novak et al. 2009; Stein et al. 2010). Compared with healthy volunteers and patients with OCD, patients with hair-pulling disorder demonstrate impaired ability to inhibit motor behaviors on tasks such as the Stop-Signal Task and the Go/No-Go Task (Bohne et al. 2008; Chamberlain et al. 2006). Finally, because very few neuroimaging studies have been conducted in subjects with hair-pulling disorder, comparisons with OCD and other related disorders are not yet possible.

Treatment

Before seeking treatment for hair pulling, many individuals with the disorder will attempt to stop the hair pulling on their own, often using barrier methods such as covering the pulling site or their fingers so that they are unable to pull. It is not clear how successful this approach is because, if successful, these individuals will not present for treatment. Nonetheless, once an individual presents for treatment, the treatment of hair-pulling disorder can include behavioral therapy, pharmacotherapy, or both. The accepted type of behavioral therapy for the treatment of hair-pulling disorder is informed by habit-reversal therapy (Azrin et al. 1980). This therapy has several components, including self-monitoring, awareness training, stimulus control, and competing response training. Three randomized, parallel-group studies demonstrated superior efficacy for habit-reversal therapy over placebo (Ninan et al. 2000; van Minnen et al. 2003; Woods et al. 2006b), providing strong evidence for habit-reversal therapy as the first-line treatment for hair-pulling disorder. Pharmacotherapy studies with SRIs have shown mixed results, with a meta-analysis failing to show any evidence of improvement with SRIs compared with placebo (Bloch et al. 2007). Encouraging initial results with antipsychotic medications (both as SRI augmentation and as monotherapy) have been reported (Grant 2015). Controlled trials in adults with hair-pulling disorder have demonstrated efficacy superior to placebo for naltrexone (Christenson et al. 1994) and for N-acetylcysteine (Grant et al. 2009), but a controlled trial in children and adolescents failed to demonstrate efficacy for N-acetylcysteine (Bloch et al. 2013).

Prognosis

An older long-term follow-up study of patients who had completed treatment with habit-reversal therapy found an 87% reduction in hair pulling at 22-month follow-up compared with pretreatment (Azrin et al. 1980). A more recent study found that hair-pulling symptoms did not significantly worsen over a 2.5-year follow-up period, although there was significant worsening in self-esteem (Keuthen et al. 2001).

Excoriation (Skin-Picking) Disorder

Definition

The diagnostic features of excoriation disorder (Wilhelm et al. 1999) are identical to those of hair-pulling disorder, with the exception that the body-focused repetitive behavior is skin picking rather than hair pulling. In DSM-5, the core diagnostic criterion of excoriation disorder is "recurrent skin picking resulting in skin lesions" (Criterion A). In addition, the individual must have made repeated attempts to decrease or stop the skin picking (Criterion B). The skin picking must cause clinically significant distress or impairment in social, occupational, or other important areas of functioning (Criterion C). Finally, the skin picking must not be attributable to the effects of a substance or another medical condition (Criterion D) or be better explained by the symptoms of another mental disorder (Criterion E).

Although patients may pick at skin anywhere on their bodies, the most common sites are the face, arms, and hands. Some people will pick at healthy skin; others will pick at real or perceived imperfections. Once picking has resulted in a scab, the scab will frequently become a recurrent target for picking. Most persons with excoriation disorder use their fingernails, but as is the case with hair-pulling disorder, some will use implements such as tweezers or knives. Some patients with the disorder may rub, squeeze, or bite their skin, and some will eat their skin after picking. Most persons with excoriation disorder report mirror checking, and many will pick skin in front of a mirror. As is the case with hair pulling, there is usually considerable shame regarding the wounds resulting from picking as well as the inability to stop the skin picking. Finally, persons with excoriation disorder often attempt to conceal their skin-picking sites with clothing or cosmetics.

Differential Diagnosis

Many individuals with BDD pick their skin in an attempt to improve their appearance. Skin picking may occur in individuals with a primary psychotic disorder (e.g., parasitosis, formication) and can be induced by certain substances (e.g., cocaine); the diagnosis of excoriation disorder would not apply in these scenarios.

Clinical Course

As is the case with hair-pulling disorder, the onset of excoriation disorder is generally in adolescence around the onset of puberty. The usual course is chronic, with waxing and waning features.

Epidemiology

Although few studies of the prevalence of excoriation disorder have been conducted, the existing studies suggest a lifetime prevalence of 2.0%–5.4%, with females more commonly affected than males (Grant and Odlaug 2009).

Etiology

Skin picking is more common in individuals with OCD and their first-degree relatives (Bienvenu et al. 2000, 2012), and there is evidence of familial transmission of excoriation disorder (Bienvenu et al. 2009; Grant and Odlaug 2009).

Treatment

Behavioral treatment of excoriation disorder is identical to that of hair-pulling disorder (i.e., based on habit-reversal therapy). The only randomized trial of habit-reversal therapy for skin picking found it to be superior to a wait-list control condition (Teng et al. 2006). To date, four double-blind, placebo-controlled trials of pharmacotherapy treatment of skin picking have been published. In one placebo-controlled trial with fluoxetine, 80% of patients assigned to fluoxetine were classified as responders (as measured with the Clinical Global Impression–Improvement scale) versus only 27.3% of those treated with placebo (Simeon et al. 1997). Another trial demonstrated efficacy for *N*-acetylcysteine (Grant et al. 2016); and two other trials failed to demonstrate efficacy for citalopram (Arbabi et al. 2008) or lamotrigine (Grant et al. 2010).

Prognosis

There are no published long-term follow-up studies in individuals with excoriation disorder. However, given the close relationship of excoriation disorder with other body-focused repetitive behavior disorders such as hair-pulling disorder, one would assume similar prognoses for excoriation disorder and hair-pulling disorder.

Substance/Medication-Induced Obsessive-Compulsive and Related Disorder

The DSM-5 diagnosis *substance/medication-induced obsessive-compulsive and related disorder* is defined as the presence of symptoms characteristic of obsessive-compulsive and related disorders (Criterion A). There must be evidence that these symptoms developed during or soon after exposure to a substance (e.g., a drug of abuse, a medication, a toxin) that is capable of producing such symptoms (Criterion B). Furthermore, the symptoms must not be better explained by an obsessive-compulsive and related disorder that is not substance/medication-induced (Criterion C); must not occur exclusively during delirium (Criterion D); and must cause clinically significant distress or impairment in social, occupational, or other important areas of functioning (Criterion E).

Clearly, it must first be determined that the individual was exposed to a substance. Once this is established, the next step is to link the onset of symptoms with exposure to or withdrawal from the substance. Once exposure to the substance has ceased, the symptoms should usually resolve over time.

The substances most commonly reported as potentially causing obsessive-compulsive and related symptoms (Table 14–3) are amphetamines, cocaine, and stimulants. Heavy metals have also been reported to cause obsessive-compulsive and related symptoms. Finally, atypical antipsychotics, when used as monotherapy, can result in the onset of OCD symptoms or exacerbate existing OCD symptoms.

Obsessive-Compulsive and Related Disorder Due to Another Medical Condition

The DSM-5 diagnosis *obsessive-compulsive and related disorder due to another medical condition* is defined as the presence of symptoms characteristic of obsessive-compulsive and related disorders (Criterion A) that are judged to be the direct pathophysiological consequence of another medical condition (Criterion B), such as a cere-

TABLE 14–3.	Substances that may cause obsessive-compulsive symptoms

Amphetamines

Cocaine

L-Dopa

Other stimulants/dopamine agonists

Heavy metals

Atypical antipsychotics

TABLE 14–4.	Medical conditions that may cause obsessive-compulsive symptoms

Cerebrovascular accident

Central nervous system (CNS) neoplasm/tumor

Head injury

CNS infection (usually, but not always, streptococcal)

brovascular accident (Table 14–4). These symptoms must not be better explained by another mental disorder (Criterion C); must not occur exclusively during delirium (Criterion D); and must cause clinically significant distress or impairment in social, occupational, or other important areas of functioning (Criterion E).

The most important step in making this diagnosis is temporally linking the onset of obsessive-compulsive and related symptoms with the onset of an illness. Obsessive-compulsive and related symptoms have been reported following viral and bacterial encephalitis. Additionally, there have been enough reports of the onset of obsessive-compulsive and related symptoms following streptococcal infection that a syndrome called pediatric acute-onset neuropsychiatric syndrome (PANS) has been defined. In PANS, children infected with *Streptococcus* may exhibit obsessive-compulsive and related symptoms that sometimes (but not always) resolve after successful treatment of the streptococcal infection. Studies have found that the basal ganglia must be affected by the infection in order for PANS to occur (Murphy et al. 2014). Finally, brain lesions due to a cerebrovascular accident, head injury, or tumor have been associated with obsessive-compulsive and related symptoms.

Other Specified or Unspecified Obsessive-Compulsive and Related Disorder

The categories *other specified obsessive-compulsive and related disorder* and *unspecified obsessive-compulsive and related disorder* may be applied to presentations that are characteristic of an obsessive-compulsive and related disorder and cause clinically significant impairment but that do not meet full criteria for any of the disorders in this diagnostic class. For an "other specified" diagnosis, the clinician provides the specific reason that full criteria are not met; for an "unspecified" diagnosis, no reason need be given.

DSM-5 describes seven examples of presentations for which an "other specified" designation might be appropriate:

- Obsessional jealousy
- Three body-focused syndromes: body dysmorphic–like disorder with actual flaws, body dysmorphic–like disorder without repetitive behaviors, and body-focused repetitive behavior disorder (e.g., nail biting, cheek chewing)
- Three disorders related to syndromes listed in the "Glossary of Cultural Concepts of Distress" in the DSM-5 appendix: *shubo-kyofu* (a variant of *taijin kyofusho* that is similar to body dysmorphic disorder), *koro* (related to *dhat syndrome*; fear that the genitals will recede into the body, possibly leading to death), and *jikoshu-kyofu* (a variant of *taijin kyofusho* characterized by fear of having an offensive body odor; also termed *olfactory reference syndrome*)

Conclusion

DSM-5 marks the separation of OCD from the anxiety disorders with the creation of a new category for "Obsessive-Compulsive and Related Disorders," which includes OCD and associated disorders that in DSM-IV were placed in other diagnostic categories. There is strong evidence supporting this change, including phenomenological similarities across OCD and related disorders, neurobiological evidence suggesting differences in pathophysiology between OCD and related disorders and anxiety disorders, and efficacy of similar treatment approaches across OCD and related disorders. The diagnoses included in "Obsessive-Compulsive and Related Disorders" all involve unwanted thoughts and/or repetitive behaviors. The pathology of these disorders does not primarily lie within the fear circuitry implicated in the pathophysiology of anxiety disorders. Several behavioral interventions, such as exposure and response prevention and habit-reversal therapy, are relatively specific to OCD and related disorders. Finally, although SRIs, commonly used to treat a variety of psychiatric illnesses, are the primary first-line pharmacotherapy intervention for OCD and some of the OCD-related disorders, the efficacy of antipsychotic augmentation and of newer glutamatergic agents also appears to differentiate OCD and related disorders from the anxiety disorders. Future studies should focus on furthering our understanding of the pathophysiology of the OCD-related disorders to the level attained regarding OCD itself, all while continuing to advance the knowledge base for the pathophysiology of OCD. Additionally, continued development of new treatments for OCD, including modifications of behavioral interventions and assessment of new therapeutic targets for psychopharmacology, should be fruitful in the coming years.

Key Clinical Points

- Although there are phenomenological and epidemiological similarities between obsessive-compulsive disorder (OCD) and its related disorders (hence their being classified together in DSM-5), it is important to recognize the differences that make them distinct disorders.

- Among the obsessive-compulsive and related disorders, OCD's pathophysiology is the best understood. The data available for OCD-related disorders suggest both similarities and differences between OCD and its related disorders.

- There appears to be a genetic component in OCD and all the related disorders for which data exist.

- If OCD and/or an OCD-related disorder is present, the clinician should screen for all other OCD-related disorders.

- Several behavioral therapy and cognitive-behavioral therapy modalities (e.g., exposure and response prevention, habit-reversal therapy) appear to be effective across OCD and its related disorders.

- Although serotonin reuptake inhibitors (SRIs) are effective in treating OCD and body dysmorphic disorder, it is less clear whether SRIs are effective in treating other OCD-related disorders.

- For all of the OCD-related disorders except OCD itself, limited data are available regarding alternative monotherapy or augmentation strategies for treatment.

References

Abramowitz JS, Franklin ME, Schwartz SA, et al: Symptom presentation and outcome of cognitive-behavioral therapy for obsessive-compulsive disorder. J Consult Clin Psychol 71(6):1049–1057, 2003 14622080

American Psychiatric Association: Diagnostic and Statistical Manual of Mental Disorders, 4th Edition. Washington, DC, American Psychiatric Association, 1994

American Psychiatric Association: Diagnostic and Statistical Manual of Mental Disorders, 4th Edition, Text Revision. Washington, DC, American Psychiatric Association, 2000

American Psychiatric Association: Diagnostic and Statistical Manual of Mental Disorders, 5th Edition. Arlington, VA, American Psychiatric Association, 2013

Arbabi M, Farnia V, Balighi K, et al: Efficacy of citalopram in treatment of pathological skin picking, a randomized double blind placebo controlled trial. Acta Medica Iranica 46(5):367–372, 2008

Azrin NH, Nunn RG, Frantz SE: Treatment of hairpulling (trichotillomania): a comparative study of habit reversal and negative practice training. Journal of Behavior Therapy and Experimental Psychiatry 11(1):13–20, 1980

Bandelow B, Zohar J, Hollander E, et al: World Federation of Societies of Biological Psychiatry (WFSBP) guidelines for the pharmacological treatment of anxiety, obsessive-compulsive and post-traumatic stress disorders—first revision. World J Biol Psychiatry 9(4):248–312, 2008 18949648

Bienvenu OJ, Samuels JF, Riddle MA, et al: The relationship of obsessive-compulsive disorder to possible spectrum disorders: results from a family study. Biol Psychiatry 48(4):287–293, 2000 10960159

Bienvenu OJ, Wang Y, Shugart YY, et al: Sapap3 and pathological grooming in humans: results from the OCD collaborative genetics study. Am J Med Genet B Neuropsychiatr Genet 150B(5):710–720, 2009 19051237

Bienvenu OJ, Samuels JF, Wuyek LA, et al: Is obsessive-compulsive disorder an anxiety disorder, and what, if any, are spectrum conditions? A family study perspective. Psychol Med 42(1):1–13, 2012 21733222

Bloch MH, Landeros-Weisenberger A, Dombrowski P, et al: Systematic review: pharmacological and behavioral treatment for trichotillomania. Biol Psychiatry 62(8):839–846, 2007 17727824

Bloch MH, Landeros-Weisenberger A, Rosario MC, et al: Meta-analysis of the symptom structure of obsessive-compulsive disorder. Am J Psychiatry 165(12):1532–1542, 2008 18923068

Bloch MH, Panza KE, Grant JE, et al: N-acetylcysteine in the treatment of pediatric trichotillomania: a randomized, double-blind, placebo-controlled add-on trial. J Am Acad Child Adolesc Psychiatry 52(3):231–240, 2013 23452680

Bloch M, Bartley C, Leckman J, et al: Meta-analysis: hoarding symptoms associated with poor treatment outcome in obsessive-compulsive disorder. Mol Psychiatry 19(9):1025–1030, 2014 24912494

Bohne A, Savage CR, Deckerbach T, et al: Motor inhibition in trichotillomania and obsessive-compulsive disorder. J Psychiatry Res 42(2):141–150, 2008 17215004

Buhlmann U, Glaesmer H, Mewes R, et al: Updates on the prevalence of body dysmorphic disorder: a population-based survey. Psychiatr Res 178(1):171–175, 2010 20452057

Chamberlain SR, Fineberg NA, Blackwell AD, et al: Motor inhibition and cognitive flexibility in obsessive-compulsive disorder and trichotillomania. Am J Psychiatry 163(7):1282–1284, 2006 16816237

Christenson GA, Mackenzie TB, Mitchell JE: Characteristics of 60 adult chronic hair pullers. Am J Psychiatry 148(3):365–370, 1991a 1992841

Christenson GA, Pyle RL, Mitchell JE: Estimated lifetime prevalence of trichotillomania in college students. J Clin Psychiatry 52(10):415–417, 1991b 1938977

Christenson GA, Crow SJ, MacKenzie TB, et al: A placebo controlled double-blind study of naltrexone for trichotillomania (NR 597), in 1994 New Research Program and Abstracts, American Psychiatric Association 147th Annual Meeting, Philadelphia, PA, May 21–26, 1994. Washington, DC, American Psychiatric Association, 1994, p 212

Dell'Osso B, Nestadt G, Allen A, et al: Serotonin-norepinephrine reuptake inhibitors in the treatment of obsessive-compulsive disorder: a critical review. J Clin Psychiatry 67(4):600–610, 2006 16669725

Dougherty DD, Rauch SL, Greenberg BD: Pathophysiology of obsessive-compulsive disorders, in Textbook of Anxiety Disorders, 2nd Edition. Edited by Stein DJ, Hollander E, Rothbaum BO. Washington, DC, American Psychiatric Publishing, 2010, pp 287–309

Duke DC, Bodzin DK, Tavares P, et al: The phenomenology of hairpulling in a community sample. J Anxiety Disord 23(8):1118–1125, 2009 19651487

Eisen JL, Pinto A, Mancebo MC, et al: A 2-year prospective follow-up study of the course of obsessive-compulsive disorder. J Clin Psychiatry 71(8):1033–1039, 2010 20797381

Feusner JD, Moody T, Hembacher E, et al: Abnormalities of visual processing and frontostriatal systems in body dysmorphic disorder. Arch Gen Psychiatry 67(2):197–205, 2010 20124119

Feusner JD, Hembacher E, Moller H, et al: Abnormalities of object visual processing in body dysmorphic disorder. Psychol Med 41(11):2385–2397, 2011 21557897

Foa EB, Kozak MJ: Psychological treatment for obsessive-compulsive disorder, in Long-Term Treatments for Anxiety Disorders. Edited by Mavissakalian MR, Prien RF. Washington, DC, American Psychiatric Press, 1996, pp 285–309

Foa EB, Liebowitz MR, Kozak MJ, et al: Randomized, placebo-controlled trial of exposure and ritual prevention, clomipramine, and their combination in the treatment of obsessive-compulsive disorder. Am J Psychiatry 162(1):151–161, 2005 15625214

Freud S: Three Case Histories: The "Wolf Man," the "Rat Man," and the Psychotic Doctor Schreber (1909). Translated by Rieff P. New York, Macmillan, 1973

Frost RO, Tolin DF: Compulsive hoarding, in Clinical Handbook of Obsessive-Compulsive Disorder and Related Problems. Edited by Abramowitz JS, Taylor S, McKay D. Baltimore, MD, Johns Hopkins University Press, 2008, pp 76–94

Frost RO, Steketee G, Tolin DF: Comorbidity in hoarding disorder. Depress Anxiety 28(10):876–884, 2011 21770000

Goodman WK: Obsessive-compulsive disorder: diagnosis and treatment. J Clin Psychiatry 60 (suppl 18):27–32, 1999 10487253

Grant JE: Review of psychopharmacological approaches for trichotillomania and other body-focused behaviors. Current Treatment Options in Psychiatry 2(4):422–431, 2015

Grant JE, Odlaug BL: Update on pathological skin picking. Curr Psychiatry Rep 11(4):283–288, 2009 19635236

Grant JE, Odlaug BL, Kim SW: N-acetylcysteine, a glutamate modulator, in the treatment of trichotillomania: a double-blind, placebo-controlled study. Arch Gen Psychiatry 66(7):756–763, 2009 19581567

Grant JE, Odlaug BL, Chamberlain SR, et al: A double-blind, placebo-controlled trial of lamotrigine for pathological skin picking: treatment efficacy and neurocognitive predictors of response. J Clin Psychopharmacol 30(4):396–403, 2010 20531220

Grant JE, Chamberlain SR, Redden SA, et al: N-acetylcysteine in the treatment of excoriation disorder: a randomized clinical trial. JAMA Psychiatry 73(5):490–496, 2016 27007062

Greist JH, Jefferson JW, Kobak KA, et al: Efficacy and tolerability of serotonin transport inhibitors in obsessive-compulsive disorder. A meta-analysis. Arch Gen Psychiatry 52(1):53–60, 1995 7811162

Grisham JR, Frost RO, Steketee G, et al: Age of onset of compulsive hoarding. J Anxiety Disord 20(5):675–686, 2006 16112837

Hettema JM, Neale MC, Kendler KS: A review and meta-analysis of the genetic epidemiology of anxiety disorders. Am J Psychiatry 158(10):1568–1578, 2001 11578982

Iervolino AC, Perroud N, Fullana MA, et al: Prevalence and heritability of compulsive hoarding: a twin study. Am J Psychiatry 166(10):1156–1161, 2009 19687130

Karno M, Golding JM, Sorenson SB, et al: The epidemiology of obsessive-compulsive disorder in five US communities. Arch Gen Psychiatry 45(12):1094–1099, 1988 3264144

Keen EC, Widge AS, Dougherty DD: Functional neurosurgery in severe and treatment-refractory OCD, in Obsessive-Compulsive Disorder: Phenomenology, Pathophysiology, and Treatment. Edited by Pittenger C. New York, Oxford University Press, 2017, pp 507–516

Keuthen NJ, Fraim C, Deckersbach T, et al: Longitudinal follow-up of naturalistic treatment outcome in patients with trichotillomania. J Clin Psychiatry 62(2):101–107, 2001 11247093

Koran LM, Abujaoude E, Large MD, et al: The prevalence of body dysmorphic disorder in the United States adult population. CNS Spectr 13(4):316–322, 2008 18408651

Mansueto CS, Stemberger RM, Thomas AM, et al: Trichotillomania: a comprehensive behavioral model. Clin Psychol Rev 17(5):567–577, 1997 9260041

Mataix-Cols D, Rauch SL, Manzo PA, et al: Use of factor-analyzed symptom dimensions to predict outcome with serotonin reuptake inhibitors and placebo in the treatment of obsessive-compulsive disorder. Am J Psychiatry 156(9):1409–1416, 1999 10484953

Mataix-Cols D, Marks IM, Greist JH, et al: Obsessive-compulsive symptom dimensions as predictors of compliance with and response to behaviour therapy: results from a controlled trial. Psychother Psychosom 71(5):255–262, 2002 12207105

Mataix-Cols D, Wooderson S, Lawrence N, et al: Distinct neural correlates of washing, checking, and hoarding symptom dimensions in obsessive-compulsive disorder. Arch Gen Psychiatry 61(6):564–576, 2004 15184236

Mataix-Cols D, Frost RO, Pertusa A, et al: Hoarding disorder: a new diagnosis for DSM-V? Depress Anxiety 27(6):556–572, 2010 20336805

Mueller A, Mitchell J, Crosby R, et al: The prevalence of compulsive hoarding and its association with compulsive buying in a German population-based sample. Behav Res Ther 47(8):705–709, 2009 19457476

Murphy TK, Gerardi DM, Leckman JF: Pediatric acute-onset neuropsychiatric syndrome. Psychiatr Clin North Am 37(3):353–374, 2014 25150567

Murray CJ, Lopez AD: The Global Burden of Disease. Boston, MA, Harvard University Press, 1996

Ninan PT, Rothbaum BO, Marsteller FA, et al: A placebo-controlled trial of cognitive-behavioral therapy and clomipramine in trichotillomania. J Clin Psychiatry 61(1):47–50, 2000 10695646

Novak CE, Keuthen NJ, Stewart SE, et al: A twin concordance study of trichotillomania. Am J Med Genet B Neuropsychiatr Genet 150B(7):944–949, 2009 19199280

Öst LG, Havnen A, Hansen B, et al: Cognitive behavioral treatments of obsessive-compulsive disorder. A systematic review and meta-analysis of studies published 1993–2014. Clin Psychol Rev 40:156–169, 2015 26117062

Pauls DL, Abramovitch A, Rauch SL, et al: Obsessive-compulsive disorder: an integrative genetic and neurobiological perspective. Nat Rev Neurosci 15(6):410–424, 2014 24840803

Perugi G, Akiskal HS, Giannotti D, et al: Gender-related differences in body dysmorphic disorder (dysmorphophobia). J Nerv Ment Dis 185(9):578–582, 1997 9307620

Phillips KA: Quality of life for patients with body dysmorphic disorder. J Nerv Ment Dis 188(3):170–175, 2000 10749282

Phillips KA: Placebo-controlled study of pimozide augmentation of fluoxetine in body dysmorphic disorder. Am J Psychiatry 162(2):377–379, 2005 15677604

Phillips KA: Body dysmorphic disorder, in Clinical Obsessive-Compulsive Disorders in Adults and Children. Edited by Hudak R, Dougherty DD. New York, Cambridge University Press, 2011, pp 191–206

Phillips KA, Diaz SF: Gender differences in body dysmorphic disorder. J Nerv Ment Dis 185(9):570–577, 1997 9307619

Phillips KA, Grant JE, Siniscalchi JM, et al: A retrospective follow-up study of body dysmorphic disorder. Compr Psychiatry 46(5):315–321, 2005 16122530

Phillips KA, Menard W, Fay C, et al: Gender similarities and differences in 200 individuals with body dysmorphic disorder. Compr Psychiatry 47(2):77–87, 2006a 16490564

Phillips KA, Pagano ME, Menard W, et al: A 12-month follow-up study of the course of body dysmorphic disorder. Am J Psychiatry 163(5):907–912, 2006b 16648334

Phillips KA, Wilhelm S, Koran LM, et al: Body dysmorphic disorder: some key issues for DSM-V. Depress Anxiety 27(6):573–591, 2010 20533368

Pittenger C, Bloch MH, Williams K: Glutamate abnormalities in obsessive compulsive disorder: neurobiology, pathophysiology, and treatment. Pharmacol Ther 132(3):314–332, 2011 21963369

Rasmussen SA, Eisen JL: The epidemiology and differential diagnosis of obsessive-compulsive disorder. J Clin Psychiatry 53 (suppl):4–10, 1992 1564054

Rief W, Buhlmann U, Wilhelm S, et al: The prevalence of body dysmorphic disorder: a population-based survey. Psychol Med 36(6):877–885, 2006 16515733

Rosa-Alcázar AI, Sánchez-Meca J, Gómez-Conesa A, et al: Psychological treatment of obsessive-compulsive disorder: a meta-analysis. Clin Psychol Rev 28(8):1310–1325, 2008 18701199

Samuels JF, Bienvenu OJ, Grados MA, et al: Prevalence and correlates of hoarding behavior in a community-based sample. Behav Res Ther 46(7):836–844, 2008 18495084

Saxena S, Bota RG, Brody AL: Brain-behavior relationships in obsessive-compulsive disorder. Semin Clin Neuropsychiatry 6(2):82–101, 2001 11296309

Simeon D, Stein DJ, Gross S, et al: A double-blind trial of fluoxetine in pathological skin picking. J Clin Psychiatry 58(8):341–347, 1997 9515971

Skoog G, Skoog I: A 40-year follow-up of patients with obsessive-compulsive disorder. Arch Gen Psychiatry 56(2):121–127, 1999 10025435

Stein DJ, Flessner CA, Franklin M, et al: Is trichotillomania a stereotypic movement disorder? An analysis of body-focused repetitive behaviors in people with hair-pulling. Ann Clin Psychiatry 20(4):194–198, 2008 19034750

Stein DJ, Grant JE, Franklin ME, et al: Trichotillomania (hair pulling disorder), skin picking disorder, and stereotypic movement disorder: toward DSM-V. Depress Anxiety 27(6):611–626, 2010 20533371

Steketee G, Frost RO, Tolin DF, et al: Waitlist-controlled trial of cognitive behavior therapy for hoarding disorder. Depress Anxiety 27(5):476–484, 2010 20336804

Teng EJ, Woods DW, Twohig MP: Habit reversal as a treatment for chronic skin picking: a pilot investigation. Behav Modif 30(4):411–422, 2006 16723422

Tolin DF, Kiehl KA, Worhunsky GA, et al: An exploratory study of the neural mechanisms of decision making in compulsive hoarding. Psychol Med 39(2):325–336, 2009 18485263

Tolin DF, Meunier SA, Frost RO, Steketee G: Course of compulsive hoarding and its relationship to life events. Depress Anxiety 27(9):829–838, 2010 20336803

van Grootheest DS, Cath DC, Beekman AT, et al: Twin studies on obsessive-compulsive disorder: a review. Twin Res Hum Genet 8(5):450–458, 2005 16212834 van Minnen A, Hoogduin KA, Keijsers GP, et al: Treatment of trichotillomania with behavioral therapy or fluoxetine: a randomized, waiting-list controlled study. Arch Gen Psychiatry 60(5):517–522, 2003 12742873

Veale D, Anson M, Miles S, et al: Efficacy of cognitive behaviour therapy versus anxiety management for body dysmorphic disorder: a randomised controlled trial. Psychother Psychosom 83(6):341–353, 2014a 25323062

Veale D, Miles S, Smallcombe N, et al: Atypical antipsychotic augmentation in SSRI treatment refractory obsessive-compulsive disorder: a systematic review and meta-analysis. BMC Psychiatry 14:317, 2014b 25432131

Wilhelm S, Keuthen NJ, Engelhard I, et al: Self-injurious skin picking: clinical characteristics and comorbidity. J Clin Psychiatry 60(7):454–459, 1999 10453800

Wilhelm S, Steketee G, Fama JM, et al: Modular cognitive therapy for obsessive-compulsive disorder: a wait-list controlled trial. J Cogn Psychother 23(4):294–305, 2009 21072138

Wilhelm S, Phillips KA, Steketee G: A Cognitive Behavioral Treatment Manual for Body Dysmorphic Disorder. New York, Guilford, 2013

Wilhelm S, Phillips KA, Didie E, et al: Modular cognitive-behavioral therapy for body dysmorphic disorder: a randomized controlled trial. Behav Ther 45(3):314–327, 2014 24680228

Wisner KL, Peindl KS, Gigliotti T, et al: Obsessions and compulsions in women with postpartum depression. J Clin Psychiatry 60(3):176–180, 1999 10192593

Woods DW, Flessner C, Franklin ME, et al: Understanding and treating trichotillomania: what we know and what we don't know. Psychiatr Clin North Am 29(2):487–501, 2006a 16650719

Woods DW, Wetterneck CT, Flessner CA: A controlled evaluation of acceptance and commitment therapy plus habit reversal for trichotillomania. Behav Res Ther 44(5):639–656, 2006b 16039603

Recommended Readings

Hudak R, Dougherty DD (eds): Clinical Obsessive-Compulsive Disorders in Adults and Children. New York, Cambridge University Press, 2011

Steketee G (ed): The Oxford Handbook of Obsessive Compulsive and Spectrum Disorders. New York, Oxford University Press, 2012

Online Resources

International OCD Foundation (IOCDF): http://www.ocfoundation.org

CHAPTER 15

Trauma- and Stressor-Related Disorders

Frederick J. Stoddard Jr., M.D.

Naomi M. Simon, M.D., M.Sc.

Roger K. Pitman, M.D.

Across the age spectrum, trauma- and stressor-related disorders represent long-lasting suffering and functional impairment for many but also offer opportunity for helpful diagnosis, early intervention, and therapeutic benefit. These disorders, and the individuals and families affected by them, are the subject of intensive research at every level—from epidemiological and clinical to genomic, translational, neurobiological, and neuropsychological. In this chapter we present the rapidly expanding, complex body of knowledge accumulated from this research (e.g., Ross et al. 2017; Saxe et al. 2016; Shalev et al. 2017; Smoller 2016; Stoddard et al. 2018; Yehuda et al. 2015) and several models for understanding trauma- and stressor-related disorders.

Although some of the historic impetus for understanding and treating the effects of psychological trauma, such as the timing in 1980 of the first inclusion of posttraumatic stress disorder (PTSD) in DSM-III (American Psychiatric Association 1980), derived from the Vietnam War and military psychiatry, much impetus came from recognition of the traumatic impacts of genocide, child abuse, the rape of women, the effects of injury or violence in the general population, and the trauma of disasters (Stoddard et al. 2011a; Ursano et al. 2017).

Several seminal writings and creative works set the stage for understanding child and adult PTSD and developing treatments. Following the Cocoanut Grove fire in Boston in 1942, Stanley Cobb, Erich Lindemann, and Alexandra Adler described symptoms, syndromes, and treatments after burn trauma and effects on grieving loved ones that are now embedded in the understanding of the diagnosis and treatment of PTSD as well as in psychiatric responses to disasters (Adler 1943; Cobb and Lindemann 1943; Lindemann 1994). In his study of survivors of Hiroshima, Robert Lifton (1967) described the horror of atomic weapons and the lasting traumatic effect on survivors.

Lenore Terr's (1991) observations of the Chowchilla children who were kidnapped on a school bus provided insights into the impact of trauma on development and informed the understanding of childhood PTSD. In *Trauma and Recovery,* Judith Herman (1992) provided direction in the psychotherapy of victims of violence and trauma, especially women. Jonathan Shay's *Achilles in Vietnam* and *Odysseus in America,* informed by Homer's epic poems, placed into a classical literary context the traumas endured by U.S. soldiers in Vietnam and after their return home (Shay 1992, 2002). More recently, the documentary film by Ken Burns and Lynn Novick, *The Vietnam War,* chronicled the searing personal and societal impacts (including PTSD) on both Americans and Vietnamese of the killings, injuries, and other traumas to adults and children, as well as their resiliency during and after that war (Burns and Novick 2017).

Overview of Trauma- and Stressor-Related Disorders

Reconceptualization of Disorders of Trauma and Stress Response

DSM-5's (American Psychiatric Association 2013) removal of PTSD from the anxiety disorder category in favor of a timely, evidence-based new categorization reflects the enormous growth in basic and clinical research on trauma- and stressor-related disorders and these disorders' broad prevalence across the age span and across cultures. This category includes disorders in which exposure to a traumatic or stressful event is required as a diagnostic criterion (PTSD, acute stress disorder, and adjustment disorders) as well as disorders that are etiologically linked to early social neglect (reactive attachment disorder and disinhibited social engagement disorder). Finally, attention is given to other trauma- and stressor-related conditions that do not meet full criteria for inclusion as a disorder in this diagnostic class, such as *persistent complex bereavement disorder* (also included in DSM-5 Section III as a condition for further study). Of note, ICD 11 has added a similar condition, *prolonged grief disorder.*

   The DSM-5 committee added a new chapter for trauma- and stressor-related disorders after scientific review to differentiate disorders related to a trauma or stressful event from anxiety disorders, which do not require such exposure. The placement of the trauma- and stressor-related disorders chapter within the DSM-5 structure preserves the close relationship between these disorders and the anxiety disorders and obsessive-compulsive and related disorders, which are addressed in the two preceding chapters in DSM-5, and also between these disorders and the dissociative disorders, which are addressed in the following chapter in DSM-5.

Psychology of Psychological Trauma and Posttraumatic Stress Disorder

The psychological theories applied to trauma and PTSD have derived primarily from learning theory–based treatment and research with rape victims and Vietnam veterans. In 1947, Mowrer proposed a two-factor theory of classical and operant conditioning to explain posttraumatic symptoms. The first factor, classical conditioning, was applied to explain the fear and distress in survivors of trauma and their exacerbation on exposure to reminders of the traumatic event. The second factor, operant conditioning, was applied to explain the development and persistence of PTSD-related avoidance symptoms. If being exposed to reminders of a traumatic event causes anxiety or other emotional distress, those who experience these symptoms are motivated to avoid such reminders. Foa et al. (2005), using Lang's (1977) emotional processing theory of anxiety development, suggested that a "fear network" forms in the memory that elicits negative emotions and cognitions as well as escape and avoidance behaviors.

Classical conditioning theory has inspired behavioral therapy approaches to PTSD. Early techniques such as systematic desensitization and stress inoculation training eventually yielded to techniques based on exposure to the traumatic event as the key therapeutic ingredient. Foa et al. (2005) based their classic controlled trial of cognitive-behavioral therapy (CBT) for rape survivors on this theory. Exposure relies on the principle of fear extinction. Unfortunately, extinction suppresses only the *expression* of the underlying fear memory, which is liable to return after a change of context (renewal), an intervening frightening event (reinstatement), or just the passage of time (spontaneous recovery). These phenomena place a theoretical limit on what exposure therapy may be able to achieve.

In contrast to the conditioning model, Mardi Horowitz in 1986 proposed social-cognitive theories that moved from psychodynamic to cognitive processing perspectives. He applied these theories to treatment aimed at resolving the conflict between the need to integrate the experience and the wish to avoid intrusive reexperiencing. Developmental psychology uses some of these perspectives and describes the effects of trauma in cognitive, affective, interpersonal, and behavioral domains from infancy through adulthood. Resick et al. (2017b) came to theorize that the key underlying problem in trauma-related disorders is the presence of dysfunctional cognitions, and they developed cognitive processing therapy as a technique for challenging and modifying such cognitions (Shalev et al. 2017).

Biology of Psychological Trauma and Posttraumatic Stress Disorder

When PTSD was first introduced into the psychiatric nomenclature nearly four decades ago, it was understood almost entirely in psychological terms. Since that time, the growth of biological knowledge has been explosive (Nemeroff and Marmar 2018; Pitman et al. 2012), to the point that more is now known about PTSD's underlying biology than about the foundations of almost any other mental disorder. Discoveries of biological abnormalities in PTSD have helped to counteract skepticism regarding a disorder whose diagnosis is based largely on self-report, sometimes in the presence of external incentives, and to promote its now-widespread acceptance.

In DSM-5, trauma- and stress-related disorders are unique in that they are defined as resulting from environmental events. These disorders are distinguished from traumatic brain injury, in which the environmental event is a physical impact, through the fact that in the former, the event is information. In PTSD and acute stress disorder, the information is that serious physical injury, sexual violence, or death is threatened or has occurred. Ultimately, the impact of an environmental event, even if it consists only of information, must be understood at the organ and molecular levels.

In classic PTSD, the traumatic event produces a response of intense fear, helplessness, or horror, which induces specific and general functional and structural changes in the nervous system that may last a lifetime (Figure 15–1). The specific change is the engraving of the memory of the traumatic event and its associated stimuli, due to the well-known potentiating effect of stress hormones and neuromodulators—including epinephrine and norepinephrine, cortisol, and neuroactive peptides—on memory consolidation. Structural manifestations of this overconsolidation include pre- and postsynaptic alterations in the amygdala and other brain areas. Epigenetic effects are almost certainly also implicated. The deeply engraved traumatic memory is the basis for DSM-5's Criterion B symptom cluster, which represents the hallmark of the disorder.

The general change following the traumatic event is the induction of a persistent state of alarm, hyperalertness, and sensitivity to threat, which is manifested in the DSM-5 PTSD Criterion D symptom cluster. This state is characterized by hyper(re)activity of the sympathetic nervous system (SNS), consisting of increased tonic and phasic levels of central nervous system, blood, and urinary catecholamines and their metabolites; increased cerebrospinal fluid corticotropin-releasing hormone; increased blood pressure and heart rate; and increased physiological responses to startling stimuli. Underlying this persistent state is hyper(re)activity of the amygdala, anterior paralimbic and dorsal anterior cingulate cortices, and insula (Hughes and Shin 2011). Through its efferent connections to the nucleus accumbens, hypothalamus, brain stem, and other structures, the amygdala represents a key structure for coordinating the behavioral, endocrine, and physiological components of the fear response.

Paralleling the heightened SNS (re)activity in PTSD is hypoactivity of the parasympathetic nervous system, manifested in decreased heart rate variability, which has been found to predict mortality. In the central nervous system, brain structures that have been found to inhibit the expression of conditioned fear, in part by facilitating extinction, including the ventromedial prefrontal cortex (vmPFC) and the anterior cingulate cortex, are hypo(re)active. The amygdala and the vmPFC have an inverse relationship—the more active the vmPFC is, the less active the amygdala is, and vice versa. An additional key inhibitory brain structure is the hippocampus, which is important in recognizing context and limiting conditioned stimulus overgeneralization. Although research to date suggests that most of the functional and structural brain abnormalities in PTSD are acquired following the traumatic event, the hippocampus appears to be at least a partial exception. Research in identical twins discordant for combat exposure suggests that lower hippocampal volume confers risk for PTSD following traumatic exposure (Gilbertson et al. 2002).

The most surprising finding in biological research of PTSD has been that cortisol is not elevated, as might be expected according to a classical stress model. If anything, cortisol is reduced (Yehuda 2002). This reduction appears to be due to hypersensitivity of the cortical hypothalamic-pituitary-adrenal (HPA) axis to negative feedback. Although cortisol is commonly understood to be a stress hormone, among its various actions is containment of the effects of the SNS. Failure of cortisol to perform this function may, in part, underlie SNS hyperactivity in PTSD.

It is becoming increasingly recognized that PTSD is associated with a variety of comorbid physical disorders, including cardiovascular disease and hypertension, type 2 diabetes mellitus, obesity, rheumatoid arthritis, and dementia (Koenen et al. 2017). Until recently, the pathophysiological mechanisms that link the brain to the periph-

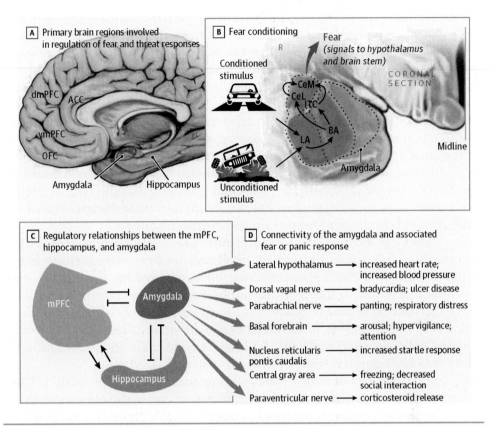

FIGURE 15–1. Schematic diagram of neural circuitry involved in fear conditioning and posttraumatic stress disorder.

(A) Primary brain regions involved in regulating fear and threat responses are the amygdala, the hippocampus, and the medial prefrontal cortex (mPFC), which consists of the dorsal (dmPFC) and ventral (vmPFC) subdivisions, the orbitofrontal cortex (OFC), and the anterior cingulate cortex (ACC).

(B) Shown are the amygdala-specific circuits involved in fear conditioning. The sensory information representing the *conditioned stimulus* (e.g., previously neutral stimulus such as driving a car) is integrated within the amygdala with the *unconditioned stimulus* information (e.g., a traumatic event such as an explosion in a car). The amygdala is central in the neural circuit involved in regulating fear conditioning. In general, input to the lateral nucleus (LA) of the amygdala leads to learning about fear, whereas the central amygdala (lateral [CeL] and medial [CeM] subdivisions) is responsible for sending output signals about fear to the hypothalamus and brain stem structures. The intercalated cell masses (ITC) are thought to regulate inhibition of information flow between the basal nucleus (BA) and the central amygdala.

(C and D) Interactions between components of the mPFC and the hippocampus constantly regulate the amygdala's output to subcortical brain regions activating the fear reflex. The mPFC (in particular, the vmPFC) is classically thought to inhibit amygdala activity and reduce subjective distress, while the hippocampus plays a role both in the coding of fear memories and in the regulation of the amygdala. The hippocampus and the mPFC also interact in regulating context and fear modulation.

To view this figure in color, see Plate 6 in Color Gallery in middle of book.

Source. Reprinted from Figure 1 in Ross DA, Arbuckle MR, Travis MJ, et al.: "An Integrated Neuroscience Perspective on Formulation and Treatment Planning for Posttraumatic Stress Disorder: An Educational Review." *JAMA Psychiatry* 74(4):407–415, 2017. Copyright 2017, American Medical Association. Used with permission. Panels C and D adapted from Parsons and Ressler 2013.

ery, in what Freud (1916–1917/1963, p. 320) called "the puzzling leap from the mental to the physical," were obscure. Recent research (Wirtz and von Känel 2017) has suggested that inflammation plays a critical role in this leap. SNS activity increases inflammation, whereas cortisol decreases it. Patients with PTSD have been found to exhibit a number of immune system changes, including increased circulating inflammatory markers and proinflammatory cytokines, increased reactivity to antigen skin tests, lower natural killer cell activity, and lower total T lymphocyte counts (Pace and Heim 2011). A recent study, the first of its kind, found that resting amygdala activity independently and robustly predicted cardiovascular disease events (Tawakol et al. 2017). This effect was mediated in part by a path that included increased bone marrow activity, presumably reflecting increased leukopoiesis, with release into the bloodstream of proinflammatory monocytes, which migrate to the arterial wall and cause arterial inflammation leading to atherosclerosis (Figure 15–2).

The finding that most, but far from all, of the key biological abnormalities in PTSD appear to be acquired after the traumatic event does not mean that pretrauma factors do not confer risk for PTSD. Hippocampal volume reduction has already been mentioned above. The finding that combat-unexposed identical twins of combat veterans with PTSD have more neurological soft signs suggests that subtle pretrauma neurological dysfunction can also confer risk for PTSD (Gurvits et al. 2006). Early-life stress, genetics, and their interaction have also been found to confer risk. Specifically, the role of the *FKBP5* gene has been implicated (Hawn et al. 2019).

Genetic factors account for approximately one-third of the vulnerability to PTSD (Banerjee et al. 2017). The risk of exposure to traumatic events also has substantial genetic determination, probably mediated through personality traits. The genes that increase PTSD risk are typically not specific, in that they also confer risk for other anxiety disorders and depression. As with other mental disorders, genetic liability to PTSD likely involves the contributions of numerous alleles of small effect, with the discouraging implication that targeting any one of them is unlikely to lead to an effective therapeutic intervention. The genetic study of PTSD may be more productive in elucidating pathogenetic mechanisms that are the final common pathways of various genetic influences, which may be targeted by therapy.

An exciting frontier of PTSD research is epigenesis, which is the ability of the environment to turn expression of the genome on or off by modifying not the DNA sequence, but rather its transcription (expression) through the macromolecular mechanisms of DNA methylation and histone deacetylation. Epigenetic effects of traumatic exposure may lie at the heart of PTSD's pathogenesis and may account for trauma's durable effects. A formidable obstacle to research is that the human tissue where the key trauma-induced epigenetic modifications are likely to reside—that is, the brain—is largely inaccessible with current technology. Overcoming this obstacle may be expected to yield exciting insights and, hopefully, novel therapeutic approaches in the years ahead.

Psychological Trauma: Role of Comorbidities

PTSD is a diagnosis that, while identifying a certain group of impaired individuals, is strongly associated in more than 50% of patients with comorbidities, including mood disorders, anxiety disorders, and substance use disorders (Shalev et al. 2017). These

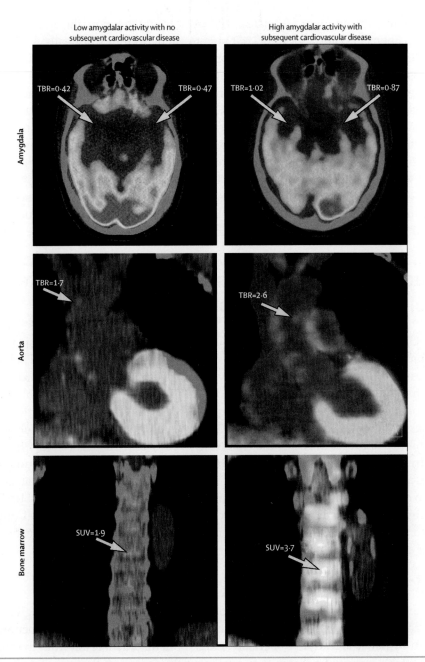

FIGURE 15–2. Pathogenic pathway linking stress to increased risk of cardiovascular disease: amygdalar, arterial, and bone-marrow uptake of ^{18}F-FDG in individuals with and without subsequent cardiovascular disease events.

Axial views of amygdala **(top,** *left and right*), coronal views of aorta **(middle,** *left and right*), and coronal views of bone marrow **(bottom,** *left and right*) are shown. ^{18}F-FDG uptake was increased in the amygdala, bone marrow, and arterial wall (aorta) in a patient who experienced an ischemic stroke during the follow-up period *(right)* compared with a patient who did not *(left).* ^{18}F-FDG = [18]F fluorodeoxyglucose; SUV=standardized uptake value; TBR=target-to-background ratio.

To view this figure in color, see Plate 7 in Color Gallery in middle of book.

Source. Reprinted from Figure 1 in Tawakol A, Ishai A, Takx RA, et al.: "Relation Between Resting Amygdalar Activity and Cardiovascular Events: A Longitudinal and Cohort Study." *Lancet* 389(10071):834–845, 2017. Copyright 2017, Elsevier Inc.

comorbidities are strongly associated with prior traumatization, the effects of which often do not meet criteria for PTSD but may result in disability or death. A transdiagnostic investigation provides a dimensional structure for the overlap of PTSD, major depressive disorder (MDD), and generalized anxiety disorder symptoms, showing differential associations with physical and mental functioning, life satisfaction, and well-being that are useful in understanding impairment status of trauma survivors. Growing evidence supports childhood trauma as a risk factor for poorer stress tolerance, difficulties with emotion regulation, and elevated incidence and severity of a range of psychiatric conditions (Stoddard 2014). Although suicidal behavior is associated with PTSD, its association with PTSD is much less robust than its association with depression, and suicidal behavior is not associated with combat or deployment in a war zone. Shalev et al. (2017) suggested that the suicide risk may be due to "protracted PTSD, life stress, loneliness or alienation" (p. 2462).

Reactive Attachment Disorder and Disinhibited Social Engagement Disorder

The DSM-IV (American Psychiatric Association 1994) childhood diagnosis reactive attachment disorder (RAD) was characterized by pervasive aberrant social behaviors that resulted from "pathogenic care." It was included in the category "Disorders Usually First Diagnosed in Infancy, Childhood, or Adolescence," with two subtypes: the emotionally withdrawn/inhibited subtype, in which the child showed little responsiveness to others and no discriminated attachments, and the indiscriminately social/disinhibited subtype, in which the child showed indiscriminate sociability or lack of selectivity in the choice of attachment figures, including attachment to unfamiliar adults and a pattern of social boundary violations. In DSM-5, RAD was recategorized as two distinct disorders within the trauma- and stressor-related disorders: RAD and disinhibited social engagement disorder (DSED). There are new empirical findings related to both disorders, and there is some consensus on the evidence base for methods of assessment and effective interventions (Zeanah et al. 2016).

Evidence Base

RAD or DSED can result from prolonged separation from a parent or caregiver at an early age, as described by John Bowlby (1951) and Rene Spitz (1946) and documented on film by James and Joyce Robertson (1952). Both disorders result from the absence of expectable caregiving; that is, they are the result of social neglect or other situations that limit a young child's opportunity to form selective attachments. Other than sharing this type of stressor affecting early development, the two disorders are phenomenologically distinct. Because of dampened positive affect, RAD (formerly known as the emotionally withdrawn/inhibited subtype of RAD) resembles internalizing disorders and converges modestly with depression. In contrast, DSED (formerly known as the indiscriminately social/disinhibited subtype of RAD) more closely resembles attention-deficit/hyperactivity disorder (ADHD) and converges modestly with it. RAD and DSED have different relationships to attachment behaviors. RAD is essentially equivalent to the lack of or incompletely formed preferred attachments to caregiving adults.

DSED, in contrast, can occur in children who lack attachments, who have established attachments, or who have secure attachments. The two disorders differ in correlates, course, and response to intervention, and for these reasons are differentiated in DSM-5 (Scott et al. 2018).

Reactive Attachment Disorder

Evaluation and Diagnosis

The diagnosis of RAD requires evidence of pervasively disturbed social relatedness before age 5 years. Several sources of information are required, including history, clinical evaluation, and confirmatory observations over time. The history usually includes prolonged separation, severe neglect and/or abuse, or living in institutional settings from an early age. Observations of the child with the parent or guardian can be made to assess the child's play behavior, acceptance of nurturance, and response to separation and other potential stressors. Videotaping and neuropsychological evaluation may be helpful.

DSM-5 describes the essential feature of RAD as absent or grossly underdeveloped attachment between the child and putative caregiving adults (Table 15–1). Children with RAD are believed to have the capacity to form selective attachments, but because of their early development, they fail to show such attachments. The disorder is associated with the absence of expected comfort seeking and response to comforting behaviors. These children show diminished or absent expression of positive emotions. Their capacity to regulate emotion is compromised, and they display episodes of fear, sadness, or irritability that are not readily explained. This diagnosis should not be made in children who are developmentally unable to form selective attachments; therefore, the child must be cognitively at least 9 months old.

Diagnosis is optimally made by interview, direct observation of behavior, and review of the child's history of or losses of primary caregiving. A validated instrument, the Relationship Problems Questionnaire (Vervoort et al. 2013), is useful for screening. Because of its etiological association with social neglect, RAD often co-occurs with delays in cognition and language. Additional features include stereotypies and other signs of severe neglect (e.g., malnutrition, signs of poor care). RAD is severe when a child exhibits all symptoms of the disorder, each at a relatively high level. It is chronic when it has been present for over 12 months.

Growing neurobiological research on RAD has demonstrated abnormalities such as decreased striatal (caudate and nucleus accumbens) neural reward activity, reduced white matter activity in the amygdala and prefrontal cortex, and reduced gray and white matter volumes. Earlier studies of institutionalized children not assessed for RAD suggested reduced blood levels of oxytocin and vasopressin and elevated cortisol.

Prevalence, Development, and Course

RAD may be more prevalent than generally recognized, with an estimate of 1.4% in a "deprived sector" of an urban center in the United Kingdom (Minnis et al. 2013). The disorder is seen relatively rarely in clinical settings. It has been found in young children exposed to severe neglect before being either placed in foster care or reared in institutions. A study of 94 maltreated toddlers evaluated 3 months after placement in foster care in New Orleans found RAD rates of 35% using ICD-10 (World Health Or-

TABLE 15–1.	Essential features of DSM-5 reactive attachment disorder

The child shows a pattern of inhibited, emotionally withdrawn behavior.

Persistent emotional and social disturbance is observed.

The child has experienced extremes of insufficient care, and this severe neglect is presumed to be the cause of the child's disturbed behavior.

Criteria are not met for autism spectrum disorder.

The disturbance is evident before age 5 years.

The child has a developmental age of at least 9 months.

Note. For the complete diagnostic criteria, please refer to pp. 265–266 in DSM-5 (American Psychiatric Association 2013).

ganization 1992) criteria (18% withdrawn type only and 17% mixed withdrawn and disinhibited type) (Zeanah et al. 2004). However, even in severely neglected children, the disorder is uncommon, occurring in fewer than 10% (Gleason et al. 2011).

Conditions of social neglect are often present in the first months of life, even before RAD is diagnosed. The clinical features of the disorder manifest in a similar fashion for children between the ages of 9 months and 5 years, but differing cognitive and motor abilities may affect how they are expressed. Without remediation and recovery through normative caregiving environments, the disorder may persist, at least for several years.

Serious social neglect is a diagnostic requirement for the disorder and is the only known risk factor, but fortunately, the majority of severely neglected children do not develop RAD. The prognosis appears to be dependent on the quality of the subsequent caregiving environment. It is unclear whether RAD occurs in older children; therefore, the diagnosis should be made with caution in children older than 5 years of age.

Disordered attachment behaviors similar to those observed in RAD have been described in young children in many different cultures. However, caution should be exercised in diagnosing RAD in cultures in which attachment has not been studied.

Differential Diagnosis

Although it is essential to distinguish autism spectrum disorder, intellectual disability (intellectual developmental disorder), and depressive disorders from RAD, evidence is increasing that comorbidity may occur. It is possible that autistic spectrum disorder should not be ruled out because it may be comorbid in children with intellectual deficiency; 14% of 102 children with intellectual disability also had RAD and autistic spectrum disorder (Giltaij et al. 2015). Conditions associated with neglect, including cognitive delays, language delays, stereotypies, and posttraumatic and depressive symptoms, may co-occur with RAD. The extent of the comorbidity of PTSD and of depressive disorders with RAD or DSED is not yet known. Zeanah et al. (2016) pointed out that "in depression, reduced positive affect and emotion regulation difficulties are similar to what is seen in RAD. There is no reason, however, to expect that the attachment behaviors of a young child with depression would be minimal to absent as is the case in RAD" (p. 993). Medical conditions (e.g., severe malnutrition) may accompany the disorder.

Interventions

The core elements of RAD treatment include facilitating the child's development through provision of emotionally available, consistent parents or other caretakers; encouraging formation of selective attachments; and providing a positively stimulating environment (Zeanah et al. 2016). Although there are no specific psychopharmacological treatments for the core features of RAD, comorbid conditions such as ADHD should be treated appropriately. For children who were previously maltreated, an assessment of the safety of their current placement is essential. Forensic involvement and foster placement may be necessary. Other intervention elements involve ensuring the child's safety with adequate housing, as well as providing pediatric care and treatment of medical illnesses; providing an appropriately nurturant caregiver to reverse the pervasive neglect and/or abuse; and, as children grow older, providing psychoeducation about the condition and psychotherapy, including various types of caregiver or parent–child dyadic therapy targeting the disturbed emotions and relationships.

Outcome

To date, children with RAD and DSED have been studied longitudinally only in the Bucharest Early Intervention Project (Nelson et al. 2014). The results showed that randomly selected young children who were removed from institutions and placed in foster care showed an early, substantial reduction in RAD symptoms compared with children who remained in institutions. After foster care placement at 22 months, the improvement by 30 months was so great that the children in the foster care group had levels of RAD symptoms comparable to those of children who had never been institutionalized and were living with their families. In contrast, children who remained in institutions continued to show stable signs of RAD through 8 years of age, and children with the longest institutional stays showed the highest levels of signs of RAD. It is not known whether RAD or DSED in childhood has long-term effects on adult development.

Despite the pervasiveness and severity of RAD, there have been few studies of treatment. Earlier interventions appear to have a greater likelihood of improving outcomes than later interventions. Cognitive and language development, motor development, and self-care are likely to improve, with less known about social development (Zeanah et al. 2016).

Disinhibited Social Engagement Disorder

Evaluation and Diagnosis

Although not as extensively studied as RAD, DSED has been described from age 1 through adolescence. As discussed in the introduction to these disorders of attachment, DSED was one of two subtypes of RAD in DSM-IV, but it is differentiated as a distinct disorder in DSM-5 (Table 15–2). Research on DSED is increasing. Lack of reticence or overly familiar social behavior forms the core of this disorder. A complicating factor is that children with DSED may or may not have selective attachment to a primary caregiver, with some studies showing none and others identifying secure attachment (Zeanah and Gleason 2015).

TABLE 15–2.   **Essential features of DSM-5 disinhibited social engagement disorder**

The child shows a pattern of behavior involving inappropriate readiness to approach and interact with strangers, exhibiting at least two of the following: reduced reticence with strangers, overly familiar behaviors, diminished checking back with adult caregiver, and willingness to go off with strangers.

The behavior is not limited to impulsivity but includes socially disinhibited behavior.

The child has experienced extremes of social neglect or deprivation (e.g., frequent changes of caregivers in foster care), and this pathogenic care is presumed to be responsible for the child's disturbed behavior.

The child has a developmental age of at least 9 months.

Note.   For the complete diagnostic criteria, please refer to pp. 268–269 in DSM-5 (American Psychiatric Association 2013).

Manifestations of DSED differ from childhood through adolescence. Across cultures, young children normally are reticent when interacting with strangers and often manifest stranger anxiety. Children with DSED fail to show reluctance to approach, engage with, and even go off with unfamiliar adults. In preschool children with DSED, verbal and social intrusiveness is prominent. Verbal and physical overfamiliarity continue throughout middle childhood. In adolescence, persons with DSED extend their indiscriminate behavior to peers, with more "superficial" peer relationships. Adult manifestations of DSED are unknown.

Prevalence, Differential Diagnosis, Interventions, and Outcome

The prevalence of DSED has been studied mainly using the DSM-IV disinhibited subtype of RAD. Among children in foster care or shared residential facilities, DSED prevalence appears to be as high as 20% (Gleason et al. 2011), may exceed that of RAD, and appears to be associated with maltreatment and out-of-home care between ages 7 and 24 months. Higher severity of DSED signs has been associated with greater numbers of disruptions in foster care placements and poorer performance in foster children with learning problems who had more school changes (Pears et al. 2010). The principal diagnostic differentiations for DSED are RAD and ADHD. In contrast to RAD, DSED occurs both in children lacking attachments and in those who have secure attachments.

As described earlier under RAD, treatment interventions are designed to provide emotionally available, consistent parents or other caretakers to improve the child's relatedness and interpersonal functioning, with the goal of eliminating this psychopathology when instituted in early life (Zeanah et al. 2016). In the absence of intervention, DSED has severe functional outcomes, including significant impairments in these children's interpersonal relationships with adults and peers. Trauma-focused therapies may be less effective in children with RAD or DSED because of these children's lack of social engagement (Overbeek et al. 2014).

Posttraumatic Stress Disorder

Diagnosis

Posttraumatic Stress Disorder in Adults, Adolescents, and Children Older Than Age 6 Years

Table 15–3 lists key features of the DSM-5 diagnostic criteria for PTSD in adults, adolescents, and children older than age 6 years. The Criterion A symptom cluster in DSM-5 describes the requisite exposure to the traumatic event. Emotional reactions to the traumatic event (e.g., fear, helplessness, horror) are no longer part of Criterion A. (Nevertheless, most PTSD patients report such reactions.) The criteria that follow A are of two types: 1) those that are specifically related to the traumatic event (the Criteria B and C symptom clusters, as well as Criteria D1 and D3) and 2) those that are not (Criteria D2, D4, D5, D6, and D7 and all of the Criterion E symptom cluster). The traumatic event–specific criteria are the more important ones. When a patient has experienced more than one traumatic event, how can one know that a specific alleged event was causative? The answer lies in the criteria that are specific to the traumatic event. Moreover, most of the criteria that are *not* specific to the traumatic event are shared by one or more other mental disorders, especially mood and anxiety disorders. In DSM-5, as in previous editions, PTSD is categorical (i.e., either PTSD is present or it is not); however, research suggests that posttraumatic psychopathology is dimensional.

Posttraumatic Stress Disorder in Children Age 6 Years and Younger

Because the evidence does not support use of adult criteria for PTSD in preschool children, diagnostic criteria for a new diagnostic subtype (PTSD for children age 6 years and younger) were added in DSM-5 (Table 15–4) (DeYoung and Scheeringa 2018). This change is an advance from the special developmental considerations provided in DSM-IV-TR (American Psychiatric Association 2000) for the specific diagnosis of PTSD in preschool children. Research with traumatized preschool children indicates that in comparison with older individuals, they require fewer criteria based on functional impairment from PTSD symptoms and they have somewhat different responses to stress. The criteria for PTSD in children younger than 6 years highlight symptom differences in this age group, such as demonstrating trauma reenactment through play and experiencing frightening dreams not clearly related to the traumatic event.

The diagnosis of PTSD in children age 6 years and younger requires fewer symptoms than for adults and older children. It requires one intrusion symptom, one avoidance or negative cognition or mood symptom, and two altered arousal and reactivity symptoms or behaviors. These diagnostic requirements reflect increasing data on behavioral signs as well as psychological symptoms in preschool children exposed to severe trauma such as sexual abuse and injuries, including burns, with significant impairment in function. It is estimated that every year, more than 30 million children age 6 years and younger are exposed to psychological trauma from injury, medical procedures, witnessing violence, and war (DeYoung and Scheeringa 2018). Worldwide,

TABLE 15–3. **Essential features of DSM-5 posttraumatic stress disorder for adults, adolescents, and children older than 6 years**

Exposure to actual or threatened death, serious injury, or sexual violence as follows:

Directly experiencing the trauma; witnessing it, in person, occurring to others; learning that it occurred to a close family member or friend; or experiencing repeated or extreme exposure to aversive details (e.g., witnessing a person with a severe burn; police exposed to details of child abuse) that are not from media, unless work related.

Presence of the following symptom types:

Intrusion symptoms (1 or more of 5 different types, including recurrent memories, dreams, dissociative reactions [e.g., flashbacks], psychological distress at reminders, marked physiological reactions to trauma cues or triggers)

Avoidance symptoms (one or both of 2 different types, including efforts to avoid distressing memories, thoughts, or feelings; or efforts to avoid external reminders)

Negative changes in cognitions and mood (2 or more of 7 different types, including inability to recall important parts of the trauma; negative beliefs about oneself, others, or the world; distorted cognitions leading to blaming oneself or others; negative emotional states; reduced interest in activities; detachment from others; inability to experience positive emotions)

Altered arousal and reactivity (2 or more of 6 different types, including irritability and anger, self-destructive behavior, hypervigilance, exaggerated startle, decreased concentration, disturbed sleep)

The disturbance has a duration greater than 1 month; causes clinically significant distress or impairment; and is not attributable to the effect of a substance or another medical condition.

Specify: Dissociative or delayed expression.

Note. For the complete diagnostic criteria, please refer to pp. 271–272 in DSM-5 (American Psychiatric Association 2013).

TABLE 15–4. **Essential features of DSM-5 posttraumatic stress disorder for children age 6 years and younger**

Exposure to death, serious injury, or sexual violence in one of the following ways:

Directly experiencing the trauma; witnessing it, in person, occurring to others, not in media, TV, movies, or pictures; learning that it occurred to a parent or caregiver.

One (or more) of the following symptoms of *intrusion* is present: recurrent distressing memories; distressing dreams; dissociation, which can occur in play reenactments; psychological or physiological distress at reminders.

One (or more) of the following symptoms is present, representing either *persistent avoidance of stimuli* or *negative changes in cognitions and mood:* avoidance of activities, places, people, or situations that arouse recollections; increased negative emotions, reduced interest in activities including constricted play, social withdrawal, or reduced positive emotions.

Two (or more) of the following symptoms of *altered arousal and reactivity* are present: irritability and anger, hypervigilance, increased startle, decreased concentration, or disturbed sleep.

The disturbance has a duration greater than 1 month; causes clinically significant distress or impairment; and is not attributable to the effect of a substance or another medical condition.

Specify: Dissociative or delayed expression.

Note. For the complete diagnostic criteria, please refer to pp. 280–281 in DSM-5 (American Psychiatric Association 2013).

this population is growing very rapidly. Significantly, most of these children do not meet adult criteria, which fail to identify many highly symptomatic young children.

Evidence Base

The formidable evidence base for the PTSD diagnosis is archived in the medical and psychological literature. A PubMed search of the medical subject heading term *stress disorders, posttraumatic* produced more than 30,000 references! Perhaps the best evidence supporting the reliability and validity of the diagnosis has come from the rigorously conducted DSM-IV PTSD field trials (Kilpatrick et al. 1998). In support of the validity of the PTSD diagnosis was the finding that few people developed the posttraumatic stress syndrome unless they had experienced one or more extremely stressful life events. Most people who developed PTSD also experienced substantial subjective emotional and physiological reactions to those events, often characterized as panic reactions. Only 11% of cases had symptom onset more than 6 months following the traumatic event (Kilpatrick et al. 1998).

The less-extensive field trials for the DSM-5 PTSD criteria focused on reliability among diagnosticians, which was quite satisfactory, with test–retest kappa results of approximately 0.66, which is better than those for most other DSM-5 disorders (Narrow et al. 2012; Regier et al. 2013). The prevalence of DSM-5 PTSD was comparable to that of DSM-IV PTSD. The four-factor (intrusion, avoidance, negative cognitions and mood, hyperarousal) symptom cluster model yielded a better fit for the data than did the previous DSM-IV three-factor model. This is not surprising, because most clinicians had already come to distinguish avoidance symptoms specific to the traumatic event from emotional numbing (the previous term for negative alterations in cognition and mood). Symptoms within each of the four clusters loaded well together (Friedman 2013).

Biological evidence (reviewed in the earlier section "Biology of Psychological Trauma and Posttraumatic Stress Disorder") also supports the validity of the PTSD diagnosis, with a number of markers significantly separating PTSD from non-PTSD subjects. For example, psychophysiological studies demonstrate the presence of "marked physiological reactions to internal or external cues that symbolize or resemble an aspect of the traumatic event(s)" (DSM-5 Criterion B5) in response to trauma-related audiovisual cues and during personal traumatic mental imagery in PTSD versus non-PTSD subjects.

Epidemiology

There are many cross-sectional studies of PTSD among special populations, including individuals who have undergone experiences such as exposure to combat, disasters, rape, or burns, but few large epidemiological studies in the general population. Most representative are those studies in the general population that set an expected baseline rate for the disorder. Studies in the United States are the most common and are cited here. The DSM versions used for diagnosis vary among the studies. The Epidemiological Catchment Area study, an early study using DSM-III criteria, found low lifetime prevalence rates of PTSD: 1.0% among 2,493 subjects in St. Louis, Missouri, and 1.3% among 2,985 subjects in North Carolina (Davidson et al. 1991; Helzer et al. 1987). However, this study employed a relatively insensitive diagnostic instrument. A U.S. telephone survey of 4,008 women using the National Women's Study PTSD module found that 12.3% of respondents (17.9% of those exposed to a traumatic event) had a lifetime history of PTSD (Resnick et al. 1993). The National Comorbidity Survey, using DSM-III-R (American Psychiatric Association 1987) criteria, found lifetime prevalence rates of 5% for males and 10.4% for females (Kessler et al. 1995). The subsequent National Comorbidity Replication Survey, using DSM-IV criteria, found a 12-month prevalence rate of 3.5% (Kessler et al. 2005). PTSD risk factors consistently identified in community studies have been female gender, low socioeconomic status, low educational levels, and exposure to physical assault or rape. In a study using data from a sample of 34,676 respondents reporting lifetime exposure to one or more traumas in the World Health Organization World Mental Health surveys, Kessler et al. () assessed the contribution of 14 lifetime DSM-IV mood, anxiety, disruptive behavior and substance disorders in predicting PTSD after subsequent trauma. They found that among the 14 disorders assessed, only a history of anxiety disorders significantly predicted PTSD in a multivariate model, with anxiety disorders showing significant interactions with three types of earlier trauma: having witnessed atrocities, having experienced physical violence in adulthood (≥18 years), and having been a victim of rape in adulthood (Kessler et al. 2018).

The incidence and prevalence of trauma- and stressor-related disorders vary depending on which diagnostic criteria are applied. Here we include available data on DSM-5 diagnostic criteria, earlier DSM criteria, and other criteria, such as those in ICD-11 (World Health Organization 2018). The World Health Organization is a primary source of epidemiological data.

The DSM-5 changes in criteria are clinically significant in that field studies indicated only a 55% correspondence between persons with DSM-5–diagnosed PTSD and persons diagnosed with PTSD by DSM-IV criteria (Hoge et al. 2014). In a study examining how well the ICD and DSM models of PTSD captured the symptoms of preadolescent children exposed to trauma, the ICD-11 model was shown in factor analysis to have the best fit, followed by the DSM-IV and DSM-5 models (La Greca et al. 2017); the analysis revealed poor overlap between DSM-5 and ICD-11, suggesting that use of only one model will likely fail to identify half of children with significant posttraumatic stress. DSM-5, ICD-11, and DSM-IV each identified children with substantial posttraumatic stress symptom severity, with DSM-5 identifying more groups with comorbidities needing clinical intervention.

Psychological traumatization and chronic stress may result in individuals who have experienced events conferring only a psychological impact (e.g., witnessing abuse), events with both psychological and physical impact (e.g., fires), and physical trauma with delayed psychological impact (e.g., traumatic brain injury). The trauma and stress may result from a single severe episode (e.g., a rape, a motor vehicle accident), or it may be continuous or complex, occurring over time (e.g., refugee trauma, a severe burn with extended treatment, chronic child or elder abuse).

Estimates of the lifetime prevalence of trauma exposure in the United States range from 39% to 90% (Breslau et al. 1991, 1998). These differences might be explained by real differences in trauma exposure across countries and cultures, but they are also attributable to differences in demographics—especially gender, income, and type of trauma—of the studied populations or in the methods of measuring or defining traumatic events. Finally, there may be cultural variations in the expression of trauma-related stress disorders, although PTSD has generally been found to be cross-culturally valid (Hinton and Lewis-Fernández 2011). Certain populations are especially at risk after traumatic events, as discussed in the following subsections. In addition, studies demonstrate psychological, social, and neurobiological factors contributing to either vulnerability or resilience to the effects of trauma (Southwick et al. 2015).

Children and Adolescents

Children and adolescents are at major risk following traumatic events. Preschool children are wholly dependent on parents and guardians for their well-being and therefore are especially vulnerable. Common traumas affecting children and adolescents include emotional and physical abuse, accidents, and the effects of war and disasters. In DSM-5, the developmental vulnerability of this population is reflected in the six trauma- and stressor-related conditions applying to children: RAD, DSED, acute stress disorder, adjustment disorder, PTSD (with a new subtype for children ages 6 years and younger), and persistent complex bereavement disorder (in DSM-5 Section III; under study).

As in adults, the prevalence of psychological trauma and stress in children and adolescents may be underreported. In studies of PTSD incidence among child survivors of disasters, rates of 30%–60% have been noted (Kaminer et al. 2005). Community studies in the United States consistently indicate that about 40% of high school students have witnessed or experienced trauma or violence, with about 3%–6% of those meeting PTSD criteria (Kaminer et al. 2005). Complex PTSD due to child maltreatment remains an area of research but is not a diagnosis in DSM-5 (Resick et al. 2012).

Women

Compared with men, women have a twofold greater overall risk of developing PTSD; among individuals deployed between 2004 and 2009, the lifetime prevalence was estimated as 8%–10% in women versus 4%–5% in men (Kessler et al. 1995; Pietrzak et al. 2011). Potential explanations for this large gender difference include differences in trauma exposure prevalence and types of trauma, such as greater exposure to sexual violence. Traumas that impair women's functioning may also undermine their capacity to care for their dependent children, compounding the impact of PTSD in mothers. Some research suggests that gender plays less of a role in occupations in which exposure levels are high, such as in military combat. Deployed female U.S. soldiers had a suicide rate that was more than three times the rate in nondeployed women in the U.S. military, whereas the rate in deployed men appeared to be similar to that in nondeployed men (Street et al. 2015). Factors hypothesized by the authors as potential contributors to the higher suicide rate in deployed women included lower levels of social support, recent (past 12 months) sexual assault victimization, and prior psychopathology. Research examining the contributions of potential differences in gender-based biological risk factors (e.g., estrogen) is ongoing (Glover et al. 2012; Maeng and Milad 2018; Ressler et al. 2011).

Injured and Medically Ill People

DSM-5 Criterion A for PTSD requires exposure to actual or threatened death, serious injury, or sexual violence. Although the presence of a life-threatening medical condition may not always meet this requirement, many acute medical experiences do, such as those involving sudden or catastrophic events. Nonetheless, increasing data suggest that PTSD symptoms are experienced by many medical and surgical patients, including those with cancer or stroke (Letamendia et al. 2012), as well as children and adults with injuries, burns, or other life-threatening illnesses (Davydow et al. 2008; Stoddard and Saxe 2001; Stoddard et al. 2017). PTSD has been reported to affect seriously injured soldiers at a rate of 12% (Grieger et al. 2006), and rates of PTSD are higher among service members with penetrating trauma (13%), blunt trauma (29%), or combination injuries (33%) (McLay et al. 2012). Behavioral and mental health stepped care for surgically hospitalized survivors of injury has been shown to reduce posttraumatic sequelae (Zatzick et al. 2013).

Older Adults

Elderly persons represent a relatively neglected, vulnerable, and growing population that is at major risk of trauma- and stress-related disorders. Epidemiological studies of trauma in the elderly are at an early stage but are increasing in response to reports of deaths and injuries in nursing facilities after hurricanes and disasters. Because of their frailty, impaired cognition, and dependence on caregivers, elderly persons may be particularly vulnerable to both psychological and physical neglect and abuse, a situation made more severe and life-threatening in the case of poverty, disaster, or war. On the other hand, research is identifying resilience in the elderly—for instance, in the Harvard Study of Adult Development, begun in 1938, which followed the emotional and physical health of 200 undergraduate men, including some who survived into their 90s (Vaillant 2012). In old age, the variability of response, continued development of character, coping skills, and often-remarkable resilience despite major difficulties in childhood and adulthood were shown in detailed longitudinal reports.

Military Populations

The military populations of the United States and its allies may be the most systematically studied regarding traumatic stressors, including both combat injury and sexual trauma. Epidemiological studies of soldiers have documented the importance of genetic factors, childhood trauma, proximity to event(s), and multiple deployments. Studies of PTSD in the U.S. military include studies of the neurobiology, epidemiology, and treatment of PTSD. Internationally, the epidemiology of PTSD and other disorders in military populations informs the need for resources dedicated to care of those in the armed services, veterans, and their families.

A study of 2,530 U.S. soldiers deployed to Iraq and 3,671 U.S. soldiers deployed to Afghanistan revealed PTSD rates of 6.2%–12.2% (Hoge et al. 2004). PTSD prevalence rates among active-duty military and veterans have varied on the basis of many factors, including the assessment methodology used (e.g., the PTSD Checklist for DSM-5 [PCL-5] vs. the Clinician-Administered PTSD Scale [CAPS]), the era of and time since service, and the DSM version of PTSD criteria used. For example, data from the National Health and Resilience Study, which used the PCL-5 in a civilian sample, found rates of probable PTSD ranging from 10.1% (sudden death of close family member or friend) to 28.0% (childhood sexual abuse) (Wisco et al. 2016). In contrast, Hoge et al. (2014), using the PCL-5 in an active-duty sample, reported that 18% screened positive for PTSD. The National Vietnam Veterans Longitudinal Study, conducted 40 years after the war, estimated a prevalence of 4.5% in male veterans based on CAPS criteria for a current PTSD diagnosis, compared with a prevalence of 11.2% based on PCL-5 criteria for current war-zone PTSD (Marmar et al. 2015). In the Millennium Cohort Study of 17,481 women in the U.S. military, those who were deployed in Iraq or Afghanistan had an increased risk (odds ratio 1.91; 95% confidence interval 1.65–2.20) of mental health conditions, including PTSD, compared with women in the army reserves or national guard, who had decreased risk (Seelig et al. 2012). Growing research is highlighting the role of military sexual assault in PTSD and its often-underrecognized or undertreated presence among both female and male service members and veterans.

Disaster Survivors

Regardless of age, survivors of disasters (natural or human-caused), including civilian war survivors, victims of terrorism, and those affected by acute climatic events, are at increased risk of traumatic stress, depending on the event's duration, the survivor's proximity to the event, and the event's impact on the community (Dodgen et al. 2016). Despite the many thousands of civilians affected by hurricanes, earthquakes, and many past and current wars, such survivors have been insufficiently studied. Nevertheless, available data indicate increased vulnerability for those with limited predisaster resources, with lasting psychological ill effects as a result of separation from loved ones; witnessing death or injury; being abused, injured, or disabled; or becoming a refugee (Stoddard et al. 2011a).

Survivors of Genocide

The effects of genocide on European Holocaust survivors and their families led the United Nations in 1948 to adopt the Universal Declaration of Human Rights. Although the United Nations has since been unsuccessful in preventing genocide in Cambodia, South Africa, Rwanda, Bosnia, Darfur, and elsewhere, international efforts continue. In the hope of preventing genocide and reducing its devastating psychological impacts, there is ongoing research on the long-term psychological and neurobiological (including epigenetic) effects on, the chronic health conditions affecting, and the resilience shown in survivors and their progeny (Yehuda et al. 2014).

People With Serious Mental Illness

Greater attention to the identification and treatment of PTSD among individuals with severe mental illnesses is needed. A racially and ethnically diverse population with severe mental illnesses had trauma exposure rates as high as 89%, with 41% of subjects meeting criteria for PTSD, which contributed to substantially poorer functioning (Subica et al. 2012). Patients with intellectual or developmental disabilities, schizophrenia, mood disorders, or other mental illnesses are vulnerable to a range of stressors, made worse in disasters if they lose access to their medications or mental health services. Traumatic stress is an important factor in the etiology of mental illnesses other than PTSD, such as borderline personality disorder. Individuals who abuse substances are also at high risk of PTSD, because use of/dependence on substances, particularly alcohol, may be involved in 34% (Zatzick et al. 2017) to 54% (Soderstrom et al. 1997) of serious physical traumas.

Developmental Considerations

The symptoms and sequelae of traumatic stress vary across the life span, with the effects being more long-lasting the younger the person is. Different stages of psychological and neurobiological development render an individual subject to differing impacts of stress on aspects such as emotion, cognitive processing, memory, motor and sensory function, neural and synaptic growth, and gene expression. Although seeking to capture some of this complexity, DSM-5 is but one step in the ongoing quest to improve categorization of the complex effects of trauma and stress on the human organism.

Evaluation

Because of the well-recognized tendency of PTSD patients to avoid painful recollections of psychologically traumatic events, superficial questioning may fail to elicit legitimate symptoms. Conversely, premature direct inquiries into the specific PTSD diagnostic criteria may be treated by some patients (who for whatever reason are motivated to obtain a PTSD diagnosis) as a series of leading questions evoking answers that too readily lead to precisely that. The interviewer should begin by asking the patient to describe the problems he or she has been experiencing, providing only as much direction as necessary to keep the information flowing and to prevent tangents. The interviewer should carefully consider the report of a patient who mentions few or no symptoms consistent with PTSD while talking at length about his problems, yet answers positively to all PTSD symptoms during subsequent direct questioning. The interviewer should ask the patient who reports nightmares or intrusive recollections to describe several of these in as much detail as possible. Convincing personal details of symptoms support the diagnosis more than do recitations from a textbook.

While eliciting the history, the interviewer should pay close attention to the patient's behavior as part of the mental status examination. Some PTSD symptoms, such as irritability, difficulty concentrating, and an exaggerated startle reflex, may be directly observed. Of special relevance is the degree to which the patient displays consistent emotion while describing the traumatic event and its consequences.

Following the nondirective portion of the interview, the interviewer should conduct a directive interview. Because of potential avoidance on the patient's part, it may be insufficient merely to ask the patient whether he or she has ever experienced a psychologically traumatic event. Rather, the interviewer may need to ask whether the patient has ever experienced any of various kinds of traumatic events that potentially cause PTSD. Checklists and questionnaires are available, for example, the Trauma History Questionnaire. A comprehensive evaluation requires that the interviewer, after identifying one or more traumatic events in the patient's history, inquire as far as possible into each PTSD diagnostic criterion for each event in question, as well as into the criteria for other mental disorders that potentially enter into the differential diagnosis. To assist in this task, structured interview instruments for clinician use (originally designed for research use) are available specifically for PTSD, such as the CAPS for DSM-5 (CAPS-5), as well as for most other mental disorders, such as the Structured Clinical Interview for DSM-5 (First et al. 2016).

In addition to instruments offering a categorical determination of the presence or absence of the PTSD diagnosis, several instruments, including the CAPS-5, have been developed to provide a continuous measure of PTSD symptom severity in the form of a total score, as well as a subscore for each PTSD symptom cluster, consistent with a dimensional approach to PTSD. Importantly, instruments administered by the clinician (as opposed to a technician) do not require the interviewer to score an item positive just because the interviewee answers affirmatively. Rather, it is the clinician's responsibility to determine through probing whether the detailed historical data satisfy the symptomatic criterion in question.

A number of self-rated psychological questionnaires and psychometric tests for PTSD are available. Foremost among these is the PCL-5. In contrast to clinician-administered instruments, which filter the patient's answers through the clinician's judgment, these paper-and-pencil or computer-administered tests generate a score for each item from the patient's response, with a diagnostic cutoff for total score suggested. These tests are highly vulnerable to either symptom exaggeration or symptom under-reporting by patients. Some of the best-known personality tests (e.g., the Minnesota Multiphasic Personality Inventory–2, the Personality Assessment Inventory) include PTSD scales as well as validity scales to detect symptom over- or underreporting. Perhaps the bottom line for self-report tests is that although they may be useful for screening and for providing ancillary information to confirm or call into question the interviewer's opinion, they should not be used as stand-alone tests for the PTSD diagnosis when time and resources are available for the use of a structured interview instrument.

An advantage of questionnaires and psychological tests is that they can be administered remotely. Telemedicine is becoming increasingly popular and widely used, especially by the U.S. Department of Veterans Affairs, to provide persons located in remote locations access to medical, including psychiatric, diagnosis and treatment. Initial studies suggest that structured interview instruments, such as the CAPS-5, can be conducted by video teleconferencing with acceptable reliability (Litwack et al. 2014).

Treatment

Psychotherapeutic Interventions

Every practice guideline emphasizes the central role of psychotherapeutic interventions (summarized later) in both the prevention and treatment of PTSD (U.S. Department of Veterans Affairs and U.S. Department of Defense 2017). Psychosocial interventions for PTSD should be the primary form of intervention, with an emphasis on evidence-based, manualized, trauma-focused therapies that include an exposure or cognitive restructuring component, assuming the patient is willing. For situations in which trauma-focused psychotherapy is not available, the U.S. Department of Veterans Affairs and U.S. Department of Defense (VA/DoD) *Clinical Practice Guideline for Management of Post-Traumatic Stress* (2017) concluded that insufficient evidence exists to determine whether non-trauma-focused therapies or pharmacotherapies are more effective; however, the guideline suggested that pharmacotherapy as a first-line intervention for PTSD should be reserved for individuals with comorbidities, targeting specific symptom clusters, or based on patient preference. For children, psychotherapy involves therapists engaging in therapeutic play targeted toward diagnostic and therapeutic goals, including trauma-focused therapies, and employing digital games and media, which are in constant use by children today with beneficial effects as well as risks (Meersand and Gilmore 2018).

Early intervention and prevention strategies. Evidence for preventive interventions for trauma survivors remains limited, and more research is needed. Although the most effective primary prevention in PTSD is clearly to reduce exposure to traumatic events such as violence, accidents, and injury, efforts to bolster resilience prior to trauma exposure may also reduce the incidence of PTSD, but more research is needed prior to recommending any specific intervention. Secondary prevention consists of early intervention following a trauma. The most studied interventions are psychological debriefing and CBT. Although once believed to be effective, psychological debriefing—particularly the form consisting of single-session critical incident stress debriefing—has been shown not to reduce PTSD incidence or symptom severity; for some, it may even be harmful, in that it may disrupt naturally occurring coping mechanisms (Rose et al. 2002; van Emmerik et al. 2002). Thus, trauma-exposed individuals who are not seeking help for symptoms should not be required to undergo debriefing of their experiences in group or individual-session formats, although psychoeducation about typical trauma responses may be helpful.

Although the preventive efficacy of CBT for asymptomatic trauma survivors has not been well studied, multisession CBT has been recommended for trauma survivors with acute trauma symptoms consistent with acute stress disorder, and there is evidence that it may provide some benefit to those with subthreshold symptoms. In a meta-analysis and systematic review of acute stress disorder, brief trauma-focused supportive therapy was found to be the most effective therapy for reducing PTSD symptom severity (Roberts et al. 2009, 2010). A randomized controlled trial of three sessions of a modified prolonged exposure intervention initiated within hours of presentation to an emergency department after a trauma regardless of symptoms also found significantly lower posttraumatic stress reactions 4 and 12 weeks posttrauma, suggesting that individually targeted CBT-based interventions may help prevent the development of PTSD (Rothbaum et al. 2012). It is worth noting, however, that implementing this intervention in an emergency setting requires the availability of well-trained and experienced therapists, not to mention willing patients.

Although there has been growing research into early intervention with pharmacotherapy, including trials with agents such as the selective serotonin reuptake inhibitor (SSRI) antidepressant escitalopram and the β-blocker propranolol, studies to date have failed to find a strong level of randomized controlled trial evidence for any specific pharmacotherapy. As a result, recent guidelines from the VA/DoD (2017) and other entities have not included such agents in their recommendations. For benzodiazepines in particular, these and other guidelines have raised concerns about potential harm, because these agents may be addictive and may interfere with trauma recovery and extinction learning. Preliminary studies (Holbrook et al. 2010; Saxe et al. 2001; Stoddard et al. 2011b) suggest that early management of pain after injury, possibly with morphine, may be protective against posttraumatic symptoms in people who have experienced physical trauma and that hydrocortisone may also be helpful acutely.

Psychotherapies.   *Adults.*   Manualized, trauma-focused individual psychotherapies that include CBT approaches such as exposure or cognitive restructuring are recommended as the first-line treatment for PTSD on the basis of the amount of currently available evidence. CBT approaches generally target emotional processing of the trauma to enhance extinction, focusing on decreasing avoidance behaviors and reducing negative emotional reactivity. CBT approaches may also include cognitive work focused on distorted beliefs about the self and safety that may arise as a result of the trauma. These treatments build on the notions that PTSD is a condition of impeded recovery from an acute reaction to trauma and that much of the psychopathology centers on failure of extinction of fear responses, as well as development of maladaptive cognitions and avoidance behaviors that interfere with recovery. In addition, growing knowledge about abnormalities in the neurocircuitry of PTSD, memory, and the stress

HPA axis suggests potential roles for trauma-focused CBT in restoring normal function to these systems (Ross et al. 2017). Psychoeducation about PTSD is an additional important initial component of all CBT approaches, and some approaches also teach stress management techniques such as breathing and relaxation skills (U.S. Department of Veterans Affairs and U.S. Department of Defense 2017).

The CBT approaches with the greatest amount of evidence supporting efficacy include prolonged exposure therapy and cognitive processing therapy; each has shown satisfactory treatment results across a range of populations with PTSD, including PTSD after sexual assault or combat trauma. Prolonged exposure therapy focuses most prominently on 1) repeated imaginal exposure to the primary trauma memories to enhance extinction, generally over the course of weekly 90-minute sessions, and 2) in vivo exposures to decrease cue reactivity and avoidance. Although not every aspect of a single trauma or every traumatic experience following multiple experiences is necessarily included in exposure work in session, the positive effects on decreased cue reactivity and overall reduction in PTSD symptoms often generalize. In some cases, however, a clinician may select more than one trauma as a target of exposure within a treatment, sequentially starting with the most disturbing one. Variations of this therapy include shorter 60-minute sessions. In addition, virtual reality–enhanced exposure, such as that involving scenes from combat situations in Iraq, has also demonstrated efficacy (e.g., see Rothbaum et al. 2014). Although the data currently do not support greater efficacy than for prolonged exposure therapy alone, virtual reality may help patients with difficulty engaging with the trauma memory and might enhance the generalization of extinction outside the therapist's office. Prolonged exposure therapy may be associated early in treatment with heightened anxiety as patients begin to expose themselves to feared and avoided memories. Extinction of reactivity to trauma cues occurs over time, as patients learn that they do not need to fear the memories or their emotional responses to them.

In contrast to prolonged exposure therapy, the original version of cognitive processing therapy used a written account of the traumatic experience and also focused on reshaping dysfunctional cognitive beliefs that often interfere with recovery. More recent data suggest that the cognitive component alone may be effective (Resick et al. 2008), and the manual has been updated (Resick et al. 2017a) without the written exposure component. Typical maladaptive thoughts targeted in cognitive processing therapy include self-blame and guilt, as well as exaggerated beliefs about safety, self-worth, and control.

Unfortunately, although prolonged exposure therapy and cognitive processing therapy are the evidence-based therapies with the greatest amount of empirical support for treating PTSD, with impressive effect sizes from a statistical standpoint, their actual benefits are only partial and tend to decrease over time. Meta-analyses (Bisson et al. 2013; Tran and Gregor 2016) are consistent in finding improvements in PTSD symptoms of less than 50%, with long-term benefits being even lower. More research is needed on bolstering the benefits of these established treatments or finding effective alternatives.

The 2017 VA/DoD guidelines suggested that other specific CBTs for PTSD, including brief eclectic psychotherapy, narrative exposure therapy, written narrative exposure, and eye movement desensitization and reprocessing (EMDR), can all be beneficial as a PTSD treatment, with EMDR having the most supporting data of these and efficacy similar to that of prolonged exposure therapy. EMDR involves trauma recall, emotional processing, and cognitive reappraisal strategies accompanied by eye movement tracking or other forms of bilateral stimulation. Results of dismantling studies, however, suggest that neither eye movements nor bilateral sensory stimulation is required for the therapeutic benefits of EMDR. EMDR purports to offer patients additional coping strategies to process and handle traumatic memories while retaining awareness of the safety of their present state. The other specific CBTs for PTSD each integrate some form of exposure and/or cognitive restructuring with additional emotion processing or narrative integration techniques (U.S. Department of Veterans Affairs and U.S. Department of Defense 2017).

Because these trauma-focused therapies are not always accessible and are sometimes not acceptable to patients, studies have identified non-trauma-focused therapies that have some but weaker support in treating PTSD. These include stress inoculation training, present-centered therapy, and interpersonal psychotherapy. Stress inoculation training aims to transform thinking patterns that lead to stress in daily life, present-centered therapy focuses on the problems in a patient's life that relate to PTSD, and interpersonal psychotherapy examines how the trauma has affected the patient's relationships. Treatment effects for these therapies are not as large as those for trauma-focused therapies, but they are better than those for the no-treatment condition and are associated with lower dropout rates. Other therapies such as skills training in affect and interpersonal regulation, acceptance and commitment therapy, dialectical behavior therapy, Seeking Safety (for comorbid PTSD and substance use), and supportive counseling may also play a role for some patients with PTSD and may address associated issues, but additional evidence is needed to determine their optimal roles.

Other psychotherapeutic interventions include group CBT, family therapy, couples therapy, and interpersonal or psychodynamic therapy. Although preferable to no therapy, group therapies have been found to be less effective than individual therapies in reducing PTSD symptoms, despite being comparably effective for reducing depression and suicidal ideation (Resick et al. 2017b). A version of cognitive processing therapy was adapted to be delivered in the context of a couple, with treatment addressing PTSD in the affected person as well as related interpersonal issues. Although it does not yet have sufficient evidence to be recommended by guidelines as a first-line treatment, cognitive-behavioral conjoint therapy for PTSD may be helpful for people who are resistant to seeking care alone, or those for whom relationship concerns are central or for whom adaptations of the partner to the PTSD symptoms (e.g., supporting avoidance behaviors) are interfering with recovery. Given the significant impact of PTSD on relationship functioning, there is a need for more research examining outcomes with trauma-focused couples interventions that integrate approaches such as emotion regulation skills.

Finally, when present, comorbid conditions such as alcohol abuse need to be addressed in the context of treatment. Available data supporting the different psychotherapy treatment approaches to PTSD, as well as a number of other treatment approaches, are summarized in the 2017 VA/DoD guidelines and in other treatment guidelines such as those of the American Psychological Association (Courtois et al. 2017). The Institute of Medicine in 2014 recommended that evidence-based treatments should be used with fidelity to their manuals. Although clinicians use a combination of evidence, clinical judgment, and patient preference in practice when matching treatments to patients, more research is needed to support an evidence-based personalized medicine approach to help guide the selection of PTSD treatments based on a patient's individual clinical and biological characteristics.

Children.   Clinical assessment and subsequent psychotherapeutic treatments are the preferred interventions for PTSD and trauma-related stress disorders in children and adolescents, as in adults. The first-line evidence-based psychotherapeutic treatments include trauma-focused CBT, prolonged exposure, Trauma Systems Therapy, EMDR, and similar therapies (Cohen et al. 2017). However, skilled clinicians able to provide some of these may not be easily accessible.

Pharmacological and Other Somatic Therapeutic Approaches

Adults.   Psychopharmacotherapy is a second-line treatment choice for PTSD after psychotherapy. Its problems include lower efficacy; adverse side effects, which sometimes lead to nonadherence; and the need, at least for most drugs, for long-term administration, sometimes indefinitely, in order for the patient to continue to reap the benefits. Nevertheless, pharmacotherapy is often tried first because of its ease of administration and/or a lack of availability of qualified psychotherapists. Pharmacotherapy is based on trial and error to find the best drug for a given patient. Once a drug is begun, it should be continued for 2 or 3 months when possible before abandoning it as a failure and trying something else. The dosage should be gradually increased as tolerated until side effects develop or until the maximum benefit has been achieved. At least 1 year of treatment is recommended before attempting discontinuation. If the patient relapses, the drug may need to be resumed.

The best-validated drugs for PTSD are the antidepressants. Despite their name, it is not necessary for the patient to have a comorbid depressive diagnosis for these drugs to work (when they do). Antidepressants include SSRIs, serotonin–norepinephrine reuptake inhibitors, tricyclic antidepressants (TCAs), monoamine oxidase inhibitors, and miscellaneous agents. SSRIs are recommended as the psychopharmacological treatment of choice for PTSD and represent the standard of care in many treatment guidelines because of their safety and (relative) efficacy. Although the SSRIs sertraline and paroxetine are the only drugs with an indication for PTSD from the U.S. Food and Drug Administration (FDA), there is no evidence to support their superiority over the numerous other SSRIs that are on the market for other indications. Guidelines and precautions for the choice and administration of an antidepressant medication for the treatment of PTSD, including warnings for possible increase in suicide risk, are the same as those for the treatment of depression and are not repeated here.

Another medication for the treatment of PTSD is the α_1-adrenergic antagonist prazosin, commonly used to treat hypertension. Given the problem of sympathetic overdrive in PTSD (reviewed in the earlier section "Biology of Psychological Trauma and Posttraumatic Stress Disorder"), this treatment would seem logical. Prazosin appears to be uniquely beneficial in the treatment of trauma-related nightmares, and it has been increasingly prescribed for this purpose. Recently, however, because of mixed evidence, the 2017 VA/DoD guidelines did not include prazosin monotherapy in its pharmacotherapy recommendations. α_2-Adrenergic agonists and β-adrenergic antagonists have not been shown to be useful in PTSD (except perhaps as described below for the latter). A nonpharmacological approach to reduce sympathetic overdrive that is receiving experimental attention is stellate ganglion block (Peterson et al. 2017).

The evidence base for other conventional nonantidepressant psychopharmacological agents for PTSD, including antipsychotics and anticonvulsants/mood stabilizers, is weak. However, unique secondary clinical manifestations of PTSD, such as agitation, violence, and mood swings, may sometimes call for their use. Also, occasionally, an individual PTSD patient may benefit from a drug even though group comparisons do not support its efficacy. Although many uninformed clinicians automatically reach for a benzodiazepine when treating a PTSD patient, this class of medication has been found to be both ineffective and problematic, with the potential for dependency and abuse, especially when taken with alcohol. Except in rare instances, benzodiazepines are generally regarded as contraindicated in PTSD.

Notable among the new classes of drugs that are being tried is the N-methyl-D-aspartate receptor antagonist ketamine, which, when administered in parenteral, subanesthetic doses, has been found to exert rapid antidepressant effects. Early results in PTSD have been promising (Kim and Mierzwinski-Urban 2017). The street drug MDMA (3,4-methylenedioxymethamphetamine), commonly known as Ecstasy, is also being tried concomitantly with psychotherapy. It has been claimed to help patients tolerate recalling their traumatic memories, but more research is needed (Schenk and Newcombe 2018).

Two novel drug treatments have been developed on the basis of neuroscientific insights into the disorder. Fear extinction is thought to be a mechanism of action of exposure therapy. PTSD has been characterized as involving a deficit in the retention of fear extinction. This theory has led to the use of the extinction memory enhancer D-cycloserine as a psychotherapy augmenter. Despite the initial excitement sparked by this clever idea, the benefit for PTSD has turned out to be small or nonexistent (Mataix-Cols et al. 2017). The second novel treatment based on neuroscientific insight derives from the discovery that when a consolidated, or stabilized, memory is activated by retrieval, it may, under certain circumstances, revert to an unstable state and need to be "reconsolidated" if it is to be retained. Propranolol is one of several so-called amnestic drugs that can block this process. Administration of propranolol simultaneously with traumatic memory retrieval has been found in open-label studies (Brunet et al. 2011) and one randomized controlled trial (Brunet et al. 2018) to reduce PTSD symptoms.

Transcranial magnetic stimulation (TMS) is a means of altering regional brain activity by applying a focused magnetic field over the scalp, producing electric currents in underlying brain tissue. It is approved by the FDA for the treatment of refractory MDD. As reviewed elsewhere in this chapter (see earlier section "Biology of Psychological Trauma and Posttraumatic Stress Disorder"), PTSD is characterized by excessive activity in certain brain regions and deficient activity in others. This suggests that the disorder might benefit from TMS. Unfortunately, most of the brain regions implicated in posttraumatic pathology are too deep to be directly accessible by TMS. Nevertheless, TMS is being used in PTSD with the dorsolateral prefrontal cortex as a target in the hope that activation of this region will have secondary effects on key brain regions implicated in PTSD, analogous to a combination shot in pocket billiards. Meta-analysis findings support TMS's efficacy in PTSD, but with a smaller effect than that for CBT (Trevizol et al. 2016). However, many patients may only be given TMS after psychotherapy has failed, which could bias against obtaining positive results for TMS (or any other second treatment) in such a population of possibly treatment-refractory persons.

Children and adolescents. Psychopharmacology is a second-line treatment for PTSD and trauma- and stressor-related disorders that is commonly used for patients with moderate to severe symptoms and functional impairment, often with accompanying comorbid conditions, in pediatric and child mental health clinics, hospitals, court clinics, detention centers, prisons, and outpatient settings. However, despite years of widespread use of medications in the treatment of PTSD and trauma- and stressor-related disorders in young and older children by pediatricians, nurses, and child psychiatrists, a robust evidence base for medications from randomized controlled trials is lacking, as described by Jani et al. (2018). A major clinical research priority is to expand the evidence base. As is the case for psychopharmacological studies in adults, most studies in children have evaluated only short-term outcomes; as a result, long-term benefits or risks of medications in children are largely unknown.

The American Academy of Child and Adolescent Psychiatry (AACAP) practice parameter (Cohen et al. 2010) noted that α- and β-adrenergic blocking agents, novel antipsychotic agents, non-SSRI antidepressants, TCAs, and mood-stabilizing agents might be effective for children on the basis of findings from open clinical trials. However, there is no updated AACAP guideline or FDA approval for a medication treatment of PTSD or trauma- and stressor-related disorders, although SSRIs such as fluoxetine and escitalopram have limited FDA approval for depression and obsessive-compulsive disorder. SSRIs do not have the risk of cardiac arrhythmia associated with TCAs, but they, and all antidepressants, have a black box warning for suicidality and mania. One trial of imipramine and chloral hydrate found that imipramine may reduce PTSD symptoms in children (Robert et al. 1999). However, risks of arrhythmia, mood change, and overdose limit the use of TCAs.

The AACAP (Cohen et al. 2010) cautioned that because of possible hyperarousal with irritability, poor sleep, or inattention, SSRIs may not be an optimal treatment for children with PTSD when used alone in the absence of psychotherapy (Robb et al. 2010). Therefore, the AACAP advised beginning with trauma-focused CBT and adding an SSRI if severity of symptoms indicates a need for more interventions (Cohen et al. 2010). Sertraline was found to have no benefit for PTSD treatment but may have a marginal benefit, on the basis of parent report, in preventing PTSD when administered soon after a burn injury in childhood (Stoddard et al. 2011c).

Other than SSRIs, there are no alternative medications for consideration. Despite wide clinical use of these agents, no evidence-based study has established the benefit of benzodiazepines, propranolol, or clonidine for PTSD. No evidence-based study supports the efficacy of antipsychotics in the treatment of childhood PTSD. Metabolic syndrome with weight gain and type 2 diabetes are among the risks associated with use of atypical antipsychotics in children. Although clonidine may be beneficial in reducing arousal and anxiety, it carries significant cardiovascular risk.

Most traumatized children, including many not diagnosed with trauma- and stressor-related disorders, require collaborative multimodal care with psychotherapists, psychopharmacologists, school, and family. Medication considerations should take into account informed consent by the parent or guardian, accompanying assent by adolescent patients when appropriate, potential short- and long-term benefits or risks for a child's well-being and development associated with lack of treatment versus providing treatment (e.g., symptom worsening vs. reduction in symptoms), potential adverse effects (e.g., metabolic syndrome), and drug interactions. New analytic methods have identified variables for targeted interventions for children, such as physiological reactivity, numbness, and exaggerated startle, and for teens, sleep difficulties, nightmares, avoidance of thoughts/feelings, and anger/irritability (Russell et al. 2017; Saxe et al. 2016).

Complementary and Alternative Medicine Therapies

Despite growing interest in complementary and alternative medicine therapies for PTSD, limited research has examined such approaches, and most of the research to date has had methodological flaws. Some findings suggest that meditation techniques may yield improvements in PTSD symptom severity and quality of life. Meditation may be a secondary or supplemental option for both clinicians and patients, partly because of its very low risks and its potential additional beneficial effects on quality of life (Benedek and Wynn 2016).

Outcome

Outcome data from longitudinal studies of PTSD are mixed. According to DSM-5, complete recovery from PTSD occurs within 3 months in approximately 50% of cases, although many individuals have symptoms lasting for more than 1 year. In contrast, the 1996 Detroit Area Survey of Trauma found that the median time to PTSD symptom remission was 24.9 months after onset (Breslau et al. 1998). A study of the U.S. general population found that PTSD symptoms persisted for longer than 60 months in more than one-third of individuals (Kessler et al. 1995).

Acute Stress Disorder

Diagnosis

Acute stress disorder (ASD) was added in DSM-IV to identify clinically significant posttraumatic symptomatology that developed within 1 month of a traumatic event. The diagnosis was introduced in 1994 because of the observation that certain symptoms appeared to predict the development of PTSD. In DSM-IV-TR, criteria for ASD required the presence of at least three of five dissociative symptoms. Otherwise, the criteria were similar to the criteria for PTSD, with one of six reexperiencing symptoms, marked avoidance, and marked anxiety or increased arousal also required. In DSM-5 (Table 15–5), the ASD diagnosis requires the presence of at least 9 of 14 symptoms in any of five categories—intrusion symptoms, negative mood, dissociative symptoms, avoidance symptoms, and arousal symptoms—beginning or worsening after the traumatic event and persisting for 3 days (instead of the 2 days required in DSM-IV) to 1 month after the trauma. (The threshold of 9 of 14 symptoms is based on an analysis of data from Israel, the United Kingdom, and Australia [Bryant et al. 2011]. Thus, the diagnosis of ASD in DSM-5 still includes, but no longer requires, dissociative symptoms.)

Evidence Base

To differentiate normal, adaptive reactions to acute stress within 48 hours of exposure to combat or disasters from ASD, the term *acute stress reaction* or *combat stress reaction*

TABLE 15–5.	Essential features of DSM-5 acute stress disorder

Exposure to actual or threatened death, serious injury, or sexual violation as follows:

Directly experiencing the trauma; witnessing it, in person, occurring to others; learning that it occurred to a close relative or friend; or extreme exposure to aversive details that is not from media, TV, movies, or pictures, unless work related.

Presence of nine (or more) posttrauma symptoms from any of the five categories of intrusion, negative mood, dissociation, avoidance, and arousal.

The disturbance has a duration of 3–30 days, starting immediately after the trauma; causes clinically significant distress or impairment; is not attributable to the effects of a substance or another medical condition; and is not better explained by a brief psychotic disorder.

Note. For the complete diagnostic criteria, please refer to pp. 280–281 in DSM-5 (American Psychiatric Association 2013).

was used to describe symptoms of stress within that early period (Friedman et al. 2011). The rationale for diagnosing ASD beginning 2 days and for up to 1 month after a traumatic event was justified, first, by the common clinical manifestation of significant acute stress symptomatology that resolves within 1 month and, second, by the acute presence of dissociation, which has been associated with the development and chronicity of PTSD. Dissociation has not, however, been demonstrated to be a necessary independent predictor of PTSD diagnosis, and the majority of people with PTSD do not meet criteria for ASD requiring dissociation. Given that the early emphasis on dissociation as the sine qua non for ASD has not been supported by subsequent research, the evidence base is dubious for even having a separate acute stress diagnosis at all, rather than just allowing PTSD to be diagnosed at any time following the traumatic event, no matter how early.

Epidemiology

The prevalence of ASD after a severe traumatic event is highly variable across studies and types of traumatic exposures and populations.

Assessment and Differential Diagnosis

Clinical assessment of the acutely traumatized patient often requires behavioral observation, careful history taking, and listening to the patient's narrative for symptomatology consistent with ASD. Therapeutic aspects of an assessment by an interested, listening clinician may contribute to the patient's feeling understood and better explaining the symptoms he or she is experiencing. After an acute traumatic event, patients may be unable for psychological or medical reasons to report their symptoms, and repeated evaluations are often necessary.

In addition to more time-consuming full diagnostic measures, several brief instruments are available for ASD screening in children or adults. One instrument used to screen children for ASD is the Child Stress Reaction Checklist, and two scales used to assess intrusive symptoms in adults are the Impact of Event Scale–Revised and the Acute Stress Disorder Scale.

Differential diagnosis should include potentially treatable contributors to posttraumatic symptoms, such as preexisting illness (including PTSD), infection, metabolic disturbance, side effects of pharmacotherapies (e.g., morphine), neurological injury after head trauma, and psychoactive substance (e.g., alcohol) use disorders or withdrawal.

Adjustment Disorders

Diagnosis

In both DSM-5 and ICD-11, adjustment disorders were classified for the first time within trauma- and-stressor-related disorders, along with PTSD and ASD. According to DSM-5 diagnostic criteria (summarized in Table 15–6), an adjustment disorder requires the development of clinically significant emotional or behavioral symptoms in response to an identifiable stressor. The symptoms must occur within 3 months of the onset of the stressor (Criterion A) and must resolve within 6 months after the stressor is removed (Criterion E). Adjustment disorders can be specified as one of six subtypes: 1) with depressed mood, 2) with anxiety, 3) with mixed anxiety and depressed mood, 4) with disturbance of conduct, 5) with mixed disturbance of emotions and conduct, and 6) unspecified.

For DSM-5, three major changes from the DSM-IV-TR adjustment disorder diagnosis were considered: 1) addition of an ASD/PTSD subtype, 2) addition of a bereavement-related subtype, and 3) removal of the bereavement exclusion (Criterion D). These changes would have required adjustments to symptom duration requirements to differentiate the acute stress and PTSD subtypes and to accommodate the extended (≥12 months) symptom persistence of the bereavement-related subtype, which was meant to identify a syndrome of prolonged or complicated grief, a new condition with a growing evidence base (Shear et al. 2016). The ASD/PTSD and bereavement-related subtypes were ultimately not added to the official diagnostic criteria (Strain and Friedman 2011). Persistent complex bereavement disorder ultimately was placed under "Conditions for Further Study" in DSM-5 Section III and was also referenced as a subtype of *other specified* or *unspecified trauma- and stressor-related disorder* (see section with that title below). Criterion D ("The symptoms do not represent normal bereavement") was also clarified as an exclusion only when symptoms are explained by normal bereavement on the basis of what would be expected when cultural, religious, or age-appropriate norms for intensity, quality, and persistence of grief reactions are taken into account. Depending on symptom duration, subsyndromal but chronic PTSD-like presentations could also potentially be assigned a diagnosis of adjustment disorder, unspecified, or could be recorded under the *other specified trauma- and stressor-related disorder* category of "adjustment-like disorders with prolonged duration of more than 6 months without prolonged duration of stressor."

Evidence Base

Despite the fact that the adjustment disorder diagnosis is commonly applied in clinical practice, the diagnosis has been a topic of debate since its initial inclusion in DSM-III-R. Points of controversy have included the absence of a specific symptom profile, the differentiation of adjustment disorders from normal responses to stressors, symptom overlap with other psychiatric disorders, difficulty standardizing assessments or interventions when the condition is not clearly defined, and the lack of stability of the

TABLE 15–6.   **Essential features of DSM-5 adjustment disorders**

Development of emotional or behavioral symptoms in response to an identifiable stressor.

The emotional or behavioral symptoms are clinically significant, with marked distress out of proportion to the severity of the stressor and/or significant impairment in important areas of functioning.

The disturbance does not meet criteria for another mental disorder; is not merely an exacerbation of a preexisting mental disorder; and does not represent normal bereavement.

The symptoms do not persist longer than an additional 6 months after the stressor has terminated.

Subtype specifiers include With depressed mood, With anxiety, With disturbance of conduct, and Unspecified.

Note.   For the complete diagnostic criteria, please refer to pp. 286–287 in DSM-5 (American Psychiatric Association 2013).

diagnosis over time. These issues have contributed to the current lack of a robust empirical evidence base supporting the adjustment disorder diagnosis.

Because an adjustment disorder, like PTSD and ASD, requires the presence of a stressful event that results in clinically significant symptoms, distress, or impairment, adjustment disorders are now classified in DSM-5 with other trauma- and stressor-related conditions to clarify that these disorders are associated with negative outcomes such as suicide and therefore may require acute intervention. This conceptualization is clinically useful, although the evidence base remains limited and the range of potential stressors and symptom profiles is broad. Also, many individuals diagnosed with adjustment disorders have symptom profiles that overlap with but are subsyndromal for DSM mood and anxiety disorder diagnoses. The stressor itself can also vary dramatically. Whereas bereavement-related depression could have been coded as an adjustment disorder in DSM-IV, the bereavement exclusion was dropped from the diagnostic criteria for MDD in DSM-5, in part because of data showing that MDD that is triggered by a loss does not differ significantly from MDD that is triggered by other life stressors. Studies examining potential differences in symptoms and associated impairment based on type of stressor are not yet available for adjustment disorders.

Epidemiology

Although robust epidemiological studies are lacking and available data have limitations, it is estimated that adjustment disorder has a prevalence of 0.9%–2.3% in the general population, with much higher rates in medical populations (Casey 2014). For example, a meta-analysis of 27 studies involving patients undergoing cancer treatment found a prevalence rate of 19% (Mitchell et al. 2011). Adjustment disorders are frequently diagnosed in clinical psychiatric and primary care populations, but more research is needed to determine definitive prevalence rates.

Evaluation

Because of the lack of specific symptom requirements for adjustment disorders (see Table 15–6), the diagnosis requires clinical judgment. Adjustment disorders provide a useful category to allow clinicians to treat clinically distressed individuals who do not meet other diagnostic criteria. Although depression scales are sometimes used, this limited specification has made standardized symptom severity assessments difficult to develop. Adjustment disorders are included in structured clinical interviews such as the Mini-International Neuropsychiatric Interview Plus 7.0 and the Structured Clinical Interview for DSM-5.

More recently, a self-report assessment instrument for adjustment disorders titled Adjustment Disorders–New Module was developed using not DSM specifically but rather the new ICD-11 diagnostic concept of adjustment disorders (Bachem et al. 2017). This instrument includes the two proposed ICD-11 core symptoms of 1) preoccupations and 2) failure to adapt, as well as questions about anxiety, depression, avoidance, and impulse disturbance. This measure has been found to be reliable and valid, but more data in clinical and research settings on optimal assessments for adjustment disorders are needed.

Treatment

Given that adjustment disorders have been associated with an elevated risk for suicide, any patient with this diagnosis should receive a careful safety assessment and treatment plan. Empirical support for the treatment of adjustment disorders is limited, however. Brief psychological interventions have been suggested as the first-line treatment and are actively being studied and developed. There is limited evidence for the benefits of pharmacological, herbal, and alternative remedies (Casey 2014). In instances in which subsyndromal subtypes of conditions such as MDD and PTSD meet DSM-5 criteria for adjustment disorders, therapies used for those conditions may be useful. Research on targeting of specific symptom clusters within adjustment disorder subtypes may provide future guidance to clinicians for treatment of adjustment disorders.

Psychological Interventions

Apart from ongoing supportive therapy for persistent stressors, brief therapies are considered the most appropriate psychological interventions for adjustment disorders (Casey 2014). Some controlled data on individuals with work-related stress suggest that cognitive therapy may be effective (van der Klink et al. 2003). However, a meta-analysis of nine studies found that among employees with adjustment disorders, cognitive therapy did not reduce the number of days out before return to work in comparison with no treatment. On the other hand, problem-solving therapy did reduce the time to partial return to work (Arends et al. 2012). Lacking an ample evidence base to guide treatment recommendations, clinicians in practice use a range of individual or group approaches, including psychodynamic, cognitive, behavioral, interpersonal, couples and family, and mindfulness-based interventions; exercise; and problem-solving approaches. It may be that some treatments best target specific types of stressors; for example, three randomized controlled trials (K. Shear et al. 2005; M.K. Shear et al. 2014, 2016) supported the efficacy of complicated grief therapy, a targeted psychotherapy, for individuals with this condition (see discussion of persistent complex bereavement disorder in the "Other Specified or Unspecified Trauma- and Stressor-Related Disorder" section near the end of this chapter). Additional research is needed to study optimal psychological interventions for each adjustment disorder subtype.

Pharmacological Interventions

Very limited data are available on pharmacological agents for adjustment disorders, although studies of pharmacotherapy approaches (e.g., antidepressants for subsyndromal depressive and anxiety disorders) may apply. Symptomatic treatment of insomnia and anxiety with benzodiazepines is common; however, some evidence suggests that benzodiazepines, in addition to having abuse potential, may worsen outcomes in trauma-exposed individuals, as noted previously, and thus are not recommended for use in patients with ASD and PTSD (Guina et al. 2015).

A few studies have focused on the anxiety subtype of adjustment disorder. For example, one randomized controlled trial found evidence that etifoxine, a nonbenzodiazepine anxiolytic, had efficacy comparable to the SSRI alprazolam (Stein 2015). Randomized controlled studies of herbal remedies and alternative interventions such as yoga suggest potential benefits from these approaches; however, no empirical data support the use of one type of treatment over another.

Outcome

Spontaneous Resolution

According to DSM-5, removal of the precipitating stressor should result in symptom remission within 6 months, with a good outcome. If symptoms persist beyond 6 months, the "adjustment-like disorder with prolonged duration" subtype could be recorded under the *other specified trauma- and stressor-related disorder* category in DSM-5.

Complications and Comorbidity

An adjustment disorder diagnosed in adolescence may eventually develop into a major mental disorder, as symptoms in the adjustment disorder may reach criteria thresholds for other mood and anxiety disorders. Adjustment disorders are associated with elevated levels of suicidal ideation and behaviors. Alcohol and other substance use disorders may be common in individuals with adjustment disorders and should be carefully assessed. The combination of substance use and maladaptive emotional responses to stressors may place individuals at even greater risk for suicide or other impulsive behaviors and therefore require careful clinical assessment and monitoring.

Other Specified or Unspecified Trauma- and Stressor-Related Disorder

The residual categories *other specified trauma- and stressor-related disorder* and *unspecified trauma- and stressor-related disorder* may be applied to presentations in which symptoms characteristic of a trauma- and stressor-related disorder are present and cause clinically significant distress or impairment but do not meet full criteria for any of the disorders in this diagnostic class. For an "other specified" designation, the clinician provides the specific reason that full criteria are not met. For an "unspecified" designation, no reason need be given, allowing use of this category in situations such as initial presentation to an emergency department.

DSM-5 lists five examples of presentations for which an "other specified" designation might be appropriate: adjustment-like disorders with 1) delayed onset of symptoms that occur more than 3 months after the stressor or 2) prolonged duration of more than 6 months without prolonged duration of stressor; 3) *ataque de nervios* and 4) other cultural syndromes defined in the "Glossary of Cultural Concepts of Distress" in the DSM-5 Appendix (see also Chapter 44 in this volume, "Culturally Diverse Patients"); and 5) persistent complex bereavement disorder (listed in "Conditions for Further Study" in Section III of DSM-5 and described in greater detail in the next section). It is possible that these categories will change or move as research adds to their evidence base. For example, substantial data support the diagnosis and targeted treatment of the persistent impairing form of grief.

Persistent Complex Bereavement Disorder

Grief after the death of a loved one may have a level of intensity and persistent symptom complications that are not consistent with normal bereavement, but rather suggest that natural recovery from acute grief has stalled. Although bereavement can trigger other conditions such as MDD or PTSD (when the death is violent or accidental), a growing literature has recognized a syndrome of persistent grief-related symptoms associated with high levels of distress, significant impairment in functioning, and elevated risk for suicide. This condition has been termed *complicated grief* and sometimes *traumatic grief* or *prolonged grief.*

A persistent and impairing form of grief has been studied in both children (Kaplow et al. 2012) and adults (e.g., M.K. Shear et al. 2011), with overlapping but not identical definitions. Although additional epidemiological research is needed, prevalence rates of prolonged grief across available studies have been estimated as 2%–4% among adults in the general population and 9.8% among those bereaved by natural causes (Lundorff et al. 2017). Furthermore, three randomized controlled trials now support the efficacy of complicated grief treatment, a targeted psychotherapy for adults, including older adults, with complicated grief; this treatment has been shown to have greater efficacy for grief and suicidal ideation than antidepressant pharmacotherapy (K. Shear et al. 2005; M.K. Shear et al. 2014, 2016). Other cognitive-behavioral grief-focused approaches also appear to be effective, suggesting that patients with the condition may benefit from a specific targeted psychotherapy.

In addition to being listed as an example of a presentation for which an "other specified trauma- and stressor-related disorder" designation might be appropriate, persistent complex bereavement disorder has been placed in Section III of DSM-5, "Conditions for Further Study," to indicate the need for additional research before its acceptance as a formal DSM diagnosis. Because of conflicting criteria proposed from previous studies, the DSM-5 Work Group developed a new criteria set, using elements of previous research, prior to full endorsement of this condition. However, growing data in this field support the likelihood that a version of this diagnosis will be advanced to formal inclusion as a trauma- and stressor-related condition in future versions of DSM. Some specifics—such as whether 6 months or 1 year is optimal as the minimum time frame for diagnosis—have remained under discussion. Recently, ICD-11 released clinically useful criteria under the name *prolonged grief disorder,* with 6 months as the minimum time frame (Killikelly and Maercker 2018); this criteria set is more inclusive than the current DSM-5 criteria set for persistent complex bereavement disorder (Boelen et al. 2019) and is similar to criteria sets for complicated grief proposals, with differences largely explained by the number of required symptoms (Cozza et al. 2019). For now, ICD-11 criteria can help clinicians identify patients presenting with persistent grief-related distress and impairment, who should be carefully assessed, monitored for suicide risk, and offered targeted treatment.

Conclusion

Although PTSD has been a formal diagnosis only since 1980, the history of trauma and stress overwhelming individuals' capacity to cope or, in some fortunate cases, stimulating resilience extends into the distant past. The biology of PTSD is well defined, and genetic determinants are being discovered. Most DSM-5 diagnoses included among the trauma- and stressor-related disorders are very prevalent, especially affecting children, women, the elderly, the injured and/or ill, members of the armed services, refugees, and disaster survivors. In DSM-5, the trauma- and stressor-related disorders category is now distinct from anxiety, obsessive-compulsive, and dissociative disorders. It is the only category of disorders directly connected to a psychologically traumatic or stressful event (even though such events may lead to alternative or comorbid disorders, such as depression). The disorders in this category are ASD, PTSD, RAD, DSED, adjustment disorders, and (under further study) persistent complex bereavement disorder.

Psychological interventions have a prominent place in the treatment of each of the trauma- and stressor-related disorders. For PTSD, psychopharmacological interventions also have a place (albeit a lesser one), with SSRIs as the first line of treatment.

Outcome studies of PTSD and related conditions indicate that these disorders often persist and, if not treated, have poor outcomes and require long-term care. There is an associated higher risk of physical morbidity and even mortality. Trajectories of individuals who are more resilient versus those at higher risk with more posttraumatic symptoms are being examined (Tsai and Pietrzak 2017), and study findings are helping to differentiate individuals with posttraumatic growth (as measured by the Posttraumatic Growth Inventory [Tedeschi and Calhoun 1996]) and more positive outcomes from those with greater functional impairment. Such studies will inform future prevention and treatment approaches. Among promising new interventions with potential broad application internationally for diagnosis and treatment of children and adults are those using telemental health (Augusterfer et al. 2015).

Key Clinical Points

- All trauma- and stressor-related disorders, especially acute stress disorder, posttraumatic stress disorder (PTSD), and adjustment disorder, are prevalent worldwide, are influenced by individual vulnerability and resilience, and may have poor outcomes without treatment.

- Evidence-based targeted psychotherapies (first line) and, if needed, psychopharmacological treatment (second line) are partially effective for PTSD.

- DSM-5 included a new subtype, PTSD for children age 6 years and younger, that highlights symptom differences in this age group based on developmental evidence.

- Two categories replaced the former diagnosis of reactive attachment disorder in infancy or early childhood: reactive attachment disorder (RAD) and disinhibited social engagement disorder (DSED).

- A bereavement-related subtype of adjustment disorders was considered for inclusion in Section II of DSM-5. Instead, however, persistent complex bereavement disorder was listed as a presentation for which an "other specified trauma- and stressor-related disorder" designation might be appropriate, and proposed criteria were placed in Section III of DSM-5 as a condition for further study.

References

Adler A: Neuropsychiatric complications in victims of Boston's Cocoanut Grove disaster. JAMA 123:1098–1101, 1943

American Psychiatric Association: Diagnostic and Statistical Manual of Mental Disorders, 3rd Edition. Washington, DC, American Psychiatric Association, 1980

American Psychiatric Association: Diagnostic and Statistical Manual of Mental Disorders, 3rd Edition, Revised. Washington, DC, American Psychiatric Association, 1987

American Psychiatric Association: Diagnostic and Statistical Manual of Mental Disorders, 4th Edition. Washington, DC, American Psychiatric Association, 1994

American Psychiatric Association: Diagnostic and Statistical Manual of Mental Disorders, 4th Edition, Text Revision. Washington, DC, American Psychiatric Association, 2000

American Psychiatric Association: Diagnostic and Statistical Manual of Mental Disorders, 5th Edition. Arlington, VA, American Psychiatric Association, 2013

Arends I, Bruinvels DJ, Rebergen DS, et al: Interventions to facilitate return to work in adults with adjustment disorders. Cochrane Database Syst Rev (12):CD006389, 2012 23235630

Augusterfer EF, Mollica RF, Lavelle J: A review of telemental health in international and post-disaster settings. Int Rev Psychiatry 27(6):540–546, 2015 26576720

Bachem R, Perkonigg A, Stein DJ, Maercker A: Measuring the ICD-11 adjustment disorder concept: validity and sensitivity to change of the Adjustment Disorder–New Module questionnaire in a clinical intervention study. Int J Methods Psychiatr Res 26(4), 2017 27862575

Banerjee SB, Morrison FG, Ressler KJ: Genetic approaches for the study of PTSD: advances and challenges. Neurosci Lett 649:139–146, 2017 28242325

Benedek DM, Wynn GH (eds): Complementary and Alternative Medicine for PTSD. New York, Oxford University Press, 2016

Bisson JI, Roberts NP, Andrew M, et al: Psychological therapies for chronic post-traumatic stress disorder (PTSD) in adults. Cochrane Database Syst Rev (12):CD003388, 2013 24338345

Boelen PA, Lenferink LIM, Smid GE: Further evaluation of the factor structure, prevalence, and concurrent validity of DSM-5 criteria for Persistent Complex Bereavement Disorder and ICD-11 criteria for Prolonged Grief Disorder. Psychiatry Res 273:206–210, 2019 30654306

Bowlby J: Maternal care and mental health. Bull World Health Organ 3(3):355–533, 1951 14821768

Breslau N, Davis GC, Andreski P, Peterson E: Traumatic events and posttraumatic stress disorder in an urban population of young adults. Arch Gen Psychiatry 48(3):216–222, 1991 1996917

Breslau N, Kessler RC, Chilcoat HD, et al: Trauma and posttraumatic stress disorder in the community: the 1996 Detroit Area Survey of Trauma. Arch Gen Psychiatry 55(7):626–632, 1998 9672053

Brunet A, Poundja J, Tremblay J, et al: Trauma reactivation under the influence of propranolol decreases posttraumatic stress symptoms and disorder: 3 open-label trials. J Clin Psychopharmacol 31(4):547–550, 2011 21720237

Brunet A, Saumier D, Liu A, et al: Reduction of PTSD symptoms with pre-reactivation propranolol therapy: a randomized controlled trial. Am J Psychiatry 175(5):427–433, 2018 29325446

Bryant RA, Friedman MJ, Spiegel D, et al: A review of acute stress disorder in DSM-5. Depress Anxiety 28(9):802–817, 2011 21910186

Burns K, Novick L: The Vietnam War. Written by Ward GC. PBS television, 2017

Casey P: Adjustment disorder: new developments. Curr Psychiatry Rep 16(6):451, 2014 24748555

Cobb S, Lindemann E: Neuropsychiatric observations. Ann Surg 117(6):814–824, 1943 17858228

Cohen JA, Bukstein O, Walter H, et al: Practice parameter for the assessment and treatment of children and adolescents with posttraumatic stress disorder. J Am Acad Child Adolesc Psychiatry 49(4):414–430, 2010 20410735

Cohen J, Mannarino A, Deblinger E: Treating Trauma and Traumatic Grief in Children and Adolescents, 2nd Edition. New York, Guilford, 2017

Courtois CA, Sonis J, Brown LS, et al: Clinical practice guideline for the treatment of posttraumatic stress disorder (PTSD) in adults. Washington, DC, American Psychological Association, 2017. Available at: https://www.apa.org/ptsd-guideline/ptsd.pdf. Accessed October 17, 2018.

Cozza SJ, Shear MK, Reynolds CF, et al: Optimizing the clinical utility of four proposed criteria for a persistent and impairing grief disorder by emphasizing core, rather than associated symptoms. Psychol Med Mar 4, 2019 [Epub ahead of print] 30829195

Davidson JR, Hughes D, Blazer DG, George LK: Post-traumatic stress disorder in the community: an epidemiological study. Psychol Med 21(3):713–721, 1991 1946860

Davydow DS, Gifford JM, Desai SV, et al: Posttraumatic stress disorder in general intensive care unit survivors: a systematic review. Gen Hosp Psychiatry 30(5):421–434, 2008 18774425

DeYoung AC, Scheeringa MS: Posttraumatic stress disorder in children six years and younger, in Trauma- and Stressor-Related Disorders. Edited by Stoddard FJ, Benedek DM, Milad MR, et al. New York, Oxford University Press, 2018, pp 85–102

Dodgen D, Donato D, Kelly N, et al: Mental health and well-being, in The Impacts of Climate Change on Human Health in the United States: A Scientific Assessment. Washington, DC, U.S. Global Change Research Program, 2016, pp 217–246

First MB, Williams JBW, Karg RS, Spitzer RL: Structured Clinical Interview for DSM-5 Disorders—Clinician Version (SCID-5-CV). Arlington, VA, American Psychiatric Association, 2016

Foa EB, Hembree EA, Cahill SP, et al: Randomized trial of prolonged exposure for posttraumatic stress disorder with and without cognitive restructuring: outcome at academic and community clinics. J Consult Clin Psychol 73(5):953–964, 2005 16287395

Freud S: Introductory Lectures on Psycho-Analysis, Part III (1916–1917), in The Standard Edition of the Complete Psychological Works of Sigmund Freud, Volume 16. Translated and edited by Strachey J. London, Hogarth Press and the Institute of Psycho-Analysis, 1963, pp 243-483

Friedman MJ: Finalizing PTSD in DSM-5: getting here from there and where to go next. J Trauma Stress 26(5):548–556, 2013 24151001

Friedman MJ, Resick PA, Bryant RA, et al: Classification of trauma and stressor-related disorders in DSM-5. Depress Anxiety 28(9):737–749, 2011 21681870

Gilbertson MW, Shenton ME, Ciszewski A, et al: Smaller hippocampal volume predicts pathologic vulnerability to psychological trauma. Nat Neurosci 5(11):1242–1247, 2002 12379862

Giltaij HP, Sterkenburg PS, Schuengel C: Psychiatric diagnostic screening of social maladaptive behaviour in children with mild intellectual disability: differentiating disordered attachment and pervasive developmental disorder behaviour. J Intellect Disabil Res 59(2):138–149, 2015 23906477

Gleason MM, Fox NA, Drury S, et al: Validity of evidence-derived criteria for reactive attachment disorder: indiscriminately social/disinhibited and emotionally withdrawn/inhibited types. J Am Acad Child Adolesc Psychiatry 50(3):216–231.e3, 2011 21334562

Glover EM, Jovanovic T, Mercer KB, et al: Estrogen levels are associated with extinction deficits in women with posttraumatic stress disorder. Biol Psychiatry 72(1):19–24, 2012 22502987

Grieger TA, Cozza SJ, Ursano RJ, et al: Posttraumatic stress disorder and depression in battle-injured soldiers. Am J Psychiatry 163(10):1777–1783; quiz 1860, 2006 17012689

Guina J, Rossetter SR, DeRhodes BJ, et al: Benzodiazepines for PTSD: a systematic review and meta-analysis. J Psychiatr Pract 21(4):281–303, 2015 26164054

Gurvits TV, Metzger LJ, Lasko NB, et al: Subtle neurologic compromise as a vulnerability factor for combat-related posttraumatic stress disorder: results of a twin study. Arch Gen Psychiatry 63(5):571–576, 2006 16651514

Hawn SE, Sheerin CM, Lind MJ, et al: GxE effects of FKBP5 and traumatic life events on PTSD: a meta-analysis. J Affect Disord 243:455–462, 2019 30273884

Helzer JE, Robins LN, McEvoy L: Post-traumatic stress disorder in the general population: findings of the Epidemiologic Catchment Area survey. N Engl J Med 317(26):1630–1634, 1987 3683502

Herman J: Trauma and Recovery: The Aftermath of Violence From Domestic Abuse to Political Terror. New York, Basic Books, 1992

Hinton DE, Lewis-Fernández R: The cross-cultural validity of posttraumatic stress disorder: implications for DSM-5. Depress Anxiety 28(9):783–801, 2011 21910185

Hoge CW, Castro CA, Messer SC, et al: Combat duty in Iraq and Afghanistan, mental health problems, and barriers to care. N Engl J Med 351(1):13–22, 2004 15229303

Hoge CW, Riviere LA, Wilk JE, et al: The prevalence of post-traumatic stress disorder (PTSD) in US combat soldiers: a head-to-head comparison of DSM-5 versus DSM-IV-TR symptom criteria with the PTSD checklist. Lancet Psychiatry 1(4):269–277, 2014 26360860

Holbrook TL, Galarneau MR, Dye JL, et al: Morphine use after combat injury in Iraq and posttraumatic stress disorder. N Engl J Med 362(2):110–117, 2010 20071700

Horowitz MJ: Stress Response Syndromes, 2nd Edition. New York, Jason Aronson, 1986

Hughes KC, Shin LM: Functional neuroimaging studies of post-traumatic stress disorder. Expert Rev Neurother 11(2):275–285, 2011 21306214

Institute of Medicine: Treatment for Posttraumatic Stress Disorder in Military and Veteran Populations: Final Assessment. Report Brief, June 2014. Washington, DC, Institute of Medicine of the National Academies, 2014. Available at: http://nationalacademies.org/hmd/~/media/Files/Report%20Files/2014/PTSD-II/PTSD-II-RB.pdf. Accessed October 17, 2018.

Jani S, Herringa R, Hursey D: Pharmacologic treatment of children with trauma and stressor-related disorders, in Trauma- and Stressor-Related Disorders. Edited by Stoddard FJ, DM Benedek DM, Milad MR, et al. New York, Oxford University Press, 2018, pp 283–309

Kaminer D, Seedat S, Stein DJ, et al: Post-traumatic stress disorder in children. World Psychiatry 4(2):121–125, 2005 16633528

Kaplow JB, Layne CM, Pynoos RS, et al: DSM-V diagnostic criteria for bereavement-related disorders in children and adolescents: developmental considerations. Psychiatry 75(3):243–266, 2012 22913501

Kessler RC, Sonnega A, Bromet E, et al: Posttraumatic stress disorder in the National Comorbidity Survey. Arch Gen Psychiatry 52(12):1048–1060, 1995 7492257

Kessler RC, Berglund P, Demler O, et al: Lifetime prevalence and age-of-onset distributions of DSM-IV disorders in the National Comorbidity Survey Replication. Arch Gen Psychiatry 62(6):593–602, 2005 15939837

Kessler RC, Aguilar-Gaxiola S, Alonso J, et al: The associations of earlier trauma exposures and history of mental disorders with PTSD after subsequent traumas. Mol Psychiatry 23(9):1–8, 2018 28924183

Killikelly C, Maercker A: Prolonged grief disorder for ICD-11: the primacy of clinical utility and international applicability. Eur J Psychotraumatol 8 (suppl 6):1476441, 2018 29887976

Kilpatrick DG, Resnick HS, Freedy JR, et al: Posttraumatic stress disorder field trial: evaluation of the PTSD construct—Criteria A through E, in DSM-IV Sourcebook, Vol 4. Edited by Widiger TA, Frances AJ, Pincus HA, et al. Washington, DC, American Psychiatric Association, 1998, pp 803–846

Kim J, Mierzwinski-Urban M: Ketamine for Treatment-Resistant Depression or Post-Traumatic Stress Disorder in Various Settings: A Review of Clinical Effectiv0eness, Safety, and Guidelines [Internet]. Rapid Response Report: Summary with Critical Appraisal. Ottawa (ON), Canadian Agency for Drugs and Technologies in Health, March 2017. Available at: https://www.ncbi.nlm.nih.gov/books/NBK487455/. Accessed January 29, 2019.

Koenen KC, Sumner JA, Gilsanz P, et al: Post-traumatic stress disorder and cardiometabolic disease: improving causal inference to inform practice. Psychol Med 47(2):209–225, 2017 27697083

La Greca AM, Danzi BA, Chan SF: DSM-5 and ICD-11 as competing models of PTSD in preadolescent children exposed to a natural disaster: assessing validity and co-occurring symptomatology. Eur J Psychotraumatol 8(1):1310591, 2017 28451076

Lang PJ: Imagery in therapy: an information processing analysis of fear. Behav Ther 8(5):862–886, 1977 27816081

Letamendia C, Leblanc NJ, Pariente J, et al: Peritraumatic distress predicts acute posttraumatic stress disorder symptoms after a first stroke. Gen Hosp Psychiatry 34(5):e11–e13, 2012 22542052

Lifton RJ: Survivors of Hiroshima. New York, Random House, 1967

Lindemann E: Symptomatology and management of acute grief: 1944. Am J Psychiatry 151 (6 suppl):155–160, 1994 8192191

Litwack SD, Jackson CE, Chen M, et al: Validation of the use of video teleconferencing technology in the assessment of PTSD. Psychol Serv 11(3):290–294, 2014 24841510

Lundorff M, Holmgren H, Zachariae R, et al: Prevalence of prolonged grief disorder in adult bereavement: a systematic review and meta-analysis. J Affect Disord 212:138–149, 2017 28167398

Maeng LY, Milad MR: PTSD in women: sex differences and gonadal hormones, in Trauma- and Stressor-Related Disorders. Edited by Stoddard FJ, Benedek DM, Milad MR, Ursano RJ. New York, Oxford University Press, 2018, pp 188–197

Marmar CR, Schlenger W, Henn-Haase C, et al: Course of posttraumatic stress disorder 40 years after the Vietnam war: findings from the National Vietnam Veterans Longitudinal Study. JAMA Psychiatry 72(9):875–881, 2015 26201054

Mataix-Cols D, Fernández de la Cruz L, Monzani B, et al: D-Cycloserine augmentation of exposure-based cognitive behavior therapy for anxiety, obsessive-compulsive, and posttraumatic stress disorders: a systematic review and meta-analysis of individual participant data. JAMA Psychiatry 74(5):501–510, 2017 [Erratum in: JAMA Psychiatry 74(5):542, 2017] 28122091

McLay RN, Webb-Murphy J, Hammer P, et al: Post-traumatic stress disorder symptom severity in service members returning from Iraq and Afghanistan with different types of injuries. CNS Spectr 17(1):11–15, 2012 22790113

Meersand P, Gilmore KJ: Play in the digital age, in Play Therapy: A Psychodynamic Primer for the Treatment of Young Children. Arlington, VA, American Psychiatric Association Publishing, 2018, pp 91–122

Minnis H, Macmillan S, Pritchett R, et al: Prevalence of reactive attachment disorder in a deprived population. Br J Psychiatry 202(5):342–346, 2013 23580380

Mitchell AJ, Chan M, Bhatti H, et al: Prevalence of depression, anxiety, and adjustment disorder in oncological, haematological, and palliative-care settings: a meta-analysis of 94 interview-based studies. Lancet Oncol 12(2):160–174, 2011 21251875

Mowrer OH: On the dual nature of learning: a re-interpretation of "conditioning" and "problem-solving." Harvard Educational Review 17:102–148, 1947

Narrow WE, Clarke DE, Kuramoto SJ, et al: DSM-5 field trials in the United States and Canada, III: development and reliability testing of a cross-cutting symptom assessment for DSM-5. Am J Psychiatry 170(1):71–82, 2012 23111499

Nelson CA, Fox NA, Zeanah CH: Romania's Abandoned Children? Deprivation, Brain Development, and the Struggle for Recovery. Cambridge, MA, Harvard University Press, 2014

Nemeroff CB, Marmar C: Post-Traumatic Stress Disorder. Oxford, UK, Oxford University Press, 2018

Overbeek MM, de Schipper JC, Lamers-Winkelman F, Schuengel C: Risk factors as moderators of recovery during and after interventions for children exposed to interparental violence. Am J Orthopsychiatry 84(3):295–306, 2014 24827024

Pace TW, Heim CM: A short review on the psychoneuroimmunology of posttraumatic stress disorder: from risk factors to medical comorbidities. Brain Behav Immun 25(1):6–13, 2011 20934505

Parsons RG, Ressler KJ: Implications of memory modulation for post-traumatic stress and fear disorders. Nat Neurosci 16(2):146–153, 2013 23354388

Pears KC, Bruce J, Fisher PA, Kim HK: Indiscriminate friendliness in maltreated foster children. Child Maltreat 15(1):64–75, 2010 19502477

Peterson K, Bourne D, Anderson J, et al: Evidence Brief: Effectiveness of stellate ganglion block for treatment of posttraumatic stress disorder (PTSD). VA Evidence-based Synthesis Program Evidence Briefs [Internet]. Washington, DC, U.S. Department of Veterans Affairs, February 2017. 28742302

Pietrzak RH, Goldstein RB, Southwick SM, et al: Prevalence and Axis I comorbidity of full and partial posttraumatic stress disorder in the United States: results from wave 2 of the National Epidemiologic Survey on Alcohol and Related Conditions. J Anxiety Disord 25(3):456–465, 2011 21168991

Pitman RK, Rasmusson AM, Koenen KC, et al: Biological studies of post-traumatic stress disorder. Nat Rev Neurosci 13(11):769–787, 2012 23047775

Regier DA, Narrow WE, Clarke DE, et al: DSM-5 field trials in the United States and Canada, II: test-retest reliability of selected categorical diagnoses. Am J Psychiatry 170(1):59–70, 2013 23111466

Resick PA, Galovski TE, O'Brien Uhlmansiek M, et al: A randomized clinical trial to dismantle components of cognitive processing therapy for posttraumatic stress disorder in female victims of interpersonal violence. J Consult Clin Psychol 76(2):243–258, 2008 18377121

Resick PA, Bovin MJ, Calloway AL, et al: A critical evaluation of the complex PTSD literature: implications for DSM-5. J Trauma Stress 25(3):241–251, 2012 22729974

Resick PA, Monson CM, Chard KM: Cognitive Processing Therapy for PTSD: A Comprehensive Manual. New York, Guilford, 2017a

Resick PA, Wachen JS, Dondanville KA, et al: Effect of group vs individual cognitive processing therapy in active-duty military seeking treatment for posttraumatic stress disorder: a randomized clinical trial. JAMA Psychiatry 74(1):28–36, 2017b 27893032

Resnick HS, Kilpatrick DG, Dansky BS, et al: Prevalence of civilian trauma and posttraumatic stress disorder in a representative national sample of women. J Consult Clin Psychol 61(6):984–991, 1993 8113499

Ressler KJ, Mercer KB, Bradley B, et al: Post-traumatic stress disorder is associated with PACAP and the PAC1 receptor. Nature 470(7335):492–497, 2011 21350482

Robb AS, Cueva JE, Sporn J, et al: Sertraline treatment of children and adolescents with posttraumatic stress disorder: a double-blind, placebo-controlled trial. J Child Adolesc Psychopharmacol 20(6):463–471, 2010 21186964

Robert R, Blakeney PE, Villarreal C, et al: Imipramine treatment in pediatric burn patients with symptoms of acute stress disorder: a pilot study. J Am Acad Child Adolesc Psychiatry 38(7):873–882, 1999 10405506

Roberts NP, Kitchiner NJ, Kenardy J, Bisson JI: Systematic review and meta-analysis of multiple-session early interventions following traumatic events. Am J Psychiatry 166(3):293–301, 2009 19188285

Roberts NP, Kitchiner NJ, Kenardy J, Bisson JI: Early psychological interventions to treat acute traumatic stress symptoms. Cochrane Database Syst Rev (3):CD007944, 2010 20238359

Robertson J: A Two-Year-Old Goes to Hospital: A Scientific Film. London, Robertson Films, 1952

Rose S, Bisson J, Churchill R, Wessely S: Psychological debriefing for preventing post traumatic stress disorder (PTSD). Cochrane Database Syst Rev (2):CD000560, 2002 12076399

Ross DA, Arbuckle MR, Travis MJ, et al: An integrated neuroscience perspective on formulation and treatment planning for posttraumatic stress disorder: an educational review. JAMA Psychiatry 74(4):407–415, 2017 28273291

Rothbaum BO, Kearns MC, Price M, et al: Early intervention may prevent the development of posttraumatic stress disorder: a randomized pilot civilian study with modified prolonged exposure. Biol Psychiatry 72(11):957–963, 2012 22766415

Rothbaum BO, Price M, Jovanovic T, et al: A randomized, double-blind evaluation of D-cycloserine or alprazolam combined with virtual reality exposure therapy for posttraumatic stress disorder in Iraq and Afghanistan War veterans. Am J Psychiatry 171(6):640–648, 2014 24743802

Russell JD, Neill EL, Carrión VG, Weems CF: The network structure of posttraumatic stress symptoms in children and adolescents exposed to disasters. J Am Acad Child Adolesc Psychiatry 56(8):669–677, 2017 28735696

Street AE, Gilman SE, Rosellini AJ, et al; Army STARRS collaborators: Understanding the elevated suicide risk of female soldiers during deployments. Psychol Med 45(4):717–726, 2015 25359554

Saxe G, Stoddard F, Courtney D, et al: Relationship between acute morphine and the course of PTSD in children with burns. J Am Acad Child Adolesc Psychiatry 40(8):915–921, 2001 11501691

Saxe GN, Statnikov A, Fenyo D, et al: A complex systems approach to causal discovery in psychiatry. PLoS One 11(3):e0151174, 2016 27028297

Schenk S, Newcombe D: Methylenedioxymethamphetamine (MDMA) in psychiatry: pros, cons, and suggestions. J Clin Psychopharmacol 38(6):632–638, 2018 30303861

Scott EL, Keary C, King JM, et al: PTSD in women: sex differences and gonadal hormones, in Trauma- and Stressor-Related Disorders. Edited by Stoddard FJ, Benedek DM, Milad MR, Ursano RJ. New York, Oxford University Press, 2018, pp 188–197

Seelig AD, Jacobson IG, Smith B, et al; Millennium Cohort Study Team: Prospective evaluation of mental health and deployment experience among women in the US military. Am J Epidemiol 176(2):135–145, 2012 22771728

Shalev A, Liberzon I, Marmar C: Post-traumatic stress disorder. N Engl J Med 376(25):2459–2469, 2017 28636846

Shay J: Achilles in Vietnam: Combat Trauma and the Undoing of Character. New York, Scribner, 1992

Shay J: Odysseus in America: Combat Trauma and the Trials of Homecoming. New York, Scribner, 2002

Shear K, Frank E, Houck PR, Reynolds CF 3rd: Treatment of complicated grief: a randomized controlled trial. JAMA 293(21):2601–2608, 2005 15928281

Shear MK, Simon N, Wall M, et al: Complicated grief and related bereavement issues for DSM-5. Depress Anxiety 28(2):103–117, 2011 21284063

Shear MK, Wang Y, Skritskaya N, et al: Treatment of complicated grief in elderly persons: a randomized clinical trial. JAMA Psychiatry 71(11):1287–1295, 2014 25250737

Shear MK, Reynolds CF 3rd, Simon NM, et al: Optimizing treatment of complicated grief: a randomized clinical trial. JAMA Psychiatry 73(7):685–694, 2016 27276373

Smoller JW: The genetics of stress-related disorders: PTSD, depression, and anxiety disorders. Neuropsychopharmacology 41(1):297–319, 2016 26321314

Southwick SM, Pietrzak RH, Charney DS, Krystal JH: Resilience: the role of accurate appraisal, thresholds, and socioenvironmental factors. Behav Brain Sci 38:e122, 2015 26786005

Soderstrom CA, Smith GS, Dischinger PC, et al: Psychoactive substance use disorders among seriously injured trauma center patients. JAMA 277(22):1769–1774, 1997 9178789

Spitz RA: Anaclitic depression: an inquiry into the genesis of psychiatric conditions in early childhood. The Psychoanalytic Study of the Child 2:313–342, 1946 20293638

Stein DJ: Etifoxine versus alprazolam for the treatment of adjustment disorder with anxiety: a randomized controlled trial. Adv Ther 32(1):57–68, 2015 25620535

Stoddard FJ Jr: Outcomes of traumatic exposure. Child Adolesc Psychiatr Clin N Am 23(2):243–256, 2014 24656578

Stoddard FJ, Saxe G: Ten-year research review of physical injuries. J Am Acad Child Adolesc Psychiatry 40(10):1128–1145, 2001 11589526

Stoddard FJ, Pandya A, Katz CL (eds): Disaster Psychiatry: Readiness, Evaluation, and Treatment. Washington, DC, American Psychiatric Publishing, 2011a

Stoddard FJ, Sheridan RL, Martyn JAJ, et al: Pain management, in Combat and Operational Behavioral Health. Edited by Ritchie EC. Washington, DC, Department of the Army, Office of the Surgeon General, Borden Institute, 2011b, pp 339–358

Stoddard FJ Jr, Luthra R, Sorrentino EA, et al: A randomized controlled trial of sertraline to prevent posttraumatic stress disorder in burned children. J Child Adolesc Psychopharmacol 21(5):469–477, 2011c 22040192

Stoddard FJ Jr, Sorrentino E, Drake JE, et al: Posttraumatic stress disorder diagnosis in young children with burns. J Burn Care Res 38(1):e343–e351, 2017 27359192

Stoddard FJ, Benedek DM, Milad MR, et al (eds): Trauma- and Stressor-Related Disorders. New York, Oxford University Press, 2018

Strain JJ, Friedman MJ: Considering adjustment disorders as stress response syndromes for DSM-5. Depress Anxiety 28(9):818–823, 2011 21254314

Subica AM, Claypoole KH, Wylie AM: PTSD's mediation of the relationships between trauma, depression, substance abuse, mental health, and physical health in individuals with severe mental illness: evaluating a comprehensive model. Schizophr Res 136(1–3):104–109, 2012 22104139

Tawakol A, Ishai A, Takx RA, et al: Relation between resting amygdalar activity and cardiovascular events: a longitudinal and cohort study. Lancet 389(10071):834–845, 2017 28088338

Tedeschi RG, Calhoun LG: The Posttraumatic Growth Inventory: measuring the positive legacy of trauma. J Trauma Stress 9(3):455–471, 1996 8827649

Terr LC: Childhood traumas: an outline and overview. Am J Psychiatry 148(1):10–20, 1991 1824611

Tran US, Gregor B: The relative efficacy of bona fide psychotherapies for post-traumatic stress disorder: a meta-analytical evaluation of randomized controlled trials. BMC Psychiatry 16:266, 2016 27460057

Trevizol AP, Barros MD, Silva PO, et al: Transcranial magnetic stimulation for posttraumatic stress disorder: an updated systematic review and meta-analysis. Trends Psychiatry Psychother 38(1):50–55, 2016 27074341

Tsai J, Pietrzak RH: Trajectories of posttraumatic growth among US military veterans: a 4-year nationally representative, prospective cohort study. Acta Psychiatr Scand 136(5):483–492, 2017 28846800

Ursano RJ, Fullerton CS, Weisaeth L, et al (eds): Textbook of Disaster Psychiatry, 2nd Edition. Cambridge, UK, Cambridge University Press, 2017

U.S. Department of Veterans Affairs, U.S. Department of Defense: VA/DoD Clinical Practice Guideline for Management of Post-Traumatic Stress (Publ No 10Q-CPG/PTSD-04). Washington, DC, Veterans Health Administration, Department of Veterans Affairs and Health Affairs, Department of Defense, Office of Quality and Performance, 2017

Vaillant GE: Triumphs of Experience: The Men of the Harvard Grant Study. Cambridge, MA, Belknap Press, 2012

van der Klink JJ, Blonk RW, Schene A, van Dijk FJ: Reducing long term sickness absence by an activating intervention in adjustment disorders: a cluster randomised controlled design. Occup Environ Med 60(6):429–437, 2003 12771395

van Emmerik AA, Kamphuis JH, Hulsbosch AM, Emmelkamp PM: Single session debriefing after psychological trauma: a meta-analysis. Lancet 360(9335):766–771, 2002 12241834

Vervoort E, De Schipper JC, Bosmans G, Verschueren K: Screening symptoms of reactive attachment disorder: evidence for measurement invariance and convergent validity. Int J Methods Psychiatr Res 22(3):256–265, 2013 24022942

Wirtz PH, von Känel R: Psychological stress, inflammation, and coronary heart disease. Curr Cardiol Rep 19(11):111, 2017 28932967

Wisco BE, Marx BP, Miller MW, et al: Probable posttraumatic stress disorder in the US veteran population according to DSM-5: results from the National Health and Resilience in Veterans Study. J Clin Psychiatry 77(11):1503–1510, 2016 27631148

World Health Organization: International Statistical Classification of Diseases and Related Health Problems, 10th Revision. Geneva, World Health Organization, 1992

World Health Organization: International Statistical Classification of Diseases and Related Health Problems, 11th Edition (ICD-11), Draft Version. Geneva, World Health Organization, June 18, 2018. Available at: http://www.who.int/classifications/icd/en/. Accessed October 17, 2018.

Yehuda R: Post-traumatic stress disorder. N Engl J Med 346(2):108–114, 2002 11784878

Yehuda R, Daskalakis NP, Lehrner A, et al: Influences of maternal and paternal PTSD on epigenetic regulation of the glucocorticoid receptor gene in Holocaust survivor offspring. Am J Psychiatry 171(8):872–880, 2014 24832930

Yehuda R, Hoge CW, McFarlane AC, et al: Post-traumatic stress disorder. Nat Rev Dis Primers 1:15057, 2015 27189040

Zatzick D, Jurkovich G, Rivara FP, et al: A randomized stepped care intervention trial targeting posttraumatic stress disorder for surgically hospitalized injury survivors. Ann Surg 257(3):390–399, 2013 23222034

Zatzick DF, Rowhani-Rahbar A, Wang J, et al: The cumulative burden of mental, substance use, and general medical disorders and rehospitalization and mortality after an injury. Psychiatr Serv 68(6):596–602, 2017 28142384

Zeanah CH, Gleason MM: Annual research review: Attachment disorders in early childhood—clinical presentation, causes, correlates, and treatment. J Child Psychol Psychiatry 56(3):207–222, 2015 25359236

Zeanah CH, Scheeringa M, Boris NW, et al: Reactive attachment disorder in maltreated toddlers. Child Abuse Negl 28(8):877–888, 2004 15350771

Zeanah CH, Chesher T, Boris NW, et al: Practice parameter for the assessment and treatment of children and adolescents with reactive attachment disorder and disinhibited social engagement disorder. J Am Acad Child Adolesc Psychiatry 55(11):990–1003, 2016 27806867

Recommended Readings

Benedek DM, Wynn GH (eds): Complementary and Alternative Medicine for PTSD. New York, Oxford University Press, 2016

Cohen J, Mannarino A, Deblinger E: Treating Trauma and Traumatic Grief in Children and Adolescents, 2nd Edition. New York, Guilford, 2017

Committee on Integrating the Science of Early Childhood Development, Youth and Families Board on Children, National Research Council, et al: From Neurons to Neighborhoods: The Science of Early Childhood Development. Washington, DC, National Academies Press, 2000

Herman J: Trauma and Recovery: The Aftermath of Violence From Domestic Abuse to Political Terror. New York, Basic Books, 1992

Lifton RJ: Survivors of Hiroshima. New York, Random House, 1967

Nemeroff CB, Marmar C: Post-Traumatic Stress Disorder. Oxford, UK, Oxford University Press, 2018

Shay J: Achilles in Vietnam: Combat Trauma and the Undoing of Character. New York, Scribner, 1992

Shay J: Odysseus in America: Combat Trauma and the Trials of Homecoming. New York, Scribner, 2002

Shear MK, Reynolds CF, Simon NM, et al: Optimizing treatment of complicated grief: a randomized clinical trial. JAMA Psychiatry 73(7):685–694, 2016

Southwick SM, Charney DS: Resilience: The Science of Mastering Life's Greatest Challenges, 2nd Edition. Cambridge, UK, Cambridge University Press, 2018

Stoddard FJ, Pandya A, Katz CL (eds): Disaster Psychiatry: Readiness, Evaluation and Treatment. Washington, DC, American Psychiatric Publishing, 2011

Stoddard FJ, Benedek DM, Milad MR, et al (eds): Trauma- and Stressor-Related Disorders. New York, Oxford University Press, 2018

Terr LC: Too Scared to Cry: How Trauma Affects Children and Ultimately Us All. New York, Basic Books, 1990

Ursano RJ, Fullerton CS, Weisaeth L, et al (eds): Textbook of Disaster Psychiatry, 2nd Edition. Cambridge, UK, Cambridge University Press, 2017

CHAPTER 16

Dissociative Disorders

José R. Maldonado, M.D., F.A.P.M., F.A.C.F.E.
David Spiegel, M.D., F.A.P.A.

The dissociative disorders involve a disturbance in the integrated organization of consciousness, memory, identity, emotion, perception, body representation, motor control, and behavior. Events normally experienced on a smooth continuum are isolated from the other mental processes with which they would ordinarily be associated. This discontinuity results in a variety of dissociative disorders depending on the primary cognitive process affected. When memories are poorly integrated, the resulting disorder is *dissociative amnesia.* If the amnesia also includes aimless wandering, the specifier "with dissociative fugue" is used. Fragmentation of identity results in *dissociative identity disorder* (DID). Disordered perception yields *depersonalization/derealization disorder* and, in conjunction with the symptoms of posttraumatic stress disorder (PTSD), produces its *dissociative subtype.* Dissociation of aspects of consciousness is also involved in acute stress disorder.

Dissociative disorders represent more a disturbance in the organization or structure of mental contents than a disturbance in the mental contents themselves. Memories in dissociative amnesia and/or identity during fugue states (as part of dissociative amnesia) are not so much distorted or bizarre as they are segregated from one another, impairing retrieval. The aspects of the self that are fragmented in DID are two-dimensional aspects of an overall personality structure. The problem is the failure of integration or the decontextualization of information, rather than the contents of the fragments. In summary, all types of dissociative disorders have in common a lack of immediate access to the entire personality structure or mental content in one form or another. Dissociative disorders are associated with negative outcomes. In fact, studies have demonstrated that those with a dissociative disorder were more prone to and showed higher indices of suicide, self-injury, and emergency consultations, as well as psychotropic drug use, compared with mood and psychotic disorders (Gonzalez Vazquez et al. 2017).

The dissociative disorders have a long history in classical psychopathology but until recently have been largely ignored. Nonetheless, the phenomena are sufficiently persistent and interesting that they have elicited growing attention from both professionals and the public. The dissociative disorders remain an area of psychopathology for which the best treatment is psychotherapy (Maldonado et al. 2002). As mental disorders, they have much to teach us about the way humans adapt to traumatic stress and about information processing in the brain.

Development of the Concept

Jean-Martin Charcot (1890), the well-known French neurologist, became interested in the dissociative symptoms experienced by some of his patients who had unusual neurological symptoms. He discovered that hypnosis could reproduce and reverse some of the deficits manifested by his patients. Charcot believed that even a normal process such as hypnosis, which could be used to access dissociated mental contents, was itself evidence of pathology—*"un état nerveux artificiel ou expérimentale"* (i.e., an artificial or experimental nervous state). He thought, for example, that once patients were cured of hysteria, they would no longer be hypnotizable. This is now known not to be the case, because many "normal" individuals are highly hypnotizable (H. Spiegel and D. Spiegel 2004).

Nevertheless, the French physician and psychologist Pierre Janet (1920) is credited with the initial description of dissociation as a disorder, a *désagrégation mentale*. The term *désagrégation* carries with it a slightly different nuance than does the English translation, *dissociation,* because the former implies a separation of certain mental contents from their general tendency to aggregate or be processed together. Janet described *hysteria* as "a malady of the personal synthesis" (Janet 1920, p. 332). Janet was probably the first to study psychological trauma as a principal cause of dissociation.

The dissociative disorders might have been studied more intensively during the twentieth century had not Janet's and Charcot's work been so thoroughly eclipsed by the psychoanalytic approach pioneered by Sigmund Freud. Freud learned the use of hypnotic techniques from Charcot and applied them in the treatment of some of his first cases. In his early writings with Breuer, Freud began an exploration of dissociative phenomena similar to those that Janet had described earlier. Cases in the *Studies on Hysteria* (Breuer and Freud 1957), such as that of Anna O., clearly involved dissociative phenomena. Indeed, Anna O. had many symptoms suggestive of DID. However, Breuer and Freud reformulated the role of the capacity to dissociate through the concept of hypnoid states, rather than the mechanism of dissociation. Indeed, they thought that dissociative symptoms should be attributed to the capacity to enter these hypnoid states rather than the reverse (Breuer and Freud 1957). However, in an effort to develop a more general theory of human psychopathology, Freud went on to study other kinds of patients, such as those with "obsessive compulsive neurosis" (i.e., obsessive-compulsive disorder) and schizophrenia. This shift in the patient population studied may well account for much of Freud's waning interest in dissociation as a defense and his increasing interest in repression as a more general model for motivated forgetting in unconscious processes. Discussion of dissociation and its relation to trauma all but disappeared after Janet. However, during World War II and the postwar period, some psychiatrists began to pay attention to two emerging phenomena: 1) a high incidence of "traumatic neurosis" among combatants and 2) dissociative symptoms such as fugue and amnesia observed among ex-inmates of concentration camps.

As a general model for keeping information out of conscious awareness, repression differs from dissociation in several important ways (Table 16–1). There has been debate about whether dissociation is a subtype of repression, or vice versa. Such a dispute is probably not resolvable, but what has become clear is that given the complexity of human information processing, the development of a sense of mental unity is an achievement, not a given (Spiegel 1986). What is remarkable is not that dissociative disorders occur but rather that they do not occur more often, given the fact that information processing comprises a variety of reasonably autonomous subsystems involving perception, memory storage and retrieval, intention, and action.

Models and Mechanisms of Dissociation

Dissociation and Information Processing

A study by Williams et al. (2006) using functional magnetic resonance imaging (fMRI) found that many of the same regions of the human brain are activated during conscious attention to signals of fear and in the absence of awareness of these signals. Through fMRI studies with connectivity analysis in healthy human subjects, the authors were able to demonstrate that level of awareness for signals of fear depends on the mode of functional connectivity in amygdala pathways rather than discrete patterns of activation in these pathways. Awareness of fear relied on negative connectivity within both cortical and subcortical pathways to the amygdala, suggesting that reentrant feedback may be necessary to allow such awareness. In contrast, responses to fear in the absence of awareness were supported by positive connections in a direct subcortical pathway to the amygdala, consistent with the view that excitatory feed-forward connections along this pathway may be sufficient for automatic responses to "unseen" fear. These findings may explain how "dissociated or unknown" memory content may exert its effects by eliciting fear or panic or by triggering altered/dissociated states in victims of trauma.

From a more clinical perspective, dissociation may be explained by one of three proposed models or combinations of these: 1) the neurological model, which suggests that some underlying neurological process, such as hemispheric disconnection or epilepsy, plays a role in promoting dissociative symptoms; 2) the role enactment model or social role demand theory, which suggests that the symptoms are an artificial social construct rather than a true psychiatric disorder; and 3) the autohypnotic model, a theory that recognizes and reconciles the connection between traumatic events, dissociative experiences, and hypnotizability. These models have been described at length elsewhere (Maldonado and Fink 2007) and are not discussed here. fMRI research has identified a dissociative subtype of PTSD that is notably different from the more common hyperarousal pattern (Lanius et al. 2010; Nicholson et al. 2017). It involves frontal hyperactivity coupled with limbic hypoactivity, consistent with cognitive suppression of emotional response, whereas hyperarousal is associated with the opposite pattern: limbic hyperactivity and hypofrontality (Brand et al. 2012). This dissociative pattern, identified by concomitant depersonalization and/or derealization (American Psychiatric Association 2013), is observed in about 14% of people with PTSD, who also report earlier and more severe childhood trauma, earlier onset of PTSD, and higher role impairment and suicidality (Stein et al. 2013). These findings

TABLE 16–1.   **Differences between dissociation and repression**

	Dissociation	Repression
Organizational structure[a]	Horizontal	Vertical
Barriers[b]	Amnesia	Dynamic conflict
Etiology[c]	Trauma	Developmental conflict over unacceptable wishes
Contents[d]	Untransformed: traumatic memories	Disguised, primary process: dreams, slips
Means of access[e]	Hypnosis	Interpretation
Psychotherapy[f]	Access, control, and working through of traumatic memories	Interpretation, transference

[a]The organizational structure of mental contents in dissociation is considered to be horizontal, with subunits of information divided from one another but equally available to consciousness (Hilgard 1977). Repressed information, on the other hand, is presumed to be stored in an archaeological manner, at various depths, and therefore, different components are not equally accessible (Freud 1923/1961).

[b]Subunits of information are presumed to be divided by amnesic barriers in dissociation, whereas dynamic conflict, or motivated forgetting, is the mechanism underlying repression.

[c]The information kept out of awareness in dissociation often involves a discrete and sharply delimited period, usually a traumatic experience, whereas repressed information may involve a variety of experiences, fears, or wishes scattered across time. Dissociation is often elicited as a defense, especially after episodes of physical trauma, whereas repression is a response to warded-off fears and wishes or a response to other dynamic conflicts.

[d]Dissociated information is stored in a discrete and untransformed manner, whereas repressed information is usually disguised and fragmented. Even when repressed information becomes available to consciousness, its meaning is hidden (e.g., in dreams, slips of the tongue).

[e]Retrieval of dissociated information often can be direct. Techniques such as hypnosis can be used to access warded-off memories. In contrast, uncovering repressed information often requires repeated recall trials through intense questioning, psychotherapy, or psychoanalysis with subsequent interpretation (i.e., of dreams).

[f]The focus of psychotherapy for dissociation is integration via control of access to dissociated states and working through of traumatic memories. The classical psychotherapy for repression involves interpretation, including working through the transference.

are consistent with fMRI indications of a dissociative pattern of inverse functional connectivity between the executive control network (dorsolateral prefrontal cortex) and the default-mode network (posterior cingulate cortex) among hypnotized individuals, indicating relative disconnection between brain regions involved in task completion and self-rumination (Jiang et al. 2017).

Modern research on memory shows that there are at least two broad categories of memory, variously described as *explicit* and *implicit* or *episodic* and *semantic*. These two memory systems serve different functions. Explicit (or episodic) memory involves recall of personal experiences identified with the self (e.g., "I was at the ball game last week"). Implicit (or semantic) memory involves the execution of routine operations, such as riding a bicycle or typing. Such operations may be carried out with a high degree of proficiency with little conscious awareness of either their current execution or the learning episodes on which the skill is based. Indeed, these two types of memory have different neuroanatomical localizations: the limbic system, especially the hippocampal formation, and mammillary bodies for episodic memory and the basal ganglia and cortex for semantic memory (Mishkin and Appenzeller 1987).

Indeed, the distinction between these two types of memory may account for certain dissociative phenomena. The automaticity observed in certain dissociative disorders may be a reflection of the separation of self-identification in certain kinds of explicit memory from routine activity in implicit or semantic memory. It is thus not at all foreign to our mental processing to act in an automatic way devoid of explicit self-identification. Were it necessary for us to retrieve explicit memories of how and when we learned all of the activities we are required to perform, it is highly unlikely that we would be able to function with anything like the degree of efficiency we have. Many athletes report focusing on some detail of the event and allowing their bodies to do what they need to, when in fact they are performing extremely well. Some have proposed that dissociation is a regulatory strategy to restrain extreme arousal in PTSD through hyperinhibition of limbic regions (van Huijstee and Vermetten 2018). There is thus a fundamental model in memory research for the dissociation between identity and performance that may well find its pathological reflection in disorders such as dissociative amnesia, dissociative fugue, and DID.

Dissociation and Trauma

In 1930, Italian psychiatrist Giovanni Enrico Morselli described the history, diagnosis, and treatment of his patient Elena, one of the most remarkable cases of DID ever published, highlighting the disorder's relationship to early childhood trauma (Schimmenti 2017). An important development in the modern understanding of dissociative disorders is the exploration of the link between trauma and dissociation. Trauma can be understood as the experience of being made into an object or a thing, the victim of someone else's rage or of nature's indifference. It is the ultimate experience of helplessness and loss of control over one's own body. Spitzer et al. (2006) postulated that the process of traumatization involves some degree of division or dissociation of psychobiological systems that constitute personality. By this theory, dissociated parts of the personality avoid traumatic memories and perform functions in daily life while one or more other parts remain fixated in traumatic experiences and defensive actions. Unfortunately, the dissociated memories may manifest themselves in the form of negative and/or positive dissociative symptoms that must be distinguished from more normal alterations of consciousness.

In fact, there is growing clinical and some empirical evidence that dissociation may occur especially as a defense during trauma, an attempt to maintain mental control at the very moment when physical control has been lost (Dalenberg et al. 2012; Kluft 1984a; Putnam and Kluft 1985; Spiegel 1984; van der Hart et al. 2005). One patient with DID reported "going to a mountain meadow full of wildflowers" when she was being sexually assaulted by her drunken father. She would concentrate on how pleasant and beautiful this imaginary scene was as a way of detaching herself from the immediate experience of terror, pain, and helplessness. Such individuals often report seeking comfort from imaginary playmates or imagined protectors or absorbing themselves in some perceptual distraction, such as the pattern of the wallpaper. Many rape victims report floating above their bodies, feeling sorry for the person being assaulted beneath them. Children exposed to multiple traumas are more likely than those without a history of trauma to use dissociative defense mechanisms, which include spontaneous trance episodes and amnesia.

A growing body of scientific literature suggests a connection between a history of physical and sexual abuse in childhood and the development of dissociative symptoms (Coons and Milstein 1986; Dalenberg et al. 2012; Freud 1946; Kluft 1984a; Şar et al. 1996; Spiegel 1984). A study by Collin-Vézina and Hébert (2005) found that sexual victimization significantly increases the odds of presenting with a clinical level of dissociation and PTSD symptoms eightfold and fourfold, respectively.

Evidence is accumulating that dissociative symptoms are more prevalent in patients with borderline personality disorder when the individuals have a history of childhood abuse (Spitzer et al. 2006). In a study of 62 women diagnosed with borderline personality disorder, Shearer (1994) found that univariate analyses demonstrated that patients with borderline personality disorder and dissociative experiences have more self-reported traumatic experiences, posttraumatic symptoms, behavioral dyscontrol, self-injurious behavior, and alcohol abuse. The findings also suggested that scores on the Dissociative Experiences Scale (DES) (Bernstein and Putnam 1986) were predicted particularly by sexual assault in adulthood, behavioral dyscontrol, and both sexual and physical abuse in childhood. Watson et al. (2006) examined 139 patients with borderline personality disorder and found that their levels of dissociation increased with levels of childhood trauma, supporting the hypothesis that traumatic childhood experiences engender dissociative symptoms later in life. More importantly, these findings suggest that emotional abuse and neglect may be at least as important as physical and sexual abuse in the development of dissociative symptoms.

A 2016 study examined the effects of child sexual, physical, and emotional abuse, as well as physical and emotional neglect, in dissociative disorder, chronic PTSD, and mixed psychiatric disorder patient samples, all with abuse and neglect histories (Dorahy et al. 2016). The results indicated that all forms of maltreatment differentiated the dissociative disorders group from the mixed psychiatric disorders group, and sexual abuse differentiated the dissociative disorders sample from the chronic PTSD group. Childhood sexual abuse was the only predictor of pathological dissociation. Emotional abuse predicted shame, guilt, relationship anxiety, and fear of relationships. Emotional neglect predicted relationship anxiety and relationship depression, whereas physical neglect was less associated with relationship anxiety.

A sample of 87 female inpatients with a history of childhood abuse and neglect was divided into two subgroups: those with no self-injurious behavior and those with nonsuicidal self-injury (NSSI) (Franzke et al. 2015). The NSSI group reported significantly more cases of childhood maltreatment and higher levels of current dissociative, posttraumatic, and depressive symptoms than the no self-injurious-behavior group. The results of a path analysis showed that only dissociation mediated the relationship between a history of child maltreatment and NSSI when all three psychopathological variables were included in the model. Similarly, in a study of psychiatric inpatients, predictive modeling accomplished with the use of conditioned random forest regression verified that PTSD symptoms were best predicted by overall severity of adverse childhood experiences (Schalinski et al. 2016). In addition, type and timing were prognostically important: physical neglect at age 5 years and emotional neglect at ages 4–5 years were related to increased symptoms of dissociation, whereas emotional neglect at ages 8–9 years enhanced symptoms of depression.

In a civilian sample of adults recruited from an urban public hospital, PTSD was measured using the Clinician-Administered PTSD Scale, emotion dysregulation was measured using the Difficulties in Emotion Regulation Scale, and dissociation was measured using the Multiscale Dissociation Inventory. A linear regression analysis showed that both PTSD and emotion dysregulation were statistically significant predictors of dissociation even after controlling for trauma exposure. Alexithymia and an inability to use emotion regulation strategies in particular were predictive of dissociation above and beyond other predictor variables and suggest that emotion dysregulation may be important in understanding the relationship between PTSD and dissociative symptoms.

Johnson et al. (2001) confirmed that peritraumatic dissociation in patients seeking treatment for childhood sexual abuse was strongly related to later development of PTSD, dissociation, and depression. Data analysis indicated that women who experienced penile penetration, who believed that someone or something else would be killed, or who were injured as a result of the abuse had more severe peritraumatic dissociation. Regression analyses indicated that peritraumatic dissociation was the only variable to significantly predict symptom severity across symptom type or disorder. Similarly, Hetzel and McCanne (2005) found that different types of childhood abuse may lead to different adult problems. For example, the combined sexual and physical abuse and sexual abuse–only groups reported significantly higher numbers of PTSD symptoms compared with the physical abuse–only and the no-abuse (control) groups. The combined sexual and physical abuse and physical abuse–only groups also reported significantly more sexual and physical victimization in adulthood than the sexual abuse–only and control groups. The results suggest that across all four groups, higher levels of peritraumatic dissociation were associated with higher levels of PTSD and adulthood sexual and physical victimization. The authors concluded that peritraumatic dissociation may have a broad effect on PTSD development and victimization in adulthood. Recent data suggest that among trauma-exposed adults, after accounting for overall symptom severity and current dissociative tendencies, peritraumatic dissociation is significantly predictive of negative beliefs about the self ($P<0.001$) (Thompson-Hollands et al. 2017).

A follow-up study of victims of the World Trade Center disaster found that baseline (peritraumatic) dissociation was the strongest predictor of *dissociation* at follow-up, whereas baseline posttraumatic stress was the strongest predictor of *PTSD* at follow-up (Simeon et al. 2005). Of the four peritraumatic distress factors generated in the original survey, loss of control and guilt/shame were significantly related to dissociation and posttraumatic stress at follow-up, whereas helplessness/anger was associated only with posttraumatic stress at follow-up. These studies confirmed previous findings by O'Toole et al. (1999) that having been wounded was not related to lifetime or current PTSD, whereas peritraumatic dissociation was related to all diagnostic components of PTSD. Similarly, Olde et al. (2005) found a 2.1% incidence of PTSD in a population of 140 women following childbirth. In their sample, both perinatal negative emotional reactions and perinatal dissociative reactions predicted PTSD symptoms at 3 months postpartum.

The presence of a concomitant dissociative disorder should be considered in victims of traumatic stress. Chronic exposure to trauma can lead not only to acute stress disorder and PTSD but also to one of the dissociative disorders (Spiegel and Cardeña 1991). In fact, it is uncommon to encounter a patient with a dissociative disorder who has not been previously exposed to intense trauma, usually physical (or sexual) abuse, to the point of also fulfilling Criterion A for the diagnosis of PTSD (American Psychiatric Association 2013). A study among war veterans confirmed a direct association between dissociation and PTSD severity and suggested that dissociation is a highly salient facet of posttraumatic psychopathology (Wolf et al. 2012).

Peritraumatic dissociation (i.e., dissociative responses at the time of or immediately after the traumatic event) may predict the development of trauma- and stressor-related disorders sometime in the future (Brewin et al. 2010). Current theories of trauma-related stress disorder suggest that peritraumatic dissociation impairs processing of traumatic experiences by preventing adequate encoding of traumatic memories and causing alterations in memory storage; and furthermore, persistent dissociation prevents memory elaboration, leading to partial amnesia, intrusive recollections, and memory fragmentation typical of these disorders (i.e., acute stress disorder, PTSD, dissociative disorders) (Bedard-Gilligan and Zoellner 2012; Feeny et al. 2000a, 2000b).

A multivariable analysis conducted in a nationally representative sample (N=1,484) from the National Health and Resilience in Veterans Study found that of the 12.0% and 5.2% of veterans who screened positive for lifetime and past-month DSM-5 PTSD (American Psychiatric Association 2013), 19.2% and 16.1% screened positive for the dissociative subtype of PTSD, respectively (Tsai et al. 2015). Among veterans with PTSD, those with the dissociative subtype reported more severe PTSD symptoms, comorbid depressive and anxiety symptoms, alcohol use problems, and hostility than those without the dissociative subtype.

Even though dissociative defenses may work well at the time of trauma, if the defense persists too long, it interferes with the working through (in Lindemann's [1994] terms, the "grief work") that is necessary to put traumatic experience into perspective and reduce the likelihood of later PTSD or other symptomatology. In fact, a study exploring the role of trauma and dissociation in psychopathology revealed that adolescents with dissociative disorders experienced higher rates of self-injurious behaviors and suicide attempts than did comparator and control groups. Dissociation was the most important variable contributing to self-injurious behavior, and female gender was the most important variable for suicide attempts. Total trauma scores were also found to be significantly higher in the dissociative disorders group, followed by the nondissociative disorder and control groups (Kiliç et al. 2017). Similarly, a recent meta-analysis of studies comparing rates of suicide attempts and NSSI in psychiatric individuals with and without dissociative disorders revealed that the presence of a dissociative disorder diagnosis or higher DES scores seems to be related to both suicide attempts and NSSI in psychiatric patients (Calati et al. 2017). These findings suggest the potential presence of a dissociative subtype in a subset of these patients, which, as a transdiagnostic factor, should be carefully assessed. Therefore, psychotherapy aimed at helping individuals acknowledge, bear, and put into perspective traumatic experience shortly after the trauma should be helpful in reducing the incidence of later PTSD.

Indeed, DSM-5 has included a dissociative subtype of PTSD. A systematic literature review of latent class and profile analytic studies of PTSD lends support to the PTSD dissociative subtype (PTSD+DS), primarily characterized by depersonalization and derealization; this highlights how the presence of dissociative symptoms in the context of PTSD may potentially interfere with treatment course or outcome (Hansen et al. 2017). These data suggest that the dissociative subtype of PTSD is as-

sociated with high PTSD severity, predominance of derealization and depersonalization symptoms, a more significant history of early-life trauma, and higher levels of
comorbid psychiatric disorders (van Huijstee and Vermetten 2018). Of note, a latent
profile analysis of cross-sectional data from an online survey of 697 trauma-exposed
military veterans yielded evidence for a small (8.3% of the sample) highly dissociative
class characterized by pronounced symptoms of derealization and depersonalization
(Wolf et al. 2017).

As noted, fMRI research has demonstrated a distinctive pattern among individuals
with the dissociative subtype of PTSD compared with those with the more common
hyperarousal pattern (Lanius et al. 2010; Nicholson et al. 2017). This pattern involves
frontal hyperactivity coupled with limbic hypoactivity in response to trauma-related
script-driven imagery, consistent with cognitive suppression of emotional response,
whereas hyperarousal is associated with the opposite pattern: limbic hyperactivity
and hypofrontality (Lanius et al. 2012). More recent research has shown that among
patients with PTSD, the PTSD+DS group exhibited greater amygdala functional connectivity to prefrontal regions involved in emotion regulation (bilateral basolateral
amygdala [BLA] and left centromedial amygdala [CMA] to the middle frontal gyrus
and bilateral CMA to the medial frontal gyrus) than the PTSD non-DS group (Nicholson et al. 2015). In addition, the PTSD+DS group showed greater amygdala connectivity to regions involved in consciousness, awareness, and proprioception implicated in
depersonalization and derealization (left BLA to superior parietal lobe and cerebellar
culmen, and left CMA to dorsal posterior cingulate and precuneus).

In comparison with data from control subjects, resting-state fMRI data from PTSD
non-DS patients displayed increased insula connectivity (bilateral anterior, bilateral
mid, and left posterior) to basolateral amygdala clusters in both hemispheres and increased insula connectivity (bilateral anterior, left mid, and left posterior) to the left
basolateral amygdala complex (Nicholson et al. 2016). Similarly, depersonalization/
derealization symptoms and PTSD symptom severity correlated with insula subregion
connectivity to the basolateral amygdala within PTSD patients. Furthermore, PTSD patients *with* dissociative symptoms exhibit aberrant psychophysiological and neural responses—namely, a decreased heart rate, increased activation of prefrontal regions,
and decreased activation of the amygdala in response to traumatic reminders (a pattern virtually opposite to that of trauma survivors without dissociation) (van Huijstee
and Vermetten 2018). In a recent study using resting-state fMRI data, increased vestibular nuclei functional connectivity with the parieto-insular vestibular cortex and the
dorsolateral prefrontal cortex (DLPFC) was observed in subjects with PTSD and in control subjects compared with those with PTSD+DS, and greater connectivity with the
posterior insula was observed in control subjects compared with those with PTSD. Interestingly, whereas PTSD symptom severity correlated negatively with DLPFC connectivity, clinical measures of depersonalization/derealization correlated negatively
with right supramarginal gyrus connectivity, thus suggesting that dysregulation of
vestibular multisensory integration may contribute to the unique symptom profiles of
each group (Harricharan et al. 2017). Using resting-state stochastic dynamic causal
modeling pairwise analyses of coupling between the ventromedial prefrontal cortex
(vmPFC), the bilateral BLA and CMA complexes, and the periaqueductal gray (PAG),
researchers found that PTSD was characterized by a pattern of predominant bottom-
up connectivity from the amygdala to the vmPFC and from the PAG to the vmPFC and

amygdala (Nicholson et al. 2017). Conversely, PTSD+DS patients exhibited predominant top-down connectivity between all node pairs (from the vmPFC to the amygdala and PAG and from the amygdala to the PAG). Interestingly, the PTSD+DS group displayed the strongest intrinsic inhibitory connections within the vmPFC, possibly explaining the hypoemotionality observed in these patients. Finally, among women with PTSD associated with a history of multiple traumas, resting-state magnetoencephalography found a relationship between dissociative symptoms and increased delta and decreased beta power (Schalinski et al. 2017). In this sample, adversity-related measures modulated theta and alpha oscillatory power (in particular, childhood sexual abuse) and differed between patients and control subjects.

DSM-5 Dissociative Disorders

Since its introduction in 1952, the *Diagnostic and Statistical Manual of Mental Disorders* has served as the standard for diagnostic classification of mental disorders. In 2013, the American Psychiatric Association unveiled the fifth edition of the manual, DSM-5. This new version contains some significant changes regarding dissociative disorders, as summarized in Table 16–2. In this section, we review the epidemiology, diagnostic criteria, and treatment of the dissociative disorders as defined in DSM-5.

Dissociative Identity Disorder

Diagnostic Features

As specified in the DSM-5 diagnostic criteria, the hallmark of DID is "disruption of identity characterized by [the presence of] two or more distinct personality states, which may be described in some cultures as an experience of possession" (American Psychiatric Association 2013, p. 292). The periods of identity disruption cause "marked discontinuity in sense of self and sense of agency, accompanied by related alterations in affect, behavior, consciousness, memory, perception, cognition, and/or sensory-motor functioning" (p. 292) and lead to gaps in memory and impairments in social and occupational functioning. By definition, individuals with DID experience recurrent gaps in their recall of routine life events and key personal information (usually of a traumatic nature) that are not consistent with ordinary forgetting (Criterion B). These symptoms are associated with clinically significant distress and functional impairment (Criterion C) and cannot be part of a broadly accepted cultural or religious practice (Criterion D) or attributable to substance use or a neurological disorder (Criterion E).

The identity temporarily lost during dissociative states or the aspects of the self that are fragmented in DID are two-dimensional aspects of an overall personality structure. In this sense, it has been said that patients with DID do not have more than one personality but rather have less than one personality. Differences between DSM-IV (American Psychiatric Association 1994) and DSM-5 diagnostic criteria for DID are itemized in Table 16–2.

Prevalence

In a study of community adults, the prevalence of DID was 1.5% (Johnson et al. 2006). In 1994, Loewenstein reported that the prevalence of DID in North America was about 1%, compared with a prevalence of 10% for all dissociative disorders as a group. Loewenstein's findings were replicated by Rifkin et al. (1998), who studied 100 randomly selected women, ages 16–50 years, who had been admitted to an acute psychiatric hospital and found that 1% of the subjects had DID. The estimated prevalence is approximately 3% among psychiatric inpatients (Ross 1991). Foote et al. (2006) carefully assessed 231 consecutive admissions to an inner-city mental health clinic and interviewed 82 of those willing to cooperate with the study. Of this sample, 29% of patients met DSM-IV criteria for a dissociative disorder (eight with dissociative amnesia, seven with dissociative disorder not otherwise specified, five with DID, and four with depersonalization disorder). Only 5% of this sample had previously been diagnosed with a dissociative disorder, suggesting systematic underdiagnosis. Furthermore, the study provided additional evidence linking both physical and sexual abuse to dissociative symptoms, determining an odds ratio of 5.86 for physical abuse and 7.87 for sexual abuse.

The number of reported DID cases has risen considerably in recent years. Factors that may account for this increase include a more general awareness of the diagnosis among mental health professionals; the availability, starting with DSM-III (American Psychiatric Association 1980), of specific diagnostic criteria; and reduced misdiagnosis of DID as schizophrenia or borderline personality disorder (Kluft 1987). Other authors have attributed the increase in reported cases to hypnotic suggestion and misdiagnosis (Dallam 2000; Merckelbach et al. 2002; Ross 2000). Proponents of this point of view argue that individuals with DID are, as a group, highly hypnotizable and therefore quite suggestible and that a few specialist clinicians usually make the vast majority of diagnoses. However, it has been observed that the symptomatology of patients diagnosed by specialists in dissociation does not differ from that of patients assessed by psychiatrists, psychologists, and physicians in more general practices, who diagnose one or two cases per year. Furthermore, a systematic review of the literature by Dalenberg et al. (2012) concluded that the evidence did not support the suggestibility model of the link between trauma and dissociation. These authors found, in accord with the trauma model, that the relationship between trauma and dissociation was consistent and moderate in strength and remained significant when objective rather than subjective measures of trauma were used (Dalenberg et al. 2012). In addition, dissociation was temporally associated with trauma and trauma-related treatment and was predictive of trauma history even when fantasy-proneness was controlled. Dissociation was not found to be reliably associated with suggestibility, nor was there evidence of greater inaccuracy of recovered versus persistent memory. This is growing evidence for dissociation as a regulatory response to fear or other extreme emotion during and after traumatic experiences, with measurable biological correlates (Dalenberg et al. 2014; Vissia et al. 2016).

Data from other countries provide further evidence that dissociation is neither culture-bound nor the product of diagnostic expectation. Akyüz et al. (1999) examined the prevalence of DID in the general population of a rural area in Turkey. Among the subjects assessed, 1.7% received a diagnosis of dissociative disorder according to a structured interview, and half of these fulfilled clinical criteria for DID, yielding a minimum prevalence of 0.4% for DID. Thus, the data of Akyüz et al. (1999), derived from a population with no public awareness of DID and no exposure to systematic psychotherapy (thus eliminating the possible "iatrogenic contamination factor"),

TABLE 16–2. **DSM dissociative disorders: comparison of DSM-IV and DSM-5**

DSM-IV disorders	DSM-5 disorders	Changes
Dissociative identity disorder	Dissociative identity disorder	Broadened cross-cultural reach of disorder by including reference to pathological possession. Detailed clinical descriptors incorporated (Criterion A) to facilitate case detection. Clarification that identity alteration does not have to be directly witnessed, but instead could be reported by the patient. Clarification of the amnesia criterion (Criterion B) to include inability to recall everyday as well as traumatic information. Inclusion of additional criteria stating that symptoms must be associated with clinically significant distress and functional impairment (Criterion C) and cannot be part of a broadly accepted cultural or religious practice (Criterion D).
Dissociative amnesia	Dissociative amnesia	Clarification of Criterion A to specify two recognized types of amnesia: selective and generalized. Addition of specifier "with dissociative fugue."
Dissociative fugue	—	Removal from DSM-5 as a diagnostic entity; fugue is now a subtype of dissociative amnesia.
Depersonalization disorder	Depersonalization/derealization disorder	Addition of "derealization." As part of Criterion A, DSM-5 allows for the presence of depersonalization, derealization, or both; the remaining criteria are identical except for minor wording changes.
Dissociative disorder not otherwise specified	Other specified or unspecified dissociative disorder	As described in DSM-IV, dissociative disorder not otherwise specified would have been a grab-all category including all dissociative phenomena not meeting one of the other formal dissociative disorders. In DSM-5 this group has been divided into "other specified" and "unspecified" dissociative disorders to allow for differentiation between syndromes where the cause is known and those in which the cause is unknown or more diagnostic information is required. Minor wording changes, including the addition of identity disturbances (dissociative) in individuals exposed to stressful events lasting less than 1 month, and modification of dissociative trance disorder were also made.

TABLE 16–2. **DSM dissociative disorders: comparison of DSM-IV and DSM-5** *(continued)*

DSM-IV disorders	DSM-5 disorders	Changes
Related disorders	Related disorders	
Acute stress disorder[a]	Acute stress disorder[b]	Some wording changes; consolidation of intrusion, dissociative, avoidance, and arousal symptoms into one criterion (B); clarification of time frame (Criterion C).
Posttraumatic stress disorder (PTSD)[a]	PTSD[b]	Some wording changes.
		Modification of Criterion A, suggesting that the disorder may be triggered by learning of a traumatic event experienced by a family member or close friend and/or exposure to aversive details of an event rather than just directly witnessing the event.
		Addition of a cluster symptom involving negative alterations in cognitions and mood associated with a traumatic event (Criterion D).
		Addition of PTSD "with dissociative symptoms" subtype.

[a]Located in the DSM-IV chapter "Anxiety Disorders."
[b]Located in the DSM-5 chapter "Trauma- and Stressor-Related Disorders."

suggest that DID cannot be considered simply an iatrogenic artifact, a culture-bound syndrome, or a phenomenon induced by media influences.

If such patients were so suggestible and subject to directive influence by diagnosticians, then it is surprising that their presenting symptoms persisted for an average of 6.5 years before the diagnosis was made (Putnam et al. 1986). Rather, it would seem likely that such patients would accept a suggestion that they have another disorder, such as schizophrenia, dysthymia, substance use disorder, or borderline personality disorder, because they encounter many clinicians who are unaware of or unfamiliar with DID.

The skepticism regarding the existence of DID is compounded in the case of criminals, because of issues of suspected malingering. In fact, peritraumatic dissociation, with or without a history of dissociative disorder, is quite frequently reported by offenders presenting for a forensic psychiatric examination, is a risk factor for violence, and is seen most often in crimes of extreme violence (Bourget et al. 2017). Lewis et al. (1997) reviewed the clinical records of 12 murderers with a DSM-IV–defined diagnosis of DID (American Psychiatric Association 1994). Data were gathered from medical, psychiatric, social service, school, military, and prison records and from records of interviews with subjects' family members. In their sample, Lewis et al. were able to independently corroborate the presence of signs and symptoms of DID in childhood and adulthood from several sources in all 12 cases. Furthermore, objective evidence of severe abuse was obtained in 11 cases. Of interest, most subjects had amnesia for most of the abuse, and thus underreported it. Marked changes in writing style and/or signatures were documented in 10 cases.

A study examined avoidance and overly general memory in patients with DID, control groups of PTSD patients, healthy control subjects, and DID simulators, using the autobiographical memory test to compare the performance of separate identity states (Huntjens et al. 2014). The authors found no significant differences in memory specificity between the separate identities in DID. Irrespective of identity state, DID patients were characterized by a lack of memory specificity that was similar to that found in PTSD patients. The converging results for DID and PTSD patients add empirical evidence for the role of overly general memory in the maintenance of posttraumatic psychopathology.

In a study using positron emission tomography, DID individuals and matched DID-simulating healthy control subjects underwent an autobiographical script-driven imagery paradigm in hypoaroused and hyperaroused identity states (Reinders et al. 2014). As in two previous studies of PTSD dissociative subtypes, Reinders et al. found activation of the rostral/dorsal anterior cingulate, the prefrontal cortex, and the amygdala and insula in the DID group. However, they also found that in DID subjects, the hypoaroused identity state activated the prefrontal cortex, cingulate, posterior association areas, and parahippocampal gyri, thereby overmodulating emotion regulation; the hyperaroused identity state activated the amygdala and insula as well as the dorsal striatum, thereby undermodulating emotion. These findings provide further evidence that DID is related to PTSD, because hypoaroused and hyperarousal states in DID and PTSD are similar.

In fact, using arterial spin labeling perfusion MRI, researchers studied two prototypical dissociative subsystems of the personality, the "emotional part" (EP) and the "apparently normal part" (ANP), among patients with DID and healthy (actors) controls (Schlumpf et al. 2014). Their findings suggested that DID involves dissociative part-dependent resting-state differences. Compared with ANP, EP activated brain structures involved in self-referencing and sensorimotor actions more. Actors had different perfusion patterns than patients with genuine ANP and EP. Comparisons of neural activity in individuals with DID and non-DID simulating control subjects suggested that the resting-state features of ANP and EP in DID are not due to imagination. These findings are consistent with the theory of structural dissociation of the personality and inconsistent with the idea that DID is caused by suggestion, fantasy-proneness, or role playing.

Given the current evidence, DID as a diagnostic entity cannot be explained as a phenomenon created by iatrogenic influences, suggestibility, malingering, or social role taking (Şar et al. 2017). On the contrary, DID is an empirically robust chronic psychiatric disorder based on neurobiological, cognitive, and interpersonal nonintegration as a response to unbearable stress. A study of brain structural MRI scans (including patients with DID, PTSD without dissociation, and healthy control subjects, all matched for age, sex, and education) found that global hippocampal volumes were significantly smaller in all patients (DID and PTSD) compared with healthy control subjects (Chalavi et al. 2015), consistent with earlier work. Of note, smaller global and subfield hippocampal volumes significantly correlated with higher severity of childhood traumatization and dissociative symptoms. PTSD–DID and PTSD-only patients with a history of childhood traumatization had significantly smaller global hippocampal volumes relative to healthy control subjects, whereas PTSD–DID patients had abnormally shaped and significantly smaller volumes in the CA2–3, CA4-DG, and (pre)subiculum compared with the healthy control group.

Course

Although DID is diagnosed in childhood with increasing frequency, it typically arises as a clinical entity between adolescence and the third decade of life (Kluft 1984b). Symptoms of DID usually appear before age 40 years, although there is often considerable delay between initial symptom presentation and diagnosis (Putnam et al. 1986). The female-to-male sex ratio of DID is 5:4 in children and adolescents and 9:1 in adults (Sno and Schalken 1999).

Untreated, DID is a chronic and recurrent disorder. It rarely remits spontaneously, but the symptoms may not be evident for some time (Kluft 1985). DID has been called "a pathology of hiddenness" (Gutheil, as quoted in Kluft 1988a, p. 575). The dissociation itself hampers self-monitoring and accurate reporting of symptoms. Many patients with the disorder are not fully aware of the extent of their dissociative symptomatology. They may be reluctant to bring up symptoms because of having encountered frequent skepticism on the part of clinicians. Furthermore, because most patients with DID report histories of sexual and physical abuse, the shame associated with such histories, as well as fear of retribution, may inhibit reporting of symptoms (Coons et al. 1988; Kluft 1988a; Putnam et al. 1986; Spiegel 1984).

Treatment

In a systematic review, Brand et al. (2009a, 2009b) included eight nonrandomized treatment outcome studies for the same patient population. These studies provided preliminary evidence that treatment is effective in reducing a range of symptoms associated with dissociative disorders, including depression, anxiety, and dissociative symptoms. Despite suggesting positive results, the findings were tempered by lack of randomization, selection bias, high dropout rates, and small sample sizes (Brand et al. 2009b). Subsequently, in a prospective study of almost 300 therapists and patients from around the world, follow-up data confirmed that patients showed decreases in dissociation, PTSD, general distress, depression, suicide attempts, self-harm, dangerous behaviors, drug use, physical pain, and hospitalizations, as well as improved functioning and higher Global Assessment of Functioning scores (Brand et al. 2009a). In addition, more patients progressed from an early stage to a more advanced stage of treatment than regressed from an advanced to an early treatment stage.

Psychotherapy. *Therapeutic guidelines.* Psychotherapy can help patients with DID gain control over the dissociative process underlying their symptoms. The fundamental psychotherapeutic stance should involve meeting patients halfway, in the sense of acknowledging that they experience themselves as fragmented, yet the reality is that the fundamental problem is a failure of integration of conflicting memories and aspects of the self. Therefore, the goal in therapy is to facilitate integration of disparate elements. This integration can be accomplished in a variety of ways.

Secrets are frequently a problem with DID patients, who attempt to use the therapist to reinforce a dissociative strategy that withholds relevant information from certain personality states. Such patients often like to confide plans or stories—for example, traumatic memories or plans for self-destructive activities—to the therapist with the idea that the information is to be kept from other parts of the self. It is important for the therapist to set clear limits and to be committed to helping all portions of a patient's personality structure to learn about warded-off information. It is wise for the therapist to clarify explicitly that he or she will not become involved in secret collusion. Furthermore, when important agreements are negotiated, such as a commitment on the part of the patient to seek medical help before acting on a thought to harm self or others, the clinician should discuss with the patient that this is an "all-points bulletin"—that is, one that requires attention from all of the relevant personality states. The patient's excuse that certain personality states were "not aware" of the agreement should not be accepted.

For example, a patient with DID who had been in treatment for many years demonstrated a new alter who threatened to arrange for an apparently accidental death. The therapist told the alter that he, the therapist, would have to share this information with the other personalities. "You can't do that," the alter replied. "That would violate doctor–patient confidentiality." Suppressing a smile, the therapist explained that confidentiality did not apply between identities.

Maldonado et al. (2002) described a series of issues (Table 16–3) to be considered in the treatment of DID. These guidelines were designed to facilitate the therapist–patient contract by establishing clear lines of communication, delineating therapeutic boundaries, eliminating splitting, and enhancing control over dissociative experiences.

Hypnosis. Hypnosis can be helpful in therapy as well as in diagnosis. The simple structure of hypnotic induction may elicit dissociative phenomena. For example, the Hypnotic Induction Profile (H. Spiegel and D. Spiegel 2004) was administered to a woman who had experienced hysterical pseudoseizures. In the middle of a routine induction, her head suddenly turned to the side, and she relived with considerable affect, as if it were happening in the present, an episode in which she had been abducted and

TABLE 16–3.	Considerations when initiating treatment of dissociative identity disorder

1. Free access to all pertinent records
2. Review of all available and pertinent records
3. Freedom to discuss all past and current pertinent information with previous therapists
4. Complete organic/neurological workup
5. Contract for safety
6. Increased communication and cooperation among alters
7. "No secrets" policy
8. Establishment of hierarchical pattern of communication
9. Establishment of hierarchical pattern of responsibility
10. Limited exploration followed by therapeutic condensation of memories
11. "All details are not needed" policy
12. Guidelines regarding contact during hospitalizations and continued therapy after discharge
13. Videotaping
14. Ultimate goal: "full integration"
15. "One day you will make me obsolete" principle

Source. Maldonado et al. 2002.

sexually assaulted. This enabled her and the clinician to reanalyze her symptoms as spontaneous dissociation, similar to the hypnotic state she had been in. The capacity to elicit such symptoms on command provides the first hint of the ability to control these symptoms. Most of these patients have the experience of being unable to stop dissociative symptoms but are often intrigued by the possibility of starting them because that carries with it the potential for changing or stopping the symptoms as well.

Hypnosis can be helpful in facilitating access to dissociated personalities. The personalities may simply occur spontaneously during hypnotic induction. An alternative strategy is to hypnotize the patient and use age regression to help the patient reorient to a time when a different personality state was manifest. An instruction later to change back to the present time usually elicits a return to the other personality state. This process then becomes an alternative means of teaching the patient control over the dissociation.

Alternatively, entering the state of hypnosis may make it possible to simply "call up" different identities or personality states. Patients can be taught a simple self-hypnosis exercise. For example, the patient can be instructed to do the following:

> Count silently from 1 to 3. On 1, do one thing: look up. On 2, do two things: slowly close your eyes, and take a deep breath. On 3, do three things: let the breath out, let your eyes relax but keep them closed, and let your body float. Then let one hand float up into the air like a balloon. Develop a pleasant sense of floating throughout your body. (H. Spiegel and D. Spiegel 2004, p. 448)

Following use of formal exercises such as this, it is often possible for the therapist to simply ask to speak with a given alter personality, without the formal use of hypnosis. After some training, a therapist may simply call up a given "identity state" (e.g., "the part of you that felt hurt") as opposed to a specific "person" (e.g., an alter who identifies herself as "Lucy" when the patient's given name is Barbara). The reason for using a particular identity state rather than a specific name to address an alter is that fostering a relationship with each personality state (which the patient identifies as a distinctive "person" or entity) serves to promote integration of these dissociated or fragmented personality states.

Memory retrieval.   Because loss of memory in DID is complex and chronic, retrieval of memory is likewise a more extended and integral part of the psychotherapeutic process. The therapy becomes an integrating experience of information sharing among disparate personality elements. In conceptualizing DID as a chronic PTSD, the psychotherapist can focus on working through traumatic memories in addition to controlling the dissociation.

Controlled access to memories greatly facilitates psychotherapy. As in the treatment of dissociative amnesia (discussed later in the "Dissociative Amnesia" section), a variety of strategies can be used to help DID patients break down amnesic barriers. Use of hypnosis to go to that place in imagination and ask one or more such parts of the self to interact can be helpful.

Once these memories of earlier traumatic experiences have been accessed and brought into consciousness, it is crucial to help the patient work through the painful affect, inappropriate self-blame, and other reactions to these memories. A model of grief work is helpful, enabling the patient to acknowledge and bear the import of such memories (Lindemann 1994). It may be useful to have the patient visualize the memories rather than relive them as a way of making their intensity more manageable. Hypnotic dissociation can be used to separate somatic from psychological distress by having the patient imagine being physically somewhere safe and comfortable, such as a bath, a lake, a hot tub, or just floating in space, and maintaining this sense of physical comfort even while imagining traumatic experiences. The balance between sympathetic arousal and parasympathetic self-soothing is closely associated with emotional arousal, so using hypnotic dissociation to separate somatic from psychological arousal is a helpful stress-modulating technique (Porges 1997). The ability to dissociate emotional from physiological arousal can help patients restructure their distress by modulating its physiological concomitants (Porges 2009). The cognitive and affective restructuring can be facilitated by having the patient separate the memories and place them on opposite sides of an imaginary screen—for example, on one side picturing something an abuser did to him or her, and on the other side picturing how the patient tried to protect himself or herself from the abuse.

> A young woman with DID remembered a particularly painful episode in hypnosis. When she was 12 years old, her stepfather smoked a good deal of marijuana and then forced her to perform oral sex on him. She recalled being repelled by what he was forcing her to do and then remembered that she had gagged and vomited all over him. "I spoiled his fun. He threw me up against a wall, but it did not bother me a bit because I knew I ruined it for him." She was instructed to picture on one side of the screen what he had done to her and on the other what she had done to him.

Such techniques can help make the traumatic memories more bearable by placing them in a broader perspective, one in which the trauma victim also can identify adaptive aspects of his or her response to the trauma.

This technique and similar approaches can help these individuals work through traumatic memories, enabling them to bear the memories in consciousness and therefore reducing the need for dissociation as a means of keeping such memories out of consciousness. Although these techniques can be helpful and often result in reduced fragmentation and integration, intense emotional distress and other complications can occur in the psychotherapy of these patients (Kluft 1992; Maldonado et al. 1998; Spiegel 1984, 1986). Given that these patients commonly have a history of trauma, usually inflicted by caretakers, it is important to discuss the therapeutic context with the patient, to deal with the understandable fear on the part of the patient that the therapist is inducing rather than trying to help with distress.

The information retrieved from memory in these ways should be reviewed, traumatic memories should be put into perspective, and emotional expression should be encouraged and worked through, with the goal of sharing the information as widely as possible among various parts of the patient's personality structure. Instructing other alter personalities to "listen" while a given alter is talking and reviewing previously dissociated material uncovered can be helpful. The therapist conveys his or her desire to disseminate the information, without accepting responsibility for transmitting it across all personality boundaries.

"Rule of thirds."   Psychotherapy with a DID patient can be a time-consuming and emotionally taxing process. The "rule of thirds" is a helpful guideline (Kluft 1988a). The therapist should spend the first third of the psychotherapy session assessing the patient's current mental state and life problems and defining a problem area that might benefit from retrieval into conscious memory and working through. The therapist should spend the second third of the session accessing and working through this memory. The therapist should allow a final third for helping the patient assimilate the information, regulate and modulate emotional and physiological responses, and discuss any responses to the therapist and plans for the immediate future.

It is wise to use this final third of the session for debriefing and helping the patient to reorient, to attempt to integrate the new material, to transmit information across personalities, and to prepare to terminate the session. The therapist may resist doing this because the intense abreacted materials are often so compelling and interesting. Also, the patient may resist sharing of information across personalities.

Given the intensity of the material that often emerges involving memories of sexual and physical abuse and the sudden shifts in mental state accompanied by amnesia, the therapist is called on to take a clear and structured role in managing the psychotherapy. Appropriate limits must be set about self-destructive or threatening behavior, agreements must be made regarding physical safety and treatment compliance, and other matters must be presented to the patient in such a way that dissociative amnesic barriers are not an acceptable explanation for failure to live up to agreements.

Traumatic transference.   Transference applies with special meaning in patients who have been physically and sexually abused. These patients have had presumed "caregivers" who acted instead in an exploitative and sometimes sadistic fashion. These patients thus expect the same from their therapists. Although their reality testing is good enough that they can perceive genuine caring, these patients expect therapists either to exploit them (with the patients viewing the working through of traumatic memories as a reinflicting of the trauma and an opportunity for the therapists to take sadistic pleasure in the patients' suffering) or to be excessively passive (with the patients identifying the therapists with some uncaring family figure who knew abuse was occurring but did little or nothing to stop it). It is important in managing the therapy to keep these issues in mind and to make them frequent topics of discussion. Attention to these issues can defuse, but not eliminate, such traumatic transference distortions of the therapeutic relationship (Maldonado et al. 1998).

Integration.   The ultimate goal of psychotherapy for patients with DID is integration of the disparate states. They might have considerable resistance to this process. Early in therapy, the patient views the dissociation as tremendous protection: "I knew my father could get some of me, but he couldn't get all of me." Indeed, the patient may experience efforts of integration as an attempt on the part of the therapist to "kill" personalities. These fears must be worked through, and the patient must be shown how to control the degree of integration, giving the patient a sense of gradually being able to control his or her dissociative processes in the service of working through traumatic memories. The process of the psychotherapy, in emphasizing control, must alter rather than reinforce the content, which involves the reexperiencing of helplessness, a symbolic reenactment of trauma.

As previously mentioned, a patient with DID often fears integration as an attempt to "kill" alter personalities, thereby making the patient more vulnerable to mistreatment by depriving him or her of the dissociative defense. At the same time, this defense represents an internalization of the abusive person or persons in the patient's memory, a kind of identification with the aggressor. Setting aside the defense also means acknowledging and bearing the discomfort of helplessness at having been victimized and working through the irrational self-blame that gave the patient a fantasy of control over events that he or she was, in fact, helpless to control. Hypnotic images of embracing oneself as a helpless child rather than blaming oneself as a willing participant in the abuse can facilitate restoration of self-esteem.

> An experienced psychotherapist in her sixties was hypnotically reliving abuse at age 8 years by her father. She initially described herself as "going along" with the abuse to avoid family problems. Only with questions about her physical size and ability to refuse did it gradually become clear that she had been helpless to stop the assaults.

Difficult as it is, the ultimate goal of psychotherapy is mastery over the dissociative process, controlled access to dissociative states, integration of warded-off painful memories and material, and a more integrated continuum of identity, memory, and consciousness (Maldonado et al. 1998). Although there have been no randomized controlled trials of psychotherapy outcome in patients with this disorder, systematic reviews of case series reports indicate a moderate to large effect size in positive outcome and demonstrate that integration is associated with better symptom reduction in most cases (Brand et al. 2009b, 2012; Kluft 1991).

Legal considerations.   The Council on Scientific Affairs of the American Medical Association convened a panel of experts to examine the research evidence relevant to the effect of hypnosis on memory and recall. The panel concluded that what evidence exists indicates that the use of hypnosis tends to increase the productivity of witnesses, resulting in new memories, some of which are true and some of which are incorrect

(Council on Scientific Affairs 1985). Furthermore, some studies showed an increase in the confidence assigned by hypnotized subjects to their memories despite the fact that the percentage of correct responses had not improved. The panel noted that the analogy between the laboratory setting in which most of the studies were done and the real-life situation in the courtroom must be drawn with great caution and that situations in which extreme emotional and physical trauma have occurred differ markedly. The panel recommended that careful guidelines similar to the ones outlined in California law be followed when hypnosis is used in the forensic setting (Kluft 1986). Similarly, the "FBI Guidelines for Use of Hypnosis" (Ault 1979) detail the parameters and rules to follow in order to maximize the yield of hypnotic recollection while preserving the integrity of the process.

Hypnosis is clearly not a truth serum, and the courts must weigh the effects of any hypnotic induction on a witness. At the same time, hypnosis may, in certain cases, help a traumatized and amnesic witness to recall details not brought forward through conventional interrogation methods. Despite the former popularity of hypnosis as a way of "improving" eyewitness memory, many courts almost always regard the use of this testimony to be inadmissible, whereas others allow it only when strict procedural guidelines have been followed. Although the U.S. Supreme Court recognized a defendant's constitutional right to admit his or her own hypnotically elicited testimony, other courts have recognized a constitutional basis to exclude hypnotically elicited testimony in most other circumstances (Newman and Thompson 1999).

Maldonado and colleagues (Maldonado and Fink 2007; Maldonado and Spiegel 2008) summarized and adapted the guidelines provided by the American Medical Association (Orne et al. 1985) and the American Society of Clinical Hypnosis (Hammond 1995) for the use of hypnosis as a method of memory enhancement. The guidelines suggest that when hypnosis or any other memory enhancement method is being used for forensic purposes or in the context of working out traumatic memories, especially those related to childhood physical and/or sexual abuse, the steps shown in Table 16–4 should be applied.

Some have proposed that DID can be simulated or that it is mediated by high suggestibility, fantasy-proneness, and sociocultural influences (Spanos 1994). However, a study comparing patients with DID, patients with PTSD, and DID-simulating healthy control subjects found that DID patients were not more fantasy-prone or suggestible and did not generate more false memories; these findings supported the trauma model of DID and challenged the core hypothesis of the fantasy model (Reinders et al. 2016; Vissia et al. 2016). Similarly, studies have demonstrated how simulators fail to adequately present the subtle and less-well-known symptoms and associated features of DID (Brand and Chasson 2015; Brand et al. 2016; Dalenberg et al. 2012; Huntjens et al. 2012; Reinders et al. 2012; Schlumpf et al. 2014).

Cognitive-behavioral approaches.   Fine (1999) summarized the tactical-integration model for the treatment of dissociative disorders. This model consists of structured cognitive-behavioral–based treatments that foster symptom relief, followed by integration of the personalities and/or ego states into one mainstream of consciousness. This approach promotes proficiency in control over posttraumatic and dissociative symptoms, is collaborative and exploratory, and conveys a consistent message of empowerment to the patient.

TABLE 16–4.	Guidelines for the use of hypnosis in memory work

1. Before hypnosis use, perform a thorough evaluation of the patient.
2. Explore the patient's expectations about treatment in general and hypnosis use in particular.
3. Obtain the patient's permission to consult with his or her attorney.
4. Clarify your role (i.e., therapist vs. forensic consultant) before initiating any assessment and/or treatment. Make sure the patient clearly understands your role in the case.
5. Obtain written informed consent regarding the nature of hypnotic retrieval (explain to the subject and his or her attorney about the nature of hypnotically retrieved memories) and possible side effects of memory work.
6. Clarify the patient's expectation regarding hypnotically enhanced or recovered memories.
7. Maintain neutrality throughout every interaction with the patient.
8. Make a video recording of the entire interview and hypnotic session.
9. Thoroughly document any and all prehypnosis memories.
10. Objectively measure hypnotizability.
11. Carefully document your discussion of hypnosis and memory, issues of accuracy of memory, informed consent, and the maintenance of a stance of neutrality and nonleading approach.
12. Use an expert as a hypnosis consultant.
13. Conduct the interview in a neutral tone; avoid leading or suggestive questions.
14. Demonstrate a balance between supportiveness and empathy while assisting the patient in critically evaluating the elicited material.
15. Do not encourage patients to institute litigation or to confront alleged perpetrators solely on the basis of information retrieved under hypnosis.
16. Carefully debrief the subject at the end of each session.
17. Carefully document and produce a report containing the following:

    Detailed prehypnotic memories

    Hypnotizability score

    Hypnotic techniques used

    Any significant behavior

    Any confirmed or new memories and details

Source. Maldonado JR: "Diagnosis and Treatment of Dissociative Disorders," in *Manual for the Course "Advanced Hypnosis: The Use of Hypnosis in Medicine and Psychiatry."* Presented at 153rd annual meeting of the American Psychiatric Association, Chicago, IL, May 13–18, 2000.

In addition, both cognitive analytic therapy (CAT) (Kellett 2005; Ryle and Fawkes 2007) and dialectical behavior therapy (DBT) (Braakmann et al. 2007) have been found to be helpful as adjunctive or primary treatment of patients with DID. In CAT, multiplicity is understood in terms of a range of self–other patterns (i.e., reciprocal role relationships) originating in childhood. These patterns alternate in determining experience and action according to the situation (i.e., contextual multiplicity). They may be restricted by adverse childhood experiences (i.e., diminished multiplicity), and severe deprivation or abuse may result in a structural dissociation of self-processes (i.e., pathological multiplicity). In CAT practice, descriptions of dysfunctional relationship patterns and of transitions between them are worked out by therapist and patient at the start of therapy and are used by both throughout its course (Ryle and Fawkes 2007).

A study using DBT found that patients with high preintervention levels of dissociation achieved the greatest relative symptom reduction (Braakmann et al. 2007). These results are explained by the DBT treatment setting, which includes specific psychoeducation and treatment concerning dissociative behavior.

Despite the challenges associated with the treatment of these individuals, analyses of a 6-year follow-up study, the Treatment of Patients with Dissociative Disorders study, revealed that dissociative disorder patients benefited from specialized treatment, experiencing significantly fewer stressors ($P<0.01$), instances of sexual revictimization ($P<0.001$), and psychiatric hospitalizations ($P<0.05$), as well as higher global functioning ($P<0.001$) (Myrick et al. 2017b). Similarly, the data show that patients receiving specialized treatment experience longitudinal and cross-sectional reductions in inpatient and outpatient costs over time, as reported by both patients and therapists (Myrick et al. 2017a, 2017b). In addition, these changes were associated with lower inpatient and outpatient treatment costs (Myrick et al. 2017a).

Psychopharmacology. To date, no good evidence shows that medication of any type has a direct therapeutic effect on the dissociative process manifested by patients with DID. In fact, most dissociative symptoms seem relatively resistant to pharmacological intervention (Loewenstein 2006). Thus, pharmacological treatment has been limited to the control of signs and symptoms afflicting patients with DID or comorbid conditions rather than the treatment of dissociation per se. In fact, a recent major review of the literature yielded 21 case studies and 80 empirical studies, presenting data on 1,171 new cases of DID, but shed no light on effective treatments (Boysen and Van Bergen 2013). Similarly, published "guidelines" add little to the pharmacological management of DID (Brand et al. 2012).

Whereas in the past, short-acting barbiturates such as sodium amobarbital were used intravenously to reverse functional amnesias, this technique is no longer used, largely because of poor results. Benzodiazepines have at times been used to facilitate recall through controlling secondary anxiety associated with retrieval of traumatic memories. However, these effects may be nonspecific at best. Furthermore, the sedative and amnestic properties of these agents and the fact that they may elicit a sudden transition in mental state may increase rather than decrease amnesic barriers and the patient's sense of lack of control and make it harder for the therapist to employ effective techniques such as hypnosis. Thus, inducing state changes pharmacologically could, in theory, add to difficulty in retrieval and behavioral dyscontrol. The only systematic study on the use of benzodiazepines in patients with DID was conducted by Loewenstein and Putnam (1988). In their study, they used clonazepam successfully to control PTSD-like symptoms in a small sample ($n=5$) of DID patients, achieving improvement in sleep continuity and a decrease in frequency of flashbacks and nightmares.

Antidepressants are the most useful class of psychotropic agents for patients with DID. Such patients frequently have dysthymic disorder or major depression as well as DID, and when these disorders are present, especially with somatic signs and suicidal ideation, antidepressant medication can be helpful. At least two studies report on the successful use of antidepressant medications (Barkin and Kluft 1986; Kluft 1984c). The use of antidepressants should be limited to the treatment of DID patients who experience symptoms of major depression (Barkin and Kluft 1986). The selective serotonin reuptake inhibitors are effective at reducing comorbid depressive symptoms and have the advantage of far less lethality in overdose compared with tricyclic antidepressants and monoamine oxidase inhibitors. Medication compliance is a problem with such patients because dissociated personality states may interfere with the taking of medication by "hiding" or hoarding pills or patients may overdose.

Antipsychotics are rarely useful in reducing dissociative symptoms. They are used occasionally for containing impulsive behavior, with varying effect. More often, they are used with little benefit when patients with DID have been given misdiagnoses of schizophrenia (Kluft 1987). In addition to the risks of side effects, such as tardive dyskinesia, the neuroleptics may reduce the range of affect, thereby making patients with DID look spuriously as though they had schizophrenia. In fact, most DID researchers have reported an extremely high incidence of adverse side effects with the use of neuroleptic medications (Barkin and Kluft 1986; Kluft 1988b; Putnam 1989).

Anticonvulsants have been used to treat seizure disorders, which have a high rate of comorbidity with DID, mood disorders, and the impulsiveness associated with personality disorders. These agents have been used to reduce impulsive behavior but are rarely definitively helpful. The high incidence of serious side effects and abuse or overdose potential also should be kept in mind. At least one study reported the effectiveness (73%) of low-dose naltrexone (0.06 mg/kg body weight) in the management of patients with severe trauma-related and dissociative disorders (Pape and Wöller 2015). Patients who responded reported experiencing a clearer perception of both their surroundings and their inner life, as well as improved self-regulation.

Dissociative Amnesia

Diagnostic Features

As specified in the DSM-5 diagnostic criteria, the hallmark of dissociative amnesia is the inability to recall important personal information, usually of a traumatic or stressful nature, that cannot be explained by ordinary forgetfulness in the absence of overt brain pathology or substance use. The main difference between the diagnostic criteria in DSM-5 and those in DSM-IV is clarification of Criterion A to allow for the presence of either 1) localized or selective amnesia for a specific event or events or 2) generalized amnesia for identity and life history. In addition, DSM-5 reduced the former diagnosis of dissociative fugue to a subtype of dissociative amnesia, designated by the specifier "with dissociative fugue" (i.e., purposeful travel or bewildered wandering). Patients with "psychogenic" or dissociative amnesia typically differ from patients with the neurological amnestic syndrome in that memory for their personal life histories is much more severely affected than is their ability to learn and retain new information; that is, they have isolated retrograde amnesia (Brandt and Van Gorp 2006).

Dissociative amnesia is considered the most common of the dissociative disorders. Amnesia is a symptom commonly found in several other dissociative and anxiety disorders, including acute stress disorder, PTSD, somatization disorder, and DID. A higher incidence of dissociative amnesia has been described in the context of war and natural and other disasters (Maldonado et al. 2002). There appears to be a direct relationship between the severity of the exposure to trauma and the incidence of amnesia. Dissociative amnesia is the classical functional disorder of memory and involves difficulty in retrieving discrete components of autobiographical–episodic memory (Kritchevsky et al. 2004; Spiegel et al. 2011). It does not, however, involve a difficulty in memory storage, as in Wernicke-Korsakoff syndrome. Because the amnesia primarily involves difficulties in retrieval rather than encoding or storage, the memory deficits are usually reversible. Once the amnesia has cleared, normal memory function is resumed. Dissociative amnesia has three primary characteristics:

1. The memory loss is episodic. The first-person recollection of certain events is lost, rather than knowledge of procedures.
2. The memory loss is for a discrete period of time, ranging from minutes to years. It is not vagueness or the inefficient retrieval of memories, but rather a dense unavailability of memories that had been clearly accessible. Unlike in the amnestic disorders, such as from damage to the medial temporal lobe in surgery, or in Wernicke-Korsakoff syndrome, there is usually no difficulty in learning *new* episodic information. Thus, the amnesia is typically retrograde rather than anterograde, with one or more discrete periods of past information becoming unavailable. However, a dissociative syndrome of continuous difficulty in incorporating new information may mimic organic amnestic syndromes.
3. The memory loss is generally for events of a traumatic or stressful nature. In one study, the majority of cases involved child abuse (60%), but disavowed behaviors such as marital problems, sexual activity, suicide attempts, criminal behavior, and the death of a relative can also be precipitants (Coons and Milstein 1986).

Dissociative amnesia is most common in the third and fourth decades of life (Coons and Milstein 1986). It usually involves one episode, but multiple periods of lost memory are not uncommon. Comorbidity with conversion disorder, bulimia, alcohol abuse, and depression is common, and diagnoses of histrionic, dependent, and borderline personality disorders occur in a substantial minority of such patients (Coons and Milstein 1986). Legal difficulties, such as driving under the influence of alcohol, also accompany dissociative amnesia in a minority of cases. Occasionally, there may be a history of head trauma. If that is the case, usually the trauma is too slight to have neurophysiological consequences. The population prevalence of dissociative amnesia is 1.8% (Johnson et al. 2006).

Dissociative amnesia can be triggered by any major incident and therefore also by brain injury, especially (mild) traumatic brain injury, or by body injury (Staniloiu et al. 2018). Even though the evidence suggests that psychological stress seems to be the major triggering factor for dissociative disorders (Bremner 2010; Dalenberg et al. 2012), substantial data suggest that somatic symptoms are, in fact, major triggers for the manifestation of dissociative amnesia, and possibly also perpetuating factors (Staniloiu et al. 2018).

Dissociative amnesia usually involves discrete boundaries around the period of time unavailable to consciousness. Individuals with such a disorder lose the ability to recall what happened during a specific time. They demonstrate not vagueness or spotty memory, but rather a loss of any episodic memory for a finite period. Such individuals initially may not be aware of the memory loss; that is, they may not remember that they do not remember. However, they may find, for example, new purchases in their homes but have no memory of having obtained them. They report being told that they have done or said things that they cannot remember. Some individuals do experience episodes of selective amnesia, usually for specific traumatic incidents, which may be more interwoven with periods of intact memory. In these cases, the amnesia is for a type of material remembered rather than for a discrete period of time.

Despite the fact that certain information is kept out of consciousness in dissociative amnesia, such information may exert an influence on consciousness. For example, a rape victim with no conscious recollection of the assault will nonetheless behave like someone who has been sexually victimized. Such individuals often show detachment and demoralization, are unable to enjoy intimate relationships, and show hyperarousal to stimuli reminiscent of the trauma. This phenomenon is similar to priming in memory research. Minutes or hours after reading a word list, individuals will complete a word stem for a word from the list (e.g., the stem *pre* for the word *prepare*) more quickly than they would for a word they have not recently seen. This phenomenon occurs even though they cannot consciously recall having recently read the word that constitutes the prime. Similarly, individuals instructed in hypnosis to forget having seen a list of words will nonetheless show priming effects from the hypnotically suppressed list. It is the essence of dissociative amnesia that material being kept out of conscious awareness is nonetheless active and may influence consciousness indirectly: out of sight does not mean out of mind.

Individuals with dissociative amnesia generally do not have disturbances of identity, except to the extent that their identity is influenced by the warded-off memory. It is not uncommon for such individuals to develop depressive symptoms as well, especially when the amnesia is in the wake of a traumatic episode. However, those with the fugue subtype of dissociative amnesia may have more pervasive amnesia for personal identity, sometimes coupled with aimless wandering or purposeful travel.

The precise mechanisms mediating dissociative amnesia are not understood. Theories vary from a self-protecting mechanism underlying the blockade of episodic memories that might also account for the extension to the semantic components of autobiographical memory (Reinhold and Markowitsch 2009) to cases of documented executive dysfunctions and reduced activation of frontal brain regions (Glisky et al. 2004) to deficits in executive functions and attention (Fujiwara et al. 2008) to prefrontal activations associated with a suppression of unwanted memories (Anderson et al. 2004). Some have theorized that in dissociative amnesia, the blocking of memory retrieval has an identity-protecting function by preserving the individual's ability to interact with his or her environment (Fujiwara and Markowitsch 2003; Reinhold and Markowitsch 2009). Markowitsch coined the term *mnestic block syndrome* to account for the phenomenon that irretrievable autobiographical memories are blocked instead of lost and to explain how the reexperiencing of sensory stimuli reminiscent of the original traumatic event may enable patients to regain further access to formerly blocked information (Markowitsch et al. 1999). In all cases, the amnestic episode is presumed to serve a protective function by offering patients a mechanism to exit a life situation that appears to them unmanageable or adverse (Staniloiu et al. 2018).

Treatment

To date, no controlled studies have addressed the treatment of dissociative amnesia. No established pharmacological treatments are available, except for the use of benzodiazepines or barbiturates for drug-assisted interviews (Maldonado et al. 2002). Most cases of dissociative amnesia revert spontaneously, especially when the individuals are removed from stressful or threatening situations, when they feel physically and psychologically safe, and/or when they are exposed to cues from the past (e.g., family members) (Loewenstein 1991; Maldonado et al. 2002). When a safe environment is not enough to restore normal memory functioning, the amnesia sometimes can be breached using techniques such as pharmacologically mediated interviews (i.e., using barbiturates and benzodiazepines), although these techniques are now rarely used.

On the other hand, most patients with dissociative disorders are highly hypnotizable on formal testing and therefore are easily able to make use of hypnotic techniques such as age regression. Patients are hypnotized and instructed to experience a time before the onset of the amnesia as though it were the present. Then the patients are reoriented in hypnosis to experience events during the amnesic period. Hypnosis can enable such patients to reorient temporally and therefore to achieve access to otherwise dissociated memories. If the warded-off memory has traumatic content, patients may abreact (i.e., express strong emotion) as these memories are elicited, and they will need psychotherapeutic help in integrating these memories and the associated affect into consciousness.

One technique that can help bring such memories into consciousness while modulating the affective response to them is the split-screen technique (H. Spiegel and D. Spiegel 2004). In this approach, patients are taught, by using hypnosis, to relive the traumatic event as if they were watching it on an imaginary movie or television screen. This technique is often helpful for individuals who are unable to relive the event as if it were occurring in the present, either because that process is too emotionally taxing or because they are not sufficiently hypnotizable to be able to engage in hypnotic age regression. The split-screen technique can also be used to provide dissociation between the psychological and the somatic aspects of the memory retrieval. Individuals can be put into self-hypnosis and instructed to get their bodies into a state of floating comfort and safety. They are reminded that no matter what they see on the screen, their bodies will be safe and comfortable.

A victim of a violent attempted rape had developed a selective amnesia for much of the physical struggle itself. She had sustained a basilar skull fracture, but she had not been rendered unconscious. She also had a generalized seizure shortly after the assault. She initially sought help with hypnosis in an attempt to improve her recollection of the assailant's face.

The woman was instructed in use of the split-screen technique and used it to relive the assault. She remembered two things that she had not previously recalled: 1) the assailant was surprised at how hard she was fighting with him, and 2) she recognized that he intended not merely to rape her but to kill her. She became convinced that had she let him drag her into her apartment, she likely would not have survived. She was tearful and frightened as she recalled this aspect of the assault that had been previously unavailable to consciousness.

She was then instructed to divide the imaginary screen in half, picturing on the left side an image of the viciousness and intensity of the assault and recognizing on the other side what she had done to protect herself. She was instructed to concentrate on these two aspects of the assault and then, when she was ready, to bring herself out of the state of self-hypnosis. She was told that she could use this as a self-hypnosis exercise several times a day if she wished, as a means of putting her memories of the rape into perspective. This cognitive and emotional restructuring of the traumatic memories made them more bearable in consciousness.

Before this psychotherapy, she had blamed herself for having fought so hard that she was seriously injured. Afterward, she recognized that she may have saved her life by fighting off the assailant so vigorously. This positive therapeutic outcome occurred despite the fact that she was unable to recall any new details about the assailant's physical appearance.

Psychotherapy for dissociative amnesia involves accessing the dissociated memories, working through affectively loaded aspects of these memories, and supporting the patient through the process of integrating these memories into consciousness.

Depersonalization/Derealization Disorder

Diagnostic Features

As specified in the DSM-5 diagnostic criteria, the essential feature of depersonalization/derealization disorder is the presence of *depersonalization* (i.e., persistent feelings of unreality, detachment, or estrangement from oneself or one's body, usually with the feeling that one is an outside observer of one's own mental processes), *derealization* (i.e., experiences of unreality or detachment with respect to surroundings), or both. Of note, Criterion A allows for the presence of either or both phenomena. Clinically, depersonalization is characterized by a profound disruption of self-awareness, mainly involving feelings of disembodiment and subjective emotional numbing (Sierra and David 2011; Spiegel et al. 2011). When derealization co-occurs with depersonalization, individuals experience an altered perception of their surroundings in which the world seems unreal or dreamlike. Affected individuals will often ruminate about this alteration and be preoccupied with their own somatic and mental functioning.

Thus, depersonalization/derealization disorder is primarily a disturbance in the integration of perceptual experience. Approximately one-third to one-half of patients with dissociative disorders will experience "hearing voices" that are described as "inner voices" and thus are distinguished from psychotic auditory hallucinations that usually seem to be coming from an external source (Coons 1998). Individuals with the disorder are usually distressed by it. Patients with dissociative disorders tend to experience these symptoms as "inexplicable and frightening" as well as indicators that they are "going crazy" (Spiegel et al. 2011). Different from those with delusional disorders and other psychotic processes, those with depersonalization/derealization disorder have intact reality testing. Patients are aware of some distortion in their perceptual experience and therefore are not delusional. The symptoms are often transient and may co-occur with a variety of other symptoms, especially anxiety, panic, or phobic symptoms. Indeed, the content of the anxiety may involve fears of "going crazy." Other than the addition of derealization as a diagnostic feature (Criterion A), there are no significant differences between the DSM-5 version and previous criteria.

Prevalence

Hunter et al. (2004) conducted a study using computerized databases and citation searches to assess the prevalence of symptoms of depersonalization and derealization in both clinical and nonclinical settings. They found that transient symptoms of depersonalization and derealization are common in the general population, with a lifetime prevalence rate of between 26% and 74% and a current prevalence rate of between 31% and 66% at the time of a traumatic event. Community surveys employing standardized diagnostic interviews revealed rates of between 1.2% and 1.7% for 1-month prevalence of symptoms of depersonalization or derealization in a U.K. sample and a 2.4%

current prevalence rate in a Canadian sample. Current prevalence rates between 1% and 16% were reported in samples of consecutive inpatient admissions, although these rates were considered to be underestimates. Prevalence rates in clinical samples of specific psychiatric disorders varied between 30% (for war veterans with PTSD) and 60% (for those with unipolar depression). There was a high prevalence of depersonalization and derealization symptoms within panic disorder samples, with rates varying from 7.8% to 82.6%.

Phenomenology and Development

Depersonalization as a symptom is seen in several psychiatric and neurological disorders. Unlike other dissociative disorders, the presence of which excludes other mental disorders such as schizophrenia and substance abuse, depersonalization disorder frequently co-occurs with such disorders. It is often a symptom of anxiety disorders and PTSD. In fact, about 69% of patients with panic disorder experience depersonalization or derealization during their panic attacks. Episodes of depersonalization may also occur as a symptom of alcohol and drug abuse, as a side effect of prescription medication, and during stress and sensory deprivation. Depersonalization is considered a disorder when it is a persistent and predominant symptom. The phenomenology of the disorder involves both the initial symptoms themselves and the reactive anxiety caused by them. In a study of community adults, the prevalence of depersonalization disorder was 0.8% (Johnson et al. 2006).

In a study of armed forces personnel ($N=184$) including subjects exposed to combat and diagnosed with PTSD, subjects exposed to combat but not diagnosed with PTSD, and healthy subjects without combat exposure, DES scores were found to be higher in the PTSD group than in any other group, and the scores positively correlated with combat exposure (Özdemir et al. 2015). In addition, combat-exposed subjects without PTSD had higher dissociation levels than healthy subjects without combat experience. In contrast, although high depersonalization/derealization factor scores were correlated with bodily injury in PTSD patients, no relationship between the presence of bodily injury and total DES scores could be demonstrated.

Treatment

Depersonalization and derealization are often transient and may remit without formal treatment. Recurrent or persistent depersonalization and derealization should be thought of both as symptoms in and of themselves and as symptoms existing within another syndrome that may require treatment, such as an anxiety disorder or schizophrenia.

Treatment modalities (Maldonado et al. 2002) include behavioral techniques such as paradoxical intention, record keeping, positive reward, flooding, psychotherapy (especially psychodynamic), cognitive-behavioral therapy (CBT), and psychoeducation. Hunter et al. (2005) reported on an open study in which 21 patients with depersonalization disorder were treated individually with CBT. The authors reported significant improvements in patient-defined measures of depersonalization/derealization severity as well as in standardized measures of dissociation, depression, anxiety, and general functioning at the end of treatment and at 6-month follow-up.

Depersonalization/derealization disorder symptoms may respond to self-hypnosis training. Often, hypnotic induction will induce transient depersonalization/derealization symptoms in susceptible subjects. This exercise is useful because by having a structure for inducing the symptoms, one provides patients with a context for understanding and controlling them. The symptoms are presented as a spontaneous form of hypnotic dissociation that can be modified. Individuals for whom this approach is effective can be taught to induce a pleasant sense of floating lightness or heaviness in place of the anxiety-related somatic detachment. Often, the use of an imaginary screen to picture problem material in a way that detaches it from the typical somatic response is also helpful (H. Spiegel and D. Spiegel 2004).

There is no known pharmacotherapy for the treatment of depersonalization/derealization disorder. Virtually all types of psychotropic medications, including psychostimulants, antidepressants, antipsychotics, anticonvulsants, and benzodiazepines, have been tried with modest success in individuals with depersonalization or derealization symptoms. Appropriate treatment of comorbid disorders—antianxiety medications for generalized anxiety, panic, or phobic disorders; antidepressants for treatment of comorbid depression or anxiety; and antipsychotic medications for true psychosis—is an important part of treatment. In an open trial of naltrexone (dosage ranged between 100 and 250 mg/day), the authors reported an average 30% reduction of symptoms of depersonalization as measured by three validated dissociation scales (Simeon et al. 2005). More recently, different authors reported on the first clinical trial of repetitive transcranial magnetic stimulation (rTMS) in depersonalization disorder (Mantovani et al. 2011). They found that after 3 weeks of right–temporoparietal junction (TPJ) rTMS, 6 of 12 patients responded. Five responders received 3 more weeks of right-TPJ rTMS, showing 68% symptom improvement. Others have reported on the successful use of rTMS applied to either the left DLPFC (Jiménez-Genchi 2004) or the right TPJ in the management of depersonalization disorder (Christopeit et al. 2014; Rachid 2017). These preliminary reports suggest that right-TPJ rTMS may be a safe and effective alternative in the management of depersonalization/derealization disorder.

Other Specified Dissociative Disorder

As described in DSM-5, the "other specified" category has been carved out to include presentations in which symptoms characteristic of a dissociative disorder cause clinically significant distress or dysfunction but do not meet full criteria for any of the disorders in the dissociative disorders diagnostic class. DSM-5 suggests that in order to facilitate communication among clinicians, the appropriate use of this category requires that following this diagnosis (i.e., "other specified dissociative disorder"), the specific syndrome exhibited is also documented (e.g., "identity disturbance due to prolonged political imprisonment"). Specific examples and details of circumstances where this diagnostic category should be used include identity disturbance associated with torture, brainwashing, and cult indoctrination. Of note, acute dissociative reactions to stressful events that are transient (lasting from a few hours up to 30 days) but fall short of meeting DSM-5 acute stress disorder diagnostic criteria are also included here. Finally, dissociative trance (i.e., an acute narrowing or complete unawareness of immediate surroundings, manifested by profound unresponsiveness to environmental stimuli, with or without involuntary stereotyped behaviors, transient paralysis, or loss of consciousness) is likewise included within this designation, as long as the trance condition does not occur solely as a normal part of a broadly accepted collective cultural or religious practice.

Unspecified Dissociative Disorder

As described in DSM-5, the "unspecified" category applies to presentations in which symptoms characteristic of a dissociative disorder cause clinically significant distress or functional impairment but do not meet full criteria for any of the disorders in the dissociative disorders diagnostic class. However, in contrast to the "other specified" category, the "unspecified" designation is used when the clinician chooses not to specify the reason that criteria are not met for a specific disorder or in cases where there is insufficient information to make a more specific diagnosis (e.g., emergency department settings). Finally, we want to remind readers that several drugs of abuse (namely 3,4-methylenedioxymethamphetamine [MDMA] and cannabis) may produce dissociative symptoms that largely exceed those observed in patients with schizophrenia and are comparable to those observed in special forces soldiers undergoing survival training but are less pronounced than dissociative symptoms induced by ketamine (van Heugten-Van der Kloet et al. 2015). In comparison, cocaine produced dissociative symptoms that were comparable to those observed in patients with schizophrenia but markedly less pronounced than those observed in special forces soldiers and ketamine users.

Conclusion

The dissociative disorders constitute a challenging component of psychiatric illness. The failure of integration of consciousness, memory, identity, emotion, perception, body representation, motor control, and behavior observed in these conditions results in symptomatology that illustrates fundamental problems in the organization of mental processes. Dissociative phenomena often occur during and after physical trauma but also may represent transient or chronic patterns of maladjustment. Dissociative disorders are generally treatable and constitute a domain in which psychotherapy is a primary modality, although pharmacological treatment of comorbid conditions such as depression can be quite helpful. The dissociative disorders are ubiquitous throughout the world, although they take a variety of forms. These disorders represent a fascinating window into the organization and processing of identity, memory, perception, and consciousness, and they pose a variety of diagnostic, therapeutic, and research challenges.

Key Clinical Points

- Dissociative disorders are often underdiagnosed.

- Dissociation is a common component of acute response to trauma, and dissociative identity disorder, dissociative amnesia, and depersonalization/derealization disorder often have a traumatic etiology.

- Dissociation represents a failure of integration of identity, memory, perception, and consciousness.

- The primary treatments for dissociative disorders involve various psychotherapies, including hypnosis, trauma-related psychotherapies, and cognitive therapies.

- Common comorbid conditions requiring treatment include depression, substance use disorders, and borderline personality disorder.

- Dissociative symptoms are ubiquitous around the world, but the content of the dissociative symptoms varies, involving presentations that are congruent with cultural idioms, such as "possession" by external entities or fragmentation of individual identity.

References

Akyüz G, Doğan O, Şar V, et al: Frequency of dissociative identity disorder in the general population in Turkey. Compr Psychiatry 40(2):151–159, 1999 10080263

American Psychiatric Association: Diagnostic and Statistical Manual: Mental Disorders. Washington, DC, American Psychiatric Association, 1952

American Psychiatric Association: Diagnostic and Statistical Manual of Mental Disorders, 3rd Edition. Washington, DC, American Psychiatric Association, 1980

American Psychiatric Association: Diagnostic and Statistical Manual of Mental Disorders, 4th Edition. Washington, DC, American Psychiatric Association, 1994

American Psychiatric Association: Diagnostic and Statistical Manual of Mental Disorders, 4th Edition, Text Revision. Washington, DC, American Psychiatric Association, 2000

American Psychiatric Association: Diagnostic and Statistical Manual of Mental Disorders, 5th Edition. Arlington, VA, American Psychiatric Association, 2013

Anderson MC, Ochsner KN, Kuhl B, et al: Neural systems underlying the suppression of unwanted memories. Science 303(5655):232–235, 2004 14716015

Ault RL Jr: FBI guidelines for use of hypnosis. Int J Clin Exp Hypn 27(4):449–451, 1979 521196

Barkin RBB, Kluft RP: The dilemma of drug therapy for multiple personality disorder, in Treatment of Multiple Personality Disorder. Edited by Braun B. Washington, DC, American Psychiatric Press, 1986, pp 107–132

Bedard-Gilligan M, Zoellner LA: Dissociation and memory fragmentation in post-traumatic stress disorder: an evaluation of the dissociative encoding hypothesis. Memory 20(3):277–299, 2012 22348400

Bernstein EM, Putnam FW: Development, reliability, and validity of a dissociation scale. J Nerv Ment Dis 174(12):727–735, 1986 3783140

Bourget D, Gagné P, Wood SF: Dissociation: defining the concept in criminal forensic psychiatry. J Am Acad Psychiatry Law 45(2):147–160, 2017 28619854

Boysen GA, VanBergen A: A review of published research on adult dissociative identity disorder: 2000–2010. J Nerv Ment Dis 201(1):5–11, 2013 23274288

Braakmann D, Ludewig S, Milde J, et al: Dissociative symptoms during treatment of borderline personality disorder [in German]. Psychother Psychosom Med Psychol 57(3–4):154–160, 2007 17523235

Brand BL, Chasson GS: Distinguishing simulated from genuine dissociative identity disorder on the MMPI-2. Psychol Trauma 7(1):93–101, 2015 25793598

Brand BL, Classen C, Lanius R: A naturalistic study of dissociative identity disorder and dissociative disorder not otherwise specified patients treated by community clinicians. Psychol Trauma 1(2):153–171, 2009a

Brand BL, Classen CC, McNary SW, et al: A review of dissociative disorders treatment studies. J Nerv Ment Dis 197(9):646–654, 2009b 19752643

Brand BL, Lanius R, Vermetten E, et al: Where are we going? An update on assessment, treatment, and neurobiological research in dissociative disorders as we move toward the DSM-5. J Trauma Dissociation 13(1):9–31, 2012 22211439

Brand BL, Chasson GS, Palermo CA, et al: MMPI-2 item endorsements in dissociative identity disorder vs. simulators. J Am Acad Psychiatry Law 44(1):63–72, 2016 26944745

Brandt J, Van Gorp WG: Functional ("psychogenic") amnesia. Semin Neurol 26(3):331–340, 2006 16791779

Bremner JD: Cognitive processes in dissociation: comment on Giesbrecht et al. (2008). Psychol Bull 136(1):1–6, discussion 7–11, 2010 20063920

Breuer J, Freud S: Studies on Hysteria. Oxford, UK, Basic Books, 1957

Brewin CR, Fuchkan N, Huntley Z, et al: Diagnostic accuracy of the Trauma Screening Questionnaire after the 2005 London bombings. J Trauma Stress 23(3):393–398, 2010 20564372

Calati R, Bensassi I, Courtet P: The link between dissociation and both suicide attempts and non-suicidal self-injury: meta-analyses. Psychiatry Res 251:103–114, 2017 28196773

Chalavi S, Vissia EM, Giesen ME, et al: Abnormal hippocampal morphology in dissociative identity disorder and post-traumatic stress disorder correlates with childhood trauma and dissociative symptoms. Hum Brain Mapp 36(5):1692–1704, 2015 25545784

Charcot J-M: Oeuvres Complètes de J.-M. Charcot. Paris, Lecrosnier et Babe, 1890

Christopeit M, Simeon D, Urban N, et al: Effects of repetitive transcranial magnetic stimulation (rTMS) on specific symptom clusters in depersonalization disorder (DPD). Brain Stimulat 7(1):141–143, 2014 23941986

Collin-Vézina D, Hébert M: Comparing dissociation and PTSD in sexually abused school-aged girls. J Nerv Ment Dis 193(1):47–52, 2005 15674134

Coons PM: The dissociative disorders. Rarely considered and underdiagnosed. Psychiatr Clin North Am 21(3):637–648, 1998 9774801

Coons PM, Milstein V: Psychosexual disturbances in multiple personality: characteristics, etiology, and treatment. J Clin Psychiatry 47(3):106–110, 1986 3949718

Coons PM, Bowman ES, Milstein V: Multiple personality disorder. A clinical investigation of 50 cases. J Nerv Ment Dis 176(9):519–527, 1988 3418321

Council on Scientific Affairs: Scientific status of refreshing recollection by the use of hypnosis. JAMA 253(13):1918–1923, 1985 3974082

Dalenberg CJ, Brand BL, Gleaves DH, et al: Evaluation of the evidence for the trauma and fantasy models of dissociation. Psychol Bull 138(3):550–588, 2012 22409505

Dalenberg CJ, Brand BL, Loewenstein RJ, et al: Reality versus fantasy: reply to Lynn et al. (2014). Psychol Bull 140(3):911–920, 2014 24773506

Dallam SJ: Crisis or creation? A systematic examination of "false memory syndrome." J Child Sex Abus 9(3–4):9–36, 2000 17521989

Dorahy MJ, Middleton W, Seager L, et al: Child abuse and neglect in complex dissociative disorder, abuse-related chronic PTSD, and mixed psychiatric samples. J Trauma Dissociation 17(2):223–236, 2016 26275087

Feeny NC, Zoellner LA, Fitzgibbons LA, et al: Exploring the roles of emotional numbing, depression, and dissociation in PTSD. J Trauma Stress 13(3):489–498, 2000a 10948488

Feeny NC, Zoellner LA, Foa EB: Anger, dissociation, and posttraumatic stress disorder among female assault victims. J Trauma Stress 13(1):89–100, 2000b 10761176

Fine CG: The tactical-integration model for the treatment of dissociative identity disorder and allied dissociative disorders. Am J Psychother 53(3):361–376, 1999 10586299

Foote B, Smolin Y, Kaplan M, et al: Prevalence of dissociative disorders in psychiatric outpatients. Am J Psychiatry 163(4):623–629, 2006 16585436

Franzke I, Wabnitz P, Catani C: Dissociation as a mediator of the relationship between childhood trauma and nonsuicidal self-injury in females: a path analytic approach. J Trauma Dissociation 16(3):286–302, 2015 25761222

Freud A: The Ego and Mechanisms of Defense. New York, International Universities Press, 1946

Freud S: The ego and the id (1923), in Standard Edition of the Complete Psychological Works of Sigmund Freud, Vol 19: The Ego and the Id and Other Works (1923–1925). Translated by Strachey J. Edited by Freud A. London, Hogarth, 1961, pp 1–66

Fujiwara E, Markowitsch HJ: The mnestic block syndrome—neural correlates of fear and stress [in German], in Neurobiologie der Psychotherapie. Edited by Schiepek G. Stuttgart, Germany, Schattauer, 2003, pp 186–212

Fujiwara E, Brand M, Kracht L, et al: Functional retrograde amnesia: a multiple case study. Cortex 44(1):29–45, 2008 18387529

Glisky EL, Ryan L, Reminger S, et al: A case of psychogenic fugue: I understand, aber ich verstehe nichts. Neuropsychologia 42(8):1132–1147, 2004 15093151

Gonzalez Vazquez AI, Seijo Ameneiros N, Díaz Del Valle JC, et al: Revisiting the concept of severe mental illness: severity indicators and healthcare spending in psychotic, depressive and dissociative disorders. J Ment Health Aug 10 2017 [Epub ahead of print] 28796557

Hammond DC: Clinical Hypnosis and Memory: Guidelines for Clinicians and for Forensic Hypnosis. Bloomingdale, IL, American Society of Clinical Hypnosis, 1995

Hansen M, Ross J, Armour C: Evidence of the dissociative PTSD subtype: a systematic literature review of latent class and profile analytic studies of PTSD. J Affect Disord 213:59–69, 2017 28192736

Harricharan S, Nicholson AA, Densmore M, et al: Sensory overload and imbalance: resting-state vestibular connectivity in PTSD and its dissociative subtype. Neuropsychologia 106:169–178, 2017 28911803

Hetzel MD, McCanne TR: The roles of peritraumatic dissociation, child physical abuse, and child sexual abuse in the development of posttraumatic stress disorder and adult victimization. Child Abuse Negl 29(8):915–930, 2005 16125234

Hilgard ER: The problem of divided consciousness: a neodissociation interpretation. Ann NY Acad Sci 296:48–59, 1977 279254

Hunter EC, Sierra M, David AS: The epidemiology of depersonalisation and derealisation. A systematic review. Soc Psychiatry Psychiatr Epidemiol 39(1):9–18, 2004 15022041

Hunter EC, Baker D, Phillips ML, et al: Cognitive-behaviour therapy for depersonalisation disorder: an open study. Behav Res Ther 43(9):1121–1130, 2005 16005701

Huntjens RJ, Verschuere B, McNally RJ: Inter-identity autobiographical amnesia in patients with dissociative identity disorder. PLoS One 7(7):e40580, 2012 22815769

Huntjens RJ, Wessel I, Hermans D, et al: Autobiographical memory specificity in dissociative identity disorder. J Abnorm Psychol 123(2):419–428, 2014 24886016

Janet P: The Major Symptoms of Hysteria: Fifteen Lectures Given in the Medical School of Harvard University, 2nd Edition. New York, Macmillan, 1920

Jiang H, White MP, Greicius MD, et al: Brain activity and functional connectivity associated with hypnosis. Cereb Cortex 27(8):4083–4093, 2017 27469596

Jiménez-Genchi AM: Repetitive transcranial magnetic stimulation improves depersonalization: a case report. CNS Spectr 9(5):375–376, 2004 15115950

Johnson DM, Pike JL, Chard KM: Factors predicting PTSD, depression, and dissociative severity in female treatment-seeking childhood sexual abuse survivors. Child Abuse Negl 25(1):179–198, 2001 11214810

Johnson JG, Cohen P, Kasen S, et al: Dissociative disorders among adults in the community, impaired functioning, and axis I and II comorbidity. J Psychiatr Res 40(2):131–140, 2006 16337235

Kellett S: The treatment of dissociative identity disorder with cognitive analytic therapy: experimental evidence of sudden gains. J Trauma Dissociation 6(3):55–81, 2005 16172082

Kiliç F, Coşkun M, Bozkurt H, et al: Self-injury and suicide attempt in relation with trauma and dissociation among adolescents with dissociative and non-dissociative disorders. Psychiatry Investig 14(2):172–178, 2017 28326115

Kluft RP: Diagnosing multiple personality disorder. Pa Med 87(9):44, 46, 1984a 6541774

Kluft RP: Multiple personality in childhood. Psychiatr Clin North Am 7(1):121–134, 1984b 6718263

Kluft RP: Treatment of multiple personality disorder. A study of 33 cases. Psychiatr Clin North Am 7(1):9–29, 1984c 6718271

Kluft RP: Using hypnotic inquiry protocols to monitor treatment progress and stability in multiple personality disorder. Am J Clin Hypn 28(2):63–75, 1985 4072949

Kluft RP: Preliminary observations on age regression in multiple personality disorder patients before and after integration. Am J Clin Hypn 28(3):147–156, 1986 3946284

Kluft RP: First-rank symptoms as a diagnostic clue to multiple personality disorder. Am J Psychiatry 144(3):293–298, 1987 3826426

Kluft RP: The dissociative disorders, in American Psychiatric Press Textbook of Psychiatry. Edited by Talbott JA, Hales RE, Yudofsky SC. Washington, DC, American Psychiatric Press, 1988a, pp 557–585

Kluft RP: On treating the older patient with multiple personality disorder: "race against time" or "make haste slowly"? Am J Clin Hypn 30(4):257–266, 1988b 3364389

Kluft RP: Multiple personality disorder, in American Psychiatric Press Review of Psychiatry, Vol 10. Edited by Tasman A, Goldfinger SM. Washington, DC, American Psychiatric Press, 1991, pp 161–188

Kluft RP: The use of hypnosis with dissociative disorders. Psychiatr Med 10(4):31–46, 1992 1289960

Kritchevsky M, Chang J, Squire LR: Functional amnesia: clinical description and neuropsychological profile of 10 cases. Learn Mem 11(2):213–226, 2004 15054137

Lanius RA, Vermetten E, Loewenstein RJ, et al: Emotion modulation in PTSD: clinical and neurobiological evidence for a dissociative subtype. Am J Psychiatry 167(6):640–647, 2010 20360318

Lanius RA, Brand B, Vermetten E, et al: The dissociative subtype of posttraumatic stress disorder: rationale, clinical and neurobiological evidence, and implications. Depress Anxiety 29(8):701–708, 2012 22431063

Lewis DO, Yeager CA, Swica Y, et al: Objective documentation of child abuse and dissociation in 12 murderers with dissociative identity disorder. Am J Psychiatry 154(12):1703–1710, 1997 9396949

Lindemann EJ: Symptomatology and management of acute grief: 1944. Am J Psychiatry 151 (6 suppl):155–160, 1994 8192191

Loewenstein R: Psychogenic amnesia and psychogenic fugue: a comprehensive review, in American Psychiatric Press Review of Psychiatry. Edited by Tasman A, Goldfinger SM. Washington, DC, American Psychiatric Press, 1991, pp 189–222

Loewenstein R: Diagnosis, epidemiology, clinical course, treatment, and cost effectiveness of treatment for dissociative disorders and MPD: report submitted to the Clinton Administration Task Force on Health Care Financing Reform. Dissociation 7(1):3–11, 1994

Loewenstein RJ: DID 101: a hands-on clinical guide to the stabilization phase of dissociative identity disorder treatment. Psychiatr Clin North Am 29(1):305–332, xii, 2006 16530599

Loewenstein RJ, Putnam FW: A comparative study of dissociative symptoms in patients with complex partial seizures, multiple personality disorder and posttraumatic stress disorder. Dissociation 1(4):17–23, 1988

Maldonado J, Fink G: Dissociation. New York, Oxford University Press, 2007

Maldonado JR, Spiegel D: Hypnosis, in Psychiatry, 3rd Edition. Edited by Tasman A, Kay J, Lieberman J. New York, Wiley, 2008, pp 1982–2026

Maldonado JR, Spiegel D, Bremner JD, et al: Trauma, dissociation, and hypnotizability, in Trauma, Memory, and Dissociation. Washington, DC, American Psychiatric Press, 1998, pp 57–106

Maldonado J, Butler L, Spiegel D: Treatment for dissociative disorders, in A Guide to Treatments That Work, 2nd Edition. Edited by Nathan PE, Gorman JM. New York, Oxford University Press, 2002, pp 463–496

Mantovani A, Simeon D, Urban N, et al: Temporo-parietal junction stimulation in the treatment of depersonalization disorder. Psychiatry Res 186(1):138–140, 2011 20837362

Markowitsch HJ, Kessler J, Russ MO, et al: Mnestic block syndrome. Cortex 35(2):219–230, 1999 10369094

Merckelbach H, Devilly GJ, Rassin E: Alters in dissociative identity disorder. Metaphors or genuine entities? Clin Psychol Rev 22(4):481–497, 2002 12094508

Mishkin M, Appenzeller T: The anatomy of memory. Sci Am 256(6):80–89, 1987 3589645

Myrick AC, Webermann AR, Langeland W, et al: Treatment of dissociative disorders and reported changes in inpatient and outpatient cost estimates. Eur J Psychotraumatol 8(1):1375829, 2017a 29038681

Myrick AC, Webermann AR, Loewenstein RJ, et al: Six-year follow-up of the treatment of patients with dissociative disorders study. Eur J Psychotraumatol 8(1):1344080, 2017b 28680542

Newman AW, Thompson JW Jr: Constitutional rights and hypnotically elicited testimony. J Am Acad Psychiatry Law 27(1):149–154, 1999 10212035

Nicholson AA, Densmore M, Frewen PA, et al: The dissociative subtype of posttraumatic stress disorder: unique resting-state functional connectivity of basolateral and centromedial amygdala complexes. Neuropsychopharmacology 40(10):2317–2326, 2015 25790021

Nicholson AA, Sapru I, Densmore M, et al: Unique insula subregion resting-state functional connectivity with amygdala complexes in posttraumatic stress disorder and its dissociative subtype. Psychiatry Res Neuroimaging 250:61–72, 2016 27042977

Nicholson AA, Friston KJ, Zeidman P, et al: Dynamic causal modeling in PTSD and its dissociative subtype: bottom-up versus top-down processing within fear and emotion regulation circuitry. Hum Brain Mapp 38(11):5551–5561, 2017 28836726

O'Toole BI, Marshall RP, Schureck RJ, et al: Combat, dissociation, and posttraumatic stress disorder in Australian Vietnam veterans. J Trauma Stress 12(4):625–640, 1999 10646181

Olde E, van der Hart O, Kleber RJ, et al: Peritraumatic dissociation and emotions as predictors of PTSD symptoms following childbirth. J Trauma Dissociation 6(3):125–142, 2005 16172085

Orne MT, Axelrad D, Diamond BL, et al: Scientific status of refreshing recollection by the use of hypnosis. JAMA 253(13):1918–1923, 1985 3974082

Özdemir B, Celik C, Oznur T: Assessment of dissociation among combat-exposed soldiers with and without posttraumatic stress disorder. Eur J Psychotraumatol 6:26657, 2015 25925021

Pape W, Wöller W: Low dose naltrexone in the treatment of dissociative symptoms [in German]. Nervenarzt 86(3):346–351, 2015 25421416

Porges SW: Emotion: an evolutionary by-product of the neural regulation of the autonomic nervous system. Ann NY Acad Sci 807:62–77, 1997 9071344

Porges SW: The polyvagal theory: new insights into adaptive reactions of the autonomic nervous system. Cleve Clin J Med 76 (suppl 2):S86–S90, 2009 19376991

Putnam FW: Diagnosis and Treatment of Multiple Personality Disorder. New York, Guilford, 1989

Putnam FW, Kluft RP: Dissociation as a response to extreme trauma, in Childhood Antecedents of Multiple Personality. Washington, DC, American Psychiatric Press, 1985, pp 65–97

Putnam FW, Guroff JJ, Silberman EK, et al: The clinical phenomenology of multiple personality disorder: review of 100 recent cases. J Clin Psychiatry 47(6):285–293, 1986 3711025

Rachid F: Treatment of a patient with depersonalization disorder with low frequency repetitive transcranial magnetic stimulation of the right temporo-parietal junction in a private practice setting. J Psychiatr Pract 23(2):145–147, 2017 28291041

Reinders AA, Willemsen AT, Vos HP, et al: Fact or factitious? A psychobiological study of authentic and simulated dissociative identity states. PLoS One 7(6):e39279, 2012 22768068

Reinders AA, Willemsen AT, den Boer JA, et al: Opposite brain emotion-regulation patterns in identity states of dissociative identity disorder: a PET study and neurobiological model. Psychiatry Res 223(3):236–243, 2014 24976633

Reinders AA, Willemsen AT, Vissia EM, et al: The psychobiology of authentic and simulated dissociative personality states: the full monty. J Nerv Ment Dis 204(6):445–457, 2016 27120718

Reinhold N, Markowitsch HJ: Retrograde episodic memory and emotion: a perspective from patients with dissociative amnesia. Neuropsychologia 47(11):2197–2206, 2009 19524087

Rifkin A, Ghisalbert D, Dimatou S, et al: Dissociative identity disorder in psychiatric inpatients. Am J Psychiatry 155(6):844–845, 1998 9619163

Ross CA: Epidemiology of multiple personality disorder and dissociation. Psychiatr Clin North Am 14(3):503–517, 1991 1946021

Ross CA: Re: The effects of hypnosis on dissociative identity disorder. Can J Psychiatry 45(3):298–299, 2000 10779893

Ryle A, Fawkes L: Multiplicity of selves and others: cognitive analytic therapy. J Clin Psychol 63(2):165–174, 2007 17173319

Şar V, Yargiç LI, Tutkun H: Structured interview data on 35 cases of dissociative identity disorder in Turkey. Am J Psychiatry 153(10):1329–1333, 1996 8831443

Şar V, Dorahy MJ, Krüger C: Revisiting the etiological aspects of dissociative identity disorder: a biopsychosocial perspective. Psychol Res Behav Manag 10:137–146, 2017 28496375

Schalinski I, Teicher MH, Nischk D, et al: Type and timing of adverse childhood experiences differentially affect severity of PTSD, dissociative and depressive symptoms in adult inpatients. BMC Psychiatry 16:295, 2016 27543114

Schalinski I, Moran JK, Elbert T, et al: Oscillatory magnetic brain activity is related to dissociative symptoms and childhood adversities—a study in women with multiple trauma. J Affect Disord 218:428–436, 2017 28505586

Schimmenti A: Elena: a case of dissociative identity disorder from the 1920s. Bull Menninger Clin 81(3):281–298, 2017 28745945

Schlumpf YR, Reinders AA, Nijenhuis ER, et al: Dissociative part-dependent resting-state activity in dissociative identity disorder: a controlled FMRI perfusion study. PLoS One 9(6):e98795, 2014 24922512

Shearer SL: Dissociative phenomena in women with borderline personality disorder. Am J Psychiatry 151(9):1324–1328, 1994 8067488

Sierra M, David AS: Depersonalization: a selective impairment of self-awareness. Conscious Cogn 20(1):99–108, 2011 21087873

Simeon D, Greenberg J, Nelson D, et al: Dissociation and posttraumatic stress 1 year after the World Trade Center disaster: follow-up of a longitudinal survey. J Clin Psychiatry 66(2):231–237, 2005 15705010

Sno HN, Schalken HF: Dissociative identity disorder: diagnosis and treatment in the Netherlands. Eur Psychiatry 14(5):270–277, 1999 10572357

Spanos NP: Multiple identity enactments and multiple personality disorder: a sociocognitive perspective. Psychol Bull 116(1):143–165, 1994 8078970

Spiegel D: Multiple personality as a post-traumatic stress disorder. Psychiatr Clin North Am 7(1):101–110, 1984 6718261

Spiegel D: Dissociating damage. Am J Clin Hypn 29(2):123–131, 1986 3535482

Spiegel D, Cardeña E: Disintegrated experience: the dissociative disorders revisited. J Abnorm Psychol 100(3):366–378, 1991 1918616

Spiegel D, Loewenstein RJ, Lewis-Fernández R, et al: Dissociative disorders in DSM-5. Depress Anxiety 28(12):E17–E45, 2011 22134959

Spiegel H, Spiegel D: Trance and Treatment: Clinical Uses of Hypnosis, 2nd Edition. Washington, DC, American Psychiatric Publishing, 2004

Spitzer C, Barnow S, Armbruster J, et al: Borderline personality organization and dissociation. Bull Menninger Clin 70(3):210–221, 2006 16981837

Staniloiu A, Markowitsch HJ, Kordon A: Psychological causes of autobiographical amnesia: a study of 28 cases. Neuropsychologia 110:134–147, 2018 29050993

Stein DJ, Koenen KC, Friedman MJ, et al: Dissociation in posttraumatic stress disorder: evidence from the world mental health surveys. Biol Psychiatry 73(4):302–312, 2013 23059051

Thompson-Hollands J, Jun JJ, Sloan DM: The association between peritraumatic dissociation and PTSD symptoms: the mediating role of negative beliefs about the self. J Trauma Stress 30(2):190–194, 2017 28449364

Tsai J, Armour C, Southwick SM, et al: Dissociative subtype of DSM-5 posttraumatic stress disorder in U.S. veterans. J Psychiatr Res 66–67:67–74, 2015 25969340

van der Hart O, Nijenhuis ER, Steele K: Dissociation: an insufficiently recognized major feature of complex posttraumatic stress disorder. J Trauma Stress 18(5):413–423, 2005 16281239

van Heugten-Van der Kloet D, Giesbrecht T, van Wel J, et al: MDMA, cannabis, and cocaine produce acute dissociative symptoms. Psychiatry Res 228(3):907–912, 2015 26003508

van Huijstee J, Vermetten E: The dissociative subtype of post-traumatic stress disorder: research update on clinical and neurobiological features. Curr Top Behav Neurosci 38:229–248, 2018 29063485

Vissia EM, Giesen ME, Chalavi S, et al: Is it trauma- or fantasy-based? Comparing dissociative identity disorder, post-traumatic stress disorder, simulators, and controls. Acta Psychiatr Scand 134(2):111–128, 2016 27225185

Watson S, Chilton R, Fairchild H, et al: Association between childhood trauma and dissociation among patients with borderline personality disorder. Aust NZ J Psychiatry 40(5):478–481, 2006 16683975

Williams LM, Das P, Liddell BJ, et al: Mode of functional connectivity in amygdala pathways dissociates level of awareness for signals of fear. J Neurosci 26(36):9264–9271, 2006 16957082

Wolf EJ, Miller MW, Reardon AF, et al: A latent class analysis of dissociation and posttraumatic stress disorder: evidence for a dissociative subtype. Arch Gen Psychiatry 69(7):698–705, 2012 22752235

Wolf EJ, Mitchell KS, Sadeh N, et al: The Dissociative Subtype of PTSD Scale: initial evaluation in a national sample of trauma-exposed veterans. Assessment 24(4):503–516, 2017 26603115

Recommended Readings

Paulsen SL, Lanius UF: Neurobiology and Treatment of Traumatic Dissociation: Towards an Embodied Self. New York, Springer, 2014

Spiegel D, Simeon D: Dissociative disorders, in Study Guide to DSM-5. Edited by Roberts L, Louie A. Washington, DC, American Psychiatric Publishing, 2015, pp 195–210

Steele K, van der Hart O, Boon S: Coping with Trauma-Related Dissociation: Skills Training for Patients and Therapists. New York, WW Norton, 2011

Vermetten E, Dorahy M, Spiegel D (eds): Traumatic Dissociation: Neurobiology and Treatment. Washington, DC, American Psychiatric Publishing, 2007

Online Resources

International Society for the Study of Trauma and Dissociation: www.isst-d.org/default.asp
Sidran Traumatic Stress Institute: www.sidran.org
Society for Clinical and Experimental Hypnosis: www.sceh.us

CHAPTER 17

Somatic Symptom and Related Disorders

Lorin M. Scher, M.D.

Erik Shwarts, M.D.

Patients with somatic symptom and related disorders chronically experience medically explained and unexplained ailments, which cause significant medical and psychiatric disability. Physicians and health systems are challenged by this patient population, because somatic symptoms are often long-lasting, are difficult to treat, and are associated with increased health care utilization. The interrelationship of mind and body is well established and increasingly accepted within medicine. However, the complexity of this interconnection creates a daunting task for physicians faced with assigning a diagnosis to and finding effective treatments for somatic symptoms. Previous DSM editions attempted to capture the pathological manifestations of the mind–body connection with many well-known diagnoses, including somatization disorder, conversion disorder, and hypochondriasis.

The DSM-5 Work Group on Somatic Symptom Disorders introduced several important changes into the organization of DSM-5 (American Psychiatric Association 2013) that have refocused classification of these disorders. The previous emphasis on absence of medical explanations for symptoms has been reduced throughout this new

This seventh edition revision of this chapter has combined diagnoses that were previously included in three different chapters, in keeping with the updated organization of DSM-5. The authors would like to acknowledge and thank the authors of the chapters in previous editions of this textbook that provided the framework for this updated chapter. Sean H. Yutzy, M.D., and Brooke S. Parish, M.D., provided the previous somatoform disorders material. Martin Leamon, M.D., and his colleagues contributed the foundation for the "Factitious Disorder" section. Much of the material included in "Psychological Factors Affecting Other Medical Conditions" stems from the fifth edition *Textbook* chapter by James Levenson, M.D., and readers are referred to that text for a more thorough discussion of the topic than is included in the current edition.

system, in recognition of the fact that the mere presence of an unexplained symptom is not a sufficient basis for assigning a psychiatric diagnosis. Furthermore, the presence of a well-documented medical symptom does not exclude the possibility of a dysfunctional psychological reaction that could be an appropriate focus for treatment. This deemphasis on medically unexplained symptoms helps to discredit dualistic mind–body concepts that may have been reinforced by previous diagnoses. Assumptions about the exact origin of the symptoms have generally been removed, in keeping with this goal. This reconceptualization aims to destigmatize illness, to prevent patients from feeling blamed for their somatic symptoms, and to improve diagnostic accuracy across medical disciplines. In DSM-5, the total number of somatic symptom and related disorders has been reduced, and efforts have been made to clarify boundaries among diagnoses, consistent with a goal of making these diagnoses more understandable and useful to nonpsychiatrist physicians. *Somatization disorder, pain disorder,* and *hypochondriasis* have been eliminated from DSM-5, and *somatic symptom disorder* and *illness anxiety disorder* have been introduced. *Factitious disorder,* formerly in a DSM chapter of its own, is now grouped with the somatic symptom and related disorders. *Psychological factors affecting other medical conditions,* which in DSM-IV (American Psychiatric Association 1994) and DSM-IV-TR (American Psychiatric Association 2000) appeared in the "Other Conditions That May Be a Focus of Clinical Attention" chapter, now appears in the DSM-5 "Somatic Symptom and Related Disorders" chapter. *Body dysmorphic disorder,* previously placed in the DSM-IV "Somatoform Disorders" chapter, has been moved to the DSM-5 "Obsessive-Compulsive and Related Disorders" chapter.

The principal features of the DSM-5 somatic symptom and related disorders are summarized in Table 17–1.

Somatic Symptom Disorder

Definition and Clinical Description

The core feature of somatic symptom disorder is the presence of one or more somatic symptoms that are distressing or that result in significant disruption of daily life.

Diagnosis

The DSM-5 diagnosis of somatic symptom disorder replaces the previous DSM-IV-TR diagnoses of somatization disorder and undifferentiated somatoform disorder. Somatic symptom disorder is defined by the presence of somatic symptoms, as in the older classifications. However, the DSM-5 criteria for somatic symptom disorder (see Table 17–1) do not require that the symptoms be medically unexplained, nor are specific numbers or types of symptoms needed to meet the diagnosis. Rather, the additional core feature of this diagnosis is the presence of abnormal thoughts, feelings, and behaviors associated with the somatic symptoms. These changes have been made in an effort to better capture the variability in the relationship between somatic symptoms and psychopathology and to shift scrutiny away from the medical plausibility of symptoms and toward the distress and maladaptive thoughts, feelings, and behaviors associated with those symptoms.

TABLE 17–1. Somatic symptom and related disorders: principal DSM-5 diagnostic criteria

	Somatic symptom disorder	Illness anxiety disorder	Conversion disorder	Psychological factors affecting medical conditions	Factitious disorder (imposed on self or another)
Core symptom	Presence of one or more somatic symptoms that are distressing or result in significant disruption to daily life	Preoccupation with having or acquiring a serious illness (no symptom need be present)	Presence of one or more symptoms of altered voluntary motor or sensory function	Presence of a medical symptom or condition	Falsification of physical or psychological signs or symptoms (or induction of injury or disease) associated with identified deception
Essential feature(s)	Individual manifests excessive thoughts, feelings, or behaviors related to the somatic symptoms or associated health concerns.	A high level of anxiety about health is present. Individual manifests excessive health-related behaviors or maladaptive avoidance.	Clinical findings provide evidence that symptoms are incompatible with recognized neurological or medical conditions.	Psychological or behavioral factors adversely affect the medical condition.	Individual presents self (or another) as being ill. Deceptive intent is evident even in the absence of obvious external rewards.
Symptom duration	Symptomatic state (as opposed to any one symptom) is persistent (typically lasting more than 6 months).	Preoccupation has been present for at least 6 months.	None specified	None specified	None specified

Note. For the complete DSM-5 diagnostic criteria, please refer to pp. 309–327 in DSM-5 (American Psychiatric Association 2013).

Hypochondriasis has been eliminated from DSM-5, but it is likely that many patients who previously met that diagnosis would now meet criteria for somatic symptom disorder. Other individuals who previously qualified for a hypochondriasis diagnosis may more appropriately receive the diagnosis of illness anxiety disorder if prominent somatic symptoms are not present. Pain disorder has been eliminated from DSM-5, but the specifier "with predominant pain" may be applied to the diagnosis of somatic symptom disorder to characterize patients whose somatic symptoms predominantly involve pain. Somatic symptom disorder is diagnosed in patients who have significant somatic symptoms. Multiple symptoms are commonly present, but a single severe symptom (such as pain) can be enough to establish the diagnosis. The diagnosis may be appropriate for some individuals in association with a medical illness.

Many of the culture-bound syndromes described in earlier DSM editions have a prominent somatic component. Culturally based somatic symptom presentations have even been described as "idioms of distress," because symptoms may have particular meanings and may be attributed to specific causes in a given cultural or ethnic group (see Chapter 44 in this volume, "Culturally Diverse Patients"). The complex and dynamic interplay between culture and expression of somatic symptoms continues to be an area of developing knowledge, but it may be safely assumed that culture will have a significant impact on the presentation and course of somatic symptom disorder. Kirmayer and Sartorius in 2007 provided a detailed review of the influence of cultural models on multiple aspects of somatic symptoms, including symptom reporting, interpretation of symptoms, modes of coping, and help-seeking behaviors (Kirmayer and Sartorius 2007).

Differential Diagnosis

The differential diagnosis for DSM-IV-TR somatization disorder included many of the "great imitator" medical disorders that were notorious for their widely varying and unpredictable symptom presentations. However, because the DSM-5 criteria for somatic symptom disorder emphasize maladaptive thoughts, feelings, and behaviors associated with symptoms, the differential diagnosis now focuses on a number of psychiatric conditions that feature similar maladaptive patterns.

Other somatic symptom and related disorders should be considered in the differential diagnosis of somatic symptom disorder. *Illness anxiety disorder* may be characterized by similar maladaptive thoughts and behaviors but would not include the presence of significant somatic symptoms. The essential feature of *conversion disorder (functional neurological symptom disorder)* is a loss of function rather than the presence of maladaptive thoughts, feelings, and behaviors related to one's symptoms.

Depressive disorders may include features similar to somatic symptom disorder. The cognitive distortions that may accompany depression in the setting of medical illness may appear similar to the "disproportionate and persistent thoughts about the seriousness of one's condition" (Criterion B1) that characterize somatic symptom disorder. Somatic symptoms and preoccupations are frequently associated with depression; however, the core depressive symptoms of low (dysphoric) mood and anhedonia must be present to establish a diagnosis of major depressive disorder.

Anxiety disorders and obsessive-compulsive disorder must be distinguished from somatic symptom disorder. Patients with *panic disorder* often experience heightened sensitivity to bodily sensations combined with catastrophic thinking about illness, resulting in frequent workups for cardiac complaints, dyspnea, and near-syncope in emergency and outpatient settings. Although panic disorder includes an intense focus on somatic concerns, such preoccupations tend to occur as acute episodes. *Generalized anxiety disorder* typically includes worries related to multiple domains, rather than solely focused on somatic symptoms. *Obsessive-compulsive disorder* could result in excessive time and energy being devoted to health concerns or somatic symptoms; however, obsessions would be accompanied by compulsions focused on reducing anxiety.

Natural History

An extensive literature on the natural history of somatic symptom disorder is not yet available. However, the DSM-IV diagnosis of somatization disorder was well studied over decades, and it can be assumed that some of its observed natural history will continue to be relevant for patients with somatic symptom disorder.

Somatization disorder, a chronic illness with fluctuations in the frequency and diversity of symptoms, was previously thought to remit only in rare cases. The most active symptomatic phase is usually early adulthood, but aging does not lead to total remission. However, newer studies have yielded much higher rates of remission, suggesting that as many as 50% of patients experience remission within 1 year (Kurlansik and Maffei 2016).

The most common and important complications of somatization disorder are repeated surgical operations, drug dependence, suicide attempts, and marital separation or divorce, according to Goodwin and Guze (1996). These authors suggested that the first two complications are preventable if the disorder is recognized and the patient's symptoms are managed appropriately. Generally, because of awareness that somatization disorder is an alternative explanation for various pains and other symptoms, invasive techniques (which have the potential to cause iatrogenic illness) can be withheld or postponed when objective indications are absent or equivocal. There is no evidence of excess mortality in patients with somatization disorder.

Avoiding the prescribing of habit-forming or addictive substances for persistent or recurrent complaints of pain should be paramount in the mind of the treating physician. Suicide attempts are common, but completed suicide is not. It is unclear whether marital or occupational dysfunction can be minimized through psychotherapy.

Epidemiology

The lifetime risk, prevalence, and incidence of somatic symptom disorder are unclear pending further research. However, in studies of DSM-IV somatization disorder, the prevalence of somatic symptom disorder in the general population was estimated at about 5%–7%; and among patients who present with acute somatic symptoms, an estimated 20%–25% will go on to develop a chronic somatic illness (Kurlansik and Maffei 2016). Somatization disorder was diagnosed predominantly in women and rarely in men, with an estimated female-to-male ratio of 10 to 1 (Kurlansik and Maffei 2016). Some suggested that this sex difference might be an artifact of bias in the diagnostic criteria, because of the inapplicability of pregnancy and menstrual complaints. The DSM-IV diagnosis of undifferentiated somatoform disorder was estimated to have a higher overall prevalence compared with somatization disorder. Studies using abridged criteria for somatization disorder found less consistent associations with female sex, with 8 of 14 studies reporting a significant effect (Creed and Barsky 2004).

Etiology

The etiology of somatic symptom disorder is not well understood. Research on the earlier DSM diagnoses of somatization disorder and undifferentiated somatoform disorder suggested several contributing factors. Temperamental characteristics, comorbid anxiety and depression, fewer years of education, psychological abuse in childhood, and recent stressful life events have been identified as important risk and prognostic factors.

A link to personality disorders has also been posited, among which avoidant, paranoid, and obsessive-compulsive personality disorders are the most commonly identified (Croicu et al. 2014). High levels of neuroticism and harm avoidance have been associated with a higher prevalence of somatic symptoms (Croicu et al. 2014). Quill (1985) postulated a social communication model based on the theory that individuals with somatization disorder learn to somatize as a means of expressing emotion (i.e., distress) in their family constellations, evoking support and care from significant individuals. Although further research is needed to more completely characterize them, these theories support the interpretation that the life course in somatization disorder is more similar to the life course in personality disorders than to that in other psychiatric disorders, considering the early onset, nonremitting nature, and pervasiveness of symptoms.

Somatic symptom disorder can be broadly viewed as a pattern of illness behavior in which bodily idioms of distress serve as symbolic means of social regulation as well as protest or contestation. As yet, however, there is little (if any) empirical evidence for such theories.

Treatment

Somatic symptom disorder is difficult to treat, and there appears to be no single superior treatment approach. In short, patients require an empathic, supportive, and functional approach to address their suffering, although physicians should be cautious about ordering repetitive, unnecessary, and invasive medical/surgical workups, which can cause iatrogenic illness.

Primary care physicians generally can manage patients with somatic symptom disorder adequately, but the expertise of a consulting psychiatrist has been shown to be useful. Cloninger (1994) provided three important general principles for treatment management for these patients: 1) establish a firm therapeutic alliance with the patient, 2) educate the patient about the manifestations of somatic symptom disorder, and 3) provide consistent reassurance. Implementation of these suggestions may greatly facilitate clinical management of somatic symptom disorder and prevent potentially serious complications, including the effects of unnecessary diagnostic and therapeutic procedures (iatrogenic illness) (Kurlansik and Maffei 2016).

During the late 1990s and early 2000s, cognitive-behavioral approaches embodying some of the principles just described were applied to "somatization" patients and yielded tentatively positive results. In 2001, the National Institute of Mental Health funded a single-blind, active-control, parallel-assignment interventional study of cognitive-behavioral therapy (CBT) for somatization disorder in the primary care setting. In this study, Allen et al. (2006) found that CBT with psychiatric consultation was more effective in improving symptoms and functioning than psychiatric consultation alone. Other studies have found that "health anxious" patients experienced sustained symptomatic benefit over 2 years, with no significant effect on total costs (Kurlansik and Maffei 2016). The clinician should develop a relationship with the patient's family so as to attain a better appreciation of the patient's social structure, which may be crucial to understanding and managing the patient's often-chaotic personal lifestyle. When appropriate, the clinician must place firm limits on excessive demands, manipulations, and attention seeking.

With regard to psychopharmacology, systematic reviews have shown that antidepressants can provide substantial benefits. Tricyclic antidepressants (TCAs) had a greater likelihood of effectiveness in comparison with selective serotonin reuptake inhibitors (SSRIs). Amitriptyline, the most studied TCA, and fluoxetine, in the SSRI class, both showed benefits in the domains of pain, functional status, global well-being, sleep, morning stiffness, and tender points (Kurlansik and Maffei 2016).

Illness Anxiety Disorder

Definition and Clinical Description

Illness anxiety disorder is a new diagnosis in DSM-5 characterized by a preoccupation with having or acquiring a serious illness (see Table 17–1). A key feature of the disorder is the absence of significant somatic symptoms; the patient's distress derives not from any specific physical complaints but rather from anxiety surrounding the possibility of having a dreaded illness. Two types of illness anxiety disorder are recognized in DSM-5: care-seeking type (in which medical care is frequently used) and care-avoidant type (in which medical care is rarely accessed). This diagnosis is expected to capture a minority of patients previously diagnosed with hypochondriasis, which is not included as a DSM-5 diagnosis.

Diagnosis

Patients with illness anxiety disorder are most commonly encountered in medical settings but may present to psychiatrists for treatment of anxiety. These patients' excessive concerns about undiagnosed disease are unlikely to be alleviated by medical reassurance or negative diagnostic tests; in some patients, this anxiety is further heightened by exposure to illness in others or medical news stories. The symptoms may reemerge periodically as a characteristic response to various stressors.

Differential Diagnosis

Various other conditions may share the diagnostic features of illness anxiety disorder, particularly mood and anxiety disorders. *Somatic symptom disorder* is characterized by the presence of at least one significant bodily symptom. *Adjustment disorder* should be considered in patients whose symptoms have not met the criteria for duration or severity and are clearly in response to a specific event. This consideration may be particularly relevant when the event leading to the adjustment disorder is health related. *Generalized anxiety disorder* typically involves persistent worrying about topics aside from those that are strictly health related. *Obsessive-compulsive disorder* would be expected to focus on a fear of getting the disease in the future as opposed to a focus on current symptoms and would also generally involve additional obsessions or compulsions. Because patients with *major depressive disorder* frequently report anxious and somatic preoccupations, depressive disorders may overlap with the symptoms of illness anxiety disorder; however, the former would include other mood, vegetative, and cognitive symptoms consistent with common mood disorders.

Natural History

The development and course of illness anxiety disorder is not well understood. Previous studies of hypochondriasis suggested that approximately one-fourth of patients with the diagnosis do poorly, two-thirds show a chronic but fluctuating course, and one-tenth recover. However, such predictions may not reflect advances in psychopharmacology. It also must be remembered that such findings pertain to the full syndrome. A much more variable course is seen in patients with some hypochondriacal concerns. Approximately 25%–50% of patients have a more transient form of hypochondriasis that is associated with less severity (American Psychiatric Association 2013).

Epidemiology

Because illness anxiety disorder is newly defined in DSM-5, detailed epidemiological studies with the exact criteria are not yet available. However, illness anxiety symptoms and the former DSM diagnosis of hypochondriasis have been studied. In a 2005 survey in the United States, 7.0% of respondents reported significant distress or impairment related to illness worry, with 6.9% of the general population reporting illness anxiety symptoms lasting 6 months or longer (Noyes et al. 2005).

Etiology

The etiology of illness anxiety disorder is unclear. However, multiple environmental factors appear to be associated with the development of excessive illness worry or hypochondriasis. These factors include early exposure to illness, parental overprotection, and exposure to childhood trauma. In considering hypochondriasis as an aspect of depressive or anxiety disorders, it has been posited that these conditions create a state of hypervigilance to bodily insult, including overperception of physical problems (Barsky and Klerman 1983).

Treatment

Treatment of illness anxiety disorder has not yet been thoroughly studied, but research on and clinical experience with hypochondriasis remain relevant. Patients referred early for psychiatric evaluation and treatment of hypochondriasis appear to have a better prognosis than those receiving only medical evaluations and treatments. As with other somatic symptom and related disorders, psychiatric referrals should be made with sensitivity and awareness of stigma related to mental illness.

Perhaps the best guideline to follow is for the referring physician to emphasize that the patient's distress is serious and that psychiatric evaluation will be a supplement to, not a replacement for, continued medical care. Patients may feel dissatisfied by reassurance that their symptoms are "not serious" and may avoid psychiatric referral due to anger over being told that the symptoms "are all in their head."

Because illness anxiety disorder shares many features with other anxiety disorders, it can be expected that SSRI pharmacotherapy may have some utility. In patients with hypochondriasis, research has suggested that SSRI treatment is useful for both acute and long-term treatment, with significant proportions of patients achieving remission (Schweitzer et al. 2011).

Investigators have tried many psychotherapeutic approaches in treating hypochondriasis. Stoudemire (1988) suggested an approach featuring consistent treatment, generally by the same primary physician, with supportive, regularly scheduled office visits not focused on the evaluation of symptoms. Hospitalization, medical tests, and medications with addictive potential are to be avoided if possible. Psychotherapeutic approaches may be greatly enhanced by effective pharmacotherapy. CBT was found to be most effective, with one study reporting that 57% of CBT-treated patients showed a reduction in hypochondriacal beliefs at 12-month follow-up (Barsky and Ahern 2004). A combined approach of medication and psychotherapy is believed to have synergistic effects. Preventing adoption of the sick role and chronic invalidism should be a guiding principle for clinicians when treating patients with illness anxiety symptoms (Harding et al. 2008).

Conversion Disorder (Functional Neurological Symptom Disorder)

Definition and Clinical Description

The essential feature of conversion disorder is the presence of symptoms of altered motor or sensory function that (as evidenced by clinical findings) are incompatible with any recognized neurological or medical condition and are not better explained by another medical or mental disorder (see Table 17–1). Specific symptoms mentioned as examples in DSM-5 include *motor symptoms* such as weakness or paralysis, abnormal movements (e.g., tremor, dystonic movements), gait abnormalities, and abnormal limb posturing and *sensory symptoms* including altered, reduced, or absent skin sensation, vision, or hearing. There may also be episodes of abnormal generalized limb shaking with apparent impairment or loss of consciousness that resemble epileptic seizures (also called *psychogenic* or *nonepileptic seizures*); episodes of unresponsiveness resembling syncope or coma; and other symptoms including reduced or absent speech volume (dysphonia/aphonia), altered articulation (dysarthria), a sensation of a lump in the throat (globus), and diplopia. Single episodes usually involve one symptom, but longitudinally, other conversion symptoms will be evident as well. Psychological factors generally appear to be involved, because symptoms often occur in the context of a conflictual situation that may in some way be resolved with the development of the symptom.

Diagnosis

In conversion disorder, the symptom or deficit cannot be fully explained by a known physical disorder. This criterion is perhaps the most important diagnostic consideration. The DSM-5 criteria for conversion disorder explicitly require neurological examination findings that are inconsistent with any known neurological disease. Many examples of these types of findings have been referenced in the literature, including the following:

- Seizures involving long duration, fluctuating course, asynchronous movement, pelvic thrusting, side-to-side head or body movement, closed eyes during the episode, ictal crying, and memory recall, features that are more consistent with a nonepileptiform etiology
- Hoover's sign, in which weakness of hip extension returns to normal strength with contralateral hip flexion against resistance
- Collapsing weakness of the affected limb
- Midline splitting of sensory modalities (light touch and temperature)
- Altered vibration sensation across the forehead
- Discrepancy of weakness in ankle plantar-flexion when tested on the bed versus walking on toes
- Tremor that changes with attention toward the limb, including tapping or distraction techniques
- The presence of rising premovement potentials on electroencephalogram/electromyelogram back-averaging in myoclonic movements that are reported to be involuntary
- For visual symptoms, a tubular visual field (i.e., tunnel vision)

The DSM-5 diagnostic criteria for conversion disorder do not include a requirement that symptoms be produced unintentionally, because absence of feigning is difficult to determine reliably. Although the symptoms of conversion disorder often occur in association with an identifiable stressor, the DSM-IV-TR criterion that required identification of associated psychological factors has been removed.

Psychogenic nonepileptic seizures (PNES) have been researched extensively, and a multitude of terms have been used to describe these events. A conversion disorder diagnosis may be appropriate for certain patients experiencing such episodes who meet the full criteria. Diagnosis of PNES is currently most reliably established by ruling out epilepsy using video electroencephalographic monitoring to capture a typical seizure event without an electrographic ictal pattern. Despite the cost and difficulty of identifying PNES in this manner, current research suggests that timely recognition of PNES yields overall cost savings and reduced utilization of services (Ahmedani et al. 2013).

Symptoms that are fully explained by culturally sanctioned behaviors or practices and that do not involve clinically significant impairment would not qualify for the diagnosis of conversion disorder. Examples of such symptoms include seizure-like episodes occurring in conjunction with certain religious ceremonies, as well as culturally expected responses from other persons present.

Differential Diagnosis

Conversion symptoms usually suggest physical illness at first, and therefore patients usually consult primary care and emergency department physicians initially. Neurologists are frequently consulted because most conversion symptom presentations suggest *neurological disease* (hence the term "functional neurological symptom disorder"). One major problem with conversion symptoms is the risk of applying a conversion disorder diagnosis when a true illness is present. Whereas earlier studies indicated that up to half of individuals initially diagnosed with conversion symptoms eventually received a neurological disorder diagnosis, more recent studies have suggested a much lower misdiagnosis rate of around 4% (Stone et al. 2005). Also noteworthy is the fact that an initial misdiagnosis may be corrected on follow-up, with patients ultimately receiving a diagnosis of conversion disorder. The trend toward less misdiagnosis may reflect growing sophistication in neurological diagnosis. Nevertheless, physicians should consider the risks of misdiagnosis when making a diagnosis of conversion disorder.

Symptoms of various neurological illnesses may seem to be inconsistent with known neurophysiology or neuropathology and may suggest conversion disorder. Diseases to be considered include multiple sclerosis (blindness secondary to optic neuritis with initially normal fundi), myasthenia gravis, periodic paralysis, myoglobinuric myopathy, polymyositis, other acquired myopathies (all of which may include marked weakness in the presence of normal deep-tendon reflexes), and Guillain-Barré syndrome (in which early weakness of the arms and legs may be inconsistent). Many actual neurological cases are diagnosed as "functional" before the elucidation of a neurological illness. Initial evidence of some neurological disease is predictive of a subsequent neurological explanation.

Complicating diagnosis is the fact that physical illness and conversion (or other apparent psychiatric overlay) are not mutually exclusive. Patients with incapacitating and frightening physical illnesses may appear to exaggerate their symptoms. Patients with documented neurological illness also may have "pseudosymptoms"; for example, patients with epilepsy may also have PNES, previously described as "pseudoseizures" (Dickinson and Looper 2012).

Longitudinal studies indicate that the most reliable predictor that a patient with apparent conversion symptoms will not later be shown to have a physical disorder is a history of conversion or other unexplained symptoms. Conversion symptoms that first occur in middle age or later warrant increased suspicion of an occult physical illness.

Several other psychiatric conditions may share features with conversion disorder. Additionally, a diagnosis of conversion disorder may be made in the presence of other DSM-5 diagnoses, such as somatic symptom and related disorders, dissociative disorders, or mood disorders. *Panic disorder* may involve neurological symptoms but would not include amnesia or tonic-clonic movements in most cases. *Depressive disorders* may feature complaints of fatigue or heaviness in the limbs but would also include prominent depressed mood or anhedonia. Although the DSM-5 criteria for conversion disorder do not include a requirement that the symptoms be unintentional, clear evidence of intentional production of symptoms would lead the clinician to a diagnosis of *factitious disorder* or malingering.

Natural History

Onset of conversion disorder is generally between late childhood and early adulthood. As previously mentioned, symptom onset in middle or late life is associated with a higher likelihood of a neurological or other medical cause.

Onset of conversion disorder is generally acute, but it may be characterized by gradually increasing symptomatology. The typical course of individual conversion symptoms is generally short; half to nearly all patients show a disappearance of symptoms by the time of hospital discharge. Factors traditionally associated with good prognosis include acute onset, presence of clearly identifiable stress at the time of onset, short interval between onset and institution of treatment, and good intelligence.

Generally, individual conversion symptoms are self-limited and do not lead to physical changes or disabilities. Occasionally, physical sequelae such as atrophy may occur, but such sequelae are rare.

Epidemiology

Research conclusions regarding the epidemiology of conversion disorder are compromised by methodological differences in diagnostic boundaries as well as by ascertainment procedures from study to study. Vastly different estimates have been reported. A marked excess of women compared with men develop conversion symptoms.

Conversion disorder has been linked with lower socioeconomic status, lower education, lack of psychological sophistication, and rural setting. The disorder appears to be diagnosed more often in women than in men. In part, this variance may relate to referral patterns, and there may be significant underreporting of some of these symptoms in men; however, more recent reports confirm that more women than men develop conversion symptoms (Bodde et al. 2009).

Etiology

An etiological hypothesis is implicit in the term *conversion*. The term, in fact, is derived from the hypothesized conversion of psychological conflict into a somatic symptom. Several psychological factors have been implicated in the pathogenesis, or at least pathophysiology, of conversion disorder. However, as the following discussion shows, such etiological relationships are difficult to establish.

Several terms have historically been used in describing aspects of conversion disorder. In *primary gain,* anxiety is theoretically reduced by keeping an internal conflict or need out of awareness by symbolic expression of an unconscious wish as a conversion symptom. However, individuals with active conversion symptoms often continue to show marked anxiety, especially on psychological tests. *Symbolism* is infrequently evident, and its evaluation involves highly inferential and unreliable judgments. Interpretation of symbolism in persons with occult medical disorder has been noted to contribute to misdiagnosis. *Secondary gain,* whereby conversion symptoms allow the person to avoid noxious activities or to obtain otherwise unavailable support, also may be apparent in persons with medical conditions, who often take advantage of such benefits. *La belle indifférence* refers to a lack of concern regarding the symptoms that has at times been observed, but this presentation is no longer thought to be of sufficient specificity to aid with a diagnosis of conversion disorder (American Psychiatric Association 2013).

If not directly etiological, many factors have been suggested as predisposing individuals to conversion disorder. In many instances, preexisting personality disorders are diagnosable and may predispose some individuals to conversion disorder. In regard to the association with personality disorders, it has been hypothesized that individuals with less healthy defense mechanisms and poorer coping are at greater risk for conversion symptoms. Several psychosocial factors in addition to a history of abuse may be involved. Preliminary functional imaging studies suggested associations among conversion disorder, depression, and posttraumatic stress disorder (Ballmaier and Schmidt 2005). Individuals with existing neurological disorders also appear to be predisposed to conversion disorder. Patients with neurological disorders are likely to observe a variety of neurological symptoms in themselves as well as in others, and they may at times simulate such symptoms as conversion symptoms.

Treatment

Generally, the initial aim in treating conversion disorder is the removal of the symptom. The urgency of this goal depends on the distress and disability associated with the symptom. If the patient is not in particular discomfort and the need to regain function is not great, direct attention may not be necessary. In any situation, direct confrontation is not recommended. Such a communication may cause a patient to feel even more isolated. A conservative approach of reassurance and relaxation is effective. Reassurance need not come from a psychiatrist but can be performed effectively by the primary physician. After physical illness is excluded, prognosis for conversion symptoms is good.

If symptoms do not resolve with a conservative approach and there is an immediate need for symptom resolution, other techniques have historically been attempted, including narcoanalysis (e.g., amobarbital interview), hypnosis, and behavior therapy. It does appear that prompt resolution of conversion symptoms is important in that the duration of conversion symptoms is associated with greater risk of recurrence and chronic disability.

Anecdotal reports exist of positive response to somatic treatments such as phenothiazines, lithium, and even electroconvulsive therapy. Of course, in some cases, such responses may also be attributable to suggestion. In others, it may be that symptom removal occurred because of resolution of another psychiatric disorder, especially a mood disorder. However, a review of all randomized controlled trials conducted in conversion disorder found no conclusive evidence for any effective treatment (Kroenke 2007).

Thus far, the discussion on treatment of conversion disorder has centered on acute treatment primarily for symptom removal. Longer-term approaches involve a pragmatic, conservative process entailing support for and exploration of various areas of conflict, particularly interpersonal relationships. Ford (1995) suggested a treatment strategy based on "three *P*s," wherein predisposing factors, precipitating stressors, and perpetuating factors are identified and addressed. A certain degree of insight may be attained, at least in terms of appreciating relationships between the onset or presence of various conflicts and stressors and the development of symptoms. More ambitious goals have been adopted by some in terms of long-term, intensive, insight-oriented psychotherapy, especially of a psychodynamic nature. Reports of such approaches date from Freud's work with Anna O. (Breuer and Freud 1955).

Psychological Factors Affecting Other Medical Conditions

Definition and Clinical Description

The relationship between psychological factors and medical illness is familiar to many clinicians and often to their patients as well. This relationship has been researched extensively, and a number of specific associations are also well known. Many of the treatment challenges faced by primary care and hospital-based physicians are further complicated by patient factors such as poor adherence to treatment plans, maladaptive coping styles, and persistent high-risk behavior. Although these factors (defined loosely) are present in many patients, the DSM-5 psychological factors affecting other medical conditions (PFAOMC) diagnosis is reserved for cases in which patient psychological factors are judged to have a clinically significant impact on a medical condition (see Table 17–1).

Many examples of common combinations that this diagnosis may take are available. Some of these combinations have been historically recognized, such as the relationship between asthma and anxiety or between stress and peptic ulcer disease. Others, such as the link between coronary artery disease and depression, have only recently become a widespread focus of clinical attention. Additional areas of mind–body connection have wide resonance and interest among laypersons, such as the role of psychological factors in cancer treatment. The management of chronic medical conditions such as diabetes requires coping with intense psychological factors for many patients. Additionally, lifestyle risk factors such as cigarette smoking, alcohol abuse, obesity, or high-risk sexual behavior are of paramount importance in the development of many medical illnesses.

Diagnosis

The core feature of the PFAOMC diagnosis is the presence of a psychological or behavioral factor that adversely affects a medical condition by increasing the risk for suffering, disability, or death. In DSM-IV, the most common types of psychological factors—mental disorders, psychological symptoms, personality traits, coping styles, and maladaptive health behaviors—were included in the criteria as specifiers. At times a given psychological factor's influence on a medical condition may be evident from the close temporal relationship between the factor and either emergence or worsened course of the condition. The factors may also directly inhibit treatment, most commonly through poor adherence to treatment plans. In other cases, the psychological factors constitute a well-established health risk for the individual. Culturally specific behaviors such as use of faith healers must be excluded when applying this diagnosis, because a variety of health practices exist as a normal pattern within certain cultures and represent attempts to treat illness rather than to perpetuate it.

Differential Diagnosis

Several other somatic symptom and related disorders must be differentiated from PFAOMC. *Somatic symptom disorder* may include the same psychological distress or maladaptive behaviors that would help to meet criteria for the PFAOMC diagnosis. However, the core of the latter diagnosis is the presence of a medical condition, the course of which has been adversely altered by the psychological factors. By contrast, a diagnosable medical condition need not be present in somatic symptom disorder; instead, the focus is on the maladaptive thoughts, behaviors, and feelings associated with a symptom. *Illness anxiety disorder* shares with PFAOMC a relationship between a psychological symptom and health concerns, but in that diagnosis, no serious medical illness is present. DSM-5 includes the diagnosis *other specified mental disorder due to another medical condition* (in the chapter "Other Mental Disorders") to capture presentations in which a medical condition is judged to be causing symptoms of a mental disorder through direct physiological means. An *adjustment disorder* diagnosis may also be appropriate in cases where the stress of coping with a medical illness has led to significant psychological or behavioral symptoms.

Factitious Disorder

Definition and Clinical Description

The essential feature in factitious disorder is falsification of physical or psychological signs or symptoms, or induction of injury or disease, with evidence of deceptive intent (see Table 17–1). This disorder has been described in medical writing throughout history (Gavin 1843) and throughout the world (Bappal et al. 2001). The concept became firmly established in modern medical thinking in 1951 when Asher (1951) described what was later classified as a subtype of factitious disorder known as Munchausen syndrome (which in DSM-5 is now classified as *factious disorder imposed on self*). Factitious disorder may remain undiagnosed, and even when recognized, it often goes untreated. Yet factitious disorder causes significant morbidity and mortality (Folks 1995), consumes an astonishing amount of medical resources, and produces significant emotional distress in the patients themselves, in their caregivers, and in their close relationships (Feldman and Smith 1996).

The DSM-5 criteria for factitious disorder have undergone minor changes from previous criteria. The DSM-IV criterion requiring that the behavior be motivated by a desire to assume the sick role has been removed. However, the requirement that identifiable external incentives for the behavior be absent has been retained in DSM-5. Additionally, the DSM-5 criteria explicitly require that the falsification of symptoms be associated with identified deception.

Diagnosis

Criterion A, falsification of physical or psychological signs or symptoms, distinguishes factitious disorder from somatic symptom disorder, in which physical symptoms are viewed as unconsciously produced. Criterion B accounts for the presentation of the symptoms in a manner designed to mimic illness, which hints at the eliminated DSM-IV Criterion B, which required that the behavior be motivated by a desire to assume the sick role. The assumption that such motivation can be reliably determined is problematic (Turner 2006), and DSM-5 Criterion B, which requires no attribution of motivation or intent, removes that obstacle. Criterion C helps to distinguish factitious disorder from malingering by excluding from the diagnosis those patients with identifiable secondary gain. The DSM-IV codes for subtyping the presentation as involving predominantly psychological, predominantly physical, or combined psychological and physical signs and symptoms were removed in DSM-5. However, the DSM-5 diagnostic criteria include separate categories for factitious disorder imposed on self and factitious disorder imposed on another (previously factitious disorder by proxy).

Illness falsification can take many forms. Patients may exaggerate symptoms, for example, by claiming that occasional tension headaches are continual crippling migraines. They may interfere with diagnostic instruments to give false readings, for example, by manipulating electrocardiogram leads or by rubbing thermometers to fake fevers. Patients may also tamper with laboratory specimens (e.g., by adding blood to urine) to falsely indicate an abnormality. They may purposefully injure themselves by active methods such as self-catheterization, self-induced infection of wounds or skin with bacteria, injection of unneeded or excessive insulin, or ingestion of thyroid hormones or anticoagulants. Finally, dissimulators may temporarily avoid necessary medical treatment to exacerbate existing conditions.

Differential Diagnosis

Given the duplicity inherent in the presentation of factitious disorder, establishing the diagnosis and differentiating this disorder from other conditions may be difficult. *Malingering* can be distinguished from factitious disorder by the presence of personal gain resulting from the symptoms. Although self-harm behaviors such as the cutting common in *borderline personality disorder* might appear similar to the deliberate induction of injury in factitious disorder, such self-injurious behaviors would not possess the required association with identified deception. Similarly, *somatic symptom disorder* lacks evidence of feigned symptoms, instead being defined by maladaptive thoughts, behaviors, and feelings associated with a symptom. *Conversion disorder* also is not characterized by duplicity and is associated with functional neurological deficits. Finally, the presence of a true medical condition does not exclude the possibility of co-occurring factitious disorder.

Natural History

Factitious disorder is thought to follow a course characterized by intermittent episodes throughout life. Onset is generally in early adulthood, often after hospitalization for a medical or psychiatric condition. Patients can be difficult to track longitudinally due to the duplicity inherent in the disorder, but the pattern of seeking medical care for falsified symptoms often continues throughout the individual's life (American Psychiatric Association 2013).

Epidemiology

Data on incidence and prevalence rates for factitious disorder are difficult to gather, vary considerably, and must be viewed with a critical eye. The covert nature of the disorder can lead to missed diagnoses and underestimation of rates or, conversely, to the same case being counted twice, thereby inflating apparent rates (Ifudu and Friedman 1993). Factitious disorder has been noted to account for between 0.6% and 3% of psychiatric consultation-liaison service referrals and between 0.02% and 0.9% of cases reviewed in specialty clinics (Yates and Feldman 2016). Whereas most reported cases have been in patients in their 20s to 40s, Munchausen syndrome has been reported in children, adolescents, and geriatric populations (Yates and Feldman 2016).

Etiology

Psychodynamic explanations for these paradoxical disorders have been provided by several authors. Many have noted the apparent prevalence of histories of early childhood physical or sexual abuse, with disturbed parental relationships and emotional deprivation. Histories of early illness or extended hospitalizations also have been noted. Nadelson (1979) conceptualized factitious disorder as a manifestation of borderline character pathology rather than as an isolated clinical syndrome. The patient becomes both the "victim and the victimizer" by garnering medical attention from physicians and other health care workers while defying and devaluing them. Projection of hostility and worthlessness onto the caregiver occurs as he or she is both desired and rejected. Plassmann (1994a, 1994b) viewed the disorders as a "symptom of a psychic problem complex." Early traumas are dealt with narcissistically and through dissociation, denial, and a type of projection. The patient's body, or part of the body, becomes perceived as an external object or as a fused symbiotic combination of self and object, which then comes to represent negative affects (hate, fear, and pain), the associated negative object concepts, and negative self-concepts. In the face of early deprivation and assaults, the "body self" is split off to preserve the "psychic self" (Hirsch 1994). When subsequent life events activate these affects or concepts, the result is extreme anxiety and growing derealization. Eventually, the patient acts out or involves the medical system in a type of countertransference identification, which leads to manipulations of the body of the patient. The manipulation results in emotional relief, albeit transient and incomplete, in the manner of most repetitious compromises. Other intrapsychic, cognitive, social learning, and behavioral theories have been advanced as well (Feldman et al. 2001; Ford 1996).

Neuropathological foundations for factitious disorder also have been suggested on the basis of abnormal findings on single photon emission computed tomography, computed tomography, and magnetic resonance imaging scans and neuropsychological testing. No consistent findings have yet been reported. Intriguing, however, is the suggestion that pseudologia fantastica may be a syndrome related to but distinct from factitious disorder, with its own associated pathology.

Although many cases of factitious disorder are chronic, the stressor of recurrent object loss, or fear of loss, occurs over and over in the literature as an antecedent to a factitious episode. For example, Carney (1980) found that 74% of his patients with factitious disorder experienced severe sexual or marital stress prior to developing factitious signs or symptoms.

Treatment

Treatment of factitious disorder can be divided into acute and long-term methods. Initially the diagnosis must be confirmed. An erroneous diagnosis of factitious disorder can itself result in trauma and may be perpetuated in medical records. Previously used methods of confirming the diagnosis, such as searching patients' belongings for paraphernalia used in producing symptoms, may continue to be tempting for clinicians, but such methods violate ethical and most likely legal boundaries. For this reason and because of the potentially strong countertransference reactions engendered by these patients, some authors have endorsed early involvement with hospital administration when a diagnosis of factitious disorder is suspected (Wise and Rundell 2005). Treatment team meetings are recommended to help coordinate efforts between providers and to allow for management of negative emotions toward patients. Countertransference can lead to several adverse consequences. "Therapeutic nihilism" on the part of the treatment system may lead to an unexamined assumption that the patient cannot or should not be treated, with subsequent failure to diagnose or refer. Anger and aversion can rupture any therapeutic alliance, undermine the unity of a treatment team, or lead to punitive acting-out against the patient. Genuine comorbid or concomitant illness may be overlooked. Nonemergent breaches of confidentiality may ensue in the diagnostic hunt or in the supposed effort to "warn" colleagues. Overidentification with the patient or activation of rescue fantasies can sabotage treatment efforts and may paradoxically reinforce continued factitious behaviors (Krahn et al. 2003).

Once the contribution of a general medical illness has been factored out, the patient must be informed of a change in the treatment plan, and an attempt must be made to enlist the patient in that plan. The literature generally refers to this process (perhaps alluding to its countertransference aspects) as containing an element of "confrontation." There is now general agreement that treatment begins at this point, and that it is best done indirectly, with minimal expectation that the patient "confess" or acknowledge the deception. Such treatment is a delicate process, with patients frequently leaving the hospital against medical advice or otherwise leaving treatment. Eisendrath (1989) described techniques for reducing confrontation, such as using inexact interpretations, therapeutic double binds, and other strategic and face-saving techniques to allow the patient tacitly to relinquish the factitious signs and symptoms.

Although the individual with Munchausen syndrome is regarded as being less likely to engage in treatment (Eisendrath 1989), and the individual with general factitious disorder is seen as being more open to intervention, there are case reports of Munchausen patients who respond favorably to treatment (Feldman 2006; Rothchild 1994).

No comparative studies of therapeutic approaches are available, although several different techniques have been described. Regardless of modality, treatment must be collaborative and involve some level of communication among all of the patient's treatment providers. The psychodynamic approach to treatment generally focuses not on the factitious behaviors themselves but rather on the underlying dynamic issues, with the therapist taking a neutral stance toward the factitious nature of the behaviors. As indicated, strategic-behavioral approaches also have been used (Teasell and Shapiro 1994), implementing standard behavioral techniques as well as the therapeutic double bind, in which the only way out is to abandon the target factitious behaviors.

Pharmacotherapy, when used, targets specific symptoms, such as depression, transient psychosis, or comorbid disorders. Some patients cease factitious behaviors on their own as a result of unanticipated life change (e.g., marriage or involvement in a church group that provides the requisite attention and support). Perceiving an "addictive" quality to these patients' factitious behaviors, others have creatively evolved personal "12-step" programs that have helped them end the deceptions.

Although insufficient studies have been conducted to address conclusively the prognostic factors in factitious disorder, children, patients with major depressive disorder, and patients without personality disorders may have better prognoses (Yates and Feldman 2016). Reviews have considered many of these treatment issues and have called for more coordination between clinicians treating this disorder in an effort to improve research of this diagnosis (Eastwood and Bisson 2008). The literature on the disorder is certainly ample, and it implies that the factitious disorder patient, although requiring considerable therapeutic skill, may be approached with a cautious hope for improvement.

Other Specified or Unspecified Somatic Symptom and Related Disorder

Two additional somatic symptom and related disorder diagnostic categories are provided in DSM-5. The categories of *other specified somatic symptom and related disorder* and *unspecified somatic symptom and related disorder* may be applied to presentations that are characteristic of a somatic symptom and related disorder and that cause clinically significant impairment but do not meet full criteria for any of the disorders in this diagnostic class. For an "other specified" diagnosis, the clinician records the specific reason that full criteria are not met; for an "unspecified" diagnosis, no reason need be given. Use of the latter category should be reserved for exceptionally uncommon situations in which there is insufficient information to make a more specific diagnosis.

DSM-5 provides four examples of presentations for which the other specified somatic symptom and related disorder designation might be appropriate:

1. Brief somatic symptom disorder—Duration of symptoms is less than 6 months.
2. Brief illness anxiety disorder—Duration of symptoms is less than 6 months.
3. Illness anxiety disorder without excessive health-related behaviors—Criterion D for illness anxiety disorder is not met.
4. Pseudocyesis—A false belief of being pregnant that is associated with objective signs and reported symptoms of pregnancy.

Conclusion

The treatment of patients with somatic symptom pathology remains challenging across medical specialties. These patients often feel blamed for their somatic symptoms, and invasive medical workups often place patients at higher risk of medically induced illness. The updated DSM-5 criteria aim to help physicians accurately diagnose these disorders and to protect patients with these conditions from undue interventions and stigma. Careful application of the updated criteria (see summary in Table 17–1, earlier in chapter) will facilitate provision of compassionate care that adheres to one of the fundamental precepts of the medical profession, *primum non nocere*, first do no harm.

Key Clinical Points

- When treating patients with somatic symptoms or factitious presentations, clinicians should use caution when considering invasive workups, as multiple workups put patients at risk for medically induced (iatrogenic) illness.

- Somatic symptoms are often present during times of psychological stress for individuals from cultures throughout the world.

- When approaching a patient with somatic symptoms, the clinician should focus on understanding and treating dysfunctional thoughts, feelings, and behaviors related to the symptoms.

- The presence or absence of a diagnosed medical illness generally does not affect the accurate diagnosis of somatic symptom disorder.

- Somatic symptoms may respond to a variety of therapeutic modalities, and psychiatric consultation and/or treatment is often beneficial.

- Clinicians should remain mindful of the varied but significant manner in which psychological factors can cause, sustain, or affect recovery from other medical conditions.

References

Ahmedani BK, Osborne J, Nerenz DR, et al: Diagnosis, costs, and utilization for psychogenic non-epileptic seizures in a US health care setting. Psychosomatics 54(1):28–34, 2013 23194931

Allen LA, Woolfolk RL, Escobar JI, et al: Cognitive-behavioral therapy for somatization disorder: a randomized controlled trial. Arch Intern Med 166(14):1512–1518, 2006 16864762

American Psychiatric Association: Diagnostic and Statistical Manual of Mental Disorders, 4th Edition. Washington, DC, American Psychiatric Association, 1994

American Psychiatric Association: Diagnostic and Statistical Manual of Mental Disorders, 4th Edition, Text Revision. Washington, DC, American Psychiatric Association, 2000

American Psychiatric Association: Diagnostic and Statistical Manual of Mental Disorders, 5th Edition. Arlington, VA, American Psychiatric Association, 2013

Asher R: Munchausen's syndrome. Lancet 1(6650):339–341, 1951 14805062

Ballmaier M, Schmidt R: Conversion disorder revisited. Funct Neurol 20(3):105–113, 2005 16324233

Bappal B, George M, Nair R, et al: Factitious hypoglycemia: a tale from the Arab world. Pediatrics 107(1):180–181, 2001 11134456

Barsky AJ, Ahern DK: Cognitive behavior therapy for hypochondriasis. JAMA 291(12):1464–1470, 2004 15039413

Barsky AJ, Klerman GL: Overview: hypochondriasis, bodily complaints, and somatic styles. Am J Psychiatry 140(3):273–283, 1983 6338747

Bodde NM, Brooks JL, Baker GA, et al: Psychogenic non-epileptic seizures—diagnostic issues: a critical review. Clin Neurol Neurosurg 111(1):1–9, 2009 19019531

Breuer J, Freud S: Studies on hysteria (1893–1895), in The Standard Edition of the Complete Psychological Works of Sigmund Freud, Vol 2. Translated and edited by Strachey J. London, Hogarth Press, 1955, pp 1–311

Carney MW: Artefactual illness to attract medical attention. Br J Psychiatry 136:542–547, 1980 7388261

Cloninger CR: Somatoform and dissociative disorders, in The Medical Basis of Psychiatry, 2nd Edition. Edited by Winokur G, Clayton P. Philadelphia, PA, WB Saunders, 1994, pp 169–192

Creed FH, Barsky A: A systematic review of the epidemiology of somatisation disorder and hypochondriasis. J Psychosom Res 56(4):391–408, 2004 15094023

Croicu C, Chwastiak L, Katon W: Approach to the patient with multiple somatic symptoms. Med Clin North Am 98(5):1079–1095, 2014 25134874

Dickinson P, Looper KJ: Psychogenic nonepileptic seizures: a current overview. Epilepsia 53(10):1679–1689, 2012 22882112

Eastwood S, Bisson JI: Management of factitious disorders: a systematic review. Psychother Psychosom 77(4):209–218, 2008 18418027

Eisendrath SJ: Factitious physical disorders: treatment without confrontation. Psychosomatics 30(4):383–387, 1989 2798730

Feldman MD: Recovery from Munchausen syndrome. South Med J 99(12):1398–1399, 2006 17236254

Feldman MD, Smith R: Personal and interpersonal toll of factitious disorders, in The Spectrum of Factitious Disorders. Edited by Feldman MD, Eisendrath SJ. Washington, DC, American Psychiatric Press, 1996, pp 175–194

Feldman MD, Hamilton JC, Deemer HN: A critical analysis of factitious disorders, in Somatoform and Factitious Disorders. Edited by Phillips KA. Washington, DC, American Psychiatric Publishing, 2001, pp 129–166

Folks DG: Munchausen's syndrome and other factitious disorders. Neurol Clin 13(2):267–281, 1995 7643825

Ford CV: Conversion disorder and somatoform disorder not otherwise specified, in Treatments of Psychiatric Disorders, 2nd Edition. Edited by Gabbard GO. Washington, DC, American Psychiatric Press, 1995, pp 1737–1753

Ford CV: Lies! Lies!! Lies!!! The Psychology of Deceit. Washington, DC, American Psychiatric Press, 1996

Gavin H: On Feigned and Factitious Diseases, Chiefly of Soldiers and Seamen, on the Means Used to Simulate or Produce Them, and on the Best Mode of Discovering Impostors: Being the Prize Essay in the Class of Military Surgery, in the University of Edinburgh, Session, 1835–1836, With Additions. London, John Churchill Princess Street Soho, 1843

Goodwin DW, Guze SB: Psychiatric Diagnoses, 5th Edition. New York, Oxford University Press, 1996

Harding KJ, Skritskaya N, Doherty E, et al: Advances in understanding illness anxiety. Curr Psychiatry Rep 10(4):311–317, 2008 18627669

Hirsch M: The body as a transitional object. Psychother Psychosom 62(1–2):78–81, 1994 7984771

Ifudu O, Friedman EA: Kidney-related Munchausen's syndrome and the Red Baron (author responses to letters). N Engl J Med 328(1):61, 1993. Available at: https://www.ncbi.nlm.nih.gov/pubmed/?term=Kidney-Related+Munchausen%27s+Syndrome+and+the+Red+Baron. Accessed January 4, 2019.

Kirmayer LJ, Sartorius N: Cultural models and somatic syndromes. Psychosom Med 69(9):832–840, 2007 18040090

Krahn LE, Li H, O'Connor MK: Patients who strive to be ill: factitious disorder with physical symptoms. Am J Psychiatry 160(6):1163–1168, 2003 12777276

Kroenke K: Efficacy of treatment for somatoform disorders: a review of randomized controlled trials. Psychosom Med 69(9):881–888, 2007 18040099

Kurlansik SL, Maffei MS: Somatic symptom disorder. Am Fam Physician 93(1):49–54, 2016 26760840

Nadelson T: The Munchausen spectrum: borderline character features. Gen Hosp Psychiatry 1(1):11–17, 1979 499769

Noyes R Jr, Carney CP, Hillis SL, et al: Prevalence and correlates of illness worry in the general population. Psychosomatics 46(6):529–539, 2005 16288132

Plassmann R: Münchhausen syndromes and factitious diseases. Psychother Psychosom 62(1–2):7–26, 1994a 7984770

Plassmann R: Structural disturbances in the body self. Psychother Psychosom 62(1–2):91–95, 1994b 7984773

Quill TE: Somatization disorder. One of medicine's blind spots. JAMA 254(21):3075–3079, 1985 4057529

Rothchild E: Fictitious twins, factitious illness. Psychiatry 57(4):326–332, 1994 7899527

Schweitzer PJ, Zafar U, Pavlicova M, et al: Long-term follow-up of hypochondriasis after selective serotonin reuptake inhibitor treatment. J Clin Psychopharmacol 31(3):365–368, 2011 21508861

Stone J, Smyth R, Carson A, et al: Systematic review of misdiagnosis of conversion symptoms and "hysteria." BMJ 331(7523):989, 2005 16223792

Stoudemire GA: Somatoform disorders, factitious disorders, and malingering, in The American Psychiatric Press Textbook of Psychiatry. Edited by Talbott JA, Hales RE, Yudofsky SC. Washington, DC, American Psychiatric Press, 1988, pp 533–556

Teasell RW, Shapiro AP: Strategic-behavioral intervention in the treatment of chronic nonorganic motor disorders. Am J Phys Med Rehabil 73(1):44–50, 1994 8305181

Turner MA: Factitious disorders: reformulating the DSM-IV criteria. Psychosomatics 47(1):23–32, 2006 16384804

Wise MG, Rundell JR: Clinical Manual of Psychosomatic Medicine: A Guide to Consultation-Liaison Psychiatry. Washington, DC, American Psychiatric Publishing, 2005

Yates GP, Feldman MD: Factitious disorder: a systematic review of 455 cases in the professional literature. Gen Hosp Psychiatry 41:20–28, 2016 27302720

Recommended Reading

Dimsdale JE, Patel V, Xin Y, et al: Somatic presentations—a challenge for DSM-V. Psychosom Med 69:829, 2007

Online Resource

http://www.dsm5.org/about/Pages/DSMVOverview.aspx

CHAPTER 18

Eating and Feeding Disorders

James Lock, M.D., Ph.D.

W. Stewart Agras, M.D.

The DSM-5 "Feeding and Eating Disorders" chapter includes the following diagnostic categories: anorexia nervosa, bulimia nervosa, binge-eating disorder (BED), avoidant/restrictive food intake disorder (ARFID), pica, rumination disorder, and other specified feeding or eating disorder (American Psychiatric Association 2013). A diagnosis of unspecified feeding and eating disorder is used when clinicians do not wish to specify a particular diagnosis. In this chapter we provide an overview of the prevalence, clinical presentation, and specific psychopathology associated with these diagnostic groups as well as descriptions of empirically supported treatments for these conditions. We begin with a discussion of the classic eating disorders (anorexia nervosa and bulimia nervosa) and move on to discuss the newer disorders, BED and ARFID, and, finally, the rarer disorders, pica and rumination disorder. We conclude with a brief discussion that considers possible future directions in furthering our understanding of the pathology and treatment of eating disorders.

Anorexia Nervosa

Psychopathology and Clinical Features

Anorexia nervosa is a serious disorder (Table 18–1), with a point prevalence of about 0.5% in female adolescents and young adults, making it the least common of the classic eating disorders (Smink et al. 2014). Anorexia nervosa usually emerges in adolescence, with peak onset at about 14 years of age. However, anorexia nervosa tends to persist if it is not treated successfully in adolescence, with high mortality rates from suicide and organ failure due to persistent starvation (Arcelus et al. 2011). Psychiatric disorders co-

TABLE 18–1.	Essential features of DSM-5 anorexia nervosa

An imbalance of energy intake to expenditure is present, leading to clinically significant weight loss for age, height, and gender.

The patient experiences severe anxiety or fear about gaining weight and/or engages in ongoing behaviors such as overexercise, dietary restriction, or purging that interfere with weight gain.

The patient has the perception that body weight is not low despite significant weight loss, or denies that the weight loss is medically serious.

The patient's self-worth is highly dependent on weight or body shape.

Note. For the complete diagnostic criteria, please refer to pp. 338–339 in DSM-5 (American Psychiatric Association 2013).

morbid with anorexia nervosa include major depressive disorder (MDD), obsessive-compulsive disorder, and anxiety disorders. Although restrictive eating based on fear of weight gain is the primary presentation of anorexia nervosa, binge eating and purging follow in about half of cases. Medical complications associated with malnutrition and purging include pericardial effusions; electrolyte abnormalities, particularly in the binge-eating and purging subtype; delayed gastric emptying; anemia; osteopenia and osteoporosis; evidence of atrophy of both gray and white matter in the brain; and sudden death due to cardiac arrest (Mehler et al. 2010). Hence, medical supervision is important in the management of anorexia nervosa regardless of the age of the patient.

Anorexia nervosa runs in families, and twin studies have shown that it is highly heritable (Clarke et al. 2012). The observation of high heritability has led to intensive genetic studies, including genome-wide association studies. Significant loci are beginning to emerge from such studies; for example, a recent study (Yilmaz et al. 2014) found a locus implicating leptin functioning as a genetic risk factor for anorexia nervosa. A further genome-wide association study (Duncan et al. 2017) implicated loci influencing metabolic pathways affecting insulin, glucose, and lipid phenotypes. Such studies may eventually shed light on the etiology of anorexia nervosa, particularly on metabolic pathways conducive to self-starvation. Both family and cultural influences are important risk factors, as illustrated by cases of anorexia nervosa occurring in cultures where the disorder was previously nonexistent but began to emerge as individuals were influenced by aspects of Western culture related to weight and appearance through television, magazines, and related media (Kuboki et al. 1996).

Clinical Presentation of Anorexia Nervosa in an Adult

Jane, a 31-year-old woman, presented to the clinic in an emaciated state, with a body mass index (BMI) of 14 kg/m^2. She had first lost weight at 14 years of age, losing for about 6 months before her parents considered treatment consisting of hospitalization aimed at weight restoration. On discharge from the hospital, she gradually lost weight again, even though she received individual psychotherapy combined with medical supervision, and she was rehospitalized. This pattern continued, with frequent inpatient admissions, partial weight restoration, and various forms of psychotherapy between hospitalizations. Over the years, weight restoration became less successful, and in Jane's better periods, her BMI hovered around 16 kg/m^2. In her mid-20s, Jane began to have periods that she characterized as overeating followed by self-induced vomiting. Physical examination on admission revealed bradycardia, low blood pressure, lanugo, and severe osteoporosis. It was noted that she had fractured a femur following a fall 3 years prior to this admission. She had never married and had worked only sporadically, being supported by and living with her family. From a psychological viewpoint, Jane stated that she continued to restrict her eating because she was afraid that she might lose control and put on too much weight. Despite her cachexia, she maintained that she felt that her lower abdomen and upper thighs were too fat. She met criteria for MDD, although whether it was due to severe malnutrition or to her restricted life was unclear.

There is evidence that anorexia nervosa symptoms may be expressed differently in childhood and adolescence compared with adulthood. Children and adolescents are often incapable of verbalizing abstract thoughts; therefore, behaviors such as food refusal that lead to malnutrition may manifest as nonverbal representations of emotional experiences. For this reason, parental reports about the child's behavior are critical, given that self-report is often unreliable due to of lack of insight, minimization, and denial by the child or adolescent. Children and adolescents with anorexia nervosa are less likely than adults with the disorder to engage in binge-eating and purging behaviors. These young patients sometimes deny any drive for thinness but often claim to be trying to eat less, avoid fattening foods, and exercise more for health reasons. Other young patients deny body image or weight concerns at assessment and insist they just are not hungry or complain of abdominal discomfort. While self-starvation persists, academic and athletic pursuits usually continue and sometimes become more compulsive and driven. Patients often appear withdrawn, depressed, and anxious. Usually they remain cognitively intact until more severe malnutrition develops. In some instances, compensatory behavior such as purging develops, but for younger patients such behavior usually occurs later in the course of the disorder.

Clinical Presentation of Anorexia Nervosa in an Adolescent

Anna is a 13-year-old who has no previous history of psychiatric problems, but her parents report that she has always been a bit anxious and socially slow to warm to other people. About 6 months ago, Anna decided to work on her health by eating better and exercising more. She had never had any problems with her weight. Over the first few months there were no real problems, but in the past several months Anna has become increasingly picky about what she eats, cutting out not only all fats but also most proteins. She has also increased her now-habitual running from 1 to 2 hours per day. As a result, Ann has lost 20 pounds, which is about 20% of her expected weight for height. Although she continues to excel in school, Anna's mood has become depressed and irritable, and she spends even less time with friends.

Treatment

Evidence-based treatment for anorexia nervosa is summarized in Table 18–7 ("Evidence-based treatments for the classic eating disorders"), at the end of this chapter.

Hospitalization and Other Intensive Treatment Settings

Despite its common use for anorexia nervosa, there is little evidence that psychiatric hospitalization is more effective than outpatient treatment (Gowers et al. 2007). A recent uncontrolled study (Twohig et al. 2016) suggested that residential and day treatment may be useful, but no randomized studies have compared residential or day treatment with outpatient treatment. However, such programs have potentially negative effects, especially for younger patients. These include separation of the developing child from family, friends, and community as well as stigma and shame. Nonetheless, hospitalization and more intensive programs are sometimes clinically necessary because of poor response to or lack of availability of appropriate specialty outpatient treatment. In those instances, negative impacts can be mitigated by keeping the length of stay short, using the lowest safe level of care, involving families in programming, and employing highly expert and experienced staff.

Hospitalization for medical complications related to severe malnutrition and purging is sometimes needed. There are no agreed-on indications for adults with persistent anorexia nervosa, but indications for medical hospitalization for children and adolescents have been published by the American Academy of Pediatrics and the Society of Adolescent Health and Medicine (Golden et al. 2003). These indications include severe abnormality of heart rate (bradycardia and orthostatic heart rate changes), blood pressure (orthostatic hypotension), and/or body temperature (hypothermia); electrolyte abnormalities; and severe malnutrition. Nasogastric tube feeding, especially for nocturnal feeds, is sometimes used with the aim of increasing the efficiency of weight gain, but the long-term benefits of this approach are not clear, and the clinical need for the approach is not established.

Evidence-Based Psychotherapy

Despite many years of research, no empirically supported psychosocial treatments are available for adults with persistent anorexia nervosa (Watson and Bulik 2013). Dropout rates from treatment trials are high, often reaching 40%–50%. Trials have included psychotherapies, such as cognitive-behavioral therapy (CBT) and interpersonal psychotherapy (IPT), that have shown efficacy in bulimia nervosa and BED. Despite different psychotherapies having differing therapeutic targets, the therapeutic equivalence of psychotherapies suggests that a common mechanism is responsible for their outcomes. The additional problem of high dropout rates has not been solved in any study.

In contrast to adult anorexia nervosa, studies of psychosocial interventions for short-duration adolescent anorexia nervosa are more promising (Lock 2015). The findings from these randomized controlled trials suggest that family approaches, particularly family-based treatment (FBT), are effective and superior to comparison individual therapies. FBT is an outpatient, manualized intervention that consists of between 10 and 20 family meetings over a 6- to 12-month treatment course (Lock and Le Grange 2013). FBT helps parents learn how to disrupt their child's starvation and overexercise and to take charge of weight restoration. Once the child is able to eat independently without parental supervision and has reached a normal weight, the treatment briefly focuses on developmental issues of adolescence. Although individual therapy was not as effective as FBT in these trials, individual approaches are nonetheless beneficial and could be offered to patients in cases in which FBT is not an acceptable or tenable option. In particular, adolescent-focused therapy (AFT), which is an individual therapy focused on individuation and self-efficacy, was found to be useful, especially for adolescents with less severe symptoms (e.g., fewer obsessions and compulsions about food and weight, less eating-related psychopathology, and no purging) (Fitzpatrick et al. 2010). AFT encourages the adolescent to manage his or her own eating and weight gain through the supportive relationship with the therapist. In addition, the main focus of AFT is to encourage an increased awareness and tolerance of emotions, particularly negative ones. To date, only a few small studies have examined CBT for adolescent anorexia nervosa in the outpatient setting (Dalle Grave et al. 2013). Although the results are preliminary, CBT for adolescents with anorexia nervosa appears to be acceptable to patients and leads to clinical improvements.

Evidence-Based Pharmacotherapy

Although a wide array of pharmacological agents, including antidepressants, antipsychotics, appetite stimulants, prokinetics, and hormonal treatments, among others, have been tested in controlled studies, no evidence-based medication for the treatment of anorexia nervosa has yet emerged (Attia et al. 2011). Several problems with this research area are apparent. Many studies have occurred in conjunction with inpatient treatment or some form of psychotherapy that may militate against the effects of medication becoming apparent (Vocks et al. 2010). Most studies have too small a sample size to provide sufficient power to differentiate the effects of medication from placebo. Finally, dropout rates are high, again threatening power to detect effects.

No systematic studies of selective serotonin reuptake inhibitors (SSRIs) have been conducted in adolescents with anorexia nervosa. Feasibility and acceptability of medication are a major problem because of fear of weight gain. A relatively recent pilot randomized controlled trial for adolescents with anorexia nervosa (Hagman et al. 2011) found few benefits from adding risperidone to standard treatment (consisting of psychotherapy and behavioral management), although the medication appeared to be well tolerated. Another small trial (Attia et al. 2011) combined treatment as usual with either placebo or olanzapine over a 10-week period and found no differential benefit with the addition of olanzapine. A small randomized study of quetiapine compared with treatment as usual (Powers et al. 2012) found some evidence of greater improvements in weight and eating-related thinking in the group randomly assigned to quetiapine, but there were no statistically significant differences between groups.

Bulimia Nervosa

Psychopathology and Clinical Features

Bulimia nervosa has a population prevalence of about 2% in women and 0.5% in men, although the female-to-male ratio in treatment-seeking samples is 10 to 1 (Smink et al. 2012). Hence, it is a relatively common disorder but is often overlooked by clinicians and underreported by patients. The disorder usually emerges in adolescence or young adulthood, often following a period of weight loss due to excessive dieting. These behaviors eventually lead to binge eating followed by compensatory purging. The disorder may have a fluctuating course, with bulimic behaviors exacerbated by stress, and often persists for many years; a 20-year follow-up study revealed that about one-third of patients with bulimia nervosa were not recovered despite having adequate access to treatment (Keel et al. 2010). The overall death rate in patients with bulimia nervosa is elevated compared with that in women without eating disorders, with a standard mortality ratio of 1.93, although it is not as high as in anorexia nervosa (Crow et al. 2009).

The primary presenting symptoms in bulimia nervosa are binge eating and compensatory behaviors such as purging, fasting, the use of diuretics, excessive exercise,

---

TABLE 18–2.   **Essential features of DSM-5 bulimia nervosa**

Repeated episodes of overeating (binge eating), which the patient feels unable to control.

The patient uses purging by vomiting; diuretics, laxatives, or other medications; or exercise in an attempt to compensate for the overeating episodes.

The overeating episodes are persistent and regular (e.g., one per week for 3 months).

The patient's self-worth is highly dependent on weight or body shape.

The patient does not have anorexia nervosa.

Note.   For the complete diagnostic criteria, please refer to p. 345 in DSM-5 (American Psychiatric Association 2013).

---

and, more rarely, chewing and spitting out food. Binge eating is defined by two characteristics: loss of control over eating and eating a large amount of food in one sitting (varying between 1,500 and 5,000 kcal or more). Binge eating is clinically subdivided into *objective binge eating*, in which large amounts of food are eaten, and *subjective binge eating*, in which loss of control is experienced but small amounts of food are consumed. Both types of binge eating may lead to purging. Secondary symptoms stemming directly from binge eating and purging behaviors range from fainting to cardiac arrhythmias and can include hypokalemia, metabolic syndrome, laxative dependence, tooth decay (sometimes associated with bone necrosis), esophageal tears with bleeding, and injuries and bone fractures. The DSM-5 diagnostic criteria (Table 18–2) specify the occurrence of one or more episodes of binge eating and compensatory behaviors per week. Comorbid psychopathology frequently seen includes MDD, anxiety disorders, and obsessive-compulsive disorder (K.S. Mitchell et al. 2012). About 25% of patients are diagnosed with current MDD.

Bulimia nervosa runs in families, and both genetics and the nonshared environment—that is, environmental factors specific to individuals—influence the development of the disorder. As in other complex disorders such as obesity, many genes, each of small effect, likely contribute to bulimia nervosa. It also appears that environmental factors are more influential early in development and that genetic contributions increase with age. At present, genetic studies have yet to reveal information useful for treatment or prevention of bulimia nervosa. Replicated risk factors for bulimia nervosa in studies meeting strict criteria include dieting, psychiatric morbidity (especially negative affect), and weight and shape concerns. Studies of appetitive regulation suggest that appetite is dysregulated in bulimia nervosa, probably at both central and peripheral levels, with disturbances of taste- and reward-processing regions of the brain likely contributing to the psychopathology. Bulimia nervosa was essentially unknown in non-Western cultures until Western influences, particularly television and other media sources, prompted the emergence of the disorder, usually among adolescent females. The critical factor transmitted appears to be preoccupation with the thin ideal weight and shape prevalent in Western settings but alien to many other cultures. Hence, cultural factors (largely Western culture), family environment, genetics, and appetitive dysregulation all contribute to the disorder.

Clinical Presentation of Bulimia Nervosa in an Adult

Jennifer, a 28-year-old software engineer, presented with a 14-year history of binge eating and vomiting, having first been treated in college when the symptoms were interfering with her studies. She also reported depression, a lack of energy, occasional dizziness, and a recent episode of fainting. She had begun to overeat during social occasions in early adolescence, but this behavior had not worried her because her friends were eating in the same way. Early in high school she began comparing herself with other classmates and began to restrict her calorie intake. This pattern led to a 10-lb weight loss, and it was at this point that she also began binge eating. A few months later she discovered self-induced vomiting via a magazine article and began to use that method as an additional way to reduce her weight. The purging behavior gradually increased in frequency until she was binge eating three or four times each week, always followed by self-induced vomiting. A typical binge would include one small plate of Chinese chicken salad, one-half cup of chicken with water chestnuts, 10 shrimps, one-third of a cup of chow mein, one cup of chicken and vegetables, a cup of steamed rice, two cokes, a cup of tea, and a cup of water. Over a period of several years, these behaviors began to take up more and more of her time, leaving less time and opportunity for socializing. Hence, she became increasingly isolated, lonely, and depressed. Moreover, she found herself preoccupied with thoughts of food and her weight and shape during the day that were interfering with her work to the point that she was beginning to worry about her job performance. She was normal weight, but her potassium level was low, at 3.0 mEq/L.

As with anorexia nervosa, there are additional challenges in diagnosing bulimia nervosa in childhood and adolescence because of developmental differences between adults and younger patients. Some studies have found that for younger patients, a feeling of a loss of control over eating is a better indicator than the amount eaten in assessing whether an eating episode should be categorized as a binge. Because parents and other adults often have greater control over the child's access to food, the number of binge episodes that young patients can engage in are likely more constrained, which may lead to fewer binge-eating episodes than might have taken place if these controls were not in place. As with younger patients with anorexia nervosa, difficulties with abstract thinking and verbal expression of emotional states, as well as minimization, are common among adolescents with bulimia nervosa. For this reason, it is usually helpful to include parental interviews to obtain a more comprehensive clinical picture.

Clinical Presentation of Bulimia Nervosa in an Adolescent

Sarah is 16 years old, is social and likable, with many friends, and is a good student. She began to feel increasingly worried about her weight and appearance after a breakup with a boy from the water polo team who said she was "too fat." Sarah began skipping breakfast and lunch. She found that she lost a few pounds using this approach, so she kept with this plan. However, after a few weeks, she felt so hungry when she returned home from school in the afternoon that she found herself snacking. Sometimes during these snacks, she could not stop eating and would rapidly eat entire bags of potato chips and a carton of ice cream. Sarah felt terrible after these episodes and felt like a failure. She also felt so full that it was easy just to bring the food up and vomit. At first, Sarah would binge-eat and vomit only once a week or so, but over time, she found she was doing it more and more. She was full of self-loathing and shame, and told no one about her behavior.

Treatment

Evidence-based treatment for bulimia nervosa is summarized in Table 18–7 ("Evidence-based treatments for the classic eating disorders"), at the end of this chapter.

Evidence-Based Psychotherapies

Among the psychotherapies, CBT currently has the largest evidence base for the treatment of adults with bulimia nervosa. CBT is based on the hypothesis that concerns about weight and shape and dietary restriction are the two processes that maintain bulimia nervosa (Fairburn et al. 2008). Treatment directly addresses these processes and consists of psychoeducation about bulimia nervosa and its maintaining factors, detailed self-monitoring of eating and purging behaviors, and the use of self-monitoring to gradually reduce dietary restriction by working toward three nutritionally adequate meals and two snacks daily, which reduces hunger and therefore loss of control over eating. Usually, self-induced vomiting requires little specific attention because it is tightly aligned with binge eating. As the diet becomes regulated, feared and avoided foods are gradually added. This phase of treatment is often accompanied by a marked reduction in binge eating and purging. The cognitive and behavioral components of concerns about weight and shape are then addressed while modifications to dietary restriction continue. In this phase of treatment, events that trigger either dietary restriction or weight and shape concerns are addressed, and alternative coping behaviors are discussed. Special attention needs to be given to diuretic and laxative use. Diuretics can usually be phased out fairly quickly, although the underlying reasons for their use, notably relief of weight and shape concerns, need to be addressed. Laxatives, because they are habit-forming, are often more difficult to stop. Patients have to choose between an abrupt withdrawal and a tapered withdrawal. Abrupt withdrawal will lead to constipation and ensuing gastrointestinal discomfort for several days and should be accompanied by increasing fruit and vegetable consumption. Gradual withdrawal is often the more difficult course because it extends discomfort over a much longer period of time.

A series of controlled trials (Svaldi et al. 2018) has shown that CBT is more effective than comparable treatments such as psychodynamic psychotherapy, IPT, weight loss treatment, and medication. Hence, CBT is regarded as the primary treatment for bulimia nervosa. However, with remission rates around 30%–40%, there is still much to improve. An enhanced version of CBT, CBT-E, has been developed and shows promise in more effectively treating patients with severe comorbid psychopathology (Fairburn et al. 2008). CBT-E has several additional modules based on the patient's specific problems, including modules targeting interpersonal problems, mood intolerance, perfectionism, and low self-esteem. Therapist-assisted CBT is a self-help version that uses brief therapy sessions but has the patient rely on a treatment manual or book. Controlled studies (Svaldi et al. 2018) suggest that this treatment may be as effective as CBT and hence is more widely usable because of the lower cost. Treatment with CBT is associated with a rapid early decrease in bulimic symptoms, such that a 50%–60% decline in purging by session 4 is a reasonably strong indicator of good outcome. This decline in purging behavior allows rapid identification of those who are less likely to improve and provides an opportunity to add adjunctive treatment such as medication or to switch to another psychotherapy.

A second-line treatment adapted from the treatment of depression, IPT, has also been shown to be effective in treating bulimia nervosa, although it is slower to work than CBT or CBT-E in the short term, and in at least in one controlled study, it was shown to be less effective than CBT in both the short and the long term (Fairburn 1997). The therapy model posits that emotional arousal from specific interpersonal interactions, rather than being handled appropriately, is dealt with by binge eating. Hence, the focus of therapy is on linking interpersonal triggering events to emotional arousal and to binge eating and helping the patient to work through better ways of adapting to such events. Treatment usually focuses on one interpersonal issue pertinent to binge eating in one of four areas: grief, role disputes, role transitions, and interpersonal deficits. A major advantage of IPT is that it is a transdiagnostic treatment, with evidence of effectiveness in treating MDD and anxiety disorders without requiring much alteration in treatment procedures.

Although a number of randomized controlled trials have examined treatment for adults with bulimia nervosa, only three examined treatment for adolescent bulimia nervosa. Schmidt et al. (2007) compared FBT and a self-help version of CBT for 85 adolescents (ages 13–20 years) who met full or partial DSM-IV bulimia nervosa criteria (American Psychiatric Association 1994), but found no differences in outcome. Le Grange et al. (2007) compared FBT and individual supportive psychotherapy in adolescents (ages 12–19) who met full or partial DSM-IV bulimia nervosa criteria. The results of this study indicated that FBT was more effective than supportive psychotherapy both at the end of treatment and at 6-month follow-up. Additionally, FBT reduced binge-eating and purging rates within a significantly shorter time compared with supportive psychotherapy. The most recent and largest treatment study was a randomized comparison of 130 adolescents with bulimia nervosa who received either FBT or CBT for bulimia nervosa (Le Grange et al. 2015). At the end of treatment, those who received FBT had significantly higher abstinence rates than those who received CBT. However, these differences were no longer statistically different at 12 months posttreatment, although both groups continued to improve.

Evidence-Based Pharmacotherapy

As noted previously, research in the use of medication to treat bulimia nervosa began contemporaneously with psychotherapy research (Aigner et al. 2011). The first controlled studies were of the tricyclic antidepressants and monoamine oxidase inhibitors, demonstrating the superiority of both to placebo in reducing binge eating and purging. These studies were eventually followed by studies demonstrating that fluoxetine (60 mg/day) was superior to placebo in treating bulimia nervosa, as are most of the serotonin reuptake inhibitors. Fluoxetine is currently the only medication approved by the U.S. Food and Drug Administration (FDA) for the treatment of bulimia nervosa. One small study of antidepressants (including SSRIs) in adolescents with bulimia nervosa (Kotler et al. 2003) found that these medications were feasible and acceptable, with few side effects in this age group. Indications for the use of antidepressants are patient preference over psychotherapy, severe MDD, and failure to respond to psychotherapy. Treatment studies in adults with bulimia have shown that adding antidepressants to CBT is more effective than the use of CBT alone; hence, the combined approach should be considered if early improvement is not seen with CBT. Overall, antidepressant medications are regarded as less effective than CBT, which remains the primary treatment of choice for bulimia nervosa. Dropout rates are also significantly higher for medication than for CBT. Antiepileptics (e.g., topiramate) are another drug class that has shown some promise, although dropout rates in controlled studies have been higher than those with antidepressants, largely because of side effects.

Binge-Eating Disorder

Psychopathology and Clinical Features

Although BED often begins in adolescence, it can also have a later onset. Hence, the BED patients seen in the clinic or enrolled in clinical trials are usually older than the patients with anorexia nervosa or bulimia nervosa. The DSM-5 criteria for the diagnosis of BED (Table 18–3) include binge eating (eating a large amount of food with loss of control over eating) at least once a week for a period of 3 months. DSM-5 criteria also specify that the binge eating is associated with at least three of five of the following behaviors: eating more rapidly than normal; eating large amounts of food when not hungry; eating until uncomfortably full; eating alone because of embarrassment about how much one is eating; and feeling guilty, disgusted, or depressed after binge eating. Unlike bulimia nervosa, BED does not involve compensatory behaviors such as self-induced vomiting, excessive exercise, or laxative and diuretic abuse.

The lifetime prevalence of BED is between 1% and 3%, with prevalence tending to increase in midlife, making BED the most common eating disorder (Swanson et al. 2011). As in the other eating disorders, the prevalence of lifetime comorbid MDD is about 60%, and that of current MDD is about 25% (Grilo et al. 2009). Patients with overvaluation of weight and shape tend to have more associated psychopathology. Because of these psychological and physical comorbidities, quality of life is generally lower in patients with BED than in comparison groups without BED. In addition to its psychological comorbidities and because of its association with obesity, BED carries a heightened risk of developing diabetes, hypercholesterolemia, and cardiovascular disease. Although studies differ, about 30% of individuals undergoing bariatric surgery have BED prior to surgery, and about one-third of that number will be diagnosed with BED postsurgery (Kalarchian et al. 1998). However, the proportion of patients reporting loss of control over eating is much higher. Moreover, studies suggest that loss of control postsurgery predicts poor outcomes in terms of weight loss (Ivezaj et al. 2017).

Because there have been few long-term observational studies, the course of BED is not well understood. There is some crossover with bulimia nervosa and, rarely, with anorexia nervosa; however, most cases of BED either remain in that diagnosis or remit (Pope et al. 2006). Longer-term follow-up studies (Hilbert et al. 2012) suggest that the disorder may fluctuate over longer periods.

Similar to the other eating disorders, BED runs in families, probably reflecting both genetic and specific family influences. Other findings implicate brain reward systems and opioid secretion (Avena and Bocarsly 2012). Environmental influences on binge eating include negative emotion, with both laboratory and naturalistic studies showing that negative emotion regularly precedes and probably triggers binge eating (Dingemans et al. 2017).

TABLE 18–3. **Essential features of DSM-5 binge-eating disorder**

Repeated episodes of overeating (binge eating), which the patient feels unable to control, associated with rapid eating; fullness; eating without hunger; and/or shame, depression, or other signs of significant emotional distress.

The overeating episodes are persistent and regular (e.g., one per week for 3 months).

The patient's self-worth is highly dependent on weight or body shape.

The patient does not have anorexia nervosa or bulimia nervosa.

Note. For the complete diagnostic criteria, please refer to p. 350 in DSM-5 (American Psychiatric Association 2013).

Clinical Presentation of Adult Binge-Eating Disorder

Susan, a 48-year-old woman, presented for treatment reporting that she had lost control of her eating, that it was affecting her weight, and that it was causing her to feel ashamed of and dissatisfied with her body and being so fat. During late adolescence, she had begun to binge-eat after repeatedly failing to lose weight through dieting—she would lose about 5 or 6 lb with every attempt, but would quickly put weight back on when she stopped whatever dieting approach she was using. Binge eating combined with occasional dieting episodes led to a gradual increase in weight and adiposity, so that at presentation, her BMI was 35 kg/m². She also noted periods of depression associated with overeating, lack of energy, and decreased libido that responded well to antidepressant treatment. She reported binge eating two to four times each day, and sometimes more frequently on the weekends, when she was alone. A typical binge consisted of 15 chocolate chip cookies, half a dozen cheese puffs, two fruit rolls, a cup of popcorn, and two cups of ice cream. She noted that when beginning a binge-eating episode, she would be thinking that "I need to do this, it will make me feel good"; however, as the binge went on, her thoughts would change to "My stomach hurts, and I feel awful."

There are similar challenges in diagnosing BED and bulimia nervosa in childhood and adolescence because of developmental differences between younger patients and adults. A sense of being out of control when eating is likely more important than eating an objectively large amount of food in younger patients because younger patients often cannot gain access to food as easily as adults. For these reasons, clinicians treating children and adolescents should consider using a lower threshold for the frequency and duration of binge-eating episodes. A suggested frequency of once per month (instead of once per week) over the previous 3-month period was recommended by a consensus group of experts in child and adolescent eating disorders (Bravender et al. 2007). In addition, as with anorexia nervosa and bulimia nervosa, children and adolescents are limited in their abstract thinking ability and self-expression. They also may minimize any discomfort or shame they experience when binge eating. Thus, parental interviews and other collateral reports are often necessary for making a definitive diagnosis of BED in children or adolescents. Bulimia nervosa usually occurs in patients who are of normal weight or who are slightly overweight; BED more often occurs in overweight and obese individuals. In bulimia nervosa, binge eating is considered to be a response to restriction of food intake, whereas in BED, binge eating occurs in the context of overall chaotic and unregulated eating patterns.

Treatment

Evidence-based treatment for binge-eating disorder is summarized in Table 18–7 ("Evidence-based treatments for the classic eating disorders"), at the end of this chapter.

Evidence-Based Psychotherapy

Before discussing the effects of treatment, it is important to understand that the placebo response is higher in BED than in bulimia nervosa; as a result, a treatment's effectiveness in BED is inflated relative to its effectiveness in bulimia nervosa. Well-designed controlled studies have shown that both CBT and IPT are effective in reducing binge eating, with 50%–60% of patients achieving remission at end of treatment (Wilson et al. 2010). Unlike the findings in bulimia nervosa, it appears that CBT and IPT are similarly effective in BED, both at the end of treatment and at follow-up. A third treatment, behavioral weight loss therapy, has also been used to treat BED on the basis of the finding that binge eating decreases with weight loss. Controlled comparisons of CBT with weight loss therapy have found that CBT is superior in reducing the frequency of binge eating; however, CBT does not reduce weight. At present, CBT and IPT are the recommended first-line treatments for BED for reducing binge eating but do not lead to weight loss. IPT has the advantage that essentially the same treatment used for BED can be used to treat depression and anxiety (for which there is an evidence base for IPT), whereas the specific applications of CBT are very different for eating disorders, depression, and anxiety disorders. In adolescents with BED, preliminary studies support the use of IPT, but BED has otherwise been relatively unexamined in younger patients.

As in bulimia nervosa, a shorter variant of CBT, therapist-guided self-help, has been shown to be as effective as full-scale CBT in reducing binge eating in the treatment of BED. As noted for bulimia nervosa, this CBT variant allows less costly treatment to be available to larger numbers of individuals needing treatment.

Evidence-Based Pharmacotherapy

Antidepressants, particularly SSRIs, used at dosages similar to those used for the treatment of depression, are effective in the treatment of BED, with response rates of about 40% (Stefano et al. 2008). Rates of dropout due to side effects tend to be higher for antidepressants than for CBT or IPT. Controlled studies suggest that CBT is more effective than antidepressants in treating BED (Ricca et al. 2001). More recently, several studies (McElroy 2017) have examined the efficacy of lisdexamfetamine (LDX), a medication used in the treatment of attention-deficit/hyperactivity disorder, resulting in FDA approval of LDX for the treatment of BED in 2015. In placebo-controlled trials of LDX (at dosages between 50 and 70 mg/day), approximately 50% of patients receiving LDX achieved abstinence from binge eating, compared with 21% of patients receiving placebo (McElroy et al. 2015). Moreover, unlike patients treated with psychotherapies such as CBT or IPT, patients on LDX showed an average weight loss of 5.0 kg, compared with little weight loss in the placebo group (McElroy et al. 2015). In a further 6-month maintenance trial (Hudson et al. 2017), only 3.7% of patient on LDX relapsed to binge eating, compared with 32.1% of patients switched to placebo. Hence, LDX appears to be a promising medication for the treatment of BED.

Avoidant/Restrictive Food Intake Disorder

Psychopathology and Clinical Features

DSM-5 diagnostic criteria for ARFID (Table 18–4) include food restriction or avoidance without shape or weight concerns or intentional efforts to lose weight that results in significant weight loss and nutritional deficiencies and is associated with disturbances in psychological development and functioning (Bryant-Waugh and Kreipe 2012). Some patients present with highly selective eating; neophobia (the fear of new things) related to food types; or hypersensitivity to food texture, appearance, and taste. For some patients, fear of swallowing or choking contributes to food avoidance; a specific event can sometimes be identified as triggering that fear. ARFID also applies to individuals who have a lack of interest in eating or low appetite. There are no epidemiological studies available for this new diagnosis. Specific etiological risk factors for ARFID are unknown. Patients with autism spectrum disorder (ASD) frequently display selective eating patterns. Anxiety disorders and anxious traits as well as depressive symptoms often predate the development of ARFID. Neglect, abuse, and developmental delays may increase the risk for chewing and spitting associated with ARFID.

ARFID can be confused with anorexia nervosa, but distinguishing features include a lack of fear of weight gain in ARFID, no shape and weight concerns in ARFID, and no specific focus on weight loss in ARFID. It is essential to obtain collateral history from parents, who will usually indicate no avoidance of high-calorie food in ARFID. Patients are aware that they are low weight and may express a wish to eat more and gain weight, but their anxiety and fear prevent them from consuming enough to do so. ARFID can sometimes be confused with ASD and other neurodevelopmental disorders.

Clinical Presentations of ARFID

Tom is an 8-year-old boy who eats only white bread, plain pasta, candy, and bananas. Tom's parents describe him as having been a picky eater ever since they began introducing solid foods into his diet when he was about 2 years old. His current food choices have become his sole menu only in the past 2 years. His parents describe many battles with Tom early on, trying to get him to try vegetables or meat, but he always complained and spit them out, saying that they tasted terrible.

Alice is a 9-year-old girl who, prior to 4 months ago, ate most foods without difficulty and, although a somewhat nervous child, otherwise had no major problems with eating until one day when she attended a birthday party of a close friend, where she choked on the thick crust of a pizza while running in a game. Alice was terrified, and when her parents picked her up, she was still crying. In the following days, Alice refused to eat any solid foods but was willing to drink milk or soups as long as there was no solid food in them.

Treatment

For children and adolescents with ARFID, there are no empirical studies to guide treatment. For the most part, ARFID requires individualized behavioral plans to ad-

TABLE 18–4.   **Essential features of DSM-5 avoidant/restrictive food intake disorder**

Problems with eating result in weight loss, malnutrition, dependence on tube feeding or other means of nutritional supplementation, or significant psychosocial problems.

The eating problems are not attributable to a lack of food or a culturally sanctioned practice.

The eating problems do not involve weight or shape concerns and are not specifically associated with anorexia nervosa or bulimia nervosa.

The eating problems are not explained by a concurrent medical or other mental disorder.

Note.   For the complete diagnostic criteria, please refer to p. 334 in DSM-5 (American Psychiatric Association 2013).

dress the specific eating problem, but use of CBT and family interventions may be helpful and are currently under study. For example, gradual desensitization procedures are often helpful, along with behavior reinforcement plans for specific types of eating problems. When eating problems are severe enough to lead to medical instability or severe malnutrition, hospitalization may be needed.

Pica

DSM-5 criteria for pica are as follows: eating of nonnutritive, nonfood substances that is persistent, occurs for at least a 1-month period, is developmentally inappropriate and not part of a culturally or socially normative practice, and is sufficiently severe to warrant clinical attention (Table 18–5). The prevalence of pica is uncertain. Onset of pica can occur at any age; however, childhood onset is most common. Putative environmental risk factors for pica include neglect, lack of supervision, and developmental delay. The most common comorbidities associated with pica are ASD, intellectual disability, and neurological syndromes or symptoms. The clinical course of pica is not well characterized, but the disorder can result in medical emergencies, including intestinal obstruction, and can be fatal. There are no known empirically supported treatments for pica. Behavioral, psychoeducational, and supportive interventions are typically offered.

Rumination Disorder

DSM-5 criteria for rumination disorder are as follows: recurrent effortless (nonretching) regurgitation of food (at least several times per week) for at least a 1-month period that is not attributable to an associated gastrointestinal or other medical condition (e.g., gastroesophageal reflux) and that is severe enough to warrant clinical attention (Table 18–6). Regurgitation behaviors may include rechewing, reswallowing, or spitting out food. Patients often report being unable to control the behavior and describe it is as habitual rather than deliberate. Although its prevalence is unknown, rumination disorder appears to occur more often in individuals with intellectual disability. Rumination disorder may begin at any age, but regardless of onset age, the course may be either episodic or continuous (Chial et al. 2003). Rumination disorder can lead to malnourishment due to reduced food intake. In younger individuals, growth and other development factors can be adversely affected, and in rare instances, rumina-

TABLE 18–5.   **Essential features of DSM-5 pica**

A pattern of consistent consumption of nonnutritive, nonfood substances (e.g., chalk, clay, paper) has been present for at least 1 month.

The behavior is not part of developmental exploration of tastes.

The behavior is not culturally normative.

If the behavior occurs as part of another disorder, it is serious enough to warrant separate clinical attention.

Note.   For the complete diagnostic criteria, please refer to pp. 329–330 in DSM-5 (American Psychiatric Association 2013).

TABLE 18–6.   **Essential features of DSM-5 rumination disorder**

A pattern of consistent regurgitation of food has been present for at least 1 month.

The behavior is not attributable to an ongoing gastrointestinal or other medical condition.

The behavior is not a part of the clinical presentation of anorexia nervosa or bulimia nervosa.

If the behavior occurs as part of another disorder, it is serious enough to warrant separate clinical attention.

Note.   For the complete diagnostic criteria, please refer to p. 332 in DSM-5 (American Psychiatric Association 2013).

tion disorder can lead to death. Lack of stimulation, neglect, stressful life events, and problems in the parent–child relationship may be risk factors for rumination disorder, although systematic studies are lacking. Ruminating sometimes appears to serve a self-soothing or self-stimulating function, especially in individuals with neurodevelopmental disorders. There are no known empirically supported treatments for rumination disorder. Gradual behavioral desensitization, slow nasogastric feeding, and low-dose serotonin reuptake inhibitors are sometimes used to disrupt persistent rumination.

Future Directions

Research into the etiology and treatment of the eating disorders has progressed rapidly in the past quarter-century but still lags behind progress in other areas, such as anxiety and depression. For the long term, research in genetics, neurobiology, and neurochemistry together with treatment research may shed light on the etiology and maintenance of eating disorders and improve treatment. However, a major problem facing the provision of mental health services is that a large proportion of the population in the United States has little or no access to effective treatment. One promising way to address this problem is to use technology to provide treatment through either the Internet or the use of mobile applications (apps) (Darcy and Lock 2017). Several controlled studies have suggested that CBT provided via telehealth is more effective in treating bulimia nervosa than no treatment but not as effective as full CBT (J. E. Mitchell et al. 2008). Apps have also been developed to assist in self-monitoring of food intake and binge eating and purging, although no controlled studies of their use in treatment have yet been reported. One problem with the use of apps in conditions such as depression

TABLE 18–7.   **Evidence-based treatments for the classic eating disorders**

	Evidence-based treatment	Strength of evidence
Anorexia nervosa	Family-based treatment (child and adolescent)	High
	Specialist care (persistent anorexia)	Low
Bulimia nervosa	Family-based treatment (child and adolescent)	Medium
	Cognitive-behavioral therapy (child and adolescent)	Medium
	Cognitive-behavioral therapy (adult)	High
	Interpersonal psychotherapy (adult)	Medium
	Fluoxetine (adult)	High; FDA approved
	Other antidepressants (adult)	Medium
Binge-eating disorder	Cognitive-behavioral therapy (adult)	High
	Interpersonal psychotherapy (adult)	Medium
	Lisdexamfetamine (adult)	Medium; FDA approved
	Antidepressants (adult)	Medium

Note.   FDA=U.S. Food and Drug Administration.

is the very high rate of nonuse and dropout. Hence, the optimal use of apps appears to be within therapy to facilitate treatment activities such as self-monitoring of symptoms and to continue therapeutic work between treatment sessions. Nonetheless, further development of more sophisticated versions of Internet CBT may eventually overcome these initial problems. Treatment via the Internet or solely via apps raises ethical and practical issues. For example, assessment via the Internet alone may not allow for detection of severe depression or suicidal ideation. Moreover, serious issues that arise during treatment may not be detected. In addition, many states do not allow therapy to be conducted across state borders by clinicians licensed in other states.

Studies have shown that many community practitioners do not use evidence-based treatments (Table 18–7) for patients with eating disorders. The reasons for this lack of use are complex and include the challenges surrounding the adoption of new psychotherapy modalities and the difficulty of implementing existing evidence-based therapies in community practice settings; for example, many community clinics cannot afford to provide the 18 sessions of treatment that most evidence-based therapies require. In addition, clinician adherence to the specific protocols of an evidence-based psychotherapy tends to fall over time, leading to lower effectiveness. These difficulties have led to efforts to better understand the factors militating against the use of new therapies and to investigate methods of training therapists in new interventions, including online training. In addition, evidence-based psychotherapies will need to be adapted to differing clinical situations.

Key Clinical Points

- Family-based treatment is effective for anorexia nervosa and bulimia nervosa in adolescents.

- Cognitive-behavioral therapy is effective for bulimia nervosa and binge-eating disorder in adults.

- No medications have yet shown systematic effectiveness for anorexia nervosa.

- Selective serotonin reuptake inhibitors are effective for adults with bulimia nervosa, especially in combination with cognitive-behavioral therapy.

- Lisdexamfetamine is FDA approved for the treatment of binge-eating disorder.

- Binge-eating disorder and avoidant/restrictive food intake disorder are new diagnoses in DSM-5.

- Access to empirically supported treatments for eating disorders is limited, and the use of technology, including telepsychiatry and mobile apps, may be helpful in overcoming this problem.

References

Aigner M, Treasure J, Kaye W, et al: World Federation of Societies of Biological Psychiatry (WFSBP) guidelines for the pharmacological treatment of eating disorders. World J Biol Psychiatry 12(6):400–443, 2011 21961502

American Psychiatric Association: Diagnostic and Statistical Manual of Mental Disorders, 4th Edition. Washington, DC, American Psychiatric Association, 1994

American Psychiatric Association: Diagnostic and Statistical Manual of Mental Disorders, 5th Edition. Arlington, VA, American Psychiatric Association, 2013

Arcelus J, Mitchell AJ, Wales J, et al: Mortality rates in patients with anorexia nervosa and other eating disorders. A meta-analysis of 36 studies. Arch Gen Psychiatry 68(7):724–731, 2011 21727255

Attia E, Kaplan AS, Walsh BT, et al: Olanzapine versus placebo for out-patients with anorexia nervosa. Psychol Med 41(10):2177–2182, 2011 21426603

Avena NM, Bocarsly ME: Dysregulation of brain reward systems in eating disorders: neurochemical information from animal models of binge eating, bulimia nervosa, and anorexia nervosa. Neuropharmacology 63(1):87–96, 2012 22138162

Bravender T, Bryant-Waugh R, Herzog D, et al; Workgroup for Classification of Eating Disorders in Children and Adolescents: Classification of child and adolescent eating disturbances. Workgroup for Classification of Eating Disorders in Children and Adolescents (WCEDCA). Int J Eat Disord 40 (suppl):S117–S1122, 2007 17868122

Bryant-Waugh R, Kreipe R: Avoidant/restrictive food intake disorder in DSM-5. Psychiatr Ann 42:402–405, 2012

Chial HJ, Camilleri M, Williams DE, et al: Rumination syndrome in children and adolescents: diagnosis, treatment, and prognosis. Pediatrics 111(1):158–162, 2003 12509570

Clarke TK, Weiss AR, Berrettini WH: The genetics of anorexia nervosa. Clin Pharmacol Ther 91(2):181–188, 2012 22190067

Crow SJ, Peterson CB, Swanson SA, et al: Increased mortality in bulimia nervosa and other eating disorders. Am J Psychiatry 166(12):1342–1346, 2009 19833789

Dalle Grave R, Calugi S, Doll HA, et al: Enhanced cognitive behaviour therapy for adolescents with anorexia nervosa: an alternative to family therapy? Behav Res Ther 51(1):R9–R12, 2013 23123081

Darcy AM, Lock J: Using technology to improve treatment outcomes for children and adolescents with eating disorders. Child Adolesc Psychiatr Clin N Am 26(1):33–42, 2017 27837940

Dingemans A, Danner U, Parks M: Emotion regulation in binge eating disorder: a review. Nutrients 9(11), 2017 29165348

Duncan L, Yilmaz Z, Gaspar H, et al; Eating Disorders Working Group of the Psychiatric Genomics Consortium: Significant locus and metabolic genetic correlations revealed in genome-wide association study of anorexia nervosa. Am J Psychiatry 174(9):850–858, 2017 28494655

Fairburn CG: Interpersonal psychotherapy for bulimia nervosa, in Handbook of Treatment for Eating Disorders, 2nd Edition. Edited by Garner DM, Garfinkel P. New York, Guilford, 1997, pp 278–294

Fairburn CG, Cooper Z, Shafran R: Enhanced cognitive behavior therapy for eating disorders ("CBT-E"): an overview, in Cognitive Behavioral Therapy and Eating Disorders. Edited by Fairburn CG. New York, Guilford, 2008, pp 23–34

Fitzpatrick KK, Moye A, Hoste R, et al: Adolescent focused therapy for adolescent anorexia nervosa. J Contemp Psychother 40(1):31–39, 2010

Golden NH, Katzman DK, Kreipe RE, et al; Society For Adolescent Medicine: Eating disorders in adolescents: position paper of the Society for Adolescent Medicine. J Adolesc Health 33(6):496–503, 2003 14642712

Gowers SG, Clark A, Roberts C, et al: Clinical effectiveness of treatments for anorexia nervosa in adolescents: randomised controlled trial. Br J Psychiatry 191(5):427–435, 2007 17978323

Grilo CM, White MA, Masheb RM: DSM-IV psychiatric disorder comorbidity and its correlates in binge eating disorder. Int J Eat Disord 42(3):228–234, 2009 18951458

Hagman J, Gralla J, Sigel E, et al: A double-blind, placebo-controlled study of risperidone for the treatment of adolescents and young adults with anorexia nervosa: a pilot study. J Am Acad Child Adolesc Psychiatry 50(9):915–924, 2011 21871373

Hilbert A, Bishop ME, Stein RI, et al: Long-term efficacy of psychological treatments for binge eating disorder. Br J Psychiatry 200(3):232–237, 2012 22282429

Hudson JI, McElroy SL, Ferreira-Cornwell MC, et al: Efficacy of lisdexamfetamine in adults with moderate to severe binge-eating disorder: a randomized clinical trial. JAMA Psychiatry 74(9):903–910, 2017 28700805

Ivezaj V, Kessler EE, Lydecker JA, et al: Loss-of-control eating following sleeve gastrectomy surgery. Surg Obes Relat Dis 13(3):392–398, 2017 27913121

Kalarchian MA, Wilson GT, Brolin RE, Bradley L: Binge eating in bariatric surgery patients. Int J Eat Disord 23(1):89–92, 1998 9429923

Keel PK, Gravener JA, Joiner TE Jr, Haedt AA: Twenty-year follow-up of bulimia nervosa and related eating disorders not otherwise specified. Int J Eat Disord 43(6):492–497, 2010 19718666

Kotler LA, Devlin MJ, Davies M, Walsh BT: An open trial of fluoxetine for adolescents with bulimia nervosa. J Child Adolesc Psychopharmacol 13(3):329–335, 2003 14642021

Kuboki T, Nomura S, Ide M, et al: Epidemiological data on anorexia nervosa in Japan. Psychiatry Res 62(1):11–16, 1996 [Erratum in: Psychiatry Res 62(3):285–286, 1996] 8739110

Le Grange D, Crosby RD, Rathouz PJ, et al: A randomized controlled comparison of family based treatment and supportive psychotherapy for adolescent bulimia nervosa. Arch Gen Psychiatry 64(9):1049–1056, 2007 17768270

Le Grange D, Lock J, Agras WS, et al: Randomized clinical trial of family-based treatment and cognitive-behavioral therapy for adolescent bulimia nervosa. J Am Acad Child Adolesc Psychiatry 54(11):886–894, 2015 26506579

Lock J: An update on evidence-based psychosocial treatments for eating disorders in children and adolescents. J Clin Child Adolesc Psychol 44(5):707–721, 2015 25580937

Lock J, Le Grange D: Treatment Manual for Anorexia Nervosa: A Family Based Approach. New York, Guilford, 2013

McElroy SL: Pharmacologic treatments for binge-eating disorder. J Clin Psychiatry 78 (suppl1):14–19, 2017 28125174

McElroy SL, Guerdjikova AI, Mori N, et al: Overview of the treatment of binge eating disorder. CNS Spectr 20(6):546–556, 2015 26594849

Mehler PS, Birmingham L, Crow SJ, et al: Medical complications of eating disorders, in The Treatment of Eating Disorders: A Clinical Handbook. Edited by Grilo CM, Mitchell JE. New York, Guilford, 2010, pp 66–82

Mitchell JE, Crosby RD, Wonderlich SA, et al: A randomized trial comparing the efficacy of cognitive-behavioral therapy for bulimia nervosa delivered via telemedicine versus face-to-face. Behav Res Ther 46(5):581–592, 2008 18374304

Mitchell KS, Mazzeo SE, Schlesinger MR, et al: Comorbidity of partial and subthreshold PTSD among men and women with eating disorders in the national comorbidity survey—replication study. Int J Eat Disord 45(3):307–315, 2012 22009722

Pope HG Jr, Lalonde JK, Pindyck LJ, et al: Binge eating disorder: a stable syndrome. Am J Psychiatry 163(12):2181–2183, 2006 17151172

Powers PS, Klabunde M, Kaye W: Double-blind placebo-controlled trial of quetiapine in anorexia nervosa. Eur Eat Disord Rev 20(4):331–334, 2012 22535517

Ricca V, Mannucci E, Mezzani B, et al: Fluoxetine and fluvoxamine combined with individual cognitive-behaviour therapy in binge eating disorder: a one-year follow-up study. Psychother Psychosom 70(6):298–306, 2001 11598429

Schmidt U, Lee S, Beecham J, et al: A randomized controlled trial of family therapy and cognitive behavior therapy guided self-care for adolescents with bulimia nervosa and related disorders. Am J Psychiatry 164(4):591–598, 2007 17403972

Smink FR, van Hoeken D, Hoek HW: Epidemiology of eating disorders: incidence, prevalence and mortality rates. Curr Psychiatry Rep 14(4):406–414, 2012 22644309

Smink FR, van Hoeken D, Oldehinkel AJ, et al: Prevalence and severity of DSM-5 eating disorders in a community cohort of adolescents. Int J Eat Disord 47(6):610–619, 2014 24903034

Stefano SC, Bacaltchuk J, Blay SL, Appolinário JC: Antidepressants in short-term treatment of binge eating disorder: systematic review and meta-analysis. Eat Behav 9(2):129–136, 2008 18329590

Svaldi J, Schmitz F, Baur J, et al: Efficacy of psychotherapies and pharmacotherapies for bulimia nervosa. Psychol Med Dec 5, 2018 [Epub ahead of print] 30514412

Swanson SA, Crow SJ, Le Grange D, et al: Prevalence and correlates of eating disorders in adolescents. Results from the national comorbidity survey replication adolescent supplement. Arch Gen Psychiatry 68(7):714–723, 2011 21383252

Twohig MP, Bluett EJ, Cullum JL, et al: Effectiveness and clinical response rates of a residential eating disorders facility. Eat Disord 24(3):224–239, 2016 26214231

Vocks S, Tuschen-Caffier B, Pietrowsky R, et al: Meta-analysis of the effectiveness of psychological and pharmacological treatments for binge eating disorder. Int J Eat Disord 43(3):205–217, 2010 19402028

Watson HJ, Bulik CM: Update on the treatment of anorexia nervosa: review of clinical trials, practice guidelines and emerging interventions. Psychol Med 43(12):2477–2500, 2013 23217606

Wilson GT, Wilfley DE, Agras WS, et al: Psychological treatments of binge eating disorder. Arch Gen Psychiatry 67(1):94–101, 2010 20048227

Yilmaz Z, Kaplan AS, Tiwari AK, et al: The role of leptin, melanocortin, and neurotrophin system genes on body weight in anorexia nervosa and bulimia nervosa. J Psychiatr Res 55:77–86, 2014 24831852

Recommended Readings

Agras WS (ed): The Oxford Handbook of Eating Disorders. New York, Oxford University Press, 2010

Fairburn CG: Cognitive Behavior Therapy and Eating Disorders. New York, Guilford, 2008

Grilo CM, Mitchell JE (eds): The Treatment of Eating Disorders: A Clinical Handbook. New York, Guilford, 2010

Lock J, Le Grange D: Treatment Manual for Anorexia Nervosa. New York, Guilford, 2013

Lock J, Le Grange D: Help Your Teenager Beat an Eating Disorder. New York, Guilford, 2015

CHAPTER 19

Elimination Disorders

Edwin J. Mikkelsen, M.D.

The term *elimination disorders* refers to the relatively common childhood disorder of enuresis and the less common problem of encopresis. Both of these disorders are self-limited and will eventually spontaneously remit. However, in the years before remission occurs, they can cause significant emotional distress to both the child and his or her family. Accordingly, it is appropriate to consider treatment approaches that have been empirically proven to be effective in limiting the duration and severity of these disorders.

Enuresis

Enuresis has been described throughout recorded history. A comprehensive summary by Glicklich (1951) found descriptions going back to the Papyrus Ebers of 1550 B.C. The history of enuresis is also rich with regard to the various treatment modalities that have been used, many of which would now appear to be sadistic in nature, given the current knowledge base.

Definition and Clinical Description

The word *enuresis* is derived from the Greek word *enourein*, meaning "to void urine." A pathological connection is not inherent in the derivation but has been acquired over time. The word has come to denote nocturnal events, but that meaning also is not inherent in the original derivation.

The phenomenology of enuresis is simply the voiding of urine, which usually occurs during sleep. However, it can also occur during the day while the individual is awake. The word *diurnal* is used to describe events that occur during the day. Individ-

The author wishes to thank Patsy Kuropatkin for her invaluable assistance with preparation of this manuscript.

uals who have episodes during both day and night are referred to as having diurnal and nocturnal enuresis. The volume of urine that is voided is not specified and technically could vary considerably while still being considered an *enuretic event*. The concrete nature of the enuretic event makes data collection relatively simple. It also makes it possible to quantify the magnitude of treatment effects by comparing the pre- and posttreatment weekly averages.

Diagnosis

There are two clinical subtypes of enuresis based on the natural history of the disorder; those individuals who have never achieved continence have the subtype called *primary enuresis,* whereas those who were able to achieve continence but then subsequently resumed wetting have the subtype called *secondary enuresis.* A time period of 6 months to 1 year is usually accepted as the length of time continence must have been maintained before secondary enuresis is diagnosed. The vast majority of children with enuresis wet involuntarily.

The objective nature of enuretic events has led to remarkable consistency in the criteria within the *Diagnostic and Statistical Manual of Mental Disorders* (DSM) throughout its evolution from DSM-III (American Psychiatric Association 1980) to the current DSM-5 (American Psychiatric Association 2013), as well as in the criteria within the *International Statistical Classification of Diseases and Related Health Problems* (ICD), soon to be released in its Eleventh Edition (ICD-11; World Health Organization 2018), although there have been some minor variations. The essential features of enuresis are summarized in Table 19–1.

Epidemiology

The epidemiology of enuresis has proven to be relatively consistent in large, cross-sectional national studies over several decades. Although these studies vary with regard to the frequency of the enuretic events and the ages of the cross-sectional samples, they are similar enough to be compared. Findings from Rutter's (1989) Isle of Wight study, the first comprehensive epidemiological investigation, clearly indicated that the prevalence of enuresis diminished with advancing age; only 1.1% of 14-year-old males and 0.5% of 14-year-old females were wetting once a week. A more recent European study, which involved a cohort of more than 8,000 children from a large prospective longitudinal follow-up of an original birth cohort of 14,000 children, indicated that the prevalence of nocturnal enuresis was 15.5% at age 7 years. However, the percentage of the sample that experienced a frequency of two or more episodes per week was 2.6% (von Gontard et al. 2011). In an epidemiological study in the United States, Shreeram et al. (2009) found that the 12-month prevalence in 1,136 children ages 8–11 years was 4.5%, with rates of 6.21% and 2.51% in males and females, respectively. All of the studies documented the disproportionate occurrence in males as well as the diminishing prevalence rate with age (Kessel et al. 2017).

Medical and Psychological Comorbidity

Various medical causes of enuresis are listed in Table 19–2. The primary concern with regard to medical comorbidity is the presence of a urinary tract infection, which can

---

TABLE 19–1.   **Essential features of enuresis**

Primary nocturnal enuresis

  A period of continence greater than 6 months has never been established.

  The frequency of enuretic events is in the range of one or two per week.

  The child has attained the chronological age by which continence could be expected to have occurred (ages 4–5 years).

  Medical causes have been excluded.

Secondary enuresis

  The criteria identified for primary enuresis have been met, but a period of continence ranging from 6 months to 1 year occurred before wetting resumed.

Diurnal enuresis

  A pattern of wetting also occurs during the day.

Note.   For the complete DSM-5 diagnostic criteria for enuresis, please refer to p. 355 in DSM-5 (American Psychiatric Association 2013).

TABLE 19–2.   **Medical causes of enuresis**

Urinary tract infection

Diabetes insipidus

Diabetes mellitus

Urethritis

Seizure disorder

Sickle cell trait

Sleep apnea

Neurogenic bladder

Sleep disorders

Genitourinary malformation or obstruction

Side effect or idiosyncratic reaction to a medication (e.g., case reports regarding SSRIs highlight the need to watch for chronological correlations)

Note.   SSRIs=selective serotonin reuptake inhibitors.

---

cause wetting, especially in females. The presence of structural urinary tract abnormalities as a primary cause of enuresis has been extensively investigated. Although some studies report a small percentage of children for whom such an abnormality may be a factor, the consensus is that there is not enough evidence to warrant routinely subjecting children to these invasive studies. Consensus guidelines suggest that a routine physical examination to rule out obvious physical causes, such as phimosis or labial agglutination, and neurological causes is sufficient and concur with the earlier observation about avoiding invasive studies, unless there is evidence to support the need for them (Vande Walle et al. 2012).

Enuresis has also been reported as a side effect of treatment with selective serotonin reuptake inhibitors (Hergüner et al. 2007) and second-generation antipsychotic agents (Barnes et al. 2012).

Children with secondary enuresis are more apt than those with primary enuresis to present with comorbid psychiatric disorders (Mikkelsen 2009). As might be expected, there is a high rate of comorbidity in children with a diagnosis of autism spectrum disorder (von Gontard et al. 2015). The psychiatric disorder with the most evidence of comorbidity is attention-deficit/hyperactivity disorder (ADHD) (von Gontard and Equit 2015). In their study from the United States referred to in the "Epidemiology" section above, Shreeram et al. (2009) also found that ADHD was "strongly associated with enuresis." These studies support the hypothesis that enuresis is comorbid with ADHD and is not secondarily related to ADHD. Other than the association with ADHD, the primary finding has been that behavioral disorders in children with enuresis are nonspecific (von Gontard et al. 2011).

Etiology, Mechanism, and Risk Factors

Etiological theories related to the phenomenon of primary nocturnal enuresis (PNE) have largely paralleled advances in treatment of the disorder. Psychodynamic theories have largely been abandoned as effective biological treatments have been developed and the role of genetic transmission has become more apparent.

The occurrence of enuretic events during sleep and the development of polysomnographic methods that permitted continuous monitoring of sleep patterns during the night initially gave rise to the concept of enuresis as a disorder of arousal, with enuretic episodes occurring as a result of the child's inability to respond to the stimuli generated from a full bladder while in deep sleep. However, larger, more systematic studies indicated that the nocturnal enuretic episodes were distributed throughout all of the sleep cycles in direct proportion to the amount of time that was spent in each phase of the sleep cycle (Mikkelsen 2001).

The first dramatically effective pharmacological treatment for enuresis was imipramine, as described in MacLean's (1960) report on its efficacy in a series of children with PNE. The initial theories related to imipramine's efficacy suggested that its positive effects were secondary to its anticholinergic effect on the urinary sphincter. However, a large, double-blind study that compared imipramine with methscopolamine, which has anticholinergic effects comparable to those of imipramine but does not cross the blood–brain barrier, indicated that imipramine was significantly more effective than methscopolamine and might have a central effect (Mikkelsen et al. 1980).

The more recent developments in the evolution of etiological theories have derived from the well-recognized efficacy of desmopressin acetate, given that desmopressin is a synthetic arginine vasopressin (antidiuretic hormone) analogue that exerts antidiuretic effects. However, a number of controlled investigations have indicated that the explanation for desmopressin's efficacy is not as straightforward as it might first appear. For example, a study that compared children with nocturnal enuresis ($n=15$) with matched control subjects ($n=11$) did not find any difference between the two groups with regard to atrial natriuretic peptide levels, although the children with nocturnal enuresis did have increased excretion of sodium and potassium as well as polyuria during the initial period of sleep. The abnormalities did not correlate with atrial natriuretic peptide levels, suggesting that the pathological processes were localized in the tubular structure within the kidneys (Mikkelsen 2009; Natochin and Kuznetsova 1999).

Abnormalities in the normal circadian variation in the production of plasma arginine vasopressin (AVP) have also been postulated. Early investigations indicated that there were significant differences between children with PNE and control subjects with regard to both the production of AVP and the circadian variation (Medel et al. 1998). However, these studies did not take into account the fact that AVP is normally secreted in a pulsatile manner. More sophisticated investigational designs have looked at the hourly secretions of AVP and other relevant variables, such as nocturnal urinary volume and osmotic pressure. Aikawa et al. (1999) suggested that there may be physiologically distinct subgroups. Specifically, there appeared to be a distinct subgroup that manifested both lower urinary production and low osmotic pressure and also had significantly lower AVP levels, which increased following treatment with desmopressin. The finding regarding lower nocturnal AVP levels in a subset of individuals was subsequently confirmed by other investigations (Rittig et al. 2008).

The observation that there is a significant hereditary component to the development of PNE is decades old, and a family history of PNE is one of the most significant risk factors. A large contemporary study by von Gontard et al. (2011) investigated family histories in a prospective, longitudinal study that involved several thousand children and their parents. The prevalence of PNE in the children at age 7 years was 15.5%, with 12.8% having only infrequent enuretic episodes and 2.6% meeting the criterion of two or more episodes per week. The percentages of parents of these children who had a similar history of PNE were 8.8% for mothers and 9.6% for fathers. Genetic linkage studies, however, have suggested that there will not be a simple, straightforward explanation for genetic transmission of enuresis, given that a number of genetic loci, including on chromosomes 12q, 13q, 13–14q, and 22q11, have been found in different pedigrees (Loeys et al. 2002).

Course and Prognosis

Perhaps the most significant observation with regard to PNE derives from the natural history of the disorder, which indicates that it is a self-limited condition that will eventually remit spontaneously. In general, the epidemiological studies cited previously (see earlier section "Epidemiology") are supportive of this observation, because they all document that the incidence of PNE decreases in each advancing age group. Yearly remission rates of 14%–16% have been reported (Fritz et al. 2004). For most children, once remission occurs, it will be sustained. However, a subgroup of children will experience transient periods of remission before final cessation of the disorder.

Clinical Evaluation

A child's developmental history, which includes a thorough review of the developmental milestones and toilet training, is obviously very important. The toilet training history should include information related to the first attempts, the duration of the trials, and the methods used by the parents. Because enuresis has a strong hereditary component, a thorough multigenerational family history with a reference to individuals who might have had PNE will be helpful. In addition, it can be helpful to ascertain the natural history of the enuretic events in family members with a childhood history of PNE. This information may lead to a better understanding of when spontaneous remission might be expected to occur in the child.

The diagnostic criteria for enuresis relate primarily to the frequency of the events, the chronological or mental age of the child, and the natural history of the disorder. It is not uncommon for the frequency of enuretic events to fluctuate from week to week, although the frequency will usually remain consistent for a given child within a general range. For example, some children will have enuretic episodes at a relatively low frequency (in the range of 1–3 nights per week), whereas other children will wet almost nightly (with a range of 5–7 nights per week). There is also a subgroup of children whose wetting episodes are much more episodic (i.e., just a few incidents per month), but these children would not meet the diagnostic criteria.

The objective nature of the enuretic event simplifies the evaluation process. It is useful to approach the problem in a nonjudgmental manner that emphasizes that the enuretic events are not voluntary. A simple calendar-tracking method can be used to record the frequency of enuretic events. This method serves both to establish the diagnosis and to provide a baseline for measuring treatment effects. It is also useful to note the time of day in addition to the date for those children with daytime wetting.

An important clinical consideration relates to whether the child ever had a period of sustained continence greater than 6 months, which is usually accepted as the time required to differentiate between primary and secondary enuresis. However, this clinically important distinction is not included in the DSM-5 diagnostic criteria, although it is discussed in the narrative material that follows the criteria. The current diagnostic criteria also specifically state that voluntary and involuntary wetting are considered to be equivalent in terms of establishing the diagnosis, although these phenomena are clearly very different with regard to both etiological and treatment considerations.

The primary medical workup consists of a physical examination to rule out any obvious rare anatomical abnormalities, as well as a urinalysis to rule out a bladder infection, which can cause wetting, particularly in females. However, a bladder infection would result in a fairly abrupt and relatively recent onset of wetting. A urine dipstick test for glucose is also indicated if there has been a recent dramatic onset of polydipsia, which could be related to new-onset diabetes mellitus. More intrusive and potentially painful diagnostic interventions are not considered necessary, unless there is reason to suspect an anatomic abnormality. Ultrasound evaluations of the bladder to assess wall thickness and other dynamics have been pursued in research investigations but are not routinely used in clinical practice.

An important part of the assessment will also include both the child's and the family's perceptions of the enuresis and the effect on both the child's self-esteem and the family's interpersonal dynamics. Other than the previously noted high comorbidity with ADHD, there are no significant correlations between other specific psychiatric disorders and PNE. The initial evaluation will also provide an opportunity to explore possible emotional and environmental contributions to the enuresis, such as whether the child is afraid of the dark and therefore avoids getting up at night to use the bathroom.

Treatment

Pharmacological Treatments

MacLean's (1960) article describing the efficacy of imipramine for treating children with PNE was followed by a number of double-blind studies in subsequent years that confirmed the findings of his initial uncontrolled case report series. Imipramine remained the primary pharmacological treatment for decades until the introduction of desmopressin. Although its use has diminished greatly, imipramine is still used for children whose symptoms do not respond to other forms of treatment. In addition to the anticholinergic side effects, the major consideration with imipramine is the potential cardiac side effects. Thus, the usual protocol for imipramine treatment is to obtain a baseline electrocardiogram and then to begin treatment at 25 mg/day, with a slow titration of 25-mg/day increments at weekly intervals until continence is achieved; a dosage of 5 mg/kg/day is considered to be the upper limit. If dosages in the 75- to 125-mg/day range have not produced a positive response, it becomes less likely that the child will be an imipramine responder. Because the disorder's rate of spontaneous remission is significant, a standard clinical protocol includes an attempt to withdraw the medication every 3 months to determine whether the enuresis has spontaneously remitted.

The form of desmopressin initially used was a nasal preparation, which was reported as being safer than imipramine. In addition, the therapeutic mechanism appeared initially to be more physiologically understandable, as discussed earlier in the "Etiology, Mechanism, and Risk Factors" section. By 1993, a review article identified 18 randomized controlled studies including 689 subjects and reported a 10%–91% range of efficacy (Moffatt et al. 1993). However, wetting almost always resumed after the desmopressin was discontinued, with only 5.7% of subjects reported as maintaining continence after medication discontinuation. During the ensuing years, a number of case reports of clinically significant hyponatremia, seizures, and related fatalities began to emerge. Eventually, excess fluid intake was identified as a contributing factor in the reported events, leading to the recommendation that children not ingest more than 8 ounces of fluid on nights when desmopressin was taken. It also appeared that younger children were at greater risk of experiencing clinically significant effects, and that these severe side effects were also more apt to occur during the initial phases of treatment. In 2007, Robson et al. reported that postmarketing data had revealed 151 cases of desmopressin-related hyponatremia, of which 145 were related to the nasal preparation and only 6 were related to the oral form. Subsequently, the U.S. Food and Drug Administration issued a safety alert, and the use of the nasal spray became contraindicated for PNE in children. The alert also recommended suspension of treatment with the oral preparation during acute illnesses that could interfere with fluid balance. A number of comparative studies have shown the oral preparation to be as effective as the nasal spray and much safer (De Guchtenaere et al. 2011).

Long-term use of oral desmopressin was found to be safe in a large Canadian study (Wolfish et al. 2003). The increased safety margin of the oral form is thought to be due to the pharmacokinetics of the tablet, which provides for a smoother disposition of the drug (Vande Walle et al. 2010).

The newest formulation of desmopressin is a sublingual oral lyophilisate formulation, referred to as MELT, which has been well tolerated and is preferred by many children. A relatively small dose (in the range of 120–240 µg) has been reported to be effective (Juul et al. 2013).

Pretreatment factors that appear to be associated with a positive response to desmopressin include lower frequency of baseline enuretic events, older age, and greater bladder capacity.

Psychotherapeutic Treatment

Psychotherapeutic interventions may be useful in ameliorating the child's embarrassment and diminished self-esteem related to enuretic events. A therapeutic education approach is also useful in helping the family to approach treatment in a nonjudgmental, supportive manner. It is extremely important that the parents realize that PNE is not volitional in nature and that a punitive response is counterproductive.

Children who have secondary enuresis are much more apt to have psychological stressors contributing to the loss of continence and therefore may be more likely to benefit from psychotherapy (Fritz et al. 2004). A psychotherapeutic approach may also be useful for comorbid psychiatric disorders.

Behavioral Treatments

Treatment with the bell-and-pad method of conditioning was initially described in 1904 and has been extensively studied over the ensuing decades (Rappaport 1997). In this treatment, the child sleeps on a pad that has wires attached to an alarm. When the enuretic event occurs, the urine completes an electrical circuit, and the alarm sounds, waking the child. A comprehensive review of the literature reported an initial response rate of approximately two-thirds with the bell-and-pad method (Glazener et al. 2005); the corresponding rate of persistent remission following this form of treatment was 50%. A recent large retrospective study reported a success rate of 76% (Apos et al. 2018). Two distinct subgroups of children experience remission with the bell-and-pad method: those who learn to wake up to urinate, and those who sleep through the night without wetting. The clinical rationale for these two subgroups has never been explained. Butler et al. (2007) undertook a pre- and postalarm treatment study to investigate possible physiological explanations for success. Seventy-five percent of their subjects met success criteria, and of these, 89% predominately slept through the night on dry nights. The children who experienced success were found to have an increase in posttreatment ability to concentrate urine, and for approximately half of these subjects, it appeared to be due to an increase in vasopressin.

Investigations that have compared the bell-and-pad method with both imipramine and desmopressin have demonstrated that the efficacy of the bell-and-pad approach is comparable to that of the pharmacological interventions, with virtually no side effects. Another advantage of the bell-and-pad method of conditioning is that the therapeutic effect is usually sustained after cessation of treatment, whereas remission almost always occurs after cessation of treatment with imipramine or desmopressin (Kwak et al. 2010).

A number of other behavioral strategies are commonly used, including retention control training, evening fluid restriction, reward systems, and nighttime awakening by the parents to toilet the child. A thorough review of the published literature on these interventions (Glazener and Evans 2004) indicated that the methodologies and small sample sizes of these reports precluded any conclusions about their efficacy. In clinical practice, parents have often attempted one or more of these treatments before seeking professional interventions.

General Treatment Considerations

Perhaps the most important factor to keep in mind when considering a treatment algorithm for a child with PNE is the spontaneous remission rate, as noted earlier in the

"Course and Prognosis" section. PNE is a self-limiting disorder. The decision to treat will primarily be related to the severity and frequency of the wetting episodes, the age of the child, and the amount of social, interpersonal distress that the disorder presents for the child and family. The distinction between primary and secondary enuresis is also important because children with secondary enuresis are much more apt to have experienced psychosocial stressors that may both require and respond to psychotherapeutic interventions.

In a large longitudinal follow-up study, Monda and Husmann (1995) compared the results of observation only with treatment with imipramine, desmopressin, or the bell-and-pad method. The results of this study clearly indicated the superiority of the bell-and-pad method of treatment with regard to the degree of relapse after cessation of active treatment. A subsequent systematic review of the literature involving the alarm, imipramine, and desmopressin confirmed this finding (Glazener et al. 2005).

On the basis of available research data, it appears that the bell-and-pad method of conditioning would be the most rational method to consider first because it is just as effective as the pharmacological approaches, it has a much safer side-effect profile, and its effects are sustained once continence has developed and been sustained for a period of time.

Encopresis

Throughout recorded history, much less literature has been published on encopresis than on enuresis. This difference most likely relates to the observation that encopresis is much less common than enuresis.

Definition and Clinical Description

The definition of *encopresis* is similar to that of *enuresis* in that it is both straightforward and empirical in nature. It simply relates to the "passage of feces."

Accordingly, as with enuresis, the diagnostic criteria for encopresis have remained relatively consistent throughout the DSM editions from DSM-III through DSM-5 and have been consistent with ICD criteria. The essential features of encopresis are summarized in Table 19–3.

Epidemiology

The prevalence of encopresis is similar to that of enuresis in that it diminishes with advancing age, and the majority of affected children are males (i.e., male-to-female ratio of 3:1). Overall, however, the incidence of encopresis is much lower than that of enuresis. An early large study involving several thousand children ages 7–8 years reported a 1.5% incidence for encopresis (Bellman 1966). More recent studies have reported similar rates (Heron et al. 2008).

Medical and Psychological Comorbidity

As with enuresis, higher rates of behavioral problems have been documented in individuals with encopresis than in the general population. However, the strong associa-

TABLE 19–3.	Essential features of encopresis

The passage of feces occurs in inappropriate places. The most common scenario is the passage of feces in one's undergarments.

Encopretic events do not need to occur as frequently as enuretic events. The criterion of at least one episode a month for 3 or more months is widely accepted.

Individuals have reached an age by which continence could be expected to have occurred (age4–5 years).

Potential medical causes have been ruled out.

Note. For the complete DSM-5 diagnostic criteria for encopresis, please refer to pp. 357–358 in DSM-5 (American Psychiatric Association 2013).

tion with ADHD that is seen with enuresis has not been documented with encopresis. Thus, although children with encopresis have been found to exhibit a greater frequency of behavioral problems than control subjects without encopresis, no specific pattern of behavioral problems has been reported (Mellon et al. 2006).

Chronic constipation is an important contributor to retentive encopresis. Although this constipation may be related to psychological factors in some children, some may also have a physiological predisposition, as discussed later in the "Retentive Encopresis" section. A simple radiographic study, the flat plate of the abdomen, can usually detect significant constipation. An ordinary digital examination of the rectum by the child's pediatrician may also reveal an impaction. Chronic physiological disorders, such as Hirschsprung's disease, will usually have manifested much earlier in life. A list of medical causes of encopresis is provided in Table 19–4.

Etiology, Mechanism, and Risk Factors

It is extremely important to subdivide encopresis into the two clinically relevant subtypes of *retentive* and *nonretentive encopresis.*

Retentive Encopresis

Clinically, retentive encopresis is more common than nonretentive encopresis, although precise figures about the relative incidence are not available. The physiological mechanism of *retentive encopresis* begins with chronic constipation, which creates a bolus of feces in the colon, and the encopretic event actually represents overflow of loose fecal matter around the impacted bolus of feces. Loening-Baucke (2004) carried out an impressive series of physiological studies over several years, and the findings suggested that children with chronic constipation may have subtle physiological abnormalities in their colon as well as in the anal sphincter. These elaborate studies were based primarily on the child's ability to expel a rectal balloon. However, it has not been possible to determine whether these deficits reflected an inherent physiological deficit or were the result of chronic constipation.

Nonretentive Encopresis

Nonretentive encopresis involves the voluntary or involuntary passing of feces in inappropriate places (e.g., clothing, floor). Voluntary nonretentive encopresis is at times associated with the hoarding of feces. Clearly, this pattern of encopresis represents underlying psychopathology that should be identified and addressed. This type of be-

TABLE 19–4. **Medical causes of encopresis**

Constipation

Hirschsprung's disease

Medical conditions producing diarrhea

Side effect or idiosyncratic reaction to a medication (maintain vigilance for chronological correlation)

Painful lesion

Hemorrhoids (contributing to constipation)

Thyroid disease

Hypercalcemia

Lactase deficiency

Pseudo obstruction

Spina bifida

Cerebral palsy with hypotonia

Rectal stenosis

Anal fissure

Anorectal trauma, including sexual abuse

havior can be seen in children who have experienced sexual abuse; however, its presence should not be considered a definite indication of sexual abuse (Mellon et al. 2006).

Children who manifest involuntary nonretentive fecal incontinence may have a deficit affecting their recognition of the need to defecate, similar to that observed in some children with enuresis. This lack of recognition may represent a lapse in attention due to an associated ADHD in some children, although a connection with ADHD has never been definitively documented for encopresis. The delayed attention could also be related to obsessive traits in children who are fearful of using bathrooms outside of the home. Fear that extends to the bathrooms in the school where the child spends several hours a day could easily become problematic and account for the episodes of soiling. The clinical interview with the child and his or her family should explore these important social ecological questions.

Course and Prognosis

The longitudinal trajectory of encopresis is similar to that of enuresis; both disorders usually resolve over time, and their incidence in adolescence is extremely low. Perhaps the best illustration of this trajectory comes from the studies of Loening-Baucke (2004), who, over several years, carried out investigations of biofeedback-based treatment for retentive encopresis. He eventually concluded that this treatment modality could not be proven to be more effective than a more traditional medical approach coupled with spontaneous remission.

Treatment

The first step in treatment involves identifying whether the encopresis is of the retentive or nonretentive subtype (see the "Etiology, Mechanism, and Risk Factors" section above), because this distinction has major treatment implications.

Nonretentive Encopresis

Obviously, children who voluntarily defecate in inappropriate places and/or hoard feces are in need of a psychological evaluation and will likely benefit from psychotherapeutic interventions. A child with nonretentive encopresis may well have a comorbid psychiatric disorder that will need to be addressed (Koppen et al. 2016). Although the sudden emergence of these symptoms in a previously asymptomatic child has been reported as a sequela of sexual abuse (see "Etiology, Mechanism, and Risk Factors" section above), it can also occur as a result of other stressors and should not be assumed to be related to childhood sexual abuse (Mellon et al. 2006).

The clinical history should include a detailed description of both the context and the frequency of these events so that the clinician can explore for the etiological factors, which may, in turn, inform the psychological or environmental interventions that are required to address them.

Retentive Encopresis

The long-standing conventional intervention for retentive encopresis involves the use of physiological, behavioral, psychological, and educational interventions (Levine and Bakow 1976). The physiological component involves bowel catharsis, coupled with the ongoing use of laxatives, for a period of time sufficient to develop a regular pattern of bowel movements. The behavioral component includes a fixed daily schedule of toileting in an effort to develop regular bowel habits. This component also involves exploration of any behavioral or psychological factors that may be contributing to the underlying constipation. The educational component is targeted toward both the parent and the child and is designed to inform them about the basic physiology of the bowel and the fundamental role of constipation. The success rate for this comprehensive treatment approach has been reported to be as high as 78% (Levine and Bakow 1976).

For the vast majority of children with retentive encopresis, a medical approach that focuses on bowel retraining coupled with psychoeducational approaches will be successful. As with enuresis, most children will experience a spontaneous remission. However, the rate at which spontaneous remission occurs is not as well documented as it is with PNE. In addition, the nature of fecal soiling is such that in almost all cases the family will elect to pursue active treatment rather than consider the possibility of a spontaneous remission. In addition, the negative physiological effects of chronic constipation argue for earlier intervention.

Other Specified or Unspecified Elimination Disorder

DSM-5 created two new categories of elimination disorders. The stated purpose of the "unspecified" category was to provide a method for noting that events consistent with an elimination disorder are present but do not meet the full criteria or the clinician is performing the evaluation in a setting that does not permit sufficient time to explore for the presence of the full criteria. The "other specified" designation provides an opportunity to specifically describe why the full criteria were not met.

Conclusion

Although the literature reviewed in this chapter indicates that both enuresis and encopresis will eventually remit without treatment in almost all children, the symptoms of these disorders are so psychologically distressing that active treatment is justified to limit their duration. However, the natural history of each disorder should figure prominently in the construction of treatment algorithms, which should always be based on risk-versus-benefit considerations. No single treatment modality will be appropriate for every child who presents with an elimination disorder. It is hoped that the information provided here will equip clinicians with the necessary tools to work with children and their families to construct individualized treatment plans that address the specific circumstances of each child's situation.

Key Clinical Points

- Enuresis is ultimately a self-limited disorder with a relatively high rate of spontaneous remission, ranging from 12% to 14% per year.

- An alert issued by the U.S. Food and Drug Administration regarding desmopressin drew attention to the risk of hyponatremia, seizures, and (in rare cases) death. The notification stated that the nasal preparation should no longer be used for enuresis and that use of the oral preparation should be interrupted during illnesses that would disrupt fluid balance.

- Behavioral treatment of enuresis with the bell-and-pad method of conditioning is as effective as pharmacological treatment, and relapse is significantly less apt to occur after the cessation of active treatment.

- Children with secondary enuresis are more likely than those with primary enuresis to have a psychological or stressful underlying condition.

- Treatment decisions for primary nocturnal enuresis should be predicated on the severity of the enuresis, the response of the child and family to the enuretic events, the possibility of spontaneous remission, the reported efficacy of the intervention, the rate of relapse after active treatment is stopped, and the side-effect risk related to the intervention. This equation will usually indicate that the bell-and-pad method of treatment is the most appropriate first choice for treatment.

- Two clinical subtypes of encopresis are recognized: retentive, which involves constipation and related overflow incontinence, and nonretentive, which does not.

- Retentive encopresis has been more extensively studied than nonretentive encopresis with regard to physiology and treatment. The most accepted form of treatment is a protocol that contains educational, psychological, behavioral, and physiological components.

- Children whose encopresis is of a voluntary nature clearly require a full psychological evaluation and may respond to psychotherapeutic interventions or treatment of the underlying and/or comorbid psychopathology.

- The natural history of encopresis is to move toward continence. However, the natural history and rate of spontaneous remission are not as well understood for encopresis as they are for enuresis.

References

Aikawa T, Kashara T, Uchiyama M: Circadian variation of plasma arginine vasopressin concentration, or arginine vasopressin in enuresis. Scand J Urol Nephrol Suppl 202:47–49, 1999 10573793

American Psychiatric Association: Diagnostic and Statistical Manual of Mental Disorders, 3rd Edition. Washington, DC, American Psychiatric Association, 1980

American Psychiatric Association: Diagnostic and Statistical Manual of Mental Disorders, 5th Edition. Arlington, VA, American Psychiatric Association, 2013

Apos E, Schuster S, Reece J, et al: Enuresis management in children: retrospective clinical audit of 2861 cases treated with practitioner-assisted bell-and-pad alarm. J Pediatr 193:211–216, 2018 29246468

Barnes TR, Drake MJ, Paton C: Nocturnal enuresis with antipsychotic medication. Br J Psychiatry 200(1):7–9, 2012 22215862

Bellman M: Studies on encopresis. Acta Paediatr Scand (suppl 170):1+, 1966 5958527

Butler RJ, Holland P, Gasson S, et al: Exploring potential mechanisms in alarm treatment for primary nocturnal enuresis. Scand J Urol Nephrol 41(5):407–413, 2007 17957577

De Guchtenaere A, Van Herzeele C, Raes A, et al: Oral lyophilizate formulation of desmopressin: superior pharmacodynamics compared to tablet due to low food interaction. J Urol 185(6):2308–2313, 2011 21511277

Fritz G, Rockney R, Bernet W, et al: Practice parameter for the assessment and treatment of children and adolescents with enuresis. J Am Acad Child Adolesc Psychiatry 43(12):1540–1550, 2004 15564822

Glazener CM, Evans JH: Simple behavioural and physical interventions for nocturnal enuresis in children. Cochrane Database Syst Rev (2):CD003673, 2004 15106210

Glazener CM, Evans JH, Peto RE: Alarm interventions for nocturnal enuresis in children. Cochrane Database Syst Rev (2):CD002911, 2005 15846643

Glicklich LB: An historical account of enuresis. Pediatrics 8(6):859–876, 1951 14911258

Hergüner S, Kilinçaslan A, Görker I, et al: Serotonin-selective reuptake inhibitor–induced enuresis in three pediatric cases. J Child Adolesc Psychopharmacol 17(3):367–370, 2007 17630870

Heron J, Joinson C, Croudace T, et al: Trajectories of daytime wetting and soiling in a United Kingdom 4- to 9-year-old population birth cohort study. J Urol 179(5):1970–1975, 2008 18355863

Juul KV, Van Herzeele C, De Bruyne P, et al: Desmopressin melt improves response and compliance compared with tablet in treatment of primary monosymptomatic nocturnal enuresis. Eur J Pediatr 172(9):1235–1242, 2013 23677249

Kessel EM, Allmann AE, Goldstein BL, et al: Predictors and outcomes of childhood primary enuresis. J Am Acad Child Adolesc Psychiatry 56(3):250–257, 2017 28219491

Koppen IJ, von Gontard A, Chase J, et al: Management of functional nonretentive fecal incontinence in children: recommendations from the International Children's Continence Society. J Pediatr Urol 12(1):56–64, 2016 26654481

Kwak KW, Lee YS, Park KH, et al: Efficacy of desmopressin and enuresis alarm as first and second line treatment for primary monosymptomatic nocturnal enuresis: prospective randomized crossover study. J Urol 184(6):2521–2526, 2010 20961574

Levine MD, Bakow H: Children with encopresis: a study of treatment outcome. Pediatrics 58(6):845–852, 1976 995511

Loening-Baucke V: Functional fecal retention with encopresis in childhood. J Pediatr Gastroenterol Nutr 38(1):79–84, 2004 14676600

Loeys B, Hoebeke P, Raes A, et al: Does monosymptomatic enuresis exist? A molecular genetic exploration of 32 families with enuresis/incontinence. BJU Int 90(1):76–83, 2002 12081775

MacLean RE: Imipramine hydrochloride (Tofranil) and enuresis. Am J Psychiatry 117:551, 1960 13764959

Medel R, Dieguez S, Brindo M, et al: Monosymptomatic primary enuresis: differences between patients responding or not responding to oral desmopressin. Br J Urol 81(suppl 3):46–49, 1998 9634019

Mellon MW, Whiteside SP, Friedrich WN: The relevance of fecal soiling as an indicator of child sexual abuse: a preliminary analysis. J Dev Behav Pediatr 27(1):25–32, 2006 16511365

Mikkelsen EJ: Enuresis and encopresis: ten years of progress. J Am Acad Child Adolesc Psychiatry 40(10):1146–1158, 2001 11589527

Mikkelsen EJ: Elimination disorders, in Kaplan and Sadock's Comprehensive Textbook of Psychiatry, 9th Edition. Edited by Sadock BJ, Sadock VA, Ruiz P. Philadelphia, PA, Lippincott, Williams and Wilkins, 2009, pp 3624–3635

Mikkelsen EJ, Rapoport JL, Nee L, et al: Childhood enuresis, I: sleep patterns and psychopathology. Arch Gen Psychiatry 37(10):1139–1144, 1980 7425798

Moffatt ME, Harlos S, Kirshen AJ, et al: Desmopressin acetate and nocturnal enuresis: how much do we know? Pediatrics 92(3):420–425, 1993 8361796

Monda JM, Husmann DA: Primary nocturnal enuresis: a comparison among observation, imipramine, desmopressin acetate and bed-wetting alarm systems. J Urol 154(2 Pt 2):745–748, 1995 7609169

Natochin YV, Kuznetsova AA: Defect of osmoregulatory renal function in nocturnal enuresis. Scand J Urol Nephrol 202:40–43; discussion 43–44, 1999 10573791

Rappaport L: Prognostic factors for alarm treatment. Scand J Urol Nephrol Suppl 183:55–57, 1997 9165609

Rittig S, Schaumburg HL, Siggaard C, et al: The circadian defect in plasma vasopressin and urine output is related to desmopressin response and enuresis status in children with nocturnal enuresis. J Urol 179(6):2389–2395, 2008 18433780

Robson WL, Leung AK, Norgaard JP: The comparative safety of oral versus intranasal desmopressin for the treatment of children with nocturnal enuresis. J Urol 178(1):24–30, 2007 17574054

Rutter M: Isle of Wight revisited: twenty-five years of child psychiatric epidemiology. J Am Acad Child Adolesc Psychiatry 28(5):633–653, 1989 2676960

Shreeram S, He JP, Kalaydjian A, et al: Prevalence of enuresis and its association with attention-deficit/hyperactivity disorder among U.S. children: results from a nationally representative study. J Am Acad Child Adolesc Psychiatry 48(1):35–41, 2009 19096296

Vande Walle J, Van Herzeele C, Raes A: Is there still a role for desmopressin in children with primary monosymptomatic nocturnal enuresis? A focus on safety issues. Drug Saf 33(4):261–271, 2010 20297859

Vande Walle J, Rittig S, Bauer S, et al: Practical consensus guidelines for the management of enuresis. Eur J Pediatr 171(6):971–983, 2012 22362256

von Gontard A, Equit M: Comorbidity of ADHD and incontinence in children. Eur Child Adolesc Psychiatry 24(2):127–140, 2015 24980793

von Gontard A, Heron J, Joinson C: Family history of nocturnal enuresis and urinary incontinence: results from a large epidemiological study. J Urol 185(6):2303–2306, 2011 21511300

von Gontard A, Pirrung M, Neimczyk J, Equit M: Incontinence in children with autism spectrum disorder. J Pediatr Urol 11(5):264.e1–264.e7, 2015 26052001

Wolfish NM, Barkin J, Gorodzinsky F, et al: The Canadian Enuresis Study and Evaluation—short- and long-term safety and efficacy of an oral desmopressin preparation. Scand J Urol Nephrol 37(1):22–27, 2003 12745738

World Health Organization: International Statistical Classification of Diseases and Related Health Problems, 11th Edition (ICD-11), Draft Version. Geneva, Switzerland, World Health Organization, June 18, 2018. Available at: http://www.who.int/classifications/icd/en/. Accessed October 17, 2018.

Recommended Readings

Heron J, Joinson C, Croudace T, et al: Trajectories of daytime wetting and soiling in a United Kingdom 4- to 9-year-old population birth cohort study. J Urol 179(5):1970–1975, 2008 18355863

Koppen IJ, von Gontard A, Chase J, et al: Management of functional nonretentive fecal incontinence in children: recommendations from the International Children's Continence Society. J Pediatr Urol 12(1):56–64, 2016 26654481

Kwak KW, Lee YS, Park KH, et al: Efficacy of desmopressin and enuresis alarm as first and second line treatment for primary monosymptomatic nocturnal enuresis: prospective randomized crossover study. J Urol 184(6):2521–2526, 2010 20961574

Shreeram S, He JP, Kalaydjian A, et al: Prevalence of enuresis and its association with attention-deficit/hyperactivity disorder among U.S. children: results from a nationally representative study. J Am Acad Child Adolesc Psychiatry 48(1):35–41, 2009 19096296

Vande Walle J, Rittig S, Bauer S, et al: Practical consensus guidelines for the management of enuresis. Eur J Pediatr 171(6):971–983, 2012 22362256

von Gontard A, Equit M: Comorbidity of ADHD and incontinence in children. Eur Child Adolesc Psychiatry 24(2):127–140, 2015 24980793

von Gontard A, Heron J, Joinson C: Family history of nocturnal enuresis and urinary incontinence: results from a large epidemiological study. J Urol 185(6):2303–2306, 2011 21511300

Online Resources

American Academy of Child and Adolescent Psychiatry: Bedwetting. Updated December 2014. Available at: www.aacap.org/AACAP/Families_and_Youth/Facts_for_Families/FFF-Guide/Bedwetting-018.aspx. Accessed September 23, 2017. (Contains Fact Sheets that can be printed.)

Boston Children's Hospital: Testing & Diagnosis for Bedwetting (Nocturnal Enuresis) in Children. Available at: www.childrenshospital.org/conditions-and-treatments/conditions/b/bedwetting-nocturnal-enuresis/testing-and-diagnosis. Accessed September 23, 2017.

Boston Children's Hospital: Clinical Consult: Evaluation and treatment of encopresis. Notes: Boston Children's Hospital's Clinical Health Blog. Posted on June 23, 2016, by Maureen McCarthy. Available at: https://notes.childrenshospital.org/clinical-consult-evaluation-treatment-encopresis/. Accessed January 9, 2019.

Mayo Clinic: Encopresis. Available at: https://www.mayoclinic.org/diseases-conditions/encopresis/symptoms-causes/syc-20354494. Accessed January 9, 2019.

CHAPTER 20

Sleep–Wake Disorders

Martin Reite, M.D.
Michael Weissberg, M.D.
Clete A. Kushida, M.D., Ph.D.

Sleep–wake disorders and disruptions of sleep are underrecognized for their impact on the health of individuals and populations. Psychiatrists, including those with subspecialty sleep medicine expertise, can play an important role in helping to elevate understanding of the health implications of sleep–wake disorders and disruptions of sleep across the fields of medicine. In their training, psychiatric practitioners should acquire an understanding of the diagnosis and treatment of sleep–wake disorders as well as knowledge of how sleep disruption may occur in many other mental and physical disorders. Psychiatrists also should be aware of the positive role of sleep on brain function and the neurocognitive, mood, and related effects of sleep deprivation and their public health consequences (Lowe et al. 2017).

The aim of this chapter is to provide essential information needed for clinicians to identify and address major sleep disorders. For psychiatrists without sleep medicine training, it is helpful to gain familiarity with the current third edition of the *International Classification of Sleep Disorders* (ICSD-3; American Academy of Sleep Medicine 2014), which is considered by many to be the definitive classification for sleep disorders. This classification includes more than 80 specific diagnoses in eight general categories.

We approach the topic of sleep–wake disorders by offering a summary of the basic science of wakefulness and sleep, introducing the various sleep–wake disorders included in DSM-5 (American Psychiatric Association 2013) and the changes from the previous edition of DSM, and presenting a four-step evaluation that informs the clinical approach to a sleep complaint.

Wake, Sleep, and Circadian Control Systems: Function and Modulation

Borbély and Achermann (1999) postulated a clinically useful two-process model for sleep and sleep regulation: Process S is the Sleep homeostatic drive, which increases in strength as a function of time awake. The opposing Process C is the Circadian arousal drive, which increases during the day, thus maintaining the state of wakefulness and preventing Process S from taking over until the normal bedtime approaches, at which point the Process C arousal drive begins to diminish and Process S is permitted to take over. Sleep ensues, with its reversal of the neurometabolic effects of the waking state. Most sleep disorders can be conceptualized as a disorder of Process C, Process S, or both.

It was previously believed that the brain can normally be in only one of three possible states: 1) wakefulness, 2) non–rapid eye movement (NREM; slow wave) sleep, or 3) rapid eye movement (REM) sleep; there are control systems (neurophysiological switches) that regulate shifting from one state to another. However, there is an emerging body of literature indicating the existence of a phenomenon called "local sleep," in which different states and stages of sleep may occur and be regulated in local brain regions (Huber et al. 2004; Siclari and Tononi 2017). This phenomenon has implications for sleep disorders, including insomnia (locally increased wake-like activity in sensorimotor areas during sleep compared with control subjects), narcolepsy (abnormal phenomena related to dissociated episodes of wakefulness, NREM sleep, and REM sleep) and parasomnias such as sleepwalking (state dissociation or an admixture of sensorimotor elements of wakefulness with NREM sleep). The probability of being in one of the different states is controlled by disruptions of the circadian timing system (Process C), which contribute to several common sleep disorders.

Our discussion of the wake–sleep control systems begins with the circadian timing system, knowledge of which is essential to understanding sleep complaints. We then discuss the wake and sleep control systems in turn.

Circadian Timing System

Circadian Physiology

The timing of sleep onset is largely controlled by a person's circadian arousal drive (Process C) and is closely associated with core body temperature, which increases during the day and early evening—maintaining wakefulness even though the homeostatic sleep drive (Process S) is increasing with time awake—and begins to decrease around the time of normal sleep onset, thus permitting sleep. Circadian rhythms are controlled by the suprachiasmatic nucleus (SCN) of the anterior hypothalamus, and the circadian clock controls many internal rhythms, including the sleep–wake cycle, which it keeps in tune with the day–night pattern of the external environment. The circadian clock also maintains temporal organization of internal physiological processes and makes sure that their changes are coordinated with one another. Circadian rhythms are hypothesized to be genetically determined and persist even in the absence of external time cues such as the day–night cycle. A number of "clock" genes have been identified as constituting the central mechanism of the brain's timekeeping system, which is central to coordination of metabolic processes, circadian rhythmicity, and sleep regulation (Wulff et al. 2009). Researchers have identified, in the pineal gland alone, more than 600 genes whose activities are modulated by the 24-hour sleep–wake rhythm and whose functions influence a diverse range of bodily processes, including inflammation, immunity, transcription, and cell signaling (Bailey et al. 2009).

The SCN is the "master clock" that controls circadian timing, and although its basic cycle is a little longer than 24 hours (mean, 24.2 hours; range, 23.8–27.1 hours in different individuals), it becomes synchronized to the 24-hour day of humans, primarily through light. Light activates nonvisual retinal photoreceptors that transmit information via the retinohypothalamic tract serving as the primary influence on the SCN; however, food, temperature, and social influences also impact SCN timing. The SCN transmits timing information to the pineal gland, which produces melatonin. Melatonin production increases in the evening as light decreases, remains elevated during the night, and falls off in the morning. The time at which melatonin increase begins— termed the *dim-light melatonin onset* (DLMO)—can be a useful biomarker of circadian timing. Maximum sleepiness occurs when body temperature reaches its lowest point (nadir) and melatonin production its highest. Melatonin is only one of a number of hormones with circadian release patterns. Cortisol, the stress hormone, and prolactin, a complex polypeptide with a multiplicity of posttranslational forms and more than 300 biological activities, also demonstrate circadian release patterns (Freeman et al. 2000). Growth hormone peaks at night during deep sleep, but this is a sleep-related rhythm, not a circadian rhythm. Figure 20–1 illustrates the release patterns of these hormones as well as body temperature.

The basic 24-hour rhythm is not present at birth but rather develops slowly over the first few months of life, first appearing as a greater-than-24-hour free-running rhythm (as new parents learn) and finally becoming entrained to the 24-hour day by about age 16 weeks, the time that most infants can begin sleeping through the night.

About 50% of blind individuals are insensitive to light and thus unable to entrain their circadian system; therefore, they have a free-running period of about 24.2 hours, which causes their sleep–wake cycle to move around the clock such that every several weeks they may sleep through the day rather than the night.

As people age, the influence of light on circadian control diminishes, the period of clock genes may decrease, and melatonin production decreases. These changes may present clinically as sleep-onset insomnia complaints in some elderly individuals, as well as a tendency toward an advanced sleep phase (Singletary and Naidoo 2011). Not all important body rhythms are circadian. Rhythms shorter than 24 hours are termed *ultradian* and include the REM sleep cycle (approximately 90–120 minutes). Rhythms longer than 24 hours, termed *infradian*, include, for example, the menstrual cycle (about 28 days).

The various disorders of circadian rhythms are listed in Table 20–1. These circadian disorders most often present as insomnia complaints, although some may present as excessive sleepiness. Sleep cycle disruption related to jet lag or shift work does not represent a primary disorder of circadian timing but rather a syndrome resulting from behaviorally induced circadian misalignment.

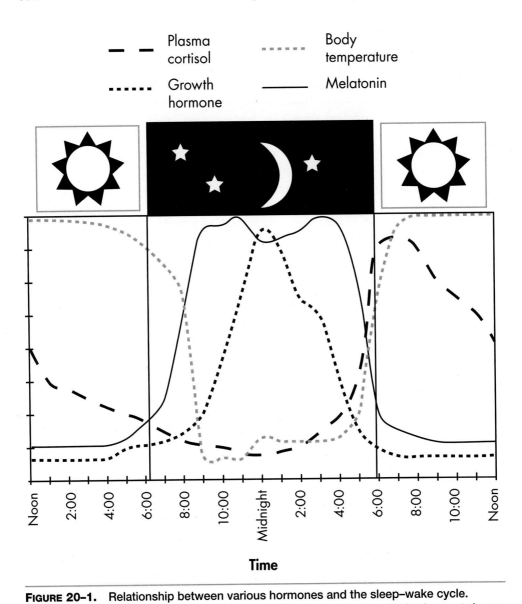

FIGURE 20–1.   Relationship between various hormones and the sleep–wake cycle.

The time scale of the x axis encompasses a 24-hour period from noon to noon, with the sleep period represented by the *dark section* (night) in the middle. Plasma cortisol secretion begins to increase before morning awakening and peaks in the early morning. Growth hormone secretion (which occurs during stage III–IV [N3] sleep) peaks early in the night. Melatonin is secreted after dark and is suppressed by light. Body temperature peaks in the late afternoon to early evening and starts to decrease before sleep onset.

Source.   Reprinted from Reite M, Weissberg M, Ruddy J: *Clinical Manual for the Evaluation and Treatment of Sleep Disorders.* Washington, DC, American Psychiatric Publishing, 2009, p. 39. Used with permission. Copyright © 2009 American Psychiatric Publishing.

TABLE 20–1. Overview of circadian rhythm sleep–wake disorders

Type	Sleep onset	Treatment	Wake/Alert	Clinical population
Delayed sleep–wake phase disorder	Later than desired	Light treatment after lowest core body temperature, melatonin in early evening, hypnotic as needed at bedtime at start of treatment	Later than desired	Most common in adolescents and young adults, but may be seen in children and older adults
Advanced sleep–wake phase disorder	Earlier than desired	Evening light treatment before lowest core body temperature	Earlier than desired	Usually the elderly and people with untreated depression
Non-24-hour sleep–wake rhythm disorder	Moves around the clock	Melatonin 5–10 mg at desired bedtime	Moves around the clock	Usually nonsighted persons with lack of light exposure due to interrupted retinohypothalamic tract
Irregular sleep–wake rhythm disorder	Erratic	Uncertain—effect of light treatment and melatonin unclear	Erratic	Persons with brain diseases, head trauma, or intellectual disability
Shift work disorder	Irregular due to work time	Modafinil 100–200 mg or caffeine for alertness; melatonin 1–3 mg 1 hour before bedtime; hypnotic (e.g., zolpidem) at bedtime	Irregular due to work time	People who work a night shift or rotating shifts
Jet lag disorder (due to circadian misalignment and sleep deprivation)	Linked to time of origin	Plot lowest core body temperature at destination and origin; time light and melatonin exposure accordingly; short-acting hypnotic on the flight	Linked to time of origin	Persons traveling rapidly across multiple time zones

Therapeutic Modulation of Circadian Timing

Treatment options for disorders of circadian timing are limited, because no effective pharmacological tools are yet available. The hypnotic agent ramelteon is a melatonin receptor agonist, but its specific use in circadian rhythm disorders is not yet clear. In 2014, the Food and Drug Administration (FDA) approved a melatonin receptor agonist, tasimelteon, for non-24-hour sleep–wake rhythm disorder in blind individuals; the sleep–wake schedules of these individuals have been shown to be re-entrained with appropriately timed exogenous melatonin (Skene and Arendt 2007).

At this time, proper timing of light exposure and appropriate use of melatonin are the two primary tools available for treatment of disorders of circadian regulation. Exposure to light before the body temperature's nadir will phase-delay the circadian system; exposure to light after the nadir will phase-advance the circadian system. Short-wavelength (blue) light is most effective in circadian timing (Lockley et al. 2006); it is important that individuals—especially those with delayed sleep–wake phase disorder—avoid use of devices that emit this wavelength of light before bedtime to avoid further delay of their sleep onset. Melatonin is also used as an adjunct in management of circadian rhythm disruptions, including those related to shift work or jet lag (Cardinali et al. 2006).

Wake–Sleep Control Systems

Several distinct neural systems control wakefulness, NREM sleep, and REM sleep. A basic understanding of these processes and control systems will help the clinician make sense of various sleep complaints that may appear to represent similar problems but in fact result from different mechanisms. When as clinicians we are attempting to treat disorders of sleep and wakefulness, we are often trying to modulate the function of the wake and/or sleep control systems with either upregulation or downregulation. For example, insomnia complaints can often be treated either by upregulating sleep control systems (the action of most common hypnotics) or by downregulating wake-promoting systems. It helps to keep in mind what one is trying to do in this regard. Both pharmacological and behavioral strategies are available for these purposes. These treatments are discussed in the following sections.

Neural Systems Promoting Wakefulness

Brain areas that support wakefulness include the ascending reticular activating system (ARAS) and cell groups near the mesopontine junction, centered around the pontine and medullary reticular formation, which have ascending projections to the forebrain and neocortex and descending projections to brain stem areas that regulate both sleep and wakefulness. The primary neurotransmitters that influence sleep–wake control systems include the catecholamines (dopamine, norepinephrine, and epinephrine) and tryptamines (serotonin and melatonin), histamine (also involved in inflammation), and orexin/hypocretin (also involved in food intake and energy expenditure). Pharmacological agents that modulate these neurotransmitter systems are generally involved in the therapeutic modulation of the sleep–wake system, as discussed later.

Waking is associated with a buildup of adenosine as a result of metabolism; increased adenosine promotes sleepiness and also serves as an activator of the ventrolateral preoptic area (VLPO)–based sleep-promoting systems. The world's most widely used stimulant, caffeine, is an adenosine antagonist.

Wake-promoting systems are extensive and redundant, such that lesions of one system will usually not eliminate the wake-promoting activity of others. During wakefulness, these arousal systems directly inhibit the activity of the sleep-promoting neurons in the VLPO, as discussed later in the section "Neural Systems Promoting Non-REM Sleep." Stress and anxiety result in increased activation or upregulation of wake-promoting systems, as do several substances of abuse (e.g., amphetamine, cocaine), and a state of hyperarousal results that leads to symptoms of insomnia.

Therapeutic Modulation of Wake-Promoting Systems

A number of pharmacological agents are used in upregulating wake-promoting systems and promoting arousal. Monoamine-active agents such as amphetamine and its derivatives, including methylphenidate, are used therapeutically to increase arousal and treat disorders of excessive daytime sleepiness (EDS), as seen with narcolepsy and primary hypersomnia, as well as some medical and psychiatric disorders (e.g., attention-deficit/hyperactivity disorder [ADHD]). Modafinil and armodafinil are agents that promote wakefulness through several mechanisms, including increasing the release of two catecholamines, norepinephrine and dopamine; elevating hypothalamic histamine levels; and possibly promoting orexinergic activity.

Downregulation of the ARAS is seen in general anesthesia, and it is possible that some antidepressant agents and atypical antipsychotics sometimes used off-label for insomnia may act in this fashion. Low-dose doxepin, a histamine H_1 and H_2 receptor antagonist, has been approved for the treatment of insomnia by the FDA and likely acts in this fashion. Most conventional sleep-promoting pharmacological agents (e.g., γ-aminobutyric acid [GABA]-ergic hypnotic agents) discussed in the following sections can also secondarily result in downregulation of the ARAS by virtue of their activation of sleep-promoting systems, which in turn decreases ARAS activity.

A number of cognitive-behavioral techniques can be used to downregulate ARAS systems and decrease arousal, thus promoting sleep. These include progressive relaxation, meditation of several types, biofeedback, and components of cognitive-behavioral therapy for insomnia (see Table 20–8, "Sleep restriction and stimulus control," later in this chapter). These nonpharmacological approaches to treating insomnia have been shown to be both safe and effective (Morin et al. 2006) and are recommended in the treatment of chronic primary and comorbid (secondary) insomnia by the American Academy of Sleep Medicine (Schutte-Rodin et al. 2008).

Neural Systems Promoting Non-REM Sleep

NREM N3 (slow wave) sleep is the state most closely associated with reversal of the neurometabolic effects of wakefulness. NREM N3 sleep is the primary component of Borbely's Process S (the homeostatic sleep drive); the role of REM sleep remains unclear. The primary neurophysiological systems responsible for promoting and maintaining NREM sleep include the output of the predominantly GABAergic and galanergic VLPO and median preoptic (MnPO) nuclei, whose neurons are primarily active during sleep and send inhibitory output to all major cell groups of the hypothalamus and brain stem that participate in arousal (Saper et al. 2005).

Activation of this GABAergic system serves to facilitate and maintain NREM sleep. These sleep-promoting systems are normally inhibited by ARAS wake-promoting activity, but after sufficient sleep debt has accumulated and after the decreasing circadian arousal drive permits, these VLPO systems are activated ("switched on") by the bistable "wake–NREM sleep" switch mechanism (see "Bistable Sleep Switches" section later in this chapter). They then begin to actively inhibit the ARAS systems, permitting entrance into and maintenance of the NREM sleep state. Important to activation of the VLPO-MnPO NREM sleep system is the buildup of adenosine associated with metabolism during the wakeful state. Adenosine appears to be an important homeostatic sleep factor acting through the adenosine A_1 and A_2 receptors, whose release is triggered by inducible nitric acid synthesis in the basal forebrain secondary to prolonged wakefulness (Stenberg 2007).

The VLPO is a sexually dimorphic region that is larger and has more cells in males. Men between ages 45 and 60 years show a decrease in cell numbers of about 3% per year until age 60 years, after which further decreases are not noted. In females, cell numbers decrease until the teen years, and then remain fairly stable until after age 50 years, when a gradual decrease begins; the decrease becomes dramatically more rapid after age 75 years. Between the ages of 75 and 85 years, cell numbers decrease in females at a rate of 4%–8% per year, leading to numbers that are only 10%–15% of the peak seen between the ages of 2 and 4 years (Hofman and Swaab 1989). As implied by these findings, both men and women have increasing difficulty in initiating and maintaining sleep beginning around age 50 years, but this difficulty stabilizes in men by age 60 years while continuing to worsen in women with increasing age. Gaus et al. (2002) have suggested that the shrinkage of the VLPO seen with advancing age may help explain sleep disturbances found in elderly individuals.

The NREM and REM sleep stages and their electroencephalographic and physiological characteristics are shown in Table 20–2. The healthy adult typically transitions through the three NREM sleep stages (N1–N3) before entering REM sleep. Infants, however, often enter REM sleep directly, as do patients with narcolepsy.

Although people are not conscious during sleep, they are able to respond to external stimuli. For example, neurons in the auditory cortex respond to auditory input during sleep (Issa and Wang 2008), and complex parasomnia behavior, including driving, can occur during sleep, indicating that the brain can respond appropriately to sensory input, as well as regulate motor output, while not conscious of it. Some of these complex parasomnias are thought to reflect the release of deep brain central pattern generators normally inhibited during sleep, which permit complex sensorimotor behaviors without cortical awareness (Tassinari et al. 2005, 2009), an example of impaired wake–sleep state control.

Therapeutic Modulation of NREM Sleep–Promoting Systems

The major sleep-promoting system is GABAergic, and most sedative-hypnotic agents approved by the FDA for insomnia treatment are GABAergic agents—that is, either benzodiazepines or the newer omega-1 active nonbenzodiazepine agonists (Table 20–3). The older benzodiazepine hypnotic agents generally nonselectively activate multiple benzodiazepine receptors and thus may have prominent muscle relaxant, anticonvulsant, and anxiolytic properties in addition to their hypnotic actions. They also have in common issues such as tolerance, habituation, and impairment of memory

TABLE 20–2. Electroencephalographic (EEG) sleep stages and their physiological correlates

Sleep stage	EEG patterns	Physiological correlates	Percentage of total sleep time in adults
N1	Loss of waking alpha frequency Increased 5–7 Hz theta frequency Occasional high voltage central sharp waves	Occasional slow rolling eye movements Heart rate and respiration more stable	5%–7%
N2	Sleep spindles (12–14 Hz) K-complexes (negative followed by positive deflection lasting 0.5 sec) Higher-voltage mixed theta <20% delta frequency (<4 Hz)	Heart rate and respiration slower, relatively stable Core body temperature declines EMG decreases	~50% Most common sleep stage
N3	Higher-voltage (>75 μV) low-frequency delta waveforms (>20%) Few spindles, rare K-complexes	Heart rate and respiration slow, stable EMG drops	~20%–25% Increased in early adolescence Decreased in elderly
REM	Low-voltage mixed-frequency activity	Very-low-voltage EMG with occasional phasic twitches Rapid eye movements Heart rate and respiration irregular Loss of body temperature control	~20% 50% in newborns 80% in premature infants Adult levels reached by about age 6 years

Note. EMG=electromyography; REM=rapid eye movement sleep.

TABLE 20–3.   **Commonly prescribed hypnotic medications**

Drug[a]	Mechanism of action	Typical dose	Half-life, hours
Temazepam	Bz GABA agonist	7.5–30.0 mg	8–12
Zaleplon	Non-Bz GABA agonist	5–20 mg	1–1.5
Zolpidem	Non-Bz GABA agonist	2.5–10 mg	1.5–2.6
Eszopiclone	Non-Bz GABA agonist	1–3 mg	6
Ramelteon	Melatonin agonist	8 mg	1–2
Suvorexant	Orexin/hypocretin antagonist	10 mg	12
Doxepin	Antihistamine	3–6 mg (generic liquid available)	15

Note.   Bz=benzodiazepine; GABA=γ-aminobutyric acid.
[a]Also sedating antidepressants and antipsychotics as appropriate for coexisting conditions.

consolidation while the drug is active. Newer nonbenzodiazepine hypnotics are more selectively hypnotic but are not free of other actions. The newest medication for insomnia is suvorexant, an orexin/hypocretin antagonist that blocks the binding of wake-promoting neuropeptides orexin/hypocretin A and orexin/hypocretin B to receptors. The most commonly used FDA-approved hypnotic agents are listed in Table 20–3.

Another GABAergic agent that promotes sleep is sodium oxybate (sodium γ-hydroxybutyrate), a drug developed under the FDA's orphan drug program as a treatment for narcolepsy.

Neural Systems Promoting REM Sleep

An epoch of NREM sleep is usually followed by a transition to REM sleep. REM sleep is associated with dreaming experiences that would be considered psychotic if they occurred during wakefulness. Abnormalities in REM sleep state control (e.g., narcolepsy) may sometimes be associated with preservation of aspects of the dream state mentation (e.g., visual hallucinations) into wakefulness, which if not recognized may be misinterpreted as psychosis. Some people with narcolepsy are misdiagnosed as having schizophrenia for this reason. In most healthy adults, the time from NREM sleep onset at night to the onset of the first REM period (termed *REM latency*) is about 60–90 minutes; however, the latency is shorter in patients with narcolepsy or depression. REM sleep constitutes about 20% of total sleep in adults and occurs in a periodic fashion, increasing in length and depth during the night. REM sleep is accompanied by low-voltage mixed-frequency electroencephalographic (EEG) activity, eye movements, loss of skeletal muscle tone (except for muscles coordinating eye movements, middle ear muscle activity, and muscles necessary to sustain life), EEG ponto-geniculo-occipital waves, and autonomic and body temperature dysregulation. People typically report dreaming when awakened from this state.

Therapeutic Modulation of REM Sleep–Promoting Systems

Transition from NREM to REM sleep is associated with the activation of predominantly cholinergic neuronal systems in the upper pontine regions, with associated decreases in monoaminergic activation. The pons has been demonstrated by pivotal early studies (Jouvet 1962) to be necessary and sufficient for the generation of REM sleep, and specific regions, such as the pedunculopontine tegmental area, laterodorsal tegmental area, and midline raphe nucleus, are particularly implicated in REM sleep generation. These regions, when activated, produce the physiological accompaniments of REM sleep. Administration of cholinergic agents accentuates REM sleep, whereas drugs promoting monoaminergic activation decrease REM sleep. Alternative REM control mechanisms have been suggested, including activity of GABAergic systems (Fort et al. 2009).

REM sleep normally appears only on a background of NREM sleep, but REM sleep phenomena may actually continue 24 hours a day in a muted form characterized by varying levels of alertness (Kripke 1972). Most catecholamine agents, as well as many antidepressants, will decrease REM sleep, whereas relatively few agents increase REM sleep, one being reserpine. It is not clear that attempts to therapeutically modulate REM sleep are clinically useful, because deviations from "normal" values in sleep recordings are of uncertain importance.

Bistable Sleep Switches

Transitions from wakefulness to NREM sleep, and vice versa, are controlled by neurophysiological systems acting in a fashion similar to bistable flip-flop switches in electrical engineering (Saper et al. 2010). These systems permit relatively rapid switching to the new state and then maintain state stability once switched, to prevent unstable back-and-forth transitions. The "wake–NREM sleep" switch is influenced primarily by VLPO activity, which when reaching critical levels (facilitated by sleep homeostatic–related adenosine buildup and decrease in circadian arousal drive) begins to actively inhibit arousal systems and triggers a transition into NREM sleep. With loss of VLPO neurons, as occurs in normal aging, the bistable switch mechanism becomes impaired, permitting the switch to "ride" closer to its transition point, resulting in more rapid transitions from wakefulness to sleep, and vice versa, with poor state control, which is often observed in elderly individuals. Orexin/hypocretin neurons contribute materially to the stability of the "wake–NREM sleep" switch, weighting the "wake" side of the switch, whereas loss of orexin neurons, as is seen in narcolepsy, results in state instability with rapid switching between states.

A similar bistable switch mechanism controls transitions from NREM to REM sleep and vice versa; this mechanism consists primarily of pontine neurons at the level of the dorsal raphe. GABAergic neurons within the pons constitute "REM sleep–off" neurons, and neurons in the sublateral dorsal nucleus adjacent to the pons are "REM sleep–on" neurons. These constitute a bistable switch mechanism, with cholinergic activity facilitating the "REM sleep–on" component and monoamine and orexin neurons again contributing to the "REM-off" state. Loss of orexin neurons (as is seen in narcolepsy) contributes to state instability and rapid switching into and out of REM sleep, including "REM sleep–awake state" instability with rapid switching into REM sleep from a wake state (e.g., cataplexy) and sometimes preservation of REM sleep (e.g., dreaming) mentation into wakefulness.

Other Important Aspects of Sleep

Delta Activity, Sleep Homeostasis, and "Local Sleep"

Delta (<4 Hz) sleep is thought to be an index of the homeostatic sleep drive (Process S). In healthy individuals, delta sleep is prominently increased after sleep deprivation. Depression and some medical conditions, including chronic fatigue syndrome and fibromyalgia, are associated with decreases in delta activity, interpreted as a deficiency in homeostatic sleep drive, which may contribute to insomnia-related sleep complaints.

Local delta activity may index synaptic "pruning and tuning" associated with the preceding day's learning; such activity has been found to be regionally increased over areas of cortex experimentally activated during wakefulness prior to sleep onset (Huber et al. 2004). This finding has led to the interesting but not yet well understood concept of "local sleep," wherein (in this case) delta activity is greater over those cortical regions that were more actively involved in information processing during preceding wakefulness (Huber et al. 2004).

Characteristics of Sequential Sleep Periods

The time from sleep onset at night to completion of the first REM sleep epoch is often termed a *sleep period;* a normal night's sleep consists of three to six sequential sleep periods. The first sleep periods at night are characterized by a greater amount of delta sleep and relatively little REM sleep, whereas sleep periods in the early morning hours have less delta and longer REM epochs, usually with more intense dream activity. Early sleep periods, with their greater delta, are more frequently accompanied by NREM-related parasomnias such as sleep terrors and sleepwalking. Later sleep periods with longer and more intense REM epochs are more often characterized by nightmares and REM-related parasomnias. As a result of REM-associated skeletal muscle hypotonia, obstructive apnea events tend to be more prominent during REM sleep.

Slow-wave activity during sleep tends to diminish throughout the night as the homeostatic sleep drive decreases, whereas REM sleep tends to increase, possibly because it is no longer being suppressed by NREM homeostatic sleep pressure. REM sleep is also homeostatically modulated, and REM suppression will be followed by REM rebound.

Sleep Across the Life Span

Sleep changes dramatically across the life span. The newborn infant, who exhibits a less-well-organized EEG response, spends approximately 50% of sleep time in REM sleep (premature infants spend even more time in REM sleep—up to 80% at 30 weeks' gestational age). Central nervous system (CNS) development in neonates and infants has been proposed as a function for REM sleep, based on their length of time spent in REM sleep. The percentage of time spent in REM sleep approaches adult levels (~20% of total sleep time) during early childhood. Newborns typically have REM sleep at the onset of their sleep periods, shifting to adult NREM-onset sleep periods by about age 4 months. Newborns' sleep is generally about equally divided into *active* (REM) sleep and *quiet* sleep, the forerunner of the later-developing N2 and N3 sleep. N2 sleep with sleep spindles and N3 (delta) sleep can usually be identified by about age 3 months.

Total sleep time diminishes with age, ranging from 16 hours per 24 hours at birth to about 9 hours at age 6, about 8 hours at age 12, and typically about 7.5 hours in adulthood. Delta activity is very prominent in sleep during early adolescence, and sleepwalking often begins around this time.

Later in adolescence a steep decline occurs in delta sleep that is thought to be associated with age-programmed synaptic pruning. This decline may be an index of brain development or maturation, and Feinberg in 1982 (cited in Feinberg et al. 2006) suggested that a defect in this brain maturational process might underlie some cases of schizophrenia with onset during adolescence. This intriguing hypothesis is still being actively investigated (Boksa 2012). Adolescents also appear to have a physiological circadian phase delay, making it more difficult for them to go to sleep early and arise early in the morning. This phase delay has led some school systems to change their schedules to start classes somewhat later for adolescents.

Typically, delta sleep again begins to decrease with advancing age, possibly due in part to loss of VLPO neurons, decline in aerobic fitness, and perhaps other yet-uncertain mechanisms. Unfortunately, in the elderly, poor sleep is often the norm, with an increased sleep latency (time from lights off to sleep onset), decreased amounts of NREM and REM sleep, advanced sleep phase, and more sleep fragmentation due to medical, psychiatric, and sleep disorders, producing significant daytime sleepiness.

Sleep and Medical and Mental Health

Psychiatrists have long been aware of the close association between sleep and mental illness. Depression is most often accompanied by disturbed sleep. Untreated insomnia can lead to depression. Disturbed sleep may be a harbinger of emerging mental illness. Sleep loss may trigger—or be an early symptom of—a manic episode. Recent research has shown that this bidirectional relationship applies to many other areas of medicine, as well as to overall health. Some examples follow:

- Difficulty falling asleep, unrefreshing sleep, and particularly loud snoring predicted the development of metabolic syndrome in adults (Troxel et al. 2010).
- Longer-term sleep restriction or deprivation has long been recognized as a major contributor to poor health and impaired function (Luyster et al. 2012).
- Adequate sleep and proper timing of sleep are essential for healthy function of the immune system (Besedovsky et al. 2012).
- Patients with obstructive sleep apnea (OSA) have evidence of coronary artery endothelial dysfunction, which may be one of the main mechanisms responsible for the higher incidence of coronary artery disease in these patients (Kadohira et al. 2011).
- Disorders of sleep and wakefulness occur in many serious and progressive neurological diseases, such as Parkinson's disease and restless legs syndrome (RLS), and in poorly understood syndromes, such as chronic fatigue syndrome and Lyme disease.
- Extended wakefulness appears to stress the endoplasmic reticulum and is associated with upregulation of the *unfolded protein response,* a mechanism designed to prevent aggregation of misfolded proteins. Normal aging may impair the adaptive unfolded protein response to sleep deprivation, leading to increased expression of pro-apoptotic proteins (Naidoo et al. 2008).
- Sleep restriction gives rise to significant negative neurocognitive processing consequences in executive functioning, sustained attention, and long-term memory (Lowe et al. 2017).

- Repeated episodes of hypoxia and reoxygenation associated with OSA increase production of reactive oxygen species, initiating inflammation and leading to impairment of endothelial function as well as early signs of clinical atherosclerosis (Lurie 2011).
- The combination of sleep restriction and circadian disruption (as seen in shift work) is especially deleterious in terms of metabolic dysregulation (Buxton et al. 2012).
- Partial sleep deprivation during only a single night induces insulin resistance in multiple metabolic pathways in healthy subjects (Donga et al. 2010).
- The restorative function of sleep may be a consequence of enhanced removal of potentially neurotoxic waste products (e.g., β-amyloid) that accumulate in the CNS during wakefulness (Xie et al. 2013).

Thus, while we have long known that sleep was essential for life, and that sleep loss was associated with impaired psychological and mental function, we now see emerging the entire complex picture of the intimate relationship between adequate sleep and proper function of multiple specific bodily systems, with significant public health impact. Perhaps it should not be surprising that a state in which we spend about one-third of our existence is so crucial to the effective functioning of the entire organism.

Overview of DSM-5 Sleep–Wake Disorders

With respect to sleep disorders, the *Diagnostic and Statistical Manual of Mental Disorders, 5th Edition* (DSM-5; American Psychiatric Association 2013), is one of three major classification systems—the other two being the ICSD-3 (American Academy of Sleep Medicine 2014), which is highly detailed and commonly used by sleep medicine specialists, and the *International Classification of Diseases, 10th Edition, Clinical Modification* (ICD-10-CM; National Center for Health Statistics 2014), which is used for billing codes in many institutions. Overall, the general classifications are in agreement in these three systems, although specifics vary.

The conceptualization and organization of sleep–wake disorders have changed substantially in DSM-5 compared with DSM-IV/DSM-IV-TR (American Psychiatric Association 1994, 2000). Previously the sleep disorders were separated by presumed etiology into three nonoverlapping groups: 1) primary sleep disorders (with subcategories dyssomnias and parasomnias), 2) sleep disorders related to another mental disorder, and 3) other sleep disorders (including sleep disorder related to a general medical condition and substance-induced sleep disorder). In DSM-5 the individual disorders are separated on the basis of comorbidity and coexisting conditions rather than on any presumptions regarding causation.

DSM-5 sleep–wake disorders now constitute 10 separate disorders or disorder groups: insomnia disorder; hypersomnolence disorder; narcolepsy; breathing-related sleep disorders; circadian rhythm sleep–wake disorders; parasomnias including NREM sleep arousal disorders, nightmare disorder, REM sleep behavior disorder, RLS; and substance-/medication-induced sleep disorder. In the insomnia domain, criteria for an insomnia diagnosis have been changed (with primary insomnia replaced by insomnia disorder), and subtypes of circadian rhythm disorders have been expanded, with jet lag removed. In the hypersomnia domain, narcolepsy has been separated from the hypersomnia group, as its association with hypocretin deficiency has been identified. The breathing disorder group has been more clearly specified and includes OSA hypopnea, central sleep apnea, and sleep-related hypoventilation. The central apnea and hypoventilation groups have several subtypes for clarification.

Two new diagnoses have been added, REM sleep behavior disorder and RLS, to limit use of the "unspecified" classification (including the former "not otherwise specified [NOS]" diagnoses in DSM-IV).

In addition to diagnostic criteria, DSM-5 provides details on differential diagnosis and available data on prevalence, development and course, risk and prognostic factors, functional consequences, comorbidity, diagnostic markers, and other information relevant to understanding the disorders. Associated codes for ICD-9-CM and ICD-10-CM are provided, and relationships with ICSD diagnostic categories are discussed.

Treatment Options and Resources

Once a diagnosis has been made, where does the clinician go to find treatment options? This chapter does not attempt to deal with the specifics of treatment for all of the various sleep disorders, nor does DSM-5. Extensive discussions of treatment options can be found in major textbooks of sleep, such as *Principles and Practice of Sleep Medicine*, 6th Edition (Kryger et al. 2016), as well as textbooks devoted to treatment (Barkoukis et al. 2012). Shorter reviews of treatment options can be found in sources such as *Clinical Manual for Evaluation and Treatment of Sleep Disorders* (Reite et al. 2009). One good treatment resource is the publications of the American Academy of Sleep Medicine (www .aasm-net.org). These practice parameters, clinical guidelines, and best-practice guides cover the general areas of insomnia, hypersomnia, circadian rhythm disorders, parasomnias, sleep-related breathing disorders, sleep-related movement disorders, and pediatric sleep disorders. Efforts are made to update these publications on a regular basis.

The Four-Step Sleep Evaluation

In this section we present an approach that we believe will help non–sleep clinicians to identify and either treat or appropriately refer common sleep disorders encountered in their practices. Sleep disorders derail health and shorten longevity. They are highly prevalent, affecting an estimated 50–70 million individuals in the United States alone. In the general population, insomnia symptoms are present in up to 33% of individuals, OSA in about 5% (although 26%–32% have symptoms suggesting risk for OSA), and RLS in 5%–15% (Senthilvel et al. 2011).

Although widespread, sleep disorders often remain unexplored if not asked about by clinicians or brought up by patients (Roth et al. 2010). Symptoms can be expressed directly by patients ("I can't sleep") or complained of by others ("her snoring/his thrashing keeps me awake"); at times, the possibility of a sleep problem can be inferred from the presence of other diagnoses known to coexist with disordered sleep, such as depression, hypertension, stroke, or other cardiac disease. However, even when a sleep disturbance is known to be present, many clinicians lack a framework for conducting a thorough evaluation.

The primary symptoms of disordered sleep—insomnia, excessive daytime sleepiness, and disturbed or disturbing sleep behavior—are usually not pathognomonic for a specific diagnosis and must be further parsed and explored. For instance, some individuals who claim to be sleepy may actually be *fatigued* (i.e., unable to either sleep at night or nap during the day). Other people are "night owls" (i.e., have a delayed sleep phase circadian rhythm disorder) who do not sleep in tune with their circadian arousal systems; these individuals can develop EDS, insomnia, or both (Ebben and Spielman 2009).

The bidirectional relationship between sleep disorders and psychiatric illness—coupled with the fact that sleep disorders often coexist with other medical, psychiatric, and sleep problems—creates a host of diagnostic pitfalls. For example, problems can arise when a clinician assumes that one disorder (e.g., comorbid depression) "causes" another (e.g., insomnia). Although depression can indeed cause sleepiness and insomnia, depression and insomnia may coexist independently and be mutually influencing; therefore, insomnia and depression each require a *separate* assessment. An insomnia disorder may have multiple roots; for instance, it may be precipitated by OSA or the circadian misalignment of sleep phase delay. In fact, it is not unusual for a patient to have all three of these conditions—OSA, insomnia disorder, and a circadian rhythm disorder, delayed sleep phase type.

Problems also arise when a clinician, having identified "the cause" of a patient's insomnia, assumes that further diagnostic evaluation is not necessary. This assumption is an error, because more than one condition is frequently present (Ebben and Spielman 2009). As John B. Hickam stated (in the medical profession's counterargument to Occam's razor that has become known as Hickam's dictum), "Patients can have as many diseases as they damn well please."

Approximately 80 sleep–wake disorders have been identified at present (American Academy of Sleep Medicine 2014). The DSM-5 sleep–wake classification encompasses considerably fewer disorders, from which we have chosen seven to demonstrate our clinical approach (the Four-Step Sleep Evaluation):

1. *Sleep phase delay ("night owl" syndrome),* a circadian rhythm sleep–wake disorder that is a frequent cause of insomnia and EDS
2. *Obstructive sleep apnea,* a breathing-related sleep disorder that is often overlooked in clinical settings because inquiring about snoring is seldom part of the review of systems; medications that cause weight gain have been implicated in the genesis of this condition
3. *Insomnia disorder,* the most prevalent sleep–wake disorder
4. *Restless legs syndrome,* a sensorimotor condition that can interfere with sleep and that also can be precipitated or worsened by commonly prescribed drugs, especially antidepressants
5. *Sleepwalking,* a potentially dangerous NREM sleep arousal disorder that likewise may be iatrogenically induced by commonly prescribed medications
6. *REM sleep behavior disorder,* another potentially dangerous disorder whose incidence appears to be increasing, possibly because of the widespread use of antidepressants
7. *Narcolepsy,* a disorder whose sleep attacks and hallucinations have been mistaken for psychosis

We strongly recommend that the first four disorders listed—delayed sleep phase circadian rhythm disorder ("night owl" syndrome), OSA, insomnia disorder, and RLS—be considered in *all* patients who present with sleep complaints, regardless of what other medical or psychiatric diagnoses are present, because they are the most prevalent sleep disorders in the general population. When symptoms suggest, the last three listed disorders should also be explored. Of high clinical importance is the fact that four of these seven disorders—OSA, RLS, sleepwalking, and REM sleep behavior disorder—can be precipitated or worsened by commonly prescribed medications.

The Four-Step Sleep Evaluation

1. Identify the complaint.
2. Clarify the complaint—Is the patient fatigued or truly sleepy?
3. Evaluate sleep habits and sleep environment—Does poor sleep hygiene contribute to the patient's sleep problems?

4a. Screen for common sleep disorders:
   - Sleep phase delay ("night owl" syndrome)
   - Obstructive sleep apnea
   - Insomnia disorder
   - Restless legs syndrome

4b. Consider the possible presence of other sleep disorders:
   - NREM sleep arousal disorders (e.g., sleepwalking)
   - REM sleep behavior disorder (e.g., "acting out" dreams)
   - Narcolepsy

Step One: Identify the Complaint

Although all patients should be screened for sleep disorders, such screening is particularly important if medical or psychiatric disorders known to coexist with sleep disorders are present. Such disorders include ADHD, cardiovascular disease, hypertension, diabetes, and depression. The following screening questions can be asked to determine the need for further exploration:

- Are you satisfied with your sleep?
- Are you excessively tired during the day?
- Has anyone ever complained about your sleep? (A "yes" answer might suggest OSA, a circadian rhythm sleep–wake disorder, an NREM sleep arousal disorder such as sleepwalking or sleep terrors, a REM sleep behavior disorder, or narcolepsy.)

Augmenting the history by interviewing someone familiar with the patient usually provides valuable insights. Reports of loud, disruptive snoring, or of snorts or gasps, in a patient who denies snoring should prompt serious consideration of sleep-related breathing disorders, whereas reports of unusual motor behaviors raise the possibility of an NREM sleep arousal disorder (e.g., sleepwalking), a REM sleep behavior disorder, OSA, or nocturnal seizures.

Step Two: Clarify the Complaint

"Sleepiness" is a common complaint of patients who *cannot stay awake* but also of those who *cannot sleep when given the opportunity*. The former is true sleepiness (EDS); the latter is fatigue/tiredness due to physiological hyperarousal, which is often accompanied by lack of energy, motivation, and mental clarity. The differential diagnosis for true sleepiness is not the same as that for fatigue (Table 20–4).

People's perceptions of sleepiness can be unreliable; some people may tolerate high degrees of sleepiness without actually "knowing" that they are sleepy. In such situations, behavioral symptoms can help identify sleepiness (Table 20–5). New digital health tools are being rapidly developed and introduced, and careful tracking of sleep and wakefulness may be helpful in the assessment of an individual patient's sleep. Sleep laboratory–based electrophysiological recordings are quite sensitive and can reliably detect sleepiness.

TABLE 20–4.   **Causes of excessive daytime sleepiness (EDS) and fatigue**

Sleepiness (behavioral symptoms[a]; elevated score on Epworth Sleepiness Scale[b])

Obstructive or central sleep apnea: 70% of patients with obstructive sleep apnea are sleepy, whereas 30% are not; central sleep apnea may be precipitated by opioid use

Circadian rhythm disorders (e.g., delayed sleep phase, shift work, jet lag)

Insufficient sleep opportunity

Narcolepsy

Idiopathic hypersomnia

Head injury

Depression: especially seasonal, atypical, and bipolar (but other causes should be considered)

Drug use or withdrawal

Restless legs syndrome (especially given the estimated 70%–80% of people with this condition who have periodic limb movement disorder, in which repetitive leg twitches disturb sleep)

Medical illness (e.g., renal or hepatic failure, brain tumors, neurodegenerative disorders)

Fatigue (low score on Epworth Sleepiness Scale[b])

Anxiety and depression

Conditioned/learned insomnia

---

[a]See Table 20–5 for behavioral symptoms of sleepiness.
[b]See Table 20–6 for Epworth Sleepiness Scale questions.

TABLE 20–5.   **Behavioral symptoms of sleepiness**

Patient does not awaken spontaneously and refreshed.

Patient depends on weekend "rescue sleep."

Patient is not generally alert throughout the day.

Patient has nodded off while driving.

Patient attempts to mask his or her sleepiness with caffeine or activity.

Patient will doze if given a chance to take an afternoon nap.

TABLE 20–6.   **Epworth Sleepiness Scale**

How likely are you to doze off or fall asleep in the following situations, in contrast to just feeling tired? This refers to your usual way of life in recent times. Even if you haven't done some of these things recently, try to work out how they would have affected you. Use the following scale to choose the most appropriate number for each situation:

0=would never doze
1=slight chance of dozing
2=moderate chance of dozing
3=high chance of dozing

Sitting and reading ____

Watching TV ____

Sitting, inactive, in a public place (e.g., a theater or a meeting) ____

As a passenger in a car for an hour without a break ____

Lying down to rest in the afternoon when circumstances permit ____

Sitting and talking to someone ____

Sitting quietly after a lunch without alcohol ____

In a car, while stopped for a few minutes in traffic ____

TOTAL ____

SCORING ____

Availability and Conditions of Use.   The developer and copyright holder of the Epworth Sleepiness Scale, Dr. Murray Johns, permits use of the scale by individual people (including clinicians and researchers) free of charge. The Epworth Sleepiness Scale is downloadable from the Web Source shown below, from which complete administration/scoring instructions and methodological data are also available.
Source.   Johns MW: "A New Method for Measuring Daytime Sleepiness: The Epworth Sleepiness Scale." *Sleep* 14:540–545, 1991. Copyright 1990, 1997, M.W. Johns.
Web Source.   Official website of the Epworth Sleepiness Scale by Dr. Murray Johns (http://www.epworthsleepinessscale.com/about-the-ess/).

Another useful tool is the Epworth Sleepiness Scale (Johns 1991; Table 20–6), a self-administered questionnaire in which the respondent is asked to rate, on a four-point scale (0–3), his or her chances of dozing off in eight different real-life situations. The summed score provides a measure of impairment and is helpful in distinguishing fatigue from true sleepiness. Some clinicians use an Epworth score of 8 as the upper limit of "normal"; others consider a score greater than 10 as an indication of pathological sleepiness. High Epworth scores may indicate EDS, possibly resulting from a sleep-related breathing disorder (Rosenthal and Dolan 2008), insufficient sleep opportunity, or a circadian rhythm sleep–wake disorder. However, a score in the "normal range" (e.g., 2–6) can be misleading, because many individuals with OSA, for instance, do not feel particularly sleepy. Epworth scores are only one piece of the diagnostic puzzle.

Very low Epworth scores (typically 0–2) may indicate that the patient is unable to relax day or night, perhaps as a result of hyperarousal secondary to anxiety, depression, or "sleep worry" (the latter is the basis of *learned* or *conditioned* psychophysiological insomnia—i.e., insomnia disorder). Hyperaroused individuals have higher core body temperatures, faster EEG responses, and elevated cortisol levels. They have trouble disengaging from the world as they try to sleep. Hypnotic medications often fail to work in such patients.

The Epworth Sleepiness Scale may yield false-negative but rarely false-positive scores. About 30% of patients with OSA, a common cause of EDS, have normal Epworth scores. Some patients in this group may have developed conditioned insomnia and are experiencing hyperarousal from sleep disruption secondary to OSA. True EDS can also be present in patients experiencing winter depression, atypical depression, or the depressed phase of bipolar illness. The bottom line is that if the Epworth score is elevated, the clinician must determine why. Epworth scores should be evaluated carefully within the patient's clinical context, including behavioral indications of sleepiness or fatigue, and should be considered a clinical guide rather than a diagnostic instrument.

Step Three: Evaluate Sleep Habits and Sleep Environment

Although not curative in itself, establishing healthy sleep habits is generally part of sleep disorder treatment (Schutte-Rodin et al. 2008). Factors that may contribute to or cause EDS or insomnia should be identified and remedied where possible. For example, does the patient:

Positive factors
- Sleep in a bedroom that is safe, dark, and quiet?
- Protect his or her genetically required sleep opportunity?
- Keep regular sleep and wake hours (even on weekends)?
- Sleep in tune with his or her circadian clock?
- Get adequate exercise and sunlight exposure?

Negative factors
- Eat large meals right before bed?
- Sleep with pets (dogs or cats) in the room or on the bed?
- Drink alcohol or smoke cigarettes a few hours before sleep?
- Read, watch television, or work in bed?
- Consume caffeinated beverages throughout the day? (Caffeine's average half-life is 4–7 hours, but half-life becomes longer with age.)
- Have a bed partner who snores ("spousal arousal") or is a night owl and comes to bed after the patient has fallen asleep?
- Go to bed hungry?

A widely held misconception is that "sleep hygiene" is the treatment for sleep complaints, not just an important part of a comprehensive approach. A thorough evaluation requires assessment of which disorders are actually present.

Step Four, Part A: Screen for Common Sleep Disorders

Sleep Phase Delay (Circadian Rhythm Sleep–Wake Phase Disorder)

Core body temperature is tightly linked with, and a proxy for, the circadian timing system that controls our sleep–wake cycle (endogenous rhythm ~24.2 hours) and oscillates independently of whether we are asleep or awake. If awake for long periods, we feel more or less alert due to these oscillations. We sleep best as the temperature drops (here around midnight) and awaken approximately 2 hours after lowest core body temperature begins to rise. We sleep poorly when not in tune with these rhythms. The sleep rhythms of "night owls" (i.e., those who stay up late) are delayed (i.e., delayed sleep–wake phase) and occur later in the 24-hour day–night cycle. In these individuals, the core body temperature may begin to drop at 2 A.M. or 3 A.M. and rise in the late morning or afternoon. If night owls sleep in phase with their rhythms, they are out of phase with social demands. If they do not, they develop insomnia, EDS, or both. Shift workers and those with jet lag also develop sleep problems when trying to sleep or stay awake at the wrong times for their internal circadian rhythms.

Circadian alerting rhythms wax and wane on their own schedules, essentially unaffected by our efforts to sleep or stay awake. When people do not follow these rhythms, symptoms of insomnia and/or EDS arise and may persist for years before misalignment of the sleep schedule with the circadian timing system is identified as their cause (Schaefer et al. 2012).

Sleep is efficiently generated when our sleep debt, which increases in a progressive, hypothetically linear fashion while we are awake, intersects with our circadian arousal system as it starts to "quiet" at night. We sleep best when our core body temperature drops (and our arousal system quiets), and we wake spontaneously about 2 hours after our temperature begins to rise. Insomnia develops if we try to initiate sleep before our core body temperature begins to drop, while our arousal system is still set to "loud"; EDS develops when our sleep period is truncated by the requirement to wake at a specific time and that hour arrives before we have gotten enough sleep.

Presentation

Misalignment of alerting rhythms with social demands is easy to identify in people who do shift work or have jet lag; it is harder to spot in people who are early risers (so-called "larks") or who stay up late ("night owls"). Sleep–wake rhythms are advanced to earlier times in about 1% of the population (larks), usually with onset in middle age; rhythms are delayed in up to 15% of adolescents and in somewhat fewer adults. When people with advanced sleep–wake rhythms are able to sleep in tune with their circadian systems, they fall asleep early, wake early, and sleep normally. However, if they stay awake to meet social demands, they still wake early and may develop EDS due to lack of sleep, and their "early morning awakening" might be misattributed to depression.

Night owls, in contrast, sleep normally when they are in phase with their internal delayed clock but can develop "insomnia" if they attempt to sleep at earlier, socially appropriate times and/or EDS if they awaken before their alerting rhythms begin to rise and adequate sleep has been obtained. Circadian rhythm sleep–wake disorder, delayed sleep phase type, is one cause of "bedtime difficulties" in children; however, such children are not really being "difficult"—they are just unable to fall asleep. These children, when put to bed before being biologically ready for sleep, also may lie in bed for hours, their minds active, developing fears of the dark, and may be diagnosed with anxiety when the issue is precipitated by parental behavior.

Although patients with mood disorders such as major depression, bipolar disorder, or seasonal depression seem to have a higher incidence of sleep phase delay, mood issues are not always present in night owls. Of course, "ersatz" sleep phase delay may be due to purely behavioral issues as well; when social demands arise, individuals with behaviorally induced sleep-phase delay have little difficulty adjusting their sleep schedules to more appropriate times.

Pathophysiology

Alerting rhythms are under the control of clock genes and light exposure (Roenneberg et al. 2007). For individuals who are in constant darkness, these rhythms typically wax and wane in 24.2-hour cycles but are reset to the 24-hour photoperiod by morning light exposure after the lowest core body temperature, which occurs about 2 hours before spontaneous wake time. Individuals sleep best by initiating sleep when their sleep debt is high and their alerting signals are waning. People wake spontaneously when sleep debt—lowered during sleep—intersects with the rising alerting system, about 2 hours after their lowest core body temperature. It is difficult to sleep on a rising temperature, a problem experienced by night-shift workers who try to sleep during the day. It is almost impossible to initiate sleep during the few hours before core body temperature begins to fall, when alerting systems are at their "loudest." This difficulty is experienced by night owls who try to initiate sleep at more conventional bedtimes, despite the fact that their core temperature will not begin to drop until hours later.

Evaluation

Morningness–eveningness questionnaires are available (Morgenthaler et al. 2007) but are cumbersome for use in clinical settings. Because measurement of circadian markers (i.e., dim-light melatonin onset and offset) is not yet clinically available, questioning about circadian propensities is necessary. A series of probes typically suffices:

- As a child, were you the last one to fall asleep at sleepovers or slumber parties?
- In high school, did you have difficult falling sleep and waking at socially appropriate times?
- In high school, at what time of the day did you become fully alert after rising? When do you become fully alert now? (This time is likely close to the internal circadian wake time.)
- What is your sleep–wake schedule on vacations?
- Are you most alert in the morning or in the evening?
- How many alarms do you use?
- Is anyone in your family a night owl?

Additionally, the completion of sleep diaries/logs by patients over a 2-week period or more can help detect abnormal sleep–wake patterns, as well as the use of actigraphy (i.e., wrist-worn devices that detect body movement and ambient light to estimate sleep–wake patterns). Consumer-wearable devices (e.g., Fitbit, Jawbone UP) can also be used to assist in the detection of abnormal sleep–wake patterns, although validation studies between such devices and medical-grade actigraphs are currently limited.

It is sometimes easier to identify circadian wake times (the time of day at which a patient becomes fully alert) and work back by 7–9 hours to get an idea of likely circadian sleep-onset times. Confusion arises when patients have high sleep debts, which can occasionally induce "normal" sleep-onset times. Some patients report gradually drifting to later sleep-onset times and ultimately not sleeping at all. The latter situation could be due to a manic episode or hypothalamic malfunction but likely occurs because of light exposure before the lowest core body temperature, which shifts the clock later. Other factors might be greater sensitivity of the phase-delay portion of the phase-response curve or lack of exposure to "morning light," which would advance rhythms to an earlier time. Some patients get no daylight at all; their clock never is reset to 24 hours and appears to "run free" on a 24.2-hour schedule. True free-running sleep disorder might be present but is rare.

Treatment

Successful treatment of circadian misalignment depends on properly timed exposure to light and a "physiological" dose of melatonin. Effective treatment of circadian rhythm disorders can be provided by clinicians other than sleep specialists (Morgenthaler et al. 2007). Melatonin taken *before* and light exposure obtained *after* the lowest core body temperature resets the alerting system to an earlier time; light exposure obtained *before* and melatonin taken *after* the lowest core body temperature pushes the alerting system to a later schedule. If the retinohypothalamic tract (the photic pathway involved in the circadian rhythms of mammals) is intact, blind people can be treated with light. Patients in whom this tract is interrupted and "free running" (i.e., controlled by the 24.2-hour endogenous rhythm) can be reentrained with melatonin given at bedtime.

The recommended treatment regimen for the delayed sleep-phase type of circadian rhythm sleep–wake disorder is as follows:

1. Have patient reduce exposure to evening light (e.g., dim computer displays).
2. Once the circadian schedule and timing of lowest core body temperature are estimated, have patient sleep in tune with his or her alerting system for 1–2 nights (i.e., initiate sleep and wake spontaneously late).
3. Advise patient to take a small dose of immediate-release melatonin (0.3–1.0 mg) 7 hours before the estimated circadian sleep-onset time, and then take melatonin 30–45 minutes earlier each night.
4. Have patients choose a melatonin regimen conducive to their schedules so that they will not forget their dose; smartphone alarms are useful in this regard. If patients "feel" the dose (e.g., feel cold or sleepy after taking it), they should take a smaller dose (0.25 mg has been shown to shift clocks, but some patients may require more).
5. Recommend that patient, upon spontaneous (not alarm clock) awakening (which should be about 2 hours after lowest core body temperature), go outside, even if

the sky is cloudy, for 45 minutes, or use a 10,000-lux light. Patient should avoid strenuous exercise or use of sunglasses during this time.

6. Recommend that patient set his or her alarm for a 30- to 45-minute earlier wake time each day, obtain light exposure upon awakening, and repeat until the desired schedule is reached.
7. If the patient must wake for school or work before the lowest core body temperature is reached, instruct him or her to wear sunglasses (or blue-blocker lenses) until 2 hours after the estimated lowest core body temperature. For instance, if estimated spontaneous wake time is noon, lowest temperature will be around 10 A.M.; thus, the patient should take off sunglasses at noon on the first day, take them off 30–45 minutes earlier on the second day, and so on.
8. Once patient reaches the desired schedule, advise him or her to keep to the same wake time (within 45 minutes or so). Such schedule stability is rarely possible for adolescents and young adults; however, they should derive reassurance from the fact that they shifted once, so they can do it again.
9. Instruct patient on recovery strategies. For example, if out late at night, patient should try to keep to his or her circadian wake time (within 45 minutes) and take a brief nap later in the day if sleepy. If patient drifts to a later wake time on weekends, a small dose of melatonin at 6 P.M. will help with "Sunday night" insomnia.

Finally, recommend that the patient keep a sleep diary/log detailing 1) timing of sleep, 2) light exposure, and 3) melatonin ingestion. Light exposure at "alarm clock" wake time, if *before* the lowest core body temperature is reached, delays rhythms and is one cause of treatment "failures." We evolved to sleep best when we sleep in tune with our circadian rhythms. Deviation from an "in phase" schedule is a common cause of poor or insufficient sleep and of sleepiness when we need to be awake.

Obstructive Sleep Apnea (Sleep-Related Breathing Disorder)

OSA is always part of the differential diagnosis of insomnia, and EDS and should be considered when conditions known to be associated with OSA are present. OSA is present in 2% of children, is common in genetic disorders such as Down syndrome, and is present in up to 15% of middle-aged adults and more than 20% of elderly persons. OSA is associated with problems in addition to insomnia and EDS—including depression and treatment-resistant depression; attentional problems in children (sometimes diagnosed as ADHD); impaired cognition; declines in work and school performance; increased risk of cardiovascular heart disease, hypertension, and stroke; gastroesophageal reflux and heartburn; morning headaches; nocturia; erectile dysfunction; and decreased libido—and is often present in sleepwalkers and people with diabetes.

Presentation

Key symptoms of snoring and daytime sleepiness are often not obvious because many patients with OSA are not subjectively sleepy, and some hardly snore. For instance, women may present with insomnia and fatigue rather than loud snoring or sleepiness. Symptoms may be subtle in children, sometimes manifesting as behavioral, attentional (ADHD), or sleep problems. Other symptoms that should trigger suspicion of OSA in children include mouth breathing, night sweats, morning head-aches, poor speech articulation and swallowing, failure to thrive, developmental de-lays, and return of enuresis after being dry.

Obesity is the strongest risk factor for OSA. The prevalence of OSA is much higher in patients with cardiac or metabolic disorders. Psychotropic medication–induced weight gain may also contribute to the development of OSA. Hypothyroidism, Cush-ing's syndrome, acromegaly, cerebral palsy, Down syndrome, Prader-Willi syndrome, neuromuscular disease, Parkinson's disease, asthma, and sickle-cell disease also in-crease the risk.

Morbidity and mortality from OSA increase with age, peaking in the mid-50s. De-spite the disorder's connection with obesity, not all people with OSA are overweight; 30% are thin and fit. Craniofacial structure (narrow chin, heart-shaped face, and over-bite), genetics, and family history play a role (the incidence is twice as high in first-degree relatives of those with the syndrome).

Although risk increases with obesity and male gender, as well as with a neck cir-cumference greater than 16 inches in women and greater than 17 inches in men, adults and children of all shapes and sizes may have symptoms for many years yet remain undiagnosed until they come to clinical attention because of one of the down-stream effects of sleep apnea (e.g., heart disease, hypertension, behavioral problems) or because of fatigue or insomnia, weight gain, or "spousal arousal" (i.e., disruption of a bed partner's sleep) (Erichsen et al. 2012).

Pathophysiology

OSA is characterized by repetitive episodes of partial to complete obstruction of the upper airway during sleep. The disorder is misnamed, because complete airway ob-struction is not necessary for pathological changes to occur. A minor collapse in-creases the work of breathing and causes a shift of brain waves to faster rhythms, termed a *respiratory effort–related arousal*; a somewhat greater collapse results in *hypo-pneas*, which are associated with a drop in oxygen or an arousal; finally, a complete collapse is an *apnea*. People prone to OSA have airways that collapse with less effort, possibly as a result of physiological characteristics (e.g., narrow airway, thick neck, large tongue, small or receding chin, larger fat pads in the neck, large tonsils and ad-enoids) or because of central respiratory control issues.

Increased work of breathing exists on a continuum from primary snoring (no evidence of collapse) to total collapse. Hypoxic stress precipitates a proinflammatory response, with oxidative stress and endothelial dysfunction, which can lead to cardiovascular dis-ease, stroke, sudden cardiac death, hypertension, and pulmonary hypertension. Primary snoring is not necessarily benign. Some children diagnosed with primary snoring were found to have abnormal nighttime blood pressure (Li et al. 2009). There is evidence that mothers who snore during pregnancy are at greater risk of having babies with lower Ap-gar scores and birth weights (Ibrahim and Foldvary-Schaefer 2012).

Evaluation

Asking about snoring, witnessed breathing pauses, gasping/gagging/choking/snort-ing during sleep, and daytime sleepiness should be part of all medical and psychiatric evaluations, as should consideration of craniofacial structure (e.g., heart-shaped face, receding chin, crowded airway, overbite). If OSA is suspected, an in-laboratory polysomnogram (sleep study) or out-of-center sleep test (home sleep test) is currently the only *definitive* way to assess its presence; nocturnal oximetry and questionnaires can result in false negatives. If the diagnosis is uncertain, the clinician should refer the patient to a sleep laboratory that scores respiratory effort–related arousals, a measure that increases diagnostic sensitivity.

Treatment

If a sleep-related breathing disorder is suspected, the workup and treatment might best be initiated and managed by a sleep specialist (i.e., a physician trained in sleep medicine). In children, removal of tonsils, adenoids, and/or tissues obstructing the airway is often necessary (Marcus et al. 2012), and that may be combined with rapid maxillary expansion (i.e., orthodontic devices to widen the upper jaw); in adults, positive airway pressure (PAP; i.e., continuous positive airway pressure [CPAP], bilevel positive airway pressure [BPAP]) is usually the preferred method of treatment (Fleetham et al. 2011). Success during the early weeks of PAP treatment is critical for long-term adherence. Patients need frequent contact with sleep technologists or respiratory therapists—who are expert in mask fitting, pressure adjustment, and PAP device downloads—to track adherence and clinical response. Use of hypnotics for the first few weeks of PAP therapy is sometimes helpful. Some patients with mild-to-moderate apnea can be managed with custom-made oral appliances that help keep the upper airway open by moving the tongue or mandible forward. The fitting of these devices is the province of sleep dentistry and requires a follow-up sleep study while wearing the appliance to gauge success of therapy. Upper airway surgery is also an option, particularly in younger patients and/or those who are nonadherent or refuse PAP treatment. These types of surgery range from soft tissue surgeries (e.g., uvulopalatopharyngoplasty) to implantable devices that electrically stimulate the tongue muscles (e.g., hypoglossal stimulation) to more advanced surgeries (e.g., bimaxillary advancement). For all of these treatments, treating the breathing disorder does not necessarily mean that the sleep problem will resolve. Patients may have developed other disorders, such as insomnia, that will need independent assessment and management.

Insomnia Disorder

Insomnia is the most complex sleep disorder that nonspecialist clinicians will encounter. It is the most frequent sleep complaint; it becomes insomnia disorder when patients experience daytime symptoms, thereby turning it into a 24-hour-a-day problem. The timing of sleeplessness may shift over time, with problems of sleep initiation, continuity, and early morning awakening present in the same patient at different points. Patients who experience true daytime sleepiness (as indicated by an elevated Epworth Sleepiness Scale score) are likely different from those who are fatigued and unable to sleep day or night (except, sometimes, when away from home). It is useful to think of such patients as having a type of "anxiety disorder" about sleep. Insomnia of more than 1 year's duration increases the risk of new-onset major depression; the presence of insomnia and nightmares increases suicide risk.

Presentation

Insomnia usually coexists with other conditions: psychiatric, sleep, and medical. Although comorbid conditions may be mutually influencing (Table 20–7), each requires

TABLE 20–7.	Disorders that may coexist with insomnia

Sleep disorders
Circadian misalignment
Obstructive/central sleep apnea
Narcolepsy
Restless legs syndrome

Medical disorders
Gastroesophageal reflux disease, nocturia, pain
Urinary, bladder issues
Movement disorders
Fibromyalgia, chronic fatigue syndrome: disrupt sleep/circadian systems
Dementia: decreases sleep–wake control

Psychiatric disorders
Anxiety: increases hyperarousal
Posttraumatic stress disorder: causes insomnia and parasomnias
Depression
   Atypical depression: can cause hypersomnia
   Bipolar disorders: can cause impaired circadian control
Substance misuse: can cause insomnia, sleep disruption

individual diagnostic attention even if it is assumed that one is causing the other (Morin and Benca 2012; Schutte-Rodin et al. 2008). Patients may report experiencing fatigue, sleepiness, cognitive or mood disturbances, and reduced social, academic, and work effectiveness.

The most common form of insomnia is transient, lasting from a day or two up to several weeks, with known causes including stress of all types, excitement, ascension to high altitudes, and circadian misalignment (e.g., due to jet lag or shift work). Such problems rarely come to the attention of clinicians in early stages and may respond to a brief course of a hypnotic (see Table 20–3, "Commonly prescribed hypnotic medications"). Transient insomnias are also common during the late luteal phase of menstruation, in women with early menses, and in perimenopausal and postmenopausal women.

Of greater concern are chronic insomnias that last for weeks, months, or years, which can be associated with medical (e.g., cardiovascular disease, hypertension, type 2 diabetes) and psychiatric (anxiety, depression, elevated suicide risk, substance use) morbidity (Pigeon et al. 2012). All patients with insomnia, regardless of the initial cause, are at risk of developing an element of conditioned (psychophysiological) insomnia, which involves physiological hyperarousal due to negative conditioning and intense worry about lack of sleep.

Pathophysiology

Patients with chronic insomnia may enter sleep faster, sleep better, and sleep longer than they think, and may even be asleep when they feel they are awake—a condition called *sleep state misperception*. One of the first observations of this phenomenon by Perlis et al. (1997) noted that these patients' EEG activity is faster than normal at sleep onset, which blurs the distinction between sleep and wakefulness. Patients with insomnia secrete high levels of stress hormones, and their brain metabolism is abnormally high during sleep, as is their heart rate and sympathetic nervous system activity. Chronic day and night hyperarousal likely plays a role in patients' increased risk of developing disorders such as depression, hypertension, or cardiac disease (Bonnet and Arand 2010). Hyperaroused patients commonly experience multiple failed medication trials but do respond to mindfulness-based interventions and cognitive-behavioral therapy for insomnia (including sleep restriction and stimulus control).

Evaluation

Figure 20–2 presents a "road map" to guide evaluation and treatment of insomnia. Identification of Spielman's "3 Ps"— the predisposing, precipitating, and perpetuating factors for insomnia—provides the framework for generating a list of potential causes, identifying coexisting conditions, and planning (or referring the patient for) treatment. One or all of the "Ps" may require clinical attention (Ebben and Spielman 2009), as detailed in the following:

- Predisposing factors: The predisposition for insomnia is increased in women; in people with a family or prior history of insomnia, anxiety, or depression; and in people who have an "active mind" and a tendency to worry or who are "light sleepers" and have trouble disengaging from the world. Predisposing factors (i.e., anxiety) may need to be addressed separately from the insomnia. However, addressing the insomnia alone sometimes moderates preexisting anxiety and depression.
- Precipitating factors: Anything that causes a sleepless night or two can precipitate insomnia (see Table 20–7). If the precipitant is still active, it and the insomnia may need individual attention. Usually when precipitants are long gone, Epworth scores tend to be low despite complaints of sleepiness.
- Perpetuating factors: At a certain point, the insomnia develops a life of its own. Concern, worry, and catastrophizing about sleep loss create difficulties for patients, who begin to view their beds as a place of defeat; their ability to sleep is derailed by performance anxiety. They may sleep better on the couch or away from home, including in the sleep laboratory. They often search for the perfect sleeping pill, as do their physicians, who may prescribe drugs in ever-increasing dosages. Patients' behaviors may further adversely affect their sleep: they may go to bed too early, lie in bed for long periods trying to sleep, or resort to alcohol or marijuana to initiate sleep. Despite feeling sleepy, these patients may be so hyperaroused that they cannot sleep even if given the chance to nap. When they finally do sleep, their sleep is unstable.

Treatment

After coexisting disorders have been or are being addressed, the general approach to patients with insomnia is as follows:

1. Acutely, consider a brief trial of hypnotic medication aimed at upregulating inhibitory systems, downregulating activating systems, or both. Remember that underlying circadian rhythm disorders respond poorly to hypnotics if aberrant circadian timing is not corrected. Discuss behavioral treatments as well.

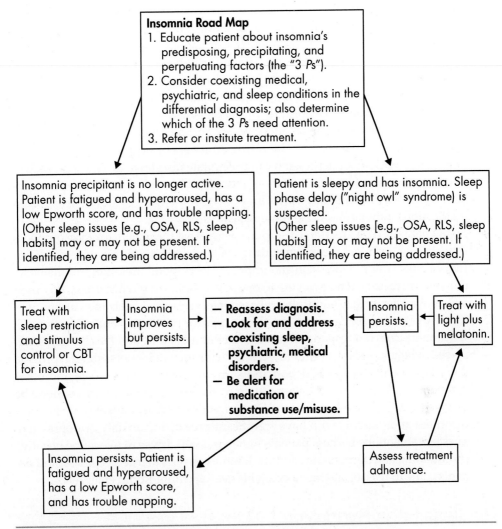

FIGURE 20–2. Insomnia road map: a guide to evaluation and treatment.

More than one problem may impact sleep; for example, the patient may be a night owl with obstructive sleep apnea who develops hyperaroused/psychophysiological insomnia and struggles with bipolar depression. When identified, all problems are amenable to treatment. CBT=cognitive-behavioral therapy; OSA=obstructive sleep apnea; RLS=restless legs syndrome.

2. Identify circadian sleep and wake times prior to insomnia onset and suggest that patient sleep on that schedule and avoid going to bed too early or remaining in bed in the morning trying capture a last ounce of sleep.

3. Patients may find this counterintuitive, but suggest that they spend *less* time in bed (i.e., observing a slightly later bedtime but keeping their pre-insomnia spontaneous wake time). This strategy has been found helpful for patients in the early stages of insomnia (Bootzin and Epstein 2011; Schutte-Rodin et al. 2008).

4. Educate patients about healthy sleep habits.

5. Help patients identify cognitive distortions and catastrophizing about lack of sleep.

6. Patients with chronic insomnia are often certain that something is physically wrong with their brain or body. Ask about any self-diagnoses so that they can be

addressed. Agreeing that something is physiologically amiss and describing physiological hyperarousal is helpful for many patients.

7. Ask the patient if he or she was a worrier or had an "active mind" prior to the onset of insomnia. For example, ask "If your tribe slept in a cave in Africa 30,000 years ago, would you be the one to be awake at night watching for lions?" Preexisting anxiety or depression may require separate attention.

8. Did the patient experience episodes of sleeplessness in response to life stressors prior to the onset of insomnia? Identify any current precipitants—often, events such as a job or social change, childbirth, an illness or hospitalization, bereavement, or an episode of depression can precipitate insomnia.

9. Suggest relaxation techniques such as abdominal breathing or progressive muscle relaxation. Patients may be willing to wean themselves slowly from sleep medications if they respond to these measures.

10. For all patients with any sleep disorder, suggest that the patient exercise outdoors three to five times per week—including walking—for 30–45 minutes, which can reduce anxiety and depression and improve sleep, blood pressure, and memory.

11. Suggest strategies patients can use to manage insomnia if it returns (e.g., go to bed later, not earlier; utilize mindfulness-based interventions or relaxation techniques; identify catastrophizing; use smart phone apps for meditation and relaxation).

12. If insomnia does not respond within a short period of time and the clinician is not versed in behavioral interventions, refer patients to practitioners who can provide these treatments. Sleep restriction and stimulus control (Table 20–8) and other components of cognitive-behavioral therapy for insomnia have been found to be as effective as sedative-hypnotic medication, even in elderly patients with medical disorders and patients who have significant preexisting anxiety or depression. These interventions harness patients' inherent sleep drives to overcome negative conditioning and perpetuating factors; fatigue converts to true sleepiness, and patients come to reassociate their beds with sleep (Schutte-Rodin et al. 2008).

Restless Legs Syndrome

RLS is rarely mentioned by patients, but its prevalence is 3%–15% and appears to be increasing, possibly because advertisements for dopamine agonists have raised public awareness of the symptoms, enabling sufferers to identify the cause of their nighttime discomfort. Depending on intensity and frequency, RLS may adversely affect sleep and have serious health consequences. RLS can be primary and familial or secondary due to a variety of other factors, including medications. It is one of several potentially iatrogenic sleep disorders, a category including NREM sleep arousal disorders (e.g., sleepwalking), REM sleep behavior disorder, and OSA, all of which can be precipitated or worsened by psychotropic medications.

Presentation

RLS is a waking diagnosis and needs to be differentiated from nervous foot shaking (unless this relieves leg discomfort) and periodic limb movements in sleep (PLMS) (although PLMS is found in the majority of patients with RLS). RLS is a neurological disorder characterized by the urge to move parts of one's body—most often the legs and/or arms—to relieve uncomfortable or unusual sensations. Patients have a hard time de-

TABLE 20–8.   **Sleep restriction and stimulus control**

Identify spontaneous sleep and wake times that existed prior to insomnia onset.

Identify catastrophizing about sleep.

Have patient keep a sleep diary for a week. Estimate mean total sleep time (TST).

Set bedtime and wake-up time to encompass only the patient's TST. If patient thinks he or she sleeps only 5 hours a night, set the time in bed to only 5 hours (do not try less than 5 hours, or less than 5.5 hours for elderly patients). For example, if patient spends 8 hours in bed and sleeps 6 hours, and spontaneous wake time is 7 A.M., ask patient to go to bed at 1 A.M. and wake at 7 A.M.

Negotiation may be necessary. Have patient go to bed earlier if he or she feels unable to stay up that late.

Tell patient that if he or she cannot sleep within approximately 10 minutes (and starts worrying), patient should get out of bed, go into another room, do something boring in dim light, and go back to bed only when sleepy. If the patient does not fall asleep, the process should be repeated.

Advise patient not to nap during the day.

Every morning, have patient call in preceding night's estimated TST.

Calculate sleep efficiency (the ratio of TST to total time in bed). When TST reaches 85% of time in bed, have patient increase time in bed by 15 minutes. Continue until sleep efficiency remains at 85% or better. TST is considered satisfactory when patient awakes feeling that he or she has slept well.

Stimulus control helps patient to reassociate bed with sleep and requires removal of clocks from patient's sight; instruction to get out of bed after approximately 10 minutes if not asleep and to return to bed only when sleepy; and learning to think of bed as being for sleep (and sex) only.

If these measures do not lead to improvement, rethink diagnosis, possibly order a polysomnogram to look for subtle sleep-disordered breathing, refer patient for cognitive-behavioral therapy for insomnia, or refer patient to a sleep physician.

scribing their symptoms, which exist on a spectrum of mild to severe and occur when patients are awake in restful situations (e.g., reading, studying, trying to sleep) and usually at night. People with RLS may use phrases such as "creeping," "runny legs," or "crawly worms" when describing symptoms; 20% of patients report pain. When seen in children, RLS may be misdiagnosed as "growing pains," and clinicians may overlook the role of RLS in precipitating attentional problems. Seventy to eighty percent of patients with RLS demonstrate PLMS, whereas 30% of patients with PLMS report symptoms of RLS. PLMS is observed on nocturnal sleep studies or noted by bed partners and is thought to correlate poorly with sleep disturbance or daytime symptoms. RLS also needs to be differentiated from akathisias attributable to antipsychotics or dopamine antagonists, nocturnal leg cramps, and peripheral neuropathy. RLS can increase the sleep pressure and sleep disruption that play a role in NREM sleep arousal disorders—sleep terrors, sleepwalking, and confusional arousals in the genetically predisposed.

Pathophysiology

Approximately 60% of RLS cases are thought to be familial, transmitted as an autosomal dominant trait with variable penetrance. Dopamine abnormalities likely play a role, and RLS is associated in some patients with low levels of serum ferritin; iron is a necessary cofactor for tyrosine hydroxylase, which is the rate-limiting step in dopamine synthesis. Risk of secondary RLS increases with age and is higher during pregnancy (third trimester). Risk is also increased in women; in persons with iron-deficiency anemia; in vegetarians; in persons with renal disease, neuropathies, ADHD, or Parkinson's disease; and in persons who abuse alcohol, use excessive caffeine, or smoke (Ibrahim and Foldvary-Schaefer 2012). Medications that precipitate or worsen RLS include most psychotropics—selective serotonin reuptake inhibitors (SSRIs), tricyclic antidepressants (TCAs), antipsychotics, and lithium—and also antihistamines. Bupropion does not cause or worsen RLS or PLMS, likely because it increases dopamine.

Evaluation

An individual who presents with an urge to move the legs that is worse at rest and worse at bedtime but is temporarily relieved by movement of the legs typically will have RLS. The RLS diagnosis can be established solely by history. A ferritin level should be obtained, and if there are conditions that might mimic RLS and need to be ruled out, further testing (i.e., electromyography/nerve conduction velocity studies to assess a peripheral neuropathy) should be obtained. If the individual states that he or she has significant daytime sleepiness and/or fragmented sleep, or the bed partner complains that the patient has leg kicking/twitching throughout the night, then a polysomnogram would be recommended to evaluate the patient for coexistent periodic limb movement disorder (as defined in the ICSD-3 [American Academy of Sleep Medicine 2014]), due to that disorder's high association with RLS. It is important to note that RLS, despite its name, has also been reported to be present in the arms and torso.

Treatment

Treatment of RLS is not necessary if symptoms rarely impact sleep. If symptoms warrant, the clinician should identify and attempt to remove offending agents such as nicotine, alcohol, or psychotropic medications.

For all patients with RLS, the clinician should obtain a serum ferritin level, which provides a measure of body iron stores. Iron needs to be replaced if levels are 50 ng/mL or less (although a level of 50 ng/mL will be reported as "normal" by laboratories). Some experts institute iron supplementation even if levels are well above 50 ng/mL, since cerebrospinal fluid ferritin levels can be lower than peripheral values. The causes of low levels need to be identified (e.g., diet). Typically, ferrous sulfate 325 mg with 100 mg vitamin C (which promotes absorption) is taken twice a day if tolerated. It should not be taken with meals. Ferritin levels should be retested every 3–4 months to avoid overtreatment and the development of hemochromatosis.

Nonmedical treatments for RLS include massage, warm baths, relaxation, exercise, and reduction of caffeine and alcohol intake. Mindfulness-based meditation has helped some patients.

Medication classes that have been found useful for treating RLS include dopamine agonists (e.g., ropinirole, pramipexole), which can provide 90%–100% relief of RLS symptoms (Earley 2003); opiates (e.g., methadone); anticonvulsants (e.g., gabapentin, gabapentin enacarbil); and benzodiazepines (e.g., clonazepam). Although widely prescribed, dopamine agonists can cause symptom rebound and augmentation; for this reason, some sleep clinicians prefer not to prescribe these agents.

Step Four, Part B: Consider Possible Presence of Other Sleep Disorders

Of the three disorder categories reviewed in this step, two—NREM sleep arousal disorders and REM sleep behavior disorder—are parasomnias (abnormal movements and behaviors associated with sleep). These disorders are potentially dangerous, can be precipitated by psychotropic medications, and may be confused with one another.

NREM Sleep Arousal Disorders (Sleepwalking, Sleep Terrors)

NREM sleep arousal disorders affect about 17% of children and typically resolve in early adolescence; these disorders are also present in about 4% of adults. In DSM-5, NREM sleep arousal events are separated into two types, which may blend into each other: sleepwalking and sleep terrors (confusional arousals are still considered by some to be part of this spectrum). Episodes typically arise out of slow-wave sleep during the first third of the sleep period, when NREM sleep predominates. Patients are hard to wake, although their eyes are open; in the morning, they have little or no recall of their activities.

Sleep-related eating and sleep-related sexual behavior (sexsomnia) are likely subtypes of sleepwalking. These disorders may be activated by sedative-hypnotics and respond to dosage reduction. Sleep-related eating should not be confused with night eating syndrome, an ill-defined condition in which awake patients binge-eat late at night. It is thought that this behavior may be due in part to circadian delays; treatment may involve sertraline and raising nighttime melatonin secretion.

Presentation

NREM sleep arousal disorder symptoms exist on a continuum: confusional arousals (sitting up, eyes open, talking), sleep terrors (usually beginning with a bloodcurdling scream), and sleepwalking all can occur in the same patient. During episodes, frontal lobes are "offline"; patients appear to be awake, with open eyes, and may be able to converse, but awareness is not present. Sleepwalkers have climbed (or fallen) out of windows, jumped off roofs, driven cars, and attacked people who got in their way or tried to wake them. In the morning, sleepwalkers are partially or totally amnestic for nighttime events.

Pathophysiology

The pathophysiology of NREM arousal disorders is poorly understood. Fragmented slow-wave sleep, sleep-state dissociation, and genetic factors are part of the story (Zadra et al. 2013). A family history is found in about 80% of patients. Arousal events occur during the first third of sleep, when slow-wave sleep (N3, which can be abnormally fragmented) predominates. They can also arise out of N2 sleep, especially if patients are extremely sleep deprived. In addition, the concept of "local sleep"—that sleep and wakefulness are not mutually exclusive but can coexist, a phenomenon that is seen in dolphins, for instance—is increasingly accepted (Huber et al. 2004).

Evaluation

Pressman's (2007) predisposing, priming, and precipitating factors can be a useful tool in evaluating NREM sleep arousal episodes. Genetically *predisposed* individuals are *primed* to sleepwalk as a result of conditions such as increased sleep pressure (from sleep deprivation, schedule changes, or poor sleep hygiene) or substances such as alcohol or medications (e.g., propranolol, antiarrhythmics, sedatives, hypnotics, antidepressants, lithium, L-dopa, antipsychotics, antihistamines). *Precipitating* triggers set episodes in motion. Sleepwalkers may have subtle OSA or RLS, which can increase sleep pressure (*priming*) and sleep fragmentation (*precipitating*). Other sleepwalking triggers include stress, anxiety, migraine, fever, gastroesophageal reflux disease, excessive caffeine intake, a full bladder, and stimuli such as noise, light, or contact with another sleeping person. Polysomnography is required if coexisting OSA is suspected, if events are frequent or stereotyped and seizures are suspected, or if patients do not respond to treatment or are injured.

Seizure disorders must also be considered with nocturnal motor behavior, especially when behaviors do not quite fit the profile of typical REM and NREM parasomnias. Seizure behaviors are usually stereotypical and repetitive, and patients often have a history of daytime epilepsy. When seizures are part of the differential diagnosis, patients require nocturnal polysomnography with a seizure montage.

Treatment

Establishing safety for the sleepwalking patient is the first step in treatment. Precautions are described in Table 20–9. Most patients can be gently redirected back to bed, but touching or attempting to wake someone in the throes of an event may trigger an aggressive response. Patients need to be screened for sleep disorders that increase sleep pressure or disrupt sleep (e.g., OSA or RLS). They should stop taking possibly offending medications. Patients should be encouraged to improve their sleep hygiene by keeping regular sleep schedules with adequate sleep opportunities. Sleep pressure can be decreased by extending sleep time (even by 20–30 minutes per night) to reduce sleep deprivation. Stress reduction at bedtime may diminish events. Relaxation techniques such as abdominal breathing, progressive relaxation, and self-hypnosis have been used with some success. Scheduled awakenings by parents before the child typically wakes can be helpful in some cases. For patients who do not respond to behavioral measures, low-dose clonazepam, TCAs, SSRIs, and melatonin have been found useful, although few studies support these treatments.

REM Sleep Behavior Disorder

Except for some skeletal muscles (e.g., eyes, diaphragm), we are paralyzed while we dream. Failure of muscle inhibition during REM sleep leads to acting out of dreams, sometimes with violent behaviors—such as punching, kicking, and tackling—that are likely to injure the patient or his or her bed partner. REM sleep behavior disorder may herald neurodegenerative disease or be induced by commonly used medications.

Presentation

In contrast to sleepwalkers, whose eyes are open and whose arousal events typically occur in the first part of the sleep period, individuals with REM sleep behavior disor-

TABLE 20–9.	Safety precautions for sleepwalkers

Put locks on doors and windows to prevent sleepwalker from leaving the safety of indoors.

Use inexpensive ultrasonic burglar alarms to alert others that sleepwalker is on the move.

Remove hazardous objects from the bedroom to avoid injury to sleepwalker or others.

Cover windows with heavy drapes to help prevent accidental falls.

Arrange for sleepwalker to sleep on first floor to avoid risk of a dangerous fall.

Make it difficult for sleepwalker to get out of bed during an event by having the person sleep in a sleeping bag placed on a mattress on the floor.

Do not try to awaken the sleepwalker. Instead, gently try to redirect the person back to bed.

der enact their dreams with eyes closed during the second half of the sleep period, when REM sleep episodes increase in length and intensity. Whereas it is dangerous to attempt to wake a sleepwalker, waking a dreamer can prevent injury, because patients with REM sleep behavior disorder wake fully alert and able to recount their dreams (unlike sleepwalkers, who might recall a snippet of a dream, if anything at all).

Pathophysiology

Loss of muscle atonia during REM sleep was previously thought to be rare and to occur primarily in men older than 50 years. Neurodegenerative diseases, such as Parkinson's disease, dementia with Lewy bodies, or multiple system atrophy, frequently coexist in older men with REM sleep behavior disorder, and REM sleep behavior disorder may precede their development, sometimes by many years. However, experts now suspect that REM sleep behavior disorder is more equally distributed in men and women and occurs in younger individuals more often than was previously reported, likely because of the widespread use of psychotropic medications. In people of all ages, REM sleep behavior disorder can be precipitated by antidepressants (TCAs, SSRIs, and monoamine oxidase inhibitors) as well as by alcohol consumption or excessive caffeine use. In addition, REM sleep behavior disorder coexists with narcolepsy in up to one-third of patients with that disease. When REM sleep behavior disorder occurs in young people or in women, the most likely causes are narcolepsy, medications, alcohol use, or excessive caffeine use.

Evaluation

Nocturnal in-lab polysomnography is needed to confirm the diagnosis of REM sleep behavior disorder. It will demonstrate increased muscle activity during REM sleep. It is sometimes difficult to distinguish REM sleep behavior disorder from NREM parasomnias by history, because some patients who have sleepwalking report some dreams or imagery during their episodes. Further evaluation of possible inciting causes or triggering conditions (e.g., OSA, periodic limb movement disorder) is also necessary.

Treatment

To protect both the dreamer and his or her bed partner, the clinician should advise them to sleep in different rooms until treatment is effective. Nightly low-dose clonazepam (0.25 mg) reduces dream enactment but does not restore atonia. Melatonin has been found to increase REM sleep atonia.

Narcolepsy

Narcolepsy is a relatively uncommon cause of EDS, although its pathophysiology—the loss of sleep-state control—is reasonably well understood. The relevance of this disorder for psychiatric clinicians is that it coexists with a variety of disorders, including depression and anxiety. It also may present with symptoms of insomnia and sleep disruption. Some reports caution that the waking dreams of narcolepsy have led to an erroneous diagnosis of schizophrenia (Walterfang et al. 2005).

Presentation

Onset of narcolepsy is typically during adolescence, more rarely in childhood or later life. Narcolepsy can present with insomnia and sleep disruption, but EDS is usually the first symptom, followed (sometimes by several years) by episodes of cataplexy in about 70% of patients. Cataplexy is a sudden, short (from a few seconds to 2 minutes), sometimes almost imperceptible episode of lost muscle tone triggered by emotions, usually laughter, and may include slight facial weakness, grimaces, a head bob or jaw drop, knee weakness, blurred vision, slurred speech, or total collapse. Narcolepsy with cataplexy is associated with low levels of cerebrospinal fluid hypocretin, typically less than one-third of the levels present in healthy control subjects ($\leq$110 pg/mL). Normal cerebrospinal fluid levels of hypocretin are present in patients who have narcolepsy without cataplexy (some of whom may experience "cataplexy-like" symptoms). Approximately 50% of patients in both groups (i.e., narcolepsy with and without cataplexy), as well as some patients without narcolepsy whose sleep is disrupted, report experiencing dreamlike imagery while falling asleep (hypnagogic hallucinations) or waking up (hypnopompic hallucinations) and sleep paralysis while falling asleep or waking due to REM sleep intrusion.

Pathophysiology

There are thought to be at least two forms of narcolepsy, which have been termed *idiopathic narcolepsy* and *symptomatic narcolepsy* (Nishino and Kanbayashi 2005). Idiopathic narcolepsy has long been known to have a genetic association with the human leukocyte antigen (HLA) *HLA-DR2*, further defined as primarily *HLA-DQB1*0602*. This association suggests a likely autoimmune etiology for at least some patients with narcolepsy who, for immunological reasons, lose hypothalamic neurons containing orexin/hypocretin and control of sleep switch mechanisms. Some cases of narcolepsy appear after infection (e.g., *Streptococcus*, H1N1 swine flu), with possible immune system stimulation. There is a strong familial incidence of narcolepsy, as well as an association with the HLA system, which supports both a genetic and an immunological component to human narcolepsy. Intravenous immunoglobulin infusions have been reported to induce transient improvement in a few patients. Symptomatic narcolepsy, although rare, can be caused by other disturbances of brain or neurological function, including brain injury (Burgess and Scammell 2012).

Evaluation

Symptoms provide a high degree of diagnostic certainty for narcolepsy if cataplexy is clearly present; however, polysomnography is necessary to rule out other potential causes of EDS and hypersomnia. The nocturnal polysomnogram may show a sleep latency of less than 10 minutes and a REM sleep latency of less than 20 minutes. The multiple sleep latency test (four or five nap attempts following the nocturnal polysomnogram) usually demonstrates a sleep latency of 8 minutes or less and at least two sleep-onset REM sleep episodes in patients with narcolepsy. Patients should not be taking drugs that affect REM sleep or sleepiness for at least 14 days prior to testing. False-positive tests can occur in patients with circadian rhythm disorders, drug withdrawal, or OSA. Urine drug screening should precede the polysomnogram; the clinician should keep in mind that some individuals may feign symptoms of narcolepsy to obtain stimulant drugs. Narcolepsy can also be diagnosed in the presence of low levels of cerebrospinal fluid hypocretin, typically less than one-third the levels found in healthy control subjects (≤110 pg/mL).

Treatment

Typically, diagnosis and treatment of narcolepsy are performed by a sleep specialist or neurologist. Treatment is symptomatic because loss of hypocretin/orexin neurons cannot currently be reversed. Education, lifestyle changes, and medication can help alleviate symptoms in most cases and permit a relatively normal life. Treatment has the following components:

1. Educate patient, family, and workplace about narcolepsy symptoms.
2. Recommend that the patient take a scheduled nap for 30–45 minutes at midday to help decrease sleep pressure.
3. Prescribe wake-promoting medications. Amphetamine derivatives and methylphenidate were previously the mainstays of treatment, but modafinil and armodafinil are now considered the first-line treatments.
4. Prescribe sodium oxybate (Xyrem), which has beneficial effects on daytime sleepiness, sleep disruption, and cataplexy. TCAs can also be helpful in treating cataplexy.

Conclusion

Once a sleep diagnosis is suspected or identified, the clinician may choose to refer the patient to a sleep specialist or clinic, proceed with further evaluation, or initiate treatment. A careful history should be obtained. Polysomnography is not necessary unless 1) sleep-related breathing disorder, narcolepsy, or REM sleep behavior disorder is suspected; 2) the causes of a patient's nocturnal movements require identification; or 3) insomnia treatment has been unsuccessful. A polysomnogram should not replace the clinical evaluation, although there are often surprises when a polysomnogram is obtained. Patients are frequently found to have more than one sleep disorder (e.g., detection of periodic limb movement disorder during a sleep study for OSA). An axiom of the sleep specialist is that the longer we live, the longer the list of things that can disturb our sleep becomes.

Disordered sleep imposes a heavy burden, especially for patients already weighed down by illness or stress; removal of this burden by identifying and treating the causes of sleep disturbance can make a tremendous difference in the lives of our patients. Failure to recognize an underlying sleep–wake disorder may contribute to poor health outcomes for individuals, and insufficient attention to the role of sleep in well-being and illness has important, negative consequences for the health of populations.

Key Clinical Points

- Sleep disorders are common and affect all aspects of health—metabolism, mood, cognition, and mortality. Therefore, all patients, no matter their age or the setting, can benefit from being queried about sleep.

- Because sleep disorders often coexist with other medical, psychiatric, and sleep problems, the diagnostic process is fraught with pitfalls. For example, a clinician may assume that a patient's insomnia is precipitated by his or her comorbid depression and, having identified "the cause," decide that further evaluation is not necessary. This assumption is an error, since more than one condition is frequently present.

- Clinician prejudices can also short-circuit clinical assessment. For example, a clinician who presumes that only obese people have obstructive sleep apnea may miss the diagnosis in a slender, fit patient.

- The four-step evaluation and insomnia road map presented in this chapter are aimed at helping clinicians to circumvent such pitfalls so that sleep disorders may be accurately identified and successfully treated.

- It is recommended that nonspecialist clinicians identify a sleep specialist in their region with whom they can consult when they have concerns about a patient's sleep.

References

American Academy of Sleep Medicine: International Classification of Sleep Disorders, 3rd Edition: Diagnostic and Coding Manual. Westchester, IL, American Academy of Sleep Medicine, 2014

American Psychiatric Association: Diagnostic and Statistical Manual of Mental Disorders, 4th Edition. Washington, DC, American Psychiatric Association, 1994

American Psychiatric Association: Diagnostic and Statistical Manual of Mental Disorders, 4th Edition, Text Revision. Washington, DC, American Psychiatric Association, 2000

American Psychiatric Association: Diagnostic and Statistical Manual of Mental Disorders, 5th Edition. Arlington, VA, American Psychiatric Association, 2013

Bailey MJ, Coon SL, Carter DA, et al: Night/day changes in pineal expression of >600 genes: central role of adrenergic/cAMP signaling. J Biol Chem 284(12):7606–7622, 2009 19103603

Barkoukis TJ, Matheson JK, Ferber R, et al (eds): Therapy in Sleep Medicine. Philadelphia, PA, Elsevier, 2012

Besedovsky L, Lange T, Born J: Sleep and immune function. Pflugers Arch 463(1):121–137, 2012 22071480

Boksa P: Abnormal synaptic pruning in schizophrenia: urban myth or reality? J Psychiatry Neurosci 37(2):75–77, 2012 22339991

Bonnet MH, Arand DL: Hyperarousal and insomnia: state of the science. Sleep Med Rev 14(1):9–15, 2010 19640748

Bootzin RR, Epstein DR: Understanding and treating insomnia. Annu Rev Clin Psychol 7:435–458, 2011 17716026

Borbély AA, Achermann P: Sleep homeostasis and models of sleep regulation. J Biol Rhythms 14(6):557–568, 1999 10643753

Burgess CR, Scammell TE: Narcolepsy: neural mechanisms of sleepiness and cataplexy. J Neurosci 32(36):12305–12311, 2012 22956821

Buxton OM, Cain SW, O'Connor SP, et al: Adverse metabolic consequences in humans of prolonged sleep restriction combined with circadian disruption. Sci Transl Med 4(129):129–143, 2012 22496545

Cardinali DP, Furio AM, Reyes MP, et al: The use of chronobiotics in the resynchronization of the sleep-wake cycle. Cancer Causes Control 17(4):601–609, 2006 16596316

Donga E, van Dijk M, van Dijk JG, et al: A single night of partial sleep deprivation induces insulin resistance in multiple metabolic pathways in healthy subjects. J Clin Endocrinol Metab 95(6):2963–2968, 2010 20371664

Earley CJ: Clinical practice. Restless legs syndrome. N Engl J Med 348(21):2103–2109, 2003 12761367

Ebben MR, Spielman AJ: Non-pharmacological treatments for insomnia. J Behav Med 32(3):244–254, 2009 19169804

Erichsen D, Godoy C, Gränse F, et al: Screening for sleep disorders in pediatric primary care: are we there yet? Clin Pediatr (Phila) 51(12):1125–1129, 2012 23203980

Feinberg I, Higgins LM, Khaw WY, et al: The adolescent decline of NREM delta, an indicator of brain maturation, is linked to age and sex but not to pubertal stage. Am J Physiol Regul Integr Comp Physiol 291(6):R1724–R1729, 2006 16857890

Fleetham J, Ayas N, Bradley D, et al: Canadian Thoracic Society 2011 guideline update: diagnosis and treatment of sleep disordered breathing. Can Respir J 18(1):25–47, 2011 21369547

Fort P, Bassetti CL, Luppi PH: Alternating vigilance states: new insights regarding neuronal networks and mechanisms. Eur J Neurosci 29(9):1741–1753, 2009 19473229

Freeman ME, Kanyicska B, Lerant A, et al: Prolactin: structure, function, and regulation of secretion. Physiol Rev 80(4):1523–1631, 2000 11015620

Gaus SE, Strecker RE, Tate BA, et al: Ventrolateral preoptic nucleus contains sleep-active, galaninergic neurons in multiple mammalian species. Neuroscience 115(1):285–294, 2002 12401341

Hofman MA, Swaab DF: The sexually dimorphic nucleus of the preoptic area in the human brain: a comparative morphometric study. J Anat 164:55–72, 1989 2606795

Huber R, Ghilardi MF, Massimini M, et al: Local sleep and learning. Nature 430(6995):78–81, 2004 15184907

Ibrahim S, Foldvary-Schaefer N: Sleep disorders in pregnancy: implications, evaluation, and treatment. Neurol Clin 30(3):925–936, 2012 22840797

Issa EB, Wang X: Sensory responses during sleep in primate primary and secondary auditory cortex. J Neurosci 28(53):14467–14480, 2008 19118181

Johns MW: A new method for measuring daytime sleepiness: the Epworth sleepiness scale. Sleep 14(6):540–545, 1991 1798888

Jouvet M: Research on the neural structures and responsible mechanisms in different phases of physiological sleep [in French]. Arch Ital Biol 100:125–206, 1962 14452612

Kadohira T, Kobayashi Y, Iwata Y, et al: Coronary artery endothelial dysfunction associated with sleep apnea. Angiology 62(5):397–400, 2011 21307000

Kripke DF: An ultradian biologic rhythm associated with perceptual deprivation and REM sleep. Psychosom Med 34(3):221–234, 1972 4338294

Kryger MH, Roth T, Dement W: Principles and Practice of Sleep Medicine, 6th Edition. St. Louis, MO, Elsevier, 2016

Li AM, Au CT, Ho C, et al: Blood pressure is elevated in children with primary snoring. J Pediatr 155(3):362–8.e1, 2009 19540515

Lockley SW, Evans EE, Scheer FA, et al: Short-wavelength sensitivity for the direct effects of light on alertness, vigilance, and the waking electroencephalogram in humans. Sleep 29(2):161–168, 2006 16494083

Lowe CJ, Safati A, Hall PA: The neurocognitive consequences of sleep restriction: a meta-analytic review. Neurosci Biobehav Rev 80:586–604, 2017 28757454

Lurie A: Endothelial dysfunction in adults with obstructive sleep apnea. Adv Cardiol 46:139–170, 2011 22005191

Luyster FS, Strollo PJ Jr, Zee PC, et al: Sleep: a health imperative. Sleep 35(6):727–734, 2012 22654183

Marcus CL, Brooks LJ, Draper KA, et al: Diagnosis and management of childhood obstructive sleep apnea syndrome. Pediatrics 130(3):576–584, 2012 22926173

Morgenthaler TI, Lee-Chiong T, Alessi C, et al: Practice parameters for the clinical evaluation and treatment of circadian rhythm sleep disorders. An American Academy of Sleep Medicine report. Sleep 30(11):1445–1459, 2007 18041479

Morin CM, Benca R: Chronic insomnia. Lancet 379(9821):1129–1141, 2012 22265700

Morin CM, Bootzin RR, Buysse DJ, et al: Psychological and behavioral treatment of insomnia: update of the recent evidence (1998–2004). Sleep 29(11):1398–1414, 2006 17162986

Naidoo N, Ferber M, Master M, et al: Aging impairs the unfolded protein response to sleep deprivation and leads to proapoptotic signaling. J Neurosci 28(26):6539–6548, 2008 18579727

National Center for Health Statistics: International Classification of Diseases, Tenth Revision, Clinical Modification (ICD-10-CM), 2011 Edition. Hyattsville, MD, National Center for Health Statistics, Centers for Disease Control and Prevention, 2014. Available at: https://www.cdc.gov/nchs/icd/icd10cm.htm. Accessed September 7, 2017.

Nishino S, Kanbayashi T: Symptomatic narcolepsy, cataplexy and hypersomnia, and their implications in the hypothalamic hypocretin/orexin system. Sleep Med Rev 9(4):269–310, 2005 16006155

Perlis ML, Giles DE, Mendelson WB, et al: Psychophysiological insomnia: the behavioural model and a neurocognitive perspective. J Sleep Res 6(3):179–188, 1997 9358396

Pigeon WR, Pinquart M, Conner K: Meta-analysis of sleep disturbance and suicidal thoughts and behaviors. J Clin Psychiatry 73(9):e1160–e1167, 2012 23059158

Pressman MR: Factors that predispose, prime and precipitate NREM parasomnias in adults: clinical and forensic implications. Sleep Med Rev 11(1):5–30, discussion 31–33, 2007 17208473

Reite M, Weissberg M, Ruddy J: Clinical Manual for the Evaluation and Treatment of Sleep Disorders. Washington, DC, American Psychiatric Publishing, 2009

Roenneberg T, Kuehnle T, Juda M, et al: Epidemiology of the human circadian clock. Sleep Med Rev 11(6):429–438, 2007 17936039

Rosenthal LD, Dolan DC: The Epworth sleepiness scale in the identification of obstructive sleep apnea. J Nerv Ment Dis 196(5):429–431, 2008 18477888

Roth T, Bogan RK, Culpepper L, et al: Excessive sleepiness: under-recognized and essential marker for sleep/wake disorder management. Curr Med Res Opin 26 (suppl 2):S3–S24; quiz S25–S27, 2010 21077746

Saper CB, Scammell TE, Lu J: Hypothalamic regulation of sleep and circadian rhythms. Nature 437(7063):1257–1263, 2005 16251950

Saper CB, Fuller PM, Pedersen NP, et al: Sleep state switching. Neuron 68(6):1023–1042, 2010 21172606

Schaefer EW, Williams MV, Zee PC: Sleep and circadian misalignment for the hospitalist: a review. J Hosp Med 7(6):489–496, 2012 22290766

Schutte-Rodin S, Broch L, Buysse D, et al: Clinical guideline for the evaluation and management of chronic insomnia in adults. J Clin Sleep Med 4(5):487–504, 2008 18853708

Senthilvel E, Auckley D, Dasarathy J: Evaluation of sleep disorders in the primary care setting: history taking compared to questionnaires. J Clin Sleep Med 7(1):41–48, 2011 21344054

Siclari F, Tononi G: Local aspects of sleep and wakefulness. Curr Opin Neurobiol 44:222–227, 2017 28575720

Singletary KG, Naidoo N: Disease and degeneration of aging neural systems that integrate sleep drive and circadian oscillations. Front Neurol 2:66, 2011 22028699

Skene DJ, Arendt J: Circadian rhythm sleep disorders in the blind and their treatment with melatonin. Sleep Med 8(6):651–655, 2007 17420154

Stenberg D: Neuroanatomy and neurochemistry of sleep. Cell Mol Life Sci 64(10):1187–1204, 2007 17364141

Tassinari CA, Rubboli G, Gardella E, et al: Central pattern generators for a common semiology in fronto-limbic seizures and in parasomnias. A neuroethologic approach. Neurol Sci 26 (suppl 3):s225–s232, 2005 16331401

Tassinari CA, Cantalupo G, Högl B, et al: Neuroethological approach to frontolimbic epileptic seizures and parasomnias: the same central pattern generators for the same behaviours. Rev Neurol (Paris) 165(10):762–768, 2009 19733874

Troxel WM, Buysse DJ, Matthews KA, et al: Sleep symptoms predict the development of the metabolic syndrome. Sleep 33(12):1633–1640, 2010 21120125

Walterfang M, Upjohn E, Velakoulis D: Is schizophrenia associated with narcolepsy? Cogn Behav Neurol 18(2):113–118, 2005 15970731

Wulff K, Porcheret K, Cussans E, Foster RG: Sleep and circadian rhythm disturbances: multiple genes and multiple phenotypes. Curr Opin Genet Dev 19(3):237–246, 2009 19423332

Xie L, Kang H, Xu Q, et al: Sleep drives metabolite clearance from the adult brain. Science 342(6156):373–377, 2013 24136970

Zadra A, Desautels A, Petit D, et al: Somnambulism: clinical aspects and pathophysiological hypotheses. Lancet Neurol 12(3):285–294, 2013 23415568

Recommended Readings

Barkoukis TJ, Matheson JK, Ferber R, et al (eds): Therapy in Sleep Medicine. Philadelphia, PA, Elsevier, 2012

Kryger MH, Roth T, Dement W: Principles and Practice of Sleep Medicine, 6th Edition. St. Louis, MO, Elsevier, 2016

Perlis ML, Aloia M, Kuhn B (eds): Behavioral Treatments for Sleep Disorders: A Comprehensive Primer of Behavioral Sleep Medicine Interventions (Practical Resources for the Mental Health Professional). London, Academic Press, 2011

Reite M, Weissberg M, Ruddy J: Clinical Manual for the Evaluation and Treatment of Sleep Disorders. Washington, DC, American Psychiatric Publishing, 2009

Online Resource

American Academy of Sleep Medicine, Practice Guidelines: http://www.aasmnet.org/practiceguidelines.aspx

CHAPTER 21

Sexual Dysfunctions

Richard Balon, M.D.

Along with eating and sleeping, sex/reproduction is one of the three basic drives. For most humans, sex and sexuality play a larger role than reproduction. Sexuality also encompasses the capacity to have erotic experiences and responses. Sexuality plays a significant role in relationships between humans, is a part of social behavior, and provides pleasure to many people. Healthy sexual functioning is considered to be a part of good overall health. Sexuality permeates many aspects of life, including relationships, physical and mental health, and reproduction, as well as moral, legal, philosophical, religious, and other aspects of life.

Sexual problems are quite prevalent. In a classic epidemiological study of sexual dysfunction by Laumann et al. (1999), 43% of women and 31% of men reported experiencing some form of sexual impairment. The prevalence estimates in a similar study organized in 29 countries (Laumann et al. 2005) were fairly similar to those reported in the earlier study. For instance, lack of interest in sex and inability to reach orgasm were the most commonly reported sexual problems across the world regions, with prevalence ranges of 26%–43% and 18%–41%, respectively. The numbers from epidemiological studies, however, should always be interpreted carefully because of the lack of universally accepted operational definitions of sexual dysfunctions. Estimates of sexual dysfunction prevalence derived from use of the new, more stringent DSM-5 criteria for sexual dysfunction (American Psychiatric Association 2013) would probably be lower than estimates from earlier studies. New studies (field or others) with these criteria are not available. Nevertheless, findings from the Laumann et al. (1999, 2005) studies point out that sexual dysfunction is a frequent problem in the general population and that its prevalence increases with age and in association with other factors, such as vascular disease and being married.

In addition to having a connection with increased age and some vascular diseases, sexual dysfunctions have also been found to be associated with other physical illnesses (e.g., diabetes mellitus, prostate illness) and with various surgeries; numerous mental disorders (e.g., depression [decreased libido], anxiety disorders); and abuse of various substances and a number of psychotropic and nonpsychotropic medications

(McCabe et al. 2016). Impairment of sexual function is frequently more complex than impairment of other functions because it usually involves more than one person. It involves relationships between people, an area not well studied and understood in present-era psychiatry. The area of sexual dysfunction constitutes the crossroads of many body systems (central nervous system [CNS], endocrine glands, vascular system, peripheral nerves) and disciplines (psychiatry, psychology, endocrinology, gynecology, urology, and a new discipline: sexual medicine). Sexual health and fulfillment do not really fall perfectly into the purview of any medical discipline and therefore can be and frequently are neglected by clinicians. Psychiatrists are (or should be) attuned to both biological and psychological aspects of human sexuality. They also understand the biopsychosocial model that fits the field of human sexual dysfunction so well. They are trained in various pharmacological and psychotherapeutic modalities used in treatment of sexual dysfunction, which makes them well qualified for managing these disorders. Finally, the complexity of relationships, the possible causal factors, and the interdisciplinary character of sexual dysfunction underscore the necessity and importance of a thorough and thoughtful clinical evaluation of patients presenting with concerns regarding impaired sexual functioning.

The cornerstone of clinical evaluation is a thorough clinical interview. In addition, psychometric assessment and laboratory tests may be used, and physical examination may help. At times, interviewing the patient's sexual partner may be indicated and quite helpful. Good clinical evaluation, especially the interview, may help to distinguish between sexual dysfunction and sexual difficulties. Physical examination and laboratory tests will help in uncovering possible biological causes of some types of dysfunction (e.g., hypogonadism, genital anomaly). Psychometric assessment (see Derogatis 2008; Derogatis and Balon 2009) may contribute to some quantification of sexual dysfunction and easier, more "objective" monitoring of treatment progress; however, such assessment will not be helpful in diagnosing sexual problems because no valid, reliable, and widely tested or used diagnostic tools are available in this area.

The focus of this chapter is primarily clinical, relational, and health-related aspects of human sexuality and its impairments. From the point of view of this chapter, it does not matter in what type of relationship the sexual dysfunctions or disorders occur. We discuss only DSM-5 diagnose and do not address other aspects of human sexuality.

Biology Versus Psychology of Sexual Function

As is the case in many other mental disorders, the area of human sexuality and sexual disorders has been entrenched in the mind–body, or psychology–biology, dichotomy. This entrenchment and the essentially unknown etiology are the reasons why the classification is atheoretical (with some exceptions) and basically consensually descriptive.

The regulation of sexual functioning is quite complex and is not fully understood. It involves the CNS, peripheral nervous system, vascular system, and endocrine glands. All of these systems interact in various ways. In addition, the role of psychological issues such as mood changes, anxiety, stress, and sexual trauma in the processes underlying the regulation of sexual functioning is unquestionable. For instance, men become aroused by visual stimuli (e.g., naked body, pictures), fantasies, or physical stimulation of the genitals. These stimuli lead to involuntary discharge in the parasympathetic nerves that control the diameter and valves of the penile blood vessels. Understanding of this process has increased in recent years with the elucidation of the mechanism of action of medications used to treat erectile disorder. The stimulation actually releases nitric oxide in the corpora cavernosa. Nitric oxide activates guanylate cyclase, leading to increased production of cyclic guanosine monophosphate (cGMP). The cGMP relaxes the smooth musculature of the corpora cavernosa and thus facilitates the blood inflow into them. Increased blood inflow into the corpora cavernosa leads to their distention, which finally produces erection. Then, continued stimulation leads to emission of semen and ejaculation, which are controlled through sympathetic fibers and the pudendal nerve. Dopaminergic systems in the CNS (particularly the nucleus accumbens, which is responsible for pleasure and other structures) facilitate arousal and ejaculation, whereas serotonergic systems inhibit these functions. (These neurotransmitter systems play similar roles in women.) In addition, androgens expedite and modulate desire and, to some extent, erection and ejaculation. This description clearly demonstrates the delicate interplay of psychology and biology: stimuli lead to a biological processes cascade, which leads to erection and ejaculation, which are usually accompanied by psychological satisfaction.

The cascade of processes is similar but not the same in women. For women, physical stimulation seems to be a more important trigger than the visual stimuli or fantasies that are more important for men. Stimulation leads to blood inflow to genitalia, resulting ultimately in lubrication of the vagina and some engorgement of the clitoris. Although estrogens and progesterone play some role in modulating these processes, it is important to note that androgens also play a role in female arousal and its maintenance (testosterone is produced in the ovaries and adrenal glands in women). Other hormones, such as oxytocin (which may be involved in orgasm and arousal and in bonding of partners), play an important role in these processes.

The study of Laumann et al. (2005), among others, further demonstrates the complexity of sexual function regulation and the interplay of various factors. As these authors noted, the significant effects of age and depression across world regions support both physiological (i.e., biological) and psychological arguments about the etiology of sexual problems. Laumann et al. (2005) also reported the impact of vascular disease (with multiple etiologies) on erectile function. Furthermore, they mentioned that mental health and stress also influence sexual function. In their study, depression was associated with increased likelihood of erectile and lubrication difficulties for people in some regions of the world, whereas stress from financial problems was positively associated with the inability to reach orgasm among women and with erectile difficulties among men. Additionally, they noted,

> Relationship also plays a role in the etiology of sexual problems. In relationships in which partners show that they care one for another in everyday matters and communicate effectively about their sexual needs, one would anticipate a relatively low risk of sexual problems. In contrast, where there are difficulties in overall relationship, one would expect this to have a negative impact on sexual functioning. In the current analysis, low expectations about the future of the relationship increased the likelihood of an inability to reach orgasm among women, while being in an uncommitted relationship was positively associated with erectile difficulties in men. Finally, having infrequent sex also increased the likelihood of erectile and lubrication difficulties. (Laumann et al. 2005, p. 55)

Impairment of sexual functioning usually cannot be reduced to one causal factor; the so-called etiology is usually a multifactorial interplay of biological, psychological, relational, and other factors. There are certainly exceptions and one-factor causes (e.g., extreme depression, severed nerves innervating the sexual organs), but even those are accompanied by other changes (e.g., physiological changes in depression, psychological reactions accompanying the nerve injury). Thus, all factors—biological, psychological, and relational—and their interplay should always be considered and evaluated in all cases of impaired sexual functioning. The effects of age on sexual functioning present a challenge of diagnosing sexual dysfunctions along the age spectrum, especially in individuals with comorbid mental and/or physical illness.

Major Changes in Sexual Dysfunction Diagnostic Criteria in DSM-5

The purpose of this section is to briefly point out the major changes in the sexual dysfunction diagnoses in DSM-5 compared with DSM-IV (American Psychiatric Association 1994) and DSM-IV-TR (American Psychiatric Association 2000). These changes have occurred in response to criticisms of the DSM-IV criteria and data regarding usage of DSM-IV diagnostic categories, as well as in response to the acquisition of new data regarding sexual function. The DSM-IV diagnostic criteria were criticized as lacking precision and as not clearly differentiating normal variations in sexual function from sexual disorders that might merit medical intervention. Epidemiological data clearly indicated that problems occurring most of the time and persisting for 6 months or longer had a much lower prevalence than disorders occurring only some of the time and lasting less than 6 months (e.g., Mercer et al. 2003). Thus, in DSM-5, most of the diagnostic criteria include the requirement that symptoms be present for at least 6 months and occur on at least 75% of occasions to meet the threshold for diagnosis. The addition of the duration criterion makes the diagnosis of sexual dysfunctions more consistent with the rest of the DSM classification system. The diagnostic criteria for substance/medication-induced sexual dysfunction represent an exception; for this diagnosis, the decision was made to leave out a duration criterion so as to encourage recognition of iatrogenic sexual dysfunction.

Research has led to other major changes in DSM-5 criteria sets for some diagnoses. Normative data concerning ejaculatory latency have permitted the introduction of a more precise definition of premature (early) ejaculation. A body of research has also indicated the major overlap of problems of desire and arousal in women, leading to a new combined diagnostic entity, female sexual interest/arousal disorder. However, the creation of this diagnostic entity has been criticized by some (e.g., Balon and Clayton 2014) as lacking validity, being poorly constructed, lacking the support of many experts, and being of questionable clinical utility.

A number of other major changes have occurred for a variety of reasons. Sexual aversion disorder was deleted as a separate diagnostic entity because of lack of prevalence data, infrequent use of this diagnosis by clinicians, and uncertainty regarding its diagnostic criteria. *Male orgasmic disorder* was changed to *delayed ejaculation* because the former term was rarely used in the literature (Segraves 2010). *Premature ejaculation* was renamed *premature (early) ejaculation* because this term is more descriptive and less pejorative. Sexual dysfunctions in DSM-IV were based on the human sexual response cycle as proposed by Masters and Johnson and subsequently modified by Lief and Kaplan (Segraves and Woodard 2006). This model assumed a parallelism between male and female sexual response disorders. This assumption, although appealing in many ways, does not have empirical validation. In DSM-5, the assumption of corresponding diagnoses in the two sexes has been abandoned. For example, desire and arousal disorders have been combined for females, whereas males can receive a diagnosis of hypoactive sexual desire disorder based solely on the absence of sexual desire, and this dysfunction is kept separate from arousal impairment (i.e., erectile disorder). Dyspareunia in the past was a unisex diagnosis, although most of the research involved female patients. As also noted, the existing data suggested a lack of reliability for the DSM-IV diagnoses of vaginismus and dyspareunia and an inability to differentiate the two disorders. The DSM-5 diagnosis genito-pelvic pain/penetration disorder (GPPPD) is descriptive and intended to reflect this situation and to provide a framework to facilitate diagnosis and assessment as well as to allow for the inclusion in DSM-5 of women who have pain and penetration difficulties.

Patients with sexual dysfunction who do not meet specific DSM-5 diagnostic criteria may be assigned a diagnosis of *other specified sexual dysfunction* or *unspecified sexual dysfunction*. Subtypes and the introduction of specifiers are other major changes in DSM-5. DSM-IV included subtypes to indicate etiological factors: dysfunctions could be subtyped as being due to psychological factors or due to combined factors (e.g., psychological factors plus the contribution of a general medical condition or substance use). With the advance in knowledge concerning etiological factors, this subtype had become less useful and thus was eliminated in DSM-5. Other changes in DSM-5 included the introduction of specifiers to indicate significant comorbid factors possibly of etiological significance and the introduction of severity specifiers.

Last but not least, DSM-5 not only introduces the duration of the dysfunction into the main diagnostic criteria (as has been done for other DSM diagnoses in the past) but also at times provides fairly detailed ratings of symptom severity and frequency for specific dysfunctions. The rationale for introducing the duration and the severity and frequency ratings was to increase the homogeneity of the diagnosis and to avoid diagnosing transitional or mild changes as a disorder.

Finally, it is important to note that most of the information used in establishing diagnoses of sexual dysfunctions comes from data collected from heterosexual individuals. Thus, although some information regarding sexual dysfunction in nonheterosexual individuals exists, establishing diagnoses of sexual dysfunction(s) along the gender spectrum may pose another diagnostic challenge.

Specific Sexual Dysfunctions: Descriptions and Treatments

Delayed Ejaculation

The major feature in delayed ejaculation is a marked delay in ejaculation or inability to achieve ejaculation in spite of adequate stimulation and the conscious desire to ejaculate. The diagnosis is usually made by patient self-report and usually involves partnered sexual activity. Some men will report prolonged thrusting that produces genital discomfort without the ability to ejaculate.

Differential Diagnosis

The major differential diagnosis involves ruling out delayed ejaculation that is fully attributable to a general medical condition or to use of a drug or substance. Another major factor to be ruled out is an idiosyncratic or paraphilic arousal pattern. The major elements in the differential diagnosis are a careful history of the presenting complaint, a thorough medical history, and a careful history of all medications or illicit drugs used. A history of a situational aspect to the problem is suggestive of a psychological aspect to the disorder. An example might be a man who can ejaculate with relative ease during masturbation alone but not during partnered sexual activity. Delayed ejaculation also needs to be differentiated from other ejaculatory complaints such as anhedonic ejaculation and retrograde ejaculation.

Etiology

Minimal evidence is available concerning the etiology of lifelong delayed ejaculation. Various psychoanalytical theorists have posited anxiety or hostility toward women as well as fear of impregnation as being of etiological significance. Other clinicians have proposed that men with delayed ejaculation may have histories of an idiosyncratic masturbatory pattern that produces much more intense stimulation than vaginal intercourse (Waldinger 2009). One large epidemiological study of twin pairs did not find evidence of a strong genetic contribution to delayed ejaculation in early sexual experiences (Jern et al. 2010).

There is more evidence concerning the etiology of late-onset delayed ejaculation. In such cases, a careful history may pinpoint the introduction of a pharmacological agent shortly before the onset of the difficulty or the presence of a disease associated with ejaculatory problems. In some cases, interpersonal stress may be found to precede the onset of the problem.

Treatment

Earlier approaches to the treatment of lifelong delayed ejaculation employed insight-oriented psychotherapy. Contemporary approaches most often involve cognitive-behavioral therapies (CBTs). These approaches might include asking the patient to refrain from all sexual activities leading to orgasm that do not include the partner and to markedly decrease the frequency of orgasmic activity with the partner. The use of a vibrator by the partner to increase stimulation may also be recommended. If the patient reports being able to achieve orgasm via masturbation but not in partnered activity, the clinician may suggest that the partners incorporate stimulation similar to the masturbatory pattern into their foreplay. There have also been isolated case reports of some pharmacological agents facilitating orgasm, such as amantadine, cabergoline, pseudoephedrine, bupropion, buspirone, cyproheptadine, and intranasal oxytocin (Abdel-Hamid et al. 2016). However, there is minimal evidence that supports the efficacy of either psychological or pharmacological interventions for lifelong delayed ejaculation.

The treatment of late-onset (acquired) delayed ejaculation is based on a careful differential diagnosis. Treatment of substance- or medication-induced delayed ejaculation involves identifying the offending agent, discontinuing it, and substituting a replacement drug if necessary. Alternatively, "antidote" therapy may be used. Many psychiatric drugs are associated with sexual side effects, especially delayed ejaculation. Such side effects are especially common with serotonergic antidepressants and are usually managed by substituting bupropion or adding an antidote medication. There is some evidence that mirtazapine, nefazodone (available only in generic formulation in the United States), duloxetine, and possibly vortioxetine may have a lower incidence of sexual dysfunction than the selective serotonin reuptake inhibitors (SSRIs). Antidotes for SSRI-induced sexual dysfunction include bupropion and buspirone (among many other agents). Antipsychotic agents, especially the traditional antipsychotics and risperidone, are associated with delayed ejaculation. This side effect can usually be managed by dosage reduction or drug substitution. Drugs such as quetiapine, ziprasidone, and aripiprazole have a lower incidence of delayed ejaculation. Some evidence also suggests that benzodiazepines may delay ejaculation.

A number of general medical conditions may be associated with delayed ejaculation. Any disease or procedure that damages either the lumbar sympathetic ganglia or their connections to the genitalia can interrupt the ejaculatory reflex. Classic examples would be surgical destruction of these nerves (e.g., abdominoperineal surgery) and any disease causing autonomic nerve neuropathy (e.g., diabetes mellitus, multiple sclerosis).

The discussion of impaired or delayed male orgasm should not omit several other orgasmic difficulties, such as retrograde ejaculation (responsive to imipramine or surgery closing the bladder neck), anesthetic ejaculation (treatment is unknown), and painful ejaculation (usually associated with medication, so the treatment would be stopping the implicated agent).

Erectile Disorder

The major DSM-5 features of erectile disorder are one or more of the following: marked difficulty in obtaining an erection during sexual activity or marked difficulty in maintaining an erection until completion of sexual activity and marked decrease in erectile rigidity.

Differential Diagnosis

Erectile disorder is a psychiatric diagnosis that is used only if the erectile problem cannot be fully explained by a general medical condition. Thus, a major issue in the differential diagnosis is whether or not the problem should be coded as a psychiatric disorder. There are classic examples in which the problem is clearly due entirely to "organic" factors (i.e., sudden onset after surgical trauma to the pelvic nerves) or to psychological factors (i.e., erectile failure in an anxious, physically healthy 17-year-old during his first sexual experience). However, most cases will have mixed etiologies. Extensive medical evaluation may reveal the presence of disease that might cause erectile problems. Nevertheless, the presence of a disease state does not prove a causal relationship (Riley and Riley 2009).

The extent to which a clinician pursues possible medical etiologies to erectile problems is dependent on the patient's age, his overall health status and risk factors, and the presentation of the problem. In general, the clinical presentation provides clues re-

The APA Publishing Textbook of Psychiatry, Seventh Edition

garding the etiology. An inconsistent problem, an acute onset following psychological stress, and a situational pattern (e.g., failure in partnered activities yet normal erections on awakening or with masturbation) are all strongly suggestive of a psychological etiology to the problem. If one suspects a peripheral neuropathy, nerve conduction studies such as somatosensory evoked potentials can be performed. If one suspects a possible vascular etiology, Doppler ultrasonography and intracavernosal injection of a vasoactive drug can be employed, as well as more invasive procedures such as dynamic infusion cavernosometry. Studies of serum lipid profiles are also indicated because studies have found that the onset of erectile problems in men age 40 years and older was highly predictive of future coronary artery disease (Osondu et al. 2018). If a patient has a history compatible with low sexual desire, either bioavailable testosterone or free testosterone levels should be obtained to rule out hypogonadism. Some clinicians would also routinely order serum glucose and thyroid-stimulating hormone levels. Measurement of nocturnal tumescence in a sleep laboratory or a RigiScan (a portable device that measures nocturnal tumescence) can be employed to provide help in the differential diagnosis on the assumption that full erections during rapid eye movement sleep indicate the probable diagnosis of psychogenic impotence. Sleep erection studies and invasive vascular studies are performed much less frequently since the introduction of oral vasoactive medications. Other factors to be considered in the differential diagnosis are major depressive and anxiety disorders, both of which can be associated with erectile problems.

As discussed in the "Delayed Ejaculation" section above, medication use and substance abuse may cause erectile problems.

Etiology

Much more is known about the etiology of late-onset erectile disorder than early-onset erectile dysfunction. Population studies have indicated that approximately 8% of men experience erectile failure on their first sexual experience. Failure on the first attempt was related to a number of environmental factors, such as being intoxicated, not knowing the partner, engaging in sex due to group pressure, and not really wanting to have intercourse (Santtila et al. 2009). Jern et al. (2012) reported a weak but significant association between failure at first coital attempt and subsequent erectile dysfunction. This study indicated that many cases of early-onset erectile problems were self-limited.

Certain personality traits have been found to be associated with erectile problems. In British students, personality traits of neuroticism (anxiety proneness) were significantly associated with the presence of erectile problems. In the Massachusetts Male Aging Study (Feldman et al. 1994), personality traits of submissiveness were associated with the subsequent development of erectile dysfunction.

Population surveys have found relationships between the presence of erectile dysfunction in men 40 years and older and aging, vascular disease, smoking, and inactivity. These studies suggest that erectile disorder in this age group may have a somatic etiology, especially vascular disease. However, some follow-up studies have found that some cases of erectile dysfunction in older men resolve without intervention. Numerous population studies have found depression to be strongly associated with erectile dysfunction. Similarly, men with depression have a high incidence of erectile dysfunction that frequently resolves with the successful treatment of the depressive disorder. It is possible that there is a complex interplay of psychological and biological factors in erectile function in aging men. If the somatic substrate underlying erectile function is partially composed of age-related factors, a psychological stress that minimally influences function in a younger male may have deleterious effects in an aging male.

Treatment

Treatment of erectile disorder should start with a thorough discussion of the dysfunction and by addressing psychological issues related to loss of erection. Marital therapy, individual therapy, reevaluation of existing medication regimens, and psychoeducation should be considered. If psychological issues are obvious, the clinician might arrange to have the patient's erectile capacity measured in a sleep laboratory (e.g., by using the RigiScan).

The next step in the management of erectile disorder should be the introduction of lifestyle changes where applicable—cessation of smoking (nicotine attenuates sexual arousal even in healthy males and constricts blood vessels); abstaining from alcohol and drugs; healthy diet (low-fat diet plus exercise may preserve endothelial function by sustaining nitric oxide synthetase); and exercise (including exercise of perineal and pelvic floor muscles). All of these changes may contribute to the restoration and preservation of erectile function.

The treatment of erectile disorder has been revolutionized by the introduction of effective oral vasoactive drugs, the phosphodiesterase type 5 (PDE-5) inhibitors such as avanafil, sildenafil, tadalafil, and vardenafil (others available outside of the United States include lodenafil and udenafil). All of these drugs inhibit the degradation of cyclic cGMP, thereby prolonging the action of cGMP in causing smooth muscle relaxation of the cavernosal muscle of the penile arteries. It is important to note that no head-to-head comparisons of these four medications have been reported to date. Their only differences are in the duration of their action: tadalafil acts longer (regular low-dose tadalafil has been approved by the U.S. Food and Drug Administration [FDA] for erectile dysfunction and symptoms of benign prostatic hypertrophy). The PDE-5 inhibitors have all been shown to be effective in the treatment of psychogenic erectile problems, as well as those due to a general medical condition or substance use. They have also been shown to be effective in reversing erectile dysfunction caused by antidepressants and other psychiatric drugs. However, several lines of evidence suggest that the use of PDE-5 inhibitors alone is insufficient. A large number of PDE-5 inhibitor prescriptions are not refilled, for unknown reasons. Also, the use of PDE-5 inhibitors is not risk free. Catastrophic hypotension can result if PDE-5 inhibitors are combined with nitrates (e.g., nitroglycerin, amyl nitrate), and there is also a risk if these drugs are combined with other hypotensive agents. The psychological consequences of using these agents for psychological erectile problems are unknown. However, one study found an association between lack of confidence in obtaining an erection and recreational use of erectile dysfunction medication (Santtila et al. 2007). Most clinicians would recommend the combination of brief psychotherapy with the use of PDE-5 in cases of psychologically based erectile problems. Consensus is lacking as to when psychotherapy alone should be used instead of combining psychotherapy with PDE-5. Cases of sexual problems clearly linked to an identifiable stress would suggest a primary use of psychotherapy.

Additional options exist if the PDE-5 agents are unsuccessful. The vacuum pump combined with constriction devices or rings is useful as a reversible intervention. Other second-line interventions include the use of intracavernosal injections or intraurethral pellets of vasoactive agents such as alprostadil, papaverine, or VIP (vasoactive intestinal polypeptide)/phentolamine. Surgical implantation of penile prosthetic devices remains an option if other treatments are unsuccessful. Patients should also be reminded that various over-the-counter preparations for erectile disorder and other male sexual dysfunctions are untested and ineffective.

Psychological treatment modalities could also be part of the comprehensive management of erectile disorder. They may address certain predisposing factors (e.g., trauma, stress, relationship problems, performance anxiety) and maintaining factors (e.g., continuous marital discord, cultural issues).

Female Orgasmic Disorder

The major diagnostic feature of female orgasmic disorder is one or both of the following: marked delay in, marked infrequency of, or absence of orgasm or markedly reduced intensity of orgasmic sensations.

Differential Diagnosis

The differential diagnosis for early-onset female orgasmic disorder (FOD) is quite different from that for late-onset disorder. Many women have trouble experiencing orgasm in their early sexual experiences but acquire this skill after repeated sexual experiences. Also, women with strong religious or cultural prohibitions against the experience of sexual pleasure may have difficulty achieving orgasm.

Because women with late-onset FOD report having previously achieved orgasm without difficulty and subsequently losing this capacity, the clinician needs to examine events that have changed. These events might include relationship discord or acute stress related to events in the extended family or the woman's profession. The clinician also needs to rule out the effects of disease (usually with insidious onset) and effects of medication use or substance abuse (usually linked temporarily to the initiation or dosage increase of a medication or substance).

Etiology

Twin studies have indicated that genetic influences account for approximately 30% of the variability in frequency of orgasm during sexual contact (Dawood et al. 2005).

Acquired FOD may be related to the effects of disease, such as spinal cord injury, multiple sclerosis, or treatment (e.g., pelvic radiation) that interrupts the innervation of the genitalia. A number of pharmacological agents, such as monoamine oxidase inhibitors (MAOIs), tricyclic antidepressants (TCAs), SSRIs, combined serotonergic–adrenergic antidepressants, and many antipsychotic agents may be associated with late-onset orgasmic disorder. Drug effects are discussed in greater detail in the "Substance/Medication-Induced Sexual Dysfunction" section later in this chapter.

There is also evidence that orgasmic function may be disrupted in women with anxiety and depressive disorders.

Treatment

Treatment of lifelong FOD is usually approached using CBT involving directed masturbatory training. Most formerly anorgasmic women are able to learn to masturbate to orgasm, and some of these women are then able to transfer this skill to partner-related activities. For women who are able to masturbate to orgasm but who cannot reach orgasm in partner-related activities, conjoint CBT is often used. Because of data indicating genetic differences in orgasmic frequency, the clinician needs to appreciate that the ability to achieve orgasm may be only partially modifiable by therapeutic intervention.

Treatment of late-onset FOD is dependent on the presumed etiology and may involve drug discontinuation, referral for drug abuse treatment, individual psychotherapy, or conjoint marital psychotherapy.

Some evidence suggests that PDE-5 inhibitor therapy may be beneficial in helping women with normal libido who are relatively sexually inexperienced to achieve orgasm. There is also mixed evidence of the efficacy of bupropion in helping women who have lifelong difficulties experiencing orgasm.

Female Sexual Interest/Arousal Disorder

The features of female sexual interest/arousal disorder (FSIAD) combine absence/reduction of interest in sexual activities and absence/reduction of sexual arousal with absence or reduction of sexual fantasies, lack of or reduced sexual activity, lack of sexual excitement or pleasure, and absence/reduction of genital and nongenital sensation during sexual activity.

Thus, the DSM-5 FSIAD diagnosis basically combines features of two DSM-IV diagnoses, female hypoactive sexual desire disorder and female sexual arousal disorder. As stated in the DSM-5 discussion of diagnostic features of the disorder, this newly introduced diagnosis reflects the common empirical finding that desire and (at least subjective) arousal strongly overlap. Many women do not clearly differentiate desire (libido) from subjective arousal (e.g., Graham 2010). Also, in some women desire precedes arousal, whereas in other women desire follows arousal (Graham 2010). There are inconsistencies in how *desire*, especially in women, is defined, with some definitions focusing on sexual behavior as an indicator of desire, others focusing on spontaneous sexual thoughts and fantasies, and still others emphasizing the responsive nature of women's desire (meaning that desire may be absent prior to the lovemaking yet may arise when the female is approached and stimulated by her partner). The definition of *desire* used in DSM-IV (i.e., sexual fantasies and desire for sexual activity) was problematic, in that some women report sexual experiences that are concordant with different models of sexual response (i.e., different from the Masters and Johnson model). Therefore, loss of anticipatory desire may be relevant only to some women. Many women also report only infrequent sexual fantasies. Nevertheless, as noted, this concept has been criticized (Balon and Clayton 2014) and is not necessarily widely accepted.

Differential Diagnosis

The differential diagnosis of FSIAD should include substance/medication-induced sexual dysfunction, various medical conditions (e.g., diabetes mellitus and other endocrine diseases, menopause, vaginitis), another mental disorder (e.g., major depressive disorder, posttraumatic stress disorder), and occasional problems (frequently relational) with sexual interest/arousal.

Treatment

Because FSIAD is a new diagnostic entity, all treatment recommendations are basically speculative and untested. Thorough examination for possible underlying causes (including laboratory testing for hormone levels) should be the starting point of the treatment process. Because the same sex therapy and cognitive interventions have been used for desire problems and arousal problems in women (Laan and Both 2011), it is probably safe to assume that sex therapy (including sex education, prohibition of intercourse at the beginning, and sensate focus exercises) and CBT (including cognitive restructuring and communication about sex) should be included in the initial treatment phase and also in continuation of treatment.

Depending on underlying etiology (e.g., a hormonal deficit determined by measuring levels of hormones such as thyroid-stimulating hormone and estrogen) and symptomatology (e.g., lack of lubrication accompanying absence of desire) and after lack of success with sex therapy and CBT, various pharmacological treatments could be implemented. These may include testosterone patches (especially in women with bilateral oophorectomy), other hormones (local and systemic estrogens), bupropion, L-arginine, and PDE-5 inhibitors (Segraves and Balon 2003). None of these preparations have been approved by the FDA for this indication (understandably, because FSIAD is a new diagnostic entity) or for other sexual dysfunctions. However, in 2015, the FDA approved flibanserin (a serotonin 1A receptor agonist and serotonin 2A receptor antagonist) for use in the treatment of hypoactive sexual desire disorder in premenopausal women (the low desire must be acquired and generalized). Although this medication is indicated for DSM-IV hypoactive sexual desire disorder, it could probably be used for premenopausal women with acquired generalized FSIAD. Because of an increased risk of hypotension and syncope due to an interaction with alcohol, flibanserin is available only through an FDA-mandated risk evaluation and mitigation strategy (REMS) program—the Addyi REMS Program. The astute clinician should not forget to recommend the use of one of the numerous commercially available lubricants and moisturizers. In addition, the only FDA-approved *device* for the DSM-IV diagnosis of female sexual arousal disorder, the EROS Clitoral Therapy Device (basically a battery-powered vacuum pump devised to increase blood flow into the clitoris), should be researched to determine whether it is also useful in the management of FSIAD.

Genito-Pelvic Pain/Penetration Disorder

The DSM-5 criteria for GPPPD basically combine and simplify two previous DSM-IV sexual pain disorder diagnoses, dyspareunia and vaginismus, into one. The main symptomatology includes one or more of the following: persistent or recurrent difficulties with vaginal penetration during intercourse, marked vulvovaginal or pelvic pain during vaginal intercourse or penetration attempts, marked fear or anxiety about this pain in anticipation of or during intercourse, and marked tensing or tightening of the pelvic floor muscles during attempted vaginal penetration.

The current diagnosis of GPPPD is descriptive and intended to reflect this situation and to provide a framework to facilitate clinical diagnosis and assessment as well as to allow for the inclusion in DSM-5 of women experiencing pain and penetration difficulties.

Differential Diagnosis

Numerous medical conditions are associated with sexual pain, including congenital anomalies, gynecological cancer, endometriosis, fistulas, hemorrhoids, pelvic prolapse, sexually transmitted diseases, vaginal atrophy, vaginal infections, and neuropathies, among others. Sexual pain could also be attributed to severe relationship distress, sexual abuse, nonsexual psychiatric disorder, and other psychological factors. Some women may have pelvic floor muscle tone dysfunction (e.g., hypertonicity). As Boyer et al. (2011) pointed out, the symptoms experienced by women with sexual pain are not purely psychological or physiological in origin, but rather "represent a complex interplay among physiological, psychological and social factors" (p. 83).

The complexity and interplay of possible etiological factors underscore the importance of a comprehensive evaluation of patients with sexual pain, which should include physical evaluation, including gynecological and/or urological evaluation. Because the presence of "organic" pathology does not exclude psychological factors, a truly comprehensive examination should include comprehensive physical and psychiatric evaluations. Therefore, a thorough psychiatric examination, focused especially on sexual functioning, the patient's fears and anxieties about sex and in general, and attitudes toward sex, should be done.

Etiology

As pointed out in the differential diagnosis discussion, the etiology of sexual pain is usually multifactorial. Because this diagnostic entity is new in DSM-5, one can only speculate about the etiology.

Boyer et al. (2011) pointed out an important issue in the development and maintenance of sexual pain: that it could be "conceptualized as cyclical in nature, usually within cognitive frameworks, whereby physiological, psychological, and interpersonal variables contribute to the exacerbation of symptoms over time" (p. 89). Interestingly, Boyer and colleagues suggested that "the relationship between the (previously classified) sexual pain disorders has also been described in a cyclical fashion, whereby symptoms of dyspareunia may lead to symptoms of vaginismus and vice versa" (pp. 89–90), thereby supporting the concept of one disorder, GPPPD. The most frequently reiterated factors in maintaining the "cyclicity" are psychological issues, pelvic floor muscle dysfunction, sexual dysfunction, and avoidance of vaginal penetration. The cyclicity of sexual pain could be an important factor in treatment planning for GPPPD.

Treatment

Our discussion of the treatment of GPPPD is, in part, speculative because there are no reports of treatment of this disorder. Our recommendations are based on the recommendations for treatment of sexual pain disorders (dyspareunia, vaginitis). A more comprehensive approach, combining various treatment methods, will probably develop gradually over time. It is important to note that most of the solid, large, randomized, and/or controlled treatment trials have been done in the area of provoked vestibulodynia (for a review, see Landry et al. 2008). Most clinicians would probably combine the available tested treatment modalities.

Unfortunately, many women with sexual pain remain undiagnosed and untreated (Boyer et al. 2011), probably because they either do not seek help or are insufficiently evaluated or treated. The cornerstone for treatment of sexual pain is a comprehensive multidisciplinary evaluation, including psychiatric, gynecological, and urological examinations, as well as a detailed self-report on pain during penetration. The evaluation could include a test to assess for pain by palpating different vestibular regions with a cotton swab (Boyer et al. 2011).

Various medical and psychological treatment modalities have been used in the management of sexual pain (for a review, see Boyer et al. 2011). An initial treatment step may involve vulvar hygiene (e.g., use of mild soap and cotton underwear). Medical modalities include systematic desensitization (e.g., in the case of vaginal spasm, by first inserting dilators of gradually increasing size and then practicing guided penetration with the partner lying on his back and the patient controlling the insertion and the following movements), pelvic floor rehabilitation (applied, usually, by specialized physical therapists), pelvic floor exercises, manual therapy techniques (massage of various areas that may increase circulation and improve motility), topical medication (botulotoxin, anesthetics such as lidocaine [the efficacy remains unclear]), systemic medications (e.g., TCAs, anticonvulsants including gabapentin [however, these medications could themselves be associated with various sexual dysfunctions]), sitz baths, biofeedback, electrotherapeutic modalities (intravaginal electrical stimulation), and surgery (removal of the hypersensitive tissue causing painful intercourse actually has the highest success rate among the current treatments for provoked vestibulodynia). Psychological modalities include using various cognitive-behavioral models (including group CBT) and sex therapy. Alternative modalities such as hypnosis and acupuncture have also been studied.

Treatment of sexual pain should probably include a carefully selected combination of medical and psychological modalities based on a patient's prevailing symptomatology (pain, spasm). Treatment should be highly individualized. Follow-up treatment is recommended to prevent the cyclicity of symptomatology (a practice that makes sense clinically but remains unproven). The involvement of clinicians (e.g., physical therapist, sex therapist) from specialty clinics is highly recommended.

Male Hypoactive Sexual Desire Disorder

The central symptomatology of male hypoactive sexual desire disorder (HSDD) involves persistently or recurrently deficient (or absent) sexual/erotic thoughts or fantasies and desire for sexual activity (the judgment of deficiency is made by the clinician, taking into account numerous factors, such as age and sociocultural context, among others).

Several things need to be noted about DSM-5 criteria. In the absence of normative data about the frequency and intensity of desire for sexual activity in the general population, an operational definition for this syndrome is not possible. The clinician typically relies on patient self-report that the patient seldom or never has a desire for sexual activity and that this lack of desire is a source of stress or that there has been a marked and persistent decrease in sexual desire. Age-related decrease in sexual desire is common, especially after age 50 years. Most studies have indicated that men have higher levels of desire for sexual activity than women and that sexual desire tends to decrease with relationship duration to a greater extent in women than men. It is also worth noting that HSDD applies only to males and that a similar category does not exist for women (Brotto 2010). In women, sexual desire and arousal are combined into a single construct.

Differential Diagnosis

The differential diagnosis of male HSDD should start by ruling out possible general medical conditions (including hypogonadism, which is assessed by measuring testosterone level) and possible substance/medication-induced HSDD. Once potential "organic" causes are ruled out, the differential diagnosis varies for men with early-onset HSDD versus men with late-onset HSDD. In men with early-onset disorder, the clinician first needs to rule out an aberrant arousal pattern by determining the frequency of masturbation and the type of fantasy. If the man masturbates frequently to a fantasy not involving his partner or to activities in which his partner will not participate, the problem is clearly not HSDD. Although some clinicians have posited that many men with low sex desire may be inhibited by strong religious beliefs, there is minimal evidence that religiosity plays an etiological role in this disorder. In many cases, there will be no clear etiology to the difficulty. The patient may report a lifelong history of low interest in sexual activity and may genuinely be puzzled by the importance that many seem to place on sexual activity.

In contrast, the major focus in the differential diagnosis of late-onset male HSDD is to rule out other treatable causes of low desire. In that regard, attention is placed on ruling out low desire as part of the presentation of a depressive disorder or of an endocrinopathy (especially hypogonadism and hyperprolactinemia). Relationship issues may be involved. Occasionally, clinicians encounter aging men who are disturbed by a normal decrease in libido with age.

Treatment

Conceptualizing male HSDD within the old framework of lifelong versus acquired and generalized versus situational may help in designing the treatment approach (Maurice 2005). Situational and acquired (or late-onset) disorder may be more amenable to various treatment modalities for this otherwise difficult-to-treat dysfunction.

Early-onset male HSDD is usually first approached by a careful exploration of any attitudes or beliefs that interfere with desire. The clinician can also focus on whether there are activities that the partner can do to engender more desire in the patient. If there is a large discrepancy in desire levels between the partners, the presence of the feeling of a constant demand to perform can dampen desire in the partner feeling pressured. In such cases, the clinician might attempt to get the couple to reach a compromise about frequency of sexual expression. When all approaches fail to increase libido, the clinician can help educate the couple about how variable levels of desire can be between individuals and help the couple learn to accept their differences.

Treatment of late-onset HSDD is dependent on etiology. If the low desire is part of the presentation of a depressive disorder, the clinician would treat the depressive disorder to determine whether desire returns as depression lifts. This depression treatment involves a psychotherapeutic approach and/or a pharmacological agent that has minimal sexual side effects.

Similarly, restoration of normal endocrine function may restore libido. Testosterone replacement should be considered only in cases of clear-cut hypogonadism. If testosterone level has been consistently below normal, one may consider administration of testosterone. However, additional testing has to be done; the level of prostate-specific antigen should generally be below 3 ng/mL. The route of testosterone administration should be carefully considered because intramuscular administration produces supraphysiological levels (which are *not* more effective) followed by subnormal levels. Oral androgens may be hepatotoxic. Thus, transdermal (patch, gel) or even transbuccal administration should probably be the administration of choice. The goal is to restore the physiological levels of testosterone. Routine monitoring of lipid, hematocrit, and prostate-specific antigen levels is recommended during regular testosterone administration.

If the decreased libido is partially a function of normal aging, one might counsel the couple after they try alternative sexual activities that might increase their arousal levels.

Premature (Early) Ejaculation

The defining symptom of the premature (early) ejaculation diagnosis is a persistent or recurrent pattern of ejaculation occurring during partnered sexual activity within approximately 1 minute following vaginal penetration and before the individual wishes it. It is important to note that the diagnosis of premature (early) ejaculation may be applied to individuals engaged in nonvaginal sexual activities; specific duration criteria have not been established for these activities.

As with most of the sexual dysfunctions, lifelong (early-onset) and acquired (late-onset) subtypes are differentiated.

Differential Diagnosis

One major factor to consider in the differential diagnosis of early ejaculation is whether the problem is transient and self-limited, in which case it would not meet the criteria for a diagnosis of early ejaculation. The other factor to consider is whether the patient has a normal ejaculatory latency but he or his partner wishes it to be much longer. Excessive expectations may require clinical intervention but do not meet the criteria for early ejaculation.

Etiology

Most of the evidence regarding the etiology of early ejaculation concerns lifelong early ejaculation, and much less evidence is available concerning acquired early ejaculation. Studies of twin pairs have indicated moderate heritability of early-onset early ejaculation and diagnostic stability of the entity (Jern et al. 2007). It occurs during early sexual experiences and persists throughout life. Much of the early research concerning the genetic basis for early ejaculation concerns polymorphism of the serotonin transporter gene (Waldinger 2011). Associations between polymorphism in the serotonin 2C receptor gene and ejaculatory latencies of less than 1 minute have been found in Han Chinese subjects (Luo et al. 2010). There is also evidence of an association of lifelong early ejaculation with social phobia (Corretti et al. 2006) and with monosymptomatic enuresis (Gökçe and Ekmekcioglu 2010).

Much less is known about acquired early ejaculation. Case reports and case series suggest that it has an onset during or after the fourth decade of life and reversal of medical conditions such as hyperthyroidism and prostatitis restores latencies to baseline values (Rowland et al. 2010). These findings suggest that early- and late-onset early ejaculation may have differing etiologies.

Treatment

A commonly employed behavioral technique to train men to delay ejaculation is the start-stop technique, which may or may not be combined with the frenulum squeeze technique. In this technique, the partner stimulates the man until he signals that ejaculation is imminent. Stimulation ceases and then is restarted once his arousal level has lowered. Over time, the man gains greater and greater control over ejaculation. Although Masters and Johnson reported high success rates utilizing this approach, there is little controlled evidence documenting the efficacy of any of the behavioral approaches (Waldinger 2009).

The only treatment approaches with proven efficacy are the pharmacotherapies. Topical anesthetic creams (e.g., EMLA [eutectic mixture of local anesthetics]), although effective, are not as commonly used as oral agents because the former can also decrease the response of one's sexual partner (thus, condoms should be used).

Outside of the United States, dapoxetine, an ultrashort-acting serotonergic agent, is used as an on-demand agent to delay ejaculation. All SSRIs delay ejaculation to some degree and are used in countries where dapoxetine is unavailable, such as the United States. Most of these agents require chronic dosing; however, an on-demand approach is also possible. Paroxetine, an SSRI with the strongest delay of ejaculation among the SSRIs, is commonly employed. The usual dosage for paroxetine is 20 mg/day. Other SSRIs whose utility in delayed ejaculation has been demonstrated in clinical studies include fluoxetine and sertraline. On the basis of research studies, citalopram and fluvoxamine do not seem to be useful for this indication. The only serotonergic drug in the United States that has been tested and appears to work on demand is clomipramine, a TCA. Clomipramine needs to be taken approximately 4 hours prior to coitus. Although PDE-5 inhibitors such as sildenafil have been reported to be helpful in the treatment of ejaculation, the evidence supporting their efficacy is weak. Interestingly, there is also evidence that tramadol may aid in ejaculatory delay (McMahon and Porst 2011). In cases of acquired early ejaculation, the clinician should search for reversible etiologies, such as prostatitis and hyperthyroidism, before employing serotonergic agents.

Substance/Medication-Induced Sexual Dysfunction

The defining symptomatology of substance/medication-induced sexual dysfunction is a clinically significant disturbance in sexual function that is known—based on evidence from the history, physical examination, or laboratory findings—to have developed during or soon after substance intoxication or withdrawal from, or after exposure to, a substance/medication that is capable of producing such a disturbance.

Differential Diagnosis

The diagnosis of a substance/medication-induced sexual dysfunction is usually made by noting a close temporal relationship between the initiation of a medication or dosage increase and the occurrence of the sexual problem. The diagnosis is substantiated if the difficulty resolves when the medication is withdrawn and reappears on reintroduction of the medication. Fortunately, most medication-induced sexual side effects appear shortly after beginning the medication and dissipate quickly on medication discontinuation. For example, the onset of sexual dysfunction secondary to SSRIs may appear within 8 days of starting the medication. There have been a small number of unconfirmed case reports of SSRI-induced sexual dysfunction persisting after the drug has been discontinued. Because many psychiatric disorders are themselves associated with sexual dysfunction, it is important to establish a pretreatment baseline of sexual function prior to initiating pharmacotherapy.

Sexual dysfunction that occurs after chronic substance abuse may be harder to diagnose. For example, the adverse effects of alcohol and nicotine on sexual function (erectile dysfunction) may not develop until after years of use.

Etiology

The largest database concerning drug-induced sexual dysfunction concerns antidepressants. MAOIs, TCAs, SSRIs, and dual-mechanism serotonergic-adrenergic antidepressants have all been reported to cause sexual dysfunction (Segraves and Balon 2003). There have been reports of differences in the incidence of sexual dysfunction with different serotonergic antidepressants (Serretti and Chiesa 2009). It is unclear whether these differences, although statistically significant in large populations of patients, are clinically meaningful. Bupropion, an antidepressant without serotonergic activity, appears to have a very low incidence of sexual dysfunction and may even augment sexual responsiveness in some individuals (Segraves 2007). Similarly, nefazodone, mirtazapine, vilazodone, and vortioxetine seem to be less frequently associated with sexual dysfunction.

Antipsychotic agents have also been reported to cause sexual problems. These side effects appear to be more frequent with prolactin-elevating antipsychotic drugs (Rettenbacher et al. 2010). It is unclear if mood stabilizers have adverse effects on sexual function. Problems with orgasm can occur with higher dosages of benzodiazepines. Sexual side effects have been reported with many nonpsychiatric drugs, including cytotoxic agents, cardiovascular drugs, and hormonal agents.

Sexual problems are common with substance abuse and appear to be more frequent with heroin and methadone than with buprenorphine. Some drugs of abuse (e.g., cocaine) may increase sexual desire in the acute phase of abuse, but their chronic abuse may result in serious impairment of sexual functioning.

Treatment

The obvious treatment of choice for medication-induced sexual dysfunction is to identify the offending agent and substitute an agent without sexual side effects, if possible. Alternatively, antidotes are known for sexual side effects produced by serotonergic antidepressants. If possible, substitution of bupropion for a serotonergic antidepressant may relieve the sexual side effect. If this is impractical, the addition of bupropion 150–300 mg or buspirone 60 mg to the serotonergic antidepressant should be considered. Sildenafil has been shown to reverse serotonergic antidepressant–induced erectile dysfunction. One study found that sildenafil had a statistically significant effect in reversing SSRI-induced sexual dysfunction in women (Nurnberg et al. 2008); however, the clinical utility of this approach is unclear. There have been isolated case reports of numerous other agents (e.g., amantadine, bethanechol, bupropion, buspirone, cyproheptadine, sildenafil, stimulants, trazodone, yohimbine) that, depending on the substance associated with the dysfunction and the character of the dysfunction, are possibly effective in managing antidepressant-induced sexual dysfunction (Segraves and Balon 2003). With antipsychotic-induced sexual dysfunction, most clinicians would first attempt a dosage reduction or shift to a prolactin-sparing antipsychotic. Additionally, there have been isolated case reports of the use of various antidotes (e.g., sildenafil) to reverse antipsychotic-induced sexual dysfunction, although none of these agents have been studied in controlled trials.

In addition to stopping the offending substance, management of sexual dysfunction associated with substances of abuse should include psychoeducation, discussion of drugs and high-risk sexual behavior leading to HIV infection and other sexually transmitted diseases, and treatment of substance abuse itself.

Other Specified or Unspecified Sexual Dysfunction

In DSM-5, a symptom presentation that does not meet criteria for a specific sexual dysfunction may be coded as other specified sexual dysfunction or unspecified sexual dysfunction. The other specified or unspecified category is applied in situations in which the clinician has concluded that a sexual dysfunction is present but 1) the symptoms are atypical, mixed, or below the threshold of a sexual dysfunction; 2) the etiology is uncertain; or 3) insufficient information is available to make a diagnosis of a specific sexual dysfunction. These dysfunctions should cause clinically significant distress but should not meet *full* criteria for any sexual dysfunction. Most patients whose symptoms would qualify for an "other specified" or "unspecified" sexual dysfunction diagnosis would probably not seek treatment. However, if such patients were to seek treatment and further workup failed to identify an underlying etiology, treatment would be guided by the symptomatology. Sex therapy and psychotherapy would probably be the treatment modalities of choice. The DSM-IV diagnosis of sexual aversion disorder could probably be classified as an other specified sexual dysfunction.

Conclusion

Impairment of sexual functioning presents a complex clinical problem requiring careful differential diagnosis, multimodal treatment, and an interdisciplinary approach. It is hoped that the DSM-5 diagnoses of sexual dysfunction represent progress toward more reliable, better delineated, and homogeneous diagnoses. Progress has been made on treatment of some, especially male, sexual dysfunctions. The advent of PDE-5 inhibitors has helped millions of males with erectile disorder. Some strides have been made in the treatment of early ejaculation using the side effect of SSRIs, that is, their ability to delay ejaculation. However, efficacious treatments are lacking for delayed orgasm for both genders. The treatment of HSDD, unless a sequel of hypogonadism, is usually also a challenge. It remains to be seen whether the newly established diagnoses of FSIAD and GPPPD will provide a better clinical framework for treatment.

While treating sexual dysfunctions, clinicians need to keep reminding themselves of the multifactorial etiology of sexual dysfunction and the complex regulation of sexual functioning. Following careful diagnosis, treatment should be framed within the biopsychosocial model and approach. We do not want to suggest that any part of the proverbial biopsychosocial model is more important than the other. However, psychiatry is becoming more medicalized, and biological factors and treatments are frequently being overemphasized. Psychological and relationship factors of human sexuality remain underappreciated. Psychiatrists need to pay more attention to relational aspects of sexual dysfunction because many so-called sexual difficulties (not full-blown dysfunctions or disorders) may have their roots in impaired dyadic relations.

Key Clinical Points

- Sexual concerns have a high prevalence in the general population.

- Sexual problems have a very high prevalence in certain psychiatric subpopulations, such as patients with depression or anxiety disorders.

- Many psychiatric drugs cause sexual dysfunction.

- Many nonpsychotropic drugs (e.g., drugs used to treat cardiovascular diseases) can cause sexual dysfunction.

- Medication-induced sexual dysfunction may be an unspoken reason for medication noncompliance.

- Evaluation and treatment of sexual dysfunction are complex tasks that should only be undertaken within the framework of a biopsychosocial model.

References

Abdel-Hamid IA, Elsaied MA, Mostafa T: The drug treatment of delayed ejaculation. Transl Androl Urol 5(4):576–591, 2016 27652229

American Psychiatric Association: Diagnostic and Statistical Manual of Mental Disorders, 4th Edition. Washington, DC, American Psychiatric Association, 1994

American Psychiatric Association: Diagnostic and Statistical Manual of Mental Disorders, 4th Edition, Text Revision. Washington, DC, American Psychiatric Association, 2000

American Psychiatric Association: Diagnostic and Statistical Manual of Mental Disorders, 5th Edition. Arlington, VA, American Psychiatric Association, 2013

Balon R, Clayton AH: Female sexual interest/arousal disorder: a diagnosis out of thin air. Arch Sex Behav 43(7):1227–1229, 2014 24496785

Boyer SC, Goldfinger C, Thibault-Gagnon S, et al: Management of female sexual pain disorders. Adv Psychosom Med 31:83–104, 2011 22005206

Brotto LA: The DSM diagnostic criteria for hypoactive sexual desire disorder in men. J Sex Med 7(6):2015–2030, 2010 20929517

Corretti G, Pierucci S, De Scisciolo M, et al: Comorbidity between social phobia and premature ejaculation: study on 242 males affected by sexual disorders. J Sex Marital Ther 32(2):183–187, 2006 16418108

Dawood K, Kirk K, Bailey J, et al: Genetic and environmental influences on the frequency of orgasm in women. Twin Res Hum Genet 8(1):27–33, 2005 15836807

Derogatis LR: Clinical and research evaluation of sexual dysfunctions. Adv Psychosom Med 29:7–22, 2008 18391554

Derogatis LR, Balon R: Clinical evaluation of sexual dysfunctions, in Clinical Manual of Sexual Disorders. Edited by Balon R, Segraves RT. Washington, DC, American Psychiatric Publishing, 2009, pp 23–57

Feldman HA, Goldstein I, Hatzichristou DG, et al: Impotence and its medical and psychological correlates: results of the Massachusetts Male Aging Study. J Urol 151(1):54–61, 1994 8254833

Gökçe A, Ekmekcioglu O: The relationship between lifelong premature ejaculation and monosymptomatic enuresis. J Sex Med 7(8):2868–2872, 2010 20233291

Graham CA: The DSM diagnostic criteria for female sexual arousal disorder. Arch Sex Behav 39(2):240–255, 2010 19777335

Jern P, Santtila P, Witting K, et al: Premature and delayed ejaculation: genetic and environmental effects in a population-based sample of Finnish twins. J Sex Med 4(6):1739–1749, 2007 17888070

Jern P, Santtila P, Johansson A, et al: Is there an association between same-sex sexual experience and ejaculatory dysfunction? J Sex Marital Ther 36(4):303–312, 2010 20574886

Jern P, Gunst A, Sandnabba K, et al: Are early and current sexual problems associated with anxiety and depression in young men? A retrospective self-report study. J Sex Marital Ther 38(4):349–364, 2012 22712819

Laan E, Both S: Sexual desire and arousal disorders in women. Adv Psychosom Med 31:16–34, 2011 22005202

Landry T, Bergeron S, Dupuis MJ, et al: The treatment of provoked vestibulodynia: a critical review. Clin J Pain 24(2):155–171, 2008 18209522

Laumann EO, Paik A, Rosen RC: Sexual dysfunction in the United States: prevalence and predictors. JAMA 281(6):537–544, 1999 10022110

Laumann EO, Nicolosi A, Glasser DB, et al: Sexual problems among women and men aged 40–80 y: prevalence and correlates identified in the Global Study of Sexual Attitudes and Behaviors. Int J Impot Res 17(1):39–57, 2005 15215881

Luo S, Lu Y, Wang F, et al: Association between polymorphisms in the serotonin 2C receptor gene and premature ejaculation in Han Chinese subjects. Urol Int 85(2):204–208, 2010 20453482

Maurice WL: Male hypoactive sexual desire disorder, in Handbook of Sexual Dysfunction. Edited by Balon R, Segraves RT. New York, Taylor and Francis, 2005, pp 67–110

McCabe MP, Sharlip ID, Lewis R, et al: Risk factors for sexual dysfunction among women and men: a consensus statement from the Fourth International Consultation on Sexual Medicine 2015. J Sex Med 13(2):153–167, 2016 26953830

McMahon CG, Porst H: Oral agents for the treatment of ejaculation: review of efficacy and safety in the context of the recent International Society for Sexual Medicine criteria for lifelong premature ejaculation. J Sex Med 8(10):2707–2725, 2011 21771283

Mercer CH, Fenton KA, Johnson AM, et al: Sexual function problems and help seeking behaviour in Britain: national probability sample survey. BMJ 327(7412):426–427, 2003 12933730

Nurnberg HG, Hensley PL, Heiman JR, et al: Sildenafil treatment of women with antidepressant-associated sexual dysfunction: a randomized controlled trial. JAMA 300(4):395–404, 2008 18647982

Osondu CU, Vo B, Oni ET, et al: The relationship of erectile dysfunction and subclinical cardiovascular disease: a systematic review and meta-analysis. Vasc Med 23(1):9–20, 2018 29243995

Rettenbacher MA, Hofer A, Ebenbichler C, et al: Prolactin levels and sexual adverse effects in patients with schizophrenia during antipsychotic treatment. J Clin Psychopharmacol 30(6):711–715, 2010 21105287

Riley A, Riley E: Male erectile disorder, in Clinical Manual of Sexual Disorders. Edited by Balon R, Segraves RT. Washington, DC, American Psychiatric Publishing, 2009, pp 213–250

Rowland D, McMahon CG, Abdo C, et al: Disorders of orgasm and ejaculation in men. J Sex Med 7 (4 Pt 2):1668–1686, 2010 20388164

Santtila P, Sandnabba N, Jern P, et al: Recreational use of erectile dysfunction medication may decrease confidence in ability to gain and hold erections in young males. Int J Impot Res 19(6):591–596, 2007 17657209

Santtila P, Sandnabba NK, Jern P: Prevalence and determinants of male sexual dysfunctions during first intercourse. J Sex Marital Ther 35(2):86–105, 2009 19266379

Segraves RT: Sexual dysfunction associated with antidepressant therapy. Urol Clin North Am 34(4):575–579, vii, 2007 17983897

Segraves RT: Considerations for a better definition of male orgasmic disorder in DSM V. J Sex Med 7 (2 Pt 1):690–695, 2010 20492418

Segraves RT, Balon R: Sexual Pharmacology: Fast Facts. New York, WW Norton, 2003

Segraves R, Woodard T: Female hypoactive sexual desire disorder: history and current status. J Sex Med 3(3):408–418, 2006 16681466

Serretti A, Chiesa A: Treatment-emergent sexual dysfunction related to antidepressants: a meta-analysis. J Clin Psychopharmacol 29(3):259–266, 2009 19440080

Waldinger M: Delayed and premature ejaculation, in Clinical Manual of Sexual Disorders. Edited by Balon R, Segraves RT. Washington, DC, American Psychiatric Publishing, 2009, pp 273–304

Waldinger M: Toward evidence-based genetic research on lifelong premature ejaculation: a critical evaluation of methodology. Korean J Urol 52(1):1–8, 2011 21344023

Recommended Readings

Balon R, Segraves RT (eds): Clinical Handbook of Sexual Disorders. Washington, DC, American Psychiatric Publishing, 2009

Ishak WW (ed): The Textbook of Clinical Sexual Medicine. New York, Springer, 2017

Levine SB, Risen CB, Althof SE (eds): Handbook of Clinical Sexuality for Mental Health Professionals, 3rd Edition. New York, Routledge, 2016

Lipschutz LI, Pastuszak AW, Goldstein AT, et al (eds): Management of Sexual Dysfunction in Men and Women: An Interdisciplinary Approach. New York, Springer 2016

Segraves RT, Balon R: Sexual Pharmacology: Fast Facts. New York, WW Norton, 2003

CHAPTER 22

Gender Dysphoria

Eric Yarbrough, M.D.

Gender dysphoria is one of the most misunderstood and infrequently treated diagnoses in the *Diagnostic and Statistical Manual of Mental Disorders* (DSM). Unlike most other DSM diagnoses, gender dysphoria is caught in the middle of an ongoing culture war. Many nonclinicians have opinions about the mental health of transgender and gender-nonconforming (TGNC) people. Historically, TGNC people were seen as mentally ill, and efforts to change or correct their diversity were employed, with little success. Although the attention that transgender people are receiving in the news is recent, the treatment of gender dysphoric symptoms is almost as old as the profession of psychiatry. Today, there are gender clinics that specialize in providing care, also known as gender-affirming treatment, to gender-diverse individuals (see Glossary at the end of this chapter).

Insurance companies are now covering treatment options for TGNC people. Treatments such as hormones and gender-affirming surgeries are now being paid for, leading to an increase in the demand for access to gender-affirming care. Despite this, there are few providers who feel comfortable and knowledgeable enough to provide safe and sufficient treatment options for TGNC patients. Efforts have been made by the American Psychiatric Association to educate providers and to advocate for gender-diverse patients to have access to the best standards of clinical practice, to have the opportunity to pursue patient-focused gender-affirming treatment decisions, and to receive scientifically established treatment (Drescher and Haller 2018).

Today, more TGNC people feel comfortable coming out and living their lives in the gender identity that fits them best. Because gender dysphoria is a DSM diagnosis, psychiatrists are asked to play a gate-keeping role in deciding who is ready for gender-affirming care. This conflict creates tension between psychiatrists and patients, making it more difficult for psychiatrists to connect to the gender-diverse community. Lack of training means that personnel at hospitals, emergency departments, and outpatient clinics are sometimes hostile to transgender people seeking care (James et al. 2016; Wise 2016). Nevertheless, individual practitioners can, with very little effort, educate themselves to become both gender-affirming providers and advocates for the community.

Case 1: The Need for Gender-Affirming Care

Tia is a 24-year-old person who is seeking psychiatric care for symptoms of depression and of chronic posttraumatic stress disorder (PTSD). When she called the psychiatrist's office to make an initial appointment, she identified herself as Tia, but when she shows up for her appointment, she has a traditional masculine appearance. She is, however, wearing some makeup, and her fingernails are painted. During her evaluation, she reports symptoms of depression, including problems with sleep, appetite, anhedonia, depressed mood, and occasional suicidal ideation. She experiences chronic symptoms of traumatic stress, which include agoraphobia and flashbacks of people bullying and attacking her in the streets, and she appears to be in a constant state of elevated physiological and psychological stress that affects all areas of her life. With her somewhat androgynous appearance, she has attracted the unwanted attention of locals, who have called her names and even progressed to physically hitting her and spitting on her, simply for showing her face in public.

Tia reports that she was assigned male at birth, but early on and throughout her childhood she knew that something was different about her identity. She was more drawn to androgynous or feminine clothes, but her family would not let her express herself in this way. Instead, they forced her to wear boys' clothing, to participate in sports, and to play only with traditional "boy's" toys, such as guns or action figures. Tia describes an ongoing theme, throughout most of her childhood, of being misunderstood and having to hide who she really was. The tension between her and her parents escalated when she reached puberty, because of her unhappiness about the way her body was developing. She was upset about the hair growing on her face and body, and she would shave her body as much as she thought she could without her parents noticing. Her body was becoming more muscular and the shape of her face more elongated, which caused her even more distress. She wanted to develop breasts, have long hair, and spend time with other girls her age. Everything felt wrong to her.

Since Tia moved to college a few months ago, she has been able to separate from her parents and individuate in a new city. She would like to explore her gender identity, obtain information about hormones, speak to a doctor about surgical options, and seek treatment for her chronic symptoms of depression and PTSD. She has been to multiple other psychiatrists and they have turned her away, saying that they do not know how to help her and cannot connect her to any of the treatments she is seeking. One psychiatrist even offered to provide therapy to "cure" her so that she could identify long-term as a male.

Case 1 Discussion

Even though this narrative is just one person's experience of gender diversity, it is a very common story in the transgender community. Psychiatrists and other clinicians typically are not trained in how to work with gender-diverse people, and the transgender population has limited access to care. Tia needs help in multiple areas. First, and most critically, she is having problems with depression and PTSD. These symptoms are likely secondary to the dysphoria she is experiencing regarding her body and how she is treated by strangers. It is still too early to know for certain the causes of her problems, however, and it may take some time to separate the multiple layers of symptoms.

The other interventions Tia is asking for are ones that most psychiatrists feel ill equipped to provide or help with. She wishes to pursue gender-affirming therapy and is asking her psychiatrist to guide her through the process. Many clinicians have turned her away when they could have at least started treating her depressive symp-

toms with therapy and/or medication. Clinicians trained in the art and practice of psychiatry are actually quite able to help with such issues, even if they lack specific
knowledge about gender-affirming care. Psychiatrists trained in psychotherapy can
help patients to process ambivalence and existential crises and can provide supportive
interventions as patients move through uncharted territory. It is often a part of their
daily work. The additional effort to understand the basics of gender-affirming treatment could be explored with the patient as long as the psychiatrist involved has an
open mind regarding gender and an eagerness to learn. If, despite a desire to help, a
psychiatrist should still feel unable to provide appropriate care, it is within the scope
of practice to connect the patient to a provider who can meet the patient's needs.

The Gender Spectrum

The most difficult conceptual benchmark that clinicians struggle with when working
with gender-diverse patients is the understanding that gender exists on a continuum
rather than as an either/or dichotomy. The phenomenon of gender has always been
built on the biological presentation of sex. Male or female sex is identified on the basis
of the external genitalia at birth, but what comes after that largely depends on when
and where one is born. Gender resides in the mind, not in the genitals. Most of our
understanding about what makes people masculine or feminine is a social construct
(Levitt and Ippolito 2014).

One way to understand the gender-diverse population is to stop thinking of people as purely masculine or feminine and instead think of people as existing on a spectrum of masculinity and femininity. Within the gender spectrum, people can be both
masculine and feminine (i.e., androgynous) (Stone 2013). The gender spectrum does
not apply only to the transgender population; it applies to all of us. Grasping that
gender is neither assigned nor constant from birth will ease the process of working
with gender-diverse people. In the end, we are all people, and we are all trying to figure out how to express ourselves and where we fit in the larger world. Gender-
diverse individuals are people who fall outside the typical cultural norms of what we
call masculine and feminine and of how we perceive these traits to relate to the male
or female sex.

Gender Dysphoria

Diagnostic concepts and terms used in thinking about and describing gender dysphoria continue to be controversial. The DSM diagnosis has evolved over time, both in the
way we understand it and in the way we conceptualize it (Drescher 2010b). In DSM-
IV (American Psychiatric Association 1994), the diagnosis of gender identity disorder
was defined as "a strong and persistent cross-gender identification accompanied by
persistent discomfort with one's assigned sex," and gender dysphoria was a specifier
applied to the diagnosis of transvestic fetishism, a paraphilia in which people dress up
as the opposite sex largely for sexual pleasure, and not because they feel themselves to
be the opposite gender. Gradually, a distinction began to be made between gender
identity and gender role—with *gender identity* being what a person views themselves

to be in their mind and *gender role* being how a person portrays themselves to the outside world. This awareness of levels of gender difference and of the fact that people can present and view themselves in a variety of ways led to a deeper understanding of the gender spectrum.

The DSM-IV diagnosis of gender identity disorder defined a person's desire to be the opposite gender through criteria that focused mainly on behaviors—on how someone dressed and presented themselves to the outside world. DSM-IV also continued to focus on the dichotomy of two genders—male and female.

In DSM-5 (American Psychiatric Association 2013), gender identity disorder was changed to gender dysphoria, in an effort to depathologize gender diversity yet still offer an avenue to care for people seeking treatment (Drescher 2010a). Gender dysphoria was given its own chapter, separate from the sexual dysfunctions and the paraphilias. The new diagnosis went a long way in separating dysphoria from transvestism, although the two are still conflated by many. The criteria also incorporated new terminology, providing expanded definitions of *gender* and many other terms. The gender dysphoria diagnosis focuses on the individual's personal, interior identity and how they view themselves. To meet criteria for the diagnosis, a person must have "a marked incongruence between their experienced/expressed gender and their assigned gender, of at least 6 months' duration" (DSM-5, p. 452). This wording still restricts our understanding of gender diversity to a gender dichotomy. Perhaps "another gender" might be used in future editions if the diagnosis remains a part of DSM.

Many people still believe that gender-diverse people are mentally ill, and given that the diagnosis appears in a manual of mental disorders (DSM), it makes sense that there is still confusion. Being diverse in one's gender presentation is not in itself a mental illness, but having dysphoric feelings about one's primary and secondary sex characteristics as well as about being labeled as "the wrong gender" can lead to psychiatric symptoms (Berlin 2016). Being uncomfortable with or experiencing distress regarding one's body or the gender that one is assigned by society will qualify for a diagnosis of gender dysphoria. It is also important to understand that certain symptoms arise because of the way that society labels and responds to gender-diverse people. These symptoms might not be present if society were more open to a spectrum of gender expression (Belluardo-Crosby and Lillis 2012).

The diagnosis of gender dysphoria will continue to evolve. In many ways, the diagnosis may be seen as mirroring the evolution of homosexuality, from its beginnings and various diagnostic incarnations to its ultimate removal from DSM (Drescher 2010a). Eventually, gender dysphoria may be removed from DSM altogether and exist only as an endocrine disorder. Although such an outcome would have positive impacts on how the world views people who are gender diverse, there might be negative repercussions for those seeking access to care. Insurance companies take the view that gender dysphoria is a mental illness and that treatments should be offered to relieve symptoms. As society continues to change, only time will tell how the diagnosis will ultimately unfold. For the foreseeable future, however, psychiatrists will be needed to help gender-diverse people obtain access to care and exist in a world that is hostile to diverse gender expressions (Griffin 2011).

History and Epidemiology

There have always been people who lived outside of traditional gender stereotypes (Stern 2009). It was just before the midpoint of the twentieth century that people first began to seek out hormonal and surgical options to change their external appearance to match the gender they felt themselves to be in their mind (Jorgensen 1967). Over time, these medical treatments became more available. Gender clinics specializing in gender-affirming care became more common in the 1970s. Harry Benjamin was one of the first physicians to specialize in providing these treatments (Yarbrough 2018). His work, and that of many others, eventually led to formation of the World Professional Association of Transgender Health, which is seen as the leading authority in regard to defining the standards of gender-affirming care (World Professional Association for Transgender Health 2018).

It was not until the current decade that the specialty of transgender medicine began to be more widely accepted. As can be seen in Figure 22–1, the number of people seeking gender-affirming treatment has skyrocketed since 2010, mainly because society has become slightly more accepting. Gender-diverse people are more comfortable coming out and publicly expressing who they are.

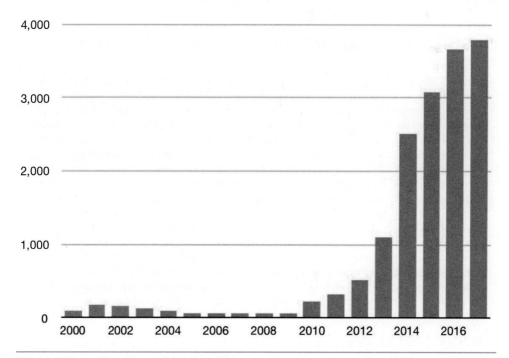

FIGURE 22–1. Numbers of gender-diverse patients served at Callen-Lorde Community Health Center, New York City, 2000–2016.

The numbers of gender-diverse people seeking care have grown significantly in the past 10 years

Source. Reprinted from Figure 4–1 (p. 44) in Yarbrough E: *Transgender Mental Health.* Washington, DC, American Psychiatric Publishing, 2018. Copyright 2018, American Psychiatric Publishing. Used with permission.

Not all gender-diverse people will seek medical or surgical interventions. People can identify as being gender diverse in some way without experiencing gender-dysphoric symptoms as defined in DSM, and this reality makes the concept of gender dysphoria more complicated to study. Some research looks at individuals who are gender diverse, whereas other research looks at individuals who meet criteria for gender dysphoria. Describing a gender-diverse person as someone who identifies as something different from the sex they were assigned at birth is one way to characterize this community. When gender diversity is defined in this way, as many as 1 in 150 people would be considered to meet the definition (Flores et al. 2016).

It is still unclear where gender diversity comes from. Many believe that gender diversity is a normal variation of the human condition, as is homosexuality (Erickson-Schroth and Jacobs 2017). Biological research examining brain morphology, prenatal hormone exposure, and fetal development has yielded little in the way of definitive evidence regarding the origins of gender diversity (Erickson-Schroth 2013). The search for reasons for diverse gender presentations prompts ethical questions—What would we do with such information were we to find it? Given the multiple variations of gender expressions within the gender-diverse community, it is unlikely that there is only one path to gender diversity. Some might say that gender diversity is part of a natural progression of humanity, and that as we evolve, the concept of gender and the presentation of gender will assume less importance.

Case 2: The Red Herring of Gender Dysphoria

Bret is a 30-year-old man of transgender experience. When he was 13 years old, he came out to his family as transgender, and they kicked him out of their home. Since then, he has been living on the streets and in a homeless shelter. He has a significant history of bipolar disorder in his family, and he first presented to a community outpatient clinic after he experienced a manic episode and was stabilized in the hospital. Because he was symptomatic for the past 6 months, he lost his job and has become homeless again.

As a result of his current medication regimen, Bret now has only minor symptoms and is doing well. He is at the clinic for continued medication management and gender-affirming therapy. He has never met a clinician who understands transgender mental health, and he would like to find such a clinician with whom he can discuss steps in treating his gender-dysphoric symptoms. He had been taking testosterone for the past 10 years, but it was stopped while he was in the hospital because of concerns that it was contributing to his manic symptoms. He has had no surgical procedures as yet but is interested in top surgery and bottom surgery (i.e., surgery that involves the breast/chest and the genitals, respectively). He is ambivalent about bottom surgery because he has heard that outcomes are generally mixed. He would like advice on what to do.

Case 2 Discussion

Bret's case is a complicated one and should be approached from a biopsychosocial stance. First, he is homeless and needs basic social supports in order to help him function and recover. Contacting the homeless shelter and ensuring that he is placed in a male-identified room might be necessary. Bret can tell you what he prefers. Furthermore, it will be necessary to look into why his testosterone was stopped. An inpatient clinician might have been quick to blame hormones for psychiatric symptoms despite the fact that Bret had been stable on hormones for a decade. Many of the concerns surrounding hormones are unwarranted, and contraindications are generally rare (Ettner et al. 2007).

Clinicians might also be quick to identify bipolar disorder as the "cause" of Bret's gender diversity. They may claim that his mania is responsible for "making him transgender." Transgender people are like anyone else in that they can develop symptoms of chronic and persistent mental illness. It is rare for a psychiatric illness to cause symptoms of gender dysphoria.

Bret is also interested in surgical treatment options. His ambivalence about surgery is a common and normal response. Anyone considering surgical treatment should weigh the pros and cons of the outcomes. Bret's diagnosis of bipolar disorder does not rule him out as a candidate for surgical procedures. A person who is stable and who understands the risks and benefits of treatment is capable of making decisions regarding care.

Comorbidity

The presence of comorbid psychiatric disorders alongside gender dysphoria is quite common. It is generally believed that the high levels of psychiatric comorbidity among gender-diverse people are largely attributable to the hostile and unaccepting environments in which many transgender people grow up. The added daily stressors, best explained by the minority stress model (Brewster et al. 2012), can lead to development and/or worsening of symptoms that might not emerge in people who are not exposed to such stressors.

Compared with the general population, transgender people report higher levels of stress, trauma, depression, anxiety, substance use, suicidal ideation, and suicide attempts. Discrimination is a common social stressor present in many areas of transgender individuals' lives—at home, at work, in the medical setting, and out in the community (Kattari and Hasche 2016). There are no "safe zones" for transgender people; their mere presence in any public place or crowded area could potentially lead to discrimination or violence. This need to continually monitor one's surroundings for potential threats can lead to the posttraumatic effects commonly seen in the transgender population.

Knowing about transgender mental health is necessary so as not to overdiagnose common experiences as a disorder. Because of the frequency of traumatic reactions and suicidal ideation, many transgender people are diagnosed with borderline personality disorder, particularly in an emergency department, where they are at their most vulnerable. Mood lability, impulsivity, and suicidal ideation are common symptoms of a personality disorder, but such symptoms could also affect anyone exposed to the daily threats faced by those in the lesbian, gay, bisexual, transgender, and queer (LGBTQ) population (Budge et al. 2013). Typically, a person who is in a stage of coming out or transitioning is more susceptible to these symptoms; however, the symptoms often resolve once the person is in a more stable place (Bariola et al. 2015). Anyone who is LGBTQ would need a more extensive observation over time before a diagnosis such as a personality disorder could be made.

Gender-Affirming Treatments

Therapy

Conceptually, gender-affirming therapy is simple to understand. It involves taking the stance that gender diversity is not pathological and that the gender spectrum has many presentations. We do not approach patients in an effort to identify who they are for them; instead, we create space for patients to identify themselves (Reisner et al. 2015).

Gender-affirming therapy becomes more complicated with the influences of the outside world. Family, friends, and work colleagues can question the person's treatment plans, creating ambivalence and triggering fears that they may be making the "wrong" choices. A gender-affirming therapist will weed through all of these external relationships and make space for the person sitting in front of them. This process largely involves exploration and validation. Patients should be called by the name they wish to be called by and identified with the pronouns they go by. Small efforts made by the psychiatrist will go a long way in validating patients who may never have encountered a clinician willing to accord them this respect (Torres et al. 2015).

In gender-affirming therapy, the social construct of gender is broken down into parts, which encompass biological influences as well as cultural norms. Psychiatrists will wade through sometimes-cloudy waters with patients to help them uncover their true self and gender. As noted regarding individuals in the LGBTQ community, many patients have spent a lifetime developing false selves in order to pass in the world and not be discovered as queer (Drescher 2001). Untangling the threads of external influences, ambivalence, and identity can be difficult and may take time.

There is no one direction that a person takes in gender-affirming therapy. An individual does not necessarily start as one gender and end up as another. Clinicians should remember that gender exists on a spectrum and that gender affirmation involves discovering masculine, feminine, androgynous, or other characteristics and expressions that fit best with one's identity. Understanding this truth and creating space is the essence of gender-affirming therapy.

Many patients also fear conversion therapy, which is an effort to "fix" someone from being transgender. Conversion therapy is considered unethical and can lead to worsening of symptoms, and even to suicide (Isay 2001). Patients should be told that the goal of gender-affirming therapy is not to change their gender identity, but rather to help them express who they feel their true self to be.

Hormones

Hormones are one way to feminize or masculinize the body. The primary hormone for feminization is estrogen; the primary hormone for masculinization is testosterone. A testosterone blocker, typically spironolactone, is typically given along with estrogen to patients who wish to feminize their body. Traditionally, hormones have fallen outside of the purview of psychiatrists, but gender dysphoria and gender-affirming care are slowly changing the psychiatrist's scope of practice regarding hormone prescribing. With an understanding of dosing and monitoring standards, psychiatrists are in a unique place to provide these types of treatment to transgender individuals who lack access to them (Thomas and Safer 2015).

Providing hormones should be viewed from an informed consent model. The clinician should ensure that the patient understands the risks and benefits of the treatment, both short-term and long-term. Armed with this information, patients can make a decision that is best for them and their bodies. Our job as psychiatrists is to make sure that the patient has understood and processed the information provided (Deutsch 2012).

The changes that take place with hormones occur over months to years. These slow changes can frustrate patients. General lab work is done prior to starting treatment and quarterly thereafter. There are a few contraindications to hormone treatment (e.g., clotting disorders, certain cancers, liver dysfunction), but they are generally rare (Ettner et al. 2007), and ultimately the patient and the prescriber must weigh the risks and benefits of treatment. Lab work and general primary care follow-up will usually identify any potential adverse reactions; however, the majority of people who take hormones are quite happy with the results (White Hughto and Reisner 2016). Hormones can change the body in such a way that strangers may start to refer to a person by the gender that they identify as. This experience can be very validating to a gender-diverse individual. Many of the concerns around hormones are unwarranted, and general lack of understanding is what makes it difficult for patients to find access to care. The most dangerous part of hormone therapy is lack of access to appropriate care, because patients may turn to nonprescribed hormones obtained from nonmedical sources. It is better that patients receive hormones under the supervision of a clinician (Mepham et al. 2014). Figures 22–2 and 22–3 show the timelines for changes that occur with transfeminine hormones and transmasculine hormones, respectively (Hembree et al. 2009).

Gender-Affirming Surgery

Understanding of gender-affirming surgical procedures is increasing, because public and private insurance companies are starting to cover the procedures. The gender dysphoria diagnosis provides surgeons with a billing code for reimbursement. With gender diversity slowly becoming more acceptable, insurance panels are beginning to approve patients' applications for gender-confirming procedures (Safer 2013).

As previously mentioned, surgery is only one of the options for gender-affirming treatment. Not every gender-diverse patient will want a surgical procedure. Although some gender-affirming surgical procedures have now been around for more than 70 years, they are still in the early stages of development and require more time and research to perfect (Schechter 2016). The decision to obtain surgery will depend on the patient's symptoms of gender dysphoria, as well as on the patient's comfort with the particular surgical procedure, the training level of the surgeon, and the cost. There is evidence that gender-affirming surgical procedures have a positive impact on a person's mental health in the long term (Ruppin and Pfäfflin 2015). Any dissatisfaction with surgical procedures may be due not to regret but rather to unhappiness with the quality of the procedure. Whereas some people may "de-transition," this phenomenon is relatively rare among those who are happy with surgical outcomes (Olsson and Möller 2006).

The gender-affirming surgical procedures are categorized into two main types— top surgery and bottom surgery. Top surgery involves the chest and/or breasts, and bottom surgery involves the genitalia. These and many other procedures are summarized in Table 22–1 (Ettner et al. 2007).

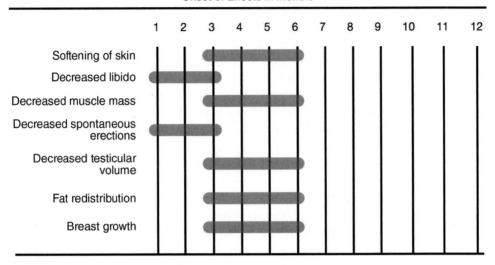

FIGURE 22–2.   Onset of effects of transfeminine hormones.

The effects of prescribing estrogen typically require months to become evident, and changes occur over the course of years.

Source.   Data adapted from Hembree et al. 2009; figure reprinted from Figure 15–1 (p. 217) in Yarbrough E: *Transgender Mental Health.* Washington, DC, American Psychiatric Association Publishing, 2018. Copyright 2018, American Psychiatric Association Publishing. Used with permission.

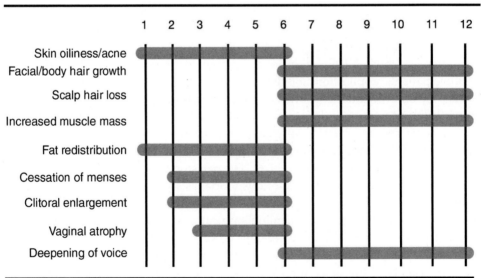

FIGURE 22–3.   Onset of effects of transmasculine hormones.

The effects of testosterone are varied, and different effects can begin to appear at different times. Time and patience are often needed when looking for results.

Source.   Data adapted from Hembree et al. 2009; figure reprinted from Figure 14–1 (p. 200) in Yarbrough E: *Transgender Mental Health.* Washington, DC, American Psychiatric Association Publishing, 2018. Copyright 2018, American Psychiatric Association Publishing. Used with permission.

TABLE 22–1. Gender-affirming procedures

Procedure	Patient	Description	Recovery and complications	Inpatient or outpatient
Top surgery for transgender men	Transgender men	Removal of breast tissue	Quick recovery; level of scarring depends on how much tissue is removed and the method of the surgery	Generally outpatient
Top surgery for transgender women	Transgender women	Breast augmentation with implants	Minimal scarring	Generally outpatient
Metoidioplasty	Transgender men	Clitoral tissue enlarges over time with the addition of testosterone; this surgery frees up clitoral tissue from ligaments so that it may become erect	Complications are minimal, with ability to experience sexual pleasure	Inpatient
Phalloplasty	Transgender men	Creation of a neo phallus, usually from forearm tissue	An invasive procedure with severe scarring; has the most complications of any gender-affirming procedure	Inpatient
Vaginoplasty	Transgender women	Creation of a neo vagina, usually from the tissue of the penis	An invasive procedure; requires frequent dilations of the neo vagina so that it will remain patent	Inpatient
Facial feminization	Transgender women	A multistep procedure that involves reshaping the face for a more feminine appearance; forehead, nose, lips, eyes, cheeks, and jawline may be altered	Minimal	Generally outpatient
Facial masculinization	Transgender men	Involves reshaping the face for a more masculine appearance; forehead, cheeks, and jawline are most commonly altered	Minimal	Generally outpatient
Tracheal shave	Transgender women	Involves removal of tissue more commonly known as the Adam's apple	Minimal	Outpatient
Vocal training	Transgender men and transgender women	Helps transgender men and women change the tone of their voice	None	Nonsurgical

Conclusion

Gender-diverse people face discrimination and health care disparities in many areas. Finding gender-affirming clinicians is just one of the struggles that gender-diverse people must endure in order to get the care they both need and deserve.

In working with gender-diverse people, psychiatrists are battling not only the current political climate but also a history of pathologizing an entire group of people. Navigating the many facets of care can be both challenging and rewarding. Psychiatrists have a unique opportunity to serve as healers and advocates to a patient population in need of help.

Going forward, we all need to continue to learn about gender-affirming treatment options, encourage research aimed at understanding and refining best practices, and begin to help heal the wounds that gender-diverse people still carry from past experiences with the psychiatric profession.

Key Clinical Points

- Gender, which is different from sex, should be thought of as existing on a continuum, with infinite presentations possible.

- One of the biggest problems facing the gender-diverse community is lack of access to competent gender-affirming care.

- The heightened risk of suicide carried by gender-diverse people is understood by gender experts as being largely due to minority stress.

- Transition is not an all-or-nothing process; people can choose which changes, if any, are best for them.

- The changes that take place from hormones occur slowly, over months to years.

References

American Psychiatric Association: Diagnostic and Statistical Manual of Mental Disorders, 4th Edition. Washington, DC, American Psychiatric Association, 1994

American Psychiatric Association: Diagnostic and Statistical Manual of Mental Disorders, 5th Edition. Arlington, VA, American Psychiatric Association, 2013

Bariola E, Lyons A, Leonard W, et al: Demographic and psychosocial factors associated with psychological distress and resilience among transgender individuals. Am J Public Health 105(10):2108–2116, 2015 26270284

Belluardo-Crosby M, Lillis PJ: Issues of diagnosis and care for the transgender patient: is the DSM-5 on point? Issues Ment Health Nurs 33(9):583–590, 2012 22957951

Berlin FS: A conceptual overview and commentary on gender dysphoria. J Am Acad Psychiatry Law 44(2):246–252, 2016 27236181

Brewster ME, Velez B, DeBlaere C, et al: Transgender individuals' workplace experiences: the applicability of sexual minority measures and models. J Couns Psychol 59(1):60–70, 2012 21875182

Budge SL, Adelson JL, Howard KA: Anxiety and depression in transgender individuals: the roles of transition status, loss, social support, and coping. J Consult Clin Psychol 81(3):545–557, 2013 23398495

Deutsch M: Use of the informed consent model in the provision of cross-sex hormone therapy: a survey of the practices of selected clinics. International Journal of Transgenderism 13(3):140–146, 2012

Drescher J: Psychoanalytic Therapy and the Gay Man. Hillsdale, NJ, Analytic Press, 2001

Drescher J: Queer diagnoses: parallels and contrasts in the history of homosexuality, gender variance, and the diagnostic and statistical manual. Arch Sex Behav 39(2):427–460, 2010a 19838785

Drescher J: Transsexualism, gender identity disorder and the DSM. Journal of Gay and Lesbian Mental Health 14(2):109–122, 2010b

Drescher J, Haller E: Position Statement on Access to Care for Transgender and Gender Variant Individuals. Revised by Yarbrough E. Washington, DC, American Psychiatric Association, 2018. Available at: https://www.psychiatry.org/File%20Library/About-APA/Organiza-tion-Documents-Policies/Policies/Position-2018-Access-to-Care-for-Transgender-and-Gender-Diverse-Individuals.pdf. Accessed February 5, 2019.

Erickson-Schroth L: Update on the biology of transgender identity. Journal of Gay and Lesbian Mental Health 17(2):150–174, 2013

Erickson-Schroth L, Jacobs L: "You're in the Wrong Bathroom!" and 20 Other Myths and Misconceptions About Transgender and Gender Nonconforming People. Boston, MA, Beacon Press, 2017

Ettner R, Monstrey S, Coleman E: Principles of Transgender Medicine and Surgery. New York, Haworth, 2007

Flores A, Herman J, Gates G, et al: How Many Adults Identify as Transgender in the United States? Los Angeles, CA, The Williams Institute, 2016

Griffin L: The other dual role: therapist as advocate with transgender clients. Journal of Gay and Lesbian Mental Health 15(2):235–236, 2011

Hembree WC, Cohen-Kettenis P, Delemarre-van de Waal HA, et al: Endocrine treatment of transsexual persons: an Endocrine Society clinical practice guideline. J Clin Endocrinol Metab 94(9):3132–3154, 2009 19509099

Isay RA: Becoming gay: a personal odyssey, in Sexual Conversion Therapy: Ethical, Clinical and Research Perspectives. Edited by Shidlo A, Schroeder M, Drescher J. New York, Haworth Medical, 2001, pp 51–67

James S, Herman J, Rankin S, et al: The Report of the 2015 U.S. Transgender Survey. Washington, DC, National Center for Transgender Equality, 2016

Jorgensen C: Christine Jorgensen: A Personal Autobiography. New York, Paul S. Eriksson, 1967

Kattari SK, Hasche L: Differences across age groups in transgender and gender non-conforming people's experiences of health care discrimination, harassment, and victimization. J Aging Health 28(2):285–306, 2016 26082132

Levitt HM, Ippolito MR: Being transgender: the experience of transgender identity development. J Homosex 61(12):1727–1758, 2014 25089681

Mepham N, Bouman WP, Arcelus J, et al: People with gender dysphoria who self-prescribe cross-sex hormones: prevalence, sources, and side effects knowledge. J Sex Med 11(12):2995–3001, 2014 25213018

Olsson SE, Möller A: Regret after sex reassignment surgery in a male-to-female transsexual: a long-term follow-up. Arch Sex Behav 35(4):501–506, 2006 16900416

Reisner SL, Bradford J, Hopwood R, et al: Comprehensive transgender healthcare: the gender affirming clinical and public health model of Fenway Health. J Urban Health 92(3):584–592, 2015 25779756

Ruppin U, Pfäfflin F: Long-term follow-up of adults with gender identity disorder. Arch Sex Behav 44(5):1321–1329, 2015 25690443

Safer JD: Transgender medical research, provider education, and patient access are overdue. Endocr Pract 19(4):575–576, 2013 23337168

Schechter LS: Gender confirmation surgery: an update for the primary care provider. Transgend Health 1(1):32–40, 2016 29159295

Shidlo A, Schroeder M, Drescher J: Becoming gay: a personal odyssey, in Sexual Conversion Therapy: Ethical, Clinical and Research Perspectives. Edited by Shidlo A, Schroeder M, Drescher J. New York, Haworth Medical, 2001, pp 51–67

Stern K: Queers in History. Dallas, TX, BenBella, 2009

Stone AL: Flexible queers, serious bodies: transgender inclusion in queer spaces. J Homosex 60(12):1647–1665, 2013 24175886

Thomas DD, Safer JD: A simple intervention raised resident-physician willingness to assist transgender patients seeking hormone therapy. Endocr Pract 21(10):1134–1142, 2015 26151424

Torres CG, Renfrew M, Kenst K, et al: Improving transgender health by building safe clinical environments that promote existing resilience: results from a qualitative analysis of providers. BMC Pediatr 15(1):187, 2015 26577820

White Hughto JM, Reisner SL: A systematic review of the effects of hormone therapy on psychological functioning and quality of life in transgender individuals. Transgend Health 1(1):21–31, 2016 27595141

Wise J: Doctors are prejudiced against transgender patients, MPs say. BMJ 352:i252, 2016 26767717

World Professional Association for Transgender Health: Mission and Vision, 2018. Available at: https://www.wpath.org/about/mission-and-vision. Accessed July 24, 2018.

Yarbrough E: Transgender Mental Health. Washington, DC, American Psychiatric Association Publishing, 2018

Recommended Readings

Barker MJ, Scheele J: Queer: A Graphic History. London, Icon Books, 2016

Erickson-Schroth L (ed): Trans Bodies, Trans Selves: A Resource for the Transgender Community. New York, Oxford University Press, 2014

Erickson-Schroth L, Jacobs LA: "You're in the Wrong Bathroom!" and 20 Other Myths and Misconceptions About Transgender and Gender Nonconforming People. Boston, MA, Beacon Press, 2017

Ettner R, Monstrey S, Coleman E (eds): Principles of Transgender Medicine and Surgery, 2nd Edition. New York, Routledge, 2016

Killermann S: The Social Justice Advocate's Handbook: A Guide to Gender. Austin, TX, Impetus Books, 2013

Makadon HJ, Mayer KH, Potter J, et al (eds): The Fenway Guide to Lesbian, Gay, Bisexual, and Transgender Health, 2nd Edition. Philadelphia, PA, American College of Physicians, 2015

Shidlo A, Schroeder M, Drescher J (eds): Sexual Conversion Therapy: Ethical, Clinical and Research Perspectives. New York, Haworth Medical, 2001

Stryker S: Transgender History. Berkeley, CA, Seal Press, 2008

Teich NM: Transgender 101: A Simple Guide to Complex Issues. New York, Columbia University Press, 2012

World Professional Association for Transgender Health: Standards of Care for the Health of Transsexual, Transgender, and Gender Nonconforming People. Available at: https://www.wpath.org/publications/soc. Accessed July 24, 2018.

Yarbrough E: Transgender Mental Health. Washington, DC, American Psychiatric Association Publishing, 2018

Appendix: Glossary of Terms

SMALL CAPS indicate a term found elsewhere in this glossary.

androgynous   Possessing both masculine and feminine qualities; somewhere in the middle.

bigender   A person who psychologically identifies as both genders and may move back and forth between genders.

cisgender   A person whose gender identity and sex assigned at birth align.

FtM   A person assigned the female sex at birth who self-identifies as male. *See also* TRANSMAN.

gender binary   The idea that there are only two genders: male and female.

gender diverse   Falling outside the typical GENDER BINARY.

gender expression   How a person presents their gender to the outside world.

gender fluid   The ability to move across the gender spectrum.

gender identity   How a person identifies their gender in their mind.

gender queer   An umbrella term that usually means that a person falls outside the typical GENDER BINARY.

intersex   Different from TRANSGENDER; refers to a person born with ambiguous genitalia.

MtF   A person assigned the male sex at birth who self-identifies as female. *See also* TRANSWOMAN.

passing   A term for GENDER-DIVERSE people that refers to their ability to be accepted or regarded as CISGENDER (can have positive and negative connotations).

queer   A term that anyone in the lesbian, gay, bisexual, and transgender community might use to describe themselves.

sex assigned at birth   Male or female sex assigned on the basis of external genitalia.

transgender   An umbrella term often used to mean someone who does not continue to identify with the gender/sex they were assigned at birth.

transman   A person assigned the female sex at birth who self-identifies as male. *See also* FtM.

transsexual   A somewhat outdated term that refers to someone who has had some form of gender-affirming surgery.

transvestite   Different from TRANSGENDER; typically refers to a person who dresses as the opposite gender for sexual pleasure.

transwoman   A person assigned the male sex at birth who self-identifies as female. *See also* MtF.

CHAPTER 23

Disruptive, Impulse-Control, and Conduct Disorders

Bonnie P. Taylor, Ph.D.

Danya Schlussel, B.A.

Eric Hollander, M.D.

The disruptive, impulse-control, and conduct disorders diagnostic class in DSM-5 (American Psychiatric Association 2013) groups together related disorders that share the underlying constructs of impulsive behavior, aggressiveness, and pathological rule breaking. Utilizing a spectrum approach to characterize related disorders with overlapping symptom presentations, one can easily conceptualize many disorders and conditions that are defined by impulsivity, aggression, and rule-breaking behaviors (Table 23–1). These disorders are found across formal DSM-5 categories, as well as among "other specified" and "unspecified" conditions, and include attention-deficit/hyperactivity disorder (ADHD), antisocial and borderline personality disorders, substance and alcohol use disorders, binge-eating disorder and bulimia nervosa, bipolar and related disorders, paraphilic disorders, excoriation (skin-picking) disorder, and Internet gaming disorder, as well as neurocognitive disorders characterized by disinhibited behaviors. Clinicians should be aware that individuals with impulsive/aggressive behaviors might indeed present with one or more of these related conditions or comorbid disorders that may contribute to their pattern of impulsive/aggressive behavior.

TABLE 23–1.	Disruptive, impulse-control, and conduct disorders and related disorders of emotional and/or behavioral dysregulation

DSM-5 Disorders

Neurodevelopmental Disorders
   Attention-deficit/hyperactivity disorder

Bipolar and Related Disorders

Disruptive, Impulse-Control, and Conduct Disorders
   Oppositional defiant disorder
   Intermittent explosive disorder
   Conduct disorder
   Antisocial personality disorder
   Pyromania
   Kleptomania
   Other specified and unspecified disruptive, impulse-control, and conduct disorder

Obsessive-Compulsive and Related Disorders
   Hoarding disorder
   Trichotillomania (hair-pulling disorder)
   Excoriation (skin-picking) disorder

Feeding and Eating Disorders
   Binge-eating disorder
   Bulimia nervosa

Substance-Related and Addictive Disorders
   Gambling disorder

Personality Disorders
   Borderline personality disorder

Paraphilic Disorders
   Voyeuristic disorder
   Exhibitionistic disorder
   Frotteuristic disorder
   Sexual masochism disorder
   Sexual sadism disorder
   Pedophilic disorder
   Fetishistic disorder
   Transvestic disorder
   Other specified and unspecified paraphilic disorder

Conditions for Further Study
   Internet gaming disorder
   Nonsuicidal self-injury

Other Disorders With Impulsivity

Impulsive-compulsive sexual disorder

Impulsive-compulsive buying disorder

Neurocognitive disorders with behavioral disturbance

Oppositional Defiant Disorder

Definition and Diagnostic Criteria

The salient characteristic of oppositional defiant disorder (ODD) is a persistent pattern of hostile, angry, argumentative, and defiant behavior that lasts at least 6 months. Although such behaviors may be displayed in all children from time to time, they are significantly more persistent and frequent in children with ODD than in peers of the same age and developmental level, and importantly, these behaviors cause considerable impairment in social functioning and/or in educational or vocational activities.

Qualitatively, children with ODD often have conflicts with authority figures, resist instruction, question rules, and are stubborn and unwilling to compromise. They may persistently test limits and deliberately ignore and/or annoy others. In addition, they may present as irritable, blame others for their mistakes or misbehaviors, and become spiteful, revenge seeking, and/or verbally aggressive when upset. Children with ODD believe that their behaviors are reasonable reactions to irrational demands or unfair circumstances, and as a result, they find their own behaviors less disturbing and upsetting than do others around them, such as family, teachers, and peers.

DSM-5 separates ODD symptoms into clusters based on whether they have an emotional component (e.g., angry, irritable, resentful behaviors), a behavioral element (e.g., argumentative, defiant behaviors), or a spiteful/vindictive aspect to them. This classification structure emerged on the basis of empirical findings suggesting that these three clusters are associated with unique predictive outcomes. Specifically, whereas the emotional symptoms of ODD (angry and irritable) are associated with the development of future mood and anxiety disorders, the headstrong symptoms (i.e., argumentative and defiant) are more likely to be predictive of a later diagnosis of ADHD, and the spiteful or vindictive behaviors (e.g., aggression) are associated with an increased risk of a conduct disorder diagnosis and development of other delinquent behaviors (Rowe et al. 2010; Stringaris and Goodman 2009). In order to meet DSM-5 criteria for ODD, a child must exhibit at least four symptoms (which may be emotional, behavioral, vindictive, or some combination) during interactions with at least one individual (who is not a sibling), with a persistence and frequency that fall outside the range typical for the individual's age or developmental level. For example, in order for a child younger than 5 years to meet the diagnostic threshold for ODD, symptoms in the emotional and behavioral categories must occur on most days for at least 6 months. In contrast, for children older than 5 years, the behaviors may occur less frequently—that is, at least once per week for at least 6 months. If spiteful/vindictive behaviors are present, they must occur at least twice within 6 months, regardless of the child's age.

It is important to note that the behaviors displayed in ODD typically first manifest in the home and over time may expand into multiple settings. The pervasiveness of the behaviors negatively affects relationships not only with family members but also with teachers, peers, and others in the community. In fact, when symptoms are reported by multiple informants (e.g., at home and by teachers), the severity of the child's impairment is greater (American Psychiatric Association 2012). Guided by the implications of this cross-situational pervasiveness of symptoms, DSM-5 provides a severity index based on the number of settings in which the oppositional behaviors are exhibited. A child categorized as having "mild" severity displays at least four symptoms that are confined to only one setting. A child whose behaviors are categorized as "severe" may similarly display only four symptoms, but they are present in three or more settings.

Epidemiology

The most recent lifetime prevalence estimates of ODD range from 3.3% to 11% (Canino et al. 2010). The National Comorbidity Survey Replication, a retrospective study of adults that used DSM-IV diagnostic criteria for ODD (American Psychiatric Association 1994), reported a similar lifetime prevalence for ODD, 10.2%, with higher rates in males than in females (11.2% vs. 9.2%, respectively) (Nock et al. 2007). A recent meta-analysis found the occurrence of ODD to be higher in boys than in girls during middle childhood (Demmer et al. 2017); however, this gender difference appears to even out after puberty (Loeber et al. 2000).

Comorbidity

The disorder that most commonly coexists with ODD is ADHD, with comorbidity rates reportedly reaching up to 39% (Speltz et al. 1999). Children with ODD comorbid with ADHD have been found to demonstrate more emotional impulsivity and deficits in executive functioning compared with children with ODD alone (Ezpeleta and Granero 2015). Other disorders that frequently co-occur with ODD are anxiety and depressive disorders (Angold et al. 1999). Learning disorders and communication disorders are also associated with ODD.

Whether ODD can manifest concurrently with conduct disorder has been a question of debate, given that ODD and conduct disorder encompass similar features. For example, both disorders consist of behaviors that are vastly negative, including disobedient, angry, defiant, rebellious, and resentful behavior. ODD differs from conduct disorder, however, in that children with conduct disorder fail to recognize societal rules and personal rights, resulting in aggression that may cause physical injury to people or animals and/or deliberate destruction of property. Table 23–2 outlines differences and similarities between ODD and conduct disorder in terms of their behavioral characteristics, age at onset, and unique specifiers. As can be seen, the age at onset for ODD is younger than that for conduct disorder, and in fact, ODD is often a precursor to a diagnosis of conduct disorder at a later age. DSM-5 allows for the concurrent diagnosis of ODD and conduct disorder and emphasizes the prognostic value of ODD symptoms in predicting future clinical outcomes (e.g., depression, anxiety, substance use, ADHD) in individuals diagnosed with conduct disorder comorbid with ODD (American Psychiatric Association 2013).

Pathogenesis

ODD is thought to be caused by a combination of risk, protective, biological, environmental, and societal factors. In regard to environmental contributions, ODD has been linked to low socioeconomic status, parental marital discord, inconsistent limit setting, low family cohesion, and parental mental disorder and/or substance use disorders (Burke et al. 2002). Biological research studies have focused on ODD comorbid with other disorders, such as ADHD and/or conduct disorder (see "Pathogenesis" in

TABLE 23–2. Comparison of DSM-5 diagnostic features for oppositional defiant disorder and conduct disorder

	Oppositional defiant disorder	Conduct disorder
Age at onset (years)	6–8	9–17
Behavioral features	Verbal arguments and temper tantrums expressed as the following: Angry/irritable mood (loses temper, easily annoyed) Argumentative/defiant behavior (argues, deliberately annoys others, defies rules/requests) Spite/vindictiveness	Lack of recognition of societal rules and personal rights, engaging in the following: Aggression toward people or animals Destruction of property Deceitfulness or theft Serious violations of rules
Specifiers	**Current severity** Mild: symptoms occur in one setting Moderate: some symptoms present in at least two settings Severe: some symptoms present in at least three settings	**Current severity** Mild: symptoms occur in one setting Moderate: some symptoms present in at least two settings Severe: some symptoms present in at least three settings **Onset type** Childhood onset: before age 10 years Adolescent onset: at or after age 10 years **With limited prosocial emotions**—persistently displays 2 or more of the following: Lack of remorse or guilt Callousness—lack of empathy Lack of concern about performance Shallow/deficient affect

Note. For the complete diagnostic criteria for oppositional defiant disorder and conduct disorder, please refer to pp. 462–463 and pp. 469–471, respectively, in DSM-5 (American Psychiatric Association 2013).

the "Conduct Disorder" section), and as a result, the unique biological underpinnings of ODD remain largely unknown. If the biological substrates of ODD without coexisting conditions are to be elucidated, studies are needed that investigate children with ODD as a single diagnosis.

Course

The age at onset of ODD is usually between 6 and 8 years, after typical normative oppositional behaviors diminish. The onset of symptoms is gradual and develops over the course of months or even years. As previously mentioned, symptoms commonly first materialize in the home setting and may then emerge in other settings and circumstances. When symptoms extend to multiple settings, they can lead to severe impairment in social, educational, and other important areas of functioning.

The stability of ODD symptoms over time correlates with the severity of the symptoms; furthermore, higher numbers of ODD symptoms are associated with greater risk for later development of conduct disorder. Early-onset ODD is likewise predictive of future conduct disorder and constitutes a risk factor for a later diagnosis of ADHD. A child with ODD is also more likely to progress to conduct disorder if he or she is of low socioeconomic status and has parents with substance use disorders. Notably, although ODD is usually a predecessor of conduct disorder, the majority of children with ODD do not go on to develop conduct disorder or antisocial behaviors in adulthood (Loeber et al. 2000).

Treatment

A comprehensive evaluation for a child presenting with symptoms of ODD should be conducted. Because oppositional behavior is normal at certain developmental stages, particularly during the preschool and adolescent years, one should be cautious in considering a diagnosis of ODD during those periods. It is likewise important to note that because oppositional behaviors generally occur during interactions with familiar adults and peers, symptoms may not materialize during the clinical interview with the child. Therefore, the interviewer may need to rely on parent, teacher, and other informant reports to make an accurate diagnosis.

In the clinical evaluation, it is essential to assess for other disorders in order to determine whether the oppositional behaviors are truly diagnostic of ODD or are a by-product of another condition. For example, a child with ODD may indeed have concurrent ADHD, or he or she may have only ADHD but appear to be oppositional and uncooperative because of inattention, impulsivity, and/or forgetfulness. Similarly, tantrums and antagonistic behaviors are common in young children with depressive and/or anxiety disorders, as well as in children with language disorders, who can become frustrated because of their impaired ability to communicate effectively. If another disorder does in fact coexist with the ODD, treating the comorbid disorder will increase the likelihood that the child will benefit from therapeutic treatment for ODD.

Psychotherapeutic interventions are generally indicated to treat children with ODD, with effective treatment targeting the unique needs of both the child and the family. Evidence-based individual approaches are cognitively based and aim to build effective anger management skills, improve problem-solving ability, develop techniques to delay impulsive responses, and improve social interactions. Parent management training is used to help parents manage their child's behavior more effectively, learn successful discipline techniques, and promote desired behaviors in their children.

When treating preschool-age children, parent management training is often recommended. There is also some evidence that programs such as Head Start and home visitation to high-risk families may prevent future oppositional behaviors and delinquency. When school age is reached, parent management training and individual cognitive-based strategies are the programs with the greatest amount of empirical support. Combining parent management training and individual problem-solving approaches has been shown to be more effective than using either treatment alone (Kazdin et al. 1992). School-based programs, such as those aimed at resisting negative peer influences and reducing bullying and antisocial behavior, may also be effective for this age group. For adolescents, cognitive-based techniques and vocational and skills training, as well as parent management tools, are recommended. Group-based treatments for adolescents can have negative outcomes, particularly if the group participants engage in discussions of oppositional behaviors (Barlow and Stewart-Brown 2000).

In regard to pharmacological treatment options, no medication has been approved to specifically treat the symptoms of ODD. Medications are nonetheless used in children with ODD to treat coexisting conditions (e.g., ADHD, depression, anxiety) and may also be effective in improving oppositional behaviors. Medications that have been helpful in this respect include stimulants (e.g., methylphenidate, dextroamphetamine) (Pappadopulos et al. 2006), atomoxetine, guanfacine, atypical antipsychotics (e.g., aripiprazole, risperidone [McKinney and Renk 2011]), buspirone, lithium, anticonvulsants (e.g., valproate), and antidepressants (e.g., selective serotonin reuptake inhibitors [SSRIs] for depression and/or anxiety and/or impulsivity).

Intermittent Explosive Disorder

Definition and Diagnostic Criteria

Intermittent explosive disorder (IED) is characterized by recurrent pathological aggressive and impulsive behavior, which may include verbal aggression (e.g., temper tantrums, tirades) and/or physical aggression that is directed toward other individuals, animals, or property. DSM-5 separates the diagnostic criteria for IED into high-frequency, low-intensity aggressive behaviors (Criterion A1) and low-frequency, high-intensity aggressive behavior (Criterion A2). Criterion A1 describes verbal and/or physical aggression that does not result in physical injury or damage (low intensity) but occurs frequently—that is, at least twice weekly for at least 3 months (high frequency). In contrast, Criterion A2 describes physically aggressive behavior that causes physical injury or property damage (high intensity) but may occur less frequently—that is, at least three times within 1 year (low frequency). According to DSM-5, individuals with IED tend to cycle between longer periods of A1 episodes and shorter periods of A2 episodes. Regardless of whether the behavioral outburst is verbal or nonverbal and physically injurious/damaging or not, the underlying trigger for all of the aggressive episodes in IED is a lack of impulse control in response to stressors. Notably, these impulsive outbursts are greatly disproportionate to the reaction that would typically be expected on the basis of the precipitating stressor, they are unplanned, and they cause marked distress and/or impairment in occupational or interpersonal functioning. A diagnosis of IED should not be made if a child is younger than 6 years of age (or similar developmental level), if a child is 6–18 years old and the aggressive outbursts occur in the context of an adjustment disorder, or if existing psychopathology or substance use may better account for the aggressive behavior (at any age) (American Psychiatric Association 2013).

Epidemiology

Lifetime prevalence rates for IED range from 1.0% to 7.3%, whereas 1-month and 12-month prevalence estimates are lower, at 1.6% and 3.9%, respectively (Coccaro et al. 2004; Scott et al. 2016). Lifetime IED is broadly defined as three or more lifetime attacks without ever having as many as three attacks in a single year. IED is prevalent in adolescents; 7.8% of adolescents polled reported a lifetime prevalence of IED, and 63.3% reported lifetime anger attacks involving property destruction or the threat or act of violence (McLaughlin et al. 2012).

Sociodemographic correlates of lifetime IED include being male, young, unemployed, and divorced or separated and having low educational attainment (Scott et al. 2016). The median age at onset of IED is 17 years (Scott et al. 2016). The age at onset for males is typically earlier than that for females, but overall, females are as likely as males to develop IED (Coccaro et al. 2005).

Comorbidity

Approximately 64% of individuals with IED meet criteria for at least one comorbid psychiatric disorder (McLaughlin et al. 2012), with depressive and anxiety disorders co-occurring most frequently (Scott et al. 2016). There are also strong correlations between IED and social phobia, other impulse-control disorders (ICDs), and bulimia (Jennings et al. 2017; Kessler et al. 2006; McLaughlin et al. 2012). A recent analysis of the National Comorbidity Survey Replication found that substance use disorders (SUDs) occurred more frequently in adults with a current diagnosis of IED than in adults without IED (Coccaro et al. 2017). Additionally, it was found that the onset of IED typically occurred before the onset of an SUD, suggesting that individuals with IED have an increased risk for SUD.

Pathogenesis

Family and Twin Studies

Relatives of probands with IED have an elevated risk of developing IED. Furthermore, first-degree relatives of children with frequent low-intensity outbursts of aggression have a greater chance of developing IED (Coccaro 2010). Studies have found that a childhood history of traumatic experiences (both physical and emotional) is more common among individuals with IED than among individuals with other psychiatric disorders and that such a history can lead to the development of IED (Coccaro 2012).

Biological Correlates

Serotonin and dopamine system.   Research supports the presence of altered serotonin function in individuals with IED. For example, subjects with IED have been shown to have decreased numbers of platelet serotonin transporters as well as differences in the availability of the serotonin transporter and serotonin type 2A receptors compared with healthy control subjects (Coccaro et al. 2010a, 2010b; Frankle et al. 2005; Rosell et al. 2010).

Psychostimulants such as methylphenidate and amphetamine are readily prescribed for the treatment of ADHD. However, more research is needed on the effects of dopamine and psychostimulants on impulsivity comorbid with aggression.

Imaging and brain localization. Research evidence points to the role of frontostriatal circuits in modulating affective aggression. Specifically, males with borderline personality disorder who also met criteria for IED were found to show reduced relative glucose metabolism in the striatum compared with both females with borderline personality disorder comorbid with IED and healthy control subjects (Perez-Rodriguez et al. 2012). Studies comparing striatal glucose metabolism in male and female populations may offer a promising path for further research in behavioral aggression.

Emerging data suggest interesting relationships between facial emotional recognition in subjects with IED and amygdala–orbitofrontal cortex dysfunction. Specifically, individuals with IED show exaggerated amygdala reactivity and diminished orbitofrontal cortex activation in response to angry faces (Coccaro et al. 2007). A study that used high-resolution 3.0 Tesla structural magnetic resonance imaging (MRI) found that IED was associated with structural abnormalities as well as a significant loss of neurons in both the amygdala and the hippocampus (Coccaro et al. 2015). The authors concluded that these changes "may play a role in the functional abnormalities observed in previous fMRI [functional MRI] studies and the pathophysiology of impulsive aggressive behavior" (Coccaro et al. 2015, p. 80).

Course

The onset of IED is abrupt and has no prodromal period. IED appears as early as prepubertal childhood and peaks in adolescence, with a mean onset from 12 to 21 years of age. Symptoms are persistent; they can last many years or can occur chronically throughout a lifetime. The severe aggressive outbursts associated with IED can have serious effects on a patient's quality of life (resulting in impairment in education, social and family function, finances, and unlawful activity) that may, in turn, promote the onset of other pathologies.

Treatment

Pharmacotherapy

Pharmacological treatment for IED is precarious because of the disorder's comorbidity with other volatile disorders. IED is highly comorbid with other disorders characterized by impulsivity, such as bipolar disorder and SUDs. Future medication studies in IED may be more likely to yield statistically significant separation from placebo if subjects are stratified a priori by predominant symptom pattern (i.e., DSM-5 Criterion A1 or Criterion A2) (Coccaro et al. 2014). An overview of pharmacotherapy for symptoms of IED is given in Table 23–3.

Symptoms of IED may respond to SSRIs, anticonvulsants, antipsychotics, phenytoin, β-blockers, and α_2-agonists (Dell'Osso et al. 2006). SSRIs show some short-term

TABLE 23–3.   Pharmacotherapy for intermittent explosive disorder

Treatment	Outcome
Selective serotonin reuptake inhibitors	
Fluoxetine (Coccaro et al. 2009)	Significant reduction in impulsive-aggressive behavior; does not reliably result in remission of core symptoms
Anticonvulsants	
Valproate (Hollander et al. 2005)	More effective than placebo in treating impulsive aggression in persons with Cluster B personality disorder features
Phenytoin, carbamazepine, valproate (Stanford et al. 2005)	Reductions in impulsive aggression with all three drugs; delayed effect for carbamazepine
Antipsychotics	
Risperidone (Buitelaar et al. 2001)	Improvement in clinical severity; relatively few side effects during risperidone treatment

effects (Dell'Osso et al. 2006) but often fail to produce long-term remission of aggressive symptoms. Certain temperamental factors, such as neuroticism and harm avoidance, may be predictive of SSRI treatment response (Phan et al. 2011).

Divalproex has shown promise as an option for the treatment of aggression because it was superior to placebo in treating impulsive aggression in persons with borderline personality disorder (Hollander et al. 2005). However, divalproex did not have significant antiaggressive effects in IED patients without Cluster B personality disorders or posttraumatic stress disorder. For this reason, divalproex may be preferentially effective in highly aggressive individuals with personality disorders (Hollander et al. 2003, 2005).

Psychotherapy

A large proportion of patients with IED seek emotional treatment (37.7%), and 17.1% of those who seek treatment do so specifically for anger (McLaughlin et al. 2012). Data on effective psychotherapeutic treatment for IED are sparse. In part, this lack of data is due to the capricious, unpredictable nature of violent outbursts in IED. Multicomponent cognitive-behavioral therapy (CBT) programs in group and individual settings produce significant posttreatment effects in measures of trait anger, hostile thoughts, anger expression, anger control, and aggression. More specifically, McCloskey et al. (2008) examined individual versus group CBT in individuals with IED. They found that both forms of CBT reduced aggression and hostile thinking. When compared with a wait-list control group, the CBT groups also demonstrated an improvement in anger control.

Conduct Disorder

Definition and Diagnostic Criteria

Conduct disorder is perhaps one of the most commonly given diagnoses within child psychiatry, both in inpatient and outpatient psychiatric pediatric settings (American

Psychiatric Association 2000), and the question of whether the diagnosis is overused and/or misused has long been debated. Nevertheless, it is believed that treatment may be inadequate for a large part of the diagnosed population. Conduct disorder is characterized by a persistent and recurrent pattern of behavior in which accepted age-appropriate rules or societal norms or the fundamental rights of other individuals are violated. DSM-5 separates the 15 behaviors that characterize conduct disorder into four groupings, as follows: 1) aggression that causes or threatens physical harm to individuals or animals (i.e., bullies others, initiates physical fights, uses a weapon that can cause physical harm, is physically cruel to people, is physically cruel to animals, steals while confronting a victim [e.g., mugging], forces another into sexual activity); 2) destruction of property (i.e., fire setting intending to cause serious damage, deliberate destruction of another's property); 3) deceitfulness or theft (i.e., breaking into someone's house or car, lying to or "conning" others to receive goods or favors, stealing without confronting the victim [e.g., shoplifting and forgery]); and 4) serious violation of rules (i.e., staying out at night despite parental rules, running away overnight, school truancy). In order to qualify for a diagnosis of conduct disorder, an individual must have exhibited at least 3 of the 15 behaviors (in any of the four groupings) listed in DSM-5 Criterion A within the past 12 months, with at least 1 of the 3 behaviors having been noted within the past 6 months. As with other disorders, the characteristic behaviors must cause functional impairment in academic, social, and/or occupational settings.

In the DSM-5 criteria, two subtypes of conduct disorder are defined on the basis of age at onset (i.e., childhood-onset type vs. adolescent-onset type; the subtype "unspecified onset" can also be used). Notably, these subtypes are prognostic of future outcomes. For example, children diagnosed with childhood-onset conduct disorder (onset before 10 years of age) are more likely to remain symptomatic and impaired and to carry the conduct disorder diagnosis into adulthood. According to DSM-5, these children are typically male, may have had ODD during early childhood, and are likely to have comorbid ADHD. By contrast, individuals with adolescent-onset conduct disorder (onset at age 10 years or older) have more typical and appropriate social relations, have less tendency to display aggression toward others, and are less likely to carry the conduct disorder diagnosis into adulthood.

"With Limited Prosocial Emotions" Specifier for Conduct Disorder

In DSM-5, the specifier "with limited prosocial emotions" (WLPE; also called the "Callous–Unemotional specifier") was introduced for conduct disorder based on findings that individuals with conduct disorder have certain traits that are associated with distinct emotional, cognitive, personality, and social characteristics; are relatively stable across time; are associated with more severe aggression, conduct problems, and delinquency; and are less responsive to behavioral treatment (Frick and Moffitt 2010). Furthermore, individuals with conduct disorder and callous-unemotional traits have poor outcomes in psychiatric and psychological treatments compared with individuals with conduct disorder without such traits (Butler et al. 2011; Vanwoerden et al. 2016).

As described in the DSM-5 diagnostic criteria (American Psychiatric Association 2013, pp. 470–471), in order to qualify for the WLPE specifier, an individual with conduct disorder must also exhibit two or more of the following characteristics persistently for at least 1 year, in more than one relationship or setting:

- *Lack of remorse or guilt:* Does not feel bad or guilty when he or she does something wrong (except when caught and/or facing punishment). There is a lack of concern or regard for the negative consequences of one's actions.
- *Callous—lack of empathy:* Disregards and is not concerned about the feelings of others. The individual is often described as uncaring and/or cold.
- *Unconcerned about performance:* Does not show concern about poor or problematic performance at school or work or in important activities. The individual does not put forth the effort necessary to perform well (even when expectations are clear), and he or she typically blames others for his or her poor performance.
- *Shallow or deficient affect:* Does not express feelings or show emotion toward others, except in ways that appear shallow, insincere, or superficial (e.g., emotions can quickly be turned on and off, are used to manipulate or intimidate others).

In assessing whether an individual meets criteria for the WLPE specifier, multiple sources should be consulted in order to determine the persistence of these traits (e.g., self-report and family member, teacher, and/or peer reports).

Epidemiology

Estimates of conduct disorder prevalence in the general population have ranged widely (fewer than 1% to greater than 10%), depending on the type of population studied and the diagnostic criteria used (Maughan et al. 2004). Prevalence estimates appear to be consistent across countries and cultures (Canino et al. 2010).

Although conduct disorder may be more common in males than in females (with ratios ranging from 2:1 to 4:1) (Moffitt et al. 2001), the lower prevalence in females is debatable, because it may reflect a gender bias against females in diagnostic criteria. Still, the childhood-onset subtype of conduct disorder has a considerable male predominance and, as previously mentioned, is predictive of a worse prognosis, with more numerous, severe, and persistent symptoms. The prevalence of conduct disorder increases from childhood to adolescence in both males and females; however, males demonstrate a more linear year-to-year increase, and females show a greater increase starting in adolescence (Maughan et al. 2004).

Differential Diagnosis

The differential diagnosis for conduct disorder includes ODD, ADHD, mood disorders, and adjustment disorder (with disturbance of conduct or with mixed disturbance of emotions and conduct) (American Psychiatric Association 2013).

Comorbidity

Conduct disorder is commonly comorbid with other psychiatric disorders, further contributing to the ambiguity of the epidemiological data for conduct disorder. Males demonstrate higher rates of comorbidity than do females (Maughan et al. 2004); comorbid ODD or ADHD is common and is associated with a poorer prognosis. Mood and anxiety symptoms, cognitive disabilities, and SUDs are also commonly comorbid with conduct disorder.

Pathogenesis

The interaction among biological, psychological, and sociological elements is thought to contribute to the development of conduct disorder. Individuals with the childhood-onset subtype of conduct disorder, which tends to be persistent and pervasive, appear to have stronger genetic influences and a more severe and prolonged course, and are more likely to develop antisocial personality disorder in adulthood (Moffitt 2005). Adoption and twin studies show that both environmental and genetic factors influence conduct disorder. There is increased risk for conduct disorder in children with an adoptive or biological parent with antisocial personality disorder or psychopathology, atypical maternal caregiving, or a sibling diagnosed with conduct disorder. Conduct disorder may be more frequent in offspring of biological parents diagnosed with mood disorders, schizophrenia, alcohol dependence, ADHD, or conduct disorder (American Psychiatric Association 1994; Moffitt 2005). Environmentally, low socioeconomic status, high degree of parental psychopathology, high level of parental conflict, absent father, greater family size, and fewer ethnic or cultural interests are all associated with a higher risk of conduct problems.

Research has identified candidate genes (e.g., gamma-aminobutyric acid A receptor α2 [*GABRA2*], monoamine oxidase A [*MAOA*], arginine vasopressin receptor 1A [*AVPR1A*]) that are associated with conduct disorder–related phenotypes, but not all of these findings have been replicated (Salvatore and Dick 2018). Studies suggest that the frequent co-occurrence of conduct disorder, ODD, and ADHD is attributable to shared genetic factors, yet this suggestion remains controversial because each individual disorder retains unique genetic elements. Genetic studies show that approximately half of the genetic influences in conduct disorder are unique to the disorder, and the other half are common to other disorders (Lahey et al. 2011). Traits that may factor into conduct disorder and that are associated with elements of antisocial personality (and thus are likely to have genetic correlates) include inattention, aggressiveness, impulsivity, and novelty seeking. Childhood conduct problems have also been correlated with specific genes for the serotonin type 1B receptor, the serotonin transporter, and adrenergic performance. Finally, aberrations in the components of serotonin function are commonly noted in individuals who have difficulty controlling impulsivity and aggression.

The relationship between hormone levels and aggression remains unclear, given the relatively small number of studies done in this area. Although higher levels of testosterone were correlated with increased aggression among boys in deviant peer groups, similar increases in testosterone were associated with greater levels of leadership among boys in nondeviant peer groups (Rowe et al. 2004).

Within the existing scant neuroimaging literature, temporal and frontal abnormalities appear to play a role in conduct disorder. Event-related potential studies indicate a reduction in P300 amplitudes in anterior brain regions when children with conduct disorder are given executive functioning tasks (Bauer and Hesselbrock 2003). fMRI studies in children diagnosed with conduct disorder have shown lower anterior cingulate reactivity to emotional stimuli, a finding that reflects deficient emotional control. Additionally, children with conduct disorder demonstrate decreased reactivity in the amygdala in response to anxiety-inducing emotional stimuli (Sterzer et al. 2005).

A meta-analysis of structural imagining studies found that youth with conduct disorder had significant gray matter reductions in the insula, amygdala, cortical frontal, and temporal regions compared with typically developing youths (Rogers and De Brito 2016). In addition, hyperintensities have been found in frontal lobe white matter (Kruesi et al. 2004). Smaragdi et al. (2017) found differential cortical thickness in the supramarginal gyrus in males and females with conduct disorder, with males showing lower and females showing higher cortical thickness compared with sex-, age-, and pubertal-status-matched control subjects. These study findings of temporal and frontal brain region structural and functional changes correlate with neuropsychological findings that suggest that children with conduct disorder have poor affective processing and executive functioning. Further studies focusing on the predictive reliability and validity of these findings are needed.

Course

Symptom onset for conduct disorder can occur in the preschool years, although more typically, significant symptoms emerge between middle childhood and middle adolescence. Symptom onset is rare after 17 years of age.

The course of conduct disorder is unpredictable. Although the behaviors usually abate by adulthood, a younger age at onset, an increased frequency of aggression, and a greater number of symptoms are each independently associated with a higher likelihood of chronicity and an increased risk for developing antisocial personality disorder and SUD. ODD, which is usually exhibited before 10 years of age, is often a precursor to the childhood-onset type of conduct disorder (Pardini et al. 2010).

It is estimated that up to 40% of children diagnosed with conduct disorder will develop antisocial personality disorder as adults, with the risk being higher for children with substance use before 15 years of age, children living in severe poverty, and children placed in foster care (Robins end Ratcliff 1978). In addition, individuals with conduct disorder have a greater risk of developing mood, anxiety, and somatic symptom disorders throughout life (American Psychiatric Association 2013). Children with conduct disorder who are categorized as "resilient" (i.e., have characteristics of high intelligence, are first born, and come from low-discord small families) are more likely to respond to treatment, as are children with symptom onset in adolescence.

Assessment of family history in children with conduct disorder is commonly used in clinical settings to enhance the calculation of conduct disorder prognosis. Such an assessment can allow better prediction of conduct disorder severity, the child's risk of developing other disorders (e.g., ADHD), and the child's (and family's) potential to respond to treatment. Family history accounts for both genetic influences and parental environmental factors, which play significant roles in children's behavioral development. For example, individuals with the childhood-onset subtype of conduct disorder have more relatives who were convicted of crimes compared with individuals with the adolescent-onset subtype (Taylor et al. 2000). Furthermore, studies have shown that parents with prior diagnoses of conduct disorder generally demonstrate inadequate parenting and disordered home environments.

Treatment

Treatment for conduct disorder varies widely, likely because of the nonspecific nature of the conduct disorder diagnosis, and can include therapy, medication, or a combination of the two. With regard to therapy, a broad range of interventions exists, which likely reflects the ambiguity of the conduct disorder diagnosis itself. Appreciation and understanding of the psychosocial components inherent in the disorder and knowledge of the resources available in the community will help direct the clinician in selection of a treatment.

Recognition and treatment of comorbid psychiatric disorders are extremely important. The most successful interventions for conduct disorder require parental participation; however, parents with antisocial traits are most likely to terminate treatment. Three main forms of therapeutic intervention for the disorder are supported by the current evidence: parent management training, problem-solving skills training, and multisystemic therapy (Farmer et al. 2002). Parent management training instructs individuals in appropriate methods of interpersonal interaction that encourage positive and discourage negative or antisocial interpersonal behaviors. This training teaches negotiating skills using negative consequences and positive reinforcement. Problem-solving skills instruction is rooted in cognitive-based methods and uses role playing and modeling to help improve the person's ability to identify and manage potentially challenging situations. Treating these symptoms in individuals with executive functioning deficits and comorbid ADHD may be difficult, a circumstance that emphasizes the necessity for correct assessment, management, and treatment of comorbidities. Not surprisingly, older children demonstrate a greater rate of success. Multisystemic therapy utilizes systems available within the individual's environment and maximizes positive interactions. Families, schools, peers, and other communities are simultaneously involved. The system is tailored to the needs of the individual. The multiple systems involved render this therapy expensive and its results difficult to replicate; nevertheless, it is very effective. A review and meta-analysis evaluating the efficacy of nonpharmacological treatments for conduct disorder found a small effect in reducing parent-, teacher-, and observer-rated problems in children with conduct disorder (Bakker et al. 2017).

Pharmacological interventions are targeted toward disruptive behaviors and symptoms. However, given the dearth of symptom specificity in conduct disorder, unambiguous replicable results are lacking. The most suitable symptom targets for pharmacological intervention are impulsivity, hyperactivity, aggression, and mood symptoms. Agents such as antidepressants, mood stabilizers, stimulants, antipsychotics, anticonvulsants, and adrenergic agents all show some efficacy, but further controlled studies are needed. Nevertheless, difficulty remains in differentiating whether the pharmacological benefit is due to amelioration of conduct disorder symptoms or of comorbid psychiatric symptoms.

Antisocial Personality Disorder

Due to its close association with conduct disorder, antisocial personality disorder has a dual listing in DSM-5 and is found in both the "Personality Disorders" and the "Disruptive, Impulse-Control, and Conduct Disorders" chapters. The DSM-5 criteria for antisocial personality disorder, and further details about the disorder, are available in the DSM-5 "Personality Disorders" chapter (American Psychiatric Association 2013; see also Chapter 26 in this volume, "Personality Pathology and Personality Disorders").

Pyromania

Definition and Diagnostic Criteria

The primary feature of pyromania is deliberate and purposeful fire setting that recurs on multiple occasions. In addition to this hallmark behavior, DSM-5 criteria require that the individual must experience tension or affective arousal before setting the fire; must have a fascination with or attraction to fire; and must feel pleasure, gratification, or relief when setting or witnessing fires or when participating in their aftermath. Furthermore, the fire setting must not be done for monetary gain, as an expression of sociopolitical ideology or anger, to conceal criminal activity, or to improve one's living circumstances. In addition, the fire setting cannot be a response to a delusion or hallucination, a result of impaired judgment, or attributable to a manic episode or another disorder. Individuals with pyromania are often regular "fire watchers," may set off false fire alarms, and derive enjoyment from being around people and items associated with fire (e.g., firefighters and firefighting equipment). When diagnosing pyromania, it is important to rule out conduct disorder, a manic episode, antisocial personality disorder, and/or a neurocognitive disorder or intellectual disability.

There has been a paucity of research examining the unique clinical characteristics of pyromania, and as a result, it is thought to be a very rare disorder (Grant and Won Kim 2007). It has been suggested that only 3%–6% of psychiatric inpatients meet diagnostic criteria for pyromania (Palermo 2015). Research in this area generally focuses on the behaviors of fire setting and arson (i.e., the crime resulting from fire setting) rather than on the psychiatric diagnosis of pyromania. Thus, many studies are skewed because they sample too broadly (i.e., surveys in the general population asking about history of fire setting) or too narrowly (i.e., focus on populations of individuals who are incarcerated or institutionalized for crimes of arson).

Adolescent fire setters disproportionately outnumber adult fire setters. Natural curiosity and experimentation with fire typically begin at 6 years of age, with certain risk factors and motivations elevating the frequency of fire-setting behaviors as children age. Juvenile fire setting is more common in males than in females, with male fire setters outnumbering female fire setters by approximately three to one (Lambie et al. 2013). Fire setting is associated with a history of physical and sexual abuse, SUDs, family dysfunction, and hostile or impulsive personality traits (MacKay et al. 2009).

Youth account for a large percentage of arson offenses in the United States, the United Kingdom, and Australia (45%, 40%, and 55.6%, respectively), and many of these offenders have high rates of recidivism (Lambie and Randell 2011; MacKay et al. 2009). Childhood fire setting is one of the strongest predictors of adult arson and is also associated with significant psychopathology. In both boys and girls, antisocial behavior and substance abuse have the strongest correlations with fire setting, with male fire setters also showing externalizing problems such as hyperactivity, thrill seeking, and cruelty to animals, and female fire setters showing internalizing problems such as anxiety and depression. Additionally, smoking was shown to correlate highly with fire-setting behaviors in children and adolescents, perhaps because the presence of and interest in fire-setting paraphernalia may increase inappropriate fire setting (MacKay et al. 2009).

Studies of fire-setting behavior and arson in adults show correlates similar to those in adolescents. In an analysis of results from the U.S. National Epidemiologic Survey on Alcohol and Related Conditions, the lifetime prevalence of fire setting was found to be 1.7% in men and 0.4% in women, and the behavior was associated with a broad range of violent and nonviolent antisocial behaviors (Lambie et al. 2013). Both male and female fire setters were shown to have higher rates of antisocial personality disorder, as well as of alcohol and drug use disorders, major depressive disorder, gambling disorder, tobacco use disorder, bipolar disorder, and obsessive-compulsive personality disorder (Hoertel et al. 2011). For this reason, some authors suggest that fire setting may be best understood in the broader context of antisocial behavior rather than as an isolated condition (Lambie et al. 2013).

Characteristics of arsonists appear to be similar to the general characteristics of fire setters. From the small amount of information known, the majority of arsonists were raised in broken homes, have lower levels of education, and have a history of psychiatric or mental health treatment. Compared with nonarson offenders, arson offenders have poorer impulse control, have significantly more alcohol misuse problems, and are less likely to be diagnosed with a major psychotic disorder. Motives for arson range from delusional thinking to revenge or property damage to excitement from fire setting. More than one motive may be behind a single act of arson. In a study of 25 arsonists, 52% of motives stemmed from delusional thinking, 36% from desire for revenge, and 12% from sexual excitement (Labree et al. 2010). It has been hypothesized that the percentage of arson committed because of sexual excitement could be higher, because arsonists may hide behind claims of delusional thinking rather than admit to this motive (Labree et al. 2010).

Epidemiology

A study of Finnish male criminals with a history of recidivist fire setting found that out of 90 arson recidivists, 12 fulfilled DSM-IV-TR (American Psychiatric Association 2000) criteria for pyromania (Lindberg et al. 2005). Of these 12 individuals, 9 were experiencing acute alcohol intoxication during the arson, which (according to DSM criteria) would exclude them from receiving a diagnosis of pyromania, suggesting a rate of 3.3% for "true" pyromania. The three men who met criteria for "true" pyromania reported experiencing tension or affective arousal before the act of fire setting, pleasure and release afterward, and an attraction or interest in fire. They also all worked as volunteer firefighters. The strong correlation between alcohol use and fire setting—and, more specifically, alcohol intoxication and pyromania—suggests that the DSM-5 Criterion E requirement that the fire setting *not* be a result of impaired judgment secondary to substance intoxication may need to be reconsidered.

A possible explanation for the rarity of pyromania could be a fallacy in epidemiological sampling, because studies tend to focus on criminal populations of individuals with pyromania, and by doing so, they exclude noncriminal fire setters from the sample. Large epidemiological studies that have examined broad samples of the population are not specific enough in their questioning to elicit answers that would yield a potential diagnosis of pyromania, because they do not ask questions that target motivation or frequency, such as "Have you ever intentionally set a fire any time in your life?" Studies of noncriminal clinical samples have found higher rates of pyromania than found in convicted criminal samples. For example, a study of 107 inpatients with depression found that 3 (2.8%) met criteria for pyromania (Lejoyeux et al. 2002). Similarly, studies of individuals with kleptomania (McElroy et al. 1991) and compulsive buying (McElroy et al. 1994) have found lifetime rates of pyromania of 15% and 10%, respectively. It has been speculated that among individuals with ICDs, one impulse disorder may be substituted for another across the individual's lifetime (Grant and Won Kim 2007).

Contrary to other studies of fire setting and arson, which have found low prevalence rates for females, Grant and Won Kim (2007) found, in a study sample of 21 adult and adolescent subjects with lifetime pyromania, that 21.4% of adults and 100% of adolescents were female. In this study, the mean age at onset of pyromania was 18.1 ($\pm$5.8) years, and the mean duration of the pyromania diagnosis was 5.6 ($\pm$4.5) years. An additional study that performed ICD screening in 102 adolescents consecutively admitted to an inpatient psychiatric service for various disorders also found a higher prevalence of pyromania in adolescent females (12.5%) compared with adolescent males (0%) (Grant et al. 2007). In a study examining differences between female and male fire setters in a prison population, female fire setters were more likely than male fire setters to be depressed and to have an internal locus of control (Alleyne et al. 2016).

Comorbidity

Pyromania has been found to be highly comorbid with major depressive disorder (47.6% prevalence [Lejoyeux et al. 2002]); with SUDs, including alcohol abuse (33.3% prevalence [Schreiber et al. 2011]); and with other ICDs (66.7% prevalence [Schreiber et al. 2011]). Fire setting has also been found to co-occur with bipolar disorder and with other disruptive, impulse-control, and conduct disorders (Grant and Won Kim 2007).

Pathogenesis

As in other areas, the etiology of pyromania has not received a significant amount of research; however, pyromania's high comorbidity with kleptomania and DSM-IV pathological gambling supports the hypothesis of a phenomenological link between pyromania and other ICDs that may indicate similarities in their etiology. Lower levels of cerebrospinal fluid (CSF) monoamine metabolites have been found in patients with ICDs, including pyromania and alcohol use disorder (Williams and Potenza 2008). Low CSF 5-hydroxyindoleacetic acid (5-HIAA) and homovanillic acid (HVA) concentrations and a family history of paternal violence and alcohol abuse are found in alcoholic male fire setters, while low CSF 5-HIAA and 3-methoxy-4-hydroxy-phenylglycol (MHPG) concentrations and a family history of paternal absence are found in recidivist alcoholic male fire setters (Virkkunen et al. 1996). Imaging studies of fire setters and individuals with pyromania have shown left inferior frontal perfusion deficits and frontal lobe dysfunction (Grant 2006a; Tyler and Gannon 2012), including a case in which the sudden onset of fire-setting behaviors was associated with a lacunar stroke (Bosshart and Capek 2011).

A history of childhood maltreatment is strongly associated with a range of psychopathology and poor prognosis. Compared with children without a history of abuse, maltreated children set more fires, have a stronger curiosity about fires, and have more emotional and behavior problems (Root et al. 2008). The distinction between normal and excessive curiosity about fire is not always evident, and there is likely a continuum between excessive interest in fire and pure pyromania. Females with pyromania frequently have a history of self-harm and psychosocial traumas, and fire setting could be a way of displacing aggression and anger and improving self-esteem.

Course

Pyromania most often begins in late adolescence or early adulthood. Notably, there are few studies that link childhood fire setting and impulsive behaviors to a diagnosis of pyromania in adolescence and adulthood. It appears that pyromania can be chronic if left untreated, although the longitudinal course of pyromania is currently unknown. Fire setting in adolescents has been found to be predictive of schizophrenia (Thomson et al. 2017). Many patients with pyromania do not commit acts of arson, but instead set controlled fires in their homes or yards; however, they report that over time, their urges increase and the time between fires decreases (Grant and Won Kim 2007). There is a possibility that these controlled fires may lead to arson, but further study is needed (Grant and Won Kim 2007).

Treatment

There have not yet been controlled treatment studies in individuals with pyromania as there have been with other ICDs, and there are currently no medications approved by the U.S. Food and Drug Administration (FDA) for any ICD. Studies of ICDs that are phenomenologically linked to pyromania, such as kleptomania, have shown benefit from opioid antagonists, including naltrexone. Medications that have been demonstrated to be effective in individual cases of pyromania include topiramate, escitalopram, sertraline, fluoxetine, and lithium (Grant and Won Kim 2007). In a case study of an 18-year-old man with an 8-month history of pyromania, including increasing intensity and urges, topiramate and CBT were prescribed concurrently (Grant 2006a). A reduction in the urge to set fires was observed after 3 weeks and continued to be observed 12 months later. An additional study comparing CBT and a fire safety intervention for child fire setters found reductions in match-playing activities, fire-setting incidents, and overall interest in fires in both groups (Kolko 2001). A follow-up study was conducted in 2006 that replicated the results and showed fire safety education and CBT to have the most influential effects (Kolko et al. 2006). A 2015 study using a CBT fire-setting intervention to treat incarcerated fire setters in U.K. prisons reported success in reducing key psychological factors associated with fire setting (Gannon et al. 2015). A wider scope of research on treatment for fire setters focuses on fire safety intervention programs and therapy, with the rationale that teaching fire knowledge and safety skills will lead to reduced interest in setting fires and increased use of alternative fire-safe behaviors (Lambie and Randell 2011). The Arson Prevention Program for Children in Toronto, Canada, is an example of a widely adopted mental health program for fire setters, although it still needs further evaluation. In summary, a multifaceted treatment, whether with CBT and medication in adults with pyromania or with CBT and fire safety interventions in at-risk child fire setters, appears to have the strongest evidence base for use in management of this ICD.

Kleptomania

Definition and Diagnostic Criteria

Kleptomania has not received much empirical study and therefore remains poorly understood. The defining feature of kleptomania is the inability to resist recurrent impulses to steal specific objects that are not required for personal use or for their monetary value (American Psychiatric Association 2013). As with pyromania, in order for an individual to meet DSM-5 criteria for kleptomania, there needs to be an increasing sense of tension immediately before stealing, as well as pleasure, gratification, or relief while committing the theft. Furthermore, the stealing is not done to express anger or vengeance or in response to a delusion or hallucination and is not better explained by conduct disorder, a manic episode, or antisocial personality disorder.

Clinically, kleptomania may have severe penalties and can be a lifelong chronic and debilitating condition if not recognized and treated. Individuals with kleptomania almost invariably can afford the stolen item, which is often given away, hoarded, hidden, thrown away, or returned secretly. It is the senselessness of the stolen item, as well as the fact that the objective of the theft is symptomatic relief rather than personal gain, that distinguishes kleptomania from ordinary shoplifting (Goldman 1991). Often, individuals keep this condition secret until they no longer can because of legal consequences and will then seek help.

Epidemiology

The lifetime prevalence of kleptomania within the general population is approximately 0.38%–0.6% (Goldman 1991; Odlaug and Grant 2010). However, many experts believe that this estimate may be too low, because the embarrassment related to shoplifting prevents many from reporting their symptoms. Although national epidemiological analyses of kleptomania have not been done, reports of kleptomania from multiple clinical samples imply a greater prevalence. As shown in Table 23–4, it appears that kleptomania is not uncommon among individuals with comorbid psychiatric conditions such as psychotic, anxiety, mood, or substance use disorders.

Kleptomania appears to be more prevalent in women than in men, with an estimated female-to-male ratio of 3 to 1 (American Psychiatric Association 2013). This reported female predominance in kleptomania may be biased, because courts are more likely to require female shoplifters to present for a psychiatric evaluation and women may be more likely to independently seek psychiatric evaluation. The severity and clinical presentation of kleptomania do not seem to differ between males and females (Grant and Kim 2002b; McElroy et al. 1991).

Comorbidity

Kleptomania is more often comorbid with affective disorders than with any other psychiatric disorders. Some studies suggest that bipolar disorder is the most common co-occurring disorder, whereas other studies suggest that unipolar depression has the highest rate of comorbidity with kleptomania. Comorbid bipolar disorder has been implicated in the high rate of suicide attempts in individuals with kleptomania (Odlaug

TABLE 23–4. **Prevalence of kleptomania in clinical samples**

Sample characteristics	Rate of kleptomania	Total sample
Adolescent inpatients with a variety of psychiatric disorders (Grant et al. 2007)	8.8%	9 of 102
Adult psychiatric inpatients with multiple disorders (Grant et al. 2005)	7.8%	16 of 204
Inpatients with alcohol dependence (Lejoyeux et al. 1999)	3.8%	3 of 79
Inpatients with depression (Lejoyeux et al. 2002)	3.7%	4 of 107
Anorexic and/or bulimic patients (Hudson et al. 1983)	28%	25 of 90
Pathological gamblers (Specker et al. 1995)	5%	2 of 40
Pathological gamblers (Grant and Kim 2003)	2.1%	2 of 96

et al. 2012). Research has also shown high rates of comorbid ICDs (20%–46%), anxiety disorders (60%–80%), eating disorders (60%), and SUDs (23%–50%) over the lifetime. Individuals with kleptomania have high rates of comorbid personality disorders, with paranoid (17.9%), schizoid (10.7%), borderline (10.7%), and histrionic (18%) personality disorders identified as the most common (Grant 2004; Grant and Kim 2002b; Kim et al. 2017; McElroy et al. 1991).

Pathogenesis

Biological Theories

Serotonin and inhibition. Patients diagnosed with kleptomania describe considerably higher rates of risk-taking behaviors and impulsivity in comparison with control subjects. Lower levels of inhibitory mechanisms could be the basis for this difference. Serotonin and the prefrontal cortex are among the most investigated inhibitory pathways. Risk-taking behaviors among adults, including pathological gambling, alcoholism, and fire setting, are associated with lower quantities of serotonin. Reduced amounts of the platelet serotonin transporter were found in patients with kleptomania in comparison with healthy control subjects (Marazziti et al. 2000). Case studies investigating pharmacological outcomes of serotonin reuptake inhibitors, including the SSRIs and clomipramine, show that these agents may reduce kleptomania-associated impulsive behavior (Durst et al. 2001).

Dopamine and reward deficiency. Dopaminergic systems that affect reinforcement and reward may influence kleptomania pathogenesis. Changes in dopaminergic pathways have been implicated as the underlying cause of increased reward-seeking behavior, such as shoplifting, which may trigger dopamine release and produce pleasurable feelings. The function and structure of dopamine neurons within the mesocorticolimbic system, concurrent with intrinsic γ-aminobutyric acid–ergic (GABAergic) and afferent glutamatergic activity, seem to adjust in response to these rewarding experiences, thereby influencing the nucleus accumbens. Later behavior may therefore be influenced by earlier rewarding experiences through neuroplastic alterations within the nucleus accumbens. These alterations may explain why many individuals with kleptomania describe shoplifting as "a habit" without feeling overt urges or cravings beforehand (Hollander et al. 2008).

Opioid system: craving and pleasure.   Urges associated with the perceived experience of pleasure and rewards are an intrinsic aspect of kleptomania in many cases. Urge regulation is thought to be controlled by the brain's μ-opioid system, at least partially through modulation of mesolimbic pathway dopamine neurons and GABA interneurons (Potenza and Hollander 2002). Moreover, studies with the opioid antagonist naltrexone have shown that this agent can reduce urges in individuals with kleptomania as well as with other ICDs (Grant et al. 2009).

Therefore, recurrent kleptomanic behavior could be due to an imbalance between a pathologically lowered inhibition and a pathologically elevated urge; that is, recurrent shoplifting could be a result of greater activity in the mesocorticolimbic dopamine pathway circuit, enhanced indirectly by the opioid system, and lower activity in cortical inhibitory processes, influenced largely by serotonin.

Neuroimaging.   In a neuroimaging study of individuals with kleptomania versus control subjects, diffusion tensor imaging findings showed that those with kleptomania had diminished microstructural coherence of white matter in the inferior frontal brain regions, which likely reflects faulty connectivity among the tracts linking the limbic area to the prefrontal and thalamus regions (Grant et al. 2006).

Psychological Theories

Some have hypothesized that kleptomania could result from attempts to alleviate depressive feelings through risk-taking behavior. Several reports suggest that antidepressants improve not only the symptoms of depression but also those of kleptomania. Behavioral models may provide insight into the pathogenesis of the disorder. According to the operant model, kleptomania is positively reinforced by the acquisition of items at no monetary cost and is intermittently reinforced through the periodic inability to shoplift due to the presence of security in the stores, therefore rendering kleptomania especially extinction resistant. Shoplifting may also produce physiological arousal, which in turn may further reinforce and perpetuate kleptomanic behavior.

Characterization of Kleptomania

Obsessive-compulsive disorder model.   Arguments that kleptomania may fall within the obsessive-compulsive disorder (OCD) spectrum are based on kleptomania's characteristic features of repetitive behaviors and faulty inhibition. However, other features of kleptomania, such as the thrill-seeking aspects of the disorder, generally speak against the OCD model because individuals with OCD are mostly harm avoidant (Hollander 1993). Moreover, studies focusing on rates of comorbid OCD in individuals with kleptomania have yielded inconsistent findings, and the co-occurrence of kleptomania in individuals with OCD is low.

Addiction model.   There is a rising wave of literature that argues that kleptomania may be better categorized as a "behavioral addiction" than as an "impulse disorder." Addiction and kleptomania share several distinct features, including comorbidity patterns, etiology, and lifetime trajectories, and frequently co-occur over the lifetime (Chamberlain et al. 2016; Kim et al. 2017; Starcevic 2016). Many individuals with kleptomania have first-degree relatives with a SUD diagnosis (Grant and Potenza 2004). Behaviorally, individuals can develop a tolerance for stealing, with the value of stolen items increasing over time. Pharmacologically, studies of individuals with kleptomania treated with naltrexone, which is used to treat addiction, have demonstrated positive response (Grant and Potenza 2004).

Affective spectrum model.　Findings that support inclusion of kleptomania within the affective spectrum include studies that show high rates of comorbid mood disorders in individuals with kleptomania (McElroy et al. 1991; Presta et al. 2002). Furthermore, kleptomanic symptoms may worsen concurrently with depression, and stealing may represent a form of antidepressant. Additionally, because of the high rates of comorbid bipolar disorder evident in various studies (McElroy et al. 1991), kleptomania is thought by some to represent a symptom of mania or subclinical hypomania.

Attention-deficit/hyperactivity model.　The ADHD model of kleptomania is only beginning to gain research attention. One study found significant comorbidity of ADHD with kleptomania (Presta et al. 2002). However, confirmatory studies supporting this finding have not yet been published. There have been a few case reports of successful use of ADHD medications in the treatment of a subset of individuals with kleptomania who appear to have inattentive and impulsive traits. This may be indicative of a category of kleptomania that is functionally related to ADHD (Grant 2006b).

Course

The onset of kleptomania generally occurs during adolescence (ages 16–20 years), although symptoms can occur in early childhood or late adulthood (Grant and Kim 2002b). The average age at which individuals first present for treatment, however, is about 35 years for females and 50 years for males (Goldman 1991). Because prevalence rates seem similar among adolescents and adults with the disorder, the course of untreated kleptomania may be better characterized as chronic. Data describing kleptomania's course are sparse, and epidemiological longitudinal studies have not been performed. Therefore, the prognosis is not clear. Three characteristic courses have been reported: sporadic with brief episodes and long periods of remission; episodic with protracted periods of stealing and periods of remission; and chronic with some degree of fluctuation (American Psychiatric Association 2013). A recent study of individuals with a DSM-IV diagnosis of kleptomania compared those who had a history of a shoplifting-related arrest and those who did not (Blum et al. 2018). Interestingly, individuals who had an arrest record rated themselves significantly higher on an impulsivity scale. There were no differences between the groups in time spent stealing, frequency of stealing, or overall functioning. The authors concluded that independent of symptom severity, kleptomania may be associated with deficits in inhibitory control (Blum et al. 2018).

Treatment

Pharmacotherapy

The FDA has not yet approved any medication for the treatment of kleptomania; therefore, patients must be informed about off-label applications of various medications for kleptomania and the evidence for treatment with medication. The literature investigating pharmacotherapy for kleptomania remains limited.

Two controlled trials of pharmacological treatment of kleptomania have been conducted. In a double-blind, placebo-controlled trial of naltrexone, individuals receiving naltrexone showed reductions in kleptomania symptoms compared with those receiving placebo (Grant et al. 2009). These findings are consistent with those of an open-label trial with naltrexone, which demonstrated a significant reduction in urge-to-steal intensity, as well as in thoughts and behaviors associated with stealing (Grant and Kim 2002a). In an open-label trial of escitalopram followed by a double-blind discontinuation phase, the response initially found in the open phase was not maintained during discontinuation, suggesting that a true drug response did not occur (Koran et al. 2007). An open trial of memantine, an N-methyl-D-aspartate receptor antagonist, in individuals with kleptomania reported a 91% response rate, with reductions demonstrated in urges to shoplift and shoplifting behavior (Grant et al. 2013). Case reports and case series have demonstrated some positive treatment response to nortriptyline, SSRIs (fluoxetine, paroxetine, fluvoxamine), trazodone, clonazepam, lithium, valproate, and topiramate.

If kleptomania is a result of both faulty urge control and impaired behavior inhibition, then both opioid antagonists and antidepressants (SSRIs) could play a significant role in alleviating these symptoms and regulating the behavior. Therefore, naltrexone may help in decreasing both the desire and the urge to steal as well as the actual behavior by diminishing the thrill related to stealing, thereby averting the positive reinforcement associated with the behavior. SSRIs may also effectively reduce kleptomania symptoms by influencing serotonergic systems thought to be associated with deficient impulse regulation.

A suggested treatment approach for kleptomania is to initiate treatment with an SSRI or a serotonin–norepinephrine reuptake inhibitor, titrated to the appropriate dosage for the appropriate duration. Nonresponse or incomplete response to this medication could be followed by a trial of naltrexone or topiramate.

Psychotherapy

Various types of psychotherapy to treat kleptomania have been attempted. However, controlled trials of psychotherapy do not exist in the literature. Case studies have reported some success for psychoanalysis as well as for behavioral therapies, including exposure and response prevention, conditioning and covert sensitization, imaginal desensitization, and CBT.

Because empirical studies are scant, further research is required to determine which psychotherapy is most efficacious for kleptomania as well as methods for combination of psychotherapy and medication in the treatment of people with kleptomania.

Other Specified Disruptive, Impulse-Control, and Conduct Disorder

The DSM-5 category of other specified disruptive, impulse-control, and conduct disorder is assigned when an individual presents with significant disruptive, impulse-control, or conduct symptoms that cause clinically significant impairment in social, occupational, or other areas of functioning but do not meet the diagnostic threshold for a specific disorder within this class. When this diagnosis is made, the clinician states a specific reason for why the presentation of symptoms does not meet full criteria for a specific diagnosis (e.g., "recurrent behavioral outbursts of insufficient frequency").

Unspecified Disruptive, Impulse-Control, and Conduct Disorder

The DSM-5 category of unspecified disruptive, impulse-control, and conduct disorder is similar to the "other specified" category in that it involves an individual who presents with significant disruptive behavior symptoms and clinical impairment but does not meet the full criteria for a disruptive, impulse-control, or conduct disorder. However, the "unspecified" category is used in situations in which the clinician does not wish to specify why an individual does not meet the threshold for a specific disorder in this diagnostic class. Thus, the unspecified category may be assigned, for example, in an emergency department setting, when there is insufficient information to make a more specific diagnosis.

Conclusion

This chapter has focused on disorders found in the DSM-5 disruptive, impulse-control, and conduct disorders diagnostic class. Pathological impulsivity, rule breaking, and aggressive behaviors may be a crucial construct in understanding a broad range of psychiatric disorders, including common psychotic disorders (e.g., bipolar disorder), personality disorders (e.g., antisocial personality disorder), and ADHD. The development of reliable diagnostic criteria has been extremely useful in promoting research on these disorders and has provided a basis for epidemiological work demonstrating their prevalence, their high comorbidity and morbidity, and their significant social costs. At the same time, advances in basic research on impulsivity and aggression, together with new methods in clinical research, have led to increased understanding of the overlapping neurocircuitry and neurochemistry that may be involved in these conditions and that in turn may ultimately lead to a revised nosology of these conditions. Developments in psychometrics and psychobiology have encouraged researchers to conduct randomized clinical trials of various medications and psychotherapies for the disruptive, impulse-control, and conduct disorders. However, the range of clinical trials in this area remains comparatively limited, and for this reason, no medications are currently approved by the FDA for treatment of disorders in this diagnostic class, nor is there an established American Psychiatric Association practice guideline for first- or second-line treatments. Instead, clinicians are required to adopt a flexible approach that includes multiple modalities of intervention in the management of these disorders. Although many patients can be helped by such an approach, much further work is needed to delineate fully the psychobiology of these disorders and to develop effective treatments.

Key Clinical Points

- Pathological impulsivity, aggression, and rule-breaking behavior are useful constructs for understanding a broad range of psychiatric symptoms and disorders.

- Disruptive, impulse-control, and conduct disorders are highly prevalent and are associated with significant disability and costs, yet these disorders receive disproportionately little attention from clinicians and researchers.

- There have been significant advances in our understanding of the neuronal circuitry that mediates impulsivity and aggression, as well as in research delineating the genes and proteins that contribute to this circuitry.

- Ultimately, a better understanding of the psychobiological underpinnings of impulsivity, aggression, and rule-breaking behavior, as well as other related constructs, may lead to changes in our classification of these disorders.

- Although no medication is approved by the FDA for the treatment of disruptive, impulse-control, and conduct disorders, a number of randomized controlled trials have demonstrated the potential value of pharmacotherapy.

- Current clinical practice emphasizes the need for a comprehensive approach to management that includes psychotherapy and family intervention. Additional work is needed to improve the efficacy of these treatments.

References

Alleyne E, Gannon TA, Mozova K, et al: Female fire-setters: gender-associated psychological and psychopathological features. Psychiatry 79(4):364–378, 2016 27997329
American Psychiatric Association: Diagnostic and Statistical Manual of Mental Disorders, 4th Edition. Washington, DC, American Psychiatric Association, 1994
American Psychiatric Association: Diagnostic and Statistical Manual of Mental Disorders, 4th Edition, Text Revision. Washington, DC, American Psychiatric Association, 2000
American Psychiatric Association: DSM-5 Development: Recent Updates to Proposed Revisions for DSM-5. American Psychiatric Association, 2012. Available at: www.dsm5.org/Pages/RecentUpdates.aspx. Accessed September 27, 2012.
American Psychiatric Association: Diagnostic and Statistical Manual of Mental Disorders, 5th Edition. Arlington, VA, American Psychiatric Association, 2013
Angold A, Costello EJ, Erkanli A: Comorbidity. J Child Psychol Psychiatry 40(1):57–87, 1999 10102726
Bakker MJ, Greven CU, Buitelaar JK, et al: Practitioner review: psychological treatments for children and adolescents with conduct disorder problems—a systematic review and meta-analysis. J Child Psychol Psychiatry 58(1):4–18, 2017 27501434
Barlow J, Stewart-Brown S: Behavior problems and group-based parent education programs. J Dev Behav Pediatr 21(5):356–370, 2000 11064964
Bauer LO, Hesselbrock VM: Brain maturation and subtypes of conduct disorder: interactive effects on P300 amplitude and topography in male adolescents. J Am Acad Child Adolesc Psychiatry 42(1):106–115, 2003 12500083
Blum AW, Odlaug BL, Redden SA, et al: Stealing behavior and impulsivity in individuals with kleptomania who have been arrested for shoplifting. Compr Psychiatry 80:186–191, 2018 29127886

Bosshart H, Capek S: An unusual case of random fire-setting behavior associated with lacunar stroke. Forensic Sci Int 209(1–3):e8–e10, 2011 21489732

Buitelaar JK, van der Gaag RJ, Cohen-Kettenis P, Melman CT: A randomized controlled trial of risperidone in the treatment of aggression in hospitalized adolescents with subaverage cognitive abilities. J Clin Psychiatry 62(4):239–248, 2001 11379837

Burke JD, Loeber R, Birmaher B: Oppositional defiant disorder and conduct disorder: a review of the past 10 years, II. J Am Acad Child Adolesc 41(11):1275–1293, 2002 12410070

Butler S, Baruch G, Hickey N, et al: A randomized controlled trial of multisystemic therapy and a statutory therapeutic intervention for young offenders. J Am Acad Child Adolesc Psychiatry 50(12):1220–1235.e2, 2011 22115143

Canino G, Polanczyk G, Bauermeister JJ, et al: Does the prevalence of CD and ODD vary across cultures? Soc Psychiatry Psychiatr Epidemiol 45(7):695–704, 2010 20532864

Chamberlain SR, Lochner C, Stein DJ, et al: Behavioural addiction—a rising tide? Eur Neuropsychopharmacol 26(5):841–855, 2016 26585600

Coccaro EF: A family history study of intermittent explosive disorder. J Psychiatr Res 44(15):1101–1105, 2010 20488459

Coccaro EF: Intermittent explosive disorder as a disorder of impulsive aggression for DSM-5. Am J Psychiatry 169(6):577–588, 2012 22535310

Coccaro EF, Schmidt CA, Samuels JF, et al: Lifetime and 1-month prevalence rates of intermittent explosive disorder in a community sample. J Clin Psychiatry 65(6):820–824, 2004 15291659

Coccaro EF, Posternak MA, Zimmerman M: Prevalence and features of intermittent explosive disorder in a clinical setting. J Clin Psychiatry 66(10):1221–1227, 2005 16259534

Coccaro EF, McCloskey MS, Fitzgerald DA, Phan KL: Amygdala and orbitofrontal reactivity to social threat in individuals with impulsive aggression. Biol Psychiatry 62(2):168–178, 2007 17210136

Coccaro EF, Lee RJ, Kavoussi RJ: A double-blind, randomized, placebo-controlled trial of fluoxetine in patients with intermittent explosive disorder. J Clin Psychiatry 70(5):653–662, 2009 19389333

Coccaro EF, Lee R, Kavoussi RJ: Aggression, suicidality, and intermittent explosive disorder: serotonergic correlates in personality disorder and healthy control subjects. Neuropsychopharmacology 35(2):435–444, 2010a 19776731

Coccaro EF, Lee R, Kavoussi RJ: Inverse relationship between numbers of 5-HT transporter binding sites and life history of aggression and intermittent explosive disorder. J Psychiatr Res 44(3):137–142, 2010b 19767013

Coccaro EF, Lee R, McCloskey MS: Validity of the new A1 and A2 criteria for DSM-5 intermittent explosive disorder. Compr Psychiatry 55(2):260–267, 2014 24321204

Coccaro EF, Lee R, McCloskey M, et al: Morphometric analysis of amygdala and hippocampus shape in impulsively aggressive and healthy control subjects. J Psychiatr Res 69:80–86, 2015 26343598

Coccaro EF, Fanning JR, Lee R: Intermittent explosive disorder and substance use disorder: analysis of the National Comorbidity Survey Replication sample. J Clin Psychiatry 78(6):697–702, 2017 28252880

Dell'Osso B, Altamura AC, Allen A, et al: Epidemiologic and clinical updates on impulse control disorders: a critical review. Eur Arch Psychiatry Clin Neurosci 256(8):464–475, 2006 16960655

Demmer DH, Hooley M, Sheen J, et al: Sex differences in the prevalence of oppositional defiant disorder during middle childhood: a meta-analysis. J Abnorm Child Psychol 45(2):313–325, 2017 27282758

Durst R, Katz G, Teitelbaum A, et al: Kleptomania: diagnosis and treatment options. CNS Drugs 15(3):185–195, 2001 11463127

Ezpeleta L, Granero R: Executive functions in preschoolers with ADHD, ODD, and comorbid ADHD-ODD: evidence from ecological and performance-based measures. J Neuropsychol 9(2):258–270, 2015 24966035

Farmer EMZ, Compton SN, Burns JB, Robertson E: Review of the evidence base for treatment of childhood psychopathology: externalizing disorders. J Consult Clin Psychol 70(6):1267–1302, 2002 12472301

Frankle WG, Lombardo I, New AS, et al: Brain serotonin transporter distribution in subjects with impulsive aggressivity: a positron emission study with [11C]McN 5652. Am J Psychiatry 162(5):915–923, 2005 15863793

Frick PJ, Moffitt TE: A proposal to the DSM-5 childhood disorders and the ADHD and Disruptive Behavior Disorders Work Groups to include a specifier to the diagnosis of conduct disorder based on the presence of callous-unemotional traits. Washington, DC, American Psychiatric Association, 2010. Available at: www.dsm5.org/Proposed%20Revision%20Attachments/Proposal%20for%20Callous%20and%20Unemotional%20Specifier%20of%20Conduct%20Disorder. pdf. Accessed March 9, 2013.

Gannon TA, Alleyne E, Butler H, et al: Specialist group therapy for psychological factors associated with firesetting: evidence of a treatment effect from a non-randomized trial with male prisoners. Behav Res Ther 73:42–51, 2015 26248329

Goldman MJ: Kleptomania: making sense of the nonsensical. Am J Psychiatry 148(8):986–996, 1991 1853988

Grant JE: Co-occurrence of personality disorders in persons with kleptomania: a preliminary investigation. J Am Acad Psychiatry Law 32:395–398, 2004 15704625

Grant JE: SPECT imaging and treatment of pyromania. J Clin Psychiatry 67(6):998, 2006a 16848668

Grant JE: Understanding and treating kleptomania: new models and new treatments. Isr J Psychiatry Relat Sci 43(2):81–87, 2006b 16910369

Grant JE, Kim SW: An open-label study of naltrexone in the treatment of kleptomania. J Clin Psychiatry 63(4):349–356, 2002a 12000210

Grant JE, Kim SW: Clinical characteristics and associated psychopathology of 22 patients with kleptomania. Compr Psychiatry 43(5):378–384, 2002b 12216013

Grant JE, Kim SW: Comorbidity of impulse control disorders in pathological gamblers. Acta Psychiatr Scand 108(3):203–207, 2003 12890275

Grant JE, Won Kim S: Clinical characteristics and psychiatric comorbidity of pyromania. J Clin Psychiatry 68(11):1717–1722, 2007 18052565

Grant JE, Potenza MN: Impulse control disorders: clinical characteristics and pharmacological management. Ann Clin Psychiatry 16(1):27–34, 2004 15147110

Grant JE, Levine L, Kim SW, Potenza MN: Impulse control disorders in adult psychiatric inpatients. Am J Psychiatry 162(11):2184–2188, 2005 16263865

Grant JE, Correia S, Brennan-Krohn T: White matter integrity in kleptomania: a pilot study. Psychiatry Res 147(2–3):233–237, 2006 16956753

Grant JE, Williams KA, Potenza MN: Impulse-control disorders in adolescent psychiatric inpatients: co-occurring disorders and sex differences. J Clin Psychiatry 68(10):1584–1592, 2007 17960976

Grant JE, Kim SW, Odlaug BL: A double-blind, placebo-controlled study of the opiate antagonist, naltrexone, in the treatment of kleptomania. Biol Psychiatry 65(7):600–606, 2009 19217077

Grant JE, Odlaug BL, Schreiber LR, et al: Memantine reduces stealing behavior and impulsivity in kleptomania: a pilot study. Int Clin Psychopharmacol 28(2):106–111, 2013 23299454

Hoertel N, Le Strat Y, Schuster JP, Limosin F: Gender differences in firesetting: results from the national epidemiologic survey on alcohol and related conditions (NESARC). Psychiatry Res 190(2–3):352–358, 2011 21684614

Hollander E (ed): Obsessive-Compulsive Related Disorders. Washington, DC, American Psychiatric Press, 1993

Hollander E, Tracy KA, Swann AC, et al: Divalproex in the treatment of impulsive aggression: efficacy in cluster B personality disorders. Neuropsychopharmacology 28(6):1186–1197, 2003 12700713

Hollander E, Swann AC, Coccaro EF, et al: Impact of trait impulsivity and state aggression on divalproex versus placebo response in borderline personality disorder. Am J Psychiatry 162(3):621–624, 2005 15741486

Hollander E, Berlin HA, Stein DJ: Impulse-control disorders not elsewhere classified, in The American Psychiatric Publishing Textbook of Psychiatry, 5th Edition. Edited by Hales RE, Yudofsky SC, Gabbard GO. Arlington, VA, American Psychiatric Publishing, 2008, pp 777–820

Hudson JI, Pope HG Jr, Jonas JM, Yurgelun-Todd D: Phenomenologic relationship of eating disorders to major affective disorder. Psychiatry Res 9(4):345–354, 1983 6580663

Jennings KM, Wildes JE, Coccaro EF: Intermittent explosive disorder and eating disorders: analysis of national comorbidity and research samples. Compr Psychiatry 75:62–67, 2017 28324677

Kazdin AE, Siegel T, Bass D: Cognitive problem-solving skills training and parent management training in the treatment of antisocial behavior in children. J Consult Clin Psychol 60(5):733–747, 1992 1401389

Kessler RC, Coccaro EF, Fava M, et al: The prevalence and correlates of DSM-IV intermittent explosive disorder in the National Comorbidity Survey Replication. Arch Gen Psychiatry 63(6):669–678, 2006 16754840

Kim HS, Christianini AR, Bertoni D, et al: Kleptomania and co-morbid addictive disorders. Psychiatry Res 250:35–37, 2017 28142063

Kolko DJ: Efficacy of cognitive-behavioral treatment and fire safety education for children who set fires: initial and follow-up outcomes. J Child Psychol Psychiatry 42(3):359–369, 2001 11321205

Kolko DJ, Herschell AD, Scharf DM: Education and treatment for boys who set fires: specificity, moderators, and predictors of recidivism. Journal of Emotional and Behavioral Disorders 14:227–239, 2006

Koran LM, Aboujaoude E, Gamel N: Escitalopram treatment of kleptomania: an open-label trial followed by double-blind discontinuation. J Clin Psychiatry 68(3):422–427, 2007 17388713

Kruesi MJP, Casanova MF, Mannheim G, et al: Reduced temporal lobe volume in early onset conduct disorder. Psychiatry Res 132(1):1–11, 2004 15546698

Labree W, Nijman H, van Marle H, Rassin E: Backgrounds and characteristics of arsonists. Int J Law Psychiatry 33(3):149–153, 2010 20434774

Lahey BB, Van Hulle CA, Singh AL, et al: Higher-order genetic and environmental structure of prevalent forms of child and adolescent psychopathology. Arch Gen Psychiatry 68(2):181–189, 2011 21300945

Lambie I, Randell I: Creating a firestorm: a review of children who deliberately light fires. Clin Psychol Rev 31(3):307–327, 2011 21382537

Lambie I, Ioane J, Randell I, et al: Offending behaviours of child and adolescent firesetters over a 10-year follow-up. J Child Psychol Psychiatry 54(12):1295–1307, 2013 23927002

Lejoyeux M, Feuche N, Loi S, et al: Study of impulse-control disorders among alcohol-dependent patients. J Clin Psychiatry 60(5):302–305, 1999 10362437

Lejoyeux M, Arbaretaz M, McLoughlin M, Adès J: Impulse control disorders and depression. J Nerv Ment Dis 190(5):310–314, 2002 12011611

Lindberg N, Holi MM, Tani P, Virkkunen M: Looking for pyromania: characteristics of a consecutive sample of Finnish male criminals with histories of recidivist fire-setting between 1973 and 1993. BMC Psychiatry 5:1–5, 2005 16351734

Loeber R, Green SM, Lahey BB, et al: Findings on disruptive behavior disorders from the first decade of the developmental trends study. Clin Child Fam Psychol Rev 3(1):37–60, 2000 11228766

MacKay S, Paglia-Boak A, Henderson J, et al: Epidemiology of firesetting in adolescents: mental health and substance use correlates. J Child Psychol Psychiatry 50(10):1282–1290, 2009 19508496

Marazziti D, Presta S, Pfanner C, et al: The biological basis of kleptomania and compulsive buying. Paper presented at the American College of Neuropsychopharmacology 39th Annual Meeting. San Juan, Puerto Rico, December 2000

Maughan B, Rowe R, Messer J, et al: Conduct disorder and oppositional defiant disorder in a national sample: developmental epidemiology. J Child Psychol Psychiatry 45(3):609–621, 2004 15055379

McCloskey MS, Noblett KL, Deffenbacher JL, et al: Cognitive-behavioral therapy for intermittent explosive disorder: a pilot randomized clinical trial. J Consult Clin Psychol 76(5):876–886, 2008 18837604

McElroy SL, Pope HG Jr, Hudson JI, et al: Kleptomania: a report of 20 cases. Am J Psychiatry 148(5):652–657, 1991 2018170

McElroy SL, Keck PE Jr, Pope HG Jr, et al: Compulsive buying: a report of 20 cases. J Clin Psychiatry 55(6):242–248, 1994 8071278

McKinney C, Renk K: Atypical antipsychotic medications in the management of disruptive behaviors in children: safety guidelines and recommendations. Clin Psychol Rev 31(3):465–471, 2011 21130552

McLaughlin KA, Green JG, Hwang I, et al: Intermittent explosive disorder in the National Comorbidity Survey Replication Adolescent Supplement. Arch Gen Psychiatry 69(11):1131–1139, 2012 22752056

Moffitt TE: Genetic and environmental influences on antisocial behaviors: evidence from behavioral-genetic research. Adv Genet 55:41–104, 2005 16291212

Moffitt TE, Caspi A, Rutter M, et al: Sex Differences in Antisocial Behaviour: Conduct Disorder, Delinquency and Violence in the Dunedin Longitudinal Study. Cambridge, UK, Cambridge University Press, 2001

Nock MK, Kazdin AE, Hiripi E, Kessler RC: Lifetime prevalence, correlates, and persistence of oppositional defiant disorder: results from the national comorbidity survey replication. J Child Psychol Psychiatry 48(7):703–713, 2007 17593151

Odlaug BL, Grant JE: Impulse-control disorders in a college sample: results from the self-administered Minnesota Impulse Disorders Interview (MIDI). Prim Care Companion J Clin Psychiatry 12(2), 2010 20694115

Odlaug BL, Grant JE, Kim SW: Suicide attempts in 107 adolescents and adults with kleptomania. Arch Suicide Res 16(4):348–359, 2012 23137224

Palermo GB: A look at firesetting, arson, and pyromania. Int J Offender Ther Comp Criminol 59(7):683–684, 2015 25977346

Pappadopulos E, Woolston S, Chait B, et al: Pharmacotherapy of aggression in children and adolescents: efficacy and effect size. J Am Acad Child Adolesc Psychiatry 15(1):27–39, 2006 18392193

Pardini DA, Frick PJ, Moffitt TE: Building an evidence base for DSM-5 conceptualizations of oppositional defiant disorder and conduct disorder: introduction to the special section. J Abnorm Psychol 119(4):683–688, 2010 21090874

Perez-Rodriguez MM, Hazlett EA, Rich EL, et al: Striatal activity in borderline personality disorder with comorbid intermittent explosive disorder: sex differences. J Psychiatr Res 46(6):797–804, 2012 22464337

Phan KL, Lee R, Coccaro EF: Personality predictors of antiaggressive response to fluoxetine: inverse association with neuroticism and harm avoidance. Int Clin Psychopharmacol 26(5):278–283, 2011 21795983

Potenza MN, Hollander E: Pathological gambling and impulse-control disorders, in Neuropsychopharmacology: The 5th Generation of Progress. Edited by Coyle JT, Nemeroff C, Charney D. Baltimore, MD, Lippincott Williams & Wilkins, 2002, pp 1725–1741

Presta S, Marazziti D, Dell'Osso L, et al: Kleptomania: clinical features and comorbidity in an Italian sample. Compr Psychiatry 43(1):7–12, 2002 11788913

Robins LN, Ratcliff KS: Risk factors in the continuation of childhood antisocial behavior into adulthood. International Journal of Mental Health 7(3–4):96–116, 1978. Available at: https://www.tandfonline.com/doi/abs/10.1080/00207411.1978.11448810. Accessed January 28, 2019.

Rogers JC, De Brito SA: Cortical and subcortical gray matter volume in youths with conduct problems: a meta-analysis. JAMA Psychiatry 73(1):64–72, 2016 26650724

Root C, Mackay S, Henderson J, et al: The link between maltreatment and juvenile firesetting: correlates and underlying mechanisms. Child Abuse Negl 32(2):161–176, 2008 18308389

Rosell DR, Thompson JL, Slifstein M, et al: Increased serotonin 2A receptor availability in the orbitofrontal cortex of physically aggressive personality disordered patients. Biol Psychiatry 67(12):1154–1162, 2010 20434136

Rowe R, Maughan B, Worthman CM, et al: Testosterone, antisocial behavior, and social dominance in boys: pubertal development and biosocial interaction. Biol Psychiatry 55(5):546–552, 2004 15023584

Rowe R, Costello EJ, Angold A, et al: Developmental pathways in oppositional defiant disorder and conduct disorder. J Abnorm Psychol 119(4):726–773, 2010 21090876

Salvatore JE, Dick DM: Genetic influences on conduct disorder. Neurosci Biobehav Rev 91:91–101, 2018 27350097

Schreiber L, Odlaug BL, Grant JE: Impulse control disorders: updated review of clinical characteristics and pharmacological management. Front Psychiatry 2:1, 2011 21556272

Scott KM, Lim CC, Hwang I, et al: The cross-national epidemiology of DSM-IV intermittent explosive disorder. Psychol Med 46(15):3161–3172, 2016 27572872

Smaragdi A, Carison GA, Christenson GA, Marcotte M: Sex differences in the relationship between conduct disorder and cortical structure in adolescents. J Am Acad Child Adolesc Psychiatry 56(8):703–712, 2017 28735700

Specker SM, Cornwell H, Toschi N, et al: Impulse control disorders and attention deficit disorder in pathological gamblers. Ann Clin Psychiatry 7(4):175–179, 1995 8721891

Speltz ML, McClellan J, Deklyen M, Jones K: Preschool boys with oppositional defiant disorder: clinical presentation and diagnostic change. J Am Acad Child Adolesc Psychiatry 38(7):838–845, 1999 10405501

Stanford MS, Helfritz LE, Conklin SM, et al: A comparison of anticonvulsants in the treatment of impulsive aggression. Exp Clin Psychopharmacol 13(1):72–77, 2005 15727506

Starcevic V: Behavioural addictions: a challenge for psychopathology and psychiatric nosology. Aust N Z J Psychiatry 50(8):721–725, 2016 27357713

Sterzer P, Stadler C, Krebs A, et al: Abnormal neural responses to emotional visual stimuli in adolescents with conduct disorder. Biol Psychiatry 57(1):7–15, 2005 15607294

Stringaris A, Goodman R: Longitudinal outcome of youth oppositionality: irritable, headstrong, and hurtful behaviors have distinctive predictions. J Am Acad Child Adolesc Psychiatry 48(4):404–412, 2009 19318881

Taylor J, Iacono WG, McGue M: Evidence for a genetic etiology of early onset delinquency. J Abnorm Psychol 109(4):634–643, 2000 11195987

Thomson A, Tiihonen J, Miettunen J, et al: Fire-setting performed in adolescence or early adulthood predicts schizophrenia: a register-based follow-up study of pre-trial offenders. Nord J Psychiatry 71(2):96–101, 2017 27670756

Tyler N, Gannon TA: Explanations of firesetting in mentally disordered offenders: a review of the literature. Psychiatry 75(2):150–166, 2012 22642434

Vanwoerden S, Reuter T, Sharp C: Exploring the clinical utility of the DSM-5 conduct disorder specifier of "with limited prosocial emotions" in an adolescent inpatient sample. Compr Psychiatry 69:116–131, 2016 27423352

Virkkunen M, Eggert M, Rawlings R, Linnoila M: A prospective follow-up study of alcoholic violent offenders and fire setters. Arch Gen Psychiatry 53(6):523–529, 1996 8639035

Williams KA, Potenza MN: The neurobiology of impulse control disorders [in Portuguese]. Revista Brasileira de Psiquiatria (Sao Paulo, Brazil) 30 (suppl 1):S24–S30, 2008

Recommended Readings

Coccaro E (ed): Aggression: Psychiatric Assessment and Treatment. New York, Informa Healthcare, 2003

Coccaro EF: Intermittent explosive disorder as a disorder of impulsive aggression for DSM-5. Am J Psychiatry 169(6):577–588, 2012 22535310

Coccaro EF, Lee R, McCloskey MS: Validity of the new A1 and A2 criteria for DSM-5 intermittent explosive disorder. Compr Psychiatry 55(2):260–267, 2014 24321204

Frick PJ, Moffitt TE: A Proposal to the DSM-V Childhood Disorders and the ADHD and Disruptive Behavior Disorders Work Groups to Include a Specifier to the Diagnosis of Conduct Disorder Based on the Presence of Callous-Unemotional Traits. Arlington, VA, American Psychiatric Association, 2010

Hollander E, Evers M: New developments in impulsivity. Lancet 358(9286):949–950, 2001 11583745

Hollander E, Stein DJ (eds): Impulsivity and Aggression. Sussex, UK, Wiley, 1995

Hollander E, Stein DJ (eds): Clinical Manual of Impulse-Control Disorders. Washington, DC, American Psychiatric Publishing, 2006

Pardini DA, Frick PJ, Moffitt TE: Building an evidence base for DSM-5 conceptualizations of oppositional defiant disorder and conduct disorder: introduction to the special section. J Abnorm Psychol 119(4):683–688, 2010 21090874

Scott KM, Lim CC, Hwang I, et al: The cross-national epidemiology of DSM-IV intermittent explosive disorder. Psychol Med 46(15):3161–3172, 2016 27572872

CHAPTER 24

Substance-Related and Addictive Disorders

Jonathan Avery, M.D.

Tarek Adam, M.D., M.Sc.

Petros Levounis, M.D., M.A.

Substance-related and addictive disorders are common, are often disabling, and frequently co-occur with other psychiatric and medical disorders. In this chapter, we present an overview of the disorders that result from the use of selected substances classified in 10 drug classes, as well as an overview of gambling disorder, which was added to this chapter in the *Diagnostic and Statistical Manual of Mental Disorders*, 5th Edition (DSM-5; American Psychiatric Association 2013).

Diagnosis

DSM-5 provides detailed criteria for establishing the diagnosis of a substance use disorder for all 10 drug classes listed in Table 24–1 except for caffeine. Other terms, including *substance dependence* and *substance abuse* (from older editions of DSM) and *substance addiction*, are commonly used in clinical practice.

All of the DSM-5 substance use disorders and gambling disorder have similar criteria, including requiring clinically significant impairment or distress and the presence of at least two physical, psychological, or social consequences of the substance use. The criteria emphasize a loss of control over the amount and duration of consumption of the substance, as well as over the time involved in obtaining, consuming, or recovering from the substance. Use of the substance continues despite impairment in social, occupational, recreational, financial, physical, or mental health domains. Tolerance to the effects of the substance results in greater quantities being used to reach a level of intoxication. Symptoms of withdrawal occur following cessation or reduction of consumption (American Psychiatric Association 2013).

TABLE 24–1.   Commonly used substances and their mechanism(s) of action

Substance	Target	Primary mechanism of action
Alcohol	Undefined	Increases DA either by direct action or possibly by disinhibition via GABAergic receptors
Caffeine	Adenosine A_{2A} antagonist	Indirectly increases glutamate release through A_{2A} receptor activation
Cannabis	Cannabinoid CB_1 receptor agonist	Increases DA by disinhibition of VTA DA neurons through CB_1 receptors on GABAergic neurons
Hallucinogens	Serotonin 5-HT_{2A} receptor agonist (numerous other targets)	Mediates hallucinogenic effects through stimulation of 5-HT_{2A} receptors; binds directly to all DA receptor subtypes, partial agonist at DA_1 and DA_2 receptors
Inhalants	Undefined	Increases DA by directly stimulating VTA DA neurons or through GABA and NMDA receptors
Opioids (morphine, heroin)	μ-Receptor agonist	Increases DA release by disinhibition of inhibitory GABAergic neurons through μ receptors
Stimulants		
Methamphetamine/ amphetamine	NET/DAT, VMAT2, MAO	Induces NE and DA presynaptic release, reverses transporters
Cocaine	DAT/NET/SERT	Binds to presynaptic monoamine transporters and blocks their reuptake, thereby increasing synaptic levels
Tobacco/nicotine	nAChR agonist	Increases firing of VTA DA neurons through nicotinic β_2 receptors; disinhibits DA neurons via $\alpha_4\beta_2$ receptors on VTA GABAergic neurons

Note.   DA=dopamine; DAT=dopamine transporter; GABA=γ-aminobutyric acid; MAO=monoamine oxidase; nAChR=nicotinic acetylcholine receptor; NE=norepinephrine; NET=norepinephrine transporter; NMDA=N-methyl-D-aspartate; SERT=serotonin transporter; VMAT2=vesicular monoamine transporter 2; VTA=ventral tegmental area.

Source.   Reprinted from Table 23–4 (p. 740) in Kosten TR, Newton TF, De La Garza R, Haile CN: "Substance-Related and Addictive Disorders," in *The American Psychiatric Publishing Textbook of Psychiatry,* Sixth Edition. Edited by Hales RE, Yudofsky SC, Roberts LW. Arlington, VA, American Psychiatric Association, 2014, pp. 735–814. Copyright 2014, American Psychiatric Association.

DSM-5 includes several specifiers to further characterize the substance use disorders; these specifiers mostly relate to *course* (e.g., early remission, sustained remission) and *severity* (based on the number of criteria endorsed). For opioid use disorder, there is also a specifier to indicate whether the individual is on maintenance therapy. DSM-5 also provides diagnostic criteria for clinical presentations that are directly related to substance use, such as intoxication and withdrawal, along with descriptive specifiers. People can also develop a substance-related disorder from many different substances not listed explicitly in DSM-5 or this chapter, and these disorders are classified under other (or unknown) substance-related disorders. Furthermore, while gambling disorder is the only behavioral addiction addressed in the substance-related and addictive disorders section of DSM-5, others have also been proposed, including Internet gaming disorder, which is listed under "Conditions for Further Study" in DSM-5. Several substance-/medication-induced mental disorders can occur from using substances as well (American Psychiatric Association 2013).

Neurobiology and Neurocircuitry of Addiction

The neurobiology and neurocircuitry of addiction are complex but not significantly different for each addictive substance or behavior (see Table 24–1 and Figure 24–1). At the simplest level, substances increase dopamine in specific areas of the brain such as the nucleus accumbens, which results in alterations in an individual's reward circuitry (Levounis 2016). We are learning, however, that many other neurotransmitters and areas of the brain play a role in substance use disorders. Animal and human models, for example, have revealed unique circuits for different stages of addiction (Koob and Volkow 2010). According to Koob's model, addiction primarily targets three brain systems:

1. The ventral tegmental area and ventral striatum, which are critical in the binge/intoxication stage.
2. The extended amygdala, which is responsible for the withdrawal/negative affect stage.
3. The final stage, preoccupation/anticipation or craving, which may involve numerous areas of the brain, including the orbitofrontal cortex–dorsal striatum, prefrontal cortex, basolateral amygdala, hippocampus, insula, cingulate gyrus, dorsolateral prefrontal, and inferior frontal cortices.

One of the reasons why gambling disorder was added to the "Substance-Related and Addictive Disorders" chapter in DSM-5 is that individuals with this disorder have brain abnormalities similar to those in people with substance use disorders.

Epidemiology

While rates vary by country and demographics, very few areas of the world are immune to substance use disorders, with tobacco being the leading global cause of preventable death and almost 5% of the global burden of disease and injury attributable to alcohol (World Health Organization 2011). In 2015, excluding tobacco, an estimated

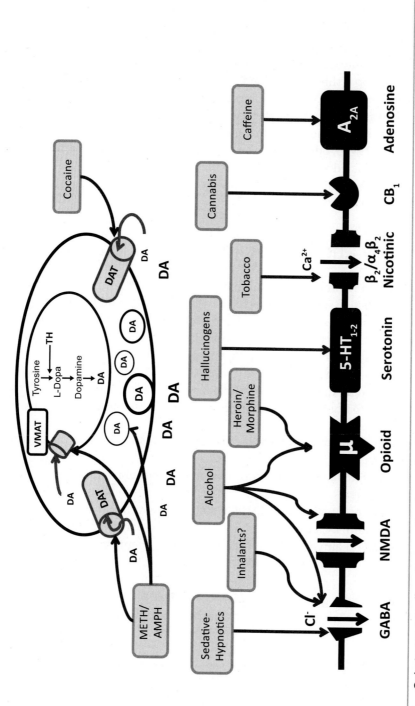

Figure 24–1.   Substance use disorders: mechanisms of action.

Note. Ca²⁺=calcium ion; CB₁=cannabinoid receptors; Cl⁻=chloride ion; DA=dopamine; DAT=dopamine transporter; GABA=γ-aminobutyric acid; METH/AMPH=methamphetamine/amphetamine; NMDA=*N*-methyl-D-aspartate; TH=tyrosine hydroxylase; VMAT=vesicular monoamine transporter.

Source.   Reprinted from Figure 23–1 (p. 741) in Kosten TR, Newton TF, De La Garza R, Haile CN: "Substance-Related and Addictive Disorders," in *The American Psychiatric Publishing Textbook of Psychiatry,* Sixth Edition. Edited by Hales RE, Yudofsky SC, Roberts LW. Arlington, VA, American Psychiatric Association, 2014, pp. 735–814. Copyright 2014, American Psychiatric Association.

21 million in the United States, or 7% of the population, met criteria for a substance use disorder in the past year, including 16 million people who had an alcohol use disorder and 8 million people who had an illicit drug use disorder (Center for Behavioral Health Statistics and Quality 2016). Overdose deaths, especially from prescription and illicit opioids, have increased dramatically in the past 20 years; in the United States alone, more than 500,000 people died from drug overdoses between 2001 and 2015 (Humphreys 2017). Statistics on gambling disorder vary, but several surveys have shown prevalence rates of Internet gaming disorder as high as 10%–15% among young people in Asian countries and 1%–10% among young people in Western countries (Saunders et al. 2017).

Assessment

The Approach

When the clinician is interviewing a patient who may have a substance-related or addictive disorder, a matter-of-fact and nonjudgmental approach is often the most effective (Levounis and Avery 2018). Many patients have been stigmatized, discriminated against, and ostracized by their families or even other treaters because of their disorder (Avery et al. 2017). Establishing a trusting and secure relationship is a key part of treatment, and special attention should be given to forging such a connection in the initial encounters with a patient.

Furthermore, as discussed in the Transtheoretical Model of Change developed by Prochaska and DiClemente (1982), patients have different levels of motivation for changing their substance use and may not always be ready to engage with the clinician. The five stages of change are listed in Table 24–2. Although patients may progress sequentially through the stages of change from precontemplation to maintenance, patients often do not follow this pattern. Clinicians often treat individuals who skip stages or sometimes go back to an earlier stage. Most—if not all—patients are ambivalent about change, and exploring this ambivalence is a critical element in enhancing their motivation and achieving a positive outcome (Levounis and Avery 2018).

Miller and Rollnick's (2013) work on motivational interviewing throughout the years has provided clinicians with an evidence-based way to assist patients in this process, although many strategies and approaches exist (see "Psychosocial Treatments" section later in chapter). The motivational interviewing approach is characterized by an empathic and supportive interviewing style that helps individuals explore and then resolve ambivalence toward making change by increasing their intrinsic motivation for change. Every interaction—including the assessment phase—aims to actively engage people in their treatment (Levounis and Avery 2018).

Family participation in the evaluation is preferred but often not an option. Patients often have strained relationships with their loved ones because of their substance use or other family dynamics. Families can become great allies in carrying out the patient's treatment plan, however, helping the patient both logistically and emotionally (Olsen and Levounis 2008).

TABLE 24–2.	The stages of change

1. Pre-contemplation—"I don't need to change."
2. Contemplation—"Maybe in the future I will quit using."
3. Preparation—"I'm considering planning to change soon."
4. Action—"I have stopped using and plan to continue sober."
5. Maintenance—"Now that I have been sober for months, I want to continue to be abstinent."

Source. Prochaska and DiClemente 1982.

Substance Use History

When taking a substance use history, clinicians should inquire about both legal and illegal substances. Asking specifically about each class of drugs, about gambling and other behavioral addictions, and about each possible source, such as dealers, friends and family, prescriptions, the Internet, herbal stores, and over-the-counter medications, can yield surprising and valuable results. For each substance, clinicians should gather information about 1) frequency of use, 2) amount used, 3) route of administration, 4) acute response to the effects of the substance, and 5) changes in use over time (Levounis and Avery 2018).

Five categories of consequences of substance use are commonly reviewed with patients as well (Levounis and Avery 2018):

1. *Medical consequences* may include gastritis, encephalopathy, hepatitis C, HIV infection, and other infections (e.g., endocarditis, abscesses), as well as injuries secondary to intoxication.
2. *Psychiatric consequences* may include depression, anxiety, and psychosis. Differentiating between substance-induced and independent psychiatric disorders can be challenging.
3. *Interpersonal and family consequences* may include separation or divorce and estrangement from parents, siblings, and children.
4. *Financial and employment consequences* may include bankruptcy, loss of job, and loss of a professional license.
5. *Legal consequences* may include arrests for driving under the influence (DUI, which refers to illicit drugs) or driving while intoxicated (DWI, which refers to alcohol), incarceration, parole or probation, and loss of custody of children.

The Alcohol Use Disorders Identification Test (AUDIT) for alcohol use disorder, the Drug Abuse Screening Test (DAST) for other substances of abuse, or similar screening tools may be useful to incorporate in the assessment as well as in ongoing treatment (Allen et al. 1997; Yudko et al. 2007). Table 24–3 presents two commonly used screens for alcohol use disorder, and Figure 24–2 presents the AUDIT.

These screening tools are often used as a part of the SBIRT (screening, brief intervention, and referral to treatment) method, which has been utilized by clinicians in many different treatment settings (Pringle et al. 2017). SBIRT provides a comprehensive, evidence-based approach to identifying patients with problematic substance use patterns with the goal of intervening early and avoiding adverse outcomes.

TABLE 24–3.   **CAGE and TWEAK brief questionnaire screens**

CAGE	TWEAK
Have you ever felt you should **C**ut down on your drinking?	Tolerance: How many drinks can you hold?
Have people **A**nnoyed you by criticizing your drinking?	Have close friends or relatives **W**orried or complained about your drinking in the past year?
Have you ever felt bad or **G**uilty about your drinking?	**E**ye opener: Do you sometimes take a drink in the morning when you first get up?
Have you ever had a drink first thing in the morning to steady your nerves or to get rid of a hangover (i.e., as an **E**ye opener)?	**A**mnesia: Has a friend or family member ever told you about things you said or did while you were drinking that you could not remember?
	Do you sometimes feel the need to C(**K**)ut down on your drinking?
Note. Two positive responses to these questions are considered a positive test and indicate that further assessment is warranted.	*Note.* The TWEAK test is scored based on a 7-point scale, 2 points each for a positive response to either one of the first two questions and 1 point for each of the last three questions. A total score of 2 or more points indicates a likely alcohol problem.
CAGE Source. Ewing 1984.	*TWEAK Source.* Russell et al. 1994.

Source.   Reprinted from Table 23–7 (p. 749) in Kosten TR, Newton TF, De La Garza R, Haile CN: "Substance-Related and Addictive Disorders," in *The American Psychiatric Publishing Textbook of Psychiatry*, Sixth Edition. Edited by Hales RE, Yudofsky SC, Roberts LW. Arlington, VA, American Psychiatric Association, 2014, pp. 735–814. Copyright 2014, American Psychiatric Association.

Previous Treatments

Some patients have participated in mutual help groups, such as Alcoholics Anonymous (AA), Narcotics Anonymous (NA), or SMART Recovery (see "Psychosocial Treatments" section later in chapter). Finding out the length of time and how often a person has been attending meetings can give the clinician an indication of the patient's engagement with recovery. If the patient has been attending mutual help meetings consistently, has formally joined a group, and has a sponsor, then she or he is more likely to be committed to the recovery process (Levounis and Avery 2018).

In reviewing previous medical treatments with the patient, the following four areas are typically addressed (Levounis and Avery 2018):

1. *Withdrawal management,* which includes inpatient hospital admissions and outpatient community-based programs
2. *Rehabilitation* in 28-day or other residential treatment facilities
3. *Outpatient counseling* or psychotherapy
4. *Long-term pharmacotherapy,* which often applies to opioid use disorder and includes maintenance with methadone (a μ opioid receptor agonist), maintenance with buprenorphine (a μ opioid receptor partial agonist), or treatment with oral or extended-release injectable naltrexone (a μ opioid receptor antagonist).

Clinicians may also ask the patient about previous periods of abstinence, how they were attained, and what worked to maintain sobriety. Inquiring about cravings and

Circle the number that comes closest to the patient's answer.

1. How often do you have a drink containing alcohol?	
(0) Never (1) Monthly or less (2) Two to four times a month (3) Two to three times a week (4) Four or more times a week	
2. How many drinks containing alcohol do you have on a typical day when you are drinking? *Code the number of standard drinks*[1]	
(0) 1 or 2 (1) 3 or 4 (2) 5 or 6 (3) 7 or 8 (4) 10 or more	
3. How often do you have six or more drinks on one occasion?	
(0) Never (1) Less than monthly (2) Monthly (3) Weekly (4) Daily or almost daily	
4. How often during the last year have you found that you were not able to stop drinking once you had started?	
(0) Never (1) Less than monthly (2) Monthly (3) Weekly (4) Daily or almost daily	
5. How often during the last year have you failed to do what was normally expected from you because of drinking?	
(0) Never (1) Less than monthly (2) Monthly (3) Weekly (4) Daily or almost daily	
6. How often during the last year have you needed a first drink in the morning to get yourself going after a heavy drinking session?	
(0) Never (1) Less than monthly (2) Monthly (3) Weekly (4) Daily or almost daily	
7. How often during the last year have you had a feeling of guilt or remorse after drinking?	
(0) Never (1) Less than monthly (2) Monthly (3) Weekly (4) Daily or almost daily	
8. How often during the last year have you been unable to remember what happened the night before because you had been drinking?	
(0) Never (1) Less than monthly (2) Monthly (3) Weekly (4) Daily or almost daily	
9. Have you or someone else been injured as a result of your drinking?	
(0) No (2) Yes, but not in the last year (4) Yes, during the last year	
10. Has a relative or friend or doctor or other health worker been concerned about your drinking or suggested you cut down?	
(0) No (2) Yes, but not in the last year (4) Yes, during the last year	

Total Score[2]: _____

[1] In determining the response categories it has been assumed that one "drink" contains 10 g alcohol. In countries where the alcohol content of a standard drink differs by more than 25% from 10 g, the response category should be modified accordingly.

[2] The AUDIT is not a diagnostic instrument. A total score of 8–15 indicates moderate problems that may respond to brief intervention. Scores of 16–19 may suggest alcohol abuse or dependence. Scores above 19 suggest alcohol dependence.

FIGURE 24–2. Alcohol Use Disorders Identification Test (AUDIT).

Source. Reprinted from Babor TF, Higgins-Biddle JC, Saunders J, et al.: AUDIT, the Alcohol Use Disorders Identification Test, 2nd Edition. Geneva, Switzerland, World Health Organization, 2001. Available at: http://www.who.int/iris/handle/10665/67205. Accessed September 30, 2018. May be reproduced without permission for noncommercial purposes.

triggers of relapse (including emotions, people, places, and things) helps the patient remember the major challenges to sobriety. The review of triggers signals to the patient that serious effort will be required to identify, avoid, and cope with these powerful culprits of relapse.

Co-Occurring Conditions

The medical history includes the direct medical consequences of substance use, acute and chronic medical illnesses, operations, allergies, and current medications. The psychiatric history consists of the review of psychiatric hospitalizations, outpatient treatments, and psychiatric medications.

Substance use disorders and other psychiatric conditions, such as depression, schizophrenia, and bipolar disorder, have significant genetic components that are at times overlapping. A detailed family history often contributes valuable information to the clinician's understanding of the patient's vulnerabilities and helps him or her to distinguish between a primary psychiatric disorder and a substance-induced psychiatric disorder (Levounis and Avery 2018).

Social History

The psychosocial history, sometimes also referred to as the personal history, completes the comprehensive history portion of the patient assessment. It consists of gathering information about the patient's childhood development; education; employment; military service; physical or sexual abuse; run-ins with the law; spouse or partner; children; housing and living situation; and religion and spirituality. For a patient with a substance use disorder, his or her function in all of these different areas is likely to be impacted.

Physical Examination and Laboratory Tests

Physical examination is sometimes necessary to determine the presence and severity of intoxication and withdrawal. This examination can also be helpful in identifying and providing care for intravenous drug use. Needle marks and sclerosed veins (track marks) on the upper extremities secondary to chronic injecting of substances can be easily concealed by clothes but become apparent on physical examination.

Certain laboratory test results can raise the clinician's level of suspicion for substance use disorders. Abnormal liver function test results (especially an elevated aspartate aminotransferase to alanine aminotransferase ratio and an elevated γ-glutamyltransferase level), elevated red blood cell mean corpuscular volume, and carbohydrate-deficient transferrin are associated with alcohol use disorder. Evidence of HIV, hepatitis B virus, and hepatitis C virus may indicate intravenous drug use.

Urine toxicology examinations are helpful in the evaluation (and often the treatment) of the substance-abusing patient, and most common substances of abuse can be detected in the urine. Blood levels are primarily used for alcohol, although the metabolites of alcohol are being increasingly tested in the urine. Detection of drugs in hair, saliva, and sweat samples has attracted increased attention as alternatives to urine toxicology tests. However, the clinical usefulness of these methods is currently limited (Levounis and Avery 2018). Table 24–4 lists the length of time that commonly used substances are detectable in the urine (Moeller et al. 2008).

TABLE 24–4. **Length of time that substances are detectable in urine**

Substance	Duration
Amphetamine	2 days
Barbiturates	1 day (i.e., short-acting pentobarbital) to 3 weeks (i.e., long-acting phenobarbital)
Benzodiazepines	3 days (i.e., short-acting lorazepam) to 30 days (i.e., long-acting diazepam)
Cocaine metabolites	2–4 days
Cannabis	3 days to 1 month (depends on amount and time course of use)
Opioids	2 days (i.e., short-acting heroin) to 4 days (i.e., long-acting methadone)
Phencyclidine	8 days

Intoxication States

Most substances produce clinically significant intoxication states, characterized by problematic behavioral and psychological changes, that develop shortly after ingestion of a substance. Type of substance, route of administration, amount consumed, and characteristics of the individual using the substance, such as body weight, determine if use of a substance results in clinically significant intoxication. For example, only 7% of people who use caffeine will ever use enough to experience clinically significant intoxication symptoms, characterized by muscle twitching and psychomotor agitation. Heroin use, on the other hand, even in small quantities, frequently produces a clinically significant intoxication in most individuals, at least at first. Table 24–5 summarizes the characteristics of intoxication from the various drug classes.

Mild to moderate intoxication syndromes typically do not require anything more than supportive care and reassurance, although more serious behavioral and psychological disturbances often require benzodiazepines or antipsychotic medications. Overdose states, especially from opioids and from mixing substances, are treated medically, often with medications that reverse the overdose (e.g., naloxone for opioids, flumazenil for benzodiazepines), and with additional medical supports as needed (e.g., intubation, telemetry).

Withdrawal States

Most drugs can also produce clinically significant withdrawal leading to impairment in social, occupational, or other important areas of functioning. These withdrawal states generally occur after the cessation of heavy and prolonged use of a substance. Table 24–6 summarizes the characteristics of withdrawal states from the different drug classes.

Severe alcohol withdrawal, opioid withdrawal, and sedative, hypnotic, and anxiolytic withdrawal often necessitate medical interventions. Acute alcohol withdrawal may lead to seizures and hallucinations (especially in the first 48 hours) and more severe states, such as delirium tremens (characterized by disorientation, agitation, psychosis, autonomic hyperactivity, and 5% mortality rate). In addition to addressing co-

TABLE 24–5.	Intoxication symptoms associated with various substances
Substance	**Intoxication signs/symptoms**
Alcohol	Slurred speech, incoordination, unsteady gait, nystagmus, impairment in attention or memory, stupor, coma
Caffeine	Restlessness, nervousness, excitement, insomnia, flushed face, diuresis, gastrointestinal distress, muscle twitching, rambling flow of thought and speech, tachycardia or cardiac arrhythmia, periods of inexhaustibility, psychomotor agitation
Cannabis	Conjunctival injection, increased appetite, dry mouth, tachycardia
Phencyclidine	Vertical or horizontal nystagmus, hyperacusis, hypertension or tachycardia, numbness or diminished responsiveness to pain, ataxia, dysarthria, muscle rigidity, seizures, coma
Hallucinogen	Pupillary dilation, tachycardia, sweating, palpitations, blurring of vision, tremors, incoordination
Inhalant	Dizziness, nystagmus, incoordination, slurred speech, unsteady gait, lethargy, depressed reflexes, psychomotor retardation, tremor, generalized weakness, blurred vision, stupor, coma
Opioid	Pupillary constriction, drowsiness, coma, slurred speech, impairment in attention or memory
Sedative, hypnotic, or anxiolytic	Slurred speech, incoordination, unsteady gait, nystagmus, impairment in cognition, stupor, coma
Stimulant	Tachycardia or bradycardia, pupillary dilation, elevated or lowered blood pressure, perspiration or chills, nausea or vomiting, evidence of weight loss, psychomotor agitation or retardation, muscular weakness, respiratory depression, chest pain, arrhythmias, confusion, seizures, dyskinesias, dystonias, coma

occurring medical conditions and providing vitamin supplementation, such as thiamine to prevent Wernicke's encephalopathy and Korsakoff's psychosis, the mainstay of treatment for alcohol withdrawal is administration of oral or intravenous benzodiazepines. Benzodiazepines are often best administered in response to rating scales, such as the Clinical Institute Withdrawal Assessment for Alcohol—Revised (CIWA-Ar), that describe the severity of alcohol withdrawal symptoms (Sullivan et al. 1989). Benzodiazepines activate the same receptor (γ-aminobutyric acid [GABA] receptor) as alcohol, and after stabilizing that system, are then slowly tapered off.

Withdrawal syndromes from sedative, hypnotic, and anxiolytic medications, such as alprazolam or phenobarbital, are similar to alcohol withdrawal syndromes and are treated similarly with long-acting benzodiazepines or barbiturates, which also activate the GABA system. The time course of the withdrawal symptoms from sedative, hypnotic, and anxiolytic medications varies based on the half-life of the drug being used.

Opioid withdrawal is treated with an induction into opioid maintenance treatment. As discussed later (see "Pharmacological Treatments" section), outcomes appear best when an individual with an opioid use disorder is provided with opioid maintenance treatment with buprenorphine (a partial opioid agonist) or methadone (a long-acting full opioid agonist). Induction to neither buprenorphine maintenance nor methadone maintenance requires medical withdrawal (what used to be called detoxification).

TABLE 24–6.   **Withdrawal symptoms associated with various substances**

Substance	Withdrawal signs/symptoms
Alcohol	Autonomic hyperactivity; hand tremor; insomnia; nausea or vomiting; transient visual, tactile, or auditory hallucinations or illusions; psychomotor agitation; anxiety; generalized tonic-clonic seizures
Caffeine	Headache, marked fatigue or drowsiness, dysphoric mood, depressed mood, irritability, difficulty concentrating, flu-like symptoms
Cannabis	Irritability, anger, aggression, nervousness, anxiety, sleep difficulty, decreased appetite, weight loss, restlessness, depressed mood, abdominal pain, tremors, sweating, fever, chills, headache
Opioid	Dysphoric mood, nausea or vomiting, muscle aches, lacrimation or rhinorrhea, pupillary dilation, piloerection, sweating
Sedative, hypnotic, or anxiolytic	Autonomic hyperactivity, hand tremor, insomnia, nausea or vomiting, transient hallucinations or illusions, psychomotor agitation, anxiety, generalized tonic-clonic seizures
Stimulant	Fatigue; vivid, unpleasant dreams; insomnia or hypersomnia; increased appetite; psychomotor retardation or agitation
Tobacco	Irritability, frustration, anger, anxiety, difficulty concentrating, increased appetite, restlessness, depressed mood, insomnia

However, for those electing against maintenance treatment, buprenorphine or methadone is commonly substituted for the opioids being used and then tapered off over a few days. There are nonopioid options for managing opioid withdrawal, including the α_2 adrenergic agonist clonidine, as well. The time course of withdrawal from opioids depends on the half-life of the opioid that was being used.

Substance Use Disorders

Most individuals who use substances will not go on to develop substance use disorders. In fact, even if a person experiences the intoxication and withdrawal symptoms just described, that does not mean that she or he has a substance use disorder. As exemplified in the alcohol use disorder criteria described, a substance use disorder occurs when a person continues to use a substance despite the significant substance-related problems. Here, we discuss the substance use disorders described in DSM-5 and review some of the risk factors for and characteristics of each of these disorders.

Alcohol Use Disorder

Alcohol use disorder impacts many people. Its 12-month prevalence is around 5% among teenagers and up to 9% in adults. Most people who have an alcohol-related disorder develop the disorder before 40 years of age. Prevalence rates are two or three times higher in men than in women, although the gender gap is narrowing with time (American Psychiatric Association 2013).

As opposed to what we understand about other substances of abuse, moderate alcohol use (one drink per day for women, two drinks per day for men) may be protective against certain diseases. For a woman, higher-risk drinking is defined as more than three drinks on any given day and more than seven drinks per week. For a man, high-risk drinking is defined as more than four drinks on a single day and more than 14 drinks per week (National Institute of Alcohol Abuse and Alcoholism 2017).

While it is often conceptualized as a condition that is difficult to treat and leads to serious consequences, the majority of individuals with this disorder have a positive outcome. Problematic medical consequences such as alcohol withdrawal or delirium tremens are not likely to occur until the alcohol use disorder is severe.

There are a number of risk factors for developing an alcohol use disorder; these include family and cultural attitudes toward alcohol, the availability of alcohol, co-occurring mental and physical disorders, and poor coping skills. Alcohol use disorder is especially known to run in families, with genetic influences thought to account for as much as 60% of the risk of developing the disorder. Certain ethnic subgroups, such as Native Americans and Alaskan Natives, are known to be especially at risk for developing an alcohol use disorder (American Psychiatric Association 2013).

Caffeine

Caffeine is a unique substance; although it can cause intoxication and withdrawal states (described in Tables 24–5 and 24–6, respectively), there is insufficient evidence that caffeine use leads to a caffeine use disorder. As a result, and despite the fact that up to 85% of children and adults consume caffeine on a regular basis, caffeine use disorder was not included among the DSM-5 substance-related disorders. Adult caffeine consumers drink on average 280 mg/day of caffeine. Rates of caffeine consumption increase with age until the 30s and 40s and then appear to level off. The use of "energy drinks" and caffeine pills with high levels of caffeine may more often lead to problems, including intoxication and withdrawal (American Psychiatric Association 2013).

Cannabis Use Disorder

Cannabis use disorder refers to disorders due to substances derived from the cannabis plant, as well as disorders due to synthetic oral formulations designed for medical use and other synthetic cannabinoid compounds designed for nonmedical use. The plant material has many names, including weed, pot, and dope, and comes in many forms, including concentrated extracts like hashish and hash oil. The potency of cannabis (i.e., delta-9-tetrahydrocannabinol or delta-9-THC concentration) varies from 1% to 25% and higher, with a steady increase of potency noted over past decades. Synthetic oral formulations of delta-9-THC are available for prescription in many countries. The non-medical synthetic cannabinoids have many names, such as K2 and spice, and are often sold illegally in the form of plant material that has been sprayed with a cannabinoid compound. While most commonly smoked (via pipes, water pipes, cigarettes, etc.), cannabis may also be ingested orally or vaporized, which involves heating the plant material to release the cannabinoids (American Psychiatric Association 2013).

Epidemiological data consistently show that cannabinoids are the most frequently used illicit substance in the United States and around the world. The 12-month prevalence rates of cannabis use disorder have risen over recent years and are approximately 3.5% in adolescents and 1.5% in adults, with rates two or three times higher in men than in women. Onset of cannabis use disorder most often occurs in adolescence or young adulthood (American Psychiatric Association 2013).

There are genetic risk factors, which are thought to account for anywhere from 30% to 80% of the risk for developing a cannabis use disorder. As is the case in other substance use disorders, a history of mental illness, including conduct disorder in adolescence, is a risk factor. There also are a number of environmental risk factors, including family and cultural attitudes, legal status and availability of the substance, and lower socioeconomic status. Cannabis is available legally in more and more countries, and the effect that legalization will have on use patterns in the coming years is hotly debated (Volkow et al. 2014).

There is a lot of debate as well on the functional consequences of cannabis use disorder for people who have the disorder. While there appears to be evidence that use may lead to an amotivational syndrome and may have a "gateway" effect, for example, the data are mixed. It does appear, however, that heavy use may impair cognitive abilities and school and work functioning, and co-occurring use of other substances is quite common (Volkow et al. 2014).

Phencyclidine Use Disorder

Phencyclidine (PCP or "angel dust") and similarly acting substances such as ketamine have been misused since the 1960s. Exact use numbers are unknown, but around 2%–3% of the population have used these substances during their life, and use is more common among younger individuals. Use of these substances is commonly associated with violence, accidents, and falls, as well as the symptoms listed in the intoxication and withdrawal sections earlier. Risk factors include other substance use and living in areas where these substances are more used and available, such as in the West and Northeast regions of the United States (American Psychiatric Association 2013).

Other Hallucinogen Use Disorder

Many substances that produce alterations in perception, mood, and cognition similar to those produced by PCP are included in this category in DSM-5. These "other hallucinogens" include the phenylalkylamines, such as mescaline; MDMA (3,4-methylenedioxymethamphetamine); the indoleamines, such as psilocybin; and the ergolines, such as lysergic acid diethylamide (LSD). Other substances included in this group are *Salvia divinorum* and jimsonweed. Most of these substances are taken orally, although some forms can be smoked or injected (American Psychiatric Association 2013).

Among the substance use disorders listed in DSM-5, other hallucinogen use disorder is the rarest, with an estimated 12-month prevalence rate of less than 0.5%. Use is most common among younger individuals. For those who do end up with this diagnosis, recovery rates are high (American Psychiatric Association 2013).

Risk factors for hallucinogen misuse include a history of using other substances, mental illness, and younger age. Of note, these substances have been used as a part of religious practices, such as the use of peyote by the Native American Church. MDMA and other hallucinogens have also been used to treat or to augment the treatment of substance use disorders and other mental disorders.

In addition to the symptoms of intoxication listed earlier, hallucinogen persisting perception disorder is a hallucinogen-caused condition that is listed as a separate diagnosis in DSM-5. Its name refers to the reexperiencing of one or more of the perceptual symptoms experienced while intoxicated following cessation of the use of the hallucinogen. This reexperiencing is not better explained by a medical or psychiatric condition and causes distress or functional impairment. Hallucinogen persisting perception disorder seems to occur primarily after using LSD, but not exclusively.

Inhalant Use Disorder

Inhalant use disorder refers to a problematic pattern of use of a hydrocarbon-based inhalant substance. Examples of these volatile hydrocarbons include toxic gases from glues, fuels, paints, and other volatile compounds. Of note, a disorder involving inhalation of nitrous oxide or any other substance would be classified as *other (or unknown) substance use disorder* (American Psychiatric Association 2013; DSM-5 p. 535 and p. 579).

Inhalant use disorder is most common among adolescents, although numbers still are low, with approximately 0.4% of adolescents in the United States qualifying for this disorder in the past year. The inhalant gases are widely available and legal, which make them readily accessible for adolescents. Inhalant use disorder is very rare in females. Risk factors include other substance use, mental illness (especially conduct disorder), trauma, and behavioral disinhibition (American Psychiatric Association 2013).

It is important to note that use of butane or propane may be fatal and can cause a host of serious problems, including arrhythmias and neurological injury, even after inhaling only one time.

Opioid Use Disorder

Opioid use disorder is a unique disorder among the substance use disorders in that it may begin with a prescription from a physician for pain relief, overdose rates are very high, and (as discussed in the "Treatment" section later in chapter) treatment often involves prescribing an individual with an opioid use disorder a long-acting opioid medication. Historically, individuals with an opioid use disorder misused heroin. Currently, however, we are in the middle of the "opioid epidemic," which, in part, was caused by the number of prescription opioids prescribed by physicians to individuals with pain over the past 3 decades (Wakeman 2017).

The 12-month prevalence of opioid use disorder is approximately 1% among adolescents and 0.5% among adults. Rates are much higher in men than in women, with a male-to-female ratio of about 15:1 for prescription opioid use disorders and 3:1 for heroin use disorder. Risk factors for developing an opioid use disorder include other substance use disorders, mental illness, pain, impulsivity, and family history of—and permissive attitudes toward—opioid use (American Psychiatric Association 2013).

Numerous public health initiatives are under way to address the opioid epidemic and the rising numbers of overdose deaths. These initiatives are targeted toward providers and individuals with opioid use disorders. Providers are learning more and more about the risks associated with prescribing opioid medications and the importance of treating opioid use disorder with medications (see "Pharmacological Treatments" section later in chapter). Individuals with opioid use disorder are increasingly being offered medications for opioid use disorder, supervised injection sites, naloxone rescue kits, and other resources.

Sedative, Hypnotic, or Anxiolytic Use Disorder

The sedative, hypnotic, or anxiolytic substances included in DSM-5 are many, and include benzodiazepines, carbamates, barbiturates, and barbiturate-like hypnotics (Table 24–7). These substances can produce clinical pictures of intoxication, withdrawal, and substance use disorder that are similar to those produced by alcohol, because they are brain depressants and have similar mechanisms of action.

The 12-month prevalence rates for sedative, hypnotic, or anxiolytic substance use disorder are estimated to be around 0.3% among adolescents and 0.2% among adults. Whereas for most other substances discussed in this chapter, rates of misuse are higher for males than for females, rates of misuse of agents in the sedative, hypnotic, and anxiolytic class are about the same for males and females. This finding is, in part, attributable to the fact that these substances are frequently—and, at times, indiscriminately—prescribed by physicians for anxiety, insomnia, and a host of other symptoms (American Psychiatric Association 2013).

The risk factors for developing a sedative, hypnotic, or anxiolytic use disorder encompass temperamental, environmental, genetic, and physiological contributions and include impulsivity, family history of use of—and permissive attitudes toward—these medications, and a history of mental illness and other substance use disorders.

Stimulant Use Disorder

Stimulant use disorder is a pattern of amphetamine-type substance, cocaine, or other stimulant use that leads to clinically significant impairment or distress. The amphetamines include amphetamine, dextroamphetamine, and methamphetamine and are consumed orally, intravenously, or by the nasal route. Cocaine has many preparations, including coca leaves, coca paste, cocaine hydrochloride, and cocaine alkaloids such as freebase and crack. Stimulants also include plant-derived stimulants such as khat, which is derived from a flowering plant native to Africa and the Middle East. Of note, amphetamines and other stimulants are prescribed for a host of conditions, and these prescribed medications are often diverted.

The 12-month prevalence rates for amphetamine-type stimulant use disorder and cocaine use disorder are about 0.2% for each disorder in adolescents and adults. Use is most common in younger adults and in males (especially for intravenous misuse). Males and females have similar rates of noninjection stimulant use disorders (American Psychiatric Association 2013).

The risk factors for developing a stimulant use disorder include impulsivity, family history of use of—and permissive attitudes toward—these medications, and a history of mental illness and other substance use disorders. Of note, people who are prescribed stimulants for treatment of attention-deficit/hyperactivity disorder (ADHD) are not more likely to develop a substance use disorder, and in fact have better outcomes overall, than individuals with ADHD who are not prescribed stimulants (Asherson 2017).

Tobacco Use Disorder

Tobacco use disorder is common and is associated with many adverse health outcomes. Historically, cigarettes were the most commonly used tobacco products, but electronic

TABLE 24–7.   Sedative-hypnotics approved for use in the United States

Generic name	Trade name	Therapeutic use
Benzodiazepines		
Alprazolam	Xanax, Niravam	Anxiety, panic disorder
Chlordiazepoxide	N/A	Anxiety, alcohol withdrawal
Clonazepam	Klonopin	Anxiety, seizure disorder, panic disorder
Clorazepate	Tranxene T-Tab	Anxiety, acute alcohol withdrawal, seizure disorder
Diazepam	Valium	Anxiety, sedation, alcohol withdrawal, muscle spasms, seizure disorder
Estazolam	N/A	Insomnia
Flurazepam	N/A	Insomnia
Lorazepam	Ativan	Anxiety, insomnia, seizure disorder, sedation
Midazolam	N/A	Sedation, general anesthesia
Oxazepam	N/A	Anxiety, alcohol withdrawal
Temazepam	Restoril	Insomnia
Triazolam	Halcion	Insomnia
Barbiturates		
Butabarbital	Butisol	Sedation, insomnia
Butalbital[a]	Fiorinal[a]	Tension headache
Phenobarbital	N/A	Seizure disorder, sedation
Pentobarbital	Nembutal	Sedation
Secobarbital	Seconal	Insomnia, sedation
Other sedative-hypnotics		
Eszopiclone	Lunesta	Insomnia
Zaleplon	Sonata	Insomnia
Zolpidem	Ambien, Edluar, Intermezzo, Zolpimist	Insomnia

[a]Butalbital is available in combination with nonopioid analgesics (Fiorinal) and opioid analgesics (Fiorinal with codeine).

Data Source.   www.fda.gov/Drugs.

Source.   Reprinted from Table 23–15 (p. 785) in Kosten TR, Newton TF, De La Garza R, Haile CN: "Substance-Related and Addictive Disorders," in *The American Psychiatric Publishing Textbook of Psychiatry,* Sixth Edition. Edited by Hales RE, Yudofsky SC, Roberts LW. Arlington, VA, American Psychiatric Association, 2014, pp. 735–814. Copyright 2014, American Psychiatric Association.

cigarettes (e-cigarettes), smokeless tobacco, and other tobacco products are increasingly being used, especially by adolescents and younger adults. Using tobacco products upon waking, using them daily, and waking at night to smoke are especially associated with having a tobacco use disorder (American Psychiatric Association 2013).

The 12-month prevalence of nicotine use disorder in the United States is approximately 13%. Most adolescents experiment with tobacco use, and by 18 years of age, almost 20% smoke at least monthly. Quitting is hard; among those who try to quit, about 60% relapse within 1 week. Only about 5% of individuals who quit remain abstinent for life. Common medical comorbidities include cardiovascular illness, lung disease, and cancer (American Psychiatric Association 2013).

Approximately 50% of the risk for developing a tobacco use disorder is thought to be due to genetic factors. As with the other substance use disorders, additional risk factors include permissive family and cultural attitudes toward tobacco, co-occurring mental and physical disorders, lower socioeconomic status, and poor coping skills. Numerous public health initiatives aimed at smoking prevention and cessation—including television ads, education in schools, and taxes on tobacco products—have been undertaken to help reduce the burden of tobacco-related disease and death.

Other (or Unknown) Substance Use Disorder

There are many other substances in addition to those listed in this chapter and DSM-5 that can lead to problematic use and result in a substance use disorder. DSM-5 mentions several noteworthy substances, including anabolic steroids; nonsteroidal anti-inflammatory drugs; cortisol; antiparkinsonian medications; nitrous oxide; amyl-, butyl-, or isobutyronitrites; betel nut; and kava. Many people—especially those who struggle with impulsivity and other substance use disorders—habitually seek out new experiences and new ways to receive a high; therefore, this list of other substances is ever expanding (American Psychiatric Association 2013).

Gambling Disorder

Gambling disorder is described as persistent and recurrent gambling behavior leading to clinically significant impairment and distress. It can take many forms, including playing card games and the slot machines and wagering on sporting events. It is characterized by increasing amounts of money spent gambling, as well as reliving gambling experiences, planning subsequent gambling experiences, and thinking about how to obtain money to gamble. This increasing time and money spent on gambling leads to, and continues despite, impairment in social, occupational, recreational, financial, and psychological domains. These domains are further jeopardized by a pattern of lying to conceal the extent of gambling and a reliance on others to relieve financial devastation caused by gambling. Similar to substance use disorders, gambling disorder can involve symptoms of tolerance and withdrawal. Tolerance to the effects of gambling results in more money gambled in order to reach excitement. Symptoms of restlessness or irritability can occur in the absence or reduction of gambling. In addition, the gambling must not be better explained as being a result of a manic episode.

The 12-month prevalence of gambling disorder is about 0.2%. Males are about three times more likely to have a gambling disorder than females. Females with a gambling disorder start later than males, have more co-occurring psychiatric disorders, and are more likely to develop problems with slot machine and bingo gambling. Risk factors for developing a gambling disorder include younger age at onset of gambling, co-occurring substance use disorders and mental illness, a family history of gambling, lower socioeconomic status, impulsivity, and poor coping skills (American Psychiatric Association 2013).

Treatment of Substance-Related and Addictive Disorders

There are many effective treatments for substance-related and addictive disorders. The right treatment for a specific patient depends on the person's motivation, the severity of the substance use, and the specific substance that is being misused. Whereas most individuals are treated as outpatients with the psychosocial interventions discussed in this section, some people require inpatient treatment, which can involve medical withdrawal services or daily psychosocial and pharmacological interventions. The American Society of Addiction Medicine Patient Placement Criteria levels and dimensions (Table 24–8) may be used to match a patient with her or his needed level of care (Mee-Lee et al. 2013).

Psychosocial Treatments

Many different psychosocial treatment options exist, and while most seem to have similar efficacy, the challenge is to match patients to the treatment that best fits their needs and that they are most likely to continue with in an ongoing way, although this is often difficult to determine (Project MATCH Research Group 1997).

AA is a free, peer-led fellowship started in 1935 by Bill Wilson and Dr. Bob Smith, which now has more than 2 million members and 115,000 registered groups (Alcoholics Anonymous 2017). AA is based on a 12-step program of spiritual and character development, along with 12 traditions to help the fellowship be stable and unified from outside influences. Following the success of AA, there was extensive growth of 12-step programs; additional fellowships now include NA, Marijuana Anonymous (MA), Cocaine Anonymous (CA), Crystal Methamphetamine Anonymous (CMA), Overeaters Anonymous (OA), Sex and Love Addicts Anonymous (SLAA), and Gamblers Anonymous (GA). These fellowships share the AA 12 steps, with minor variations. While historically 12-step programs have been the only option for persons seeking free, peer-led psychosocial treatment for substance use disorders, other treatments have emerged, which may also benefit persons with co-occurring psychiatric disorders. These include SMART Recovery and Moderation Management, among others (Ascher et al. 2013).

As discussed earlier in the chapter (see "Assessment" section), Miller and Rollnick's (2013) work on motivational interviewing throughout the years has provided clinicians with an evidence-based way to assist patients. The motivational interviewing approach involves an empathic and supportive interviewing style that helps individuals resolve ambivalence toward making change by attempting to increase intrinsic motivation for change and is often used in combination with other psychosocial and psychopharmacological interventions.

Other evidence-based psychosocial treatments include relapse prevention, cognitive-behavioral therapy (CBT), dialectical behavior therapy, and contingency management (Table 24–9 briefly describes these modalities). Among these options, relapse prevention strategies, which conceptualize relapse as a process while improving the ability to identify its warning signs, are often incorporated into everyday clinical practice. CBT, in addition to also addressing co-occurring psychiatric disorders, has been

TABLE 24–8.   American Society of Addiction Medicine Patient Placement Criteria levels and dimensions

Patient assessment dimensions

1. Intoxication/withdrawal potential
2. Biomedical conditions and complications
3. Emotional, behavioral, or cognitive conditions and complications
4. Readiness to change
5. Relapse, continued use, or continued problem potential
6. Recovery environment

Levels of care[a]

Level 0.5 Early intervention

Level I Outpatient treatment

Level II Intensive outpatient/partial hospitalization

Level III Residential/inpatient treatment

Level IV Medically managed intensive inpatient treatment

[a]Within each general level of care are a number of more refined sublevels.
Data Source.   Mee-Lee et al. 2013.
Source.   Reprinted from Table 23–3 (p. 739) in Kosten TR, Newton TF, De La Garza R, Haile CN: "Substance-Related and Addictive Disorders," in *The American Psychiatric Publishing Textbook of Psychiatry,* Sixth Edition. Edited by Hales RE, Yudofsky SC, Roberts LW. Arlington, VA, American Psychiatric Association, 2014, pp. 735–814. Copyright 2014, American Psychiatric Association.

TABLE 24–9.   Psychosocial treatments for substance-related and addictive disorders

Relapse prevention	Conceptualizes relapse as a process while improving the ability to identify its warning signs
Cognitive-behavioral therapy (CBT)	Utilizes cognitive and behavioral techniques to help clients identify and cope with the thoughts, feelings, behaviors, and high-risk situations that can lead to relapse
Dialectical behavior therapy	Combines the above CBT techniques for relapse with distress tolerance, acceptance, and mindfulness
Contingency management	Uses contingent-based reinforcements to change behaviors

shown to benefit individuals with multiple substance use disorders and is one of the most effective treatments for gambling disorder (Choi et al. 2017).

Pharmacological Treatments

Medications have been essential in the successful treatment of tobacco use disorder and opioid use disorder and helpful in the treatment of alcohol use disorder. To date, unfortunately, there is limited evidence that medications are helpful in the treatment of other substance use disorders and gambling disorder. Naltrexone, however, is sometimes used for gambling disorder and may be more effective than other options (Rosenberg et al. 2013). Table 24–10 provides a complete list of U.S. Food and Drug Administration (FDA)–approved medications to treat substance use disorders. (Note that, in addition to FDA-approved agents, we have also included topiramate and

TABLE 24–10. **Medications for substance use disorders (with typical target dosages)**

Tobacco use disorder	Alcohol use disorder	Opioid use disorder
Varenicline (Chantix) 1 mg PO bid	Naltrexone (ReVia) 50 mg PO qd	Buprenorphine[a] (Suboxone) 8–16 mg SL qd
Bupropion (Wellbutrin, Zyban) 150 mg PO bid	Naltrexone (Vivitrol) 380 mg IM monthly	Methadone 60–120 mg PO qd
Nicotine replacement therapies Gum (Nicorette) Inhaler (Nicotrol Inhaler) Lozenge (Commit) Patch (Nicotine CQ) Spray (Nicotrol NS)	Acamprosate (Campral) 666 mg PO tid	Naltrexone (ReVia) 50 mg PO qd
	Disulfiram (Antabuse) 125–500 mg PO qd	Naltrexone (Vivitrol) 380 mg IM monthly
	Topiramate (Topamax)[b] 75–150 mg PO bid	
	Gabapentin (Neurontin)[b] 300–600 mg PO tid	

Note. bid=twice per day; CQ=cigarette quit; IM=intramuscular injection; NS=nasal spray; PO=oral tablets or capsules; qd=once per day; SL=sublingual; tid=three times per day.
[a]Usually combined with naloxone, and available in several forms and preparations (film, tablet, subcutaneous injection, implants).
[b]Not U.S. Food and Drug Administration approved; included in table on the basis of currently available scientific evidence.

gabapentin for the treatment of alcohol use disorder in this table based on our review of the currently available scientific evidence.)

Tobacco Use Disorder

The first-line pharmacological interventions for tobacco use disorder are nicotine replacement therapy (available in many forms [e.g., gum, patch]), varenicline (a partial nicotinic receptor agonist), and bupropion (an antidepressant that inhibits the reuptake of dopamine and norepinephrine). These pharmacological options can more than double the chance of quitting, especially when used in combination with psychosocial treatments (Cahill et al. 2013).

Alcohol Use Disorder

There are several medications for alcohol use disorder. Disulfiram is an aldehyde dehydrogenase inhibitor, which blocks the metabolism of alcohol. If a person drinks alcohol while taking disulfiram, she or he experiences the disulfiram reaction, an agonizing and (ultimately) aversive syndrome characterized by increased heart rate, flushing, headache, nausea, and vomiting. Disulfiram has been integrated into substance use treatments for many years and seems to work best when individuals are highly motivated to maintain abstinence and supervised when they take it to ensure adherence. Oral naltrexone and long-acting injectable naltrexone, which are opioid antagonists, help to reduce craving and increase the ability to maintain abstinence or moderation. Acamprosate, an *N*-methyl-D-aspartate (NMDA) receptor modulator, has the advantage of being metabolized by the kidney, although the evidence supporting its use is not as strong as that for naltrexone (Gueorguieva et al. 2010). The use of gabapentin and topiramate for alcohol use disorder is especially promising for persons with co-occurring disorders because these medications also have evidence for treating mental illnesses. Both are thought to potentially help with mood stabilization and anxiety, although they are not supported by the same level of evidence as the antidepressants or the more classic mood stabilizers. Topiramate may also be helpful for people with borderline personality disorder or cocaine use disorder (Johnson et al. 2013; Stoffers et al. 2010).

Opioid Use Disorder

For opioid use disorder, buprenorphine, methadone, and naltrexone are the standard of treatment, with the evidence being strongest for buprenorphine and methadone. Methadone for the treatment of opioid use disorder can be administered only in federally accredited opioid treatment programs (OTPs, previously known as methadone clinics), as part of a comprehensive treatment program (Baxter et al. 2013). As with any other full agonist opioid, methadone carries a risk of respiratory depression and overdose, especially when taken in combination with other central nervous system depressants such as benzodiazepines or alcohol. Methadone is metabolized by enzymes in the cytochrome P450 (CYP) system (particularly CYP3A4) and interacts with many medications. Higher doses of methadone prolong the QT interval, increasing the risk of torsades de pointes. Ideally, a clinician treating an individual receiving methadone will be in close contact with the individual's treatment team at the opioid treatment program for optimal patient care coordination.

Buprenorphine is a partial opioid agonist that can be prescribed by any clinician who has obtained permission from the U.S. Drug Enforcement Administration to provide office-based buprenorphine treatment (Kraus et al. 2011). Buprenorphine is also metabolized by the CYP3A4 system but does not appear to prolong the QT interval in any clinically significant manner. Buprenorphine may be administered alone or in combination with the opioid antagonist naloxone, which becomes active if opioids are used intravenously and protects against such abuse. Unlike drug interactions with methadone, drug–drug interactions with the buprenorphine/naloxone combination are of limited clinical significance, and the risk for respiratory depression is very low. Table 24–11 lists considerations helpful in making the choice between methadone and buprenorphine (Levounis and Avery 2018).

Substance-/Medication-Induced Mental Disorders and Co-Occurring Disorders

Substances of abuse have a complex relationship with mood, behavior, memory, and all the variables that go into making us human. It can be challenging to determine whether a patient's presentation (e.g., depression, mania, confusion) is a manifestation of a primary psychiatric disorder or of substance intoxication, withdrawal, or chronic use. Furthermore, people with co-occurring disorders often face complex psychosocial situations, have murky histories, and show a pattern of failed treatments (Avery and Barnhill 2017).

TABLE 24–11. **Selection considerations: buprenorphine vs. methadone**

	Buprenorphine in office-based treatment	Methadone in opioid treatment program
Criteria	Current diagnosis of opioid use disorder	Current diagnosis of opioid use disorder and 1-year history of addiction
Age (years)	16 and older	18 and older
Reliability	Higher	Lower
Motivation	Higher	Lower
Social needs	Lower	Higher
Level of function	Higher	Lower

Within psychiatry, co-occurring disorders are more the rule than the exception. People with substance use disorders often have one or more co-occurring psychiatric and medical disorders, while people with a primary psychiatric disorder often have one or more co-occurring substance use disorders (Avery and Barnhill 2017).

The general rule is that all disorders should be addressed when treating a patient, yet this is often not done. In a study in the U.S. Veterans Affairs health care system, for example, only 7%–11% of patients received medications for their alcohol use disorder, while 69%–82% received medications for a co-occurring psychiatric disorder (Rubinsky et al. 2015). Reasons behind this reluctance to address substance use disorders include lack of knowledge about such substance use treatment, rejection of the disease model of addiction, and stigmatizing attitudes toward individuals with substance use disorders.

Medical conditions are frequently associated with substance use disorders, both as antecedents of addiction (e.g., opioid addiction secondary to inappropriate treatment of chronic back pain) and as consequences of addiction (e.g., cirrhosis secondary to alcoholism). In addition to Wernicke's encephalopathy and Korsakoff's syndrome (discussed earlier in "Withdrawal States" section), alcohol consumption can impact almost every system in the body (cardiomyopathy, gastritis, stroke, neurocognitive disorders). Tobacco use is the leading global cause of preventable death and is associated with lung disease, cardiovascular disease, and multiple cancers. Cannabis use has more medical and neurological complications than is often believed as well (Volkow et al. 2014). Intravenous drug use comes with many risks, including hepatitis C, HIV, and other infections. Substance use also is a significant risk factor for trauma resulting from motor vehicle accidents and domestic violence.

Substance use during pregnancy can lead to a host of complications and adverse outcomes for both the pregnant woman and the fetus. One of these outcomes, neurobehavioral disorder associated with prenatal alcohol exposure, is included among the Conditions for Further Study in DSM-5. This disorder is characterized by childhood onset of impaired neurocognitive functioning; impaired self-regulation of mood, attention, or impulse; and impaired adaptive functioning, as well as clinically significant distress or impairment in important areas of functioning—all associated with confirmed exposure to alcohol during gestation (American Psychiatric Association 2013).

Conclusion

Clinicians will frequently encounter individuals with substance-related and addictive disorders. While these patients may be complex and challenging at times, safe and effective psychosocial and pharmacological treatments have revolutionized the care of the addicted patient in the twenty-first century.

Key Clinical Points

- To diagnose a substance use disorder, DSM-5 requires the presence of clinically significant impairment or distress and the presence of at least two physical, psychological, and social consequences of the substance use.

- When the clinician is interviewing a patient who has a substance-related or addictive disorder, a matter-of-fact, nonjudgmental, and respectful approach often works best.

- The Alcohol Use Disorders Identification Test (AUDIT) for alcohol use disorder and the Drug Abuse Screening Test (DAST) for other substances of abuse are often helpful in the assessment and ongoing treatment of patients with substance use disorders.

- Severe alcohol withdrawal, opioid withdrawal, and sedative, hypnotic, and anxiolytic withdrawal often necessitate medical interventions.

- The American Society of Addiction Medicine Patient Placement Criteria levels and dimensions may be used to match a given patient with the most appropriate level of care.

- Many different psychosocial treatment options exist, including 12-step groups, cognitive-behavioral therapy, and dialectical behavior therapy. Although most of these options are similar in efficacy, the challenge is to match the patient to the treatment that best fits his or her needs.

- The first-line pharmacological intervention for tobacco use disorder is varenicline (a partial nicotinic receptor agonist). Nicotine replacement therapy and bupropion (an antidepressant that inhibits the reuptake of dopamine and norepinephrine) are also safe and effective.

- There are several effective medications for alcohol use disorder, including disulfiram, naltrexone, and acamprosate.

- For opioid use disorder, buprenorphine, methadone, and naltrexone are the standard of treatment, with the evidence being strongest for buprenorphine and methadone.

- People with substance use disorders often have at least one co-occurring psychiatric or medical disorder, while people with a primary psychiatric disorder often have at least one co-occurring substance use disorder.

References

Alcoholics Anonymous: A.A. Fact File. New York, Alcoholics Anonymous World Services, 2017. Available at: http://www.aa.org/assets/en_US/m-24_aafactfile.pdf. Accessed August 21, 2017.

Allen JP, Litten RZ, Fertig JB, et al: A review of research on the Alcohol Use Disorders Identification Test (AUDIT). Alcohol Clin Exp Res 21(4):613–619, 1997 9194913

American Psychiatric Association: Diagnostic and Statistical Manual of Mental Disorders, 5th Edition. Arlington, VA, American Psychiatric Association, 2013

Ascher M, Wittenauer J, Avery J: Alternatives to 12-step groups. Current Psychiatry 12(9):E1–E2, 2013. Available at: https://www.mdedge.com/psychiatry/article/77225/practice-management/alternatives-12-step-groups. Accessed August 1, 2018.

Asherson P: Drug treatments for ADHD reduce risk of substance use disorders. Am J Psychiatry 174(9):827–828, 2017 28859502

Avery J, Barnhill J: Co-occurring Mental Illness and Substance Use Disorders: A Guide to Diagnosis and Treatment. Arlington, VA, American Psychiatric Association Publishing, 2017

Avery J, Han BH, Zerbo E, et al: Changes in psychiatry residents' attitudes towards individuals with substance use disorders over the course of residency training. Am J Addict 26(1):75–79, 2017 27749984

Baxter LE Sr, Campbell A, Deshields M, et al: Safe methadone induction and stabilization: report of an expert panel. J Addict Med 7(6):377–386, 2013 24189172

Cahill K, Stevens S, Perera R, et al: Pharmacological interventions for smoking cessation: an overview and network meta-analysis. Cochrane Database Syst Rev (5):CD009329, 2013 23728690

Center for Behavioral Health Statistics and Quality: Key Substance Use and Mental Health Indicators in the United States: Results From the 2015 National Survey on Drug Use and Health (HHS Publ No SMA 16-4984, NSDUH Ser H-51). Rockville, MD, Substance Abuse and Mental Health Services Administration, 2016

Choi SW, Shin YC, Kim DJ, et al: Treatment modalities for patients with gambling disorder. Ann Gen Psychiatry 16:23, 2017 28465711

Ewing JA: Detecting alcoholism. The CAGE questionnaire. JAMA 252(14):1905–1907, 1984 6471323

Gueorguieva R, Wu R, Donovan D, et al: Naltrexone and combined behavioral intervention effects on trajectories of drinking in the COMBINE study. Drug Alcohol Depend 107(2–3):221–229, 2010 19969427

Humphreys K: Avoiding globalisation of the prescription opioid epidemic. Lancet 390(10093):437–439, 2017 28792397

Johnson BA, Ait-Daoud N, Wang XQ, et al: Topiramate for the treatment of cocaine addiction: a randomized clinical trial. JAMA Psychiatry 70(12):1338–1346, 2013 24132249

Koob GF, Volkow ND: Neurocircuitry of addiction. Neuropsychopharmacology 35(1):217–238, 2010 19710631

Kraus ML, Alford DP, Kotz MM, et al: Statement of the American Society Of Addiction Medicine Consensus Panel on the use of buprenorphine in office-based treatment of opioid addiction. J Addict Med 5(4):254–263, 2011 22042215

Levounis P: Bench to bedside: from the science to the practice of addiction medicine. J Med Toxicol 12(1):50–53, 2016 26553278

Levounis P, Avery J: Patient assessment, in Office-Based Buprenorphine Treatment of Opioid Use Disorder, 2nd Edition. Edited by Renner JA Jr, Levounis P, LaRose AT. Arlington, VA, American Psychiatric Association Publishing, 2018, pp 73–88

Mee-Lee D, Shulman MJ, Gastfriend DR, et al: The ASAM Criteria: Treatment Criteria for Addictive, Substance-Related, and Co-Occurring Conditions, 3rd Edition, 2013. Available at: https://www.asam.org/resources/the-asam-criteria. Accessed August 21, 2017.

Miller WR, Rollnick S: Motivational Interviewing: Helping People Change, 3rd Edition. New York, Guilford, 2013

Moeller KE, Lee KC, Kissack JC: Urine drug screening: practical guide for clinicians. Mayo Clin Proc 83(1):66–76, 2008 18174009

National Institute of Alcohol Abuse and Alcoholism: Drinking Levels Defined (website). Washington, DC, National Institute of Alcohol Abuse and Alcoholism, 2017. Available at: https://www.niaaa.nih.gov/alcohol-health/overview-alcohol-consumption/moderate-binge-drinking. Accessed September 7, 2017.

Olsen PR, Levounis P: Sober Siblings: How to Help Your Alcoholic Brother or Sister—and Not Lose Yourself. Cambridge, MA, Da Capo Lifelong Books (Perseus), 2008

Pringle JL, Kearney SM, Rickard-Aasen S, et al: A statewide screening, brief intervention, and referral to treatment (SBIRT) curriculum for medical residents: differential implementation strategies in heterogeneous medical residency programs. Subst Abus 38(2):161–167, 2017 28332942

Prochaska JO, DiClemente CC: Transtheoretical therapy: toward a more integrative model of change. Psychotherapy: Theory, Research, and Practice 19(3):276–288, 1982

Project MATCH Research Group: Matching alcoholism treatments to client heterogeneity: Project MATCH posttreatment drinking outcomes. J Stud Alcohol 58(1):7–29, 1997 8979210

Rosenberg O, Dinur LK, Dannon PN: Four-year follow-up study of pharmacological treatment in pathological gamblers. Clin Neuropharmacol 36(2):42–45, 2013 23503545

Rubinsky AD, Chen C, Batki SL, et al: Comparative utilization of pharmacotherapy for alcohol use disorder and other psychiatric disorders among U.S. Veterans Health Administration patients with dual diagnoses. J Psychiatr Res 69:150–157, 2015 26343607

Russell M, Martier SS, Sokol RJ, et al: Screening for pregnancy risk-drinking. Alcohol Clin Exp Res 18(5):1156–1161, 1994 7847599

Saunders JB, Hao W, Long J, et al: Gaming disorder: its delineation as an important condition for diagnosis, management, and prevention. J Behav Addict 6(3):271–279, 2017 28816494

Stoffers J, Völlm BA, Rücker G, et al: Pharmacological interventions for borderline personality disorder. Cochrane Database Syst Rev (6):CD005653, 2010 20556762

Sullivan JT, Sykora K, Schneiderman J, et al: Assessment of alcohol withdrawal: the revised clinical institute withdrawal assessment for alcohol scale (CIWA-Ar). Br J Addict 84(11):1353–1357, 1989 2597811

Volkow ND, Baler RD, Compton WM, et al: Adverse health effects of marijuana use. N Engl J Med 370(23):2219–2227, 2014 24897085

Wakeman SE: Medications for addiction treatment: changing language to improve care. J Addict Med 11(1):1–2, 2017 27898497

World Health Organization: Global Status Report on Noncommunicable Diseases 2010: Description of the Global Burden of NCDs, Their Risk Factors and Determinants. Geneva, World Health Organization, 2011. Available at: http://www.who.int/nmh/publications/ncd_report2010/en/. Accessed August, 20, 2017.

Yudko E, Lozhkina O, Fouts A: A comprehensive review of the psychometric properties of the Drug Abuse Screening Test. J Subst Abuse Treat 32(2):189–198, 2007 17306727

Recommended Readings

Ascher M, Levounis P: The Behavioral Addictions Casebook. Arlington, VA, American Psychiatric Publishing, 2015

Avery J, Barnhill J: Co-occurring Mental Illness and Substance Use Disorders: A Guide to Diagnosis and Treatment. Arlington, VA, American Psychiatric Publishing, 2017

Kleber HD, Weiss RD, Anton RF Jr, et al: Practice Guidelines for the Treatment of Patients with Substance Use Disorders, 2nd Edition. Arlington, VA, American Psychiatric Association, 2006

Koob GF, Volkow ND: Neurocircuitry of addiction. Neuropsychopharmacology 35:217–238, 2010

Levounis P, Avery J: Patient assessment, in Office-Based Buprenorphine Treatment of Opioid Dependence, 2nd Edition. Arlington, VA, American Psychiatric Association Publishing, 2018, pp 73–88

Levounis P, Arnaout B, Marienfeld C: Motivational Interviewing for Clinical Practice. Arlington, VA, American Psychiatric Association Publishing, 2017

Levounis P, Zerbo E, Aggarwal R: The Pocket Guide to Addiction Assessment and Treatment. Arlington, VA, American Psychiatric Association Publishing, 2016

Renner JA, Levounis P, LaRose AT: Office-Based Buprenorphine Treatment of Opioid Use Disorder, 2nd Edition. Arlington, VA, American Psychiatric Association Publishing, 2018

Volkow ND, Baler RD, Compton WM, et al: Adverse health effects of marijuana use. N Engl J Med 370:2219–2227, 2014

Zerbo EA, Schlechter A, Desai S, et al: Becoming Mindful: Integrating Mindfulness Into Your Psychiatric Practice. Arlington, VA, American Psychiatric Association Publishing, 2017

CHAPTER 25

Neurocognitive Disorders

Allyson C. Rosen, Ph.D., ABPP-CN
Thomas A. Hammeke, Ph.D., ABPP-CN
Steven Z. Chao, M.D., Ph.D.

The neurocognitive disorders category includes diagnoses conceptualized as likely having underlying brain pathology, or what historically was referred to as "organic" mental disorders. Grouping these disorders together positions them to leverage the exciting advances in brain imaging and biomarkers that will be integrated into clinical diagnosis and treatment as evidence grows. The DSM-5 (American Psychiatric Association 2013) Neurocognitive Disorders category replaces and extends the DSM-IV (American Psychiatric Association 1994) category "Dementia, Delirium, Amnestic, and Other Cognitive Disorders," which traditionally focused on age-related disorders. The neurocognitive disorder (NCD) formulations represent an attempt both to simplify the neuropathology-based diagnostic categories and to allow greater precision in linking neurobehavioral symptoms with specific neuropathological conditions. For example, the diagnosis of dementia has commonly been associated with neurodegenerative conditions and can still be used where contextually appropriate (e.g., Alzheimer's disease). NCD can likewise represent a similar collection of neurobehavioral features in patients with the residuals of severe traumatic brain injury without having implications of age-related degeneration. The NCD formulations additionally recognize that there are grades of severity in neurobehavioral manifestations associated with the natural course of many neurodegenerative diseases, and therefore further subdivide the NCDs into mild and major NCDs. Early DSM editions similarly distinguished between *organic mental disorders*, conceptualized

The authors wish to acknowledge Myron F. Weiner, M.D., who was author of this chapter in the previous edition of *The American Psychiatric Publishing Textbook of Psychiatry*. This chapter is an update and revision of that chapter (Weiner MF: "Neurocognitive Disorders," in *The American Psychiatric Publishing Textbook of Psychiatry*, Sixth Edition. Edited by Hales RE, Yudofsky SC, Roberts LW. Arlington, VA, American Psychiatric Association, 2014, pp. 815–850).

as the product of structural or physiological brain changes in brain tissue, and *functional disorders,* thought to represent mental aberrations occurring in the context of normal brain functioning. For example, although nonspecific attentional problems and subjective experiences of memory loss commonly occur in mood disorders and anxiety states, these disruptions in cognitive functioning were considered to be incidental to the emotional distress and introspective processes associated with those conditions rather than brain dysfunction per se. With the advent of brain imaging and other techniques for identifying biomarkers of brain pathology, there is broad recognition that the line between many "organic" and "functional" disorders has become less clear, and that this line will undoubtedly be the focus of future research and conceptualizations. For example, many disorders previously conceptualized as being "functional" (e.g., schizophrenia) were subsequently found to also involve abnormalities of brain integrity, and psychiatric symptoms are sometimes the first signs of an incipient dementia. The NCD categories adopted in DSM-5 (American Psychiatric Association 2013) thus represent the latest stage of an evolution in diagnosis and treatment that is advancing in concert with discoveries in brain sciences.

Overview of Neurocognitive Disorder Categories

The major categories within the NCD category are delirium and mild and major NCDs. Table 25–1 lists the most common DSM-5 subtypes within these categories of NCDs. *Delirium* refers to a cause of mental dysfunction that is usually acute and reversible. Ruling out the presence of delirium is critical prior to determining major or mild NCD diagnoses that are presumed to be more stable neurocognitive conditions. The major and mild NCDs differ in severity. Until DSM-5, psychiatrically diagnosable conditions needed to cause "clinically significant distress or impairment in social, occupational, or other important areas of functioning" (American Psychiatric Association 2000, p. 8). This level of disability is now classified as *major NCD.* In contrast, *mild NCD* describes symptoms that are minimally disabling or disruptive. A significant benefit of including a mild NCD category is that there is now a method of formally diagnosing patients with the early stages of degenerative dementias, during which there is subtle brain and cognitive dysfunction that progresses over time to meet the threshold of social or occupational disability (e.g., DSM-IV-TR dementia [American Psychiatric Association 2000]). Depending on the diagnosis, it is possible to specify whether a behavioral disturbance (e.g., delusions, hallucinations, mania, agitation, wandering) is present. It is also possible to specify level of severity, or the amount of functional disability as a result of the NCD. *Mild* denotes difficulties with instrumental activities of daily living (e.g., managing money). *Moderate* denotes difficulties with basic activities of daily living (e.g., dressing). *Severe* denotes full dependency.

Because there frequently will be varying levels of uncertainty in regard to the brain pathology underlying the cognitive symptoms, DSM-5 allows for the diagnosis to be designated as either *probable* or *possible.* For example, the presence of causative genetic factors (e.g., mutations associated with tau neuropathology) or distinctive neuroimaging abnormalities (e.g., frontal brain atrophy or hypometabolism) would increase diagnostic certainty and hence move frontotemporal lobar degeneration (FTLD) from *possible* to *probable.* In contrast, mild NCD due to Alzheimer's disease without signif-

TABLE 25–1.   **DSM-5 categories and subtypes of neurocognitive disorders**

Delirium

  Substance intoxication or withdrawal delirium

  Medication-related delirium

  Delirium due to other medical conditions or to multiple etiologies

Major neurocognitive disorders (specify due to [presumed etiology*])

Mild neurocognitive disorders (specify due to [presumed etiology*])

*Due to Alzheimer's disease, frontotemporal lobar degeneration, Lewy body disease, vascular disease, traumatic brain injury, substance/medication use, other neurodegenerative or medical conditions, or multiple etiologies; either with or without behavioral disturbance.

icant evidence of the presence of a causative gene (e.g., genetic testing, autosomal dominant inheritance pattern) can only be described as *possible*, given the current level of uncertainty for progression. A careful examination of the "Diagnostic Features" section for each subtype is important in making this distinction.

Diagnostic Issues

A critical task in identifying an NCD, particularly a mild NCD, is detecting change from a healthy, premorbid state. This task typically involves determining that a change has occurred in an individual's neurocognitive profile relative to an estimation of the individual's premorbid status, and/or determining that a change has occurred on psychometric testing or activities of daily living. The diagnostic task is made more difficult by several factors:

1. Substantial heterogeneity in cognitive function exists among neurologically healthy adults, which complicates reliance on a simple test score cutoff to detect NCD.
2. Many neurocognitive abilities decline substantially with age, and changes simply represent normal aging.
3. As noted, many primary psychiatric states (e.g., depression, anxiety, chronic pain, sleep disorders) are commonly associated with a subjective sense of memory loss that is incidental to the nonspecific attention disruptions inherent in the psychiatric conditions.

These nonspecific attentional disruptions, while real, are not due to underlying brain neuropathology, and thus are not considered to represent an NCD. In the following subsections we discuss several other issues of particular relevance to diagnosis of NCDs.

Cognitive Functioning

NCD refers to acquired brain dysfunction; however, clinicians do not typically have the luxury of conducting repeated assessments to track cognitive decline for every patient; therefore, dysfunction is often inferred by a deviation from a normative group. To the extent that patients with NCD differ from healthy control subjects, these comparisons are problematic. For example, movement problems from arthritis, orthopedic injury, Parkinson's disease, or stroke may confound interpretation of tests of different abilities;

hence, neuropsychological assessments often have multiple measures to capture these differences. Cultural and education differences from a normative group have a strong effect on language measures, particularly for non-native English speakers. These effects can be pervasive, particularly when test materials are highly unfamiliar.

Because many of the NCDs occur in older adults, the clinician's familiarity with known patterns of typical age-related cognitive dysfunction is important. Whereas there is a vast amount of individual variability in age-related declines, there are certain typical patterns (Institute of Medicine 2015). Vocabulary and general knowledge tend to remain stable with aging, although word-finding difficulty is common. Speed of information processing and psychomotor performance decline with age. Older adults typically take longer to respond to and process information; therefore, clinicians must adjust their evaluations to accommodate patients and to ensure that they understand what is expected of them. Often older patients have perceptual or motor limitations that interfere with clinical interactions; hence, checking for acuity and hearing difficulty should occur early in evaluations.

Daily Functioning and Independence

Conducting a careful history of a patient's occupation, current environmental demands, and description of functional changes prior to diagnosis is important, particularly in mild NCD. Patients with complex and demanding jobs may struggle with subtle cognitive difficulties; for example, a college student with new-onset inattentiveness following a head injury may fail in school. In contrast, patients with minimal responsibilities and interactions, such as a retired older adult with Alzheimer's disease who lives alone, may be found in a delirium state because they have lost interest in food and forgotten to take their medications. For patients with obvious cognitive difficulties and progressive degenerative NCDs, it may be important to conduct a formal assessment of performance of activities of daily living, as well as to identify any contributors to functional disability, such as wandering behavior. As with cognitive assessments, significant motor or sensory limitations often make it difficult to identify functional declines related to cognition, but the distinction between functional declines due to cognitive problems and functional declines due to motor or sensory symptoms is important. For example, a patient with Parkinson's disease may be unable to dress him- or herself because of rigidity and bradykinesia, not because of motor apraxia, a neurologically based difficulty with complex motor planning.

The Complaint of Impairment

Identifying the chief complaint and the informant is a crucial aspect of an evaluation. Older adults with cognitive concerns but without objective neuropsychological dysfunction are receiving increasing attention in studies of mild NCD, because there is evidence that this phenomenon, termed *subjective cognitive decline* (SCD) (Jessen et al. 2014), may represent an early sign of disease. In fact, studies have found that SCD, when accompanied by selected risk factors, does have an increased likelihood of developing into mild NCD, and thus the diagnostic entity of mild NCD will likely evolve with further research on SCD. Insensitivity of standardized cognitive tests to subtle cognitive dysfunction may be another potential reason why a person's subjectively reported cognitive dysfunction is not detected by objective measures, and research to improve the sensitivity of cognitive assessment is ongoing. Gathering information from an informant may provide additional insights, because there are a variety of reasons why patients may be unaware of or forget the problems they experience in everyday life. For patients who live alone, finding an informant may be difficult. Concerns about cognition may be expressed by the patient, the family, or perhaps by an employer. Persons with NCDs who are employed may be fired because of poor performance, but they may not become aware of their cognitive dysfunction until later—too late for continued insurance coverage and disability compensation. Unfortunately, a substantial percentage of persons with Alzheimer's disease are unaware of their cognitive deficits, and persons with the behavioral variant of FTLD are invariably unaware of such deficits. Some cultures may be more stigmatizing or less accepting of age-related dementia; as a result, patients and families may delay seeking help. Difficulties related to cognitive impairment are often dismissed by family members or physicians as normal aging. Complaints of memory decline are common, but a careful interview to identify examples of dysfunction is critical, because many different types of cognitive dysfunction can be mislabeled as memory loss—for example, patients may refer to word-finding difficulty (a language problem) as a problem "remembering" words. A report of confusion, memory loss, or poor judgment warrants active investigation, with the extent of the investigation dependent on the history, physical/neurological findings, and mental status examination.

Comorbidity

Several disorders are often present simultaneously or serially in the same patient with an NCD. Persons with major or mild neurocognitive impairment often experience delirium. Vascular NCD and Alzheimer's disease are often comorbid in the same individual. In addition, psychiatric and neurocognitive disorders may coexist. Major depressive disorder may coexist with an NCD. In addition, an NCD such as Alzheimer's disease may complicate schizophrenia, bipolar disorder, or recurrent depression. The most common diagnostic issue in the evaluation for NCD in older adults is distinguishing between normal aging and disease.

Base Rates and Prevalence

Clinicians should be generally familiar with prevalence statistics so that when deciding among possible diagnoses, they are able to assign appropriate weights based on likelihoods. Up-to-date statistics for degenerative diseases are summarized yearly in *Alzheimer's and Dementia*, the journal of the Alzheimer's Association (see the annual report "Alzheimer's Disease Facts and Figures"), and head-injury statistics are reported by the Centers for Disease Control and Prevention (2017). In this chapter we focus on the more common forms of NCD that are challenging to differentiate, and only briefly discuss epidemiology, given its extensive coverage elsewhere.

Cognitive Domains

Table 1 ("Neurocognitive Domains") in the DSM-5 Neurocognitive Disorders chapter (American Psychiatric Association 2013, pp. 593–595) clearly defines multiple domains of cognitive dysfunction with respect to symptoms/observations and examples of psychometrically based tests. Examples of major versus mild levels of severity are also provided. We review these domains briefly here, but each domain could be the subject of volumes. Blumenfeld (2010) and Purves et al. (2017) have written helpful textbooks that relate neural substrates to neurobehavioral deficits.

Complex Attention and Executive Function

Whereas DSM-5 separates the domains of complex attention and executive function, they overlap and hence are discussed together here. Classically, attention involves the ability to select, divide, and maintain a mental focus in the face of distraction. One example of a psychometric measure of attention is a continuous performance task. The task entails viewing a series of items (e.g., letters or symbols) one at a time and pressing a button in response to a particular item. Another attentional measure involves searching through a complex array of items and counting the numbers of a particular item. Executive function involves control of prepotent/impulsive responses, planning, decision making, and mental flexibility. Examples of psychometric tests to evaluate executive function include tasks involving shifting between rules (e.g., looking for numbers and then letters in order), navigating through mazes, learning from mistakes, and figuring out new rules. Difficulties in the domains of complex attention and executive function can alter performance in other cognitive domains. For example, a patient being tested in a noisy room may fail to attend to a list of words because of difficulty screening out the distracting noises, and thus may appear to have a memory disorder; however, if the test were conducted in a quiet room, the patient's performance might instead be normal.

Learning and Memory

There are many forms of memory, and asking patients about their memory will often elicit multiple cognitive complaints related to other mental abilities. Declines in memory for recent events (i.e., episodic or "recent memory") are the most common difficulties for older adults, particularly adults in the early stages of NCD due to Alzheimer's disease. The most sensitive and the most commonly used test of episodic memory in clinical examinations involves presenting the patient with a list of words to learn and asking the patient to recall the words after a long delay. Often distinctions are made between recalling versus recognizing information given in an evaluation. Patients with selective and significant dysfunction in episodic memory were described in DSM-IV as having an amnestic disorder rather than an NCD. DSM-5 contrasts episodic memory with other forms of "very-long-term memory," such as semantic (e.g., knowledge of word meaning or facts) and implicit memory (e.g., learning a skill, such as how to play the piano). Whereas DSM-5 states that tests involving immediate recall of a series of numbers are tests of immediate memory or working memory span, such tests are also often classified as measures of attention, because they require a great deal of attentional focus.

Language

Language abilities involve verbal expression and comprehension (often referred to as "reception"). Loss of the ability to understand or use speech is called *aphasia*. A distinction is made between *fluent aphasia*, in which patients produce words easily, and *nonfluent aphasia*, in which patients have difficulty producing words. A patient may have difficulty producing words and thus uses word approximations (paraphasias). Phonemic paraphasic errors involve substituting words with similar sounds, such as "meek" for "meat." Semantic paraphasic errors involve substituting words with similar meanings, such as "writer" for "pencil." One of the most common complaints in older adults and patients with brain damage is word-finding problems, and when these patients are shown pictures of objects to name (a confrontation naming test), they struggle to recall the word names. Aphasias typically manifest as syndromes of associated symptoms across a variety of language domains with accompanying non-language-related neurological deficits. For example, for a patient with a nonfluent aphasia, speech requires great effort and is agrammatical, with omission of function words such as articles, prepositions, and conjunctions. A patient who wants to go to a particular place, such as a restaurant, might say, "Want...go...you know...eat...," with great effort and great relief after having expressed him- or herself. These patients generally understand what is said to them and can obey simple commands (although they may make errors when performing complex sequential motor tasks for reasons unrelated to comprehension), but they have difficulty with repetition, reading aloud, and writing. Aphasia can affect speech (phonology/the sound/articulation system), grammar and syntax, lexical access (word retrieval), and semantic representation (meaning). Different patterns of aphasia are often associated with specific neurological deficits that are unrelated to the language dysfunction. For example, patients with nonfluent aphasia often have motor apraxia (i.e., difficulty executing complex symbolic movements, such as pretending to comb one's hair) or right-sided limb weakness/rigidity. In patients with fluent aphasia, spontaneous speech is well articulated and may sound like it *should* be understandable, but it is meaningless. The pattern of change in deficits over time is also important for differential diagnosis. In general, symptoms that worsen over time suggest neurodegenerative disease; symptoms that have an acute onset and improve over time generally result from acute brain injury. Traditionally, tests of general knowledge and vocabulary were believed to be relatively resilient against most degenerative disorders (except semantic dementia); however, word-retrieval difficulties can depress performance on these measures. For example, on a test that displays a picture of an object, the patient may fail to recall the word "broom" but can still use pantomime to indicate that he or she understands the meaning of the object.

Perceptual–Motor Abilities

In the perceptual–motor domain, a distinction is typically made between perception and construction/production, similar to the language domain's distinction between comprehension and expression. For example, a patient may be able to recognize (perceive) but not draw (visuoconstruction) a clock. There may be deficits of higher-order perception, such as prosopagnosia, a selective inability to recognize faces. *Praxis* refers to the ability to execute learned movements. A patient with praxis deficits who is asked to pretend to blow out a candle may say the word "blow" rather than producing the appropriate breath. Perceptual–motor deficits reflect difficulty in tasks involving integration of perception with movement—for example, brushing one's teeth or using tools that were previously familiar.

Social Cognition

Whereas the NCDs are described as primarily involving cognition, inappropriate behavior is an early sign of social cognitive dysfunction. Patients may lose the ability to recognize facial expressions or to understand social emotional aspects of a situation, such as sarcasm, humor, or the perspective of another person.

Assessment

A comprehensive assessment for the presence and differential diagnosis of an NCD involves history taking, mental status examination, and physical and neurological examination, including relevant laboratory screening, brain imaging, and neuropsychological testing. Assessment often requires the skills and cooperation of a psychiatrist/neurologist and neuropsychologist. A careful history and mental status examination are important for ruling out a delirium prior to considering a mild or major NCD, because delirium may involve an urgently treatable condition. Furthermore, formal neuropsychological tests will be unreliable in a patient with delirium.

History Taking

Assessment begins with history taking, which involves the patient, a knowledgeable caretaker, friend, or relative, and all pertinent medical information. Direct access to medical records is important because patients and informants often do not accurately recall medical events or the results of various laboratory tests.

In addition to elicitation of information concerning patients' cognitive abilities, evidence is sought of emotional or interpersonal contributions to the cognitive complaint, concomitants of the cognitive complaint, and its emotional or interpersonal impact. Patients' emotional responses to their mental difficulties are evaluated, and an attempt is made to determine family strengths and weaknesses. Patients' personality patterns are also considered. All of this information helps shape the plan of management.

It is important for the clinician to know what medications the patient is taking, including any over-the-counter (OTC) medications, and in the case of an older adult, to request that the patient bring all prescribed and OTC medications to the appointment. A patient (with his or her permission) can be interviewed in the presence of a family member to ensure the accuracy of factual information and to ascertain how the patient's performance during the examination compares with his or her daily performance. A patient is interviewed alone if unaccompanied or if he or she objects to having others in the examination room. When possible, the clinician should allow enough time to interview the accompanying person alone, because if interviewed only with the patient present, he or she might withhold information that may humiliate or anger the patient. Information withheld typically relates to paranoid thinking, hallucinations, or incontinence.

Having a friend or relative present is a comfort to most persons with cognitive impairment. In this situation, history taking can be a three-way conversation rather than a formal interview. However, effort should be focused on directly communicating with the patient in most cases. In the flow of the conversation, many clues emerge concerning the relationship between patients and significant others, the impact of patients on their families, and the impact of others on the patients. Husbands often resent their wives' diminished ability to maintain their household. Dependent spouses may resent being responsible for their formerly dominant spouses. In many cases, there is tension between spouses because one does not believe that the other truly cannot learn, remember, or understand. Examining one spouse in the presence of the other can also be helpful in dealing with the caregiver spouse's denial and in demonstrating how to deal with the other's inability to remember, plan, and cooperate.

Symptom onset over minutes or hours suggests delirium and the possibility of infectious, toxic/metabolic, drug-induced, vascular, traumatic, psychiatric, or multiple converging factors. Onset over days or weeks suggests infectious, toxic/metabolic, or neoplastic origin. Gradual decline over months to years is more typical of degenerative disorders, except in vascular/multi-infarct dementia, where decline has a more stepwise pattern, with abrupt onset related to a stroke. Dating the onset of cognitive or behavioral difficulties is often difficult. Chronic cognitive impairment may be perceived as an acute decline when a supportive spouse becomes ill or dies.

Symptomatic improvement is often reported with brain trauma, acute vascular disorders, and acute toxic and metabolic disorders. Marked fluctuations in cognitive dysfunction over hours or days are more likely to occur in Lewy body disease than in other NCDs (e.g., NCD due to Alzheimer's disease). In most NCDs, cognitive impairment fluctuates depending on the complexity of environmental/emotional demands, fatigue, general physical health, and time of day.

Frequently reported first symptoms of an NCD are loss of initiative and loss of interest in the family, the surroundings, and activities that were formerly pleasurable. Individuals with impaired frontotemporal lobe function may become either apathetic or disinhibited. Suspiciousness, irritability, and depression may manifest early on. Well-formed visual hallucinations are often seen in Lewy body disease. Visual and tactile hallucinations and illusions are common in delirium and in Lewy body disease. Auditory hallucinations in persons with NCDs tend to be of familiar persons speaking or music playing, whereas accusatory or threatening voices are more typical of schizophrenia and psychotic depression. Rapid eye movement (REM) sleep behavior disorder may precede the onset of Parkinson's or Lewy body disease. Generalized seizures can cause intermittent periods of staring blankly into space accompanied by motor stereotypy and postictal confusion. Diabetes, hypertension, strokes, and heart disease are risk factors for vascular cognitive impairment and may hasten the clinical progression of Alzheimer's disease. Acute renal or hepatic decompensation may lead to delirium. HIV seropositivity raises the possibility of viral brain pathology or an opportunistic brain infection.

Certain genetic mutations increase the likelihood of an NCD to varying degrees. For example, in autosomal dominant familial disorders such as Huntington's disease, having one copy of an affected gene from a parent leads to inheritance of the disorder. Having mutations in the presenilin 1 and 2 genes or an additional copy of the amyloid precursor protein gene (as occurs in Down syndrome) leads to early-onset Alzheimer's disease.

Many medications may impair cognition, including anticholinergic agents such as bowel and bladder relaxants, the antihistamine diphenhydramine (a common ingredient in over-the-counter sleep aids), benzodiazepine hypnotics and sedatives, barbiturates, anticonvulsants, propranolol, and cardiac glycosides. Episodes of confusion in persons with porphyria may be induced by various medications, including barbiturates and benzodiazepines. A history of a serious reaction to antipsychotic medication in a patient with visual hallucinations raises the possibility of NCD due to Lewy body disease.

Alcohol abuse with severe malnutrition or episodes of delirium tremens may be followed by an NCD. Toxic chemical exposures—either through recreational drug use or from the environment, such as arsenic, mercury, lead, organic solvents, and organophosphate insecticides—can produce neurocognitive syndromes, but sometimes the cognitive-behavioral impairment is overshadowed by severe systemic symptoms.

The list of conditions and agents that can cause NCDs is long. One mnemonic for remembering the reversible causes of NCDs makes use of the word *DEMENTIAS* (Table 25–2).

Mental Status Examination and Cognitive Screening

Cognitive disorders are often overlooked, especially when patients are well dressed and well groomed and give appropriate social responses, as is common in Alzheimer's disease. It is common for persons with slowly progressive disorders to retain social graces until well along in the course of the illness. Developing a positive relationship with patients and their families is critical for a careful evaluation. The mental status examination can be stressful for patients; therefore, the clinical interaction should probably not begin with the physician administering a cognitive screening examination. The examination should be performed with consideration for the patient's frustration tolerance and is tailored to his or her level of cognitive performance. For example, when it becomes obvious that a patient is not oriented to year and month, there is little point in inquiring about orientation to day and date unless malingering is suspected. Each category of inquiry should be abbreviated when the patient is irritable or easily frustrated. All responses—whether correct or not—should be treated as equally valid, and the patient should be praised for effort.

Several standardized cognitive screening measures are available, which vary in depth and sensitivity. Use of a standardized measure (e.g., the Montreal Cognitive Assessment [MoCA], which is in the public domain and freely available) facilitates communication between professionals and establishes a sensitive and stable baseline for longitudinal follow-up. Before we discuss screening measures (see "Psychometric Screening for Cognitive Impairment" below), we will first briefly review some of the cognitive processes that these measures evaluate.

Attention/working memory is tested by digit span, forward and backward. Most English speakers with 12 years of education and a clear sensorium can repeat seven digits forward and five backward. Memory is screened by asking patients to recall three to five words after a 5-minute distraction. This test can be performed with objects presented verbally or, in the case of aphasic subjects, objects shown to the patient without naming them. Patients' responses to cueing are also important, because they help to distinguish retrieval deficits from failure to encode or amnesia. Remote memory is more difficult to test than working memory. Patients with little formal education can be asked about events that fall within their range of interest; such questioning is most effective if the examiner, before questioning the patient, first takes aside the accompanying person and asks him or her about recent events in the patient's life (e.g., birthdays, other family events).

Routine examination of language includes assessment of articulation, fluency, comprehension, repetition, naming, reading, and the ability to write sentences. Language dysfluencies include delays in word finding, paraphasias, and neologisms. Word fluency (the ability to generate a list of words for a given category), a very sensitive indi-

TABLE 25–2. **"DEMENTIAS" mnemonic for common "reversible/treatable" causes of neurocognitive disorders and delirium**

Drugs (medications that cause dementia/delirium [e.g., analgesics, sedatives, antipsychotics])

Emotional symptoms (e.g., depression/anxiety)

Metabolic disorders (e.g., hyperammonemia, uremia, hyper-/hypoglycemia, Wilson's disease)

Endocrine disorders (e.g., hypo-/hyperthyroidism, parathyroid disease, pituitary insufficiency, Cushing's disease, Addison's disease)

Nutrition (vitamin deficiencies: B$_1$, B$_6$, B$_{12}$, and folate); also **N**ormal-pressure hydrocephalus

Trauma (e.g., subdural hematoma, hypoxic/anoxic brain injury), **T**oxins (e.g., ethanol, heavy metals), or **T**umors (e.g., intracranial tumors)

Infectious disease (e.g., central nervous system or systemic infection, Lyme disease, neurosyphilis, Whipple's disease, HIV, herpes, fungal infection, tuberculosis)

Autoimmune disorders (e.g., paraneoplastic syndrome–limbic/Hashimoto's encephalopathy, central nervous system vasculitis, sarcoidosis, multiple sclerosis, systemic lupus erythematosus)

Sensory deficits (vision/hearing impairment); also **S**eizures (e.g., subclinical seizure) and **S**troke (vascular disease)

cator of cognitive impairment, can be tested by asking patients to name all of the animals (for example) they can think of in 1 minute.

Comprehension tests begin with graded tasks, such as asking patients to point to one, two, and three objects in the room. These are followed by simple logic questions, such as "Is my cousin's mother a man or a woman?" or "When you are dressing, which do you put on first, your shirt (blouse) or your coat?"

To increase difficulty/sensitivity, naming tests can include the parts of objects, such as the parts of a shirt (sleeve, collar, pocket, buttonhole). Reading and naming ability should be considered in the context of the patient's level of education and acculturation. Writing ability is assessed by asking patients to write a dictated sentence and then to compose a sentence of their own.

Praxis is evaluated by asking patients to imitate an action performed by the examiner, to perform simple motor acts in response to the examiner's request, and to copy a set of simple geometric figures (e.g., intersecting pentagons). For a well-educated person who is mildly impaired, the patient's drawing of a three-dimensional cube can be used to detect constructional dyspraxia.

Fund of information is assessed by using a standard set of questions, ranging from simple to difficult, and by evaluating the responses in relation to the patient's level of education and work achievement.

Assessment of the ability to think abstractly requires consideration of the patient's education, cultural background, and native language. Impairment in abstract reasoning can be inferred from evidence of concrete thinking, such as indicating the time "ten after eleven" on a clock drawing by placing the number 10 after the number 11. Judgment may be estimated by asking patients questions about how they would manage certain life situations, such as "What would you do if the electric company called and told you that your last check was returned because of insufficient funds?" However, judgment is best assessed from history elicited from the informant.

Elements of the mental status examination designed to detect executive dysfunction include abstract reasoning and judgment. Executive function is also assessed by portions of the neurological examination, including go/no-go tasks and reciprocal motor tasks (e.g., instructing the patient to "tap the desk twice when I tap it once, and tap once when I tap twice"). Clock drawing is another useful test of executive function. Executive dysfunction is also reflected in the patient's history, such as mistakes in social judgment (e.g., inappropriate sexual advances), and in the course of the mental status examination, such as through inappropriate handling of objects (utilization behavior), inappropriate laughter, flirtation, or inability to maintain appropriate social and physical distance from the examiner.

Psychometric Screening for Cognitive Impairment

Screening is particularly important for degenerative conditions because the early signs are often missed. A detailed discussion of these measures can be found in Ashford (2008). The MoCA (Nasreddine et al. 2005) is one of the most commonly used screening tools for detecting mild cognitive impairment (e.g., mild NCD). It requires about 15 minutes to administer and assesses executive function in addition to other cognitive domains. The score range is 0–30 (with a suggested cutoff of <27 points for detection of mild NCD). Population-based norms developed for this instrument suggest that a more appropriate cutoff score in the United States is 23 points (Rossetti et al. 2011). The MoCA is available at no cost from the author's website (www.mocatest.org).

The Mini-Mental State Examination (MMSE; Folstein et al. 1975), traditionally the most widely used brief screening tool for cognitive impairment, requires 10–15 minutes to administer. The MMSE is confounded by premorbid intelligence and education and has limited capability to assess executive function. A perfect score is 30 points. Varying MMSE cutoff scores, ranging from 18 to 27, identify a major NCD with varying sensitivity and specificity. The cutoff chosen typically depends on what is optimal for the patient cohort and the NCD. The MMSE is protected by copyright and must be ordered from Psychological Assessment Resources (www.parinc.com).

Screening for psychiatric symptoms in older patients with an underlying NCD can be problematic, because symptoms that occur with NCDs are similar to symptoms associated with other, unrelated disorders (e.g., apathy/anhedonia of NCD and depression). The most commonly used measure of psychiatric symptoms in persons with a major NCD is the Neuropsychiatric Inventory (Cummings 1997; Cummings et al. 1994), a brief instrument that identifies dementia-related behavioral symptoms. The test is administered to a person who knows the patient well. Addressing treatable psychiatric illness in persons with NCDs can improve their quality of life. Patients with NCDs can be screened for comorbid depression or anxiety by means of the Geriatric Depression Scale (Yesavage 1988) or the Geriatric Anxiety Inventory (Pachana et al. 2007).

Physical and Neurological Examination

Physical examination may suggest a specific disease or condition. Evidence of severe malnutrition suggests an avitaminosis such as thiamine deficiency. Argyll-Robertson pupils suggest neurosyphilis. Atrial fibrillation raises the possibility of a cerebral embolic infarct. Gait apraxia and urinary incontinence are associated with normal-pressure hydrocephalus. Limited range of voluntary downward gaze suggests progressive supranuclear palsy. Unilateral limb apraxia suggests corticobasal ganglionic degeneration. Bradykinesia and rigidity may indicate Parkinson's or Lewy body disease, and patients with these symptoms often appear to be depressed. Early autonomic dysfunction is commonly seen in multiple system atrophy. Choreiform movements frequently accompany Huntington's disease. Myoclonic jerks may suggest Creutzfeldt-Jakob disease or Wilson's disease. Focal neurological signs and symptoms suggest a possible vascular origin. Cortical release signs such as the palmomental reflex, grasp reflex, and suck and snout reflexes are nonspecific indicators of severe cortical dysfunction, as are performance abnormalities on programmed motor tasks such as the Luria three-step test.

Laboratory Studies

A list of laboratory studies that are potentially useful in diagnosing NCDs is presented in Table 25–3. Although a clinician may be tempted to use fixed panels, decisions concerning laboratory studies should be based on the individual's clinical picture. Suspected drug use or abuse calls for a toxicology battery. It is especially important to detect alcohol, barbiturate, or benzodiazepine use to prevent severe withdrawal delirium. Determination of electrolyte concentrations is primarily useful in the workup for acute changes in cognition. A serological test for syphilis used to be performed as a matter of routine, but it is not indicated unless the history and clinical presentation suggest exposure to syphilis or the presence of neurosyphilis. Low blood ceruloplasmin and high urinary copper aid in the diagnosis of Wilson's disease. Vitamin B_{12} levels are recommended as a screening study in a dementia workup (Warren and Weiner 2012). A cerebrospinal fluid (CSF) study can yield critical information in the clinical diagnosis of multiple sclerosis, neurosyphilis, or other opportunistic central nervous system infections. HIV testing may be indicated if there is a history of sexual exposure or blood transfusion. The American Academy of Neurology guidelines (Muayqil et al. 2012) recommend that clinicians order a CSF 14-3-3 assay in clinically unclear cases to reduce uncertainty in diagnosing Creutzfeldt-Jakob disease.

Currently, the functional brain imaging study most widely used in clinical diagnosis of degenerative NCDs is fluorodeoxyglucose–positron emission tomography (FDG-PET). The tracer FDG is capable of detecting patterns of cerebral glucose uptake and is approved by U.S. Food and Drug Administration (FDA). This technology has also been approved by the Centers for Medicare and Medicaid Services (2004) for use in differentiating Alzheimer's disease from FTLD. Single-photon emission computed tomography (SPECT) has the advantage of lower cost; however, PET has higher resolution, and thus SPECT is rarely used. Three PET imaging radiotracers have been approved by the FDA for evaluating cerebral amyloid deposition and are now being used to rule out non-Alzheimer's NCD (Figure 25–1). New research guidelines from the National Institute on Aging and the Alzheimer's Association—the NIA-AA Research Framework—have been proposed for classifying imaging biomarkers of Alzheimer's disease (Jack et al. 2016, 2018). This biomarker classification scheme, known as the AT(N) system, focuses on three types of pathological processes in Alzheimer's disease that biomarkers can measure: (A) β-amyloid deposition on PET, (T) tau aggregation on tau PET, and (N) neurodegeneration/neuronal atrophy on structural MRI. Each biomarker category is rated as positive or negative, and the resulting biomarker profile can be integrated into the diagnostic process. It should be noted that this framework is intended for use in research only, not routine clinical care, and it is not currently part of DSM-5.

TABLE 25–3.   Laboratory aids to diagnosis of neurocognitive disorders

General screening	Additional tests and procedures
Complete blood count	Lumbar puncture
Liver function tests/ammonia	14-3-3 protein for Creutzfeldt-Jakob disease
Blood urea nitrogen/creatinine	Oligoclonal bands for multiple sclerosis
Blood glucose	HIV testing
Calcium	Fluorodeoxyglucose–PET
Thyroid function tests	Cerebral amyloid imaging
Serological test for syphilis	Genetic testing
Folic acid	Presenilin 1 and 2 for dominantly inherited AD
Vitamin B_{12}	Trinucleotide repeats in Huntington's disease
Brain CT or MRI	Wilson's disease

Note.   AD=Alzheimer's disease; CT=computed tomography; MRI=magnetic resonance imaging; PET=positron emission tomography.

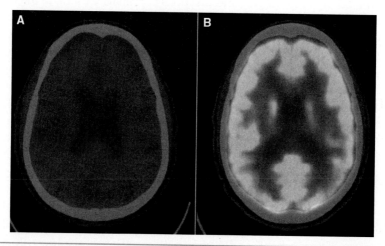

FIGURE 25–1.   Florbetapir F 18 (^{18}F-AV-45) positron emission tomography scans for β-amyloid in two patients with a diagnosis of dementia.

The negative scan **(A)** suggests an underlying pathology other than Alzheimer's disease, whereas the positive scan **(B)** suggests that Alzheimer's pathology is the cause of cognitive decline.

To view this figure in color, see Plate 8 in Color Gallery in middle of book.

Source.   Images courtesy of Steven Z. Chao, M.D., Ph.D.

Genetic testing can help to confirm the diagnosis of dominantly inherited familial Alzheimer's disease (mutations in presenilin 1 and 2 genes), Huntington's disease (more than 40 cytosine-adenine-guanine repeats in DNA), and Wilson's disease and can be used to ascertain risk in asymptomatic persons. Whereas the apolipoprotein E (*APOE*) gene on chromosome 19—specifically the ε4 allele (*APOE 4*) of the gene—has been associated with increased risk of sporadic Alzheimer's disease, DSM-5 does not include that carrier status as providing evidence of a causative Alzheimer's disease genetic mutation, because *APOE 4* status is not highly predictive. For example, the risk of developing Alzheimer's disease with an ε4/ε4 genotype (odds ratio [OR]=14.9) is greater than the risk with an ε2/ε2 genotype (OR]=0.6) (Farrer et al. 1997) but is not at the level of the risk with a Down syndrome–associated mutation (trisomy 21), in which the patient will be certain to develop Alzheimer's disease in middle age (Castro et al. 2017). Genetic counseling is highly recommended for any individuals who discover that they have a genetic mutation associated with an elevated risk for dementia, and such counseling is particularly important for individuals who discover their genotypes through nonclinical means (e.g., direct-to-consumer genetic testing).

Neuropsychological Testing

The clinical neuropsychologist often plays an important role in several tasks: determining adequacy of effort on testing for reliable assessment, establishing the presence of an NCD, conducting the differential diagnosis, quantifying impairment, and assessing patient cognitive strengths and weaknesses. Serial testing provides information on disease progression, treatment effects, and/or degree of recovery from brain insults such as stroke or traumatic brain injury. In addition to the cognitive domains of formal testing described earlier in the chapter (see subsections "Mental Status Examination and Cognitive Screening" and "Psychometric Screening for Cognitive Impairment"), excellent comprehensive textbooks on neuropsychological assessment are available (Lezak et al. 2012; Strauss et al. 2006). After confirming that the effort expended by the patient in the tests was adequate for reliable assessment, the neuropsychologist will interpret the test results. Determining abnormality in a set of neuropsychological test findings typically involves use of several strategies, often simultaneously (Table 25–4). Determining *absolute skill impairment* involves comparing the patient's performance on neuropsychological tests with the average performance of appropriately matched healthy control subjects. Performance below a specific cutoff (e.g., 1.5 standard deviations below the average of controls) indicates the relative gradation of absolute deficit in comparison with a reference population. Determining *relative skill impairment* involves comparing a test score with an estimate of the individual's baseline ability level, which might be derived from demographics (e.g., academic achievement, vocational success), external sources (e.g., academic transcripts), or performance on tests that are resistant to most forms of acquired brain injury (e.g., reading skills). For example, a patient who performs in the average range could be considered normal; however, if the patient's educational and other demographic information suggests that his or her premorbid level should be in the superior range, an average score could be used to support the evidence of dysfunction. Some normative datasets enable determination of *statistical pattern improbability* (i.e., how rare it is for a difference between two scores to occur in neurologically normal populations). Determining *clinical syndrome consistency* involves looking for patterns of skill impairment that are consistent with a known clinical syndrome (e.g., aphasia, dementia of the Alzheimer's type, dominant parietal lobe syndrome). Finally, some neuropsychological tests aim to detect *pathognomonic signs of brain dysfunction*—that is, neurobehavioral signs (e.g., indications of unilateral neglect or unrestrained repetitions in figure drawing) that occur rarely in normal populations but frequently in patients with neurocognitive disorders. Collectively, these interpretive strategies are used to determine when there is abnormality in a set of test findings. Typically, test performance more than two standard deviations below the population

TABLE 25–4.	Strategies for interpreting neuropsychological test data
1.	Method of absolute skill impairment
2.	Method of relative skill impairment
3.	Method of statistical pattern improbability
4.	Method of clinical syndrome consistency
5.	Method of pathognomonic signs

norm would qualify for major NCD, and performance one to two standard deviations below the norm would quality for mild NCD (Lezak et al. 2012; Strauss et al. 2006).

Main Neurocognitive Disorder Categories

There are three categories of NCDs in DSM-5: delirium, major NCD, and mild NCD. We first discuss delirium and then move on to major and mild NCD.

Delirium

Delirium is a state of altered consciousness and cognition, usually of acute onset (hours or days) and brief duration (days or weeks). The hallmark of delirium is impaired attention. Many persons with delirium remain oriented to person, place, and time but demonstrate impairment on tests of sustained attention such as digit span and months of the year in reverse. Sleep–wake disturbances are common, as are reduced or increased psychomotor activity. Misidentifications, illusions, and visual hallucinations are also frequent. Because of these symptoms, delirious patients are often thought by nonpsychiatrists to have schizophrenia, but visual hallucinations in delirium have a different quality from those of schizophrenia. They tend to be mundane and nonthreatening rather than bizarre. They often consist of animals or persons whose presence is not understood and are sometimes frightening to the patient and are not explained by an organized delusional system. Tactile hallucinations in the presence of clouded sensorium are almost invariably due to delirium. When they occur with clear sensorium, tactile hallucinations may be part of psychotic syndromes such as delusional parasitosis.

Essential features of DSM-5 delirium are listed in Table 25–5. Of note, the listed symptoms represent what is typical and should not be rigidly applied if the preponderance of the evidence is inconsistent with a delirium diagnosis. For example, a patient with mild NCD, such as NCD due to Lewy body disease, could appear to be disoriented because he is talking to nonexistent people, but on more extensive questioning, the patient could instead be found to have a consistent and systematized delusion. Delirium is common in general hospital patients, and fears regarding the risk of postoperative cognitive decline following delirium often lead older adults to avoid surgical interventions.

In many individuals, the first sign of an NCD may be postoperative delirium. Episodes of delirium commonly herald Lewy body disease. Delirium has a greater degree of personality disorganization and clouding of consciousness than mild or major NCD. Fluctuations in cognitive ability occur in many persons with impaired cognition, but

TABLE 25–5.	Essential features of DSM-5 delirium

A. Impaired attention and orientation.

B. Abrupt onset (over hours to days) and fluctuating severity over the day.

C. Impairment in an additional cognitive domain (e.g., memory, language, visuospatial functioning, perception).

D. Dysfunction in A and C is not explained by another disorder of arousal (e.g., coma).

E. Evidence that dysfunction is a consequence of another medical condition.

Note. For the complete diagnostic criteria, please refer to pp. 596–598 in DSM-5 (American Psychiatric Association 2013).

not to the extent or with the rapidity of onset (minutes or hours) seen in patients with delirium. Persons with NCDs usually give their best cognitive performance early in the day, when they are not fatigued, and under circumstances in which they do not feel challenged or anxious. Toward the end of the day, many persons with cognitive impairment become transiently delirious, a phenomenon often referred to as *sundowning*. The diagnosis of mild or major NCD cannot be made in the presence of delirium.

Etiology

Delirium can be conceptualized as an acute failure of the brain's ability to process information. In recent years there has been much speculation about the pathophysiological processes underlying delirium, and innovative neuroimaging studies hold promise in elucidating the brain mechanisms. For example, research has suggested that a functional disconnection between the dorsolateral prefrontal cortex and the posterior cingulate gyrus may underlie the pathophysiology of delirium (Choi et al. 2012). Delirium has many potential causes, the most common of which are probably acute infections, brain trauma, and prescribed or over-the-counter medications, and the brain mechanisms that lead from these causes to delirium may similarly vary. In fact, there are many medications that can cause delirium. Thus, in the evaluation of a patient with delirium, all drugs should be suspected. The most common culprits are highly anticholinergic drugs, including over-the-counter diphenhydramine, which is often taken as a sleep aid and is not seen as a potentially toxic drug. Over-the-counter antidiarrheal drugs such as loperamide are potently anticholinergic, as are drugs commonly prescribed for overactive bladder, including tolterodine and oxybutynin. In elderly persons, dopamine agonists or dopamine reuptake inhibitors are common causes of delirium, especially in cognitively compromised persons with Parkinson's disease.

Treatment

In the general hospital setting, treatment of delirium is indicated if the patient's delirium significantly interferes with sleep or medical treatment or causes the patient extreme fear and discomfort. Mild delirium that does not cause sleep loss, interfere with medical treatment, or lead to great fear and discomfort does not require pharmacological treatment. The inpatient management of delirium is outlined in Table 25–6.

Prevention

The best treatment for delirium is prevention, which means attending to the needs of vulnerable populations—that is, cognitively impaired persons with poor hearing and

TABLE 25–6.   Inpatient management of delirium

Identify and reverse all medical cause of delirium.

Presume withdrawal delirium if symptoms begin 1–3 days after admission.

Review use of substances with family member(s).

Consider neuroleptic malignant syndrome in persons receiving chronic antipsychotic treatment.

Consider serotonergic syndrome in persons taking serotonin reuptake inhibitors.

Avoid use of mechanical restraint if possible; instead, use nonpharmacological interventions to support the patient.

Ideally, arrange for a well-liked family member to sit with the patient.

Provide frequent physical contact (e.g., holding patient's hand or placing hand on patient's shoulder).

Assist orientation to time, place, and staff members.

Provide clocks and large calendars near patient.

Ensure that staff members reintroduce themselves at each visit.

Keep room well lit to minimize misperceptions.

Place patient in a room with a window for day/night orientation.

Optimize stimulation.

If television helps with reality contact, keep it on; if it agitates the patient, turn it off.

Use pharmacological approaches only after environmental methods have failed.

Avoid benzodiazepines, except for withdrawal deliria.

Use oral or parenteral high-potency conventional antipsychotics only when needed to ensure the patient's safety, and only after environmental measures have failed.

Avoid use of prophylactic antiparkinsonian drugs.

Do not administer conventional antipsychotics to hyperthyroid patients.

Return patient to home environment as rapidly as possible.

---

vision. Ideally, these vulnerable persons should be identified prior to hospitalization. For patients in long-term care facilities, cognitive impairment is the norm. Most often, consultation is requested after delirium becomes severe enough to endanger patients or to interfere with their treatment. Delirium also occurs in outpatient settings, as illustrated in the following example:

> A young boy was brought in by his mother for psychiatric evaluation because of the acute onset of visual hallucinations. On the child's medication history, the mother reported the use of a topical nasal decongestant. However, an examination of the label indicated that he was actually taking atropine drops the mother had been given for treatment of an eye disorder; the hallucinations cleared soon after the medication was discontinued.

Major and Mild Neurocognitive Disorders

There are two categories of DSM-5 NCDs: major and mild. Major NCD is equivalent to the DSM-IV diagnosis of dementia: an impairment of multiple cognitive abilities sufficient to interfere with self-maintenance, work, or social relationships. The diagnosis of mild NCD indicates that the person is able to maintain independence despite the presence of impaired cognition. The diagnosis of NCD is complicated by the enormous variation among individuals. Many persons with a high functional baseline who are experiencing cognitive decline may still function at a level comparable to that of an average person their own age. Therefore, clinicians must compare a person's current abilities with his or her past abilities, typically by using retrospective accounts furnished by patients or their families, supplemented with simple scales assessing activities of daily living. The distinctions among mild, moderate, and severe major NCD are as follows. *Mild* denotes difficulty with instrumental activities of daily living (e.g., managing finances). *Moderate* denotes difficulty with basic activities of daily living (e.g., eating, toileting). *Severe* denotes full dependency on others for performance of activities of daily living.

Essential features of DSM-5 major NCD and mild MCD are listed in Tables 25–7 and 25–8, respectively. Cognitive impairment that is mild in severity, especially when due to medications or metabolic disorders, is frequently reversible, but a full-blown major NCD is rarely reversible. Treatments are available for many causes of NCD, including neurosyphilis, central nervous system infection, tumor, alcohol use disorder, subdural hematoma, normal-pressure hydrocephalus, Alzheimer's dementia, HIV-related illness, Lewy body dementia, and vascular dementia. Reversible NCDs include depression, drug toxicity, metabolic disorders, vitamin B_{12} deficiency, and hypothyroidism.

Mild Cognitive Impairment Versus Mild Neurocognitive Disorder

The term *mild cognitive impairment* (MCI; Petersen et al. 1997) was adopted by ICD-10 and is roughly equivalent to DSM-5 mild NCD. MCI is extensively described elsewhere (Smith and Bondi 2013), and hence only a few points are made here. Although individuals with amnestic MCI (as defined by Petersen and colleagues) have complaints of poor memory and show objective evidence of abnormal memory function for age, their general cognitive functioning and performance of activities of daily living are normal, and they do not meet criteria for major NCD but are at increased risk. In the early days (Petersen et al. 1997), the study of this diagnosis focused on preclinical Alzheimer's disease. There was often a belief that there should be strictly applied psychometric definitions of severity of cognitive dysfunction (i.e., a memory performance two standard deviations below the population norm was required for MCI); however, this psychometric approach was not sensitive under several circumstances in detecting certain patients with cognitive decline. For example, patients with well above average performance who declined to the average range would not be identified by this definition. Psychometric data are now interpreted in a more thoughtful and nuanced manner, with an eye toward estimating decline relative to a previously healthy state. The definition of MCI has been expanded to include amnestic and nonamnestic types, with the former likely to progress to Alzheimer's disease (approximately 50% over 5 years) and the latter likely to progress to other NCDs. There are, however, many cases of nonprogressive MCI. Imaging biomarkers associated with increased risk of progression from MCI to Alzheimer's disease include accumulation of brain amyloid detected on PET scanning and low hippocampal volume detected on magnetic resonance imaging (MRI). Beyond DSM-5, MCI due to other etiologies is extensively described in Smith and Bondi (2013).

TABLE 25–7.	Essential features of DSM-5 major neurocognitive disorder

A. Decline in cognition from a previous level of performance in one or more cognitive domains based on:

    1. Concern of the patient, an informant, or the clinician; and

    2. Significant impairment in cognitive performance on formal tests.

B. Cognitive deficits interfere with independence in everyday activities (i.e., at least affecting independence in complex instrumental activities of daily living such as managing medications).

C. Not accounted for by delirium.

D. Not explained by another disorder.

Specify

    1. Presumed etiology (e.g., due to Alzheimer's disease).

    2. Presence of behavioral disturbance (i.e., with or without).

    3. Severity (i.e., mild, moderate, severe).

Note. For the complete diagnostic criteria, please refer to pp. 602–605 in DSM-5 (American Psychiatric Association 2013).

TABLE 25–8.	Essential features of DSM-5 mild neurocognitive disorder

A. Mild cognitive decline in one or more cognitive domains based on:

    1. Concern of the patient, informant, or the clinician; and

    2. Mild impairment in cognitive performance verified by quantified psychometric assessment, preferably neuropsychological testing.

B. Cognitive dysfunction is not disabling, but there is some difficulty with independence in everyday activities (i.e., activities of daily living still performed but greater effort is required).

C. Not accounted for by delirium.

D. Not explained by another disorder.

Specify

    1. Presumed etiology (e.g., due to Alzheimer's disease).

    2. Presence of behavioral disturbance (i.e., with or without).

Note. For the complete diagnostic criteria, please refer to pp. 605–606 in DSM-5 (American Psychiatric Association 2013).

Etiology and Differential Diagnosis

A discussion of the many conditions that can cause NCDs is beyond the scope of this chapter but is presented in Miller and Boeve (2017). In this section we consider the more common causes of major NCDs—for example, those due to degenerative disorders in adults, including Alzheimer's disease, FTLD, Lewy body disease, and cerebrovascular disease—as well as some general distinctions among them (Table 25–9). For other examples of the NCD framework we briefly discuss traumatic brain injury, postoperative cognitive decline, and a less common subtype of substance/medication-induced major NCD that is classically known as Korsakoff's amnestic disorder (i.e., alcohol-induced major NCD, amnestic confabulatory type [ICD-10-CM code F10.26]).

TABLE 25–9. Diagnostic features of the most common neurocognitive disorders in adults

	Alzheimer's disease	Frontotemporal lobar degeneration	Lewy body disease	Cerebrovascular disease
Clinical onset	Insidious	Insidious	Insidious	Sudden
Initial symptom	Recent memory impairment	Poor judgment or language impairment	Memory impairment Visual hallucinations	Related to stroke site
Progression	Insidious	Insidious	Fluctuating	Stepwise
Rapid eye movement sleep behavior disorder present	No	No	Often precedes cognitive symptoms	No
Computed tomography / magnetic resonance imaging findings	Normal to global and/or hippocampal atrophy	Frontotemporal atrophy	Normal to global and/or hippocampal atrophy	Cortical stroke(s) or subcortical lacunes
Positron emission tomography findings	Reduced temporoparietal and posterior cingulate metabolism	Reduced frontotemporal metabolism	Reduced temporoparietal and occipital metabolism	Reduced metabolism in area of stroke(s)
Cerebrospinal fluid findings	Low β-amyloid 42, high tau and phosphorylated tau	Normal	Normal, unless coincident with Alzheimer's disease	Depends on recency of stroke
Extrapyramidal signs	Late	In corticobasal ganglionic degeneration, progressive supranuclear palsy, multisystem degeneration	Resting tremor and cogwheel rigidity	Related to site of stroke(s)
Motor / sensory signs	None	None	Resting tremor	Related to site of stroke(s)

Alzheimer's Disease

Alzheimer's disease is highly prevalent, occurring most commonly as the sporadic form. Its prevalence increases with age, to the point that among people ages 85 years and older, up to 30% have Alzheimer's disease. In rare cases, the disease is dominantly inherited may have onset as early as the twenties. The most commonly presumed etiology is overabundance in the brain of the dimeric form of β-amyloid 42 (Aβ$_{42}$), a peptide that is derived from amyloid precursor protein by the joint actions of enzymes β and γ secretase. This overabundance of Aβ$_{42}$ may be due to overproduction (as occurs in trisomy 21 [Down syndrome]) or to inadequate clearance from the brain and leads to the designation of Alzheimer's disease as an amyloidopathy. Two of the major risk factors for Alzheimer's disease are older age and carriage of the ε4 allele of the cholesterol-transporting molecule APOE (Genin et al. 2011). The histopathology of the disease includes extracellular neuritic plaques with an amyloid core surrounded by dystrophic neuritis and intracellular tangles consisting of phosphorylated tau protein. This pathology usually appears first in the medial temporal lobes and later involves the parietal and frontal lobes. The clinical illness usually manifests in the late 60s or early 70s with impairment of short-term memory that may or may not be noticed by the patient. In many cases, the disease first comes to medical attention with the advent of executive impairment. It is possible to function well if one's only cognitive problem is impaired short-term memory (e.g., amnestic MCI), but not if one develops concomitant impairment of attention and other aspects of executive function. The course of the disease is in terms of years but is highly variable, with survival up to 20 years and with life expectancy dependent on quality of nursing care. Apparent sudden onset may occur with the loss of a protective spouse who has been compensating for the patient's declining functioning. Disease onset in the ninth decade with very slow progression is suggestive of the tangle-only variant of Alzheimer's disease (Yamada 2003). Essential features of DSM-5 major or mild NCD due to probable or possible Alzheimer's disease are listed in Table 25–10.

In addition to impaired recent memory, common additional findings on mental status examination are reduced attention and verbal fluency, word (noun)–finding difficulties, ideational dyspraxia (e.g., when asked to "show me how you turn a key in a lock"), constructional dyspraxia (e.g., when copying a drawing of intersecting pentagons), impaired clock drawing, and impaired abstract reasoning. Neuropsychiatric symptoms in early disease tend to be apathy and depression. Psychotic symptoms may occur in midstage disease, and a common symptom is delusions of theft, but these psychotic symptoms are rarely systematized. Visual hallucinations can occur in moderate to severe Alzheimer's disease and may point to the coexistence of Lewy body pathology.

Neurological examination findings are mostly normal in patients with mild Alzheimer's disease. Later in the course of the disease, myoclonus and mild extrapyramidal signs may appear. Seizures may occur late in the course of the disease. Computed tomography (CT) and MRI scans of the brain are frequently normal in early disease, as are electroencephalograms, although reduced hippocampal volume and slightly enlarged ventricular temporal horns may be found. FDG-PET scans may show reduced uptake of FDG in temporoparietal regions. Low CSF Aβ$_{42}$ and high phosphorylated tau protein are found in research settings. The FDA has approved several radioligands for use in detecting amyloid deposition in the brain, and imag-

TABLE 25–10. **Essential features of DSM-5 major or mild neurocognitive disorder due to Alzheimer's disease**

A. Criteria are met for major or mild neurocognitive disorder.

B. Insidious onset and gradual progression of impairment in one or more cognitive domains (for major neurocognitive disorder, at least two domains must be impaired).

C. Criteria are met for either probable or possible Alzheimer's disease, as follows:

For major neurocognitive disorder:

Probable Alzheimer's disease is diagnosed if either of the following is present; otherwise, **possible Alzheimer's disease** should be diagnosed.

 1. Evidence of a causative Alzheimer's disease (e.g., family history suggestive of genetic mutation or genetic testing results).

 2. Presence of all three of the following:

   a. Evidence of decline in memory and one other cognitive domain (based on history or longitudinal neuropsychological data).

   b. Progressive, gradual cognitive decline without periods of stability.

   c. Absence of other etiology that could explain the cognitive decline suggesting a mixed disorder (e.g., cerebrovascular or systemic disease).

For mild neurocognitive disorder:

Probable Alzheimer's disease is diagnosed if there is evidence of a causative Alzheimer's disease genetic mutation (based on genetic testing or family history).

Possible Alzheimer's disease is diagnosed if there is insufficient evidence to support probable Alzheimer's disease, and all three of the following are present:

 1. Evidence of decline in memory and one other cognitive domain (based on history or longitudinal neuropsychological data).

 2. Progressive, gradual cognitive decline without periods of stability.

 3. Absence of other etiology that could explain the cognitive decline suggesting a mixed disorder (e.g., cerebrovascular or systemic disease).

D. The dysfunction is not better explained by another disorder.

Note. For the complete diagnostic criteria, please refer to pp. 611–612 in DSM-5 (American Psychiatric Association 2013).

ing with these new radiotracers is now gaining wider use in both clinical and research settings to help exclude non-Alzheimer's dementia.

Frontotemporal Lobar Degeneration

FTLD is one of the leading causes of dementia in adults younger than 60 years. The term *frontotemporal lobar degeneration* is applied to a number of conditions—including Pick's disease, semantic aphasia, and progressive nonfluent aphasia. (Essential features of DSM-5 major or minor NCD associated with probable or possible FTLD are listed in Table 25–11.) Some individuals with FTLD have mutations in the genes for tau (leading to the term *tauopathies*) and progranulin proteins. Of these disorders, the most likely to come to psychiatric attention are those with predominant behavioral symptoms, the so-called behavioral variant of FTLD. In addition, corticobasal degeneration and progressive supranuclear palsy overlap with FTLD clinically and pathologically. Genetic mutations consistent with probable FTLD include those in the microtubule-associated protein tau gene (*MAPT*), the granulin gene (*GRN*), and the *C9orf72* gene.

TABLE 25–11. **Essential features of DSM-5 major or mild frontotemporal neurocognitive disorder**

A. Criteria are met for major or mild neurocognitive disorder.

B. Insidious onset and gradual progression.

C. Either (1) or (2):

    1. Behavioral variant requires

        a. Three or more of the following:

            i. Disinhibition.

            ii. Apathy or inertia.

            iii. Loss of empathy.

            iv. Perseverative, stereotyped, or compulsive/ritualistic behavior.

            v. Hyperorality and dietary changes.

        b. Disproportionate decline in social cognition and/or executive abilities.

    2. Language variant requires aphasic symptoms (e.g., declines in speech production or comprehension ability, difficulty in word finding).

D. Memory and perceptual–motor function are relatively preserved.

E. The dysfunction is not better explained by another disorder.

Probable frontotemporal neurocognitive disorder is diagnosed if one of the following is present; otherwise, **possible frontotemporal neurocognitive disorder** is diagnosed:

    1. Evidence of a causative frontotemporal disorder (e.g., family history suggestive of genetic mutation or genetic testing results).

    2. Evidence of disproportionate frontal and/or temporal lobe involvement from neuroimaging.

Note. For the complete diagnostic criteria, please refer to pp. 614–615 in DSM-5 (American Psychiatric Association 2013).

Behavioral Variant

The prototypical behavioral variant of FTLD is often caused by Pick's disease and presents as personality change with progressive impairment of judgment, loss of social graces, disinhibition, stimulus boundedness, and a craving for sweets. Patients' impaired judgment, irritability, impulsiveness, and total lack of self-awareness often lead to a misdiagnosis of bipolar disorder.

Language Variant

A diagnosis of language-variant FTLD requires that the most prominent feature be difficulty with language, that the language impairment be the principal cause of impaired performance in activities of daily living, and that aphasia be the most prominent deficit at symptom onset and in the initial stage of the disease. The language variant includes the subtypes semantic aphasia and progressive nonfluent aphasia (PNFA). Semantic aphasia usually begins as a fluent dysphasia involving such severe difficulty in naming and in understanding that these patients at first may appear to be malingering. Patients are often unable to describe or demonstrate the use of common objects, such as door keys. Less frequently used words will be the most difficult to retrieve. PNFA involves difficulties with verbal expression, characterized by apraxia of speech, agrammatism (i.e., sentences contain few or inaccurately used function words such as "if," "the," and "have"), and phonemic paraphasias (e.g., "cluck" or "click" for *clock*). Often, functional or behavioral symptoms do not appear until late in the disease. A third language-variant subtype, not included in DSM-5, has been proposed. This form, known as the logopenic/phonological variant, is mostly associated with Alzheimer's pathology, and it is characterized by impaired single-word retrieval in spontaneous speech and writing as well as impaired repetition of sentences and phrases.

The clinical presentations of these language variant subtypes relate to the loci of brain pathology. Patients with the semantic form have prominent anterior temporal atrophy in the language-dominant hemisphere, patients with the PNFA form have left posterior frontoinsular atrophy in the dominant hemisphere, and those with the logopenic form have posterior perisylvian or parietal atrophy in the dominant hemisphere. SPECT and PET studies show corresponding areas of decreased blood flow and glucose uptake (Gorno-Tempini et al. 2011).

Lewy Body Disease

Essential features of DSM-5 major or mild NCD associated with probable or possible Lewy body disease are listed in Table 25–12. Lewy bodies are round, often haloed cytoplasmic inclusions composed largely of alpha synuclein (leading to the designation of Lewy body disease as a *synucleinopathy*). Up to 20% of persons with clinically diagnosed Alzheimer's disease also have numerous cortical Lewy bodies (Weiner et al. 1996). Lewy body disease often clinically resembles Alzheimer's disease; however, there are certain key features that can aid in the differential diagnosis. These include visual and tactile hallucinations with sudden onset and frequent remission and recurrence; marked fluctuations in cognition, with episodes of confusion lasting hours or days followed by relative clarity; and motor features of Parkinson's disease that occur early in the disease. In addition, REM sleep behavior disorder is a frequent concomitant that can precede the cognitive symptoms by decades. Further confirmation of Lewy body disease is provided by low levels of dopamine transporter (DaT) in the basal ganglia, as revealed on DaT PET imaging with the [123I] ioflupane tracer. In most cases, disturbing psychotic symptoms can be ameliorated by cholinesterase inhibitors. In general, the extrapyramidal motor symptoms of Lewy body disease may not respond well to treatment with dopaminergic drugs. Antipsychotic medications should be avoided, since they place patients at risk for neuroleptic sensitivity or neuroleptic malignant syndrome, a condition characterized by worsening cognition, sedation, and increased or possibly irreversible acute-onset parkinsonism.

Cerebrovascular Disease

NCD associated with vascular disease is diagnosed when the patient has cognitive impairment with evidence on imaging, history, or clinical examination of cerebrovascular disease that is judged to be responsible for the cognitive impairment. Memory impairment, if present, is characteristically of the nonamnestic type, with impaired initial registration and recall and often with impaired remote memory. There may be focal neurological signs consistent with stroke (with or without a history of stroke) and brain imaging evidence of cerebrovascular disease, such as multiple large-vessel infarcts or a single strategically placed infarct (angular gyrus, thalamus, basal fore-

TABLE 25–12.   **Essential features of DSM-5 major or mild neurocognitive disorder with Lewy bodies**

A.   Criteria are met for major or mild neurocognitive disorder.

B.   Insidious onset and gradual progression.

C.   Major or mild neurocognitive disorder meets core and suggestive diagnostic features for either probable or possible neurocognitive disorder with Lewy bodies.

For **probable:** Two core features OR one suggestive feature with one or more core features.

For **possible:** One core feature OR one or more suggestive features.

    1.   Core diagnostic features:

        a.   Fluctuating attention, alertness, and cognition.

        b.   Recurrent, stereotyped, detailed visual hallucinations.

        c.   Parkinsonian features 1 year after cognitive impairment (for major neurocognitive disorder).

    2.   Suggestive diagnostic features:

        a.   Rapid eye movement behavior disorder of sleep.

        b.   Severe neuroleptic sensitivity.

        c.   Imaging (e.g., positron emission tomography) indicates low dopamine transporter uptake in basal ganglia.

D.   The disturbance is not better explained by cerebrovascular disease, another neurodegenerative disease, the effects of a substance, or another mental, neurological, or systemic disorder.

Note.   For the complete diagnostic criteria, please refer to pp. 618–619 in DSM-5 (American Psychiatric Association 2013).

TABLE 25–13.   **Essential features of DSM-5 major or mild vascular neurocognitive disorder**

A.   Criteria are met for major or mild neurocognitive disorder.

B.   Dysfunction consistent with vascular etiology, as defined by either 1 or 2:

    1.   Cerebrovascular event and associated cognitive dysfunction.

    2.   Decline in executive/complex attention and/or processing speed.

C.   Medical/neurological/historical/imaging evidence that accounts for dysfunction.

D.   The dysfunction is not better explained by another disorder.

For **probable vascular neurocognitive disorder:** One of the following is required:

    1.   Neuroimaging supports vascular insult consistent with dysfunction.

    2.   Temporal association between cerebrovascular and functional changes.

    3.   Clinical and genetic evidence of cerebrovascular disease.

For **possible vascular neurocognitive disorder:**

Clinical criteria evident but neuroimaging is unavailable; and

Insufficient evidence of a temporal relationship between the onset of a cerebrovascular event and a functional deficit.

Note.   For the complete diagnostic criteria, please refer to p. 621 in DSM-5 (American Psychiatric Association 2013).

brain, or anterior or posterior communicating territories), as well as multiple basal ganglia and white matter lacunes, extensive periventricular white matter lesions, or combinations of these. Essential features of DSM-5 major or mild NCD associated with probable or possible vascular disease are listed in Table 25–13. The probable versus possible distinction depends on the degree of certainty that brain damage from vascular disease underlies the cognitive dysfunction. For example, a finding of cerebral autosomal dominant arteriopathy with subcortical infarcts would support the third criterion (i.e., clinical and genetic evidence) for NCD associated with probable vascular disease.

Traumatic Brain Injury

Whereas NCD due to traumatic brain injury (TBI) has in common with the other NCDs evidence of brain dysfunction, the field of study is vast and expanding to include subspecialization based on type of injury, populations, dementia risk, stage of insult, and recovery, and the field strives to characterize increasingly subtle neuropsychological and neuropsychiatric symptoms (e.g., Sherer and Sander 2014). An understanding of the location and severity of the trauma can be highly informative. The Glasgow Coma Scale (Royal College of Physicians and Surgeons of Glasgow N.D.) is used to grade severity of the injury. The scale captures three categories of response—eye opening, verbal functioning, and motor functioning—observed in a person who has experienced head trauma (e.g., does patient open his/her eyes in response to hearing a voice? can patient orient to sounds?). *Posttraumatic amnesia*—the length of time that memory is lost for events surrounding the time of a head injury—is an important predictor of recovery, with longer periods of amnesia being associated with worse functional outcomes among survivors. Populations of TBI survivors are changing, and now include increasing numbers of young and middle-aged adults. Advances in the treatment of both closed and open head injuries have led to substantial increases in survival after TBI, with outcomes ranging from complete recovery to major NCD.

Amnestic Disorders (Memory Impairment Without Other Significant Cognitive Dysfunction)

Persistent amnesia may result from many types of brain injury, the best known being bilateral hippocampal lesions, which impair recent memory and prevent additional storage while sparing memories that were stored before the injury (Zola-Morgan et al. 1986). An individual with persistent impairment in memory caused by brain damage, whether induced by TBI, a toxic substance, or a tumor, would receive a DSM-5 diagnosis of major NCD due to the underlying medical condition. The DSM-IV amnestic disorders were subsumed under the DSM-5 major and minor NCDs and their etiological subtypes. In DSM-5, the amnestic confabulatory disorder known as Korsakoff's syndrome would receive a diagnosis of alcohol-induced major NCD, amnestic-confabulatory type, persistent. Korsakoff's syndrome results from thiamine deficiency, typically associated with malnutrition accompanying long-term alcohol abuse, and is often preceded by the delirium, ophthalmoplegia, and ataxia of Wernicke's encephalopathy. In contrast to the persistence of Korsakoff's syndrome, the amnestic episodes that occur with short-acting benzodiazepines are transient; however, they may confound diagnosis of other disorders. It is important to consider substance/medication-induced amnestic syndromes in the differential diagnosis of NCDs, because drug-induced amnestic symptoms are reversible.

Postoperative Cognitive Dysfunction

Postoperative cognitive dysfunction is a common cause of mild NCD. This NCD is characterized as a chronic level of dysfunction that manifests after a medical/surgical procedure that is followed by a delirium. Postoperative cognitive dysfunction would meet criteria for a diagnosis of major or mild NCD due to another medical condition without or with behavioral disturbance. Some authors have speculated that delirium and underlying degenerative processes are likely the major contributors to postoperative cognitive dysfunction, rather than exposure to surgical procedures per se, although this remains a topic of active research (Dokkedal et al. 2016; Fink et al. 2014). If it is true that surgery is not the primary cause of this condition, healthy older adults may not need to forgo necessary interventions because of fears of postoperative cognitive dysfunction.

Complicating or Confounding Disorders

In an evaluation of a person with a cognitive complaint, depression must be considered as the cause or as an aggravating factor. Many depressed persons experience cognitive impairment, although the severity of their impairment does not correlate with the severity of their depressive symptoms. Persistent deficits in cognitive function often remain after remission of depressive symptoms (Snyder 2013). The level and frequency of depressive comorbidity with Alzheimer's disease is highly controversial, partly due to the similarity between the symptoms of each illness. Depression is common after stroke (Robinson and Jorge 2016) and hence is often comorbid with NCD due to vascular disease. Depression is also common in Parkinson's disease and Huntington's disease.

Structural brain scans are not usually helpful in differentiating depression from an NCD without neurological signs, but functional imaging techniques such as PET may be useful when there are signs characteristic of a disorder such as Alzheimer's or Pick's disease. Neuropsychological testing can help in distinguishing between mood disorders and NCDs and in detecting comorbid mood disorders or NCDs, in addition to characterizing and quantifying cognitive deficits in domains such as memory and executive function.

A general medical condition may exaggerate preexisting personality traits or cause a change in personality. There are many possible patterns, but emotional instability, recurrent outbursts of aggression or rage, impaired social judgment, apathy, suspiciousness, and paranoid ideation are frequently noted. Encephalitis, brain tumor, head trauma, multiple sclerosis, frontotemporal degenerative disease, and stroke are common causes of personality changes. It is important in this population, as in all others, to seek remediable causes of functional decline.

Drug Treatment of Neurocognitive Disorders

Cognitive Enhancement Pharmacotherapy

A number of symptom-targeted drug treatments—including cholinesterase inhibitors and an *N*-methyl-D-aspartate (NMDA) receptor antagonist—are used clinically in NCDs. There is little evidence of a salutary drug treatment effect on cognition after traumatic brain injury. Treatment of Alzheimer's disease with selegiline, estrogen, prednisone, nonsteroidal anti-inflammatory drugs, statins, rosiglitazone, chelating agents, and the naturally occurring substances huperzine and Ginkgo biloba have not been shown to be successful in slowing cognitive deterioration in clinical trials. Treatments addressing the amyloid-related pathology have been successful in mouse models of Alzheimer's disease but have not yet been demonstrated to be effective and safe in humans with NCDs. Such treatments include active and passive immunization against $A\beta_{42}$ (the toxic product of abnormal amyloid precursor protein processing) and inhibitors of γ secretase (the enzyme co-responsible with β secretase for abnormal cleavage of amyloid precursor protein). These and a number of other strategies—including use of the naturally occurring antioxidants curcumin and resveratrol and of intranasal insulin—have failed to show efficacy in enhancing cognitive functioning. Development of treatments directed at tau protein is now in progress.

Cholinesterase Inhibitors

Acetylcholinesterase inhibitors have been used with some success in patients with all stages of Alzheimer's disease and Lewy body disease, as well as in cognitive impairment associated with vascular disease. Results in the treatment of traumatic brain injury are not clear. Patients with Alzheimer's disease have deficient cholinergic input to the neocortex. Patients with Lewy body disease have even greater cholinergic deficits. Individuals with vascular dementia often have a component of Alzheimer's disease. Cholinesterase inhibitors have modest effects on cognition in these disorders but can reduce or eliminate visual hallucinations in Lewy body disease. Most commonly, patients and caregivers report increased attention and comprehension. This class of drugs raises baseline cognitive performance but does not slow the rate of decline. All cholinesterase inhibitors are available in once-a-day preparations. Donepezil and galantamine are administered orally; rivastigmine is available in a transdermal formulation as patches. Both donepezil and rivastigmine have been marketed as high-dose preparations for moderate to severe Alzheimer's disease. Dosing for commonly used cholinesterase-inhibiting agents is presented in Table 25–14. Side effects of these drugs are dosage related and include nausea, vomiting, diarrhea, muscle cramps (from nicotinic effects), and postural hypotension and syncope due to bradycardia. A resting pulse below 50 and severe bronchopulmonary disease are relative contraindications, but the treatment decision should be made on a case-by-case basis. Many athletic individuals with a resting pulse in the 40s tolerate cholinesterase inhibitors well.

N-Methyl-D-Aspartate Receptor Antagonist

Memantine theoretically blocks the action of NMDA-type glutamate receptors, improving synaptic transmission and/or preventing calcium release, which may pro-

TABLE 25–14. Dosages of commonly used cholinesterase inhibitors

Generic name	Trade name	Initial dosage	Final dosage	Instructions
Donepezil	Aricept	5 mg	10–23[a] mg	Daily
Rivastigmine	Exelon patch	4.6 mg	9.5–13.3[b] mg	Daily
Galantamine	Razadyne ER	8 mg	24 mg	Daily with food

Note. Dosage should be adjusted on individual basis, and 4–6 weeks should be allowed between dosage escalations.
[a]Use only if patient can tolerate donepezil 10 mg/day or equivalent.
[b]Use only if patient can tolerate rivastigmine 9.5 mg/day or equivalent.

vide neuroprotection. Memantine is well absorbed and has a half-life of 70 hours or greater but is given twice per day because that was the dosage scheme used in the studies establishing the drug's efficacy. Memantine has been approved by the FDA for use in the treatment of moderate to severe Alzheimer's disease. Dosing starts at 5 mg/day and is titrated up 5 mg/day weekly to a final dosage of 10 mg twice a day. There may be transient confusion or sedation during the titration phase, but memantine generally has few adverse effects. Although it is frequently used in patients with early Alzheimer's disease, there are no convincing efficacy data for this use of memantine.

Combination Therapy With Cholinesterase Inhibitors and Memantine

Cholinesterase inhibitors and memantine have different mechanisms of action; thus, combination therapy could confer additional benefits (Tariot et al. 2004). This combination has become the standard of care in clinical practice for patients with moderate to severe Alzheimer's disease.

Vitamin E

Vitamin E is known to act as an antioxidant to scavenge toxic free radicals, and it has been studied extensively in the treatment of MCI and Alzheimer's dementia. However, evidence for its benefit in MCI or Alzheimer's disease is lacking, with the exception of a study that reported that vitamin E may slow functional decline in Alzheimer's disease (Dysken et al. 2014). Because long-term vitamin E supplementation was found to be associated with a small increased risk of cardiovascular events in a large trial involving older patients with vascular disease or diabetes mellitus (Lonn et al. 2005), vitamin E has become less popular as a treatment option.

Treatment of Superimposed Mental Disorders

Persons with any NCD may develop delirium, paranoid psychosis, or depression, all of which can be treated in the same manner as in persons without dementia. For example, electroconvulsive therapy can be used to treat severe depression. As expected, the cognitive side effects of such therapy are more severe for persons with dementia than for cognitively intact persons, but such effects do not represent an absolute contraindication. In addition, medications with significant anticholinergic side effects are generally avoided in patients with delirium or dementia.

Treatment of Behavioral and Emotional Symptoms of Neurocognitive Disorders

An important part of treatment involves managing the behavioral and emotional symptoms of NCDs, which can include psychosis, depression, apathy, aggression and violence, and/or inappropriate sexuality. Ideally, the first step in addressing a patient's behavioral symptoms should focus on modifying the behavior of the caregiver or reducing environmental triggers. For example, caregivers can be trained to "fill in the gaps" for patients' defective memory rather than asking patients to remember, or can be coached to answer repetitive questions directly rather than saying, "I already told you that." They can avoid violence by easing patients into frightening activities such as showering or bathing instead of trying to force them. The level of noise or interpersonal stimulation in the environment can be reduced. Caregivers can help alleviate apathy by initiating activities and setting up daily routines. Family caregivers can learn much from dementia support groups as well as from the wealth of publications and information available online (e.g., from the Alzheimer's Association, the Lewy Body Dementia Association, the Association for Frontotemporal Degeneration, and the Brain Injury Association of America). Nevertheless, rather than increasing demands on exhausted caregivers, patients' behavioral and emotional symptoms are often managed with medication.

No drug treatment has received FDA approval for use in treating any of the behavioral and emotional symptoms (except major depressive disorder and mania) that may arise during the course of an NCD. Pharmacological treatments that have been employed include antipsychotics, serotonin reuptake inhibitors, mood stabilizers, cholinesterase inhibitors, and anticonvulsants. Drug dosages presented in this chapter are those appropriate for elders. Because virtually all drugs used to treat behavioral disturbances in persons with NCDs are administered off label, the general guideline for younger adults is to escalate the dosage until the behavior is controlled or until untoward side effects occur. (See Chapter 29 in this volume, "Psychopharmacology," for recommended adult dosages of psychotropic drugs.)

The generally adopted psychopharmacological approach is that of Tariot (1999), which can be summarized as follows:

1. Use a drug with known efficacy in the symptom complex that most closely resembles the presenting symptoms.
2. Employ low dosages and escalate slowly, assessing both target symptoms and toxicity.
3. If a psychotropic medication is helpful, attempt to withdraw it at an appropriate time and monitor for recurrence of the problem. Several medications may need to be tried, either serially or conjointly. Sometimes no medication is useful.

Antipsychotic Medications

Antipsychotic medications should not routinely be used to treat neuropsychiatric symptoms related to dementia because these agents are associated with an increased risk of mortality (Reus et al. 2016). For antipsychotics used to treat agitation with psychotic features, therapeutic effects are often small and inconsistent. The potential side effects (e.g., akathisia, parkinsonism, tardive dyskinesia, sedation, neuroleptic malignant syndrome, peripheral and central anticholinergic effects, postural hypotension, cardiac conduction defects, falls) must be weighed against the potential benefits. There is no overall difference in efficacy between typical and atypical antipsychotic drugs, and little distinguishes them from each other except their side-effect profiles. It is important to note that FDA warnings have been issued about increased cardiac disease and increased mortality with both typical and atypical antipsychotics in elderly dementia patients (U.S. Food and Drug Administration 2008). Although use of an atypical antipsychotic in dementia patients increases the risk of mortality, the absolute increased risk to a given individual, at least with short-term treatment, is likely small (approximately 1%–2%) (Steinberg and Lyketsos 2012).

Typical antipsychotics.   The typical antipsychotic drug in widest use for psychiatric symptoms of NCDs is haloperidol, usually at dosages ranging from 0.5 mg/day to 1 mg twice a day orally. In cases of severe agitation, haloperidol may be given parenterally. Toxicity consists largely of dystonias and extrapyramidal symptoms. Larger haloperidol dosages have little therapeutic advantage, and extrapyramidal effects become much more frequent. The concomitant use of prophylactic diphenhydramine or benztropine mesylate is not recommended because of potential anticholinergic toxicity.

Atypical antipsychotics.   In view of the considerable toxicity of many typical agents, there was great hope that atypical antipsychotic drugs would have special utility in patients with NCDs. Due to the medications' side effects, however, careful selection for individual patients is necessary. A review of eight randomized controlled trials of atypical antipsychotics in adults with dementia concluded that aripiprazole, risperidone, and olanzapine—but not quetiapine—resulted in modest (standardized mean difference <0.5 standard deviation) improvement in neuropsychiatric symptoms relative to placebo (Farlow and Shamliyan 2017). Aripiprazole, risperidone, quetiapine, and olanzapine are associated with an increased risk of acute myocardial infarction, and risperidone and olanzapine are associated with an increased risk of hip fracture (Farlow and Shamliyan 2017).

Serotonin Reuptake Inhibitors

Serotonin reuptake inhibitors can reduce agitation and irritability in depressed or nondepressed persons with Alzheimer's disease (Porsteinsson et al. 2014). Serotonin reuptake inhibitors should be preferred over other antipsychotic medication and sedative medication for treating behavior problems. However, some selective serotonin reuptake inhibitors have potential cardiac side effects in elderly patients at higher dosages.

Stimulants

There is inadequate clinical trial evidence to support the use of stimulants in individuals with NCDs. The potential of stimulants to increase blood pressure and heart rate and to lead to irritability, agitation, and psychosis makes their usage in this population extremely rare.

Anticonvulsants/Mood Stabilizers

There is evidence supporting the use of valproic acid to reduce aggression in young to middle-aged adults with brain injury, but not in older adults. Generally administered once or twice a day, the drug is titrated upward from a total initial dosage of 250 mg/day. Use of carbamazepine is less desirable due to its propensity for producing agranulocytosis. There is no targeted therapeutic blood level for anticonvulsants used in the treatment of aggression. Patients are generally treated with increasing dosages until their behavior is controlled or they become somnolent or ataxic. Lithium is relatively contraindicated in older adults because of the frequency of tremor but has been used with success in younger adults with brain injury.

Hypnotics

Although hypnotic drugs may be administered to patients, these agents are generally prescribed so that caregivers can get adequate sleep and are not optimal for the patients. Conventional hypnotics (i.e., benzodiazepines) are generally avoided because of their tendency to oversedate and to cause confusion. For patients with insomnia, melatonin should be tried first, given its minimal side effects. However, if there are no other alternatives, the drugs commonly employed as hypnotics are trazodone (25–100 mg at bedtime) and mirtazapine (15–30 mg at bedtime). For treatment of the REM sleep behavior disorder that accompanies Lewy body disease, melatonin should be given before conventional hypnotics. Because treatment of insomnia in older adults is a complex and evolving field, clinicians should monitor the literature for new developments.

Prevention of Neurocognitive Disorders

The most preventable cause of NCDs in young adults is traumatic brain injury. The use of helmets for bicycle and motorcycle riders significantly reduces mortality and morbidity from head injuries, as do helmets in situations in which military personnel are exposed to blast injury. Efforts to prevent sports-related concussions are increasing, given that these injuries are no longer believed to be benign (Schneider et al. 2017).

A meta-analysis and consensus report estimated that one-third of dementia risk is related to lifestyle factors (Livingston et al. 2017). Protective factors include higher levels of education in childhood, increased exercise, maintenance of social engagement, reduction or cessation of smoking, and management of hearing loss, depression, diabetes, hypertension, and obesity. Epidemiological studies are observational, and not all risk factors are amenable to alteration through interventions or have treatments that demonstrate effectiveness in clinical trials. For example, nonsteroidal anti-inflammatory drugs have been associated with decreased dementia risk, but randomized clinical trials have not supported their preventive ability (Wang et al. 2015). Evidence that cognitive exercises have a preventive effect is mixed at best, with the strongest criticism being that skills fail to generalize beyond the tasks learned (Simons et al. 2016). In contrast, there appear to be a variety of cognitive and brain-based benefits from physical exercise that endure if exercise is maintained (Erickson et al. 2014; Oberlin et al. 2016). There is no evidence that NCD due to Lewy body disease is preventable, but avoidance of antipsychotic medication is critical to prevent a serious condition called neuroleptic sensitivity (Aarsland et al. 2005). Primary prevention of NCD due to vascular disease involves the general approach used in prevention of cardiovascular disease, including management of cholesterol levels and weight, good control of diabetes and hypertension, avoidance of smoking, and moderate exercise.

Legal and Ethical Issues

Legal and ethical issues abound in the clinical care of persons with impaired cognition (see also Chapter 7, "Ethical Considerations in Psychiatry," and Chapter 8, "Legal Considerations in Psychiatry"). How much disclosure should be made of the potential harmful effects of psychotropic drugs? Is written consent needed, and is consent valid if given by the patient alone? Is it safe for the patient to continue driving? If not, how should this issue be presented to the patient? When and how should the issue of long-term care be raised? When is it reasonable to institutionalize a family member against his or her will? Is the patient able to manage financial affairs? To make contracts (including marriage contracts)? To make medical decisions? To consent to treatment? To be liable for criminal acts? Who will act for patients when they become unable to act for themselves?

Ethical practice with patients having NCD involves understanding a patient's capacity for independence and balancing respect for the patient's autonomy against the obligation to act in the patient's best interests. In degenerative illnesses (and particularly in mild NCD), patients have a window of opportunity during which they can advocate for their future needs before their disease progresses; thus, it is useful during this period to raise the question of medical and/or financial power of attorney and to initiate a discussion of wills. Patients with major NCD or delirium are considered to be potentially vulnerable to undue influence and therefore require special protection. Clinicians must be able to assess how well patients understand decisions surrounding their care and financial best interests and must be alert to signs that patients' judgment may be compromised. If patients lack the capacity to comprehend the risks or benefits of a specific procedure, then, at a bare minimum, clinicians need to obtain assent from the patient and consent from the caregiver. The assent process essentially involves explaining the proposed treatment to the patient in simple language and asking for the patient's voluntary affirmative agreement to participate in the treatment. For patients with compromised judgment, clinicians must work closely with caregivers. Clinicians should be vigilant for signs that caregivers may not be acting in the patient's best interest. They should check whether the appropriate person has power of attorney. When a family member or a close friend is clearly incapable of serving in this role, guardianship could be considered, but this approach is frequently adversarial and may alienate patients from other family members. It should be emphasized that the large majority of patients with NCD have loving, supportive caregivers, and that this population of caregivers is at significant risk of depression. There is a vast body of literature devoted to caregiver support, as well as advocacy organizations to link caregivers with appropriate information and resources.

Clinicians often feel unable or reluctant to discuss a diagnosis of degenerative NCD with the family, or the patient resists following up on concerns surrounding the diagnosis. The result is that families suffer and worry without support and without the knowledge to help them cope. Armed with this knowledge, clinicians can serve a vital role in helping families to adapt to NCDs, obtain legal guidance in preparing documents to protect and care for patients, and make use of all of the resources available from society.

Conclusion

The neurocognitive disorders represent a broad category of illnesses in which there is presumed to be underlying brain pathology. In DSM-5, there are three major categories: delirium, and major and mild neurocognitive disorder. Identification of delirium with a careful history and mental status examination is imperative, because this NCD is often caused by an urgently treatable condition. The major and mild NCDs differ both in severity of cognitive dysfunction and, most critically, in severity of functional limitations. The mild NCDs are conceptualized as being much like mild cognitive impairment, a classification that was ultimately adopted by ICD-10, in which patients have cognitive dysfunction but are functionally independent. A diagnosis of mild or major NCD should include specification of subtype based on the presumed neuropathological etiology. In this chapter we focused on the most common subtypes—Alzheimer's disease, cerebrovascular disease, frontotemporal lobar degeneration, and Lewy body disease—and also touched on head injury and amnestic syndromes. We additionally provided a brief overview of treatment and clinical management considerations. Because of the risk of neuroleptic malignant syndrome, it is best to avoid use of antipsychotic medications in patients with Lewy body disease. Anticholinergic and antipsychotic medications should also be avoided in patients with Alzheimer's disease. The neuroscience of brain disorders is rapidly advancing, and clinicians must closely follow research in the field for discoveries that may lead to practice changes.

Key Clinical Points

- Neurocognitive disorders (NCDs) are detected by history and mental status examination; laboratory tests serve as supportive or exclusionary measures.

- Neuropsychiatric symptoms (e.g., behavioral, emotional, vegetative, ideational, perceptual disturbances) are common components of NCDs.

- Instruments are available for both clinical and research purposes to identify and quantify the cognitive and neuropsychiatric symptoms of NCDs.

- Neuropsychological testing is useful in early detection and quantification of impairment in NCDs.

- Neuroimaging is becoming an increasingly important tool in NCD diagnosis.

References

Aarsland D, Perry R, Larsen JP, et al: Neuroleptic sensitivity in Parkinson's disease and parkinsonian dementias. J Clin Psychiatry 66(5):633–637, 2005 15889951

American Psychiatric Association: Diagnostic and Statistical Manual of Mental Disorders, 4th Edition. Washington, DC, American Psychiatric Association, 1994

American Psychiatric Association: Diagnostic and Statistical Manual of Mental Disorders, 4th Edition, Text Revision. Washington, DC, American Psychiatric Association, 2000

American Psychiatric Association: Diagnostic and Statistical Manual of Mental Disorders, 5th Edition. Arlington, VA, American Psychiatric Association, 2013

Ashford JW: Screening for memory disorders, dementia, and Alzheimer's disease. Aging Health 4(4):399–432, 2008

Blumenfeld H: Neuroanatomy Through Clinical Cases, 2nd Edition. Sunderland, MA, Sinauer Associates, 2010

Castro P, Zaman S, Holland A: Alzheimer's disease in people with Down's syndrome: the prospects for and the challenges of developing preventative treatments. J Neurol 264(4):804–813, 2017 27778163

Centers for Disease Control and Prevention: Traumatic Brain Injury and Concussion Statistics. Atlanta, GA, Centers for Disease Control and Prevention, 2017. Available at: https://www.cdc.gov/traumaticbraininjury/data/index.html. Accessed November 11, 2018.

Centers for Medicare and Medicaid Services: Decision Memo for Positron Emission Tomography (FDG) and Other Neuroimaging Devices for Suspected Dementia (CAG-00088R). September 15, 2004. Available at: https://www.cms.gov/medicare-coverage-database/details/nca-decision-memo.aspx?NCAId=104. Accessed February 8. 2019.

Choi S-H, Lee H, Chung T-S, et al: Neural network functional connectivity during and after an episode of delirium. Am J Psychiatry 169(5):498–507, 2012 22549209

Cummings JL: The Neuropsychiatric Inventory: assessing psychopathology in dementia patients. Neurology 48 (5 suppl 6):S10–S16, 1997 9153155

Cummings JL, Mega M, Gray K, et al: The Neuropsychiatric Inventory: comprehensive assessment of psychopathology in dementia. Neurology 44(12):2308–2314, 1994 7991117

Dokkedal U, Hansen TG, Rasmussen LS, et al: Cognitive functioning after surgery in middle-aged and elderly Danish twins. Anesthesiology 124(2):312–321, 2016 26785430

Dysken MW, Guarino PD, Vertrees JE, et al: Vitamin E and memantine in Alzheimer's disease: clinical trial methods and baseline data. Alzheimers Dement 10(1):36–44, 2014 23583234

Erickson KI, Leckie RL, Weinstein AM: Physical activity, fitness, and gray matter volume. Neurobiol Aging 35 (suppl 2):S20–S28, 2014 24952993

Farlow MR, Shamliyan TA: Benefits and harms of atypical antipsychotics for agitation in adults with dementia. Eur Neuropsychopharmacol 27(3):217–231, 2017 28111239

Farrer LA, Cupples LA, Haines JL, et al: Effects of age, sex, and ethnicity on the association between apolipoprotein E genotype and Alzheimer disease. A meta-analysis. JAMA 278(16):1349–1356, 1997 9343467

Fink HA, Hemmy LS, MacDonald R, et al: Cognitive outcomes after cardiovascular procedures in older adults: a systematic review [Internet]. AHRQ Technology Assessments Nov 2014 25905147

Folstein MF, Folstein SE, McHugh PR: "Mini-mental state." A practical method for grading the cognitive state of patients for the clinician. J Psychiatr Res 12(3):189–198, 1975 1202204

Genin E, Hannequin D, Wallon D, et al: APOE and Alzheimer disease: a major gene with semi-dominant inheritance. Mol Psychiatry 16(9):903–907, 2011 21556001

Gorno-Tempini ML, Hillis AE, Weintraub S, et al: Classification of primary progressive aphasia and its variants. Neurology 76(11):1006–1014, 2011 21325651

Institute of Medicine: Cognitive Aging: Progress in Understanding and Opportunities for Action. Washington, DC, National Academies Press, 2015

Jack CR Jr, Bennett DA, Blennow K, et al: A/T/N: an unbiased descriptive classification scheme for Alzheimer disease biomarkers. Neurology 87(5):539–547, 2016 27371494

Jack CR Jr, Bennett DA, Blennow K, et al: NIA-AA Research Framework: toward a biological definition of Alzheimer's disease. Alzheimers Dement 14(4):535–562, 2018 29653606

Jessen F, Amariglio RE, van Boxtel M, et al: A conceptual framework for research on subjective cognitive decline in preclinical Alzheimer's disease. Alzheimers Dement 10(6):844–852, 2014 24798886

Lezak MD, Howieson DB, Bigler ED, et al: Neuropsychological Assessment, 5th Edition. New York, Oxford University Press, 2012

Livingston G, Sommerlad A, Orgeta V, et al: Dementia prevention, intervention, and care. Lancet 390(10113):2673–2734, 2017 28735855

Lonn E, Bosch J, Yusuf S, et al; HOPE and HOPE-TOO Trial Investigators: Effects of long-term vitamin E supplementation on cardiovascular events and cancer: a randomized controlled trial. JAMA 293(11):1338–1347, 2005 15769967

Miller BL, Boeve BF: The Behavioral Neurology of Dementia, 2nd Edition. Cambridge, UK, Cambridge University Press, 2017

Muayqil T, Gronseth G, Camicioli R: Evidence-based guideline: diagnostic accuracy of CSF 14-3-3 protein in sporadic Creutzfeldt-Jakob disease: report of the guideline development subcommittee of the American Academy of Neurology. Neurology 79(14):1499–1506, 2012 22993290

Nasreddine ZS, Phillips NA, Bedirian V, et al: The Montreal Cognitive Assessment, MoCA: a brief screening tool for mild cognitive impairment. J Am Geriatr Soc 53(4):695–699, 2005 15817019

Oberlin LE, Verstynen TD, Burzynska AZ, et al: White matter microstructure mediates the relationship between cardiorespiratory fitness and spatial working memory in older adults. Neuroimage 131:91–101, 2016 26439513

Pachana NA, Byrne GJ, Siddle H, et al: Development and validation of the Geriatric Anxiety Inventory. Int Psychogeriatr 19(1):103–114, 2007 16805925

Petersen RC, Smith GE, Waring SC, et al: Aging, memory, and mild cognitive impairment. Int Psychogeriatr 9 (suppl 1):65–69, 1997 9447429

Porsteinsson AP, Drye LT, Pollock BG, et al: Effect of citalopram on agitation in Alzheimer disease: the CitAD randomized clinical trial. JAMA 311(7):682–691, 2014 24549548

Purves D, Augustine GJ, Fitzpatrick D, et al (eds): Neuroscience, 6th Edition. Sunderland MA, Sinauer Associates, 2017

Reus VI, Fochtmann LJ, Eyler AE, et al: The American Psychiatric Association practice guideline on the use of antipsychotics to treat agitation or psychosis in patients with dementia. Am J Psychiatry 173(5):543–546, 2016 27133416

Robinson RG, Jorge RE: Post-stroke depression: a review. Am J Psychiatry 173(3):221–231, 2016 26684921

Rossetti HC, Lacritz LH, Cullum CM, et al: Normative data for the Montreal Cognitive Assessment (MoCA) in a population-based sample. Neurology 77(13):1272–1275, 2011 21917776

Royal College of Physicians and Surgeons of Glasgow: The Glasgow Structured Approach to Assessment of the Glasgow Coma Scale. N.D. Available at: https://www.glasgowcomascale.org/. Accessed January 22, 2019.

Schneider DK, Grandhi RK, Bansal P, et al: Current state of concussion prevention strategies: a systematic review and meta-analysis of prospective, controlled studies. Br J Sports Med 51(20):1473–1482, 2017 27251896

Sherer M, Sander AM: Handbook on the Neuropsychology of Traumatic Brain Injury. New York, Springer-Verlag, 2014

Simons DJ, Boot WR, Charness N, et al: Do "brain-training" programs work? Psychol Sci Public Interest 17(3):103–186, 2016 27697851

Smith GE, Bondi MW: Mild Cognitive Impairment and Dementia: Definitions, Diagnosis, and Treatment. New York, Oxford University Press, 2013

Snyder HR: Major depressive disorder is associated with broad impairments on neuropsychological measures of executive function: a meta-analysis and review. Psychol Bull 139(1):81–132, 2013 22642228

Steinberg M, Lyketsos CG: Atypical antipsychotic use in patients with dementia: managing safety concerns. Am J Psychiatry 169(9):900–906, 2012 22952071

Strauss E, Sherman E, Spreen O: A Compendium of Neuropsychological Tests, 3rd Edition. New York, Oxford University Press, 2006

Tariot PN: Treatment of agitation in dementia. J Clin Psychiatry 60 (suppl 8):11–20, 1999 10335667

Tariot PN, Farlow MR, Grossberg GT, et al; Memantine Study Group: Memantine treatment in patients with moderate to severe Alzheimer disease already receiving donepezil: a randomized controlled trial. JAMA 291(3):317–324, 2004 14734594

U.S. Food and Drug Administration: Information for Healthcare Professionals: Conventional Antipsychotics, FDA ALERT [6/16/2008]. Silver Spring, MD, U.S. Food and Drug Administration, June 16, 2008. Available on FDA Archive at: http://wayback.archive-it.org/7993/20170112032513/http://www.fda.gov/Drugs/DrugSafety/PostmarketDrugSafetyInformationforPatientsandProviders/ucm124830.htm. Accessed December 31, 2018.

Wang J, Tan L, Wang HF, et al: Anti-inflammatory drugs and risk of Alzheimer's disease: an updated systematic review and meta-analysis. J Alzheimers Dis 44(2):385–396, 2015 25227314

Warren MW, Weiner MF: Is routine testing of vitamin B12 cost-effective in workup for cognitive impairment? Am Fam Physician 85(8):e1, author reply e1–2, 2012 22534395

Weiner MF, Risser RC, Cullum CM, et al: Alzheimer's disease and its Lewy body variant: a clinical analysis of postmortem verified cases. Am J Psychiatry 153(10):1269–1273, 1996 8831433

Yamada M: Senile dementia of the neurofibrillary tangle type (tangle-only dementia): neuropathological criteria and clinical guidelines for diagnosis. Neuropathology 23(4):311–317, 2003 14719548

Yesavage JA: Geriatric Depression Scale. Psychopharmacol Bull 24(4):709–711, 1988 3249773

Zola-Morgan S, Squire LR, Amaral DG: Human amnesia and the medial temporal region: enduring memory impairment following a bilateral lesion limited to field CA1 of the hippocampus. J Neurosci 6(10):2950–2967, 1986 3760943

Recommended Readings

Blazer DG, Steffens DC: The American Psychiatric Publishing Textbook of Geriatric Psychiatry. Washington, DC, American Psychiatric Publishing, 2009

Blumenfeld H: Neuroanatomy Through Clinical Cases, 2nd Edition. Sunderland, MA, Sinauer Associates, 2010

Lezak MD, Howieson DB, Bigler ED, et al: Neuropsychological Assessment, 5th Edition. New York, Oxford University Press, 2012

Purves D, Augustine GJ, Fitzpatrick D, et al: Neuroscience, 4th Edition. Sunderland MA, Sinauer Associates, 2008

Smith GE, Bondi MW: Mild Cognitive Impairment and Dementia: Definitions, Diagnosis, and Treatment. New York, Oxford University Press, 2013

Weiner MF, Lipton AM (eds): The Dementias: Diagnosis, Treatment and Research. Washington, DC, American Psychiatric Publishing, 2009

Online Resource

Alzheimers & Dementia: For the latest epidemiology on degenerative dementias, see http://www.alzheimersanddementia.com/ yearly facts and figures

CHAPTER 26

Personality Pathology and Personality Disorders

Andrew E. Skodol, M.D.

Donna S. Bender, Ph.D.

John M. Oldham, M.D.

Personality pathology is associated with significant problems in self-appraisal and self-regulation as well as with impaired interpersonal relationships. Clinicians frequently encounter patients with personality pathology in both outpatient and inpatient settings. Studies indicate that at least 50% of patients evaluated in clinical settings have a personality disorder (Zimmerman et al. 2005), often co-occurring with other mental disorders, and many more patients have significant personality problems that do not meet criteria for a personality disorder diagnosis, making personality pathology one of the most common psychopathologies encountered by mental health professionals. Personality disorders are also common in the general population, with an estimated prevalence of about 11% (Torgersen 2014). Personality pathology can be complex and challenging to assess and to treat, and it affects many of the symptom disorders (e.g., depressive or anxiety disorders) that are targeted in treatment, often without attention to the possibility of underlying personality factors.

General Considerations

Essential Features of Personality Disorders

Personality disorders in Section II ("Diagnostic Criteria and Codes") of DSM-5 (American Psychiatric Association 2013) are defined by general criteria exactly as they were in DSM-IV-TR (American Psychiatric Association 2000), despite the absence of either theoretical or empirical justification for key aspects of these criteria. According to DSM-5 Section II, personality disorders are enduring patterns of inner experience and behavior that are inflexible and pervasive and cause clinically significant distress or impairment in social, occupational, or other areas of functioning. These patterns deviate markedly from the expectations of an individual's culture and are said in DSM-5 Section II to manifest in two or more of the following areas: cognition, affectivity, interpersonal functioning, and impulse control. These features are not specific to personality disorders, however, and may characterize other chronic mental disorders, contributing to problems in differential diagnosis. To address the limitations of the Section II categorical approach and to respond to the original DSM-5 call for dimensional solutions, an innovative assessment approach with a revised set of general criteria—the Alternative DSM-5 Model for Personality Disorders (AMPD)—was included in Section III (Emerging Measures and Models) of the manual. The alternative criteria focus on 1) impairments in aspects of *personality functioning* (Criterion A), including identity, self-direction, empathy, and intimacy, that have been shown to be core features of personality psychopathology (Bender et al. 2011) and have been empirically demonstrated to have specificity for personality disorders (Morey et al. 2011), thereby facilitating differential diagnosis; and 2) *pathological personality traits* (Criterion B) that describe the myriad variations in personality pathology.

Pervasiveness and Stability of Personality Disorders

According to both the Section II and the Section III definitions, the manifestations of personality pathology are relatively pervasive—that is, they are exhibited across a broad range of contexts and situations rather than in only one specific triggering situation or in response to a particular stimulus or person. Whereas the DSM-5 Section II personality disorder criteria specify that the patterns must have been stably present and enduring since adolescence or early adulthood, the alternative criteria in Section III require that the core impairments in personality functioning and pathological personality traits must have been *relatively* stable across time and consistent across situations. This change from stability to *relative* stability was motivated by data from prospective longitudinal follow-along studies (Gunderson et al. 2011; Zanarini et al. 2012) that consistently showed that the stability of disorder constructs is considerably lower than that implied by DSM-5 Section II and that personality disorders have a clinical course that tends toward improvement or remission. In addition, both normal and pathological personality traits, while more stable than disorders, still change across the life span. Thus, although shifting to a more trait-based set of criteria is expected to increase the stability of personality disorder constructs, allowance for some change in clinical course is also warranted.

A schematic of the Section III AMPD general criteria for personality disorder is presented in Table 26–1.

History of DSM Personality Disorders

Personality disorders have been included in every version of DSM, but only obsessive-compulsive personality disorder and antisocial personality disorder have been consistently defined across time. Some current categories (e.g., borderline personality disorder) were added in later editions, whereas others (e.g., passive-aggressive per-

TABLE 26–1. Alternative DSM-5 Model for Personality Disorders: general criteria

1. Moderate or greater impairment in personality functioning

+

2. Presence of one or more pathological personality traits

+

3. Relative stability and consistency; developmental, cultural, substance, and medical exclusions

=

4. General criteria for personality disorder

sonality disorder) were dropped. The theoretical underpinnings of the DSM personality disorder categories have also changed over the years.

DSM-I (American Psychiatric Association 1952) defined personality disorders not as stable and enduring patterns but rather as traits that malfunctioned under stressful circumstances, leading to inflexible and maladaptive behavior. DSM-II (American Psychiatric Association 1968) emphasized that personality disorders involved distress and impairment in functioning, not merely socially deviant behavior. In DSM-III (American Psychiatric Association 1980), several major changes in personality disorder conceptualization and classification were made. There was a shift away from a somewhat psychoanalytically informed orientation and toward a more atheoretical, descriptive approach. Specific diagnostic criteria were assigned, and personality disorders were placed on a separate assessment "axis," which highlighted their importance.

The changes made in DSM-III-R (American Psychiatric Association 1987) and DSM-IV (American Psychiatric Association 1994) attempted to increase the reliability and validity of the personality disorder categories by incorporating findings from the growing empirical literature. For DSM-5, an attempt was made to further increase the validity of personality disorders by developing a hybrid dimensional–categorical model that more faithfully captured the continuous, dimensional nature of personality pathology while preserving continuity with the current clinical practice of diagnosing personality disorders as categories. Ultimately, this hybrid model was placed in Section III of DSM-5 (the section for "Emerging Measures and Models") as an "official" alternative method for describing personality pathology and diagnosing personality disorders. The familiar 10-category system of DSM-IV was retained in DSM-5 Section II. The Axis II designation for personality disorders was eliminated from DSM-5, however.

Classification Issues

An unresolved issue over the past 35-plus years has been whether the personality disorders (and other mental disorders) are better classified as dimensions or categories. Addressing this question was a major motivation for undertaking the DSM-5 revision. Do personality disorders exist along dimensions that reflect variants of personality functioning and pathological personality traits, or are they distinct categories that are qualitatively different and clearly demarcated from normal personality traits and from one another? Categorical diagnoses of personality disorders have been criticized for many reasons. First, excessive diagnostic co-occurrence among personality disorders has been observed in many studies: most patients with personality disorders meet criteria for more than one disorder. Second, there is considerable heterogeneity of features among patients receiving the same diagnosis. For example, given that a diagnosis of borderline personality disorder requires any five or more of nine criteria from its polythetic criteria set, there are 256 separate ways to meet the criteria for the disorder. The thresholds for making a personality disorder diagnosis are arbitrary in that they were decided based on expert consensus and not based on empirical research. How different is a patient who meets four of seven criteria for avoidant personality disorder (the diagnostic threshold) from one who meets only three of seven (subthreshold)? Finally, despite the listing of 10 specific personality disorder types in DSM-IV-TR, the residual category of *personality disorder not otherwise specified* has been the most commonly applied personality disorder diagnosis in clinical practice, which suggests inadequate coverage of personality psychopathology by the DSM classification—or else reflects the secondary importance accorded to personality disorders by psychiatrists and the inordinate amount of time required to accurately diagnose them with the DSM-IV-TR criteria (e.g., 79 adult and 15 childhood [for antisocial personality disorder] criteria).

Several different dimensional approaches to personality disorder assessment have been proposed as alternatives to DSM categories. The most direct approach has been to simply transform the categories into dimensions by counting criteria or rating the degree to which patients meet criteria on a continuous scale. Another "person-centered" dimensional approach is prototype matching. Using this approach, the clinician rates on a continuous scale the degree to which a patient meets the written description of a prototypical patient with each personality disorder. This approach has been shown to have clinical utility and to be very "clinician friendly." Other dimensional approaches require the clinician to rate a patient's pathological personality traits on a scale of severity, whereas still other "spectrum" models attempt to bring together so-called Axis I and Axis II disorders that seem to share fundamental underlying dimensions of psychopathology, such as internalizing versus externalizing or cognitive/perceptual versus affective disturbances.

The most widely used dimensional approaches describe personality according to several broad trait factors, or *domains,* and more narrow trait dimensions, or *facets,* and assess the degree to which these personality trait domains and facets are present for a given patient. These models may more comprehensively cover both normal and pathological personality traits. Of special significance are the widely accepted "Big Five" dimensions of the five-factor model (FFM) of personality: neuroticism, extraversion, openness, agreeableness, and conscientiousness (Costa and McCrae 1990). Cloninger's seven-dimension psychobiological model of temperament and character (Cloninger et al. 1993)—which encompasses four temperament dimensions (novelty seeking, harm avoidance, reward dependence, and persistence) and three character dimensions (self-directedness, cooperativeness, and self-transcendence)—has also generated a large body of research. The pathological personality trait model developed for DSM-5, which is based on these and other existing trait models, consists of five domains—negative affectivity, detachment, antagonism, disinhibition, and psychoticism—each composed of 3–8 trait facets (for a total of 25) (Table 26–2).

Dimensional models vary in the empirical support each has received. The genetic and phenotypic structure of the basic traits delineating personality disorders, however, has been shown to be consistent (Livesley et al. 1998). Nonetheless, dimensional

TABLE 26–2. Alternative DSM-5 Model for Personality Disorders: personality trait domains[a] and component facets[a]

Negative affectivity	Detachment	Antagonism	Disinhibition	Psychoticism
Emotional lability	Withdrawal	Manipulativeness	Irresponsibility	Unusual beliefs and experiences
Anxiousness	Intimacy avoidance	Deceitfulness	Impulsivity	Eccentricity
Separation insecurity	Anhedonia	Grandiosity	Distractibility	Cognitive and perceptual dysregulation
Submissiveness	Depressivity[b]	Attention seeking	Risk taking	
Hostility[b]	Restricted affectivity	Callousness	Rigid perfectionism (lack of)[c]	
Perseveration	Suspiciousness[b]	Hostility[b]		
Depressivity[b]				
Suspiciousness[b]				
Restricted affectivity (lack of)[c]				

[a]For the complete definitions of all trait domains and facets, please refer to pp. 779–781 in DSM-5 (American Psychiatric Association 2013).
[b]Some trait facets loaded on two trait domains in factor analyses leading to the AMPD pathological trait model. These facets are listed under both trait domains in the table.
[c]The *lack of* this trait facet is consistent with *higher levels of* the superordinate trait domain.

approaches are unfamiliar to those trained in a medical model of diagnosis and can appear complex to use. Categories enable clinicians to summarize patients' difficulties succinctly and facilitate communication about them, but often at the expense of describing more specific elements that are clinically meaningful with respect to treatment.

The Alternative DSM-5 Model for Personality Disorders

In 2007, a Personality and Personality Disorders Work Group was appointed to consider the future of personality disorder assessment and classification in DSM-5. Key questions were articulated to inform potential revisions: What is the core definition of a personality disorder that distinguishes it from other types of psychopathology? Is personality psychopathology better described by dimensional representations of diagnostic categories or by extremes on dimensions of general personality functioning than by the categories themselves? Is a separate Axis II for personality assessment valuable? What is the clinical importance (for risk, treatment, or prognosis) of assessing personality or personality disorders in other diagnostic domains, such as mood, anxiety, substance use, eating, or psychotic disorders?

Although the categorical approach to personality disorders and their specific criteria did not change in DSM-5 Section II, the new hybrid dimensional–categorical approach to personality pathology referred to earlier was placed in DSM-5 Section III. The AMPD was designed around core features of personality functioning and pathological traits and presents a "telescoping" approach to personality assessment—that is, clinicians or researchers may choose to use only one part of the model, such as to focus solely on the level of personality functioning or on prominent personality traits, or they may choose to evaluate whether criteria are met for one of the six newly defined categorical personality disorder diagnoses or for personality disorder–trait specified (PD-TS).

For the general criteria for personality disorder (see Table 26–1), a revised personality functioning criterion—Criterion A, encompassing self (identity and self-direction) and interpersonal (empathy and intimacy) functioning—was developed on the basis of a literature review of reliable clinical measures of core impairments central to personality pathology (Bender et al. 2011), and was validated as specific for semistructured interview diagnoses of personality disorders in samples of more than 2,000 patients and community subjects (Morey et al. 2011). A recent meta-analysis of 127 studies (Wilson et al. 2017) confirmed that disturbances in self and interpersonal functioning are at the core of personality psychopathology. In the creation of the AMPD, the moderate-severity level of impairment in personality functioning—as measured by the Level of Personality Functioning Scale (LPFS; Figure 26–1)—that was required for a personality disorder diagnosis in DSM-5 Section III was set empirically to maximize the ability of clinicians to identify personality disorder pathology accurately and efficiently (Morey et al. 2013). With a single assessment of level of personality functioning, a clinician can determine whether a full assessment for personality disorder is necessary.

The diagnostic criteria for specific DSM-5 personality disorders in the Section III model are consistently defined across disorders by typical impairments in personality functioning (Criterion A) and by characteristic pathological personality traits (Crite-

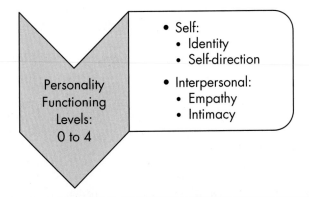

FIGURE 26–1. Alternative DSM-5 Model for Personality Disorders Level of Personality Functioning Scale.

Note. For the complete Level of Personality Functioning Scale, please refer to pp. 775–778 in DSM-5 (American Psychiatric Association 2013).

rion B) that have been empirically determined to be related to the personality disorders they represent (Morey et al. 2016). Diagnostic thresholds for both the A and the B criteria have been set empirically to minimize change in disorder prevalence (from DSM-IV) and overlap with other personality disorders and to maximize relations with psychosocial impairment (Morey and Skodol 2013). A greater emphasis on personality functioning and trait-based criteria strengthens the evidence base and increases the stability and predictive validity of the disorders (Hopwood et al. 2013; Wright et al. 2016).

The six specific personality disorders included in the AMPD on the basis of existing empirical evidence and clinical utility are antisocial, avoidant, borderline, narcissistic, obsessive-compulsive, and schizotypal personality disorder (Skodol et al. 2011a, 2014). The diagnosis of PD-TS, denoting moderate or greater impairment in personality functioning and the presence of pathological personality traits, replaces personality disorder not otherwise specified and provides a much more informative diagnosis for patients who are not optimally described as having a specific personality disorder. The four Section II personality disorders not included as specific personality disorders in the AMPD (i.e., paranoid, schizoid, histrionic, and dependent), as well as any other personality disorder presentations (e.g., passive-aggressive, depressive), would be diagnosed as PD-TS, with the level of impairment in personality functioning and the pathological personality traits present noted (Table 26–3).

The DSM-5 AMPD combines major paradigms of personality assessment and has been described as facilitating case conceptualization, being easy to learn and use, assisting in providing patient feedback, and enriching clinical thinking and practice (Waugh et al. 2017). New measures have been developed for the assessment of the AMPD, such as the Personality Inventory for DSM-5 (PID-5; Krueger et al. 2012), the Level of Personality Functioning Scale—Self Report (LPFS-SR; Morey 2017), and the Structured Clinical Interview for the DSM-5 Alternative Model for Personality Disorders (SCID-5-AMPD; First et al. 2018), but some existing measures already in common use can also inform assessment (see Waugh et al. 2017).

TABLE 26–3.   Defining features of DSM-5 Section III and Section II personality
               disorders

Personality disorder	Section III features	Section II features
Antisocial	Failure to conform to lawful and ethical behavior and an egocentric, callous lack of concern for others, accompanied by deceitfulness, irresponsibility, manipulativeness, and/or risk taking	History of conduct disorder before age 15 years; pervasive pattern of disregard for and violation of the rights of others; current age at least 18 years
Avoidant	Avoidance of social situations and inhibition in interpersonal relationships related to feelings of ineptitude and inadequacy, anxious preoccupation with negative evaluation and rejection, and fears of ridicule or embarrassment	Pervasive pattern of social inhibition, feelings of inadequacy, and hypersensitivity to negative evaluation
Borderline	Instability of self-image, personal goals, interpersonal relationships, and affects, accompanied by impulsivity, risk taking, and/or hostility	Pervasive pattern of instability of interpersonal relationships, self-image, and affects, and marked impulsivity
Narcissistic	Variable and vulnerable self-esteem, with attempts at regulation through attention and approval seeking, and either overt or covert grandiosity	Pervasive pattern of grandiosity (in fantasy or behavior), need for admiration, and lack of empathy
Obsessive-compulsive	Difficulties in establishing and sustaining close relationships, associated with rigid perfectionism, inflexibility, and restricted emotional expression	Pervasive pattern of preoccupation with orderliness, perfectionism, and mental and interpersonal control at the expense of flexibility, openness, and efficiency
Schizotypal	Impairments in the capacity for social and close relationships, and eccentricities in cognition, perception, and behavior that are associated with distorted self-image and incoherent personal goals and accompanied by suspiciousness and restricted emotional expression	Pervasive pattern of social and interpersonal deficits marked by acute discomfort with, and reduced capacity for, close interpersonal relationships, as well as by cognitive or perceptual distortions and eccentricities of behavior
Dependent	Moderate or greater impairment in personality functioning; traits of submissiveness, anxiousness, and separation insecurity (PD-TS)	Pervasive and excessive need to be taken care of that leads to submissive and clinging behavior and fears of separation
Histrionic	Moderate or greater impairment in personality functioning; traits of emotional lability, attention seeking, and manipulativeness (PD-TS)	Pervasive pattern of excessive emotionality and attention seeking

TABLE 26–3. **Defining features of DSM-5 Section III and Section II personality disorders** *(continued)*

Personality disorder	Section III features	Section II features
Paranoid	Moderate or greater impairment in personality functioning; traits of suspiciousness and hostility (PD-TS)	Pervasive distrust and suspiciousness of others such that their motives are interpreted as malevolent
Schizoid	Moderate or greater impairment in personality functioning; traits of withdrawal, intimacy avoidance, anhedonia, and restricted affectivity (PD-TS)	Pervasive pattern of detachment from social relationships and restricted range of emotions in interpersonal settings

Note. PD-TS=personality disorder—trait specified.
Source. Adapted from American Psychiatric Association 2013 and from Skodol AE: "Manifestations, Assessment, and Differential Diagnosis," in *The American Psychiatric Publishing Textbook of Personality Disorders,* 2nd Edition. Edited by Oldham JM, Skodol AE, Bender DS. Washington, DC, American Psychiatric Publishing, 2014, pp 131–164. Copyright © 2014 American Psychiatric Publishing. Used with permission.

Assessment Issues

The assessment of personality pathology is in some ways more complex than the assessment of other mental disorders. Because clinicians often are not trained to attend to personality in their patient evaluations, they may find it difficult to assess multiple aspects of personality pathology and to determine whether these aspects are distressing or impairing, of early onset, and sufficiently pervasive and enduring. Nonetheless, an assessment of personality pathology is essential for comprehensive evaluation and adequate treatment of all patients.

Case Vignette

Ms. K, a 24-year-old graduate student in public health, was recommended for treatment at a university counseling center by her primary care physician, who was concerned that she might have clinically significant depression and substance use. In the initial meeting with a therapist, Ms. K confirmed that she did feel depressed at times, but she attributed that to her unhappy relationship. Ms. K and her boyfriend, who lived together, had been having many heated arguments for quite a while, often with Ms. K storming out afterward and disappearing for several hours. Ms. K explained that she currently hates her boyfriend, feeling very controlled by him. However, she sees herself as utterly dependent on him as well, which makes her feel worthless and loathe him even more. She also was experiencing intermittent suicidal thoughts but said she would not act on them because of her family.

During the consultation, Ms. K revealed that when she leaves the house after an argument with her boyfriend, she sometimes goes to bars and drinks quite a lot. During one of these outings, she started hooking up with another man. She described this man, Mr. Q, as "an angel," and said that he had everything her boyfriend did not have, except money. Sometimes, in the middle of the night, she would sneak out of her house to meet this man, because she felt as if "I won't be able to live unless I have sex with Q."

However, after these nights out, she feels horrible guilt and remorse, becomes depressed, and makes herself throw up. When trying to reflect on her behavior, she said, "I don't know why I act this way. My boyfriend really is a good person. I am such a loser." On the other hand, when her boyfriend tries to talk to her about how it upsets him when she disappears for hours, she becomes angry and defensive and cannot really consider what he is trying to communicate about his experience. When her emotions become too much for her, she takes pain medication that she had received after a back injury. She reports that lately she has been taking these drugs on occasion to "numb out."

When asked about school, Ms. K began to weep. She apparently is quite intelligent, having done well as an undergraduate, but she is dismissive of her accomplishments. She said, "I only had a 3.5 GPA, not great." Now, as a public health student, she said she wants to help the world "more than my life," but she doesn't exactly know what she means by that and feels so distressed at times that it is hard for her to focus on her studies. She recently "screamed" at her research partner when her partner did not have time to work on their project on the night that Ms. K was available. Ms. K is sometimes able to do her work adequately, but other times, when she is feeling too stressed and overwhelmed, her boyfriend must step in and take care of her. She saw a therapist while in college, about whom she said, "I really loved her, she helped me so much, but sometimes I thought she was a bitch. That's how it is with people, you really can't trust them."

Ms. K was a music minor as an undergraduate, reportedly a very skilled pianist, but described herself as being too emotionally fragile—frequently upset by something in her personal life or easily offended by her professors' comments—to really excel with her talents. She has not touched the piano in several years and feels envious of the choir at her church because they are making music, while she feels she cannot. She has successfully taught children's Sunday school at church, but she denigrates her contribution. She also belongs to a women's prayer group. She likes a few of the group members but cannot become friends with any of them because, "they will find out what a disgusting person I am inside."

Ms. K was at first aloof and somewhat defensive. As the discussion went on, she became tearful. When the idea of possibly being referred to a therapist in the community for longer-term therapy was raised, she became haughty and said, "So, I'm too much for you to handle?" The consulting therapist went significantly over the time allotted for the session and scheduled a follow-up for the next week.

Options for Evaluation

A skilled clinical interview is the mainstay of the assessment of personality pathology and requires the clinician be attuned to gathering information about how the individual thinks about her- or himself and his or her interpersonal relationships and to inquire about the individual's typical approaches to interacting with others and situations of living. The DSM-5 AMPD can be used for assessment in a stepwise fashion, addressing each aspect of the general criteria for a personality disorder in turn (Skodol et al. 2015). A common place to begin an AMPD assessment is to consider personality functioning by asking questions to yield information to score the LPFS. Central to functioning and adaptation are individuals' characteristic ways of thinking about and understanding themselves and their interactions with other people. An optimally functioning person has a complex, fully elaborated, and well-integrated psychological world that includes a mostly positive, volitional, and effective self-concept; a rich, broad, and appropriately regulated emotional life; and the capacity to function as a productive member of society, with reciprocal, enduring, and fulfilling interpersonal relationships. At the opposite end of the continuum, an individual with severe personality pathology has an impoverished, disorganized, and/or conflicted psychological world that includes a weak, unclear, and maladaptive self-concept; a propensity to experience negative, dysregulated emotions; and a deficient capacity for adaptive interpersonal functioning and social behavior. Questions such as "How would you describe yourself as a person?" and "Who are the most important people in your life? How do you get along with them?" often can encourage a patient to speak freely about him- or herself and may provide a clinician with clues about an individual's personality functioning.

In the case vignette, the interviewer was successful in eliciting key aspects of Ms. K's personality pathology that underlie her depression and substance use. Ms. K struggles intensely with figuring out who she is and what she would like to do with her life. She sees herself as "disgusting" inside and uses drinking, pain medications, and sexual infidelity to attempt to regulate her self-esteem and emotions. She has little insight about her behaviors, however. She feels utterly dependent on her boyfriend and either despises him while idealizing her lover or idealizes him while denigrating herself. She would like to have some meaningful life goals—she has some talents that she has successfully cultivated in the past but is fearful she will be a failure because of her ongoing instability. It is also difficult for her to clearly see the potential impact of her destructive actions on others, particularly when she becomes preoccupied with fleeing her "controlling" boyfriend. Other people are important to Ms. K, as evidenced by her attempts to be a productive member of her church community, but her problems with self-loathing and emotional fragility make it very difficult for her to establish fulfilling relationships. Ms. K's personality functioning would be described as severely impaired (Level 3 on the LPFS).

Ms. K might also be understood by considering the AMPD trait domains and facets. Personality traits are tendencies to feel, perceive, behave, and think in relatively consistent ways across time and across situations. A comprehensive personality trait assessment serves as a personality trait "review of systems" and describes the myriad manifestations of personality and personality disorder encountered by clinicians in practice. The comprehensive assessment of personality trait facets across all five broad personality domains in the DSM-5 AMPD allows for identification of multiple areas of personality variation present in all people, rather than focusing on identification of one and only one optimal diagnostic label.

When considering Ms. K from a trait perspective, it is readily apparent that she exhibits several traits from the negative affectivity domain. Her interpersonal reactivity and frequently shifting emotions are emblematic of the trait of emotional lability. There are many times when she feels very down about her life and attacks herself and her self-worth, which are tendencies associated with the depressivity trait. When talking about her relationship with her boyfriend, she describes feeling completely stuck and dependent on him, which reflects her underlying separation insecurity. Ms. K attempts to cope with her fluctuating emotions, low self-esteem, and relationship troubles by precipitously fleeing the house, abusing substances, and having affairs. These behaviors are encompassed by the impulsivity trait from the disinhibition domain. She exhibits aloofness with the interviewer and asserts, about her previous therapist, "That's how it is with people, you really can't trust them." These observations and her obvious difficulty trusting and becoming emotionally intimate with her boyfriend point to a level of suspiciousness, a trait that is part of both the detachment and the negative affectivity domains.

Research has shown that reliable and valid ratings of level of personality functioning can be made by raters with little or no formal training, following the guidance provided in the DSM-5 AMPD LPFS (Morey 2018; Zimmermann et al. 2014). However, an open-ended interview approach may often elicit insufficient information to assess personality pathology; thus, the addition of a self-report or semistructured (i.e., interviewer-administered) personality disorder assessment instrument may be helpful to augment the clinical interview. Such instruments systematically assess each aspect of personality pathology and each personality disorder criterion with standard questions or probes. Although self-report instruments have the advantage of saving the interviewer time and being free of interviewer bias, they may yield false-positive results. Semistructured interviews—which require the interviewer to use certain questions, but allow further probing—facilitate accurate diagnosis in several ways: they ensure coverage of relevant domains of personality psychopathology, allow the interviewer to attempt to differentiate traits from states, encourage clarification of contradictions or ambiguities in the patient's responses, and provide the opportunity to determine whether traits, for example, are relatively pervasive (i.e., by eliciting multiple examples of trait expression) or are limited to a specific situation.

A new semistructured interview, the Structured Clinical Interview for the DSM-5 Alternative Model for Personality Disorders (SCID-5-AMPD), is available to assist in the evaluation of the three essential parts of the AMPD: 1) the level of impairment in personality functioning (Module I), 2) the AMPD's 25 pathological personality traits (Module II), and 3) the criteria for the six specific personality disorders in the AMPD and PD-TS (Module III) (First et al. 2018). Self-report instruments with adequate psychometric properties (Al-Dajani et al. 2016; Morey 2017) are also available for the trait and functioning components of the AMPD—the Personality Inventory for DSM-5 (Krueger et al. 2012) and the LPFS–Self Report (Morey 2017). With or without the use of a semistructured interview or a self-report scale, the interviewer must use his or her judgment to make the determinations and discriminations critical for personality pathology assessment and disorder diagnosis.

State Versus Trait

The presence of another mental disorder can complicate the assessment of personality traits. For example, a person with social withdrawal, low self-esteem, and lack of motivation or energy associated with major depressive disorder (MDD) might also meet criteria for avoidant personality disorder, which may be the underlying factor giving rise to the depression. A hypomanic person with symptoms of grandiosity or hypersexuality might appear narcissistic. In some cases, assessment of personality disorders may need to wait until the other condition, such as severe depression or a manic episode, has subsided. However, the clinician can often differentiate personality traits from states during an episode by asking the patient to describe his or her usual personality when not experiencing an episode; the use of informants who have observed the patient over time with and without a disorder can also be helpful. A longitudinal study showed that personality disorders could be accurately diagnosed in the presence of MDD, in that their outcomes were almost identical to those of personality disorders diagnosed in the absence of MDD (Morey et al. 2010). Furthermore, while it may be important to identify personality disorder, it is always clinically advisable to more broadly consider personality factors that may serve to help or hinder treatment interventions and the individual's adaptation to life's responsibilities and events.

Medical Illness Versus Trait

Similarly, the interviewer must ascertain that apparent personality traits are not in fact symptoms of a medical illness. For example, aggressive outbursts caused by a seizure disorder should not be misattributed to borderline or antisocial personality disorder, and the unusual perceptual experiences that can accompany temporal lobe epilepsy should not be misattributed to schizotypal personality disorder. On the other hand, it is possible for a personality disorder to co-occur with a medical disorder, so that possibility should not be ruled out. A thorough medical evaluation is essential if a medical causation is suspected.

Situation Versus Trait

The interviewer should also determine whether personality disorder features are sufficiently pervasive—that is, not limited to only one situation or occurring in response to only one specific trigger or person—to qualify for a disorder diagnosis. Similarly, personality traits should be relatively enduring rather than transient. Asking the patient for behavioral examples of the expression of a trait can help determine whether the trait is indeed present in a wide variety of situations and is expressed in many relationships. Specific behaviors, such as suicidal or other self-destructive actions, may be evident only at specific times or in specific situations, but the trait of impulsivity would need to be more persistent for a personality disorder diagnosis.

Gender and Cultural Bias

Although most research suggests that existing personality disorder criteria are relatively free of gender bias, interviewers can unknowingly allow such bias to affect their assessments. It is important, for example, that borderline and avoidant personality disorders be assessed as carefully in men as they are in women and that obsessive-compulsive, antisocial, and narcissistic personality disorders be assessed as carefully in women as they are in men. Interviewers should also be careful to avoid cultural bias when diagnosing personality disorders, especially when evaluating traits such as emotional lability, suspiciousness, risk taking, perfectionism in work, or unusual beliefs and experiences, which may reflect different norms in diverse cultures.

Diagnosis of Personality Disorders in Different Age Groups

Because the personalities of children and adolescents are still developing, personality disorders should be diagnosed sparingly in this age group. At the same time, clinicians should take care to consider personality strengths and challenges contributing to a young person's functioning. Although children and young adolescents frequently manifest significant personality disorder characteristics, it is often preferable to defer diagnosis until early adulthood, at which time a personality disorder diagnosis may be appropriate if the features appear to be more pervasive and stable. Early diagnosis may prove to be wrong, given that stage-specific difficulties of childhood or adolescence, such as submissiveness and dependency or hostility and risk taking, often resolve as the person matures. A meta-analysis of 152 longitudinal studies of personality traits showed that change was the rule until about age 22 years (Roberts and DelVecchio 2000). Nonetheless, adolescents with elevated levels of personality psychopathology are at greater risk of developing personality disorders in early adulthood; therefore, early identification may provide an opportunity for early intervention. In early adulthood, transitions such as leaving home, becoming economically self-sufficient, and becoming intimately involved with people outside of one's family of origin are important developmental tasks. Consequently, personality pathology most often becomes evident when young people attempt these transitions. No minimum age for the diagnosis of a personality disorder is included in either DSM-5 Section II or Section III criteria, with the exception of antisocial personality disorder, for which criteria specify a minimum age of at least 18 years in both sections.

Personality disorder diagnostic criteria have poor face validity in older adults because they often refer to occupational or interpersonal activities that may no longer be relevant to this population. The few existing longitudinal studies of personality disorders over the life span (Gunderson et al. 2011; Zanarini et al. 2012) suggest a decrease in personality disorder prevalence in older adults, but it is not known how much this is dependent on inapplicable criteria. Some argue that personality traits are generally stable across the age span, with slight decreases in FFM neuroticism, extraversion, and openness and slight increases in agreeableness and conscientiousness over time. However, trait expression in later life might be a function not only of underlying neurobiology but also of different (from youth) contextual factors over the life span. Thus, the degree of social, physical, occupational, or economic stress experienced by an individual over time may determine how stable or unstable his or her personality appears.

Clinical Significance of Personality Pathology

Personality functioning and traits have relevance for every individual and should be considered in all clinical assessments. If personality disturbances exist at the level of disorder impairment, significant problems of living and adjustment will be apparent. Persons with personality disorders often suffer, and their relationships with others are typically problematic. They have difficulty responding flexibly and adaptively to the environment and to the changes and demands of life, and they lack resilience when under stress. Instead, their usual ways of responding tend to perpetuate and intensify their difficulties. However, individuals with personality disorders often blame others for their difficulties or even deny that they have any problems at all.

Studies that have compared patients with personality disorders with patients without personality disorders or with other mental disorders have found that those with personality disorders were more likely than patients in the two latter categories to be separated, divorced, or never married and to have experienced frequent unemployment, job changes, or periods of disability (Skodol et al. 2002). Studies that have examined quality of functioning in patients with personality disorders have found poorer social functioning or interpersonal relationships and poorer work functioning or occupational achievement and satisfaction (Skodol et al. 2002). Among patients with personality disorders, those with severe types, such as schizotypal or borderline, have been found to have significantly more impairment at work, in social relationships, and in leisure activities compared with patients with less severe types, such as obsessive-compulsive, or patients with an impairing mental disorder such as MDD in the absence of personality disorder (Skodol et al. 2002).

In patients with personality disorders, impairments in functioning tend to persist even after apparent improvements in personality disorder psychopathology (Gunderson et al. 2011). The persistence of impairment is understandable because personality disorder psychopathology usually is relatively long standing and therefore has disrupted a person's work and social development over an extended period of time.

Personality pathology often causes problems for others and is costly to society. It is associated with elevated rates of separation, divorce, conflict with family members and romantic partners, child custody proceedings, homelessness, high-risk sexual behavior, and perpetration of child abuse. Individuals with personality disorders have increased rates of accidents; police contacts; emergency department visits; medical hospitalization and treatment utilization; violence and criminal behavior, including homicide; self-injurious behavior; attempted suicide; and completed suicide. A high percentage of individuals with criminal convictions, alcoholism, or drug abuse have a personality disorder.

DSM-5 Section III pathological personality traits have been found to incrementally predict psychosocial impairment over normal-range personality traits, personality disorder criterion counts, and common psychiatric symptoms (Simms and Calabrese 2016). In contrast, the incremental effects of normal traits, personality disorder criterion counts, and common symptoms were substantially smaller than those of pathological personality traits. In the Collaborative Longitudinal Personality Disorders study follow-along, personality disorder criteria counts were strongly associated with impairment in psychosocial functioning at intake (more strongly than categorical personality disorder diagnoses), but the strength of this relationship diminished over time (Morey et al. 2012). The best longitudinal predictors of impairment were models that combined normative traits and maladaptive variables (i.e., the Schedule for Nonadaptive and Adaptive Personality [SNAP] model or a model composed of DSM-IV personality disorder criteria counts and FFM domains). At 6-, 8-, and 10-year follow-ups, the SNAP continued to be most predictive, and DSM personality disorder criteria and FFM domains tended to provide substantial incremental validity to one another, supporting a hybrid model (Morey et al. 2012). Also, in another study using the Collaborative Longitudinal Personality Disorders sample, general personality disorder features representing "disorder" severity were more strongly related to psychosocial functioning concurrently and prospectively than were specific features representing personality "style" (Wright et al. 2016).

Finally, personality and personality pathology should be identified because of their implications for the development of other disorders and for treatment planning, including working to enlist and enhance an individual's personality strengths in the clinical process. Personality and personality pathology often need to be a focus of treatment or, at the very least, need to be considered when other co-occurring mental disorders are treated, because personality features often affect another disorder's prognosis and treatment response. For example, patients with depressive disorders, bipolar disorder, panic disorder, obsessive-compulsive disorder, or substance use disorders often respond less well to pharmacotherapy when they have a co-occurring personality disorder. The presence of a co-occurring personality disorder is also associated with poor adherence to pharmacotherapy. Furthermore, personality disorders have been shown to predict the development and relapse of MDD, and individuals with a personality disorder are less likely to experience remission of MDD (Skodol et al. 2011b) and substance use disorders (Hasin et al. 2011). As most clinicians are aware, the characteristics of patients with personality disorders are likely to be manifested in the treatment relationship regardless of whether the personality disorder is the focus of treatment. For example, some patients may be overly dependent on the clinician, others may not follow treatment recommendations, and still others may experience significant conflict about getting well. Although individuals with personality disorders tend to use psychiatric services extensively, they are more likely than persons without personality disorders to be dissatisfied with the treatment they receive.

Clinical Utility

In the DSM-5 field trials, clinicians were asked to rate the usefulness of tested diagnostic criteria for all DSM-IV disorders with proposed changes. In both the academic centers and the routine clinical practice field trials, more than 80% of clinicians rated the DSM-5 Section III AMPD as being "moderately," "very," or "extremely" useful. In utility ratings in the field trials, the DSM-5 Section III model was more often rated by clinicians as being "very" or "extremely" useful relative to its DSM-IV counterpart than were all other disorder categories, with the exceptions of somatic symptom and related disorders and feeding and eating disorders in the academic centers field trial, and of neurocognitive disorders and substance use and addictive disorders in the routine clinical practice field trial.

In a separate investigation, clinicians rated their perceptions regarding the utility of the DSM-5 AMPD's rendering of personality pathology compared with the DSM-IV personality disorder conceptualization (Morey et al. 2014). Although the participating clinicians were much more familiar with DSM-IV personality disorders, they rated all DSM-5 Section III components to be generally "as useful as" or "more useful than" DSM-IV for clinical description and treatment planning. Furthermore, compared with the DSM-IV personality disorder conceptualization, the DSM-5 pathological trait system was rated by both psychiatrists and psychologists as being easier to use and more useful for communicating with other clinicians and with patients about patients' problems and treatment planning.

In addition to the positive ratings of perceived utility given by clinicians in the field trials to the DSM-5 AMPD impairments in personality functioning and personality traits, the AMPD conceptualization of self–interpersonal functioning problems (e.g., intimacy avoidance and maladaptive self-schemas) has been shown to be significantly associated with personality disorder psychopathology and impairments in psychosocial functioning, as well as to affect clinical outcomes. Self–other dimensions have helped to discriminate different types of personality disorder pathology, have been used to predict various areas of psychosocial functioning, and have been shown to be moderators of the treatment alliance and treatment outcome. The single-item LPFS rating has been shown to predict variance in clinician ratings of psychosocial functioning, prognosis, and treatment needs over and above that predicted by all 10 DSM-IV personality disorder diagnoses combined (Morey et al. 2013).

On top of the findings that DSM-5 AMPD pathological personality traits and personality functioning showed independent utility in identifying and describing personality pathology and in planning and predicting the outcome of treatment, other studies (e.g., Hopwood and Zanarini 2010; Morey et al. 2012) have provided further support for a model of personality psychopathology that specifically combines ratings of disorder and trait constructs. Each of these two construct types has been shown to add incremental value to the other in predicting important antecedent (e.g., family history, history of child abuse), concurrent (e.g., functional impairment, medication use), and future (e.g., functioning, hospitalization, suicide attempts) variables (Morey et al. 2012).

Etiology and Pathogenesis

What causes personality pathology remains a central and challenging question. As is the case with other psychiatric disorders, all available data suggest that personality psychopathology (as well as normal personality traits) results from a complex combination of, and interaction between, temperament (genetic and other biological factors) and psychological (developmental or environmental) factors. There is growing evidence supporting a developmental perspective on personality pathology that implicates early and ongoing adverse experiences, particularly with caregivers, as key factors shaping the development of disturbed views of self and others (Luyten and Blatt 2013). In addition, an attachment paradigm has been used to synthesize the developmental and neurobiological influences on the evolution of personality and personality psychopathology. Although the degree to which genetic and environmental factors contribute to etiology may vary for different personality disorders, twin studies show that both factors are important in these disorders (Ma et al. 2016). A recent twin-based study (South et al. 2017) found moderate genetic influence (19%–37%) across AMPD trait domains.

Investigation of the underlying neurobiology of personality disorders is rapidly increasing. A growing body of evidence supports the importance of various neurobiological abnormalities in persons with personality disorders—abnormalities in dopaminergic systems in individuals with schizotypal personality disorder and in the serotonin system (which appears to mediate behavioral inhibition) in individuals with impulsive aggression. Of note is the growing interest in neurobiological correlates of personality disorders, including the contribution of neuropeptide system dysregulation to the disturbed interpersonal relationships seen in borderline personality disorder (Herpertz and Bertsch 2015). Molecular genetic analyses have suggested associations between neuroticism and the short allele of the serotonin transporter gene *5-HTTLPR* and between novelty seeking and the long allele of the dopamine receptor gene *DRD4*. Although these studies have opened a new frontier in research on personality traits and disorders, early results have generally not been replicated or the gene polymorphisms in question have been found to be less specific than originally thought (Ma et al. 2016).

Increasing numbers of studies of environmental antecedents of personality psychopathology (Carlson and Ruiz 2016), such as family environment and sexual and physical abuse, are substantiating a likely role for such factors in the development of certain personality disorders, particularly borderline personality disorder (Stepp et al. 2016). Of note has been the growing literature on the relationship of caregiver factors and disturbed early attachment to later development of personality pathology. Research in these areas is expected to continue to increase rapidly. In addition to providing information about the origins of personality pathology, such findings are expected to further inform approaches to treatment.

Treatment

Significant developments in the treatment of personality pathology include the use of multiple modalities, the growth of the evidence base on the results of treatment studies, and greater optimism about treatment effectiveness. Reviews of psychotherapy outcome studies, including psychodynamic/interpersonal, cognitive-behavioral, mixed, and supportive therapies, have found that psychotherapy was associated with a significantly faster rate of recovery compared with the natural course of personality disorders (Leichsenring and Leibing 2003). Historical therapeutic pessimism and reluctance to assess, diagnose, and/or treat patients with personality pathology has yielded to a widespread (albeit sometimes inconsistent) use of the spectrum of potentially valuable treatment modalities. Opportunities to build a constructive alliance with individuals presenting with a broad range of personality pathology can be cultivated if a clinician is mindful of the nature of the personality issues at play (Bender 2014).

Although psychotherapy remains the mainstay of treatment for personality disorders, the uses of pharmacotherapy are being explored because biological dimensions of personality psychopathology have been identified. For example, research has increasingly suggested that impulsivity and aggression may respond to serotonergic medications; that mood instability and lability may respond to serotonergic or dopaminergic medications; and that psychotic-like experiences may respond to antipsychotics, particularly newer-generation antipsychotics. There is a clear consensus in the literature, however, that studies to date have not shown that medications constitute the primary, or core, treatment for personality disorders, but they may be helpful in a symptom-targeted, adjunctive role (Mazza et al. 2016).

Specific Personality Disorders

A clinically oriented overview of the DSM-5 AMPD follows. We discuss in detail only the six disorders retained in Section III of DSM-5, because growing evidence suggests that the other four categories—dependent, histrionic, paranoid, and schizoid personality disorders—might be better represented as impairments in personality functioning and pathological personality traits (i.e., as PD-TS). Furthermore, the extensive co-occurrence among DSM personality disorders provides additional evidence that the categorical representation of personality psychopathology may be an inaccurate and limited model. Therefore, we explain how the disorders are represented by the alternative DSM-5 personality functioning and trait-based model. The defining features of DSM-5 Section III and Section II personality disorders are compared in Table 26–3.

Empirically based diagnostic algorithms were successful in rendering DSM-IV personality disorder diagnoses according to personality functioning impairments and pathological personality traits and with very good fidelity (correlations between DSM-IV categorical and DSM-5 AMPD dimensional criterion counts were 0.80 for antisocial personality disorder, 0.80 for borderline personality disorder, 0.77 for avoidant personality disorder, 0.74 for narcissistic personality disorder, 0.60 for schizotypal personality disorder, and 0.57 for obsessive-compulsive personality disorder) (Morey and Skodol 2013).

Antisocial Personality Disorder

Clinical Features

Antisocial personality disorder (ASPD) is included as a specific personality disorder in the alternative DSM-5 model. The disorder is characterized by specific impairments in personality functioning at a moderate or greater level and by six or more of the following seven pathological personality traits: manipulativeness, callousness, deceitfulness, hostility, risk taking, impulsivity, and irresponsibility.

Problems with identity include egocentrism, with self-esteem derived from personal gain, power, or pleasure. Goal setting is based on personal gratification. The individual with ASPD exhibits an absence of prosocial internal standards, associated with failure to conform to lawful or culturally normative ethical behavior. In the interpersonal domain of empathy, the individual lacks concern for the feelings, needs, or suffering of others and lacks remorse after hurting or mistreating another person. The individual is incapable of mutually intimate relationships because exploitation is a primary means of relating to others, including by deceit and coercion. Dominance and intimidation are used to control others.

Manipulativeness is evidenced by the frequent use of subterfuge to influence or control others or the use of seduction, charm, glibness, or ingratiation to achieve one's own ends. Callousness is reflected by a lack of concern for the feelings or problems of others, a lack of guilt or remorse about the negative or harmful effects of one's actions on others, aggression, and sadism. Dishonesty and fraudulence, misrepresentation of self, and embellishment or fabrication when relating events reflect the trait of deceitfulness. Hostility is exhibited by persistent or frequent angry feelings; anger or irritability in response to minor slights and insults; and mean, nasty, or vengeful behavior. Risk taking involves engagement in dangerous, risky, and potentially self-damaging activities, unnecessarily and without regard for consequences; boredom proneness and thoughtless initiation of activities to counter boredom; and lack of concern for limitations and denial of the real possibility of personal danger. Acting on the spur of the moment in response to immediate stimuli, acting on a momentary basis without a plan or consideration of outcomes, or difficulty establishing and following plans is reflective of the trait of impulsivity. Finally, the antisocial person's irresponsibility is demonstrated by disregard for—and failure to honor—financial and other obligations or commitments as well as lack of respect for—and lack of follow-through on—agreements and promises.

According to the AMPD, a history of conduct disorder in childhood is no longer a requirement for the diagnosis of ASPD. This change was prompted by the practical difficulty of documenting such a history in many cases (e.g., when juvenile court records are "sealed") and because evidence indicates that antisocial individuals without a childhood history of conduct disorder (so-called adult antisocial behavioral syndrome) are not substantially different with respect to sociodemographic and psychiatric correlates and disability from those who have such a history (Goldstein et al. 2017). Antisocial personality syndromes are associated with high rates of substance abuse, which may contribute to the persistence of antisocial behavior over time.

Epidemiology

ASPD occurs in about 1.8% of the general population (Torgersen 2014). It is much more common among men than among women.

Etiology

The early family lives of individuals with ASPD often involve severe environmental handicaps in the form of absent, inconsistent, or abusive parenting and poverty (Cohen et al. 2012). Indeed, many family members of individuals with ASPD also have significant externalizing psychopathology, such as substance abuse or ASPD itself. Modern behavioral genetic research is focusing on interactions between genes and the environment to explain the genesis of antisocial behavior (Hicks et al. 2013).

Twin and adoption studies indicate that genetic factors can predispose to the development of ASPD (Lyons et al. 1995). Nonetheless, it is unclear how much variance is accounted for by genetic factors and whether the nature of the predisposition is relatively specific or is best conceptualized in terms of relatively nonspecific traits such as impulsivity or hostility. Conduct problems, stimulus seeking, and callousness are antisocial traits that have substantial heritability. Psychopathic traits of fearless dominance and impulsive antisocial behavior also show significant genetic influences (Rautiainen et al. 2016). Growing evidence indicates that impulsive and aggressive behaviors may be mediated by abnormal serotonin transporter functioning in the brain. Different psychophysiological patterns may characterize aggression, psychopathy, and antisocial behavior, however (Lorber 2004). In comparison with healthy control subjects, persons with ASPD have been found to have smaller whole-brain volumes and temporal lobe volumes (Barkataki et al. 2006). Brain activation in the limbic–prefrontal circuit during fear conditioning has been shown to be deficient in psychopathic criminal offenders (Birbaumer et al. 2005). Neurocognitive impairments in spatial and memory functions have been found in adolescents with persistent antisocial behavior (Raine et al. 2005).

Treatment

It is important to recognize antisocial personality characteristics; because these individuals may appear to be cooperative and to have good intentions, clinicians may fail to discern their underlying motivations, leading to disruptive effects on treatment teams and other patients. However, there is little evidence to suggest that this disorder can be successfully treated with the usual clinical interventions. Nonetheless, there are reports suggesting that in confined settings, such as the military or prisons, depressive and introspective concerns may surface. Under these circumstances, confrontation by peers may bring about changes in the antisocial person's social behaviors. It is also notable that some patients with ASPD do demonstrate an ability to form a therapeutic alliance with psychotherapists, which augurs well for these patients' future course. Some success in addressing antisocial tendencies has been noted in the context of psychoeducational treatment for co-occurring substance abuse (Thylstrup et al. 2017). These findings contrast with the clinical tradition that emphasizes the inability of these persons to learn from harmful consequences. Yet longitudinal follow-up studies have shown that the prevalence of ASPD diminishes with age, as these individuals become more aware of the harmful effects of their maladaptive social and interpersonal behaviors. Preventive efforts with at-risk individuals (e.g., siblings of children with conduct disorder) have also shown promise.

Avoidant Personality Disorder

Clinical Features

Avoidant personality disorder has also been identified as a specific personality disorder in the alternative DSM-5 model. It is characterized by specific impairments in personality functioning that are at a moderate level and by three or more of the following four pathological personality traits: anxiousness (required), withdrawal, anhedonia, and intimacy avoidance.

The identity of the person with avoidant personality disorder is characterized by self-appraisal as socially inept, personally unappealing, or inferior, associated with low self-esteem and feelings of shame. The individual is reluctant to pursue goals, take personal risks, or engage in new activities involving interpersonal contact. There is preoccupation with, and sensitivity to, criticism or rejection, with a distorted inference that others' perspectives are negative. The avoidant person is reluctant to get involved with others unless certain of being liked, and intimacy with another person is quite difficult because of a fear of being shamed or ridiculed.

The person with avoidant personality disorder experiences intense feelings of anxiety—nervousness, tenseness, or panic—often in reaction to social situations and worries about the negative effects of past unpleasant experiences and future negative possibilities. Fear, apprehension, and the perceived threat of uncertainty are frequent concerns. Embarrassment and shame lead to reticence and avoidance in social situations and a failure to initiate social contact. Lack of enjoyment from, engagement in, or energy for life's experiences may be apparent. There may be a deficit in the capacity to feel pleasure or take interest in things. History reveals avoidance of close or romantic relationships, interpersonal attachments, and intimate sexual relationships.

Epidemiology

The prevalence of avoidant personality disorder, based on epidemiological studies, is about 2.7% (Torgersen 2014). Avoidant personality disorder may be more common among women.

Etiology

Research on childhood experiences of avoidant persons has revealed negative childhood memories (e.g., of isolation, rejection); poorer athletic performance, less involvement in hobbies, and less popularity; and parental neglect. Research in the biological sphere has highlighted the importance of inborn temperament in the development of avoidant behavior. Some children as young as 21 months manifest increased physiological arousal and avoidant traits in social situations (e.g., retreat from the unfamiliar and avoidance of interaction with strangers), and this social inhibition tends to persist for many years. Family studies have demonstrated elevated rates of trait and social anxiety, as well as personality traits such as harm avoidance, in the first-degree relatives of patients with generalized social phobia (Stein et al. 2001), suggesting that social anxiety lies on a continuum that may be influenced by familial factors.

Treatment

Because of their excessive fear of rejection and criticism and their reluctance to form relationships, individuals with avoidant personality disorder may be difficult to engage in treatment. Engagement in psychotherapy may be facilitated by the therapist's use of supportive techniques, attunement to the patient's hypersensitivity, and gentle discussion about the underlying thoughts and feelings contributing to avoidance. Although early in treatment these patients may tolerate only supportive techniques, they may eventually respond well to all kinds of psychotherapy. Clinicians should be aware of the potential for countertransference reactions such as overprotectiveness, hesitancy to adequately address core issues, or excessive expectations for change.

Promising empirical findings have supported psychodynamic interventions for avoidant personality (Neumann et al. 2014). Although few data exist, it seems likely also that assertiveness and social skills training may increase patients' confidence and willingness to take risks in social situations. Cognitive techniques that sensitively illuminate patients' pathological assumptions about their sense of ineptness may also be useful. Group experiences—in particular, homogeneous supportive groups that emphasize the development of social skills—may prove useful for avoidant patients.

Preliminary data suggest that avoidant personality disorder may improve with treatment with monoamine oxidase inhibitors or serotonin reuptake inhibitors. Anxiolytics sometimes help patients better manage anxiety (especially severe anxiety) caused by facing previously avoided situations or trying new behaviors.

Borderline Personality Disorder

Clinical Features

Borderline personality disorder (BPD) is a specific personality disorder in the alternative DSM-5 model. It is defined by characteristic impairments in personality functioning that are at a severe level and by four or more of the following seven pathological personality traits: emotional lability, anxiousness, separation insecurity, depressivity, impulsivity, risk taking, and hostility. The diagnostic algorithm requires at least one of the latter three traits, because BPD has traits from both the negative affectivity and the disinhibition or antagonism domains and is not typically represented by only emotional dysregulation.

Patients with borderline personality pathology have a markedly impoverished, poorly developed, or unstable self-image, often associated with excessive self-criticism. They experience chronic feeling of emptiness and may exhibit dissociative states under stress. Instability also characterizes life goals, aspirations, values, and career plans, which appear to be constantly changing. The ability to recognize the feelings and needs of others is compromised. Interpersonal hypersensitivity is prominent (marked by a tendency to feel slighted or insulted), and perceptions of others are biased toward negative attributes or vulnerabilities. Close interpersonal relationships are typically intense, unstable, and conflicted—troubled by mistrust, neediness, and anxious preoccupation with real or imagined abandonment. Relationships may be viewed in extremes of idealization and devaluation and alternate between overinvolvement with others and withdrawal.

Individuals with borderline personality pathology have unstable emotions and frequent mood changes. Emotions are easily aroused, intense, and often out of proportion to actual events or circumstances. Intense feelings of nervousness, tenseness, or panic arise, often in reaction to interpersonal stresses, and there is worry about the past and about anticipated future negative possibilities. Fear of rejection by and/or separation from significant others on whom they depend can be acute, yet fear of excessive dependency and complete loss of autonomy may punctuate relationships as well. Borderline pathology is frequently associated with depression, misery, and hopelessness, with difficulty recovering from such moods. Pessimism about the future is often present, along with pervasive shame and feelings of inferiority. Frequent suicidal thoughts and behaviors are common. Impulsivity, interpersonal reactivity, and difficulty establishing or following plans are also prominent. Self-harm under emotional distress and dangerous, risky, and potentially self-damaging activities without regard to consequences may occur. Frequent or persistent angry feelings may be present, although sometimes not readily acknowledged or understood.

Roughly half of patients with BPD experience significant remissions of their overt psychopathology within 2 years of follow-up. Higher levels of social dysfunction, greater severity of childhood trauma, and persistence of substance abuse are predictive of a worse prognosis. Overall, the longer-term course of BPD may be more benign than was previously thought (Gunderson et al. 2011; Zanarini et al. 2012), and may be predicted from historical, clinical, functional, and personality features. About 10% of patients with the disorder die by suicide, however.

Epidemiology

BPD is estimated to occur in 1.6% of the general population (Torgersen 2014) and in about 20% of hospital and clinical admissions. Although BPD is more commonly diagnosed among women than among men in clinical settings, this difference is not found in community-based studies (Torgersen 2014).

Etiology

Several theories and lines of research have emphasized the importance of early parent–child relationships in the etiology of BPD. These theories are gradually being explored and modified by direct observations of these early dyads with long-term follow-ups. Research has generally confirmed the theories that inconsistent or absent feedback from caretakers predicts insecure attachments and that certain parents may not be cognitively and emotionally able to adequately respond to the particular needs and temperament of their infant (Sturrock and Mellor 2014). A considerable body of empirical research has also documented a high frequency of traumatic early abandonment, physical abuse, and sexual abuse among individuals with BPD (Infurna et al. 2016; Temes et al. 2017). These experiences have enduring traumatic effects when they occur in particularly sensitive children or in children who do not have opportunities to process the events. Impediments to secure attachment to caretakers during development result in problems in creating and maintaining a stable sense of self and others, and this troubled internal world has been shown to be the overriding basis for the emotional dysregulation, negative affect, and impulsivity associated with border-line difficulties (Huprich et al. 2017).

Evidence of 69% overall heritability for BPD in one twin study (Torgersen et al. 2000) has mobilized efforts to identify genetic contributions to the etiology of specific borderline traits. Fundamental dimensions of affective instability and impulsive aggression have been posited to underlie BPD. Heritability of about 50% for borderline traits such as affective lability and insecure attachment and later for the broader domains of emotional dysregulation and dissocial behavior has been found (Livesley et al. 1993). There is evidence of serotonergic dysfunction in the borderline trait of impulsivity. Structural and functional neuroimaging studies (Lieb et al. 2004) have shown reductions in frontal and orbitofrontal lobe volumes, altered metabolism in prefrontal brain regions, and failure of activation of these brain regions under stress. Because these brain regions are important in serotonergic function and mediate affective control, the observed deficits may be the source of the disinhibited impulses and affects characteristic of patients with BPD. Other studies (Gunderson et al. 2018) have shown hyperactivity of the amygdala, which also plays a significant role in emotion regulation. Patients with BPD perform poorly in multiple neurocognitive domains, particularly in functions lateralized to the right hemisphere. It is unknown, however, whether neurobiological dysfunctions are due to genetics, pre- or postnatal factors, or adverse events during childhood or are the consequences of the disorder (Ruocco and Carcone 2016).

Some current theories about the etiology of BPD posit that genetic vulnerabilities underlie the poor emotional, behavioral, and interpersonal control that characterizes the disorder, with the recognition that the expression of these vulnerabilities—that is, whether children with these vulnerabilities develop BPD—depends on adverse childhood environments and on triggering stressors. Thus, although the specific factors in the etiology of BPD are yet to be determined, the pathways to these difficulties are complex and multifactorial.

Treatment

Patients with BPD are high utilizers of outpatient, inpatient, partial hospital, and psychopharmacological treatment. Almost all modalities can be helpful, depending on the clinical presentation of the given patient and the training and sensitivity of the treater. The extensive literature on the treatment of BPD universally notes the extreme difficulties that clinicians encounter in their efforts to help patients with this challenging condition. These problems derive from the patients' appeal to their treaters' wishes to rescue and from the patients' angry accusations when they perceive their treaters to have failed them. Many clinicians do not like working with these patients despite their generally good prognosis. Therapists often develop intense countertransference reactions that lead them to attempt to re-parent or, conversely, to reject patients with BPD. Regardless of the treatment approach used, personal maturity and considerable clinical experience are important assets for clinicians.

Treatment of patients with BPD typically requires good case management. Essential aspects of case management include skill in managing suicidal or self-destructive threats and behaviors alongside calm and knowledgeable psychoeducational discussion of the individuals' challenges and vulnerabilities and their treatment. Case management is usually accompanied by psychotherapeutic and pharmacological interventions, provided within a frame of realistic goals and a good therapeutic alliance.

Much of the historical treatment literature has focused on the value of intensive exploratory psychotherapies directed at modifying the basic character structure of patients with BPD. However, it has been increasingly suggested that improvement may be related not to the acquisition of insight but rather to the corrective experience of developing a stable, trusting relationship with a therapist who refrains from retaliating in response to these patients' angry and disruptive behaviors. Paralleling this development has been the suggestion that supportive psychotherapies or group therapies may bring about similar changes. Research evidence has provided support for the effectiveness of several forms of psychodynamic treatment. The first, *mentalization-based treatment*, involves a nondirective discussion of the interactions between patient and therapist (Bateman and Fonagy 1999). The second, *transference-focused psychotherapy*, involves more traditional interventions (Clarkin et al. 1999). Both forms attribute change to an improved ability to mentalize. Psychoanalytic–interactional psychotherapy is another psychodynamic approach that is being studied for BPD as well (Leichsenring et al. 2010).

Behavioral treatment consisting of once-weekly individual psychotherapy and twice-weekly group skills training can effectively diminish the self-destructive behaviors and hospitalizations of patients with BPD (Linehan et al. 2006). The success and cost benefits of this treatment, called *dialectical behavior therapy*, have led to its widespread adoption and to modifications that can be used in a variety of settings. *Schema-focused therapy* is another cognitive therapy that has been shown to be efficacious (Giesen-Bloo et al. 2006). It has also been suggested that treatment might proceed in phases, perhaps beginning with a supportive, skills-focused, or mentalization-based approach, depending on the clinical picture, and transitioning to more insight-oriented work later once basic capacities have been improved (Choi-Kain et al. 2017). A recent systematic review and meta-analysis of randomized clinical trials to assess the efficacy of psychotherapies for BPD (Cristea et al. 2017) found that psychotherapies of various types—most notably dialectical behavior therapy and psychodynamic approaches—were effective in improving several borderline-relevant outcomes.

Although no one class of medication has been found to have dramatic or predictable effects in BPD, studies indicate that medications from certain classes may sometimes be beneficial for specific problems, such as depression, impulsivity, affective lability, or intermittent cognitive and perceptual disturbances, as well as for reducing irritability and aggressive behavior. In general, the profusion of options and the often-unclear benefits have encouraged polypharmacy, with sometimes unfortunate side effects (Stoffers and Lieb 2015).

Narcissistic Personality Disorder

Clinical Features

The proposed criteria for narcissistic personality disorder in the alternative DSM-5 model explicitly note that self-appraisal may be either inflated or deflated and that feelings of entitlement can be either overt or covert. Typical impairments in personality functioning are at the moderate level, and relevant traits include grandiosity and attention seeking.

The patient with narcissistic personality disorder excessively relies on others for self-definition and for self-esteem regulation. Self-appraisal is either inflated or deflated or may vacillate between extremes of the two. The ability to regulate emotions mirrors fluctuations in self-esteem. Goals are set to gain approval from others, while personal standards may be unreasonably high so as to create the illusion of exceptionalism or too low based on a sense of entitlement. Awareness of personal motivations may be elusive, and there is impaired ability to recognize or identify with the needs of others. At the same time, there may be a dependence on others' reactions to regulate self-esteem but a deficit in understanding the impact of one's behaviors on others. Interpersonal relationships are largely superficial, with little genuine interest in others' experiences. The need to gain personally from others constrains mutuality.

Grandiosity is evident from feelings of entitlement (which may be either overt or covert), self-centeredness, the belief that one is better than others, and condescension toward others. Excessive attempts to attract and be the focus of the attention of others are prominent, as is the need for admiration.

Epidemiology

Narcissistic personality disorder had a mean prevalence of 0.8% in 13 community studies (Torgersen 2014), and it appears to be more common among men.

Etiology

Little scientific evidence is available about the pathogenesis of narcissistic personality disorder. Reconstructions based on developmental history and observations in psychotherapies suggest that this disorder develops in persons who have had their needs, aspirations, talents, fears, failures, or dependency responded to with criticism, disdain, or neglect during their childhood years. Such experiences lead to being cut off from genuine internal experience and may result in contempt for, lack of awareness of, or shame about personal vulnerabilities while desperately seeking others' admiration, validation, and appreciation. Early deprivation may result in an attempted veneer of invulnerability and self-sufficiency that masks underlying emptiness and constricts the capacity to feel deeply. Another theory of the etiology of narcissistic personality disorder is that it results from the parenting of "stage" or "beauty contest" mothers or "sports hero" fathers who convey to their child from an early age that she or he is special, remarkable, or a future famous figure, reflecting a view of the child as an ornamental enhancement of the parent(s).

Treatment

Clinicians need to be able to look beyond the alienating exterior of the individual with narcissistic difficulties and understand the vulnerabilities that lie within (Bender 2012). Individual psychodynamic psychotherapy, including psychoanalysis, is the cornerstone of treatment for persons with narcissistic personality disorder. Following Kohut's (1971) lead, some therapists believe that the vulnerability to narcissistic injury indicates that intervention should be directed at conveying empathy for the patient's sensitivities and disappointments. This approach, in theory, allows a positive idealized transference to develop that will then be gradually disillusioned by the inevitable frustrations encountered in therapy—disillusionment that will clarify the excessive nature of the patient's reactions to frustrations and disappointments. An alternative view, explicated by Kernberg (1975), is that the vulnerability should be addressed earlier and more directly to assist with the recognition of compensatory grandiosity and its maladaptive consequences. With either approach, the psychotherapeutic process usually requires a relatively intensive schedule over a period of years, during which the therapist needs to keep foremost in his or her mind and interventions the narcissistic patient's hypersensitivity to slights and self-protective tendency to perceive the therapist through the lens of whether he or she gratifies the patient's needs. There may be an extended period of time requiring the therapist to tolerate with good grace being used mostly as an audience for the patient, as therapeutic trust slowly is built. In the absence of an opportunity for long-term psychoanalytic treatment with an appropriately trained clinician, several approaches that are more time-limited have been studied (Caligor et al. 2015).

Obsessive-Compulsive Personality Disorder

Clinical Features

Obsessive-compulsive personality disorder (OCPD) is another of the six personality disorders featured in the alternative DSM-5 model. It is characterized by specific impairments in personality functioning that are at a moderate level and by three or more of the following four pathological personality traits: rigid perfectionism (required), perseveration, intimacy avoidance, and restricted affectivity.

The sense of self for a person with OCPD is derived predominantly from work or productivity, with experience and expression of emotions usually constricted. Sometimes there is difficulty completing tasks and realizing goals because of rigid and unreasonably high and inflexible standards of behavior and overly conscientious and moralistic attitudes. Empathy is somewhat impaired: there may be some understanding of others' perspectives, but not much interest in or appreciation of the ideas, feelings, or behavior of others. Intimacy is impaired because relationships are seen as secondary to work and productivity, and rigidity and stubbornness negatively affect relationships.

In persons with OCPD, rigid perfectionism is evidenced by an insistence on everything being flawless, perfect, and without errors or faults, including their own and others' performance. Individuals with OCPD will sacrifice timeliness to ensure correctness in every detail, believing that there is only one right way to do things. They have difficulty changing their personal point of view and are preoccupied with details, organization, and order. They show persistence at tasks or in particular activities long after the behavior has ceased to be functional or effective, and despite repeated failures. Relationships are often part of life but are characterized by a certain amount of emotional distance and need for control. Emotionally arousing situations are avoided when possible, with constricted emotional experience and expression. Indifference or coldness is sometimes perceived by others.

Epidemiology

OCPD is one of the most common personality disorders in the general population, with a prevalence of about 2.5% (Torgersen 2014). OCPD is more common in men than in women.

Etiology

Constitutional factors may play a role in the formation of OCPD. Compulsivity, oppositional behavior, restricted expression of emotion, and intimacy problems have all been shown to be moderately heritable. An increase in serotonin activity has been associated with perfectionism and compulsivity. As is the case in other personality disorders, more empirical studies are needed to clarify this disorder's sources.

Treatment

Persons with OCPD may seem difficult to treat because of their excessive intellectualization and difficulty expressing emotion. However, these patients often respond well to psychoanalytic psychotherapy or psychoanalysis. The level of active presence and interventions employed by the therapist should be predicated upon the patient's ability to tolerate such engagement. Clinicians should also avoid being drawn into interesting but affectless discussions that are unlikely to have therapeutic benefit. In other words, rather than intellectualizing with patients, therapists should focus on the feelings these patients usually avoid. Power struggles that may occur in treatment offer opportunities to address the patient's excessive need for control.

Cognitive techniques may also be used to diminish the patient's excessive need for control and perfection. Although patients may resist group treatment because of their need for control, dynamically oriented groups that focus on feelings may provide insight and increase patients' comfort with exploring and expressing new affects.

Schizotypal Personality Disorder

Clinical Features

Schizotypal personality disorder has been retained in the alternative DSM-5 model. It is characterized by specific impairments in personality functioning that are at an extreme level and by four or more of the following six pathological personality traits: cognitive and perceptual dysregulation, unusual beliefs and experiences, eccentricity, restricted affectivity, withdrawal, and suspiciousness.

The person with schizotypal personality disorder has confused boundaries between self and others, a distorted self-concept, and emotional expression that is often not congruent with the context of what is happening or even his or her own internal experience. Personal goals are unrealistic or incoherent, with no clear set of internal standards guiding behavior. There is pronounced difficulty understanding the impact of one's own behavior on others and frequent misinterpretation of others' motivations and behaviors. Severe impairments exist in the capacity to develop close relationships because of mistrust.

The person with schizotypal personality disorder shows multiple signs of cognitive and perceptual dysregulation, including odd or unusual thought processes; vague, circumstantial, metaphorical, overelaborate, or stereotyped thought or speech; and odd sensations reported in various sensory modalities. Thought content and views of reality are bizarre or idiosyncratic, possibly along with odd, unusual, or bizarre behavior or appearance. Restricted affectivity is common, with little reaction to emotionally arousing situations, constricted emotional experience and expression, indifference, and coldness. The preference for being alone manifests as significant discomfort in social situations and avoidance of social contact and activity. Suspiciousness drives expectations of interpersonal ill-intent or harm, doubts about the loyalty and fidelity of others, and feelings of persecution.

Epidemiology

Schizotypal personality disorder occurs in 1.3% of the general population (Torgersen 2014). No gender difference in prevalence has been found for this disorder.

Etiology

Schizotypal personality disorder is considered a schizophrenia spectrum disorder—that is, related to schizophrenia. Phenomenological as well as genetic, biological, treatment, and outcome data support this link. For example, family history studies show an increased prevalence of schizophrenia-related disorders in relatives of schizotypal probands and, conversely, an increased prevalence of schizotypal personality disorder in relatives of probands with schizophrenia (Siever and Davis 2004). Both the positive and the negative components of schizotypal personality disorder are moderately heritable, although it may be that only the deficit symptoms are genetically related to schizophrenia.

At least some forms or aspects of schizotypal personality disorder involve abnormalities of brain structure, physiology, chemistry, and functioning characteristic of schizophrenia—for example, increased cerebrospinal fluid and reduced cortical volume; temporal lobe volume reductions and dysfunctions; and evidence pointing to problems with brain physiological functions that modulate attention and inhibit sensory input, such as deficient P50 suppression, reduced prepulse inhibition, impaired smooth-pursuit eye movements, and poor performance on the continuous performance task. Higher cerebrospinal fluid and plasma homovanillic acid concentrations correlated with psychotic-like symptoms, and lower concentrations correlated with deficit-like symptoms, have been found in patients with schizotypal personality disorder as well as in patients with schizophrenia. Patients with schizotypal personality disorder have also been shown to have impaired performance on tests of executive function and other tests of visual or auditory attention, such as the Wisconsin Card Sorting Test and the backward masking task, and deficits on verbal learning and working memory tasks, attention-orienting tasks, and instrumental motor tasks. Because of this evidence, schizotypal personality disorder is classified with schizophrenia rather than with the personality disorders in the *International Statistical Classification of Diseases and Related Health Problems*, 10th Revision (ICD-10; World Health Organization 1992). Differences between schizophrenia and schizotypal personality disorder do exist, however, particularly with respect to frontal lobe structure and functioning, and these differences may account for the infrequency of overt psychosis in patients with schizotypal personality disorder. Genetic or environmental factors that promote greater frontal lobe capacity and reduced striatal dopaminergic reactivity might protect persons with schizotypal personality disorder from developing psychosis and the severe social and cognitive deterioration of chronic schizophrenia.

Treatment

Because they are socially anxious and somewhat paranoid, persons with schizotypal personality disorder usually avoid treatment. They may, however, seek such treatment—or be brought for treatment by concerned family members—when they become depressed or overtly psychotic. It may be difficult to establish an alliance with patients who have schizotypal personality disorder, and they are unlikely to immediately tolerate exploratory techniques that emphasize interpretation or confrontation. A supportive relationship that addresses cognitive distortions and ego-boundary problems may be useful. It has been suggested that schizotypal phenomena may be best understood and treated by using a conflict and deficit model and employing supportive psychodynamic therapy (Ridenour 2016). A case study of schizotypal personality disorder treatment demonstrated positive results from emphasizing various aspects of functioning, including psychotherapy targeting positive self-statements, social skills training, and anxiety reduction (Nathanson and Jamison 2011). If the patient is willing to participate, cognitive-behavioral therapy and highly structured educational groups with a social skills focus may also be helpful.

Several studies support the usefulness of low-dosage antipsychotic medications, including atypical antipsychotics such as risperidone (Koenigsberg et al. 2003) and olanzapine (Keshavan et al. 2004), in the treatment of schizotypal personality disorder. These medications may ameliorate the anxiety and psychotic-like features associated with this disorder, and they are particularly indicated in the treatment of the more overt psychotic decompensations that these patients can experience.

Personality Disorder—Trait Specified

A diagnosis of PD-TS is applicable for individuals whose personality pathology is characterized by moderate or greater impairment in personality functioning and one or more DSM-5 pathological personality traits. The PD-TS diagnosis may be assigned when a clinician or researcher prefers not to assign a specific personality disorder category, or when none applies. PD-TS also can be used to capture phenomena associated with one of the four DSM-5 Section II personality disorders—dependent, histrionic, paranoid, and schizoid—that are not included in DSM-5 Section III and that have not been discussed in the preceding sections here, as well as phenomena associated with any other non–DSM-5 personality disorder presentation, such as passive-aggressive personality disorder, depressive personality disorder, or some other specified personality disorder.

For example, DSM-5 Section II *dependent personality disorder* would typically involve impairments in personality functioning at the moderate level and pathological traits including submissiveness, separation insecurity, and anxiousness. In *histrionic personality disorder,* the level of impairment in personality functioning would typically be moderate, and relevant pathological personality traits would include attention seeking, emotional lability, and manipulativeness. The level of impairment in personality functioning associated with *paranoid personality disorder* typically would be severe or extreme, and relevant pathological personality traits would include suspiciousness and hostility. In *schizoid personality disorder,* the level of impairment in personality functioning would typically be extreme, and relevant pathological personality traits would include withdrawal, intimacy avoidance, anhedonia, and restricted affectivity. In the case of non–DSM-5 personality disorder constructs, the listed traits for *passive-aggressive personality disorder* might include submissiveness and hostility, and those for *depressive personality disorder* might include depressivity, anxiousness, and anhedonia. A presentation that had features of several personality disorders but did not meet the full criteria for any one ("mixed personality disorder") would also be diagnosed as PD-TS according to the AMPD. The Section III model provides considerable flexibility in describing the myriad presentations of personality pathology that do not fit one of the specific types.

For any patient given the diagnosis of PD-TS, the clinician would designate both the level of impairment in personality functioning and the pathological personality traits present. Both of these components have important implications for treatment planning and treatment outcome.

- Excessively *dependent* patients often enter therapy with complaints of depression or anxiety that may be precipitated by the threatened or actual loss of a dependent relationship. These patients often respond well to various types of individual psychotherapy. Treatment may be particularly helpful if it explores the patients' fears of independence; uses the transference to explore their dependency; and is directed toward increasing patients' self-esteem, sense of effectiveness, assertiveness, and independent functioning. These patients often seek an excessively dependent relationship with the therapist, which can lead to countertransference problems that may reinforce their dependence. The therapist, for example, may overprotect or be overly directive with the patient, give inappropriate reassurance and support, or prolong the treatment unnecessarily. He or she may also have excessive expectations for change or withdraw from a patient who is perceived as too needy. Group therapy and cognitive-behavioral therapy aimed at increasing independent functioning, including assertiveness and social skills training, may be useful for some patients with excessive dependence. If the patient is in a relationship that is maintaining and reinforcing his or her excessive dependence, couples or family therapy may be helpful.
- For persons with relationship and social functioning challenges associated with "*histrionic* personality" traits, individual psychodynamic psychotherapy, including psychoanalysis, remains the cornerstone of most treatments. This treatment is directed at increasing patients' awareness of 1) how their self-esteem is maladaptively tied to their ability to attract attention at the expense of developing other skills and 2) how their shallow relationships and emotional experiences reflect unconscious fears of real commitments. Much of this increase in awareness occurs through analysis of the here-and-now doctor–patient relationship rather than through reconstruction of childhood experiences. Therapists should be aware that the idealization and eroticization that such patients typically bring into treatment are material for exploration, and thus, therapists should be aware of countertransference gratification.
- Because they mistrust others, *paranoid* individuals will usually avoid psychiatric treatment. If they do seek treatment, the clinician likely will encounter the challenge of engaging them and keeping them in treatment. This can best be accomplished by maintaining a respectful, straightforward, and unobtrusive style aimed at building trust. If a rupture develops in the treatment relationship (e.g., the patient accuses the therapist of some fault or some perceived betrayal), it is best simply to offer a straightforward apology, if warranted, rather than to respond evasively or defensively. It is also best to avoid an overly warm style, especially if this is not the characteristic approach of the therapist, because excessive and less-than-genuine warmth and expression of interest may intensify the patient's mistrust of the therapist's motives. A supportive individual psychotherapy that incorporates such approaches may be the best treatment for these patients. Although group

treatment or cognitive-behavioral treatment aimed at anxiety management and development of social skills can occasionally be of benefit, these patients tend to resist such approaches because of their suspiciousness, hypersensitivity to criticism, and misinterpretation of others' comments. Although seldom studied, antipsychotic medications may sometimes be useful in the treatment of paranoid symptoms. Patients may view such treatment with mistrust; however, these medications are clearly indicated in the treatment of the overtly psychotic decompensations that these patients sometimes experience.

- Individuals with *schizoid* tendencies are very inhibited in genuinely connecting with others, so they may not easily form relationships, including with a therapist. Occasionally these persons may seek treatment for an associated problem, such as depression, or they may be brought for treatment by others. Whereas some patients can tolerate only a supportive therapy or treatment aimed at the resolution of a crisis or associated other mental disorder, other patients may do well with insight-oriented psychotherapy aimed at bringing about a basic shift in their comfort with intimacy and affects. Development of a therapeutic alliance may be difficult with schizoid patients but can be facilitated by assuming an interested and caring attitude to address the possibility of underlying neediness and by avoiding early interpretation or confrontation. Some authors have suggested the use of so-called inanimate bridges, such as writing and artistic productions, to ease the patient into a therapy relationship. Incorporation of cognitive-behavioral approaches that encourage gradual increases in social involvement may be of value. Although many patients with schizoid tendencies may be unwilling to participate in a group, group therapy may help facilitate the development of social skills and relationships.

Conclusion

Clinical interest and research in personality pathology have grown over the past several decades, prompting investment in research and increased attention to effective treatment strategies and a better understanding of phenomenology, prognosis, and etiology. Even more dramatic than the knowledge gained are the heightened awareness of the clinical impact and potential research significance of personality psychopathology and the new and more informed questions that this awareness has generated. With the advent of the Alternative DSM-5 Model for Personality Disorders, there is a richer, more flexible, and more clinically informative approach to considering the central role of personality difficulties in the lives of individuals.

Key Clinical Points

- Personality psychopathology is common in clinical settings and in the community.
- Personality pathology requires thoughtful and informed assessment.
- Personality pathology causes significant problems for those who are affected and for others, and is costly to society.

- Most personality pathology is treatable but often complicates the treatment of other mental disorders.

- Although personality disorders are defined in Section II of DSM-5 exactly as they were in DSM-IV, DSM-5 Section III provides an alternative model of personality disorders with the promise of greater clinical utility.

References

Al-Dajani N, Gralnick TM, Bagby RM: A psychometric review of the Personality Inventory for DSM-5 (PID-5): current status and future directions. J Pers Assess 98(1):62–81, 2016 26619968

American Psychiatric Association: Diagnostic and Statistical Manual: Mental Disorders. Washington, DC, American Psychiatric Association, 1952

American Psychiatric Association: Diagnostic and Statistical Manual of Mental Disorders, 2nd Edition. Washington, DC, American Psychiatric Association, 1968

American Psychiatric Association: Diagnostic and Statistical Manual of Mental Disorders, 3rd Edition. Washington, DC, American Psychiatric Association, 1980

American Psychiatric Association: Diagnostic and Statistical Manual of Mental Disorders, 3rd Edition, Revised. Washington, DC, American Psychiatric Association, 1987

American Psychiatric Association: Diagnostic and Statistical Manual of Mental Disorders, 4th Edition. Washington, DC, American Psychiatric Association, 1994

American Psychiatric Association: Diagnostic and Statistical Manual of Mental Disorders, 4th Edition, Text Revision. Washington, DC, American Psychiatric Association, 2000

American Psychiatric Association: Diagnostic and Statistical Manual of Mental Disorders, 5th Edition. Arlington, VA, American Psychiatric Association, 2013

Barkataki I, Kumari V, Das M, et al: Volumetric structural brain abnormalities in men with schizophrenia or antisocial personality disorder. Behav Brain Res 169(2):239–247, 2006 16466814

Bateman A, Fonagy P: Effectiveness of partial hospitalization in the treatment of borderline personality disorder: a randomized controlled trial. Am J Psychiatry 156(10):1563–1569, 1999 10518167

Bender DS: Mirror, mirror on the wall: reflecting on narcissism. J Clin Psychol 68(8):877–885, 2012 22729995

Bender DS: Therapeutic alliance, in Textbook of Personality Disorders, 2nd Edition. Edited by Oldham JM, Skodol AE, Bender DS. Washington, DC, American Psychiatric Publishing, 2014, pp 189–216

Birbaumer N, Veit R, Lotze M, et al: Deficient fear conditioning in psychopathy: a functional magnetic resonance imaging study. Arch Gen Psychiatry 62(7):799–805, 2005 15997022

Bender DS, Morey LC, Skodol AE: Toward a model for assessing level of personality functioning in DSM-5, I: a review of theory and methods. J Pers Assess 93(4):332–346, 2011 22804672

Caligor E, Levy KN, Yeomans FE: Narcissistic personality disorder: diagnostic and clinical challenges. Am J Psychiatry 172(5):415–422, 2015 25930131

Carlson EA, Ruiz SK: Transactional processes in the development of adult personality disorder symptoms. Dev Psychopathol 28(3):639–651, 2016 27427797

Choi-Kain LW, Finch EF, Masland SR, et al: What works in the treatment of borderline personality disorder. Curr Behav Neurosci Rep 4(1):21–30, 2017 28331780

Clarkin JF, Yeomans FE, Kernberg OF: Psychotherapy for Borderline Personality. New York, Wiley, 1999

Cloninger CR, Svrakic DM, Przybeck TR: A psychobiological model of temperament and character. Arch Gen Psychiatry 50(12):975–990, 1993 8250684

Cohen P, Crawford T, Chen H, et al: Predictors, correlates, and consequences of trajectories of antisocial personality disorder symptoms from early adolescence to mid-30s, in Trauma,

Psychopathology, and Violence: Causes, Consequences, or Correlates? Edited by Widom CS. New York, Oxford University Press, 2012, pp 109–129

Costa P, McCrae RR: Personality disorders and the five-factor model of personality. Journal of Personality Disorders 4(4):362–371, 1990

Cristea IA, Gentili C, Cotet CD, et al: Efficacy of psychotherapies for borderline personality disorder: a systematic review and meta-analysis. JAMA Psychiatry 74(4):319–328, 2017 28249086

First MB, Skodol AE, Bender DS, et al: User's Guide for the Structured Clinical Interview for the DSM-5 Alternative Model for Personality Disorders (SCID-5-AMPD). Arlington, VA, American Psychiatric Association Publishing, 2018

Giesen-Bloo J, van Dyck R, Spinhoven P, et al: Outpatient psychotherapy for borderline personality disorder: randomized trial of schema-focused therapy vs transference-focused psychotherapy. Arch Gen Psychiatry 63(6):649–658, 2006 16754838

Goldstein RB, Chou SP, Saha TD, et al: The epidemiology of antisocial behavioral syndromes in adulthood: results from the National Epidemiologic Survey on Alcohol and Related Conditions–III. J Clin Psychiatry 78(1):90–98, 2017 27035627

Gunderson JG, Stout RL, McGlashan TH, et al: Ten-year course of borderline personality disorder: psychopathology and function from the Collaborative Longitudinal Personality Disorders study. Arch Gen Psychiatry 68(8):827–837, 2011 21464343

Gunderson JG, Herpertz SC, Skodol AE, et al: Borderline personality disorder. Nat Rev Dis Primers 4:18029, 2018 29795363

Hasin D, Fenton MC, Skodol A, et al: Personality disorders and the 3-year course of alcohol, drug, and nicotine use disorders. Arch Gen Psychiatry 68(11):1158–1167, 2011 22065531

Herpertz SC, Bertsch K: A new perspective on the pathophysiology of borderline personality disorder: a model of the role of oxytocin. Am J Psychiatry 172(9):840–851, 2015 26324303

Hicks BM, Foster KT, Iacono WG, et al: Genetic and environmental influences on the familial transmission of externalizing disorders in adoptive and twin offspring. JAMA Psychiatry 70(10):1076–1083, 2013 23965950

Hopwood CJ, Zanarini MC: Borderline personality traits and disorder: predicting prospective patient functioning. J Consult Clin Psychol 78(4):585–589, 2010 20658814

Hopwood CJ, Morey LC, Donnellan MB, et al: Ten-year rank-order stability of personality traits and disorders in a clinical sample. J Pers 81(3):335–344, 2013 22812532

Huprich SK, Nelson SM, Paggeot A, et al: Object relations predicts borderline personality disorder symptoms beyond emotional dysregulation, negative affect, and impulsivity. Pers Disord 8(1):46–53, 2017 27176498

Infurna MR, Brunner R, Holz B, et al: The specific role of childhood abuse, parental bonding, and family functioning in female adolescents with borderline personality disorder. J Pers Disord 30(2):177–192, 2016 25905734

Kernberg OF: Borderline Conditions and Pathological Narcissism. New York, Jason Aronson, 1975

Keshavan M, Shad M, Soloff P, Schooler N: Efficacy and tolerability of olanzapine in the treatment of schizotypal personality disorder. Schizophr Res 71(1):97–101, 2004 15374577

Koenigsberg HW, Reynolds D, Goodman M, et al: Risperidone in the treatment of schizotypal personality disorder. J Clin Psychiatry 64(6):628–634, 2003 12823075

Kohut H: The Analysis of the Self: A Systematic Approach to the Psychoanalytic Treatment of Narcissistic Personality Disorders. New York, International Universities Press, 1971

Krueger RF, Derringer J, Markon KE, et al: Initial construction of a maladaptive personality trait model and inventory for DSM-5. Psychol Med 42(9):1879–1890, 2012 22153017

Leichsenring F, Leibing E: The effectiveness of psychodynamic therapy and cognitive behavior therapy in the treatment of personality disorders: a meta-analysis. Am J Psychiatry 160(7):1223–1232, 2003 12832233

Leichsenring F, Masuhr O, Jaeger U, et al: The effectiveness of psychoanalytic-interactional psychotherapy in borderline personality disorder. Bull Menninger Clin 74(3):206–218, 2010 20925484

Lieb K, Zanarini MC, Schmahl C, et al: Borderline personality disorder. Lancet 364(9432):453–461, 2004 15288745

Linehan MM, Comtois KA, Murray AM, et al: Two-year randomized controlled trial and follow-up of dialectical behavior therapy vs. therapy by experts for suicidal behaviors and borderline personality disorder. Arch Gen Psychiatry 63(7):757–766, 2006 16818865

Livesley WJ, Jang KL, Jackson DN, Vernon PA: Genetic and environmental contributions to dimensions of personality disorder. Am J Psychiatry 150(12):1826–1831, 1993 8238637

Livesley WJ, Jang KL, Vernon PA: Phenotypic and genetic structure of traits delineating personality disorder. Arch Gen Psychiatry 55(10):941–948, 1998 9783566

Lorber MF: Psychophysiology of aggression, psychopathy, and conduct problems: a meta-analysis. Psychol Bull 130(4):531–552, 2004 15250812

Luyten P, Blatt SJ: Interpersonal relatedness and self-definition in normal and disrupted personality development: retrospect and prospect. Am Psychol 68(3):172–183, 2013 23586492

Lyons MJ, True WR, Eisen SA, et al: Differential heritability of adult and juvenile antisocial traits. Arch Gen Psychiatry 52(11):906–915, 1995 7487339

Ma G, Fan H, Shen C, et al: Genetic and neuroimaging features of personality disorders: state of the art. Neurosci Bull 32(3):286–306, 2016 27037690

Mazza M, Marano G, Janiri L: An update on pharmacotherapy for personality disorders. Expert Opin Pharmacother 17(15):1977–1979, 2016 27487174

Morey LC: Development and initial evaluation of a self-report form of the DSM-5 Level of Personality Functioning Scale. Psychol Assess 29(10):1302–1308, 2017 28240933

Morey LC: Application of the DSM-5 Level of Personality Functioning Scale by lay raters. J Pers Disord 32(5):709–720, 2018 28758883

Morey LC, Skodol AE: Convergence between DSM-IV-TR and DSM-5 diagnostic models for personality disorder: evaluation of strategies for establishing diagnostic thresholds. J Psychiatr Pract 19(3):179–193, 2013 23653075

Morey LC, Shea MT, Markowitz JC, et al: State effects of major depression on the assessment of personality and personality disorder. Am J Psychiatry 167(5):528–535, 2010 20160004

Morey LC, Berghuis H, Bender DS, et al: Toward a model for assessing level of personality functioning in DSM-5, II: empirical articulation of a core dimension of personality pathology. J Pers Assess 93(4):347–353, 2011 22804673

Morey LC, Hopwood CJ, Markowitz JC, et al: Comparison of alternative models for personality disorders, II: 6-, 8- and 10-year follow-up. Psychol Med 42(8):1705–1713, 2012 22132840

Morey LC, Bender DS, Skodol AE: Validating the proposed Diagnostic and Statistical Manual of Mental Disorders, 5th Edition, severity indicator for personality disorder. J Nerv Ment Dis 201(9):729–735, 2013 23995027

Morey LC, Skodol AE, Oldham JM: Clinician judgments of clinical utility: a comparison of DSM-IV-TR personality disorders and the alternative model for DSM-5 personality disorders. J Abnorm Psychol 123(2):398–405, 2014 24886013

Morey LC, Benson KT, Skodol AE: Relating DSM-5 section III personality traits to section II personality disorder diagnoses. Psychol Med 46(3):647–655, 2016 26515656

Nathanson B, Jamison S: Psychotherapeutic and pharmacologic treatment of schizotypal personality disorder: the heuristic utility of stressing function over form. Clinical Case Studies 10(5):395–407, 2011

Neumann E, Kanyi C, Wulf M-A, Tress W: Psychodynamic short-term therapy for dependent and avoidant personality disorders [in German]. Psychotherapeut 59(5):392–398, 2014

Raine A, Moffitt TE, Caspi A, et al: Neurocognitive impairments in boys on the life-course persistent antisocial path. J Abnorm Psychol 114(1):38–49, 2005 15709810

Rautiainen MR, Paunio T, Repo-Tiihonen E, et al: Genome-wide association study of antisocial personality disorder. Transl Psychiatry 6(9):e883, 2016 27598967

Ridenour J: Psychodynamic model and treatment of schizotypal personality disorder. Psychoanalytic Psychology 33(1):129–146, 2016

Roberts BW, DelVecchio WF: The rank-order consistency of personality traits from childhood to old age: a quantitative review of longitudinal studies. Psychol Bull 126(1):3–25, 2000 10668348

Ruocco AC, Carcone D: A neurobiological model of borderline personality disorder: systematic and integrative review. Harv Rev Psychiatry 24(5):311–329, 2016 27603741

Siever LJ, Davis KL: The pathophysiology of schizophrenia disorders: perspectives from the spectrum. Am J Psychiatry 161(3): 398–413, 2004 14992962

Simms LJ, Calabrese WR: Incremental validity of the DSM-5 section III personality disorder traits with respect to psychosocial impairment. J Pers Disord 30(1):95–111, 2016 25905731

Skodol AE, Gunderson JG, McGlashan TH, et al: Functional impairment in patients with schizotypal, borderline, avoidant, or obsessive-compulsive personality disorder. Am J Psychiatry 159(2):276–283, 2002 11823271

Skodol AE, Bender DS, Morey LC, et al: Personality disorder types proposed for DSM-5. J Pers Disord 25(2):136–169, 2011a 21466247

Skodol AE, Grilo CM, Keyes KM, et al: Relationship of personality disorders to the course of major depressive disorder in a nationally representative sample. Am J Psychiatry 168(3):257–264, 2011b 21245088

Skodol AE, Bender DS, Morey LC: Narcissistic personality disorder in DSM-5. Pers Disord 5(4):422–427, 2014 23834518

Skodol AE, Morey LC, Bender DS, et al: The Alternative DSM-5 Model for Personality Disorders: a clinical application. Am J Psychiatry 172(7):606–613, 2015 26130200

South SC, Krueger RF, Knudsen GP, et al: A population-based twin study of DSM-5 maladaptive personality domains. Pers Disord 8(4):366–375, 2017 27797545

Stein MB, Chartier MJ, Lizak MV, Jang KL: Familial aggregation of anxiety-related quantitative traits in generalized social phobia: clues to understanding "disorder" heritability? Am J Med Genet 105(7):79–83, 2001 11425006

Stepp SD, Lazarus SA, Byrd AL: A systematic review of risk factors prospectively associated with borderline personality disorder: taking stock and moving forward. Pers Disord 7(4):316–323, 2016 27709988

Stoffers JM, Lieb K: Pharmacotherapy for borderline personality disorder—current evidence and recent trends. Curr Psychiatry Rep 17(1):534, 2015 25413640

Sturrock B, Mellor D: Perceived emotional invalidation and borderline personality disorder features: a test of theory. Pers Ment Health 8(2):128–142, 2014 24700736

Temes CM, Magni LR, Fitzmaurice GM, et al: Prevalence and severity of childhood adversity in adolescents with BPD, psychiatrically healthy adolescents, and adults with BPD. Pers Ment Health 11(3):171–178, 2017 28786232

Thylstrup B, Schrøder S, Fridell M, et al: Did you get any help? A post-hoc secondary analysis of a randomized controlled trial of psychoeducation for patients with antisocial personality disorder in outpatient substance abuse treatment programs. BMC Psychiatry 17(1):7, 2017 28068951

Torgersen S: Prevalence, sociodemographics, and functional impairment, in Textbook of Personality Disorders, 2nd Edition. Edited by Oldham JM, Skodol AE, Bender DS. Washington, DC, American Psychiatric Publishing, 2014, pp 109–130

Torgersen S, Lygren S, Øien PA, et al: A twin study of personality disorders. Compr Psychiatry 41(6):416–425, 2000 11086146

Waugh MH, Hopwood CJ, Krueger RF, et al: Psychological assessment with the DSM-5 Alternative Model for Personality Disorders: tradition and innovation. Prof Psychol Res Pr 48(2):79–89, 2017 28450760

Wilson S, Stroud CB, Durbin CE: Interpersonal dysfunction in personality disorders: a meta-analytic review. Psychol Bull 143(7):677–734, 2017 28447827

World Health Organization: International Statistical Classification of Diseases and Related Health Problems, 10th Revision. Geneva, World Health Organization, 1992

Wright AGC, Hopwood CJ, Skodol AE, et al: Longitudinal validation of general and specific structural features of personality pathology. J Abnorm Psychol 125(8):1120–1134, 2016 27819472

Zanarini MC, Frankenburg FR, Reich DB, et al: Attainment and stability of sustained symptomatic remission and recovery among patients with borderline personality disorder and Axis II comparison subjects: a 16-year prospective follow-up study. Am J Psychiatry 169(5):476–483, 2012 22737693

Zimmerman M, Rothchild L, Chelminski I: The prevalence of DSM-IV personality disorders in psychiatric outpatients. Am J Psychiatry 162(10):1911–1918, 2005 16199838

Zimmermann J, Benecke C, Bender DS, et al: Assessing DSM-5 level of personality functioning from videotaped clinical interviews: a pilot study with untrained and clinically inexperienced students. J Pers Assess 96(4):397–409, 2014 24224740

Recommended Readings

American Psychiatric Association: Practice guideline for the treatment of patients with borderline personality disorder. Am J Psychiatry 158 (suppl):1–52, 2001

American Psychiatric Association: Practice Guidelines for the Treatment of Psychiatric Disorders: Compendium 2006. Washington, DC, American Psychiatric Publishing, 2006. Available at: https://psychiatryonline.org/guidelines. Accessed November 30, 2018.

Bateman A, Fonagy P: Mentalization-Based Treatment for Borderline Personality Disorder: A Practical Guide, 2nd Edition. New York, Oxford University Press, 2016

Beck AT, Davis DD, Freeman A: Cognitive Therapy of Personality Disorders, 3rd Edition. New York, Guilford, 2015

Clarkin JF, Fonagy P, Gabbard GO: Psychodynamic Psychotherapy for Personality Disorders: A Clinical Handbook. Washington, DC, American Psychiatric Publishing, 2010

Gabbard GO: Gabbard's Treatments of Psychiatric Disorders, 5th Edition. Washington, DC, American Psychiatric Publishing, 2014

Gunderson JG, Links PS: Handbook of Good Psychiatric Management for Borderline Personality Disorder. Arlington, VA, American Psychiatric Publishing, 2014

Livesley W: Integrated Modular Treatment for Borderline Personality Disorder: A Practical Guide to Combining Effective Treatment Methods. New York, Cambridge University Press, 2017

Luyten P, Mayes, L, Fonagy P, et al: Handbook of Psychodynamic Approaches to Psychopathology. New York, Guilford Press, 2015

Ogrodniczuk JS (ed): Understanding and Treating Pathological Narcissism. Washington, DC, American Psychological Association, 2013

Oldham JM, Skodol AE, Bender DS (eds): Essentials of Personality Disorders. Washington, DC, American Psychiatric Publishing, 2009

Oldham JM, Skodol AE, Bender DS (eds): The American Psychiatric Publishing Textbook of Personality Disorders, 2nd Edition. Washington, DC, American Psychiatric Publishing, 2014

Sharp C, Tackett J: Handbook of Borderline Personality Disorder in Children and Adolescents. New York, Springer Science + Business Media, 2014

Widiger TA (ed): The Oxford Handbook of Personality Disorders. New York, Oxford University Press, 2012

Widiger TA, Costa PT Jr (eds): Personality Disorders and the Five-Factor Model of Personality, 3rd Edition. Washington, DC, American Psychological Association, 2012

CHAPTER 27

Paraphilic Disorders

Richard Balon, M.D.

Paraphilias and paraphilic disorders have been an "unwanted child" of psychiatry, mostly because of their social stigma and legal implications but also because of the lack of information we have about them. The term *paraphilia(s)* is about 100 years old and is derived from the Greek words *para,* which means, among other things, "beyond," and *philia,* which means "love" or "friendship." Thus, we can translate it as "love beyond the usual." Previous editions of DSM used the category name *paraphilias,* whereas DSM-5 (American Psychiatric Association 2013) uses the category name *paraphilic disorders.* In DSM-5,

> The term *paraphilia* denotes any intense and persistent sexual interest other than sexual interest in genital stimulation or preparatory fondling with phenotypically normal, physiologically mature, consenting human partners. In some circumstances, the criteria "intense and persistent" may be difficult to apply, such as in the assessment of persons who are very old or medically ill and who may not have "intense" sexual interests of any kind. In such circumstances, the term *paraphilia* may be defined as any sexual interest greater than or equal to normophilic sexual interests. There are also specific paraphilias that are generally better described as *preferential* sexual interests rather than intense sexual interests. Some paraphilias primarily concern the individual's erotic activities, and others primarily concern the individual's erotic targets. (p. 685)

In contrast to the paraphilias category in DSM-IV (American Psychiatric Association 1994), DSM-5 delineated a more strict term and category of *paraphilic disorders:* "A *paraphilic disorder* is a paraphilia that is currently causing distress or impairment to the individual or a paraphilia whose satisfaction has entailed personal harm, or risk of harm, to others. A paraphilia is a necessary but not a sufficient condition for having

---

This chapter is an update and revision of Becker JV, Johnson BR, Perkins A: "Paraphilic Disorders," in *The American Psychiatric Publishing Textbook of Psychiatry,* Sixth Edition. Edited by Hales RE, Yudofsky SC, Roberts LW. Arlington, VA, American Psychiatric Association, 2014, pp. 895–925.

a paraphilic disorder, and a paraphilia by itself does not necessarily justify or require clinical intervention" (American Psychiatric Association 2013, pp. 685–686).

Because the area of assessing, diagnosing, and treating paraphilic disorders has become a specialty in the field of psychiatry, most psychiatrists will have little exposure to patients with paraphilic disorders in the course of their training and career. Psychiatrists should, of course, as part of a standard diagnostic interview, ask questions regarding sexual functioning, such as "Are you having difficulty with sexual functioning?" or "Do you engage in sexual behavior that is of concern?" Because paraphilic disorders are most frequently associated with sexual offenses, these disorders may be more commonly seen by psychiatrists practicing in the forensic arena. However, paraphilic disorders are not always associated with sexual offenses. In fact, many people commit sexual offenses that do not meet the criteria for a paraphilic disorder; likewise, some people diagnosed with a paraphilic disorder never commit a sex crime.

The paraphilic disorders are characterized by experiencing, over a period of at least 6 months, recurrent, intense sexually arousing fantasies, sexual urges, or behaviors generally involving nonhuman objects or nonconsenting partners. In diagnosing any of the paraphilic disorders, the clinician should also consider whether the person has acted on the urges or is markedly distressed by them. Although an individual may have engaged in a behavior that may be sexually inappropriate or even illegal, he or she may only have the urges or fantasies associated with the paraphilic disorder and never act on them. Many of the paraphilic disorders have specifiers unique to that particular disorder, and most have to do with the target of the fantasy, urge, or behavior. Additionally, DSM-5 has added the following two specifiers to the paraphilic disorders in general (with the exception of pedophilic disorder): 1) "in a controlled environment," which applies to individuals living in institutional or other settings that limit their opportunities to engage in the behavior, and 2) "in remission," which indicates a lack of distress, impairment, or recurrence of the behavior with a nonconsenting partner for 5 years in an uncontrolled environment. "In remission" does not necessarily mean that the interest no longer exists; rather, it indicates that the behavior is not currently problematic.

Paraphilic Disorders

Voyeuristic Disorder

Voyeuristic disorder is commonly viewed as the act of becoming sexually aroused by fantasy or the actual viewing of unsuspecting and nonconsenting people who are naked, disrobing, or engaging in sexual activity when they do not realize they are being watched or have not given permission (Långström 2010). The behavior may lead to sexual excitement, but generally there is no sexual activity between the voyeur and the victim, although the voyeur may masturbate at the time or later to the memory of the event. This type of behavior often has an onset in adolescence and can become persistent (American Psychiatric Association 2013); however, according to DSM-5, the diagnosis cannot be made until an individual is at least age 18 years. The desire to view naked individuals is not necessarily unusual, but in the case of this diagnosis, the professional should be looking for qualitative and quantitative differences from normal behavior, fantasy, or urges. This information either can be freely offered by the individual or can be inferred in some cases by a pattern of recurrent behavior (based on significant objective evidence), even in individuals who do not admit a sexual interest in voyeuristic behavior. The term *voyeurism* as used in this chapter should not be confused with the popular-culture definition of voyeurism (i.e., the practice of taking pleasure in observing something private, sordid, or salacious) and should also not be used for watching pornography or striptease.

Exhibitionistic Disorder

Exhibitionistic disorder is identified as either the exposure of one's genitals to an unsuspecting person or the manifestation of urges to do so in the form of fantasy. When the behavior does occur, it may involve masturbation during the exposure, and in some cases the individual tries to surprise or shock the observer. The exhibitionistic individual may hope or desire that the observer will become sexually aroused or join in sexual activity. Exhibitionistic disorder is generally thought to be a disorder of males, sometimes has an early onset (before age 18 years), and is directed primarily at females. Victims can be adults, children, or adolescents. DSM-5 criteria provide specifications for exposing to prepubertal or early pubertal children, to physically mature individuals, or to both. As with many types of paraphilic disorders, there are no good personality profiles for those with exhibitionistic disorder. Långström and Seto (2006) found that individuals who admitted to having engaged in exhibitionistic behavior also tended to have higher levels of sexual activity in general.

DSM-5 provides for the diagnosis of exhibitionistic disorder both in situations where an individual freely admits to the sexual fantasy, urge, or behavior and in situations where an individual may deny such attraction, as long as there is substantial objective evidence that the individual has engaged in the behavior.

Frotteuristic Disorder

Frotteuristic disorder involves touching or rubbing against a nonconsenting person, or having fantasies about or urges to do so (Långström 2010). When the behavior does occur, it frequently takes place in crowded areas, such as a bus, subway, hall, or sidewalk. Although there are many different ways in which a person can engage in frotteuristic activity, one of the more common is for a male to rub his genitals against the unsuspecting victim; however, the behavior may include touching or rubbing the genitals or sexual organs (including breasts) of the victim without the victim knowing that he or she has been intentionally offended against. Freund et al. (1997) found that this disorder is quite comorbid with other paraphilic behaviors, most typically the other "courtship disorders" (so called because they resemble distorted components of human courtship behavior), which include voyeuristic disorder and exhibitionistic disorder. Single acts of frotteurism, however, may not be sufficient to qualify for a diagnosis of frotteuristic disorder in a nonadmitter.

Sexual Masochism Disorder

The DSM-5 diagnostic criteria for sexual masochism disorder require intense sexually arousing fantasies, urges, or behaviors involving the act of being humiliated, beaten, bound, or otherwise made to suffer. Such acts may include restraint, blindfolding, paddling, spanking, whipping, beating, electrical shocks, cutting, piercing, and being urinated or defecated on (Krueger 2010a). It is important to note that an individual can meet criteria for a diagnosis of sexual masochism disorder only if he or she indicates distress or impairment. Behaviors associated with sexual masochism disorder are typically practiced in a consenting, nondistressing, nonpathological way (Baumeister and Butler 1997). For this reason, sexual masochism disorder should only be diagnosed in individuals who freely admit to the behavior and express clinically significant distress or psychosocial role impairment from the behavior. In extreme instances, associated behaviors can be dangerous or even life-threatening. Therefore, a new specifier has been added to indicate whether these behaviors or fantasies occur with asphyxiophilia (sexual arousal by asphyxiation). This is a particularly important specification to make, considering that asphyxiation, whether with a partner or alone, can be particularly dangerous and even life-threatening. On the other hand, it is important to realize that bondage, discipline, dominance, sadism, and masochism (BDSM) are frequent erotic behaviors (nondistressing) among consenting adults of all social strata.

Sexual Sadism Disorder

According to DSM-5, sexual sadism involves real acts (not simulated) in which sexual arousal is achieved from the psychological or physical suffering of another nonconsenting individual. Like sexual masochism disorder, this behavior can occur between consenting individuals who are neither distressed nor impaired by the behavior and who practice it in a safe manner; these individuals may be considered to have sadistic sexual interest but not a disorder (Krueger 2010b). Sexual sadism disorder is more likely to be seen in a mental health context when it involves a nonconsenting person. As with the other paraphilic disorders that involve nonconsenting individuals, sexual sadism disorder can be diagnosed in the face of nonadmission of the fantasy, urge, or behavior if there is substantial objective evidence from the person's psychosocial or legal history that he or she has engaged in this behavior on a recurrent basis. The sadistic acts may involve such things as controlling or dominating the person but may also include, for example, restraint, blindfolding, paddling, spanking, whipping, pinching, beating, burning, electrical shocks, rape (simulated or actual), cutting, stabbing, strangulation, torture, mutilation, or even killing. In individuals with sexual sadism disorder, such fantasies may have begun in childhood but are usually present by early adulthood.

Pedophilic Disorder

Pedophilic disorder is defined as intense, recurrent, sexually arousing fantasies, urges, or behaviors involving a prepubescent child or children (generally age 13 years or younger) over a period of at least 6 months. A diagnosis is suggested if an individual has acted on these urges or if the urges or fantasies caused marked distress. To receive a diagnosis of pedophilic disorder, the individual must have been at least age 16 years and at least 5 years older than the child. The criteria also provide specifiers for an exclusive type (only attracted to children) versus a nonexclusive type (attracted to both adults and children), as well as a specifier for the gender of the child (male, female, or both) and a specifier indicating whether the diagnosis is limited to incest. In contrast to the other DSM-5 paraphilic disorders (as previously noted), the diagnostic criteria for pedophilic disorder do not include the specifiers "in a controlled environment" and "in full remission."

It is also important to realize that the legal and medical definitions of what constitutes paraphilic behavior and what constitutes pedophilia/pedophilic disorder can sometimes differ. DSM-5 specifies that the individual diagnosed with pedophilic disorder is at least 16 years of age and at least 5 years older than the child or children he or she is sexually involved with. This criterion, especially the age difference, does not necessarily hold in the legal system, and thus a 16- or 17-year-old person who has sex with a 15-year-old child may still be labeled as a sexual offender.

A large spectrum of inappropriate sexual activity can occur between adults and children and be indicative of a pedophilic disorder, ranging from undressing and looking at the child to penetration of different forms and even torture. There have been cases in which pedophilic disorder started during adolescence, and other cases in which the disorder did not seem to begin until middle adulthood (Seto 2008). Notably, however, a subset of individuals who have this desire do not act on their urges and may seek treatment without having committed a sex offense. Additionally, the Internet has created a new problem in the form of child pornography, viewing of which may be indicative of pedophilia/pedophilic disorder. Although this disorder is most often seen in males, and most of the available information is based on the study of males, there are females who meet criteria for this disorder.

Fetishistic Disorder

The main feature of fetishistic disorder is sexual arousal that often involves the use of nonliving objects, such as women's underpants, bras, stockings, shoes, boots, or other apparel, but may also include a highly specific focus on nongenital body parts (Kafka 2010). The inclusion of nongenital body parts is new in DSM-5, and a specifier is now included so that a clinician can indicate on which body part(s) or nonliving object(s) a specific individual focuses. In this disorder, the individual might masturbate while holding, rubbing, or smelling an item. Objects used exclusively for the purpose of cross-dressing or objects designed for genital stimulation (e.g., vibrators) are not included in this diagnosis. In general, the person may have difficulty in becoming sexually aroused in the absence of the item. One of the most important features of this diagnosis is that the individual must experience clinically significant distress or impairment. If an individual experiences strong fantasies, urges, and behaviors involving the use of nonliving objects but experiences no distress or psychosocial role impairment, then a diagnosis would not be appropriate.

Despite a paucity of research on fetishistic disorder, some trends do emerge. Fetishistic disorder, like many of the paraphilic disorders, is primarily found in males, and the most common foci are feet and their associated objects (i.e., footwear, socks) and female undergarments (American Psychiatric Association 2013).

Transvestic Disorder

DSM-5 transvestic disorder involves cross-dressing, in most cases producing sexual arousal (American Psychiatric Association 2013). In comparison with the DSM-IV criteria, several specifiers have been added to and others removed from the DSM-5 criteria. The "with gender dysphoria" specifier has been removed to reduce the overlap between this diagnosis and that of gender dysphoria. The specifier "with fetishism" has been added to identify individuals who experience arousal in response to the garments, materials, or fabrics, and the specifier "with autogynephilia" has been added to indicate that the cross-dressing is accompanied by sexually arousing thoughts or images of the self as female (Blanchard 2010). Although the diagnosis is no longer restricted to heterosexual males, it has most typically been described in heterosexual male. In the differential diagnosis, the clinician needs to rule out fetishistic disorder and gender dysphoria. Transvestic disorder may begin in childhood or adulthood, may be temporary or chronic, and may lead to gender dysphoria in some cases (it is often at this point that the individual seeks treatment). Transvestic disorder should be diagnosed only in the presence of clinically significant distress or impairment on the part of the individual.

Other Specified and Unspecified Paraphilic Disorders

The *other specified* and *unspecified* diagnoses represent a change that has been applied throughout DSM-5. The other specified and unspecified diagnostic categories replace the *not otherwise specified* (NOS) category as a method for recording presentations in which symptoms do not meet criteria for any specific paraphilic disorder or there is insufficient information to make a specific diagnosis. The diagnosis *other specified paraphilic disorder* is used in cases where the clinician can specify the reason that full criteria are not met. Presentations for which the "other specified" designation would be appropriate include—but are not limited to—recurrent and intense sexual arousal involving telephone scatologia (obscene phone calls), necrophilia (corpses), zoophilia (animals), coprophilia (feces), klismaphilia (enemas), or urophilia (urine). *Unspecified paraphilic disorder* is used in situations where a paraphilic disorder appears to be present but does not meet full criteria for any of the listed disorders and either the clinician chooses not to specify why the disorder does not meet full criteria or there is not enough information to make a more specific diagnosis.

Epidemiology

Because the DSM-5 diagnostic concept of paraphilic disorders is new, epidemiological data on paraphilic disorders do not yet exist. All studies on prevalence refer rather to prevalence of paraphilias, and thus because paraphilic behaviors do not typically cause personal distress, scant data are available on the prevalence or course of many of these disorders. In addition, paraphilias/paraphilic disorders tend to be underreported by patients because of the associated legal implications and societal stigma. Historically, information on paraphilic disorders that involve victims (e.g., pedophilic disorder, exhibitionistic disorder) has been obtained from studies of incarcerated sex offenders. However, such data are limited in that many sex offenders are not arrested, and those who are tend to underreport their deviant behavior for fear of further prosecution.

The vast majority of individuals with paraphilic disorders are men, with the possible exception of sexual masochism disorder. For example, among reported cases of sexual abuse, more than 90% of offenders were men (Browne and Finkelhor 1986). Across studies, the prevalence of identified female perpetrators has varied from 5% to 44%, depending on the specific study and the sex of the victim (Bunting 2005; Faller

1995; Peter 2009). However, the low rates of female offenders could in part be due to bias on the part of professionals and the public; sociocultural norms leave little room for women to be diagnosed with paraphilic disorders.

Paraphilic Disorders and Comorbid Psychiatric Diagnoses

The study of comorbidity in regard to paraphilic disorders suffers from the same drawbacks as more general epidemiological research. However, the research does suggest that comorbid psychiatric disorders (especially personality disorders) are likely to be present in individuals with paraphilic disorders and should be addressed. Interestingly, the Tenth Revision of the *International Classification of Diseases* (ICD-10; World Health Organization 1992) classified paraphilias as disorders of sexual preference under disorders of adult personality and behavior. The psychiatric disorders most commonly comorbid with paraphilic disorders are mood disorders, anxiety disorders, substance use disorders (especially alcohol use disorder), and personality disorders (American Psychiatric Association 2013).

Etiology

Various theories have been put forth to explain the development of paraphilic disorders. Most of the theories center on those paraphilic disorders that involve victims and are considered criminal behaviors. Some of these theories are specific to the development of paraphilic disorders in general, but most are applied to the development of paraphilic interest and subsequent illegal behavior.

Biological factors have been postulated. Destruction of parts of the limbic system in animals causes hypersexual behavior (Klüver-Bucy syndrome), and temporal lobe diseases such as psychomotor seizures or temporal lobe tumors have been implicated in some persons with paraphilic disorders. It also has been suggested that abnormal levels of androgens may contribute to inappropriate sexual arousal. Most studies, however, have dealt only with violent sex offenders and have yielded inconclusive results.

According to learning theory, sexual arousal develops when a person engages in a sexual behavior that is subsequently reinforced through sexual fantasies and masturbation. It is thought that there are certain vulnerable periods (e.g., puberty) in which the development of paraphilic sexual arousal can occur. For example, if an adolescent boy is sexual with a 7-year-old boy and there are no negative consequences, the adolescent may continue to fantasize about having sex with the boy and masturbate to those fantasies, developing arousal to young boys (i.e., pedophilia).

Cognitive distortions are often referenced to explain the maintenance of paraphilic behaviors that cause harm to others. Distortions in thinking, or thinking errors, provide a way for an individual to give him- or herself permission to engage in inappropriate or deviant sexual behaviors (Abel et al. 1984).

Some theories attempt to provide comprehensive models of sex offending. Freund (e.g., Freund et al. 1997) suggested that several paraphilias—voyeurism, exhibitionism, frotteurism, telephone scatophilia, and preferential rape—could be explained in terms of a disturbance/impairment of one of the four phases of the normal courtship process in males: 1) finding phase (voyeurism), 2) affiliative phase (exhibitionism), 3) tactile phase (frotteurism), and 4) copulatory phase (preferential rape). Although this is a fairly comprehensive theory, it is only a theory and does not explain all paraphilias.

More recent studies suggest that pedophilia specifically may arise from neuropsychological differences. Certain features suggestive of early-occurring brain differences have been found to be more prevalent among men with pedophilia; these include non-right-handedness, lower IQ, childhood head injuries, and a history of placement in special education programs (e.g., Blanchard et al. 2003; Cantor et al. 2004). Additionally, Cantor et al. (2008) and Cantor and Blanchard (2012) found evidence using robust methods that pedophiles have lower volumes of white matter in the temporal lobes bilaterally and the parietal lobes bilaterally.

Diagnosis

As noted, it is important to make a distinction between paraphilia and paraphilic disorder (in simplistic terms, the latter equals paraphilia plus distress and/or impairment). Diagnoses of paraphilic disorders are typically made only when 1) these activities are the exclusive or preferred means of achieving sexual excitement and orgasm and this behavior is distressing, or 2) the sexual behavior is not consensual. In some cases, the identified client may not be distressed, but his or her partner may be. In such cases, it is important to tread carefully and not make diagnostic conclusions before a thorough evaluation can be conducted. Additionally, depending on the situation—forensic, pretreatment, risk, inpatient, outpatient, and so forth—the clinician may need to obtain collateral data before making a diagnosis. It is important to distinguish between some paraphilic disorders such as fetishistic disorder and transvestic disorder and normal variations of sexual behavior. Some couples occasionally augment their usual sexual activities with, for example, bondage or cross-dressing.

Obviously, nonconsensual sexual activities, such as sexual contact with children or exhibitionism, can never be appropriate; children can never give consent for sexual activity with an adult. Notably, the DSM-5 criteria give considerably more leeway in diagnosing a paraphilic disorder in situations where an individual is denying interest in the behavior. This latitude is no doubt useful, but evaluators should also use caution and ensure that any diagnosis is based on a solid foundation of objective data.

Inappropriate sexual behavior is not always the result of a paraphilia. A psychotic patient may cross-dress because of a delusional belief that God wishes her to hide her true sex. A manic patient may expose himself to women because of his hypersexuality and belief that he will be able to "pick them up." A patient with dementia can behave in a sexually inappropriate manner (e.g., masturbate in a room full of people) because of cognitive impairment. An individual with intellectual developmental disorder may engage in a sexually inappropriate behavior because of cognitive impairment, poor impulse control, and lack of sexual knowledge. Some individuals with antisocial personality disorder also commit deviant sexual acts; such behaviors usually are part of the individuals' overall disregard for societal norms and sanctions and are not necessarily indicative of a deviant sexual interest. Last but not least, the term *sexual offender* is not a psychiatric diagnosis. It is a legal term, whereas *paraphilic disorder* is a psychiatric/medical term and diagnosis.

Evaluation and Assessment

Clinical Evaluation

In evaluating an individual for paraphilic behavior, the clinician must perform a careful psychiatric evaluation to exclude other possible causes of this behavior (see previous section, "Diagnosis"). Evaluation of paraphilic behavior should not be done in isolation but as a part of a comprehensive sexual history. The clinician should take a detailed sexual history, noting the onset and course of paraphilic and appropriate sexual fantasies and behavior and the present degree of control over the deviant behavior. In addition, the individual should be evaluated for faulty beliefs (i.e., cognitive distortions) about his or her sexual behavior, social and assertive skills with appropriate adult partners, sexual dysfunctions, and sexual knowledge. Table 27–1 lists specific details that may be covered in the sexual history portion of the evaluation. As discussed in "Diagnosis" earlier, it is important to consider the purpose of the evaluation and possibly obtain collateral data before making a diagnosis.

Phallometric Assessment

Phallometric assessments (i.e., measurements of penile erection) have been used to objectively assess the sexual arousal of individuals who have engaged in paraphilic behavior. This assessment is important because persons with paraphilic disorders, especially those in trouble with the law, are reluctant to disclose the full extent of their deviant behavior and fantasies. A transducer (either a thin metal ring or mercury-in-rubber strain gauge) is placed around the penis, and the degree of erection is recorded while the individual is exposed to various sexual stimuli (audiotapes, slides, videotapes) depicting paraphilic and appropriate sexual scenes (of note: the ownership of naked child pictures, including child pornography, may be problematic in the United States because it is illegal). This information is then recorded on a polygraph or computer, and the degree of arousal to deviant sexual scenes is compared with arousal to nonparaphilic scenes.

Phallometric assessments of sexual age and gender preferences have excellent discriminant validity with extrafamilial child molesters (Freund and Blanchard 1989). Although phallometric assessments attempt to measure the degree of sexual preference among stimulus categories, they do not detail whether someone has engaged in paraphilic behavior or has committed a sexual offense. Furthermore, some individuals are able to influence their responses to appear to have nonparaphilic preferences (Freund et al. 1988).

As with the interpretation of most physiological procedures, caution is necessary in interpreting results from plethysmography because the setting in which the data are obtained is quite different from the real world. Also, because variation can occur within subjects over time, the interpretation must take into account the context of the offender's history, available records, and psychological characteristics.

TABLE 27–1.	**Sexual history**

When puberty began

When the person as an adolescent first became aware of his or her own sexuality (e.g., for a male, when he became aware of obtaining erections and when the erections correlated with sexual stimuli or fantasies)

Personal beliefs about sex

Perception of one's sexual orientation

How the person's sexual relationships developed (e.g., when the person experienced his or her first crush and romantic kiss and how the person first learned about sex)

The nature of his or her first type of sexual contact (e.g., prolonged kissing, touching, oral sexual contact, anal sexual contact, intercourse)

Number of sexual contacts

Age range of sexual fantasies and contacts

Gender of sexual fantasies and contacts

Exposure to sexually stimulating materials (e.g., magazines, videos, books, Internet, sexting, sexual telephone calls, adult bookstores, strip clubs)

Specific focus on Internet use and exposure to paraphilic materials

Personal feelings about his or her body and sexual organs and any sexual dysfunctions

Fantasies and behaviors regarding common as well as serious sexual paraphilic disorders and related topics (e.g., voyeurism, exhibitionism, frotteurism, sexual masochism, sexual sadism, pedophilia, fetishism, transvestism, zoophilia, necrophilia, rape, killing, torture, control)

History of sexual abuse

History of incest

History of gender identity concerns or disorder

Any other pertinent sexual issue not covered previously

Visual Reaction Time

Some instruments have been developed based on the assumption that the length of viewing time of stimuli may correlate to the measure of sexual interest. The Abel Assessment for Sexual Interest is used to measure the subject's viewing time of specially designed photographs of clothed models. Although this seems like a less invasive and simple method compared with the plethysmograph, the procedure and its reliability, sensitivity, and specificity must be corroborated (Krueger et al. 1998). Abel et al. (2001) reported, however, that data support the use of their instrument.

Self-Report Measures and Other Sources of Data

Other assessments and data sources are used at times to gain additional information. A useful reference is *Assessing Sexual Abuse: A Resource Guide for Practitioners* (Prentky and Edmunds 1997). In addition to administering sex-specific self-report instruments, the clinician would be wise to administer measures of personality, trauma, and other areas of psychopathology. The clinician should be careful to correlate assessment results to the clinical evaluation, and *not depend on them for diagnosis*. Collateral sources of information may be quite helpful to corroborate claims from the person if an offense has been committed. This task may require reviewing such items as police reports, victim statements, prior mental health records, jail or prison records, sex offender treatment records, and school records. In some cases, the clinician may also consider interviewing family members, friends, or even victims to obtain additional information.

Risk Assessment of Sex Offenders

Paraphilic disorders typically come to clinical attention in the context of illegal sexual activity. A mental health professional may be asked not only to determine an appropriate diagnosis but also to address whether or not the individual is at risk to reoffend. This determination is especially important in states with sexually violent predator legislation where individuals may potentially be petitioned for civil commitment. Although the wording of the statutes may vary from state to state, in general the commitment criteria pertain to an individual who has been convicted or adjudicated guilty of a sexually violent offense and has been determined to have a mental disorder—typically a paraphilic disorder or personality disorder—that predisposes him or her to commit dangerous sexual acts. Taken together, these factors identify the individual as a danger to the health and safety of others.

Most models of risk assessment are not very successful or reliable. Risk assessment should be left to forensic experts or experts in the field, rather than being attempted in routine clinical practice.

Treatment

Therapeutic Treatment of Paraphilic Disorders

Nonpharmacological Interventions

Historically, psychoanalysis and psychodynamic therapy have been used in treating paraphilic disorders, although there is general consensus in the field that this approach alone is not effective in treating deviant sexual arousal. Currently, most sex offender treatment programs—the most common context for paraphilic disorder treatment—identify as having a cognitive-behavioral focus (McGrath et al. 2010). Cognitive-behavioral treatments typically involve skills training and cognitive restructuring to change an individual's maladaptive beliefs that lead to sex offenses. Empathy and social skills training are also often components in these types of treatment programs. Some treatments also use behavior therapies that focus on aversive conditioning to deviant fantasy as well as changes to masturbatory behavior.

Marques et al. (2005) conducted the only large-scale, randomized controlled outcome study to date with incarcerated sex offenders, utilizing a cognitive-behavioral program within a relapse prevention framework. On the basis of a follow-up period of 8 years, the study found no significant differences between treated and untreated groups. However, despite these findings, in a meta-analysis involving a total of 22,181 offenders, Schmucker and Lösel (2008) found that reoffending rates were 37% lower in treated offenders than in untreated offenders. Newer models are seeking to integrate etiological research on the maintenance of sex offending behavior; knowledge about the general therapeutic factors that contribute to change; and the risk, needs, and responsivity principles shown to be effective with antisocial populations (Andrews and Dowden 2007). Many of these newer models include a greater focus on motivation, goals, self-regulation, and criminogenic needs than on sexual deviance per se. One example is the Good Lives Model, which focuses on shared goals, values, and characteristics as well as on positive principles toward living more productive lives (Stinson and Becker 2012).

Biological Treatments of Paraphilic Disorders

Biological treatments, especially hormonal therapy, have been traditionally used for individuals with pedophilic, sexual sadism, or exhibitionistic disorder, although occasionally individuals with other paraphilic disorders receive treatment with medications (Bradford and Kaye 1999). Medication treatments are often reserved for more severe cases, especially for individuals who are at high risk to reoffend and do not respond adequately to other interventions. The general consensus is that medication treatments should not be used as the sole form of treatment for sex offenders.

No medications on the market in the United States have been approved by the U.S. Food and Drug Administration for treating paraphilic disorders or for reducing paraphilic fantasy and behavior. However, the off-label use of medications is not unusual in the treatment of psychiatric disorders, and it is accepted in the field that the use of off-label medications that have been shown in the literature to be successful in some cases may be appropriate (Ali and Ajmal 2012). The use of off-label medications is considered a current standard of care for some individuals with paraphilic disorders who do not adequately respond to first-line cognitive-behavioral therapies.

Hormonal preparations.   The main target of hormonal treatment has been the lowering of testosterone levels. Some studies (e.g., Studer et al. 2005) demonstrated a relationship between high testosterone and sexual violence. These results suggest that there may be cases in which medical lowering of testosterone levels may be helpful in decreasing the risk of recidivism in men with paraphilic disorders. Of course, one has to keep in mind that even if sexual desire is decreased pharmacologically, this does not necessarily change the patients' sexual interest or their behavior, and an unwilling patient can easily reverse the situation through testosterone replacement (Berlin 2003; Weinberger et al. 2005).

Surgical castration was used in Europe and some U.S. states in the past as a method for reducing testosterone with incarcerated sex offenders. However, some have suggested that the results from this procedure are variable, unpredictable, and irreversible, and furthermore many view it not only as highly intrusive but also as cruel and unusual punishment. Weinberger et al. (2005) reviewed the relationship of surgical castration and sexual recidivism in a sexually violent predator/sexually dangerous person population, concluding that surgically castrated sex offenders had a very low incidence of sexual recidivism. However, these authors also pointed out that although orchiectomy can reduce sexual desire, it does not completely eliminate the ability to obtain an erection in response to sexually stimulating material, and the effects can be reversed by testosterone replacement. Berlin (2005) suggested that from a treatment standpoint, although lowering testosterone can provide a decrease in sexual appetite in this population, there seems to be little reason to use surgical castration because the same effects can be achieved with testosterone-lowering medications. Surgical castration as a treatment modality for paraphilia has gradually stopped being used in most countries (it is still allowed in some countries, such as Germany [where it is permitted but not practiced] and the Czech Republic [on a voluntary basis while under the review of a special panel]).

Cyproterone acetate (CPA), a progestin derivate, was introduced in Europe and Canada, but it has never been made available in the United States. Medroxyprogesterone acetate (MPA) is available in the United States, and now gonadotropin-releasing hormone (GnRH) agonists, including leuprolide acetate, are being used. Each of these medications works because of its effect on sexual libido by ultimately, although by different mechanisms, lowering testosterone levels. Both MPA and CPA may be given orally or via long-acting intramuscular depot injection (to improve compliance). The MPA intramuscular dosages vary from 100 mg to 400 mg either weekly or less frequently (every 2–4 weeks) during the acute phase of treatment and 100–400 mg/week during the maintenance phase (oral dosing is also possible). CPA dosages range from 50 to 200 mg/day orally or 200 to 600 mg/week or less frequently intramuscularly. Importantly, these preparations do not appear to influence the direction of sexual drive toward appropriate adult partners; rather, they act to decrease libido. MPA and CPA thus work best in those persons with paraphilia who have a high sexual drive and less well in those with a low sexual drive or antisocial personality disorder (Cooper 1986). Other hormonal preparations include GnRH agonists, the pure antiandrogen flutamide, and the long-acting analogue of GnRH triptorelin.

A few researchers (Cooper et al. 1992; Hill et al. 2003) demonstrated that many sex offenders are reluctant to use hormonal treatment and that these medications can be the cause of numerous side effects, some of which are serious (Krueger et al. 2006). Hormonal treatment should not be viewed as a guarantee against recidivism, and therefore these medications should never be the sole form of treatment (Briken et al. 2004).

The most significant long-term side effects of hormonal treatment are weight gain, increased blood pressure, impaired glucose tolerance (and diabetes), deep venous thrombosis, nausea, vomiting, and decreased sperm production. Clinicians should also be aware of medical contraindications to the use of hormonal treatments; such contraindications include preexisting pituitary disease, liver disease, and thromboembolic disorders. Hormonal treatments have also been associated with cardiac complications. Osteoporosis has also been associated with each of the hormonal medications and has also been seen in surgically castrated individuals. Clinicians are advised to consult with an endocrinologist and/or internist before and during hormonal treatment.

Treatment protocols often include monitoring of blood pressure, weight, testosterone level, follicle-stimulating hormone, luteinizing hormone, prolactin, liver function, electrolytes, glucose, and complete blood count, with laboratory tests being repeated every 2–3 months until the patient is stable and then every 6 months thereafter. Bone scans of pelvis and long bones should be repeated annually, and the patient should be monitored with a physical examination yearly. One could consider also performing baseline and follow-up electrocardiographic monitoring.

The use of hormonal or antiandrogen preparations is often referred to as *chemical castration*, although we do not think this is necessarily a very helpful terminology to use.

Some U.S. states and several countries have laws regarding chemical or surgical castration of sexual offenders. Such laws in the United States have withstood legal challenge thus far, but many experts in the field have written about the ethics of such treatments with sex offenders, although it is accepted that some sex offenders can be offered medical treatments ethically (e.g., Harrison and Rainey 2009).

Serotonergic antidepressants (selective serotonin reuptake inhibitors and clomipramine). There have been a number of case reports and open-label studies reporting on the use of serotonergic antidepressants (selective serotonin reuptake inhibitors [SSRIs] and clomipramine) in treating paraphilic disorders (see Balon 1998). One pathway through which SSRIs have been proposed to be effective is by decreasing the libido due to a side effect, thus making paraphilic urges more manageable. One has to keep in mind, however, that there may be multiple reasons for their possible effectiveness. SSRIs have been helpful in treating depression, generalized anxiety disorder, panic disorder, and obsessive-compulsive disorder. Studies also have shown their benefit in such off-label uses as aggression, self-injurious behavior, and impulsivity (Goedhard et al. 2006). It is possible that the combined effects of serotonergic agents on helping to improve mood, decrease impulsivity, decrease sexual obsessions, and lead to sexual dysfunction might increase the ability of these individuals to control their paraphilic behaviors.

For various reasons (e.g., difficulty in recruitment, stigma, ethical issues), there have been no double-blind, placebo-controlled studies to test the efficacy of SSRIs in treating paraphilic disorders. However, case reports and open-label studies dating back to as early as 1990 have concluded that SSRIs can be helpful in treating paraphilic disorder and related disorders (for reviews, see Balon 1998; Greenberg and Bradford 1997). Other serotonergic agents such as clomipramine have also been studied (Clayton 1993), as has nefazodone (Coleman et al. 2000). Treatment using SSRIs may be applicable to different types of sexually inappropriate behaviors.

Kafka (2000) noted that both men with paraphilic disorders and men with nonparaphilic hypersexuality benefited from SSRI treatment and speculated that enhancement of central serotonin neurotransmission by SSRIs may ameliorate symptoms of mood disorder, heightened sexual desire, compulsivity, and impulsivity associated with these disorders. The antidepressant dosages used in treating paraphilias/paraphilic disorders have usually been higher than typical dosages—for example, in small studies, clomipramine up to 400 mg/day, desipramine up to 250 mg/day, fluoxetine up to 80 mg/day, fluvoxamine up to 300 mg/day, nefazodone up to 400 mg/day, and sertraline up to 250 mg/day (paroxetine up to 30 mg/day in one case report) (Balon 1998; Segraves and Balon 2003).

Kafka and Hennen (2000) described an open trial in which psychostimulants were added to SSRI treatment in men with paraphilic disorders. They concluded that sustained-release methylphenidate combined with SSRIs can be effective in ameliorating paraphilia/paraphilic disorder in selected cases. However, there have been no known follow-up studies to this initial investigation.

Antipsychotics. Several case reports and one study (Bourgeois and Klein 1996; Segraves and Balon 2003) described use of antipsychotics in the treatment of paraphilias (antipsychotics may decrease sexual desire via blockade of dopamine receptors). These reports included use of chlorpromazine, clozapine, risperidone, and two depot antipsychotics not available in the United States (fluphenazine enanthate and oxyprothepine decanoate). However, antipsychotics are usually not recommended for treatment of paraphilias/paraphilic disorders for various reasons, such as side effects and availability of other, safer medications such as serotonergic antidepressants.

Various other medications.   Several case reports have described use of mood stabilizers such as lithium (Cesnik and Coleman 1989) and carbamazepine (Goldberg
and Buongiorno 1982–1983). One retrospective case series of 17 patients described the
usefulness of divalproex sodium in sex offenders with bipolar disorder and comorbid
paraphilias (Nelson et al. 2001). Some clinicians reported use of buspirone (Fedoroff
1988) or cimetidine in complicated cases with comorbid disorders. Finally, the opioid
receptor antagonist naltrexone was used in a small, open-ended prospective study
(Ryback 2004).

Other Pharmacotherapy Issues (Algorithms, Special Populations)

Several treatment algorithms developed for paraphilias could be used to guide treatment of paraphilic disorders. Bradford (2000, 2001) proposed an algorithm consisting
of six levels of increasing treatment intensity, starting with Level 1, which—regardless
of the severity of the paraphilia—advocated use of cognitive-behavioral therapy and
relapse prevention treatment. Level 2 involved starting pharmacotherapy with antidepressants. If serotonergic antidepressants alone were not effective, Level 3 involved
adding a small dose of an antiandrogen to the regimen. Levels 4 and 5 involved use of
various combinations of hormonal preparations administered orally and intramuscularly (IM), respectively; and Level 6 involved implementing complete suppression of
androgens and sex drive using either CPA (200–400 mg IM once weekly) or a luteinizing hormone–releasing hormone (LHRH) agonist.

Hill et al. (2003) proposed a similar algorithm for progressive-intensity pharmacotherapy of paraphilic disorders in sex offenders, starting with SSRIs for mild paraphilias and progressing to LHRH in combination with CPA for severe cases. In this
algorithm, Hill et al. (2003) also suggested that all patients at all levels receive psychotherapy and pharmacotherapy for comorbid disorders. With that said, many clinicians begin with the use of SSRI medications, and only if the SSRIs fail to help the
patient do the clinicians progress to using hormonal treatments, which have more serious side effects.

Because adolescents are estimated to commit up to 20% of rapes and 50% of child
molestations (Hunter 2000), some have proposed using medication treatments in this
younger population. Notably, however, the majority of adolescents who commit sex-
related crimes would not typically be diagnosed with a paraphilic disorder; therefore,
reduction of sexual arousal will likely not be the primary issue of concern in most situations. However, some clinicians do feel that biological treatments may be called for
in severe cases. The use of SSRIs in the adolescent population is quite limited (Galli et
al. 1998) but may be considered with informed consent from parents or guardians.
The use of hormonal agents in the adolescent population is not without controversy,
given that these agents can suppress levels of androgens that promote the physiological changes occurring in puberty, including growth. If a trial with a hormonal agent
is deemed necessary for an adolescent, the treatment should be prescribed only for a
short period of time and only if the individual's sexual aggression has not responded
to any other treatments (Saleh and Grasswick 2005).

Conclusion

Although significant advances have been made in the risk assessment and treatment of the paraphilic disorders, many questions remain to be answered for us to be able to help patients with these disorders. By successfully treating those individuals who have paraphilic disorders that involve the victimization of children, adolescents, and adults, clinicians will also make society safer.

Key Clinical Points

- The paraphilic disorders are characterized as experiencing, over a period of at least 6 months, recurrent and intense sexually arousing fantasies, sexual urges, or behaviors, generally involving nonhuman objects or nonconsenting partners.

- If paraphilic behaviors involve only consenting partners, the diagnosis of a disorder should only be made in the presence of significant distress or psychosocial role impairment.

- If paraphilic behaviors involve nonconsenting partners, the diagnosis of a disorder may be made in the presence of objective evidence of recurrent behaviors, even when an individual denies a sexual interest in the behavior.

- It is important to keep in mind the purpose of the assessment, whether it is forensic or strictly clinical, because this may impact the methods used.

- Assessment of paraphilic disorders should be comprehensive and utilize not only self-report but also, when possible, standardized assessment instruments, physiological assessment tools, and sources of collateral information.

- A variety of behavioral therapies, hormonal treatments, and psychopharmacological treatments have been used to manage paraphilic disorders.

- In the treatment of paraphilic disorders that involve nonconsenting partners and illegal behavior, the clinician should conduct a thorough risk assessment and tailor the intensity of the intervention to the risk level.

- Treatment should focus not only on deviant sexual arousal but also on comorbid psychiatric disorders, criminogenic needs, self-regulatory deficits, and prosocial goals that lead to stability in the community.

References

Abel GG, Becker JV, Cunningham-Rathner J: Complications, consent, and cognitions in sex between children and adults. Int J Law Psychiatry 7(1):89–103, 1984 6519869

Abel GG, Jordan A, Hand CG, et al: Classification models of child molesters utilizing the Abel Assessment for sexual interest. Child Abuse Negl 25(5):703–718, 2001 11428430

Ali SI, Ajmal SR: When is off-label prescribing appropriate? Curr Psychiatr 11(7):23–27, 2012

American Psychiatric Association: Diagnostic and Statistical Manual of Mental Disorders, 4th Edition. Washington, DC, American Psychiatric Association, 1994

American Psychiatric Association: Diagnostic and Statistical Manual of Mental Disorders, 5th Edition. Arlington, VA, American Psychiatric Association, 2013

Andrews DA, Dowden C: The risk-need-responsivity model of assessment and human service in prevention and corrections: crime-prevention jurisprudence. Canadian Journal of Criminology and Criminal Justice 49(4):439–464, 2007

Balon R: Pharmacological treatment of paraphilias with a focus on antidepressants. J Sex Marital Ther 24(4):241–254, 1998 9805285

Baumeister R, Butler JL: Sexual masochism: deviance without pathology, in Sexual Deviance: Theory, Assessment, and Treatment. Edited by Laws DR, O'Donohue W. New York, Guilford, 1997, pp 225–239

Becker JV, Johnson BR, Perkins A: Paraphilic disorders, in American Psychiatric Publishing Textbook of Psychiatry, 6th Edition. Edited by Hales R, Yudofsky S, Roberts LW. Washington, DC, American Psychiatric Publishing, 2014, pp 895–925

Berlin FS: Sex offender treatment and legislation. J Am Acad Psychiatry Law 31(4):510–513, 2003 14974807

Berlin FS: Commentary: the impact of surgical castration on sexual recidivism risk among civilly committed sexual offenders. J Am Acad Psychiatry Law 33(1):37–41, 2005 15809236

Blanchard R: The DSM diagnostic criteria for transvestic fetishism. Arch Sex Behav 39(2):363–372, 2010 19757010

Blanchard R, Kuban ME, Klassen P, et al: Self-reported head injuries before and after age 13 in pedophilic and nonpedophilic men referred for clinical assessment. Arch Sex Behav 32(6):573–581, 2003 14574100

Bourgeois JA, Klein M: Risperidone and fluoxetine in the treatment of pedophilia with comorbid dysthymia. J Clin Psychopharmacol 16(3):257–258, 1996 8784662

Bradford JMW: The treatment of sexual deviation using a pharmacological approach. J Sex Res 37(3):248–257, 2000

Bradford JMW: The neurobiology, neuropharmacology, and pharmacological treatment of the paraphilias and compulsive sexual behaviour. Can J Psychiatry 46(1):26–34, 2001 11221487

Bradford J, Kaye NS: Pharmacological treatment of sexual offenders. American Academy of Psychiatry and the Law Newsletter 24:16–17, 1999

Briken P, Hill A, Berner W: A relapse in pedophilic sex offending and subsequent suicide attempt during luteinizing hormone-releasing hormone treatment. J Clin Psychiatry 65(10):1429, 2004 15491250

Browne A, Finkelhor D: Impact of child sexual abuse: a review of the research. Psychol Bull 99(1):66–77, 1986 3704036

Bunting L: Females Who Sexually Offend Against Children: Responses of the Child Protection and Criminal Justice Systems—Executive Summary. London, National Society for the Prevention of Cruelty to Children (NSPCC), 2005

Cantor JM, Blanchard R: White matter volumes in pedophiles, hebephiles, and teleiophiles. Arch Sex Behav 41(4):749–752, 2012 22476520

Cantor JM, Blanchard R, Christensen BK, et al: Intelligence, memory, and handedness in pedophilia. Neuropsychology 18(1):3–14, 2004 14744183

Cantor JM, Kabani N, Christensen BK, et al: Cerebral white matter deficiencies in pedophilic men. J Psychiatr Res 42(3):167–183, 2008 18039544

Cesnik JA, Coleman E: Use of lithium carbonate in the treatment of autoerotic asphyxia. Am J Psychother 43(2):277–286, 1989 2502035

Clayton AH: Fetishism and clomipramine. Am J Psychiatry 150(4):673–674, 1993 8465891

Coleman E, Gratzer T, Nesvacil L, et al: Nefazodone and the treatment of nonparaphilic compulsive sexual behavior: a retrospective study. J Clin Psychiatry 61(4):282–284, 2000 10830149

Cooper AJ: Progestogens in the treatment of male sex offenders: a review. Can J Psychiatry 31(1):73–79, 1986 2936441

Cooper AJ, Sandhu S, Losztyn S, et al: A double-blind placebo controlled trial of medroxyprogesterone acetate and cyproterone acetate with seven pedophiles. Can J Psychiatry 37(10):687–693, 1992 1473073

Faller KCJ: Clinical sample of women who have sexually abused children. Journal of Child Sexual Abuse 4(3):13–30, 1995

Fedoroff JP: Buspirone hydrochloride in the treatment of transvestic fetishism. J Clin Psychiatry 49(10):408–409, 1988 3271001

Freund K, Blanchard R: Phallometric diagnosis of pedophilia. J Consult Clin Psychol 57(1):100–105, 1989 2925958

Freund K, Watson R, Rienzo D: Signs of feigning in the phallometric test. Behav Res Ther 26(2):105–112, 1988 3365200

Freund K, Seto MC, Kuban M: Frotteurism: the theory of courtship disorder, in Sexual Deviance: Theory, Assessment, and Treatment. Edited by Laws DR, O'Donohue W. New York, Guilford, 1997, pp 111–130

Galli VB, Raute NJ, McConville BJ, et al: An adolescent male with multiple paraphilias successfully treated with fluoxetine. J Child Adolesc Psychopharmacol 8(3):195–197, 1998 9853694

Goedhard LE, Stolker JJ, Heerdink ER, et al: Pharmacotherapy for the treatment of aggressive behavior in general adult psychiatry: a systematic review. J Clin Psychiatry 67(7):1013–1024, 2006 16889443

Goldberg RL, Buongiorno PA: The use of carbamazepine for the treatment of paraphilias in a brain damaged patient. Int J Psychiatry Med 12(4):275–279, 1982–1983 7166459

Greenberg DM, Bradford JM: Treatment of the paraphilic disorders: a review of the role of the selective serotonin reuptake inhibitors. Sex Abuse 9(4):349–360, 1997

Harrison K, Rainey G: Suppressing human rights? A rights-based approach to the use of pharmacotherapy with sex offenders. Legal Studies 29(1):47–74, 2009

Hill A, Briken P, Kraus C, et al: Differential pharmacological treatment of paraphilias and sex offenders. Int J Offender Ther Comp Criminol 47(4):407–421, 2003 12971182

Hunter JA: Understanding Juvenile Sex Offending: Research Findings and Guidelines for Effective Treatment. Juvenile Justice Fact Sheet. Charlottesville, VA, Institute of Law, Psychiatry, and Public Policy, University of Virginia, 2000

Kafka MP: Psychopharmacologic treatments for nonparaphilic compulsive sexual behaviors. CNS Spectr 5(1):49–59, 2000 18311100

Kafka MP: The DSM diagnostic criteria for fetishism. Arch Sex Behav 39(2):357–362, 2010 19795202

Kafka MP, Hennen J: Psychostimulant augmentation during treatment with selective serotonin reuptake inhibitors in men with paraphilias and paraphilia-related disorders: a case series. J Clin Psychiatry 61(9):664–670, 2000 11030487

Krueger RB: The DSM diagnostic criteria for sexual masochism. Arch Sex Behav 39(2):346–356, 2010a 20221792

Krueger RB: The DSM diagnostic criteria for sexual sadism. Arch Sex Behav 39(2):325–345, 2010b 19997774

Krueger R, Bradford J, Glancy G: Report from the Committee on Sex Offenders: the Abel Assessment for Sexual Interest—a brief description. J Am Acad Psychiatry Law 26(2):277–280, 1998 9664263

Krueger RB, Hembree W, Hill M: Prescription of medroxyprogesterone acetate to a patient with pedophilia, resulting in Cushing's syndrome and adrenal insufficiency. Sex Abuse 18(2):227–228, 2006 16868842

Långström N: The DSM diagnostic criteria for exhibitionism, voyeurism, and frotteurism. Arch Sex Behav 39(2):317–324, 2010 19924524

Långström N, Seto MC: Exhibitionistic and voyeuristic behavior in a Swedish national population survey. Arch Sex Behav 35(4): 427–435, 2006 16900414

Marques JK, Wiederanders M, Day DM, et al: Effects of a relapse prevention program on sexual recidivism: final results from California's Sex Offender Treatment and Evaluation Project (SOTEP). Sex Abuse 17(1):79–107, 2005 15757007

McGrath RJ, Cumming GF, Burchard BL, et al: Current Practices and Emerging Trends in Sexual Abuser Management. Brandon, VT, Safer Society Press, 2010

Nelson E, Brusman L, Holcomb J, et al: Divalproex sodium in sex offenders with bipolar disorders and comorbid paraphilias: an open retrospective study. J Affect Disord 64(2–3):249–255, 2001 11313091

Peter T: Exploring taboos comparing male- and female-perpetrated child sexual abuse. J Interpers Violence 24(7):1111–1128, 2009 18701747

Prentky RA, Edmunds SB: Assessing Sexual Abuse: A Resource Guide for Practitioners. Brandon, VT, Safer Society Press, 1997

Ryback RS: Naltrexone in the treatment of adolescent sexual offenders. J Clin Psychiatry 65(7):982–986, 2004 15291688

Saleh FM, Grasswick LJ: Juvenile sexual offenders. American Academy of Psychiatry and the Law Newsletter 30:12–13, 2005

Schmucker M, Lösel F: Does sexual offender treatment work? A systematic review of outcome evaluations. Psicothema 20(1):10–19, 2008 18206060

Segraves RT, Balon R: Sexual Pharmacology: Fast Facts New York, WW Norton, 2003, pp 287–311

Seto MC: Pedophilia: psychopathology and theory, in Sexual Deviance: Theory, Assessment, and Treatment, 2nd Edition. Edited by Laws DR, O'Donohue WT. New York, Guilford, 2008, pp 164–182

Stinson JD, Becker JV: Treating Sex Offenders: An Evidence-Based Manual. New York, Guilford, 2012

Studer LH, Aylwin AS, Reddon JR: Testosterone, sexual offense recidivism, and treatment effect among adult male sex offenders. Sex Abuse 17(2):171–181, 2005 15974423

Weinberger LE, Sreenivasan S, Garrick T, et al: The impact of surgical castration on sexual recidivism risk among sexually violent predatory offenders. J Am Acad Psychiatry Law 33(1):16–36, 2005 15809235

World Health Organization: International Statistical Classification of Diseases and Related Health Problems, 10th Revision. Geneva, World Health Organization, 1992

Recommended Readings

Balon R: Practical Guide to Paraphilia and Paraphilic Disorders. New York, Springer, 2016

Laws DR, O'Donohue WT (eds): Sexual Deviance: Theory, Assessment, and Treatment, 2nd Edition. New York, Guilford, 2008

PART III

Treatments

CHAPTER 28

Precision Psychiatry

Leanne M. Williams, Ph.D.
Tali M. Ball, Ph.D.
Catherine L. Kircos, M.A.

A revolution is under way in psychiatry. We are witnessing the emergence of precision medicine for psychiatry: "precision psychiatry." Precision psychiatry is an integrative approach, one that pulls together the scientific foundations of the discipline and recent technological advances and directs them toward closing the gap between discovery and clinical translation. Today, although many effective treatments are available, finding the right treatment for the right patient is largely a matter of trial and error, and treatment selection is not linked to a precise understanding of an individual patient's pathophysiology. In addition, efforts to prevent psychiatric conditions are in their infancy. The goals of precision psychiatry are threefold: *precise classification* (i.e., a specific understanding of the pathophysiology of each individual patient—what has gone wrong?), *precise treatment planning* (i.e., tailoring treatment plans in a personalized manner—how can we fix what has gone wrong?), and *precise prevention* (i.e., targeted and tailored prevention strategies—how can we keep things from going wrong?).

The first of these three goals, precise classification, hinges on identification of subtype profiles (or "biotypes") that coherently map neurobiological disruptions onto symptoms and behaviors, take into account life experience and context, and are relevant to guiding treatment choices (Williams 2016). These profiles and biotypes may in some instances align with our rich symptom classifications, currently defined by the *Diagnostic and Statistical Manual of Mental Disorders*, 5th edition (DSM-5; American Psychiatric Association 2013); in other cases may cut across diagnostic classifications; and in still others may reflect unforeseen, novel subtypes. Precision psychiatry, a rapidly emerging field, encompasses the discovery of these new subtypes as well as their application to treatment and prevention. Although the scientific insights and treatment models on which precision psychiatry is based are well established, the dissemination of scientific insights into clinical practice is now on the horizon.

In this chapter we present our view of precision psychiatry and why it is needed. Our primary focus is on the organ of dysfunction in psychiatry: the brain. At the same time, we recognize the complementary importance of other domains, such as genetics, life history, and cognition. We review emerging findings that form the foundations of precise classification, initial results for precise treatment planning, and promising directions for precise prevention. Mood disorders, anxiety and traumatic stress disorders, and psychosis receive the most representation in this review due to the predominance of research in these disorder classes. We conclude by highlighting what is needed to accelerate precision psychiatry from vision to reality.

Precision Psychiatry in the National Spotlight

The urgent need for precision medicine in general, and for precision psychiatry in particular, is in the national spotlight. The emergence of precision psychiatry is part of a new national focus on precision medicine (Hudson et al. 2015). Federal initiatives focus on three important and interrelated aspects of a precision approach to psychiatry and other complex disorders: 1) precise classification—acquiring a more precise understanding of the characteristics that contribute to a person's experience of a given disorder, 2) precise treatment planning—learning how to use this more precise understanding to tailor treatments in a more personalized way, and 3) precise prevention—learning how to use this precise understanding to develop more targeted prevention strategies. Precision medicine encompasses other interchangeably used terms: *stratified medicine, personalized medicine,* and *precision health,* respectively (Fernandes et al. 2017; FORUM Academy of Medical Sciences 2015). *Stratified medicine* focuses on identifying subgroups of patients who will benefit from treatments as a step toward a fully personalized approach that tailors treatments to individual people. *Personalized medicine* has focused on harnessing new advances in genomics to identify treatment options with the greatest likelihood of success. *Precision health* can be thought of as a major new frontier, expanding our breakthroughs in precision medicine to a wider concept of health and prevention that goes beyond a focus on disease.

In 2015, the Obama administration launched the Precision Medicine Initiative, a major research effort aimed at improving health and changing the way we treat disease (Office of the Press Secretary 2015a). In the press release announcing this initiative, precision medicine was defined as "an innovative approach that takes into account individual differences in people's genes, environments, and lifestyles," thereby allowing doctors to tailor treatment to individual patients (Office of the Press Secretary 2015a, para. 2). In his remarks at the launching of the Precision Medicine Initiative, President Obama said: "Precision medicine—in some cases, people call it personalized medicine—gives us one of the greatest opportunities for new medical breakthroughs that we have ever seen" (Office of the Press Secretary 2015b, para. 11).

This federal Precision Medicine Initiative is paralleled by two federal research efforts focused specifically on psychiatry and neurosciences. First, the "BRAIN Initiative" is aimed at developing neurotechnologies for demystifying brain disorders, including psychiatric disorders (Markoff 2013). This depth of understanding of the brain will strengthen our ability to precisely identify dysfunction at the level of a single patient. Second, the National Institute of Mental Health (NIMH) is pioneering the

Research Domain Criteria (RDoC) project (Insel et al. 2010), which has initiated a research approach to generating a neurobiologically valid framework for classifying psychiatric disorders and for generating novel interventions related to neurobiological underpinnings. Together, the Precision Medicine, BRAIN, and RDoC initiatives will support and promote significant advances in precision psychiatry.

Forecasting the Path of Precision Psychiatry by Analogy With Other Revolutions in Precision Medicine

An analogy can be made between the new advances on the path of precision psychiatry and the path traversed by other areas of medicine that are further along in closing the gap between scientific and technological advances and their clinical applications. For example, just 70 years ago, the tools to measure the unobservable aspects of heart structure and function—such as fluoroscopy, multidetector computed tomography, ultrasound, magnetic resonance imaging (MRI), myocardial perfusion scintigraphy, echocardiography, and positron emission tomography (PET)—were not available. Physicians would have attempted to personalize their assessments to each patient, yet they were not able to observe the heart's behavior or how it related to observable symptoms prior to the incorporation of measurements. Today this ability is taken for granted. The shift began in 1948 with the Framingham study, which was inspired by Franklin Delano Roosevelt's death from cardiovascular disease (Mahmood et al. 2014). The Framingham study spawned the assessment of standard vital signs and a subsequent range of imaging techniques capable of linking precise insights about the organ of interest (the heart) to treatment indications and even prevention. It is now routine to take serial images to provide a baseline from which to assess each individual's progress toward recovery and subsequent risk for relapse or new problems. These measurements also inform the development of a personalized plan that considers the whole individual, including lifestyle and diet alongside medical interventions. For example, the echocardiogram can be used to identify types of arrhythmia (e.g., too fast, too slow, irregular) and to indicate specific treatments (e.g., pacemaker), and the angiogram can confirm the presence of blockage (e.g., emboli, stroke, myocardial infarction) and indicate other treatments (e.g., lifestyle changes, medications, surgery) (Gladding et al. 2013).

More recently, a similar revolution in precision medicine has been under way in oncology. Scientific and technical advances in personalized genomics have revolutionized care by enabling physicians to test a person's cancer to find out if a certain type of treatment will work on it, to know from the patient's genetic code whether he or she will be able to cope with the treatment, and to undertake genetic testing to identify the person's future risks for cancer. Because testing of the genetic makeup of tumors has become a relatively quick and low-cost procedure, it has rapidly become one of the catalysts propelling progress in personalized cancer care. To enhance precision, genetic information is increasingly being integrated with tumor imaging findings to further characterize each patient's cancer profile and to tailor treatment needs accordingly (Letai 2017).

A major challenge for precision medicine in psychiatry is that psychiatry does not yet use measurement to track the equivalent of vitals (Harding et al. 2011) or to image the organ of interest (the brain). Although modern neuroimaging techniques have generated many insights about types of brain circuit dysfunction that underlie psychiatric disorders, these insights have not been systematically linked to prediction of clinical outcomes and have not been delivered into the hands of clinicians as a usable system for improving people's lives. That precision psychiatry is "new to the game" in precision medicine is not surprising, given the complexity of the organ and behavior of interest. However, psychiatry can benefit tremendously by incorporating advanced diagnostic and therapeutic technologies that form an integral part of other clinical specialties.

Envisioning New Models for Precision Psychiatry

Paradigm shifts in the integration of psychiatry with neuroscience and neurotechnology are set to accelerate the development of precision psychiatry. The integration of psychiatry and neuroscience is motivated by the search for a model that connects a neurobiological understanding of psychiatric disorders with clinical phenomenology in order to improve the precision of classification, treatment decisions, and prevention efforts. Thus far, clinicians and clinical researchers have tended to be oriented toward precision in terms of predictors of treatment outcomes or disease progression, independent of disease mechanism. In contrast, neuroscientists and other basic researchers have been oriented toward precision in terms of mechanistic understanding, independent of meaningful clinical outcomes. Precision psychiatry requires effective interdisciplinary collaboration between these orientations.

In addition to the integration of clinical and basic research agendas, precision psychiatry also requires an integration of multimodal data over time. An important direction for precision psychiatry is not only to identify the neurobiological bases of disorders in order to build out the scientific foundations of our discipline but also to understand the mechanisms by which disorders develop and change over time. With the advent of noninvasive functional neuroimaging (e.g., PET, functional MRI), we now have more precise methods for quantifying the brain in action, and synthesizing multiple sources of complex data over time becomes feasible.

A dimensional framework is pertinent for conceptualizing these mechanisms. Within a dimensional framework, we could consider psychiatric disorders as disorders of functional systems and their underlying neural circuits. Variables such as brain activation and connectivity may be considered to serve a dual function; on the one hand, they contribute to normal variation in brain capacities, and on the other, they also confer vulnerability to mental disorders. Observable discontinuities in behavior may occur when neural trait vulnerabilities are coupled with other risk factors, such as environmental hazards (e.g., stress), and pushed to their extreme. An analogous variable in cardiovascular disease would be blood pressure, which has a fairly wide range of normal distribution but also can confer vulnerability to pathological conditions when higher levels are reached. Furthermore, observable discontinuities such as stroke may occur when high blood pressure (producing hypertension) is coupled with the effects of other risk factors (e.g., stress, diet). Although this analogy does not capture the complexity of brain circuits and their interactions, it serves as an illustration of how extremes of brain activation and connectivity can produce identifiable failures of function and result in psychiatric disorders.

Overall, there has been a tremendous accumulation of knowledge regarding brain circuitry and genomics in psychiatric disorders. This knowledge has formed the foundation of large biomarker discovery trials using neuroimaging and genetic measures (Dunlop et al. 2012; Tamminga et al. 2014; Trivedi et al. 2016; Williams et al. 2011). In the following discussion, we highlight emerging literature on the foundational neuroimaging and genetic markers and provide examples of their use in achieving precise classification, as well as in tailoring treatment and prevention efforts.

Foundations for Precise Classification: Neuroimaging

Psychiatric disorders have not always been considered "brain diseases"; rather, the term *brain disease* has been more consistently used to refer to neurological conditions associated with a discrete lesion or degenerative process. This usage may reflect our limited understanding of the dynamics of the brain and the fact that psychiatric disorders are functional expressions of subtler pathologies. With the advent of brain imaging techniques with sufficient spatial and temporal resolution to quantify neural connections in vivo, particularly functional MRI, we can begin to reformulate our understanding of mental illnesses as disorders of brain *functioning* (Tretter and Gebicke-Haerter 2011). Modern imaging technologies allow researchers to see the brain at work, examine differences in how an individual's brain is functioning, and use those differences to predict what treatments may work best for that individual.

Researchers using these technologies have identified an intrinsic neural architecture of large-scale circuits (e.g., Cole et al. 2014). The universality of this intrinsic architecture has been demonstrated with meta-analyses of the relationships among brain regions in the brain at rest, termed *functional connectivity* (Cole et al. 2014). There is also converging evidence that these same intrinsic circuits are disrupted in psychiatric disorders (Williams 2016).

Of particular interest are the default mode, salience, and attention (sometimes called *central executive* or *frontoparietal*) circuits. The default mode circuit has core nodes in the anterior and posterior cingulate cortex and has been implicated in self-reflective thought. High functional connectivity in this circuit is thought to reflect maladaptive self-referential thought such as rumination and worry (Hamilton et al. 2015). The salience circuit has core nodes in the anterior cingulate cortex, amygdala, and anterior insula and is thought to detect salient internal sensations and external changes. Low functional connectivity in this circuit has been associated with social anxiety disorder and may reflect anxious avoidance (reviewed in Williams 2016). The attention circuit has core nodes in the medial superior frontal cortex, anterior inferior parietal lobe, anterior insula, and precuneus. Low functional connectivity in this circuit is thought to reflect the inattention symptoms common across psychiatric disorders (Williams 2016).

In addition to this intrinsic architecture, large-scale circuits related to specific processing of threat, reward, and cognitive load have been identified. The extent to which these circuits are engaged by threatening, rewarding, or cognitively challenging tasks varies across individuals and may relate to specific biomarkers of psychopathology.

For example, increased activation in the amygdala in response to threatening stimuli has been associated with heightened anxiety (Shin and Liberzon 2010), whereas decreased activation in the ventral striatum, a core node of the reward circuit, has been associated with anhedonia (Der-Avakian and Markou 2012).

Several promising findings provide proof-of-concept illustrative examples of subtypes of disorders based on specific dysfunctions in brain circuits. By synthesizing research findings on the circuits just described, we have identified eight biotypes that may underlie different subtypes of affective psychopathology (Williams 2016). Although these biotypes are anchored in brain circuits, we anticipate that they can be refined based on genetic variation and specific symptom profiles. The ultimate test of this brain circuit biotype model will be its ability to differentially predict treatment outcomes. Data-driven approaches have similarly identified subtypes for depression based on resting-state brain imaging data and for psychotic disorders based on electroencephalographic data (e.g., Clementz et al. 2016).

Foundations for Precise Classification: Genetics

Over the past decade there has been significant progress in research on the genetics of mental disorders, as there has been for imaging. Psychiatric disorders that have been studied intensively in genome-wide analyses (Sullivan et al. 2012) and in studies of candidate genetic variants (Gatt et al. 2015) include major depressive disorder, bipolar disorder, schizophrenia, attention-deficit/hyperactivity disorder, and autism spectrum disorder (Psychiatric Genomics Consortium 2016). The results across studies indicate that the etiology of psychiatric disorders involves both rare and common genetic variants. Results also highlight the polygenic nature of psychiatric disorders, just like other complex biomedical diseases. Indeed, former NIMH director Thomas Insel noted that precision medicine for mental disorders will likely "not come from a single genomic glitch. Rather, like many other areas of medicine, many genes each contribute only a small amount of vulnerability as part of an overall risk profile that includes life experiences, neurodevelopment, and social and cultural factors" (Insel 2015, para. 3).

The rigor of large-scale genetic studies has been laudable, and the findings have accelerated insights into the neurobiology of psychiatric disorders. Possibly because of the genetic complexity and polygenic nature of these disorders, however, the current findings are not directly applicable to precision diagnostics. Nonetheless, the findings on the shared versus specific genetic contributions to psychiatric disorders are important for developing new models for precise classification, and for forging ahead with initiatives such as RDoC (Doherty and Owen 2014). For example, insights into the genetic architecture of psychiatric disorders promise to yield a comprehensive understanding of pathways contributing to the onset, prognosis, and functional management of psychiatric illnesses (Sullivan et al. 2012). It is also worth noting one area of direct clinical application: for autism spectrum disorder, there is active pursuit of the translation of genetic insights into genetic tests for screening and diagnosis (Schaefer et al. 2008), especially in regard to genomic structural variation.

As we develop computational horsepower, there are exciting opportunities to integrate our current knowledge with next-generation "omics" to expand our insights into precision classification and treatment prediction. For example, analysis of metabolomes (i.e., the set of small-molecule metabolites within human tissue) provides a window into changes in body biochemistry as a function of treatment response and allows us to correlate changes in the metabolome with genes in relevant pathways. Analysis of human microbiomes (i.e., the genomes of microorganisms within the body) provides a window into certain bacterial species that have the capacity to modulate the stress response and have shown antidepressant effects in animal models (Wang and Kasper 2014).

Foundations for Precise Treatment Planning

Precise classification based on etiologically relevant biomarkers such as neuroimaging and genetic factors is valuable only to the extent that it improves patients' lives. Precisely diagnosing a problem allows precise tailoring of treatment choices—for example, identifying which patients may benefit from pharmacotherapy and which patients may not, selecting among types of pharmacotherapy, and limiting side effects. Several biomarker trials have yielded potential predictors relevant to precise treatment planning, and more are under way (Trivedi et al. 2016).

The international Study to Predict Optimized Treatment for Depression (iSPOT-D) trial (Williams et al. 2011) uncovered several promising predictors of treatment response. This study randomly assigned more than 1,000 adults with major depressive disorder to escitalopram, sertraline, or venlafaxine. All participants received a comprehensive baseline assessment of symptoms, cognitive function, electroencephalography, and genetics, and a subset received functional neuroimaging. The iSPOT-D trial found that clinical variables such as early-life stress (Williams et al. 2016) and high levels of anxious arousal (Saveanu et al. 2015) predicted poorer treatment response to any medication, while higher body mass index predicted better response specifically to venlafaxine (Green et al. 2017). Functional neuroimaging analyses have suggested that intact cognitive control circuitry (Gyurak et al. 2016) and less-responsive threat circuitry (Williams et al. 2015) are predictive of good antidepressant outcomes. Importantly, interactions and combinations of predictors are beginning to be examined (Goldstein-Piekarski et al. 2016) so that recommendations can be made for patients with more than one predictive marker.

The iSPOT-D trial, as well as other efforts, also identified genetic predictors of antidepressant outcomes. A single-nucleotide polymorphism in the *ABCB1* gene (which plays a role in controlling antidepressant concentrations in the brain) predicts good response to escitalopram and sertraline for individuals with the common variant and good response to venlafaxine for those with the more rare variant (Schatzberg et al. 2015). Hypothalamic-pituitary-adrenal (HPA) axis and cortisol genes have also been implicated in determining who is likely to experience symptom remission with antidepressants (O'Connell et al. 2018). Finally, Mayo Clinic researchers are working with industry partners to evaluate the utility of individualized genetic prediction of antidepressant choice in practice and have focused on candidate genes identified in the literature, including *SLC6AF* and *HTR2A* (Hodgson et al. 2012). These efforts have the potential to address needs at the population level, given that major depressive disorder is now the leading cause of disability in the United States, that antidepressants are the second most frequently prescribed pharmacotherapy in the United States after cholesterol-lowering drugs (IMS Institute for Healthcare Informatics 2015), and that the antidepressant decision process is otherwise one of trial and error.

In addition to treatment selection, precise treatment planning must also consider side-effect burden and when to layer multiple treatment modalities. For example, a review of potential biomarkers of psychosis identified a pharmacogenetic biomarker in the *HLA-DQB1* gene that predicts significantly greater risk for clozapine-induced agranulocytosis (Prata et al. 2014). In addition, impaired cognition has been highlighted as a key predictor of poor functional outcomes in both psychosis (Nuechterlein et al. 2011) and depression (Etkin et al. 2015), suggesting that a cognitive rehabilitation program could be a valuable treatment component to include for patients with this profile.

The majority of these biomarker studies have found 70% predictive accuracy or greater, suggesting that these markers have clinical utility. Although these estimates may diminish following external validation studies (i.e., in which replications are attempted in completely independent samples), they still reflect great promise. Given that current treatment-matching approaches essentially involve trial and error and that most patients do not respond to their first medication, even a small increase in predictive accuracy would be worthwhile. Furthermore, there is minimal risk in a novel strategy to select between U.S. Food and Drug Administration (FDA)–approved treatments of comparable overall efficacy.

Foundations for Precise Prevention

The truly transformative potential of precision psychiatry lies in a precise understanding of risk and resilience that can ultimately prevent psychiatric disorders from occurring in the first place. A longer-term goal for precision psychiatry is therefore to detect problems earlier and to deploy targeted strategies for prevention. Most work in this area has focused on secondary or tertiary prevention, such as identifying risk factors to more precisely and efficiently predict conversion from prodromal schizophrenia to full psychosis (Lawrie et al. 2016). These risk factors include clinical symptoms such as odd behaviors, negative symptoms, sensorimotor dysfunction, and social isolation, as well as biomarkers such as polygenic risk scores, white matter integrity, and D_2 dopamine receptor occupancy (Millan et al. 2016). The promise of precision psychiatry is that these risk factors could be used to target early intervention strategies (e.g., Kreyenbuhl et al. 2016) based on each individual's specific constellation of risk and protective factors.

Precision psychiatry can also apply to the prevention of comorbidities. For example, ongoing research at Stanford University is applying precision psychiatry to the prevention of premature mortality. People with serious mental illness on average die a decade or more earlier than people without psychiatric disorders, due to a combination of illness sequelae (e.g., suicide, substance abuse), social and economic consequences of psychiatric disorders, and increased burden of co-occurring medical conditions (Roberts et al. 2017). Researchers are working to identify at-risk individuals and families and to develop interventions to preempt and prevent problems.

Precision prevention efforts are most likely to succeed when they are grounded in data from large-scale prospective, longitudinal studies. For example, the Army Study To Assess Risk and Resilience in Servicemembers (STARRS) and its newer longitudinal counterpart, Army STARRS–LS, are Department of Defense–funded large-scale projects ($N > 70,000$) that aim to provide information that can be acted upon to prevent major negative outcomes in U.S. Army service members. This project has already identified complex combinations of clinical and demographic variables (e.g., anger outbursts, insomnia, low education, high religiosity, childhood maltreatment) that predict negative outcomes such as psychiatric diagnoses, suicide attempts, violent behavior, or victimization (Bandoli et al. 2017; Rosellini et al. 2017; Stein et al. 2018). Genetic risk for suicidal behavior and posttraumatic stress disorder are also being explored (Stein et al. 2016, 2017).

Closing the Clinical Translational Gap

Despite the admirable progress described in the preceding section, precision psychiatry is not yet a clinical reality. In order to escalate progress toward a clinically applicable precision psychiatry model of mental disorders, there is a need for standardized protocols, inclusion of multiple diagnoses, normative data, multimodal data integration, new computational models, and application of precision psychiatry to optimize existing interventions and develop novel interventions (Figure 28–1).

Standardized Protocols

Currently, our understanding of the role that brain circuits and their activation play in clinical dysfunction is limited in part by inconsistent findings stemming from a lack of standardization across research protocols. To advance the field of precision psychiatry, it will be necessary to undertake larger, multisite, multidiagnostic investigations made possible by the use of standardized protocols, integrative analytic models, and databases (reviewed in Siegle 2011). This approach has been implemented with success in several imaging studies to date (e.g., Trivedi et al. 2016). While novel imaging protocols are important for new scientific discoveries, standardized protocols will be essential for the future viability of routine scans for mental health assessment. With use of standardized protocols, it becomes feasible to pursue multidiagnostic samples and to thus parse the features and phenotypes that characterize individuals in common across as well as within diagnoses (see Figure 28–1).

Norms and Clinical Thresholds

In order to incorporate pathophysiology into psychiatric diagnoses, we must be able to define for each person whether they have normal or abnormal functioning. This is straightforward for self-report scales and cognitive testing, for which population norms are often available. Genomic data, being inherently categorical, can also be clearly separated into normal and abnormal risk/variants. Neuroimaging, however, poses more of a challenge. It will therefore be important to define the normative distribution of neural circuit function in healthy individuals (as in Ball et al. 2017) and to identify thresholds for overt disorder and failures of function. Methods for establishing the reproducibility of imaging data across people, sites, and time are also needed.

Integration Across Modalities Within the Same Patients

Currently, our insights about the neurobiological, genetic, behavioral, and experiential characteristics of psychiatric disorders are typically derived from studies that have focused on the individual contributions of these characteristics rather than their

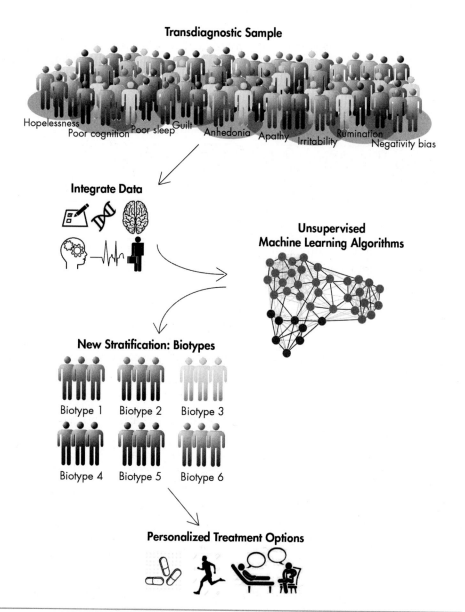

Transdiagnostic Sample

Hopelessness
Poor cognition   Poor sleep   Guilt   Anhedonia   Apathy   Irritability   Rumination   Negativity bias

Integrate Data

Unsupervised Machine Learning Algorithms

New Stratification: Biotypes

Biotype 1   Biotype 2   Biotype 3

Biotype 4   Biotype 5   Biotype 6

Personalized Treatment Options

FIGURE 28–1. One path toward closing the clinical translational gap between research insights and clinical practice.

To view this figure in color, see Plate 9 in Color Gallery in middle of book.

This flow diagram illustrates a proposed framework for escalating progress toward a clinically applicable precision psychiatry model of mental disorders: **(1) Transdiagnostic Sample**—Use standardized protocols and assessments that apply across multidiagnostic clinical samples and normative samples, allowing for a focus on features that are common to individuals across as well as within diagnoses; **(2) Integrate Data**—Gather and integrate data across clinical, genomic, imaging, cognitive behavior, physiological, and life history domains; **(3) Unsupervised Machine Learning Algorithms**—Harness new computational approaches to learn from the integrated data; **(4) New Stratification: Biotypes**—Identify coherent relations between clinical features and integrated domains of data that define new ways to stratify patients that may cut across some traditional diagnostic boundaries; for example, the term *biotype* is used to refer to coherent relations between profiles of brain function assessed by neuroimaging and profiles of symptoms and behavior; **(5) Personalized Treatment Options**—Use these data-derived stratification approaches in prospective and target-driven trials to optimize the choice of existing interventions and develop.

combined effects. Correspondingly, within each of these domains of characteristics, the focus has typically been on a particular modality (such as functional imaging or structural imaging) rather than on the integration of information across modalities. Of course, this modality-specific focus has been necessary for building the requisite scientific and technological foundations. Yet an integrated understanding of a patient across modalities will be essential to advance precision psychiatry.

Systematic mapping of combinatorial and interactive insights across modalities is a significant challenge and requires purposeful interdisciplinary effort (see Figure 28–1). We could consider imaging as just one starting point for directing such effort. To refine classifications based on neural circuits, there is a need to consider the relations among activation, connectivity, and structure within a circuit, as well as the more nuanced interactions between circuits. In parallel, there is a need to dig more deeply to elucidate the precise ways in which brain circuits relate to behavior and symptoms—for example, which specific symptoms reflect the activation of particular circuits? Are there symptoms that reflect a "final common pathway" as the outcome of multiple different types of circuit disruptions? Does a change in a brain circuits predict a change in symptoms? An integrated understanding of how neural circuit dysfunctions are modulated by more distal factors, such as genetic variation, genetic expression, and life events and their interaction, will also be paramount. These multimodal efforts will necessarily accumulate increasingly "big data." In turn, big data require computational innovation.

Computational Innovation

Handling large integrated datasets in a manner that translates insights into clinically meaningful outcomes requires special attention to computational approaches (see Figure 28–1). Broadly speaking, there are two complementary approaches to computational psychiatry: data driven and theory driven (for a review and synthesis, see Huys et al. 2016). Results from previously mentioned classification studies highlight the value of data-driven approaches, for which there are no priors from existing knowledge (e.g., Drysdale et al. 2017). By contrast, theoretical approaches are based on mathematical specifications and include algorithmic, biophysical, and Bayesian learning models (for a review, see Huys et al. 2016). Regardless of the exact approach, it is increasingly recognized in psychiatry (as it is in other areas of medicine) that demonstrating the reproducibility of findings is key to ultimately having sufficient confidence to warrant clinical translation.

Optimizing Existing Interventions and Generating New Ones

Short-term progress can be made using precision psychiatry to better match patients to existing treatments and/or prevention strategies (see Figure 28–1); however, longer-term progress in precision psychiatry will come from improving existing interventions and generating new ones. As etiologically based subtypes of psychiatric disorders are discovered, new medications can be developed to target specific deficits. For example, based on results from genome-wide association studies, Drs. Michael Ostacher and Roy Perlis and their colleagues are evaluating the "re-purposing" of isradipine (an FDA-approved antihypertensive drug that interacts with the protein product of *CAC-*

NA1C) for the treatment of bipolar disorder. Preliminary proof-of-concept findings are promising (Ostacher et al. 2014).

New medications designed to boost psychotherapy efficacy are also being developed; several compounds (e.g., D-cycloserine, glucocorticoids, cannabinoids) are candidates that may improve learning in exposure therapy for anxiety disorders based on their ability to induce cellular learning in animal models. Initial findings in humans have been mixed but suggest that such augmentation strategies may be used effectively as part of a precision approach, whereby augmentation is offered specifically to the patients who are most likely to benefit from its use (e.g., Smits et al. 2013).

In addition, new technological advances, such as repetitive transcranial magnetic stimulation (rTMS), allow for new intervention strategies that can capitalize on emerging neurobiological insights and iteratively increase precision. rTMS, a noninvasive high-frequency stimulation of the cortex, is an FDA-approved intervention for depression when applied to the left dorsolateral prefrontal cortex. It was initially conceptualized as an intervention for treatment-resistant depression due to the low response and remission rates for rTMS in early trials. However, applications of rTMS are rapidly expanding to allow precise tailoring based on individual patients' circuit-level dysfunction, with corresponding increases in response and remission rates (Downar and Daskalakis 2013). The rTMS clinic of the future may precisely match the location, frequency, and intensity of stimulation to individual patients' needs in order to minimize side effects and optimize efficacy.

Considering the Impacts on Society and the Challenges for Application

Even if all of the preceding issues are resolved and the scientific grounding of precision psychiatry is accelerated, realizing the promise of precision psychiatry will rely on a variety of societal and systems-level factors. Even after a consensus is reached about which evidence is "field ready," translating precision models from the laboratory to the clinic will require the capacity to provide access to new assessment techniques such as neuroimaging and genetics on a greater scale, integrate these new techniques with existing workflow and reimbursement models, develop training for new approaches, and carefully consider social and ethical issues.

Scale and Access Issues

Many promising findings in precision psychiatry rely on techniques—such as genetic assays and functional neuroimaging—that are currently not widely available, in part because of relatively high costs and other logistical hurdles. Similar hurdles in other branches of medicine have been overcome through a stepped approach; for example, in cardiovascular medicine, imaging tools that require intensive on-site testing may be indicated when symptoms are present and function is being disrupted, whereas field-accessible tests such as blood pressure cuffs are available for routine screening, and commercially available sensors can track fitness and heart health indicators over time to monitor patients' adherence to treatments or to detect changes that may need further assessment. With the technology and app revolution has come a panoply of opportunities for such monitoring and collection of real-time mental health–related information about individuals. The challenge is how to tie this information to routine clinical screenings and ultimately to electronic medical records. New research that integrates easy-to-scale technologies with more intensive lab-based neurobiological tests is also needed, in order to embed both in a common understanding of the mechanisms of psychiatric disorders. Such research will rely on interdisciplinary communication across clinical, neurobiological, engineering, and data science disciplines to develop systems that are clinically meaningful and valid, that can integrate with interventions, and that can readily increase the scale and scope of their reach. Without such collaborations, we run the risk of escalating the fragmentation of psychiatry rather than binding together important threads of information and data.

The integration of neuroscience insights with natural-world sensors has the added-value capacity for yielding richer temporal information about the trajectory of each patient's risk, recovery, and adherence to interventions. Of course, sensor technology also entails accumulation of massive datasets that will rely on the innovative computational approaches outlined earlier for their analysis. Clinical utility of sensors and large datasets would rely on close-to-real-time data-crunching and delivery (in the form of reports, individualized profiles, and so forth) rather than the time frame of months that is more typical of laboratory settings.

Workflow and Reimbursement Issues

Application of precision psychiatry in practice will require consideration of how testing information and precision measurement–based management are incorporated into workflow and reimbursement models. One barrier to routine application of imaging is the presumption that such use would be too expensive, but the economic case for how such costs might be offset by savings due to reduced utilization and disability has not been tested. Because psychiatric disorders confer significant disability and often involve prolonged periods of trial and error to find effective treatments, it would not be surprising if the costs of introducing precision testing in the short term were dwarfed by the benefits of reducing this toll over the longer term. Furthermore, when imaging can reliably refine diagnosis, help decide among treatment options, and monitor treatment progress, imaging is routinely reimbursed without question (for a broken bone or torn ligament, for example). Integrating imaging or genetic testing into the clinical workflow will require resolving challenges such as introducing new referral, reimbursement, and reporting systems as tests for imaging, genetics, and other information become part of the psychiatric toolkit.

Ethical Issues

It will be important for researchers to partner with patients, providers, and key stakeholders at every phase of discovery and translation to ensure that new models are relevant, culturally centered, and effective across populations. Too often, innovative new technologies and biomedical advances initially widen disparities in health outcomes, such that individuals with resources are able to take advantage of these advances while those without resources are left out. Because serious mental illnesses are often poorly understood by patients and families; because many of the treatments involve decision making based on personal values and because gathering of personal health information, including genetic data, may have unanticipated psychosocial consequences, attention to the distinct ethical issues in personalized genomics in depression is also essential.

Furthermore, precision psychiatry as we are envisioning it requires continuous integration and updating of disease models and treatment planning based on emerging neuroscience and other research findings. A major challenge to this continual updating is that researchers are often hesitant to disseminate findings without an extremely high level of certainty, and providers are often hesitant to adopt new approaches. Caution is certainly warranted; adopting new scientific results into clinical practice too early has the potential for causing harm to patients, particularly if novel and invasive interventions are attempted without adequate safety testing. On the other hand, adopting new scientific results into clinical practice too late also has the potential to cause great harm, as patients miss the opportunity to receive intervention or assessment procedures that could have helped them.

Training the Future Generation of Leaders

Research efforts must be deeply intertwined with educational programs. It is of no use to patients if providers are not competent to utilize precision psychiatry models in their practices. Case-based learning (in which educational content is delivered through case examples) is especially useful, because it affords the opportunity to discuss how individual patients' treatment plans can be precisely optimized based on specific patient characteristics. However, as genetic, neuroimaging, and other biological markers become incorporated into routine clinical assessments, additional curricula that more thoroughly address the integration of neuroscience and psychiatry will be critical.

One example of such integration is a unique "discovery clinic" collaboration among researchers, educators, and clinicians in the Stanford Psychiatry Department (http://med.stanford.edu/williamslab/research/current/PPCC.html). Patients entering a training clinic within the department are offered a thorough assessment of symptoms, cognition, genetics, and brain circuit functioning. For half of participating patients, their doctor will receive information from the assessment prior to their first appointment. The remaining patients receive the information 12 weeks later, to allow the research team to test the impact of receiving information from neuroscience-based assessments relative to usual care. The research team also provides advanced training in neuroscience models and their applicability to clinical care to the residents rotating in the clinic. This trial is the first of its kind to integrate assessments for precision psychiatry into routine clinical care and will provide valuable insights into the pragmatics and benefits of such integration as it progresses. This "discovery clinic" model builds on a 3-year program involving development of a closed-loop process for integrating multimodal testing insights into a clinically relevant report format (Figure 28–2) and providing this report as feedback directly to clinicians and their patients, in a series of more than 50 case conferences.

At the national level, the National Neuroscience Curriculum Initiative (NNCI) was established in 2013 to promote the inclusion of a modern neuroscience prospective in psychiatry training. The aim of the NNCI is to create learning modules and resources that can be integrated into residency programs. These resources provide residents with an understanding of the fundamentals and importance of neuroscience and tools for communicating neuroscientific concepts with their patients. NNCI resources

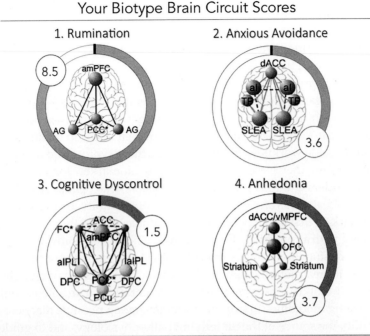

FIGURE 28–2. Example of patient-facing precision psychiatry report.

ACC=anterior cingulate cortex; AG=angular gyrus; aI=anterior insula; aIPL=anterior inferior parietal lobule; amPFC=anterior medial prefrontal cortex; dACC=dorsal anterior cingulate cortex; DPC=dorsal parietal cortex; FC=frontal cortex; OFC=orbitofrontal cortex; PCC=posterior cingulate cortex; PCu=precuneus; SLEA=superior lateral extended amygdala; TP=temporal parietal junction; vmPFC=ventromedial prefrontal cortex.

have already been incorporated into dozens of residency curricula across the United States and internationally.

Social Impacts and a New Narrative

Because precision psychiatry is based on a deep biological understanding of psychiatric disorders, it offers a model for patients to understand their experiences from an external perspective, rather than as an internal character flaw. This potential for alternate perspective-taking is not typically raised in discussions about the emergence of a precision medicine for psychiatry; however, it is likely one impact that could be transformative for patients. A tangible model of understanding that is shared by the patient and the clinician can lead to a new perspective on the illness that diminishes the patient's shame and self-blame. Brain-based models of mental illness are rapidly being infused into the public consciousness, fostering more open and less stigmatizing discussions about psychiatry and mental health. If the brain-based model is a shared understanding between patient and clinician, it has the potential to provide a mutual narrative that strengthens the therapeutic alliance and patient adherence to interventions.

In this chapter, we have stressed the need for a holistic approach in which an understanding of neurobiology is integrated with an understanding of life history and subjective experience. We restate this need here in order to make the point that a biologically based model has the potential to be empowering for both patients and clinicians, without reducing patients' experience to a deterministic sum of their biological parts.

Conclusion

We are at an exciting moment when a new paradigm for precision psychiatry is being realized. We envision a future that overcomes the gaps between research advances and their application in practice. New knowledge about brain circuits will be incorporated into models of assessment, care delivery, and prevention; residency programs will prepare graduates with training in brain circuit and genetic markers; and clinicians will have access to neuroscience-based tools to inform their decision making as part of the routine, reimbursable workflow. Findings such as those synthesized in this chapter are encouraging because they indicate that we can use biomarkers to identify subtypes of psychiatric disorders and thus predict with precision which patients are likely to benefit from which treatments and why. We have the opportunity to develop clinically applicable biomarkers that also have an understandable basis in the brain. To extend our earlier analogy, with a concerted effort we can envision a taxonomy for psychiatry that links different dysfunctions in the organ of interest, the brain, to specific symptom expressions and to treatment indications.Thus, we can imagine having at hand an expanded clinical toolkit—the psychiatry equivalent of the cardiology toolkit—with multiple imaging modalities to help differentiate among possible diagnoses and ultimately identify the source of the underlying pathophysiology, and to guide choice of treatments accordingly, including lifestyle changes, medications, behavioral therapies, neuromodulation, and their combination. With such a precision approach that translates brain insights into tools that can guide clinical decision making, we will have the opportunity to improve and save the lives of many.

Key Clinical Points

- We are witnessing the emergence of precision medicine for psychiatry: "precision psychiatry." Precision psychiatry is an integrative approach, one that pulls together the scientific foundations of the discipline and recent technological advances and directs them toward closing the gap between discovery and clinical translation.

- There is a clinical need for this new approach because although many effective treatments are available, finding the right treatment for the right patient remains largely a matter of trial and error.

- Reflecting the goal for its development, DSM provides a system for clinicians and researchers to communicate reliably about observed diagnostic signs and symptoms. Yet we do not have a nosology for diagnosis and for guiding treatment choices that is based in an understanding of the underlying pathophysiology.

- The goal of precision psychiatry, informed by neuroscience, is to provide precise measurement and neurological markers for classification, tailored treatment planning (i.e., using the biomarkers to select the best treatment for each person—how can we fix what has gone wrong?), and precise prevention (i.e., targeted and tailored prevention strategies—how can we keep things from going wrong?).

- As precision psychiatry develops, and to achieve this goal, clinicians will need to have a working knowledge of the evidence that forms the current state of knowledge about precise classification and treatment planning as well as the promise for future directions in precise prevention.

References

American Psychiatric Association: Diagnostic and Statistical Manual of Mental Disorders, 5th Edition. Arlington, VA, American Psychiatric Association, 2013

Ball TM, Goldstein-Piekarski AN, Gatt JM, et al: Quantifying person-level brain network functioning to facilitate clinical translation. Transl Psychiatry 7(10):e1248, 2017 29039851

Bandoli G, Campbell-Sills L, Kessler RC, et al: Childhood adversity, adult stress, and the risk of major depression or generalized anxiety disorder in US soldiers: a test of the stress sensitization hypothesis. Psychol Med 47(13):2379–2392, 2017 28443533

Clementz BA, Sweeney JA, Hamm JP, et al: Identification of distinct psychosis biotypes using brain-based biomarkers. Am J Psychiatry 173(4):373–384, 2016 26651391

Cole MW, Bassett DS, Power JD, et al: Intrinsic and task-evoked network architectures of the human brain. Neuron 83(1):238–251, 2014 24991964

Der-Avakian A, Markou A: The neurobiology of anhedonia and other reward-related deficits. Trends Neurosci 35(1):68–77, 2012 22177980

Doherty JL, Owen MJ: Genomic insights into the overlap between psychiatric disorders: implications for research and clinical practice. Genome Med 6(4):29, 2014 24944580

Downar J, Daskalakis ZJ: New targets for rTMS in depression: a review of convergent evidence. Brain Stimulat 6(3):231–240, 2013 22975030

Drysdale AT, Grosenick L, Downar J, et al: Erratum: Resting-state connectivity biomarkers define neurophysiological subtypes of depression. Nat Med 23(2):264, 2017 28170383

Dunlop BW, Binder EB, Cubells JF, et al: Predictors of remission in depression to individual and combined treatments (PReDICT): study protocol for a randomized controlled trial. Trials 13(1):106, 2012 22776534

Etkin A, Patenaude B, Song YJC, et al: A cognitive-emotional biomarker for predicting remission with antidepressant medications: a report from the iSPOT-D trial. Neuropsychopharmacology 40(6):1332–1342, 2015 25547711

Fernandes BS, Williams LM, Steiner J, et al: The new field of "precision psychiatry." BMC Med 15(1):80, 2017 28403846

FORUM Academy of Medical Sciences: Stratified, personalised or P4 medicine: A new direction for placing the patient at the centre of healthcare and health education. 2015. Available at: https://acmedsci.ac.uk/viewFile/564091e072d41.pdf. Accessed October 7, 2018.

Gatt JM, Burton KLO, Williams LM, et al: Specific and common genes implicated across major mental disorders: a review of meta-analysis studies. J Psychiatr Res 60(October):1–13, 2015 25287955

Gladding PA, Cave A, Zareian M, et al: Open access integrated therapeutic and diagnostic platforms for personalized cardiovascular medicine. J Pers Med 3(3):203–237, 2013 25562653

Goldstein-Piekarski AN, Korgaonkar MS, Green E, et al: Human amygdala engagement moderated by early life stress exposure is a biobehavioral target for predicting recovery on antidepressants. Proc Natl Acad Sci U S A 113(42):11955–11960, 2016 27791054

Green E, Goldstein-Piekarski AN, Schatzberg AF, et al: Personalizing antidepressant choice by sex, body mass index, and symptom profile: an iSPOT-D report. Personalized Medicine in Psychiatry 1–2(March–April):65–73, 2017

Gyurak A, Patenaude B, Korgaonkar MS, et al: Frontoparietal activation during response inhibition predicts remission to antidepressants in patients with major depression. Biol Psychiatry 79(4):274–281, 2016 25891220

Hamilton JP, Farmer M, Fogelman P, et al: Depressive rumination, the default-mode network, and the dark matter of clinical neuroscience. Biol Psychiatry 78(4):224–230, 2015 25861700

Harding KJK, Rush AJ, Arbuckle M, et al: Measurement-based care in psychiatric practice: a policy framework for implementation. J Clin Psychiatry 72(8):1136–1143, 2011 21295000

Hodgson K, Mufti SJ, Uher R, et al: Genome-wide approaches to antidepressant treatment: working towards understanding and predicting response. Genome Med 4(6):52, 2012 22738351

Hudson K, Lifton R, Patrick-Lane B, et al: The Precision Medicine Initiative Cohort Program—Building a Research Foundation for 21st Century Medicine. Precision Medicine Initiative (PMI) Working Group Report to the Advisory Committee to the Director, NIH, 2015. Available at: https://acd.od.nih.gov/documents/reports/DRAFT-PMI-WG-Report-9-11-2015-508.pdf. Accessed October 7, 2018.

Huys QJM, Maia TV, Frank MJ: Computational psychiatry as a bridge from neuroscience to clinical applications. Nat Neurosci 19(3):404–413, 2016 26906507

IMS Institute for Healthcare Informatics: Medicines Use and Spending Shifts: A Review of the Use of Medicines in the U.S. in 2014. Parsippany, NJ, IMS Institute for Healthcare Informatics, April 2015. Available at: https://www.iqvia.com/-/media/iqvia/pdfs/institute-reports/medicines-use-and-spending-shifts-in-the-us-in-2014.pdf. Accessed January 16, 2019.

Insel TR: Post by Former NIH Director Thomas Insel: Precision Medicine for Mental Disorders. National Institute of Mental Health website, February 2, 2015. Available at: https://www.nimh.nih.gov/about/directors/thomas-insel/blog/2015/precision-medicine-for-mental-disorders.shtml. Accessed March 14, 2018.

Insel T, Cuthbert B, Garvey M, et al: Research domain criteria (RDoC): toward a new classification framework for research on mental disorders. Am J Psychiatry 167(7):748–751, 2010 20595427

Kreyenbuhl JA, Medoff DR, McEvoy JP, et al: The RAISE connection program: psychopharmacological treatment of people with a first episode of schizophrenia. Psychiatr Serv 67(12):1300–1306, 2016 27364816

Lawrie SM, O'Donovan MC, Saks E, et al: Improving classification of psychoses. Lancet Psychiatry 3(4):367–374, 2016 27063387

Letai A: Functional precision cancer medicine-moving beyond pure genomics. Nat Med 23(9):1028–1035, 2017 28886003

Mahmood SS, Levy D, Vasan RS, et al: The Framingham Heart Study and the epidemiology of cardiovascular disease: a historical perspective. Lancet 383(9921):999–1008, 2014 24084292

Markoff J: Obama seeking to boost study of human brain. The New York Times, February 17, 2013. Available at: http://www.nytimes.com/2013/02/18/science/project-seeks-to-build-map-of-human-brain.html. Accessed March 14, 2018.

Millan MJ, Andrieux A, Bartzokis G, et al: Altering the course of schizophrenia: progress and perspectives. Nat Rev Drug Discov 15(7):485–515, 2016 26939910

Nuechterlein KH, Subotnik KL, Green MF, et al: Neurocognitive predictors of work outcome in recent-onset schizophrenia. Schizophr Bull 37 (suppl 2):S33–S40, 2011 21860045

O'Connell CP, Goldstein-Piekarski AN, Nemeroff CB, et al: Antidepressant outcomes predicted by genetic variation in corticotropin-releasing hormone binding protein. Am J Psychiatry 175(3):251–261, 2018 29241359

Office of the Press Secretary: Fact Sheet: President Obama's Precision Medicine Initiative. Washington, DC, The White House, January 30, 2015a. Available at: https://obamawhitehouse.archives.gov/the-press-office/2015/01/30/fact-sheet-president-obama-s-precision-medicine-initiative. Accessed March 14, 2018.

Office of the Press Secretary: Remarks by the President on Precision Medicine. Washington, DC, The White House, January 30, 2015b. Available at: https://obamawhitehouse.archives.gov/the-press-office/2015/01/30/remarks-president-precision-medicine. Accessed March 14, 2018.

Ostacher MJ, Iosifescu DV, Hay A, et al: Pilot investigation of isradipine in the treatment of bipolar depression motivated by genome-wide association. Bipolar Disord 16(2):199–203, 2014 24372835

Prata D, Mechelli A, Kapur S: Clinically meaningful biomarkers for psychosis: a systematic and quantitative review. Neurosci Biobehav Rev 45:134–141, 2014 24877683

Psychiatric Genomics Consortium: Psychiatric Genomics Consortium: What is the PGC? (website). Chapel Hill, University of North Carolina School of Medicine, 2016. Available at: http://www.med.unc.edu/pgc/. Accessed March 14, 2018.

Roberts LW, Louie AK, Guerrero APS, et al: Premature mortality among people with mental illness: advocacy in academic psychiatry. Acad Psychiatry 41(4):441–446, 2017 28585124

Rosellini AJ, Stein MB, Benedek DM, et al: Using self-report surveys at the beginning of service to develop multi-outcome risk models for new soldiers in the U.S. Army. Psychol Med 47(13):2275–2287, 2017 28374665

Saveanu R, Etkin A, Duchemin AM, et al: The international Study to Predict Optimized Treatment in Depression (iSPOT-D): outcomes from the acute phase of antidepressant treatment. J Psychiatr Res 61:1–12, 2015 25586212

Schaefer GB, Mendelsohn NJ; Professional Practice and Guidelines Committee: Clinical genetics evaluation in identifying the etiology of autism spectrum disorders. Genet Med 10(4):301–305, 2008 18414214

Schatzberg AF, DeBattista C, Lazzeroni LC, et al: ABCB1 genetic effects on antidepressant outcomes: a report from the iSPOT-D trial. Am J Psychiatry 172(8):751–759, 2015 25815420

Shin LM, Liberzon I: The neurocircuitry of fear, stress, and anxiety disorders. Neuropsychopharmacology 35(1):169–191, 2010 19625997

Siegle GJ: Beyond depression commentary: wherefore art thou, depression clinic of tomorrow? Clin Psychol (New York) 18(4):305–310, 2011 24634570

Smits JAJ, Rosenfield D, Otto MW, et al: D-cycloserine enhancement of exposure therapy for social anxiety disorder depends on the success of exposure sessions. J Psychiatr Res 47(10):1455–1461, 2013 23870811

Stein MB, Chen C-Y, Ursano RJ, et al: Genome-wide association studies of posttraumatic stress disorder in 2 cohorts of US army soldiers. JAMA Psychiatry 73(7):695–704, 2016 27167565

Stein MB, Ware EB, Mitchell C, et al: Genomewide association studies of suicide attempts in US soldiers. Am J Med Genet B Neuropsychiatr Genet 174(8):786–797, 2017 28902444

Stein MB, Campbell-Sills L, Ursano RJ, et al; Army STARRS Collaborators: Childhood maltreatment and lifetime suicidal behaviors among new soldiers in the US army: results from the Army Study To Assess Risk and Resilience in Servicemembers (Army STARRS). J Clin Psychiatry 79(2), 2018 28541647

Sullivan PF, Daly MJ, O'Donovan M: Genetic architectures of psychiatric disorders: the emerging picture and its implications. Nat Rev Genet 13(8):537–551, 2012 22777127

Tamminga CA, Pearlson G, Keshavan M, et al: Bipolar and schizophrenia network for intermediate phenotypes: outcomes across the psychosis continuum. Schizophr Bull 40 (suppl 2):S131–S137, 2014 24562492

Tretter F, Gebicke-Haerter PJ: Systems biology in psychiatric research: from complex data sets over wiring diagrams to computer simulations, in Psychiatric Disorders: Methods and Protocols. Edited by Kobeissy FH. New York, Humana Press, 2011, pp 567–589

Trivedi MH, McGrath PJ, Fava M, et al: Establishing moderators and biosignatures of antidepressant response in clinical care (EMBARC): rationale and design. J Psychiatr Res 78:11–23, 2016 27038550

Wang Y, Kasper LH: The role of microbiome in central nervous system disorders. Brain Behav Immun 38:1–12, 2014 24370461

Williams LM: Precision psychiatry: a neural circuit taxonomy for depression and anxiety. Lancet Psychiatry 3(5):472–480, 2016 27150382

Williams LM, Rush AJ, Koslow SH, et al: International Study to Predict Optimized Treatment for Depression (iSPOT-D), a randomized clinical trial: rationale and protocol. Trials 12(1):4, 2011 21208417

Williams LM, Korgaonkar MS, Song YC, et al: Amygdala reactivity to emotional faces in the prediction of general and medication-specific responses to antidepressant treatment in the randomized iSPOT-D trial. Neuropsychopharmacology 40(10):2398–2408, 2015 25824424

Williams LM, Debattista C, Duchemin A-M, et al: Childhood trauma predicts antidepressant response in adults with major depression: data from the randomized international study to predict optimized treatment for depression. Transl Psychiatry 6:e799, 2016 27138798

Recommended Readings

Fernandes BS, Williams LM, Steiner J, et al: The new field of "precision psychiatry." BMC Med 15(1):80, 2017

FORUM Academy of Medical Sciences: Stratified, personalised or P4 medicine: a new direction for placing the patient at the centre of healthcare and health education. 2015. Available at: https://acmedsci.ac.uk/download?f=fileandi=32644. Accessed March 14, 2018.

Hudson K, Lifton R, Patrick-Lane B, et al: The Precision Medicine Initiative Cohort Program—Building a Research Foundation for 21st Century Medicine. Precision Medicine Initiative (PMI) Working Group Report to the Advisory Committee to the Director, NIH, 2015. Available at: http://www.nih.gov/precisionmedicine/. Accessed March 14, 2018.

Insel TR: Post by Former NIH Director Thomas Insel: Precision Medicine for Mental Disorders. National Institute of Mental Health website, February 2, 2015. Available at: https://www.nimh.nih.gov/about/directors/thomas-insel/blog/2015/precision-medicine-for-mental-disorders.shtml. Accessed March 14, 2018.

Williams LM: Precision psychiatry: a neural circuit taxonomy for depression and anxiety. Lancet Psychiatry 3(5):472–480, 2016

CHAPTER 29

Psychopharmacology

James L. Levenson, M.D.

Ericka L. Crouse, Pharm.D.

Kevin M. Bozymski, Pharm.D.

Psychopharmacology is critical to the management of all major psychiatric disorders. Since the serendipitous discovery of the psychotropic effects of antidepressants, antipsychotics, and lithium in the early 1950s, the pharmacological armamentarium and evidence for efficacy have grown dramatically, yet many of these original agents remain relevant today. Despite decades of progress, many challenges remain. Our practice of psychiatry is hampered by lack of explanatory biological specificity for the major disorders, making precise diagnosis and medication choice dependent on observation, best application of available evidence, and trial and error. Even with an appropriate diagnosis, medications have limited ability to induce remission, there is significant inter- and intra-individual difference in response, and cure is usually not possible. Further complicating treatment are psychiatric, substance use, and medical comorbidities.

This chapter provides an overview of basic psychopharmacological principles as well as of the major classes of psychotropics, including antipsychotics, antidepressants, anxiolytics and sedative-hypnotics, mood stabilizers, psychostimulants, and cognitive enhancers. Pharmacological treatment guidelines for specific disorders are covered in the respective chapters. It is implicit that psychopharmacology should be combined, when appropriate, with evidence-based psychosocial and psychotherapeutic treatments in order to enhance medication adherence, reduce symptom burden and relapse, and increase function. Finally, the overview of psychopharmacology presented in this chapter is not exhaustive; therefore, the reader is referred to one of the many comprehensive texts (e.g., Levenson and Ferrando 2017; Schatzberg and Nemeroff 2017) for a more detailed review of selected topics.

General Principles

Choice of Medication

In general, all drugs indicated for the treatment of a particular psychiatric disorder have similar therapeutic efficacy. However, individual patients may better respond to or tolerate one agent over another because of differences in each drug's pharmacokinetics (absorption, distribution, metabolism, and excretion), spectrum of secondary pharmacological effects, or drug interactions. A patient's personal or family history of response to and tolerance of a drug can guide future drug selection. Drug choice is further influenced by the potential for interaction with a medical condition, concurrent medications, or patient preference.

Comorbid medical conditions may influence drug choice. For example, hypotensive patients should avoid medications with substantial α_1-adrenergic blockade that exacerbate hypotension. Patients with compromised hepatic function are better able to eliminate those drugs primarily metabolized by conjugation or renal excretion. Conversely, in patients with renal impairment, drugs undergoing oxidative metabolism, with no active metabolites, are preferred. Comorbid psychiatric conditions may be exacerbated by certain psychiatric and nonpsychiatric agents. Medically compromised patients, including those with severe nausea and vomiting, dysphagia, or malabsorption, or patients unable or unwilling to take medications by mouth may prefer a drug delivered by a nonoral route such as transdermal, sublingual, or intramuscular. Several psychotropics are available in nonoral formulations (see Levenson and Ferrando 2017 for additional information).

Polypharmacy increases the risk of drug–drug interactions and should be minimized or avoided if possible. Drugs with less potential to cause drug interactions are preferred (see "Drug Interactions" subsection below). Often, the number of medications can be reduced by making constructive use of a drug's secondary pharmacological effects. For example, a depressed patient with insomnia may benefit from a sedating antidepressant administered at bedtime rather than an additional hypnotic.

Where possible, clinicians should involve patients in medication selection. Patients may find the side effect of one drug (e.g., weight gain) preferable to that of another (e.g., sexual dysfunction). Treatment adherence is improved when the patient takes part in the treatment process. Other strategies for improving adherence are listed in Table 29–1.

Drug Interactions

A *drug interaction* is the alteration of the pharmacological effect of one drug by another concurrently administered drug or substance. A *pharmacokinetic interaction* occurs when an interacting substance alters a drug's concentration due to a change in its absorption, distribution, metabolism, or excretion. These interactions are most likely to be clinically meaningful when the drug involved has a low therapeutic index or active metabolites. *Pharmacodynamic interactions* alter the body's responses to a drug by altering drug binding to a receptor site or indirectly through other mechanisms (see Levenson and Ferrando 2017 for a more extensive review of this topic).

TABLE 29–1.   **Strategies to maximize medication adherence**

Provide patient education.

Inform patient about potential adverse effects, their speed of onset, and whether tolerance will develop over time.

Indicate the time for onset of the therapeutic effect. For many psychotropics, adverse effects occur immediately but therapeutic effects may be delayed by weeks.

Generic medications may differ in appearance from each other and from the nongeneric product. Patients may avoid taking different-appearing medications unless informed of the change.

Arrange a convenient dosing schedule.

Compliance is maximized with once-daily dosing.

Long-acting formulations with dosing intervals of several weeks are available for some antipsychotics.

Minimize adverse effects.

Select drugs with minimal pharmacokinetic interactions where possible.

Gradually increase drug dosage over several days/weeks ("start low, go slow").

Use the minimum effective dosage.

Select a drug with an adverse effect profile the patient can best tolerate.

Reduce peak concentration–dependent adverse effects by taking drug with food, taking in divided doses, or using extended-release formulations to reduce/delay peak drug levels.

Schedule dose so that side effect is less bothersome. If possible, prescribe activating drugs in the morning and sedating drugs or those that cause gastrointestinal distress in the evening.

Check for patient adherence.

Schedule office or telephone visits to discuss adherence and adverse effects for newly prescribed drugs.

Pharmacokinetic Drug Interactions

Metabolism.   The majority of drugs are substrates for phase I (oxidative) metabolism by one or more cytochrome P450 (CYP) enzymes. The most common pharmacokinetic drug–drug interaction involves changes in the CYP-mediated metabolism of the *substrate* drug by an interacting drug. The interacting drug may be either an inducer or an inhibitor of the specific CYP enzymes involved in the substrate drug's metabolism. In the presence of an *inducer*, CYP enzyme activity and the rate of metabolism of the substrate are increased. Enzyme induction is not an immediate process but occurs over several weeks. Induction will decrease the amount of circulating parent drug and may reduce or abolish therapeutic efficacy. Consider a patient stabilized on olanzapine (a CYP1A2 substrate) who begins to smoke (a CYP1A2 inducer). Smoking will increase olanzapine metabolism, and unless the drug dosage is adjusted, olanzapine levels will fall and psychotic symptoms may worsen. Metabolism of drugs that are not CYP1A2 substrates will not be affected. If the interacting drug is a metabolic *inhibitor,* drug metabolism mediated through the inhibited CYP isozymes will be impaired. The resulting rise in substrate drug levels may increase drug toxicity and prolong the pharmacological effect. Although enzyme inhibition is a rapid process, substrate drug levels respond more slowly, taking five half-lives to restabilize.

Not all combinations of substrate drug and interacting drug will result in clinically significant drug–drug interactions. For a drug eliminated by several mechanisms, including multiple CYP enzymes or non-CYP routes (e.g., renal elimination), the inhibition of a single CYP isozyme only serves to divert elimination to other pathways, with little change in overall elimination rate. Generally, for these interactions to be clinically relevant, a *critical substrate* drug must have a narrow therapeutic index and one primary CYP isozyme mediating its metabolism. For example, metoprolol, like all β-blockers, is primarily metabolized by the CYP2D6 isozyme. The addition of a potent CYP2D6 inhibitor, such as paroxetine, will inhibit metoprolol metabolism. Without a compensatory reduction in metoprolol dosage, drug levels will rise and toxicity (hypotension) may result. When prescribing in a polypharmacy environment, clinicians should attempt to avoid medications that significantly inhibit or induce CYP enzymes and instead choose medications that are eliminated by multiple pathways and that have a wide safety margin. In a polypharmacy environment, clinicians should consult drug information resources or a drug interaction database to screen for clinically significant drug interactions. Many computer systems used by pharmacists and physicians are equipped with drug interaction software. Extensive tables of drug interactions are provided in Levenson and Ferrando (2017).

The abundance of clinically significant pharmacokinetic interactions involving monoamine oxidase inhibitors (MAOIs), especially inhibitors of MAO-A, has limited their therapeutic use. Many of these interactions involve foods containing high levels of tyramine, a pressor amine metabolized by gut MAO-A. Several drugs, including some sympathomimetics and triptan antimigraine medications, are also metabolized by MAO. In the medically ill population, the antibiotics linezolid and tedizolid are also MAOIs and may increase risk of serotonin syndrome if combined with antidepressants or other serotonergic medications.

The role of phase II (conjugative) metabolism is increasingly being recognized in clinical pharmacology, although surprisingly few clinically significant drug interactions are known to involve conjugation systems.

Absorption.   Many orally administered drugs, including a number of psychotropics, have poor bioavailability due to extensive first-pass metabolism. In the gut wall, drug metabolism by gut CYP3A4 and drug transport back into the gut lumen by the P-glycoprotein efflux transporter system form a barrier to absorption. Inhibitors of CYP3A4 and P-glycoprotein can lead to drug toxicity due to dramatic increases in the oral bioavailability of poorly bioavailable drugs. Psychotropics with poor bioavailability include buspirone, selegiline, venlafaxine, ramelteon, zaleplon, rivastigmine, and quetiapine. Common CYP3A4 and/or P-glycoprotein inhibitors include grapefruit juice, verapamil, diltiazem, quinidine, progestogen oral contraceptives, and proton pump inhibitors. Furthermore, CYP3A4 and P-glycoprotein inducers, such as St. John's wort, may significantly reduce the oral bioavailability of already poorly bioavailable drugs.

Distribution.   Changes in drug protein binding, either disease-induced or the result of a protein-binding drug interaction, were once considered a common cause of drug toxicity because therapeutic and toxic effects increase with increasing concentrations of free drug. In the absence of changes in metabolism or excretion, these interactions are now seen as clinically significant only in very limited cases involving rapidly acting, highly protein-bound (>80%), low-therapeutic-index drugs with high hepatic extraction.

Excretion. Drug interactions altering renal drug elimination are clinically significant only if the parent drug or its active metabolite undergoes appreciable renal excretion. By reducing renal blood flow, some drugs, including many nonsteroidal anti-inflammatory agents and antihypertensive agents (e.g., thiazide diuretics, angiotensin-converting enzyme inhibitors), decrease the glomerular filtration rate and impair renal elimination. These interactions are often responsible for lithium toxicity.

Pharmacodynamic Drug Interactions

Pharmacodynamic interactions occur when drugs with similar or opposing effects are combined. The nature of the interaction relates to the addition or antagonism of the pharmacological and toxic effects of each drug. Generally, pharmacodynamic interactions are most apparent in individuals with compromised physiological function such as cardiovascular disease or the elderly. For example, drugs with anticholinergic activity cause a degree of cognitive impairment, an effect exacerbated when several anticholinergic agents are combined (see Table 29–16, later in this chapter). Unfortunately, anticholinergic activity is often an unrecognized property of many common drugs such as antispasmodics, antiparkinsonian agents, and antihistamines. This additive interaction is most disruptive in cognitively compromised patients, such as the elderly or those with Alzheimer's disease, and forms the basis for many cases of delirium. Recent warnings have focused on reducing the combination of opioids with benzodiazepines, given their additive respiratory depressant effects.

Additive pharmacodynamic interactions are often employed therapeutically to enhance a drug response—this is the purpose of adjunctive medications. Antagonistic pharmacodynamic interactions are sometimes used deliberately to diminish a particular adverse effect. Unintentional antagonistic interactions may be countertherapeutic; for example, addition of an anticholinergic agent such as diphenhydramine to a cholinesterase-inhibiting medication will reduce the cognitive benefit obtained from the cholinesterase inhibitor.

Knowledge of a drug's therapeutic and adverse effects is essential to avoid unwanted pharmacodynamic drug interactions, such as additive or synergistic toxicities, or countertherapeutic effects.

Antipsychotics

The antipsychotics (also known as neuroleptics) have as their core application the treatment of psychosis in schizophrenia; however, they are playing an increasing role in the treatment of bipolar and unipolar mood disorders. There are two major categories of antipsychotics: the first-generation antipsychotics (FGAs; also known as typical or conventional antipsychotics) and the second-generation antipsychotics (SGAs; also called atypical antipsychotics). The FGAs, most prominently the phenothiazines (e.g., chlorpromazine) and the butyrophenones (e.g., haloperidol), have heterogeneous receptor effects; however, their primary therapeutic effect is via nonspecific blockade of the dopamine D_2 receptor subtype. The SGAs (clozapine, olanzapine, risperidone, paliperidone, ziprasidone, quetiapine, asenapine, lurasidone, and iloperidone) are a heterogeneous group of medications that are thought to exert more specific mesolimbic dopamine receptor blockade compared with the FGAs, combined with 5-hydroxytryptamine (5-HT; serotonin) type 2 (5-HT_{2A}) receptor antagonism. Three SGAs—aripiprazole, brexpiprazole, and cariprazine—work as partial agonists at both D_2 receptors and 5-HT_{1A} receptors and as antagonists at 5-HT_{2A} receptors. SGAs and FGAs appear to be equally efficacious for the treatment of schizophrenia and other psychoses, with the exception of clozapine, which has superior effects in treatment-refractory illness. The receptor profile of SGAs is thought to confer a lower risk of extrapyramidal side effects (EPS). In recent years, SGAs have played a more significant role in the treatment of bipolar disorder (mania, bipolar depression) and refractory unipolar depression, particularly as adjuncts to mood stabilizer and antidepressant medications, respectively. Generally, the SGAs have the advantage of less common EPS, including parkinsonism, neuroleptic malignant syndrome (NMS), and tardive dyskinesia (TD); however, like many FGAs, the SGAs have significant long-term metabolic (e.g., weight gain, hyperglycemia) and other side effects (e.g., sedation, hypotension). Pimavanserin is a new SGA approved in the United States for the treatment of hallucinations and delusions associated with Parkinson's disease psychosis. It has no affinity for dopamine receptors, but instead acts as a highly selective 5-HT_{2A} inverse agonist. Whether pimavanserin may be effective for other psychiatric disorders has not yet been established.

Indications and Efficacy

Table 29–2 summarizes the U.S. Food and Drug Administration (FDA)–approved[1] indications, dosages, formulations, routes of administration, and key distinguishing characteristics of currently available antipsychotics.

There are multiple "off label" uses for antipsychotics, with variable evidence in the literature. Such uses include (but are not limited to) treatment of substance-induced psychotic symptoms, agitation and psychosis in delirium, delusional disorders, severe anxiety/agitation, insomnia, psychosis and mood instability in borderline and schizotypal personality disorders, and adjunctive treatment of refractory obsessive-compulsive disorder (OCD). Use of antipsychotics for elderly patients with dementia-related psychosis carries an FDA black box warning for increased risk for mortality secondary to cardiovascular events and infections, particularly pneumonia. Because of their dopamine-blocking effects, antipsychotics are also used as antiemetics in medically ill patients. Clinicians considering off-label use of antipsychotics must carefully weigh the potential benefits against the substantial short- and long-term side effects. The risks and benefits should be discussed with patients or their families, and the fact that this discussion took place should be documented in the medical record.

Dosage, Response, and Routes of Administration

Recommended dosages for antipsychotics with given indications are outlined in Table 29–2. It is important to note that treatment response may take days to weeks, and

---

[1] It is important to note that presence of an FDA-approved indication for a given disorder is not an indicator of a drug's superiority, and lack of a labeled indication is not necessarily proof of its inferiority, especially for drugs that have long been available in generic form. Many of the FGAs have been used for years for conditions in which the SGAs have received specific FDA approval (e.g., bipolar mania) but have never been FDA approved for these uses.

TABLE 29–2. Antipsychotic agents

Generic name	Trade name	Dosage forms and strengths, mg	FDA-approved indications	Recommended dosage range (mg/day unless otherwise noted)	Comments
Second-generation antipsychotics					
Aripiprazole	Abilify	PO: 2, 5, 10, 15, 20, 30 L: 1 mg/mL ODT: 10, 15	SZ (acute, maintenance) BP mania (acute, maintenance; monotherapy, adjunct) MDD refractory—adjunctive to antidepressants Autism spectrum disorder—irritability (ages 6–17 years) Tourette's disorder	15–30 10–30 5.25–15 2–5 5–15 2–20	Dosage depends on weight
Aripiprazole lauroxil	Aristada	LAI: 441, 662, 882, 1,064; 675 (initial)	SZ	441–882 monthly 882 every 6 weeks 1,064 every 2 months	Dosage adjustment if on concurrent CYP2D6 and 3A4 inhibitors
Aripiprazole monohydrate	Abilify Maintena	LAI: 300, 400	SZ (acute, maintenance) BP maintenance as monotherapy	400 monthly	Dosage adjustment if on concurrent CYP2D6 and 3A4 inhibitors
Asenapine	Saphris	SL: 2.5, 5, 10	SZ (acute, maintenance) BP mania (ages 10 years–adult; acute, maintenance [adult only]; monotherapy, adjunct)	C, T: 5–20 10–20	Oral mucosal absorption is unique

TABLE 29–2.   Antipsychotic agents *(continued)*

Generic name	Trade name	Dosage forms and strengths, mg	FDA-approved indications	Recommended dosage range (mg/day unless otherwise noted)	Comments
Second-generation antipsychotics *(continued)*					
Brexpiprazole	Rexulti	PO: 0.25, 0.5, 1, 2, 3, 4	SZ (acute, maintenance) MDD—adjunctive to antidepressants	2–4 2	
Cariprazine	Vraylar	PO: 1.5, 3, 4.5, 6	SZ (acute, maintenance) BP mania (acute)	1.5–6 3–6	
Clozapine	Clozaril	PO: 25, 100, 200	SZ—refractory	250–500	Weight gain, neutropenia, seizure risk
	FazaClo (ODT)	ODT: 12.5, 25, 100, 150, 200	Suicidality in SZ and SZAD		
	Versacloz	L: 50 mg/mL			
Iloperidone	Fanapt	PO: 1, 2, 4, 6, 8, 10, 12	SZ (acute, maintenance)	12–24	Administer bid Prolongs QTc
Lurasidone	Latuda	PO: 20, 40, 60, 80, 120	SZ (ages 13 years–adult; acute, maintenance) BP depression as monotherapy or adjunct	40–160 C, T: 40–80 20–120	Administer with food (≥350 kcals)

TABLE 29–2. Antipsychotic agents *(continued)*

Generic name	Trade name	Dosage forms and strengths, mg	FDA-approved indications	Recommended dosage range (mg/day unless otherwise noted)	Comments
Second-generation antipsychotics *(continued)*					
Olanzapine	Zyprexa	PO: 2.5, 5, 7.5, 10, 15, 20 ODT: 5, 10, 15, 20 IM: 10	SZ (acute, maintenance) BP mania (acute, maintenance; monotherapy, adjunct) Acute agitation in SZ and BP (IM preparation)	10–20 5–20 2.5–10	CATIE findings showed fewest discontinuations for lack of efficacy but most discontinuations for side effects; mostly weight gain
	Symbyax (olanzapine/ fluoxetine combination)	Symbyax: 3/25, 6/25, 6/50, 12/25, 12/50	MDD refractory—in combination with fluoxetine Bipolar depression—in combination with fluoxetine	6/25–18/50 3/25–12/50	
Olanzapine pamoate	Zyprexa Relprevv	LAI: 210, 300, 405	SZ (acute, maintenance)	150–405 every 2–4 weeks	Boxed warning for PDSS
Paliperidone	Invega	PO: 1.5, 3, 6, 9	SZ (acute, maintenance) SZAD (acute) as monotherapy or adjunct to mood stabilizers or antidepressants	3–12 3–12	Risperidone metabolite, once-daily dosing Ghost tablet excreted in feces
Paliperidone palmitate depot injection	Invega Sustenna	LAI: 39, 78, 117, 156, 234	SZ (acute, maintenance)	39–234 monthly	Recommended to establish tolerability with PO paliperidone or risperidone
	Invega Trinza	LAI: 273, 410, 546, 819	SZ (maintenance)	273–819 every 3 months	Recommended to be treated with Invega Sustenna for 4 months; dosage is 3.5 times Sustenna dosage

TABLE 29–2. Antipsychotic agents *(continued)*

Generic name	Trade name	Dosage forms and strengths, mg	FDA-approved indications	Recommended dosage range (mg/day unless otherwise noted)	Comments
Second-generation antipsychotics *(continued)*					
Quetiapine	Seroquel	PO: 25, 50, 100, 200, 300, 400	SZ (adult, adolescent; acute, maintenance)	A: 150–800; T: 400–800	Significant sedation, hypotension
			BP mania (ages 10 years–adult; acute, maintenance; monotherapy, adjunct)	A: 400–800; C, T: 400–600	
			BP depression	300	
Quetiapine extended-release	Seroquel XR	PO: 50, 150, 200, 300, 400	SZ (acute, maintenance)	400–800	Once-daily dosing
			BP mania (ages 10 years–adult; acute, maintenance; monotherapy, adjunct)	400–800	
			BP depression	300	
			MDD—refractory (adjunct to antidepressant)	150–300	
Risperidone	Risperdal	PO: 0.25, 0.5, 1, 2, 3, 4 ODT: 0.25, 0.5, 1, 2, 3, 4 L: 1 mg/mL	SZ (A, T; acute, maintenance)	A: 4–8; T: 1–3	Highest EPS and hyperprolactinemia risk among SGAs
			BP mania (ages 10 years–adult; acute, maintenance; monotherapy, adjunct)	A: 1–6; ages 10–17 years 1–2.5	
			Autism spectrum disorder—irritability (ages 5–17 years)	0.5–3.0	
Risperidone long-acting injection	Risperdal Consta	LAI: 12.5, 25, 37.5, 50	SZ and BP (maintenance)	25–50 mg IM every 2 weeks	

TABLE 29–2. Antipsychotic agents *(continued)*

Generic name	Trade name	Dosage forms and strengths, mg	FDA-approved indications	Recommended dosage range (mg/day unless otherwise noted)	Comments
Second-generation antipsychotics *(continued)*					
Ziprasidone	Geodon	PO: 20, 40, 60, 80 IM: 20 mg/mL	SZ (acute, maintenance) BP mania (acute, maintenance; monotherapy, adjunct) Acute agitation in SZ (IM preparation)	80–160 80–160 10 every 2 hours or 20 every 4 hours; max. 40 mg/day	Risk for prolonged QTc and torsades de pointes Administer with food (≥500 kcals)
First-generation antipsychotics					
Butyrophenones					
Haloperidol	Haldol	PO: 0.5, 1, 2, 5, 10, 20 CL: 2 mg/mL IM: 5 mg/mL	SZ (A, C >3 years) Tourette's tics (A, C >3 years) Refractory hyperactivity and severe disruptive behavior (C >3 years)	5–15 PO 2–5 mg IM every 4–8 hours 0.5–10	High-potency D$_2$ blockade, EPS risk Risk for prolonged QTc and torsades de pointes with high-dose intravenous use[a] (off label)
Haloperidol decanoate	Haldol decanoate	D: 50, 100 mg/mL	SZ (A; maintenance)	10–20 times daily PO dose monthly	Monthly IM injection for patients with medication nonadherence
Dibenzoxazepines					
Loxapine	Loxitane Adasuve	PO: 5, 10, 25, 50 Oral inhalation: 10	SZ (acute, maintenance) Acute agitation in SZ and BP	60–100 10 single doses every 24 hours	Contraindicated in asthma, COPD, or other lung disease

TABLE 29–2. Antipsychotic agents (continued)

Generic name	Trade name	Dosage forms and strengths, mg	FDA-approved indications	Recommended dosage range (mg/day unless otherwise noted)	Comments
First-generation antipsychotics (continued)					
Phenothiazines: Aliphatics					
Chlorpromazine	Thorazine	PO: 10, 25, 50, 100, 200 IM: 25 mg/mL	SZ (acute, maintenance) BP mania (acute) Refractory hyperactivity and severe disruptive behavior (C >3 years)	300–600 300–600 0.25–0.5 mg/lb. body weight every 4–6 hours	Low-potency D_2 blockade; risk for prolonged QTc and torsades de pointes,[a] hypotension
Phenothiazines: Piperazines					
Fluphenazine	Prolixin	PO: 1, 2.5, 5, 10 L: 0.5 mg/mL CL: 5 mg/mL IM: 2.5 mg/mL	SZ (acute, maintenance)	5–20	Medium-potency D_2 blockade, moderate EPS risk
Fluphenazine decanoate	Prolixin decanoate	D: 25 mg/mL	SZ (maintenance)	25–50 mg every 2–4 weeks	To convert PO to D dosing, use the following formula: 10 mg/day PO≈12.5 mg D every 3 weeks
Perphenazine	Trilafon, Etrafon Triavil (perphenazine/ amitriptyline combination)	PO: 2, 4, 8, 16 PO: 2/10, 4/10, 2/25, 4/25, 4/50	SZ (acute, maintenance) Depression with anxiety SZ with depression	12–64 2/10–16/200	Comparison FGA in CATIE: efficacy similar to SGAs, increased EPS risk
Trifluoperazine	Stelazine	PO: 1, 2, 5, 10	SZ (acute, maintenance; A, C, T) Anxiety (nonpsychotic)	A: 15–30; C, T: 1–15 1–6	

TABLE 29–2. Antipsychotic agents *(continued)*

Generic name	Trade name	Dosage forms and strengths, mg	FDA-approved indications	Recommended dosage range (mg/day unless otherwise noted)	Comments
First-generation antipsychotics *(continued)*					
Phenothiazines: Piperidines					
Thioridazine	Mellaril	PO: 10, 25, 50, 100	SZ (acute, maintenance; A, C, T)	200–600	Risk for prolonged QTc, torsades de pointes[a]
Phenothiazines: Diphenylbutylpiperidine					
Pimozide	Orap	PO: 1, 2	Tourette's tics (A, C, T)	0.05–0.2 mg/kg/day, max. 10 mg/day	Risk for prolonged QTc, torsades de pointes[a]
Thioxanthenes					
Thiothixene	Navane	PO: 1, 2, 5, 10	SZ (acute, maintenance)	5–30	Medium-high potency D_2 blockade, significant EPS risk

Note. A=adult; acute=acute treatment; adjunct=adjunctive treatment; BP=bipolar disorder; C=child; CATIE=Clinical Antipsychotic Treatment Effectiveness Trial (Lieberman et al. 2005); CL=concentrated liquid; COPD=chronic obstructive pulmonary disease; CYP=cytochrome P450; D=decanoate; EPS=extrapyramidal side effects; FDA=U.S. Food and Drug Administration; FGA=first-generation antipsychotic; IM=intramuscular injection; L=liquid; LAI=long-acting injection; maintenance=maintenance treatment; MDD=major depressive disorder; ODT=oral disintegrating tablets; PO=oral tablets or capsules; PDSS=post-injection delirium/sedation syndrome; R=rectal suppository SGA=second-generation antipsychotic; SL=sublingual; SZ=schizophrenia; SZAD=schizoaffective disorder; T=adolescent.
[a]Risk for prolonged QTc may be associated with fatal arrhythmias, including torsades de pointes. Obtain baseline electrocardiogram. Avoid use in patients with prolonged QTc, hypokalemia, hypomagnesemia, or concomitant use of other drugs that inhibit metabolism or themselves prolong QTc.
Source. U.S. Food and Drug Administration: Orange Book: Approved Drug Products with Therapeutic Equivalence Evaluations (website). Silver Spring, MD, U.S. Food and Drug Administration, August 2018. Available at: https://www.accessdata.fda.gov/scripts/cder/ob/. Accessed October 7, 2018.

it may be tempting for clinicians to rapidly escalate dosages in the hope of hastening clinical response. However, rapid dosage titration and use of high antipsychotic dosages may lead to unwanted dosage-related toxicity with little or no additive benefit.

Fortunately, multiple routes of administration are available for antipsychotics, which allow for clinical versatility (e.g., emergency control of psychotic agitation, difficulty with swallowing) and serve to enhance adherence (e.g., orally dissolving and depot preparations) (see Levenson and Ferrando 2017 for a review of alternative routes of administration for all psychotropics). Orally dissolving formulations are available for aripiprazole, clozapine, olanzapine, and risperidone, but they require swallowing and are absorbed enterally. Because it has no significant enteral absorption, asenapine is the only antipsychotic available as a sublingual preparation. Liquid formulations are commercially available for aripiprazole, clozapine, risperidone, fluphenazine, and haloperidol. Olanzapine and ziprasidone each have an intramuscular formulation approved for use in treating acute agitation in schizophrenia and bipolar disorder. Haloperidol, chlorpromazine, and fluphenazine also have short-acting intramuscular formulations. Long-acting injectable formulations are available for aripiprazole, olanzapine, risperidone, paliperidone, haloperidol, and fluphenazine. Haloperidol is often given intravenously for the control of severe psychosis and agitation in medically hospitalized patients with delirium, although haloperidol is not FDA approved for this route of administration and purpose. This use of haloperidol intravenously carries a black box warning for QTc prolongation and torsades de pointes. Parenteral formulations of olanzapine and ziprasidone should not be given intravenously.

Adverse Effects

There are numerous potential adverse effects of antipsychotics, ranging from mild nuisance effects to severe, life-threatening conditions. These adverse effects can significantly impair quality of life, can pose potential short- and long-term health risks, and, importantly, may impede adherence, leading to relapse of the underlying psychiatric condition. These adverse effects are outlined in Table 29–3. As stated earlier, SGAs as a class generally have a lowered risk for EPS (detailed below) as well as for NMS and TD. However, it is important to note that SGAs are not free of these effects, and risk varies based on D_2 receptor potency, which is highest for risperidone. The partial D_2 agonist aripiprazole is associated with increased impulse-control behaviors (e.g., pathological gambling).

Extrapyramidal Side Effects

EPS include acute dystonic reactions, parkinsonian syndrome, akathisia, TD, and NMS. In general, high-potency FGAs carry the greatest risk, whereas low-potency phenothiazines and SGAs (except risperidone) carry a significantly lower risk.

Acute dystonic reactions are perhaps the most disturbing EPS for patients and may be life-threatening in the case of laryngeal dystonia. Patients who experience acute dystonia are at risk of medication nonadherence. Patients with a history of or risk factors for dystonia may be treated prophylactically. The need for prophylactic medication to prevent antipsychotic-induced dystonia is generally averted by SGA use. Medications used to treat EPS are outlined in Table 29–4. With the exception of akathisia, which is responsive to propranolol or benzodiazepines, most EPS are responsive to anticholinergic agents or amantadine.

TABLE 29–3. Antipsychotic adverse effects

Adverse effect	Proposed causal mechanism(s)	Clinical manifestation(s)	Management[a]
Extrapyramidal effects			
Acute dystonia	Nigrostriatal DA receptor blockade	Muscular spasm in neck (torticollis), back (opisthotonus), tongue, ocular muscles (oculogyric crisis), larynx (laryngeal dystonia)	See Table 29–4 for available medications
Parkinsonism	Nigrostriatal DA receptor blockade	Cogwheel rigidity, masked facies, bradykinesia, sialorrhea, micrographia, pill-rolling tremor, rabbit syndrome	See Table 29–4 for available medications
Akathisia	Nigrostriatal DA receptor blockade	Internal sense of restlessness, inability to sit still	Propranolol (poorly responsive to anticholinergics, sedatives, amantadine)
Tardive dyskinesia	Prolonged DA receptor blockade, oxidative damage, glutamatergic neurotoxicity	Involuntary choreoathetoid movements of the face, trunk, or extremities	Spontaneous resolution may occur with discontinuation Clozapine Valbenazine, deutetrabenazine (see Table 29–4)
Neuroleptic malignant syndrome	Sudden, marked reduction in DA activity, either from withdrawal of DA agonists or from blockade of DA receptors	Muscle rigidity (may be absent with SGAs), fever, autonomic instability, increased WBC count (>15,000/mm^3), increased creatine kinase levels (>300 U/mL), delirium	Discontinue antipsychotic Supportive care (hydration, antipyretic agents, blood pressure) Bromocriptine, dantrolene, benzodiazepines, ECT (all with anecdotal support in the literature)
Dysphagia	Nigrostriatal DA receptor blockade or muscarinic cholinergic receptor blockade	Esophageal dysmotility, aspiration, choking, weight loss	Reduce dosage or discontinue antipsychotic
Anticholinergic effects	Muscarinic cholinergic receptor blockade	Dry mouth, blurred vision, constipation, urinary retention, tachycardia, cognitive impairment (especially in elderly), anticholinergic delirium	Bethanechol (urecholine) Physostigmine (for anticholinergic delirium)

TABLE 29–3. Antipsychotic adverse effects *(continued)*

Adverse effect	Proposed causal mechanism(s)	Clinical manifestation(s)	Management[a]
Weight gain	Increased appetite and food intake from hypothalamic histaminergic H_1 receptor blockade; alterations in serum leptin levels	May lead to metabolic syndrome, elevated cardiovascular risk	Use care in selecting antipsychotic (greatest risk for olanzapine, clozapine; least risk for aripiprazole, ziprasidone) Weight monitoring ?Metformin
Sedation	Hypothalamic histaminergic H_1 receptor blockade	Daytime sleepiness, impaired motor and cognitive performance	Dose in late evening or at bedtime, switch to less-sedating drug Prescribe wakefulness agents (modafinil, armodafinil—limited evidence) or psychostimulants (limited evidence, may exacerbate psychosis)
Impaired thermoregulation	Hypothalamic histaminergic H_1 receptor blockade	Hypothermia or hyperthermia may be life threatening	Recommend avoidance of extreme temperatures Prescribe wakefulness agents (modafinil, armodafinil—limited evidence) or psychostimulants (limited evidence, may exacerbate psychosis)
Orthostatic hypotension	α_1-Adrenergic receptor antagonism	Dizziness, syncope, falls (with or without fractures)	Provide education regarding sudden postural changes Ensure adequate hydration If nonadherence is an issue, reduce dosage when restarting (especially with clozapine and iloperidone)

TABLE 29–3. Antipsychotic adverse effects *(continued)*

Adverse effect	Proposed causal mechanism(s)	Clinical manifestation(s)	Management[a]
Endocrine effects			
Hyperprolactinemia	Tuberoinfundibular DA receptor blockade	Gynecomastia, galactorrhea, amenorrhea, sexual dysfunction, osteoporosis	Lower dosage or switch to a drug with less propensity to elevate prolactin DA agonist (may exacerbate psychosis) Least risk with aripiprazole
Metabolic syndrome (hyperglycemia, dyslipidemia, hypertension)	Weight gain associated with histaminergic H_1-receptor blockade, 5-HT_{2C} blockade; dysfunction of pancreatic islet cells, hepatic and skeletal muscle glucose transport	Weight gain, hyperglycemia, diabetes, elevated cardiovascular risk	Use care in selecting antipsychotic (greatest risk for olanzapine, clozapine; least risk for aripiprazole, ziprasidone, lurasidone) Close laboratory monitoring Metformin
Lowering of seizure threshold	Unknown, dose-dependent effect for clozapine; small underlying risk with other antipsychotics; patient factors important	Predominantly generalized tonic-clonic seizures	Avoid high-risk agents in patients with epilepsy or brain injury Greatest risk for clozapine, dosage dependent (lower dosage, add anticonvulsant if dosage exceeds 600 mg/day)
Hematological side effects	Bone marrow suppression	Decreased absolute neutrophil count; agranulocytosis (usually early in treatment, greatest risk with clozapine); fever, stomatitis, pharyngitis, lymphadenopathy, malaise	Initiate regular WBC monitoring early in antipsychotic therapy Follow guidelines for clozapine monitoring

TABLE 29–3. Antipsychotic adverse effects (continued)

Adverse effect	Proposed causal mechanism(s)	Clinical manifestation(s)	Management[a]
Cardiac side effects	Delayed atrioventricular conduction, quinidine-like effects, calcium channel blockade Myocarditis with clozapine	Prolonged QTc,[b] ventricular arrhythmias, torsades de pointes, sudden cardiac death; heart failure	Obtain baseline and regular electrocardiograms for patients with cardiac risk factors (e.g., long-QT syndrome, hypokalemia, hypomagnesemia, concurrent metabolic inhibitors), higher-risk antipsychotics
Mortality risk in elderly patients with dementia-related psychosis	Cardiac conduction effects, excessive sedation	Cardiovascular arrest; infections (pneumonia)	Conduct careful risk–benefit assessment in elderly patients with dementia-related psychosis; antipsychotics are not approved for use in this condition
Dermatological effects	Unknown	Sun sensitivity	Recommend avoidance of excessive sun exposure and use of sunscreen
Ocular effects	Retinal pigment deposition	Pigmentary retinopathy is a rare effect of thioridazine Cataracts is a rare effect of cariprazine Cataracts found in dogs exposed to quetiapine Cataracts not found in human trials or in clinical use of quetiapine	Periodic ocular examination for patients on thioridazine or cariprazine Slit-lamp examination for patients on chronic quetiapine treatment

Note. 5-HT=5-hydroxytryptamine (serotonin); DA=dopamine; ECT=electroconvulsive therapy; SGA=second-generation antipsychotic; WBC=white blood cell.

[a]Most of the adverse effects listed will respond to dosage reduction or discontinuation of medication and switch to an alternative agent with less propensity to cause the effect in question. Therefore, this strategy is not listed for each adverse effect. If an adverse effect is not dose-related, that circumstance is indicated.

[b]Highest risk associated with thioridazine, chlorpromazine, quetiapine, ziprasidone, intravenous haloperidol, pimozide, and iloperidone. Increased risk associated with coadministration of metabolic inhibitors of antipsychotics. Lowest-risk agent is aripiprazole.

TABLE 29–4. Medications used to treat extrapyramidal side effects (EPS)

Generic name	Trade name	Drug type (mechanism)	Usual adult dosage	Indications for EPS
Amantadine	Symmetrel	Dopaminergic agent	100 mg PO bid	Parkinsonian syndrome
Benztropine	Cogentin	Anticholinergic agent	1–2 mg PO bid 2 mg IM or IV[a]	Dystonia, parkinsonian syndrome Acute dystonia
Deutetrabenazine	Austedo	VMAT2 inhibitor	6–24 mg PO bid	Tardive dyskinesia
Diphenhydramine	Benadryl	Anticholinergic agent	25–50 mg PO tid 25 mg IM or IV[a]	Dystonia, parkinsonian syndrome Acute dystonia
Propranolol	Inderal	β-blocker	20 mg PO tid	Akathisia
Trihexyphenidyl	Artane	Anticholinergic agent	5–10 mg PO bid	Dystonia, parkinsonian syndrome
Valbenazine	Ingrezza	VMAT2 inhibitor	80 mg PO qd	Tardive dyskinesia

Note. bid=twice per day; IM=intramuscular injection; IV=intravenous injection; PO=oral medication; qd=once per day; tid=three times per day; VMAT2=vesicular monoamine transporter 2.
[a]Follow with oral medication.

Tardive dyskinesia.   TD is a disorder characterized by involuntary choreoathetoid movements of the face, trunk, or extremities as well as by tardive akathisia, dystonias, and tics. TD is associated with prolonged exposure to high-potency FGAs; however, the disorder has also been reported with SGAs and dopamine antagonist antiemetics (especially metoclopramide). TD often emerges abruptly after antipsychotic discontinuation and is mitigated or masked by resumption of the same or an alternative antipsychotic. Risk factors include older age, female sex, EPS early in treatment, history of drug holidays, presence of other brain disorders, diabetes mellitus, substance abuse, and a diagnosis of a mood disorder (Salem et al. 2017).

The Abnormal Involuntary Movement Scale (AIMS) may be used to assess and monitor patients at risk of TD. An evaluation for abnormal movements should be conducted before treatment begins and every 6 or 12 months thereafter. Patients often tend to minimize or be unaware of TD symptoms.

Although TD often resolves within weeks or months of antipsychotic discontinuation and may improve by switching the patient to an SGA with a lower propensity to cause TD, such as ziprasidone in mild TD and clozapine in more severe and progressive TD, the disorder may persist indefinitely. Many drugs have been used off-label for treatment of TD (e.g., amantadine, benztropine, clonazepam, ginkgo biloba, propranolol), despite limited evidence of their efficacy. In 2017, two vesicular monoamine transporter 2 (VMAT2) inhibitors, valbenazine and deutetrabenazine, became the first agents to receive FDA approval specifically for use in treatment of TD, based on their performance in short phase III trials. Longer studies are needed to elucidate the place of these drugs in clinical practice (Salem et al. 2017).

Neuroleptic malignant syndrome.   The incidence of NMS is about 0.02% among patients treated with antipsychotics (Caroff 2003b). Classic signs are hyperthermia, generalized rigidity with tremors, altered consciousness with catatonia, and autonomic instability (Caroff 2003a). Laboratory findings include muscle enzyme elevations (primarily creatine phosphokinase, levels >800 IU/L), myoglobinuria, leukocytosis, metabolic acidosis, hypoxia, and low serum iron levels. Risk factors include dehydration, exhaustion, agitation, catatonia, previous episodes, and high dosages of high-potency antipsychotics given parenterally at a rapid rate of titration. NMS may develop within hours but usually evolves over days, with two-thirds of cases occurring during the first 1–2 weeks after antipsychotic initiation. Once dopamine-blocking drugs are withheld, two-thirds of NMS cases resolve within 1–2 weeks, with an average duration of 7–10 days (Caroff 2003b). Patients may experience more prolonged symptoms (up to 4 weeks) if injectable long-acting antipsychotics are implicated. Occasional patients develop a residual catatonic and parkinsonian state that can last for weeks unless electroconvulsive therapy (ECT) is administered. NMS is potentially fatal in some cases due to renal failure, cardiorespiratory arrest, disseminated intravascular coagulation, pulmonary emboli, or aspiration pneumonia.

Treatment of NMS consists of early diagnosis, discontinuation of dopamine antagonists, and supportive medical care. Benzodiazepines, dopamine agonists, dantrolene, and ECT have been described in clinical and case reports as being helpful; however, there are no data from randomized controlled trials to support these approaches. These agents may be considered empirically in individual cases based on symptoms, severity, and duration of the episode.

Endocrinological Effects

Metabolic syndrome. Most antipsychotics are associated with metabolic syndrome. Metabolic syndrome is defined by five criteria: abdominal obesity, triglycerides 150 mg/dL or greater (≥1.7 mmol/L), high-density lipoprotein less than 40 mg/dL (<1.03 mmol/L) for men or less than 50 mg/dL (<1.28 mmol/L) for women, blood pressure 130/85 mm Hg or higher, and fasting glucose 100 mg/dL or higher (≥5.6 mmol/L) (Grundy et al. 2005). Metabolic syndrome is an independent risk factor for diabetes (including ketoacidosis) and for cardiovascular, cerebrovascular, and peripheral vascular disease. The extent to which metabolic syndrome is solely a function of antipsychotic treatment is controversial. Compared with the general population, medication-naive patients with schizophrenia, bipolar disorder, and schizoaffective disorder have been found to have impaired glucose tolerance. Weight gain is common with SGAs; clozapine and olanzapine cause the greatest weight gain, whereas quetiapine, risperidone, and paliperidone cause mild to moderate weight gain. Ziprasidone and lurasidone tend to be the most weight-neutral. Aripiprazole is considered weight-neutral, yet some patients do gain weight. Elevations in serum triglycerides and low-density lipoprotein cholesterol and decreases in high-density lipoprotein cholesterol usually occur in parallel, but these changes may occur in the absence of weight gain. Patients taking antipsychotics should be monitored for weight gain, hypertension, glucose intolerance, and lipid derangements. Guidelines for patient monitoring are summarized in Table 29–5.

Treatment of metabolic syndrome begins with dosage adjustment (when feasible) or cross-tapering to a more weight-neutral medication. Techniques including dietary education, exercise, and cognitive-behavioral interventions are effective for either maintaining or losing weight in patients treated with SGAs. A meta-analysis of 12 studies found that the addition of metformin to an antipsychotic regimen showed benefit in reducing weight gain and insulin resistance (de Silva et al. 2016).

Hyperprolactinemia may cause impotence, menstrual dysregulation, amenorrhea, infertility, galactorrhea, gynecomastia, and sexual dysfunction. Emerging evidence suggests long-term sequelae, including loss of bone mineral density, osteoporosis, and breast cancer (Grigg et al. 2017). Hyperprolactinemia is most likely to occur with risperidone, paliperidone, and high-potency FGAs and is least likely with aripiprazole. Relevant American Psychiatric Association guidelines recommend routine monitoring of prolactin serum levels only in symptomatic patients (Lehman et al. 2004). Treatment strategies include decreasing the dosage of the offending agent, switching the patient to an agent less likely to affect prolactin, and preventing bone demineralization by addressing insufficient exercise, poor nutrition, smoking, alcohol use, and low vitamin D levels.

Cardiac Effects

All antipsychotics may prolong the QT interval, with the possible exception of aripiprazole. Haloperidol, droperidol, thioridazine, sertindole, ziprasidone, and iloperidone tend to produce greater-magnitude QT prolongation than other agents (Beach et al. 2013). QT interval prolongation corrected for heart rate (QTc) greater than 500 msec is associated with increased risk of polymorphic sustained ventricular tachycardia (torsades de pointes), which can degenerate into ventricular fibrillation. Women,

TABLE 29–5. Consensus guidelines for monitoring metabolic status in patients taking antipsychotic medications

Metabolic risk parameter	Baseline	4 weeks	8 weeks	12 weeks	Quarterly	Annually	Every 5 years
Personal and family history of diabetes mellitus, cardiovascular disease	X					X	
Weight (body mass index)	X	X	X	X	X		
Waist circumference	X					X	
Blood pressure	X			X		X	
Fasting plasma glucose	X			X		X	
Fasting lipid profile	X			X			X

Source.   Adapted from American Diabetes Association et al. 2004.

patients with chronic heavy alcohol consumption, and patients with anorexia nervosa are at increased risk. Other noted risk factors for torsades de pointes include familial long-QT syndrome, severe heart disease, hypokalemia, hypomagnesemia, and concurrent treatment with other drugs that prolong the QT interval or that inhibit antipsychotic metabolism (Beach et al. 2013).

In elderly patients with behavioral disturbances, both FGAs and SGAs are associated with about a 1.9% absolute increase in short-term mortality (4.5% vs. 2.6%, or about a 70% increase in adjusted relative risk [Kuehn 2008]), due mostly to cardiovascular events and infections. This associated increase in mortality resulted in an FDA-mandated black box warning about off-label treatment of agitation and psychotic symptoms in elderly patients with dementia. A review of Tennessee Medicaid data found that antipsychotics were associated with an approximate doubling of the risk for sudden death, but the absolute risk was only about 0.0015 deaths per person-year, yielding a number needed to treat to cause 1 additional sudden death annually of 666 persons (Ray et al. 2009).

Clozapine is associated with risk of myocarditis and cardiomyopathy, which can be life-threatening if unaddressed (for more information, see "Clozapine" section later in this chapter).

Dermatological Effects

Most phenothiazines are associated with increased photosensitivity and risk of sunburn. Additionally, skin pigmentation changes to a grayish color have been observed with chlorpromazine. The FDA issued a warning regarding risk of serious skin reactions, including drug reaction with eosinophilia and systemic symptoms (DRESS), for olanzapine and ziprasidone. DRESS is characterized by a severe rash and systemic symptoms including fever (38°C to 40°C [100.4°F to 104°F]), malaise, lymphadenopathy, and symptoms related to visceral involvement. Asenapine is associated with reports of type I hypersensitivity reactions, including anaphylaxis and angioedema.

Drug Interactions (See Also "General Principles" Section at Beginning of Chapter)

Most antipsychotics are metabolized by the hepatic CYP2D6 isoenzyme. Exceptions include ziprasidone and quetiapine, which are metabolized mainly by the CYP3A4 enzyme. Thus, metabolism may be affected by inhibition or induction of these enzymes. For example, the addition of fluoxetine can increase serum haloperidol concentrations, although sources disagree as to whether this increase occurs to a clinically significant degree. Two categories of potential drug–drug interactions are of particular concern: 1) interactions that can increase serum concentrations of antipsychotics to dangerous levels, and 2) interactions that can reduce serum concentrations of antipsychotics, rendering them ineffective. As an example of the first category of interaction, clozapine is metabolized primarily by CYP1A2 (major), in addition to CYP2D6 and CYP3A4 (both minor) isoenzymes. Coadministration of potent CYP1A2 inhibitors (e.g., ciprofloxacin, fluvoxamine) can lead to toxic serum clozapine concentrations (Meyer et al. 2016). As an example of the second category, reductions in serum clozapine and haloperidol concentrations have been reported with the addition of enzyme inducers of CYP3A4 and CYP1A2, such as carbamazepine (Tsuda et al. 2014). Cigarette smoking, via

CYP1A2 induction, can likewise affect antipsychotic metabolism; serum concentrations of clozapine and olanzapine are reduced with smoking and increased after smoking cessation (Tsuda et al. 2014).

Clozapine

Clozapine, the first and a uniquely important SGA, has been shown in multiple clinical trials to be efficacious for treatment-resistant schizophrenia, to significantly reduce negative symptoms of schizophrenia, and to reduce suicidal ideation and attempts in patients with schizophrenia and related disorders. Clozapine rarely causes EPS, especially TD.

Because clozapine is associated with a risk of severe neutropenia (defined as an absolute neutrophil count less than 500/μL), its use is usually reserved for patients who have not adequately responded to or who have not tolerated treatment with at least two other antipsychotics. Clozapine's efficacy in patients with a history of nonresponse to previous antipsychotic treatment has been documented in the literature, with up to 30% of such patients responding (Lewis et al. 2006).

Clozapine therapy is usually begun by cross-titrating clozapine with the previous agent that has shown insufficient efficacy. Clozapine is initiated at a dosage of 12.5 mg/day, with a rapid increase to 12.5 mg twice daily. The dosage is then increased as tolerated, generally in 25- or 50-mg increments every day or every other day. It is important to monitor for sedation, orthostatic hypotension, tachycardia and bradycardia, and syncope. Clozapine dosages can be increased much more rapidly in an inpatient setting with monitoring of vital signs. The typical target dosage is 300–500 mg/day given in divided doses. Serum levels should be ascertained in nonresponders. Gradual titration up to 900 mg/day may be necessary for patients who have not responded to clozapine after 6 months and who have no other viable options.

The cumulative incidence of severe neutropenia is estimated as 0.8% of patients receiving clozapine over a 15-month period, with a peak incidence in the first 6–18 weeks of treatment (Raja 2011). The FDA mandated implementation of a Risk Evaluation and Mitigation Strategy (REMS) program to ensure optimal patient monitoring for and management of clozapine-induced severe neutropenia. All prescribers (or their designees), dispensing pharmacies, and patients must be enrolled in the program, and prescribers and pharmacies must be certified. Clozapine dispensing is linked to weekly absolute neutrophil counts during the first 6 months of treatment, biweekly (every 2 weeks) counts for the next 6 months, and monthly counts thereafter. White blood cell (WBC) counts are no longer required, and lower absolute neutrophil count thresholds are allowable for patients with benign ethnic neutropenia. These required guidelines for clozapine use based on absolute neutrophil count are shown in Table 29–6.

If severe neutropenia develops, prompt consultation with a hematologist is indicated. Granulocyte colony–stimulating factors or lithium may be considered for counteracting or preventing severe neutropenia when using clozapine, although these strategies carry their own safety concerns (Raja 2011). Once an individual has developed severe neutropenia while taking clozapine, he or she should not be rechallenged unless the prescriber determines that the potential benefits outweigh the risk of recurrence. Clozapine is relatively contraindicated in patients who have myeloproliferative disorders and/or who are immunocompromised, because of their increased risk for se-

Source. Adapted from Clozapine REMS Program: "Recommended Monitoring Frequency and Clinical Decisions by ANC Level," from *Clozapine and the Risk of Neutropenia: An Overview for Healthcare Providers*, Version 2.0, December 23, 2014. Available at: https://www.clozapinerems.com/CpmgClozapineUI/rems/pdf/resources/ANC_Table.pdf. Accessed November 11, 2018.

TABLE 29–6. **Monitoring guidelines for clozapine**

Baseline absolute neutrophil count (ANC) must be at least 1,500/μL in the normal population. If the individual has benign ethnic neutropenia (BEN), initial ANC must be at least 1,000/μL (at least two baseline ANC levels required).

Weekly ANC is required for the first 6 months of treatment. From 6 to 12 months, monitoring is required every 2 weeks. After 12 months, monitoring is required monthly.

If ANC is 1,000–1,499/μL (500–999/μL if BEN), continue treatment with clozapine and obtain ANC three times weekly until ANC is at least 1,500/μL (at least 1,000/μL if BEN). Once the specified ANC threshold is met, return to the individual's previous ANC monitoring interval if clinically appropriate.

If ANC is 500–999/μL (less than 500/μL if BEN), interrupt clozapine treatment and recommend a hematology consultation. Obtain daily ANCs until at least 1,000/μL (at least 500/μL if BEN), then obtain ANC three times weekly until at least 1,500/μL (at least established ANC baseline if BEN). Do not rechallenge any patient with an ANC less than 500/μL unless benefits clearly outweigh risks.

vere neutropenia. Concomitant administration of medications that are associated with bone marrow suppression, such as carbamazepine, is also relatively contraindicated.

Clozapine is associated with a dose-dependent risk of seizures. Dosages of less than 300 mg/day are associated with a 1% risk of seizures, those of 300–600 mg/day with a 2.7% risk, and those of greater than 600 mg/day with a 4.4% risk (Raja 2011). Care should be taken to avoid drug interactions that inhibit the CYP1A2-mediated metabolism of clozapine. Reports have described use of anticonvulsant drugs (e.g., valproate, gabapentin, lamotrigine, topiramate) to prevent clozapine-associated seizures (Raja 2011).

Clozapine is associated with fatal myocarditis and cardiomyopathy. Estimates of the incidence of myocarditis range from 0.015% to 0.19%, but the incidence is likely higher, given diagnostic and reporting limitations. Although 90% of myocarditis cases occur within the first 8 weeks of treatment, cardiomyopathy can occur in the absence of acute myocarditis months to years after clozapine initiation (Raja 2011). The clinical presentation of myocarditis is often nonspecific; therefore, performing a baseline cardiac evaluation and monitoring patients for cardiac signs and symptoms are encouraged. Rechallenging of a patient who develops myocarditis or cardiomyopathy on clozapine is not recommended.

Clozapine can cause hypersalivation, constipation, and nocturnal enuresis. Clozapine-induced constipation can lead to fatal complications (e.g., bowel obstruction, toxic megacolon) if not treated appropriately (Raja 2011).

Mood Stabilizers

Three primary classes of medications have efficacy in the treatment of bipolar mania: lithium, selected anticonvulsants (covered in this section), and antipsychotics (covered previously). The approved indications and documented efficacy of these drugs vary for different targets of bipolar disorder treatment, including acute mania, maintenance treatment (prevention of mania and depression relapse), mixed manic states, and bipolar depression. Table 29–7 outlines the indications, dosing, serum drug level monitoring (as applicable), and adverse effects of the approved mood stabilizers. Table 29–2 outlines the indications and dosing of the antipsychotics used to treat mood disorders.

Lithium

The tranquilizing properties of lithium have been known for millennia; however, its toxicity with unregulated use limited its application in medicine. The modern use of lithium for the treatment of mania was described by Cade in 1949 (Richardson and Macaluso 2017). He and others studied the pharmacological use of lithium in manic-depressive patients during the 1950s and 1960s, and the FDA approved lithium for the treatment of mania in 1970. It remains the gold standard medication for mania.

Lithium is approved for acute manic episodes and maintenance treatment of bipolar disorder and is a first-line choice for treatment of bipolar depression. Patients with rapid-cycling bipolar disorder may respond to lithium, but lithium is less likely to prevent mood episode recurrence in these patients (Richardson and Macaluso 2017). Lithium is also effective as an adjunct to antidepressants in treating refractory unipolar depression and in reducing suicidality in mood disorder patients, and in combination with antidepressants may be useful in maintaining remission of depression after ECT (Richardson and Macaluso 2017).

Clinical Use

Lithium carbonate is completely absorbed in the gastrointestinal tract, reaches peak plasma levels in 1–2 hours, has an elimination half-life of approximately 24 hours, and reaches steady state in approximately 5 days. It is excreted unaltered through the urine. Lithium is dosed according to clinical response, side effects, and serum levels. When used for acute treatment, lithium is generally started at 900–1,200 mg/day in divided doses, and the dosage may be raised as high as 1,500–1,800 mg/day based on serum levels. A serum level of 0.8–1.2 mEq/L (sometimes up to 1.5 mEq/L) is generally necessary for treatment of acute mania; however, side effects must be monitored closely when levels are at the higher end of this target range. During the initiation of lithium treatment, it is often combined with an antipsychotic and/or a benzodiazepine until lithium has a chance to take effect. Once sustained remission of mania is achieved, adjunctive medications are tapered if possible.

For most patients with bipolar disorder, a lithium serum concentration in the range of 0.8–1.0 mEq/L is the target for maintenance treatment to reduce risk of relapse, but some patients can maintain remission with lower lithium levels (0.4–0.6 mEq/L). A relapse may be more likely to be triggered by a sudden rather than a gradual drop in lithium level.

Lithium is often given in divided doses at the initiation of treatment; however, once stability is achieved and side effects have been assessed, it may be preferable to give lithium once daily in the evening or at bedtime. Once-daily administration helps to increase adherence and to minimize adverse effects and possibly renal impairment.

Lithium levels should be measured about 12 hours after the last lithium dose. After therapeutic lithium levels have been established, levels should usually be measured every month for the first 3 months and every 3–6 months thereafter. Renal function should be determined before lithium therapy and periodically thereafter, more frequently if adverse effects increase or if there are signs of or risks for renal insufficiency.

Lithium is almost entirely excreted by the kidneys. It is contraindicated in patients with acute renal failure but not in chronic renal failure. For patients with stable partial renal insufficiency, clinicians should dose conservatively and monitor renal function frequently. For patients on dialysis, lithium is completely dialyzed and may be given as a single oral dose (300–600 mg) following hemodialysis treatment. Lithium levels should not be checked until at least 2–3 hours after dialysis, because re-equilibration from tissue stores occurs in the immediate postdialysis period. Lithium may prolong the QTc interval and may increase the risk of cardiac arrhythmias in patients with electrolyte disturbances.

Adverse Effects

Lithium has a number of concentration-dependent side effects that, if present, can be a significant impediment to adherence and at worst may cause severe toxicity. Lithium has a narrow therapeutic index (i.e., a small difference between therapeutic and toxic levels). Fluid and electrolyte disturbances as well as concurrent medications that modify renal function (discussed in the "Drug Interactions" section that follows) may reduce elimination and increase adverse effects. Children, the elderly, and patients with medical or neurological comorbidity are at heightened risk. Table 29–8 outlines the adverse effects of lithium according to serum level in adults. Common adverse effects in the therapeutic range include gastrointestinal disturbances (nausea, vomiting), fine motor tremor, cognitive slowing, weight gain, cardiac effects (benign flattening of T wave, QTc prolongation), benign leukocytosis, and dermatological complications including acne, folliculitis, psoriasis, and alopecia. Fine motor tremor is successfully treated in most patients with propranolol up to 120 mg/day in divided doses. If β-blockers are ineffective or not tolerated, primidone, benzodiazepines, and vitamin B_6 have been used (Gitlin 2016). Patients may complain of impaired cognition and psychomotor slowing while on lithium, effects that may precipitate nonadherence in individuals who are accustomed to the rapid thoughts and perceived clarity associated with mania. It is important to note that bipolar disorder is itself associated with neuropsychological impairment, independent of medications.

Acute lithium toxicity occurs at serum levels above 1.5 mEq/L and can involve moderate to severe gastrointestinal, neurological, and cardiovascular effects, outlined in Table 29–8.

Lithium and the kidney. Lithium causes water and sodium diuresis and may precipitate nephrogenic diabetes insipidus (NDI). Most patients receiving lithium have polydipsia and polyuria, reflecting mild benign NDI. Lithium-induced NDI sometimes has persisted long after lithium discontinuation and varies from mild polyuria to hyperosmolar coma. Amiloride is considered the treatment of choice for lithium-induced NDI.

The effects of lithium on renal function are controversial; some studies report that a longer duration of lithium therapy is predictive of a progressive decrease in the estimated glomerular filtration rate ("creeping creatinine"), whereas others do not (Cukor et al. 2019). Although long-term lithium treatment is the only well-established factor associated with lithium-induced nephropathy, changes in renal function are often associated with other factors, including age, episodes of lithium toxicity, other medications (analgesics, substance abuse), and the presence of comorbid disorders

TABLE 29–7.   Mood stabilizers

Generic name	Dosage forms and strengths, mg	FDA-approved indications	Recommended dosage range	Therapeutic serum level	Adverse effects
Lithium					
Lithium carbonate	Tablet: 300 Capsule: 150, 300, 600 ER tablet: 300, 450	Acute manic episodes and maintenance treatment of bipolar disorder	Mania: 900–1,800 mg/day Maintenance: 600–1,200 mg/day	Mania: 0.8–1.5 mEq/L Maintenance: 0.6–1.0 mEq/L	Nausea, vomiting, fine tremor, leukocytosis, weight gain, hypo- and hyperthyroidism, hyperparathyroidism, nephrogenic diabetes insipidus, Ebstein's anomaly in first-trimester pregnancy
Lithium citrate	Liquid: 8 mEq/5 mL				
Valproate					
Divalproex sodium	Delayed-release capsule, tablet: 125, 250, 500 Delayed-release sprinkle capsule: 125 ER (24-hour) tablet: 250, 500	Acute manic or mixed episodes in bipolar disorder	10–60 mg/kg/day divided (loading strategy: 20 mg/kg of delayed-release day 1; 25 mg/kg of ER formulation)	Mania: 85–125 mg/L	Nausea, vomiting, diarrhea, tremor, weight gain, reversible alopecia, polycystic ovary syndrome, thrombocytopenia, blood dyscrasias (rare), hepatotoxicity, pancreatitis, neural tube defects from first-trimester exposure
Valproate sodium	Injection: 100 mg/5 mL				
Valproic acid	Capsule: 250 Oral solution: 250 mg/5 mL				

TABLE 29–7. Mood stabilizers *(continued)*

Generic name	Dosage forms and strengths, mg	FDA-approved indications	Recommended dosage range	Therapeutic serum level	Adverse effects
Lamotrigine	Tablet: 25, 100, 150, 200 ER tablet: 25, 50, 100, 200, 250, 300 Chewable tablet: 2, 5, 25 Orally dissolving tablet: 25, 50, 100, 200	Maintenance treatment of bipolar I disorder	200 mg/day (100 with valproate; 400 with carbamazepine) Strict titration schedule to reduce risk of severe rash	N/A	Headache, dizziness, diplopia, benign to severe Stevens-Johnson syndrome (rare) rash, nausea, diarrhea, abnormal dreams, pruritus, aseptic meningitis (rare)
Carbamazepine	ER capsule: 100, 200, 300 Chewable tablet: 100, 200 ER tablet: 100, 200, 400 Oral solution: 100 mg/ 5 mL Tablet: 200	Acute manic or mixed episodes associated with bipolar I disorder (ER capsule)	400–1,600 mg/day	N/A in bipolar disorder; 4–12 mg/L for epilepsy; useful for monitoring toxicity and drug interactions	Dizziness, sedation, nausea, ataxia, constipation; severe dermatological reactions, especially with HLA-B*1502 allele; agranulocytosis; aplastic anemia, DRESS syndrome; hyponatremia

Note. DRESS=drug reaction with eosinophilia and systemic symptoms; ER=extended release.
Table excludes antipsychotics that are U.S. Food and Drug Administration (FDA) approved for use in bipolar disorder (aripiprazole, asenapine, cariprazine, lurasidone, olanzapine, quetiapine, risperidone, and ziprasidone). See Table 29–2 for details regarding use of antipsychotics in bipolar disorder.

TABLE 29–8.   Signs of lithium toxicity

Mild to moderate intoxication (lithium level=1.5–2.0 mEq/L)

Gastrointestinal symptoms

Nausea, vomiting, diarrhea, abdominal pain, dry mouth, polydipsia, polyuria

Neurological symptoms

Ataxia, dizziness, slurred speech, nystagmus, muscle weakness, lethargy or excitement, worsening tremor, poor concentration

Moderate to severe intoxication (lithium level=2.1–2.5 mEq/L)

Gastrointestinal symptoms

Anorexia, persistent nausea and vomiting

Neurological symptoms

Blurred vision, muscle fasciculations, clonic limb movements, hyperactive deep tendon reflexes, choreoathetoid movements, seizure, delirium/confusion, gross tremor

Cardiovascular symptoms

Electrocardiogram changes: QT prolongation, T-wave flattening, arrhythmias

Circulatory failure (decreased blood pressure, tachycardia), syncope

Severe intoxication (lithium level>2.5 mEq/L)

Generalized seizures, oliguria and renal failure, death

(hypertension, diabetes). Lithium dosage has not been strongly related to nephrotoxic effects, but recent studies suggest that there are lower rates of end-stage renal disease with lower mean therapeutic lithium levels (Gitlin 2016). The progression of lithium nephrotoxicity to end-stage renal disease is rare and requires lithium use for several decades. With regular monitoring of renal function, the benefits of long-term lithium maintenance for bipolar disorder far outweigh the risks to renal function.

Lithium-induced thyroid disorders.   Lithium-induced hypothyroidism is common, developing in 5%–35% of patients with varying degrees of severity, from subclinical effects to myxedema. The risk is three times higher in women than in men. Subclinical hypothyroidism (i.e., elevated thyroid-stimulating hormone [TSH] with normal thyroxine and no symptoms) is more prevalent than clinical hypothyroidism.

TSH should be measured prior to initiating lithium therapy and 3 months into treatment. If TSH is normal, it should be rechecked every 6–12 months. If clinically significant hypothyroidism develops or subclinical effects persist after 4 months of lithium treatment, thyroxine replacement or a switch to an alternative mood stabilizer is recommended.

Approximately 1%–2% of lithium-treated patients may develop hyperthyroidism. Lithium-induced hyperthyroidism may be missed because it is often transient, asymptomatic, and followed by hypothyroidism, or mistaken for hypomania.

Lithium and hyperparathyroidism.   Hyperparathyroidism is an underrecognized side effect of long-term lithium therapy, and it is prudent to screen patients undergoing chronic lithium therapy for hypercalcemia. Cessation of lithium may not correct the hyperparathyroidism, necessitating parathyroidectomy. Although hyperparathyroidism is a risk factor for osteoporosis, patients taking lithium who have normal calcium and parathyroid hormone levels do not have an increased risk of osteoporosis.

Drug Interactions (See Also "General Principles" Section at Beginning of Chapter)

Lithium is renally excreted. Thiazide diuretics, loop diuretics, nonsteroidal anti-inflammatory drugs, angiotensin-converting enzyme inhibitors, and angiotensin receptor blockers increase lithium levels. Ideally, these combinations should be avoided; however, if a thiazide diuretic is added to lithium, the lithium dosage should be reduced by 25–50% and the level rechecked when the new steady state is reached. Toxicity resulting from addition of an angiotensin-converting enzyme inhibitor or angiotensin receptor blocker to lithium is usually delayed. Carbonic anhydrase inhibitors, osmotic diuretics, methylxanthines, and caffeine reduce lithium levels (Richardson and Macaluso 2017).

Valproate

Clinical Use

Divalproex sodium is approved for the treatment of acute mania. Several valproate preparations are available in the United States, including valproic acid, sodium valproate, divalproex sodium, and an extended-release preparation of divalproex sodium. Divalproex sodium, a dimer of sodium valproate and valproic acid with an enteric coating, is the best tolerated. The half-life of valproate is 9–16 hours.

There are two primary strategies for initiation of valproate: gradual dosage titration and valproate loading. Gradual dosage titration is appropriate for patients with hypomania or mild manic symptoms, with treatment initiated at 250 mg three times daily, then adjusted upward every 3–4 days to a target range of 1,000–2,000 mg/day. Valproate loading is used for patients with acute mania, with treatment initiated at a dosage of 20 mg per kilogram of body weight (Keck et al. 1993). Plasma levels of 85–125 mg/L are recommended for the treatment of acute mania (see Table 29–7); however, dosing should be based on clinical response and side-effect burden.

Adverse Effects

The most common adverse effects of valproate are gastrointestinal and include indigestion, nausea, vomiting, and diarrhea, which can be reduced with enteric-coated and extended-release formulations. Sedation, mild ataxia, benign tremor, and weight gain are also common. Weight gain does not appear to be dose dependent, and attention to diet and exercise should always be recommended. Valproate treatment can cause alopecia, which is generally but not always reversible.

Valproate has been associated with rare hepatic failure and is considered to be relatively contraindicated for patients with severe liver disease. Risk of fatal hepatotoxicity is highest in young children (especially those on multiple anticonvulsants), and risk decreases with age. Baseline liver function tests are prudent prior to initiation of valproate, and liver function tests should be monitored during valproate therapy. Elevated liver enzymes two or three times the upper limit of normal may not require discontinuation of therapy if levels remain stable and are not associated with clinical signs of liver toxicity. Serum ammonia and γ-glutamyltransferase levels may also be transiently elevated. Valproate can cause asymptomatic hyperammonemia and hyperammonemic encephalopathy (symptomatically similar to hepatic encephalopathy). Routine ammonia-level monitoring is not recommended unless a patient is symptomatic.

In rare cases, valproate can cause pancreatitis. If vomiting and severe abdominal pain develop during valproate therapy, serum amylase levels should be measured immediately and valproate discontinued. Valproate has been associated with dose-dependent thrombocytopenia and should be given with caution in patients requiring anticoagulation. Valproate has also in rare cases been associated with hyponatremia. Finally, valproate has been associated with polycystic ovary syndrome, which is characterized by menstrual irregularity and hyperandrogenism, including hirsutism; this syndrome occurs in about 10% of women taking valproate (Bilo and Meo 2008).

Valproate overdose results in sedation, confusion, and ultimately coma. Hyperreflexia or hyporeflexia, seizures, respiratory suppression, and supraventricular tachycardia can also be present. Treatment should include activated charcoal, electrocardiographic monitoring, treatment of emergent seizures, and respiratory support.

Drug Interactions (See Also "General Principles" Section at Beginning of Chapter)

Valproate can inhibit hepatic enzymes (UDP-glucuronosyltransferase [UGT] and CYP), leading to increased levels of other medications, particularly lamotrigine, thereby increasing the risk of lamotrigine-induced rash (current lamotrigine product labeling provides specific lamotrigine dosing guidelines for patients who are taking valproate). Valproate may increase concentrations of phenobarbital, ethosuximide, and the active 10,11-epoxide metabolite of carbamazepine, increasing the risk of toxicity. Valproate is also highly bound to plasma proteins and may displace other highly bound drugs from protein-binding sites, which may lead to toxicity with low-therapeutic-index drugs. Drugs that may increase valproate levels include cimetidine, macrolide antibiotics (e.g., erythromycin), and felbamate. Valproate metabolism may be induced by other anticonvulsants, including carbamazepine, phenytoin, primidone, and phenobarbital, resulting in an increased total clearance of valproate and perhaps decreased efficacy. Carbapenem antibiotics significantly reduce valproic acid concentrations (by approximately 60%), which can lead to subtherapeutic levels within 24 hours of antibiotic initiation (Wu et al. 2016).

Carbamazepine

Clinical Use

The carbamazepine extended-release capsule (Equetro) formulation is approved by the FDA for the treatment of acute manic and mixed episodes of bipolar I disorder; however, efficacy data are available for other carbamazepine formulations and for use of carbamazepine in maintenance treatment. Carbamazepine should be initiated at a dosage of 200 mg twice daily. The dosage is increased in increments of 200 mg/day every 3–5 days to a maximum of 1,600 mg/day. A therapeutic serum level of 4–12 mg/L is documented in patients with epilepsy, but the upper limit of this range is more useful for monitoring toxicity in patients with bipolar disorder. During the titration phase, patients may experience sedation, dizziness, and ataxia, necessitating a more gradual increase in dosage. Carbamazepine induces its own metabolism, which may cause downward fluctuations in serum levels and clinical response in the early stages of treatment, necessitating careful upward dose adjustment. Autoinduction typically begins 3–5 days after initiating treatment and reaches steady state after 3–5 weeks of continuous dosing.

Adverse Effects

Gastrointestinal (e.g., nausea, vomiting) and mild neurological (e.g., dizziness, drowsiness, ataxia) side effects are common with carbamazepine, particularly early in treatment. The most serious toxic hematological side effects of carbamazepine are agranulocytosis and aplastic anemia, which can be fatal. Fortunately, these effects are rare compared with other hematological effects, such as leukopenia (defined as a total WBC count <3,000 cells/mm^3), thrombocytopenia, and mild anemia. The onset of carbamazepine-induced agranulocytosis is rapid when it occurs, making periodic hematological monitoring of limited benefit. Therefore, it is important to educate patients about early signs and symptoms of agranulocytosis and thrombocytopenia.

Carbamazepine may cause hepatotoxicity, usually a hypersensitivity hepatitis. Cholestasis is also possible. Mild transient increases in transaminase levels (two or three times the upper limit of normal) generally do not necessitate discontinuation of carbamazepine.

Rash is a common side effect of carbamazepine, occurring in 3%–17% of patients within the first 6 months of treatment. If rash develops, dermatological consultation and cessation of carbamazepine should be considered because of the risk of Stevens-Johnson syndrome and toxic epidermal necrolysis. A strong association has been found between this risk and the *HLA-B*1502* allele; therefore, genetic testing should be performed prior to initiating carbamazepine in patients with a higher likelihood of carrying this allele (i.e., certain Asian ancestries).

Carbamazepine can cause the syndrome of inappropriate antidiuretic hormone secretion (SIADH), with resultant hyponatremia. The elderly, patients with alcohol use disorder, and patients receiving selective serotonin reuptake inhibitors (SSRIs) may be at greater risk of developing carbamazepine-induced SIADH.

Carbamazepine overdose presents with neurological signs, such as nystagmus, myoclonus, and hyperreflexia, and may progress to seizures and coma. Cardiac conduction changes, nausea, vomiting, and urinary retention may also occur. Blood pressure, respiratory function, and kidney function should be monitored for several days after a serious overdose.

Drug Interactions (See Also "General Principles" Section at Beginning of Chapter)

Carbamazepine induces multiple CYP enzymes and may reduce levels of other medications, including itself (autoinduction) and oral contraceptives. Therefore, women initiating carbamazepine therapy should be advised to consider alternative forms of birth control. Concomitant use of medications or substances that inhibit CYP3A4 may result in significant increases in plasma carbamazepine levels.

Oxcarbazepine

Oxcarbazepine is a keto derivative of carbamazepine that is often used as an alternative to carbamazepine because it has a milder side-effect profile; however, it is not FDA approved for use in bipolar disorder, and evidence for its efficacy is lacking.

Lamotrigine

Clinical Use

Lamotrigine is approved by the FDA for maintenance treatment of bipolar I disorder; no data are available on its use as monotherapy for acute mania. It is considered a first-line option for bipolar depression, although it is not FDA approved for acute use. Lamotrigine treatment is usually initiated at 25 mg taken once daily. Because the risk of a serious rash increases with rapid titration, it is essential to follow the recommended titration schedule. After 2 weeks, the dosage is increased to 50 mg/day, which is maintained for another 2 weeks. At week 5, the dosage can be increased to 100 mg/day, and at week 6, to 200 mg/day. In patients who are taking valproate, the dosing schedule and target dosage are reduced by half to compensate for the decreased lamotrigine clearance. Conversely, the titration rate and dosage are increased in patients who are taking carbamazepine, phenytoin, phenobarbital, primidone, or other CYP enzyme–inducing medications (without valproate). In the absence of these inducers, lamotrigine dosages greater than 200 mg/day are typically not recommended.

Adverse Effects

Lamotrigine is well tolerated and is not associated with hepatotoxicity, weight gain, or significant sedation. Common early side effects include headache, dizziness, gastrointestinal distress, and blurred or double vision.

Lamotrigine has been associated with both benign and severe rashes. A maculopapular rash develops in 5%–10% of patients taking lamotrigine, usually within the first 8 weeks. Lamotrigine has been associated with severe, life-threatening rashes, including Stevens-Johnson syndrome and toxic epidermal necrolysis; in clinical trials of lamotrigine in bipolar and other mood disorders, the rate of serious rash was approximately 0.1% in adult patients receiving lamotrigine as adjunctive therapy (Seo et al. 2011). Risk for serious rashes may increase with concurrent use of valproate. Before initiating lamotrigine, patients must be advised of the potential risk of developing a serious rash and the need to call the clinician immediately if a rash emerges, especially if it is accompanied by systemic symptoms (e.g. fever, malaise). However, benign rashes are much more common.

Drug Interactions (See Also "General Principles" Section at Beginning of Chapter)

Concurrent treatment with valproate will increase lamotrigine levels, and concurrent treatment with carbamazepine will decrease lamotrigine levels. Many other anticonvulsants interact with lamotrigine as well. Concurrent use of oral contraceptives can result in decreased lamotrigine concentrations, but lamotrigine does not affect the availability of oral contraceptives. Dosage adjustments of lamotrigine are required when an interacting medication is being discontinued.

Antidepressants

Antidepressants include several different types of medications, categorized largely by their neurotransmitter effects. To date, all antidepressants appear to be similarly effective for treating major depressive disorder, although individual patients may respond preferentially to one agent or another. There are significant differences among agents with regard to side effects, lethality in overdose, pharmacokinetics, drug–drug interactions, and ability to treat comorbid disorders.

All antidepressants are effective for and FDA approved for treatment of major depressive disorder (clomipramine is approved only for OCD). Additionally, some antidepressants are effective in OCD (SSRIs and clomipramine), panic disorder (tricyclic antidepressants [TCAs] and SSRIs), generalized anxiety disorder (venlafaxine, duloxetine, and SSRIs), bulimia (TCAs, SSRIs, and MAOIs), dysthymia (SSRIs), bipolar depression (in combination with a mood stabilizer), social phobia (SSRIs, venlafaxine, MAOIs), posttraumatic stress disorder (SSRIs), irritable bowel syndrome (TCAs for diarrhea predominant, SSRIs for constipation predominant), enuresis (TCAs), neuropathic pain (TCAs, duloxetine), fibromyalgia (TCAs, milnacipran, duloxetine), migraine headache (TCAs, venlafaxine), attention-deficit/hyperactivity disorder (bupropion), autism spectrum disorder (SSRIs), late luteal phase dysphoric disorder (SSRIs), vasomotor symptoms (venlafaxine, paroxetine), borderline personality disorder (SSRIs), and smoking cessation (bupropion). However, the FDA has not evaluated or approved the use of antidepressants to treat many of these conditions. We refer the reader to current product labeling for information regarding indications for use approved by the FDA for a specific medication. Clinicians should exercise caution when using antidepressants in bipolar depression, because antidepressants can increase the risk of switching to mania and rapid cycling.

Information on dosing is summarized in Table 29–9, and a list of key features and side effects is presented in Table 29–10. The choice of a specific antidepressant medication is based on several factors, including the patient's psychiatric symptoms, history of previous treatment response and tolerability, family members' history of response, medication side-effect profiles, potential drug–drug interactions, and presence of comorbid disorders that may respond to (or preclude the use of) specific antidepressants. In general, SSRIs and other newer antidepressants are preferred as initial treatment options because they are better tolerated and safer than TCAs, nefazodone, and MAOIs, although many patients benefit from treatment with the older drugs.

Selective Serotonin Reuptake Inhibitors and Novel/Mixed-Action Agents

Mechanisms of Action

SSRIs selectively inhibit serotonin reuptake and are largely devoid of other major pharmacological properties, resulting in relatively few serious side effects. Duloxetine, venlafaxine, desvenlafaxine, and levomilnacipran selectively inhibit uptake of both serotonin and norepinephrine (i.e., they are serotonin–norepinephrine reuptake inhibitors [SNRIs]). Bupropion is a relatively weak reuptake inhibitor of dopamine and norepinephrine. Mirtazapine modulates the actions of norepinephrine and serotonin, whereas trazodone modulates serotonin. Vilazodone is considered to be both an SSRI and a partial 5-HT$_{1A}$ receptor agonist. Vortioxetine is considered to be an SSRI, a 5-HT$_{1A}$ receptor agonist, and a 5-HT$_3$ receptor antagonist.

TABLE 29–9. Antidepressant medications: dosing and half-life information

Generic name	Trade name	Usual starting dosage, mg/day[a]	Usual daily dosage, mg	Available oral doses, mg	Mean half-life, h (active metabolites)[b]
Monoamine oxidase inhibitors					
Irreversible, nonselective monoamine oxidase inhibitors					
Isocarboxazid	Marplan	20	20–60	10	2
Phenelzine	Nardil	45	15–90	15	11.6
Tranylcypromine	Parnate	10	30–60	10	2.5
Transdermal monoamine oxidase inhibitors					
Transdermal selegiline	EMSAM	6	6	None for depression Transdermal doses: 6 mg/24 hours, 9 mg/24 hours, 12 mg/24 hours	18–25
Reversible inhibitors of monoamine oxidase A					
Moclobemide[c]	Aurorix, Manerix	150	300–600	100, 150	2
Tricyclic antidepressants					
Tertiary-amine tricyclic antidepressants					
Amitriptyline	Elavil	25–50	100–300[d]	10, 25, 50, 75, 100, 150	16 (27)
Clomipramine	Anafranil	25	100–250	25, 50, 75	32 (69)
Doxepin	Sinequan	25–50	100–300[d]	10, 25, 50, 75, 100, 150, L	17
Imipramine	Tofranil	25–75	100–300	10, 25, 50, 75, 100, 125, 150	8 (17)
Trimipramine	Surmontil	25–50	100–300	25, 50, 100	24
Secondary-amine tricyclic antidepressants					
Desipramine	Norpramin	25–50	100–300	10, 25, 50, 75, 100, 150	17
Nortriptyline	Pamelor	25	50–150	10, 25, 50, 75, L	27
Protriptyline	Vivactil	10–20	20–60	5, 10	79

TABLE 29–9. Antidepressant medications: dosing and half-life information (continued)

Generic name	Trade name	Usual starting dosage, mg/day[a]	Usual daily dosage, mg	Available oral doses, mg	Mean half-life, h (active metabolites)[b]
Tetracyclic antidepressants					
Amoxapine	Asendin	50	100–400[d]	25, 50, 100, 150	8
Maprotiline	Ludiomil	50	100–225[d]	25, 50, 75	43
Selective serotonin reuptake inhibitors					
Citalopram	Celexa	20	20–40	10, 20, 40, L	35
Escitalopram	Lexapro	10	10–20	5, 10, 20, L	27–32
Fluoxetine	Prozac	20	20–60[d]	10, 20, 40, L	72 (216)
Fluoxetine Weekly	Prozac Weekly	90	NA	90	—
Fluvoxamine[e]	Luvox	50	50–300	25, 50, 100	15
Fluvoxamine CR	Luvox CR	100	100–300[d]	100, 150	16.3
Paroxetine	Paxil, Pexeva, Brisdelle	20	20–60	10, 20, 30, 40, L	20
Paroxetine CR	Paxil CR	25	25–62.5	12.5, 25, 37.5	15–20
Sertraline	Zoloft	50	50–200	25, 50, 100, L	26 (66)
Serotonin–norepinephrine reuptake inhibitors					
Desvenlafaxine	Pristiq, Khedezla	50	50	25, 50, 100	10
Duloxetine	Cymbalta	30	60–120	20, 30, 60	12
Levomilnacipran	Fetzima	20	40–120	20, 40, 80, 120	12
Venlafaxine	Effexor	37.5	75–225	25, 37.5, 50, 75, 100	5 (11)
Venlafaxine XR	Effexor XR	37.5–75	75–225	37.5, 75, 150, 225	5 (11)

TABLE 29–9. Antidepressant medications: dosing and half-life information *(continued)*

Generic name	Trade name	Usual starting dosage, mg/day[a]	Usual daily dosage, mg	Available oral doses, mg	Mean half-life, h (active metabolites)[b]
Serotonin modulators					
Nefazodone	Serzone	50–200	150–600[d]	50, 100, 150, 200, 250	4
Trazodone	Desyrel	50	75–300[d]	50, 100, 150, 300	7
Vilazodone	Viibryd	10	40	10, 20, 40	25
Vortioxetine	Trintellix	10	5–20	5, 10, 20	66
Norepinephrine–serotonin modulator					
Mirtazapine	Remeron	15	15–45	7.5, 15, 30, 45, SolTab	20–40
Norepinephrine–dopamine reuptake inhibitors					
Bupropion	Wellbutrin	150	300–450	75, 100	14
Bupropion SR	Wellbutrin SR	150	300–400	100, 150, 200	21
Bupropion XL	Wellbutrin XL, Forfivo XL	150	300	150, 300, 450	21
Bupropion XL	Aplenzin[f]	174	348	174, 345, 522	21

Note. CR=controlled release; L=liquid; SolTab=orally disintegrating tablets; SR=sustained release; XL or XR=extended release.
[a]Lower starting dosages are recommended for elderly patients and patients with panic disorder, significant anxiety, or hepatic disease.
[b]Mean half-lives of active metabolites are given in parentheses.
[c]Not available in the United States due to incidents of severe hepatotoxicity.
[d]Dosage varies with diagnosis. See text for specific guidelines.
[e]Generic only.
[f]Hydrobromide salt.

Source. Product information. U.S. National Library of Medicine: DailyMed (website). Available at: https://dailymed.nlm.nih.gov/dailymed/. Accessed October 7, 2018. U.S. Food and Drug Administration: Orange Book: Approved Drug Products with Therapeutic Equivalence Evaluations (website). Silver Spring, MD, U.S. Food and Drug Administration, August 2018. Available at: https://www.accessdata.fda.gov/scripts/cder/ob/. Accessed October 7, 2018.

TABLE 29–10. Key side effects of major antidepressant drugs

Medications	Sedation	Weight gain	Sexual dysfunction	Other key side effects
Tricyclic antidepressants (TCAs)	Most, yes	Yes	Yes	Anticholinergic effects, orthostasis, quinidine-like effects on cardiac conduction; lethal in overdose
Selective serotonin reuptake inhibitors (SSRIs)	Minimal	Yes	Yes	Initial: nausea, loose bowel movements, headache, insomnia; paroxetine sedation, anticholinergic
Serotonin–norepinephrine reuptake inhibitors (SNRIs)	Minimal	Rare	Yes	Initial: nausea; side effects similar to those of SSRIs; dose-dependent hypertension (duloxetine may be the exception), sweating; levomilnacipran—urinary hesitation
Bupropion	Rare	Rare	Rare	Initial: nausea, headache, insomnia, anxiety or agitation, dry mouth, constipation, tachycardia, sweating, tremor; seizure risk
Trazodone	Yes	Rare	Rare	Sedation, priapism, dizziness, orthostasis
Vilazodone	Moderate	Rare	Yes	Diarrhea, nausea, dizziness, insomnia, anxiety
Vortioxetine	No	Rare	Yes	Nausea, dizziness, diarrhea, pruritus
Mirtazapine	Yes	Yes	Rare	Anticholinergic effects; may increase serum lipid levels; rare effects: orthostasis, hypertension, peripheral edema, agranulocytosis
Monoamine oxidase inhibitors (MAOIs)	Rare	Yes	Yes	Orthostatic hypotension, insomnia, peripheral edema; avoid in patients with congestive heart failure; avoid phenelzine in patients with hepatic impairment; potentially life-threatening drug interactions; dietary restrictions

Source. Product information. Lexicomp Online, Hudson, OH, Lexi-Comp, 2017; and U.S. National Library of Medicine: DailyMed (website). Available at: https://dailymed.nlm.nih.gov/dailymed. Accessed October 7, 2018.

Indications and Efficacy

Despite their highly selective pharmacological activity, SSRIs have a broad spectrum of action. They are efficacious in the treatment of depression and many other psychiatric disorders, including many anxiety disorders. All of the SSRIs have similar spectra of efficacy and side-effect profiles. However, they are structurally distinct, and response or nonresponse to one SSRI does not necessarily predict a similar reaction to another SSRI. Likewise, allergy or intolerance to one SSRI does not necessarily predict allergy or intolerance to another. SSRIs have distinct pharmacokinetic properties, including differences in half-life and drug–drug interaction potential. Fluoxetine, fluvoxamine, and paroxetine are more likely that sertraline, citalopram, or escitalopram to have clinically significant drug interactions. SNRIs have indications similar to those of SSRIs; in addition, they are effective in some forms of chronic pain (e.g., neuropathic, fibromyalgia). Bupropion is the one antidepressant that is generally ineffective for treatment of anxiety disorders. Because of their sedating properties, trazodone and mirtazapine are often used to treat insomnia, especially insomnia caused by a more activating antidepressant.

Adverse Effects

Adverse effects of SSRIs and novel/mixed-action agents are common, but they are usually mild and dose related, and most abate over time (see Table 29–10). However, serotonergic agents, especially when used in combination, can induce the potentially fatal serotonin syndrome (see "Serotonin Syndrome" subsection below).

Common short-term side effects of SSRIs and SNRIs include nausea, vomiting, anxiety, headache, sedation, tremors, and anorexia. Common long-term side effects include sexual dysfunction, dry mouth, sweating, impaired sleep, and potential weight gain. Trazodone causes sedation in 20%–50% of patients and is often used for its sedating properties. In rare cases, it causes priapism.

Side effects commonly associated with SNRIs include nausea, dry mouth, fatigue, dizziness, constipation, somnolence, decreased appetite, and increased sweating. Mirtazapine is associated with a high incidence of sedation, increased appetite, and weight gain. Patients treated with reboxetine (used only in Europe) often report dry mouth, insomnia, constipation, sweating, and hypotension. Milnacipran, an SNRI approved for depression in Europe and Japan and approved for fibromyalgia in the United States, is associated with the same side effects as other SNRIs.

Central nervous system effects.   In May 2007, the FDA concluded that all antidepressants increase the risk of suicidal thinking and behavior in young adults (age <24 years) during initial treatment and required manufacturers to include in their labeling a warning statement that recommends close observation for worsening depression or the emergence of suicidality in young adult and pediatric patients treated with these agents (Stone et al. 2009). There is no evidence that antidepressants increase the risk of completed suicide in children or adults.

Bupropion causes a dose-related lowering of the seizure threshold and may precipitate seizures in susceptible patients receiving dosages greater than 450 mg/day. The incidence of seizure rises with increasing dosage, from 0.1% at 100–300 mg/day to 0.4% at 300–450 mg/day (McEvoy 2017). Sustained-release dosage forms are associated with a lower seizure risk than are immediate-release bupropion products. The seizure incidence reported for other antidepressants ranges from 0.04% for mirtazapine to 0.5% for clomipramine (Harden and Goldstein 2002; Rosenstein et al. 1993). Given that the annual incidence of first unprovoked seizure is 0.06% in the general population, the seizure risk for most antidepressants is not appreciably elevated. However, it is clear that certain antidepressants, including bupropion, clomipramine, maprotiline, and venlafaxine, are associated with a greater seizure risk than are other antidepressants (Harden and Goldstein 2002; Whyte et al. 2003), although this risk is rarely significant except at toxic doses.

Potential side effects of SSRIs include SSRI-induced EPS, likely resulting from serotonergic antagonism of dopaminergic pathways in the central nervous system (CNS). Akathisia, dystonia, parkinsonism, and TD-like states have been infrequently reported, with akathisia being the most common effect and TD-like states being the least common. Elderly patients, patients with Parkinson's disease, and patients being concurrently treated with dopamine antagonists appear to be at increased risk.

Serotonin syndrome. Serotonin syndrome is an uncommon but potentially life-threatening complication of treatment with serotonergic agents (Boyer and Shannon 2005). Overall, there is considerable heterogeneity in the reported clinical features and severity of serotonin syndrome (Table 29–11). The incidence of the syndrome is unknown because of diagnostic uncertainty. Virtually all medications that potentiate CNS serotonergic neurotransmission have been reported in association with serotonin syndrome, including medications that enhance serotonin synthesis (e.g., L-tryptophan), increase serotonin release (e.g., cocaine, amphetamine, dextromethorphan, lithium), stimulate serotonin receptors (e.g., triptans, trazodone), inhibit serotonin catabolism (e.g., MAOIs, linezolid), and inhibit serotonin reuptake (e.g., SSRIs, SNRIs, TCAs, mirtazapine, trazodone). The antidepressant combinations most commonly implicated have been MAOIs (reversible and irreversible) taken concurrently with other antidepressants.

Currently there is no formal consensus regarding diagnostic criteria for serotonin syndrome. The first operationalized criteria, proposed by Sternbach (1991), were found to have low specificity. The Hunter Serotonin Toxicity Criteria subsequently gained acceptance as a simple set of highly sensitive and specific decision rules; these criteria are listed in Table 29–12 (Dunkley et al. 2003). Laboratory findings have not been commonly reported in cases of serotonin syndrome, but some reports have noted the presence of leukocytosis, rhabdomyolysis with elevated creatine phosphokinase, serum hepatic transaminase elevations, electrolyte abnormalities (hyponatremia, hypomagnesemia, hypercalcemia), and disseminated intravascular coagulopathy. The differential diagnosis includes CNS infection, delirium tremens, poisoning with anticholinergic or adrenergic agents, NMS, and malignant hyperthermia. Differentiating serotonin syndrome from NMS can be very difficult in patients receiving both serotonergic medications and antipsychotics (see "Neuroleptic Malignant Syndrome" under "Antipsychotics" earlier in this chapter).

Serotonin syndrome is often self-limited and usually resolves quickly after discontinuation of serotonergic agents and provision of supportive care. Severe cases will require admission to an intensive care unit, but most cases will show improvement within 24 hours with supportive care alone. There are no specific antidotes. The antihistamine cyproheptadine has some antiserotonergic activity and may reduce symp-

TABLE 29–11.   Clinical features of serotonin syndrome

Category	Clinical features
Mental status and behavioral	Delirium, confusion, agitation, anxiety, irritability, euphoria, dysphoria, restlessness
Neurological and motor	Ataxia/incoordination, tremor, muscle rigidity, myoclonus, hyperreflexia, clonus, seizures, trismus, teeth chattering
Gastrointestinal	Nausea, vomiting, diarrhea, incontinence
Autonomic nervous system	Hypertension, hypotension, tachycardia, diaphoresis, shivering, sialorrhea, mydriasis, tachypnea, pupillary dilation
Thermoregulation	Hyperthermia

Source.   Compiled in part from Boyer and Shannon 2005; Dunkley et al. 2003.

TABLE 29–12.   Hunter Serotonin Toxicity Criteria for serotonin syndrome

Use of a serotonergic agent PLUS any of the following symptoms:

Spontaneous clonus

Inducible clonus PLUS either agitation or diaphoresis

Tremor PLUS hyperreflexia

Muscle rigidity PLUS elevated body temperature PLUS either ocular clonus or inducible clonus

Exclude the following conditions:

Infection, metabolic, endocrine, or toxic causes

Neuroleptic malignant syndrome

Delirium tremens

Malignant hyperthermia

Source.   Compiled from Boyer and Shannon 2005; Dunkley et al. 2003.

toms; however, it can only be administered orally. For adults, the recommended dose is 4–8 mg, which may be repeated every 1–4 hours, up to a maximum daily dosage of 32 mg. There is limited information on drug rechallenge in patients who have developed serotonin syndrome. General guidelines include reevaluating the necessity for drug therapy, switching the patient to a nonserotonergic medication, using single-drug therapy when serotonergic medications are required, and implementing an extended (6-week) serotonin "drug-free" period before restarting a serotonergic agent.

Autonomic and cardiovascular effects.   The SSRIs and the novel/mixed-action antidepressants have a much safer cardiovascular profile than do the TCAs and MAOIs. In general, the SSRIs have little effect on blood pressure or cardiac conduction. In rare cases, SSRIs have been reported to cause mild bradycardia in elderly patients with preexisting cardiac arrhythmias. In 2011, the FDA announced that there had been reports of citalopram causing dosage-dependent QTc interval prolongation and torsades de pointes (Vieweg et al. 2012). The FDA advised that citalopram should no longer be prescribed at dosages greater than 40 mg/day, and that the dosage should not exceed 20 mg/day for patients who have hepatic impairment, who are older than

60 years, who are CYP2C19 poor metabolizers, or who are taking concomitant CYP2C19 inhibitors. Many clinicians feel that this risk has been overestimated. A large Veterans Health Administration study involving more than 600,000 patients did not find an elevated risk of ventricular arrhythmia or all-cause mortality (cardiac or noncardiac) with use of citalopram dosages exceeding 40 mg/day (Zivin et al. 2013). Citalopram should not be prescribed in patients with the congenital long-QT syndrome. Caution is also advised in patients who have other risk factors for QTc prolongation (e.g., hypocalcemia, hypomagnesemia) or who use other QTc-prolonging drugs.

The novel/mixed-action agents venlafaxine, desvenlafaxine, duloxetine, bupropion, mirtazapine, trazodone, vilazodone, vortioxetine, and reboxetine have little effect on cardiac conduction but may affect blood pressure or heart rate. Venlafaxine causes dosage-related increases in heart rate and blood pressure, typically at dosages greater than 300 mg/day. Similar effects would be expected for desvenlafaxine and levomilnacipran. Duloxetine and bupropion may also cause elevations in blood pressure. Bupropion is more likely to cause blood pressure increases when used in combination with nicotine replacement products. Trazodone lacks significant effects on cardiac conduction but in rare cases has been reported to cause ventricular ectopy and ventricular tachycardia. The most common cardiovascular adverse effect of trazodone is postural hypotension, which may be associated with syncope. Mirtazapine does not have significant effects on cardiac conduction but is associated with a 7% incidence of orthostatic hypotension. Hypotension and elevated heart rate have been reported in patients receiving reboxetine. Vilazodone and vortioxetine have minimal effects on cardiac conduction and blood pressure.

Gastrointestinal effects.   Nausea is the most common adverse effect associated with the serotonergic antidepressants. Nausea is most likely to occur with fluvoxamine, venlafaxine, and duloxetine (e.g., 30%–40% of patients report this effect at a starting duloxetine dosage of 60 mg/day [Detke et al. 2002]). Other serotonergic antidepressants have a lower incidence of nausea (20%–25%), but the rates of occurrence are still much higher than rates reported with placebo (9%–12%). Loose stools and diarrhea are also common with SSRIs. Nausea and vomiting are much less common with bupropion or mirtazapine than with SSRIs or SNRIs. Mirtazapine may be a preferred agent in patients with significant nausea from other serotonergic antidepressants.

Although most adverse gastrointestinal effects of serotonergic antidepressants are dosage related and generally diminish with continued treatment, sometimes severe side effects require antidepressant discontinuation. Potential severe hepatotoxicity with nefazodone led to its removal from the market in a number of countries, and it should not be used in patients with preexisting liver disease. Among newer antidepressants, duloxetine is associated with significant hepatotoxicity, with an estimated incidence of 26 cases per 100,000 patient-years (Bunchorntavakul and Reddy 2017). Therefore, duloxetine should be avoided in patients with substantial alcohol use, hepatic insufficiency, chronic liver disease, or severe renal impairment.

Hematological effects.   SSRIs have the potential to cause hemorrhage by interfering with serotonin-induced platelet aggregation through depletion of platelet serotonin stores. The absolute effects are modest and about equal to those of low-dose ibuprofen. The relative risk of gastrointestinal bleeding increases if patients are receiving an SSRI and a nonsteroidal anti-inflammatory drug, and even more so if in conjunction with a third drug interfering with platelet function (e.g., clopidogrel), but the absolute risk remains low in patients not otherwise at increased risk for gastrointestinal bleeding. Increased risk would be expected in patients with thrombocytopenia, clotting disorders, or platelet dysfunction (e.g., von Willebrand's disease).

Weight gain or loss.   Weight gain is a relatively common problem during both acute and long-term treatment with antidepressants. Among the antidepressants, mirtazapine and TCAs are the most likely to cause significant weight gain. Although SSRIs are weight-neutral in most patients, they can cause considerable weight gain in a minority of patients. Bupropion is the only antidepressant that has not been associated with weight gain.

Sexual dysfunction.   Most antidepressants have been reported to cause sexual dysfunction. Delayed orgasm/anorgasmia is most common with SSRIs, SNRIs, and TCAs, with diminished libido less so. Sildenafil may reverse SSRI-related sexual side effects in men and women. Other strategies, such as dosage reduction and drug holidays, must be approached with caution, given the risk for depression relapse. Trazodone causes priapism in about 1 in 5,000 men. Bupropion and mirtazapine do not cause sexual side effects.

Serotonin reuptake inhibitor discontinuation syndrome.   Abrupt discontinuation of SSRIs or SNRIs, especially agents with short half-lives (e.g., fluvoxamine, paroxetine, venlafaxine), may give rise to a discontinuation syndrome characterized by a wide variety of symptoms, including psychiatric, neurological, sensory (e.g., electric shock–like symptoms) and flulike symptoms (nausea, vomiting, sweats); sleep disturbances; and headache, usually resolving within 3 weeks. Some patients experience discontinuation symptoms even with very gradual withdrawal over months. Antidepressants, like all psychoactive medications, should be gradually withdrawn when possible. Discontinuation symptoms can lead to misdiagnosis and inappropriate treatment, particularly in a patient with an active medical illness, as well as erode future medication adherence. During cross-titration, discontinuation symptoms may be misinterpreted as being an adverse effect of the new antidepressant.

Tricyclic Antidepressants

TCAs are now viewed as second-line treatments for depression because their adverse-effect profile is less benign than that of other antidepressant classes.

Adverse Effects

Many adverse effects of TCAs are due not to their effects on serotonin or norepinephrine reuptake inhibition but rather to their secondary pharmacological actions. TCAs are antagonists at histamine H_1, α_1-adrenergic, and muscarinic receptors and have class Ia antiarrhythmic (quinidine-like) effects. Adverse effects of TCAs include sedation, anticholinergic effects (e.g., dry mouth, dry eyes, constipation, urinary retention, decreased sweating, confusion, memory impairment, tachycardia, blurred vision), and postural hypotension. Tolerance to these effects usually develops over time. TCAs at or just above therapeutic plasma levels frequently prolong PR, QRS, and QTc intervals, but rarely to a clinically significant degree in patients without preexisting cardiac disease or conduction defects. TCAs can cause heart block, arrhythmias, palpitations, tachycardia, syncope, and heart failure and should be used with caution in patients with preexisting cardiovascular disease or at risk of suicide. Given the discovery that class I antiarrhythmic drugs can increase mortality in patients after myocardial infarction, it is prudent to assume that TCAs may carry the same risk.

Toxicity/Overdose

TCA overdose carries a risk of death from cardiac conduction abnormalities that result in malignant ventricular arrhythmias. Initial symptoms of overdose involve CNS stimulation, in part due to anticholinergic effects, and include hyperpyrexia, delirium, hypertension, hallucinations, seizure, agitation, hyperreflexia, and parkinsonian symptoms. The initial stimulation phase is typically followed by CNS depression, with drowsiness, areflexia, hypothermia, respiratory depression, severe hypotension, and coma. Risk of cardiotoxicity is high if the QRS interval exceeds 100 msec or if the total TCA plasma concentration is greater than 1,000 ng/mL; concentrations greater than 2,500 ng/mL are often fatal.

Abrupt discontinuation of TCAs may give rise to a discontinuation syndrome characterized by dizziness, lethargy, headache, nightmares, and symptoms of anticholinergic rebound, including gastrointestinal upset, nausea, vomiting, diarrhea, excessive salivation, sweating, anxiety, restlessness, piloerection, and delirium. This syndrome can be avoided by gradual withdrawal.

Monoamine Oxidase Inhibitors

MAOIs, with the possible exception of moclobemide (not available in the United States), are seen as third-line antidepressants because of their significant drug interactions and the dietary restrictions that are required with their use. Phenelzine and tranylcypromine are irreversible inhibitors of MAO-A and MAO-B. Hypertensive crisis can occur in patients taking MAOIs who take sympathomimetic drugs, including over-the-counter decongestants, atomoxetine, dopamine agonists (e.g., stimulants), or foods containing tyramine. MAOIs may trigger serotonin syndrome when combined with other medications (see "Serotonin Syndrome" subsection earlier in chapter). MAOIs may greatly potentiate the hypotensive effects of antihypertensive agents. Common adverse effects of MAOIs include orthostatic hypotension, dizziness, headache, sedation, insomnia or hypersomnia, tremor, and hyperreflexia.

Selegiline, a semiselective MAO-B inhibitor, is available as an oral formulation used for treatment of Parkinson's disease and as a transdermal patch indicated for treatment of depression. At oral dosages greater than 10 mg/day, and with patch strengths greater than 6 mg/24 hours, selegiline also inhibits MAO-A, thereby acquiring the same risks for adverse effects and drug–food interactions associated with the antidepressant MAOIs. Moclobemide, a short-half-life reversible inhibitor of MAO-A, is less susceptible to dietary interactions provided that it is taken after meals.

Anxiolytics and Sedative-Hypnotics

Many psychotropics have antianxiety properties and sedative effects that promote sleep. In early years of use, the antipsychotics were frequently called "major tranquilizers" owing to these properties and were often prescribed for anxiety states. Nonetheless, these drugs are seldom used as monotherapy for anxiety disorders today because of their risk for adverse effects. Drugs that are used primarily to treat anxiety symptoms and disorders (i.e., anxiolytics) include the benzodiazepines, buspirone, and many serotonergic antidepressants, which are covered in the previous section. Drugs that are indicated for the treatment of insomnia (i.e., hypnotics) include the benzodiazepines, nonbenzodiazepine γ-aminobutyric acid (GABA) receptor agonist hypnotics, melatonin MT_1 and MT_2 receptor agonists, orexin (OX1R and OX2R) antagonists, and low dosages of the TCA doxepin. The benzodiazepines, buspirone, and the abovementioned hypnotics are discussed in this section and are summarized in Table 29–13.

Benzodiazepines

Benzodiazepines are used to treat both short-term and long-term anxiety and insomnia. Although these medications may provide rapid relief of anxiety symptoms, their use is limited by the development of tolerance and withdrawal as well as by their abuse liability and propensity to impair judgment, cognition, and motor performance. In general, benzodiazepines are best for short-term use (e.g., for episodic stress-related anxiety and insomnia). Despite these concerns, many patients receive chronic benzodiazepine therapy and do not experience deleterious effects. Patients should be counseled regarding the potential liabilities of chronic benzodiazepine use and should be monitored closely.

Benzodiazepines enhance the inhibitory effects of GABA by binding to the benzodiazepine site on the $GABA_A$ receptor. Choice of benzodiazepine agent is based primarily on pharmacokinetic properties, including half-life, rapidity of onset, metabolism, and potency. In general, longer-acting agents possess active metabolites and tend to produce a steady serum drug concentration and few rebound effects between doses, whereas shorter-acting agents are associated with emergence of symptoms between doses. All benzodiazepines are metabolized by the liver and thus increase the risk of sedation, confusion, and hepatic encephalopathy in patients with hepatic failure. In patients with liver failure, lorazepam, oxazepam, and temazepam are the preferred agents because they undergo hepatic conjugation and renal excretion and have no active metabolites, whereas other benzodiazepines undergo phase I hepatic metabolism and may have long-acting active metabolites.

Adverse effects of benzodiazepines are dose dependent and include sedation, impaired cognitive function and judgment, amnesia, impaired motor performance, and disinhibition. Elderly patients are at higher risk of adverse effects. Benzodiazepines also cause respiratory suppression and may produce respiratory arrest in overdose, especially in combination with other sedatives, opioids, or alcohol. Abrupt cessation of benzodiazepine use after sustained administration may result in withdrawal symptoms that include anxiety, agitation, tremor, autonomic hyperactivity, insomnia, nausea and vomiting, hallucinations, seizure, and delirium. Benzodiazepine withdrawal is best managed by resumption of an intermediate- to long-acting benzodiazepine to stabilize the patient, followed by gradual taper under supervision.

Buspirone

Buspirone is a 5-HT_{1A} receptor partial agonist. Because it does not affect GABA receptors or chloride ion channels, buspirone does not possess many of the major concerns associated with benzodiazepines—namely, the potential for abuse, tolerance, and with-drawal. Buspirone is not cross-tolerant with benzodiazepines; thus, a rapid switch from a benzodiazepine to buspirone is likely to precipitate benzodiazepine withdrawal.

Buspirone is indicated for the treatment of generalized anxiety disorder. Limited literature supports its use as an augmentation agent in refractory depression and OCD.

Buspirone is administered in divided doses three times daily. It has a very short half-life and may precipitate a discontinuation reaction much like that of SSRIs if abruptly stopped. Buspirone has a relatively slow onset of therapeutic action, similar to that of antidepressants. Buspirone works best for benzodiazepine-naive patients. Adverse effects include nausea, headache, nervousness, and insomnia. Buspirone is not lethal in overdose. Its metabolism is decreased by CYP3A4 inhibitors.

Eszopiclone, Zopiclone, Zolpidem, and Zaleplon

Eszopiclone, zopiclone, zolpidem, and zaleplon are selective agonists at the ω_1 modulatory site of the GABA$_A$ receptor complex, producing sedation. Zolpidem and zaleplon do not have significant anxiolytic, muscle-relaxant, or anticonvulsant properties.

Eszopiclone and zopiclone (the latter not available in the United States) are well-tolerated short-half-life hypnotics with only a few dose-related adverse effects, which include bitter taste, dry mouth, difficulty arising in the morning, sleepiness, nausea, and nightmares. Zolpidem is a short-acting hypnotic with established efficacy in inducing and maintaining sleep. Because of zolpidem's short half-life, most patients taking the drug report minimal daytime sedation. Zolpidem is available in an extended-release formulation to assist with sleeping through the night, as well as a sublingual formulation for middle insomnia. Zaleplon is an ultra-short-acting hypnotic with minimal residual sedative effects. For both zolpidem and zaleplon, short-term or intermittent use is recommended to avoid tolerance.

Side effects of zopiclone, eszopiclone, zolpidem, and zaleplon are similar to those of benzodiazepines. Daytime sedation, impaired cognitive performance, amnesia, and nocturnal activity such as wandering, eating, and driving that is not recalled the next day have been reported. Elderly patients are at increased risk for amnesia and falls with zolpidem. Because of these side effects, the FDA has recommended reducing by half the dosage of products containing zolpidem, especially in women and the elderly (U.S. Food and Drug Administration 2013). Caution is also advised in patients with hepatic dysfunction. Zopiclone, eszopiclone, zolpidem, and zaleplon may be abused. Unless combined with other drugs or alcohol, they do not appear to be fatal in overdose.

Ramelteon and Tasimelteon

Ramelteon is a melatonin agonist that is FDA approved for treatment of insomnia. It has demonstrated efficacy for sleep-onset insomnia with no next-morning residual effects and adverse effects similar to those of placebo, no abuse potential, and minimal withdrawal symptoms upon discontinuation. Tasimelteon, another melatonin agonist, is FDA approved for non-24-hour sleep–wake disorder; it is not approved for insomnia. Ramelteon, tasimelteon, and herbal melatonin are all substrates of CYP1A2 and should not be combined with strong CYP1A2 inhibitors (e.g., fluvoxamine).

TABLE 29–13. Benzodiazepines, buspirone, and sedative-hypnotics

Name	Dose equivalence, mg	Typical daily dosage range in adults,[a] mg/day	Half-life of parent drug (active metabolite), h
Anxiolytic medications			
Antihistamines used as anxiolytics			
Hydroxyzine pamoate (Vistaril)	N/A	25–400 (divided)	20–29
Benzodiazepines used as anxiolytics			
Alprazolam (Xanax)	0.5	0.75–4 (divided); 1–6 for panic	9–20
Alprazolam extended-release (Xanax XR)	N/A	3–6	11–16
Chlordiazepoxide (Librium)	10	15–100 (divided tid or qid)	5–30 (36–200)
Clonazepam (Klonopin)	0.25	1–4 (divided)	18–50
Clorazepate (Tranxene)	7.5	T-tab: 15–60 (divided) SD: 22.5 qd to replace T-tab 7.5 tid	36–100
Diazepam (Valium)	5	4–40 (divided)	20–100 (36–200)
Lorazepam (Ativan)	1	2–4 (divided)	10–20
Oxazepam (Serax)	15	30–120 (divided)	4–15
Nonbenzodiazepines used as anxiolytics			
Buspirone (BuSpar)	N/A	30–60 (divided)	2–3
Hypnotic medications			
Benzodiazepines used as hypnotics			
Estazolam (ProSom)	—	1–2	10–24
Flurazepam (Dalmane)	—	15–30	40–250
Quazepam (Doral)	—	7.5–15	39–120
Temazepam (Restoril)	—	15–30	8–22
Triazolam (Halcion)	—	0.125–0.25	2

TABLE 29–13. Benzodiazepines, buspirone, and sedative-hypnotics *(continued)*

Name	Dose equivalence, mg	Typical daily dosage range in adults,[a] mg/day	Half-life of parent drug (active metabolite), h
Hypnotic medications *(continued)*			
Nonbenzodiazepine GABA–benzodiazepine receptor agonists used as hypnotics			
Eszopiclone (Lunesta)	N/A	1–3	6
Zaleplon (Sonata)	N/A	5–10	1.5–2
Zolpidem (Ambien)	N/A	5–10	1–5
Zolpidem extended-release (Ambien CR)	N/A	6.25–12.5	1–5
Zolpidem sublingual (low dose) (Intermezzo)	N/A	1.75–3.25	1.4–3.6
Zopiclone[b] (Imovane)	N/A	5–7.5	5
Nonbenzodiazepine melatonin MT$_1$ and MT$_2$ receptor agonists used as hypnotics			
Ramelteon (Rozerem)	N/A	8	1–6
Orexin (OX1R and OX2R) antagonists used as hypnotics			
Suvorexant (Belsomra)	N/A	10–20	10–22
Tricyclic antidepressant used as hypnotic (via H$_1$ antagonism)			
Doxepin (Silenor)	N/A	3–6	15.3 (31)

Note. CR=extended release; GABA=γ-aminobutyric acid; SD=single dose; T-tab=T-shaped tablet.
[a]Lower dosages may be required in special populations, such as elderly, debilitated, or hepatically or renally impaired patients; use of certain agents may also be precluded in such patients.
[b]Not available in the United States.

Suvorexant

Suvorexant is the only orexin receptor antagonist currently FDA approved for insomnia (both sleep onset and sleep maintenance). It carries a potential for abuse.

Suvorexant is associated with side effects similar to those of many hypnotics, including parasomnias, somnolence, and next-day drowsiness. Rare side effects unique to suvorexant include dose-dependent narcolepsy-like effects such as sleep paralysis, cataplexy-like symptoms, and hypnagogic/hypnopompic hallucinations. Use of suvorexant is contraindicated in patients with narcolepsy. The dosage should be reduced if suvorexant is combined with a moderate CYP3A4 inhibitor. Use of suvorexant is not recommended in combination with strong CYP3A4 inhibitors or in patients with severe hepatic impairment.

Psychostimulants

Psychostimulants are used to treat attention-deficit/hyperactivity disorder (ADHD), excessive sleepiness due to narcolepsy, shift work sleep disorder, and obstructive sleep apnea. Psychostimulant agents are also used off-label to augment treatments for depression, apathy, and analgesia.

Although all psychostimulant medications have CNS-stimulant properties, they are often subclassified as stimulant or nonstimulant agents based roughly on their degree of stimulation and time to onset of effect. Agents classified as stimulants have strong effects with rapid onset (i.e., within hours) and include methylphenidate, dexmethylphenidate, amphetamines (i.e., mixed amphetamine salts, dextroamphetamine), and the amphetamine prodrug lisdexamfetamine. Agents categorized as nonstimulants include atomoxetine, clonidine, guanfacine, modafinil, and armodafinil (Table 29–14).

Stimulants: Methylphenidate, Dexmethylphenidate, Amphetamine, and Lisdexamfetamine

All stimulant formulations are indicated for first-line treatment of ADHD, but only short- and intermediate-duration formulations (4–10 hours) are indicated for treatment of narcolepsy. Amphetamine, methylphenidate, and atomoxetine increase synaptic concentrations of catecholamines in the prefrontal cortex via one or more mechanisms, including inhibition of presynaptic norepinephrine reuptake (amphetamine, methylphenidate, atomoxetine) and inhibition of dopamine reuptake (methylphenidate and amphetamine). Amphetamine also increases presynaptic dopamine release by reversing the action of the dopamine reuptake transporters. Meta-analyses of studies examining response in children and adolescents with ADHD provide strong evidence for the efficacy of short- and long-acting stimulants.

Stimulants, except for lisdexamfetamine, are available in a variety of formulations, providing a range of drug-release profiles differing in time to onset of action (0.5–2 hours) and duration of effect (4–12 hours). Specific formulations are described in Table 29–14. Because of variations in drug-release profiles, different formulations are generally not interchangeable.

TABLE 29–14. Selected psychostimulants

Generic name	Trade name	Release profile	Onset of action, h	Duration of action, h[a]	Indications	Usual dosage range, mg/day	Dosing interval[b]
Stimulants—amphetamine derivatives							
Amphetamine mixed salts	Adderall	Immediate	1.5	4–6 (longer with higher dose)	ADHD	C: 3–5 years: 2.5–40 C: >6 years: 5–40	bid–tid
					Narcolepsy	C: 5–60 T, A: 5–60	bid–tid
	Adderall XR	Bimodal—immediate and delayed	1.5–2	8–12	ADHD	C: 5–30 T: 10–30 A: 20–30 Capsule taken whole or sprinkled on applesauce; do not crush	qam
Amphetamine sulfate	Dyanavel XR	Oral suspension containing immediate and extended	1	13	ADHD	C, T, A: 2.5–20 Shake well	qam
Dextroamphetamine	Dexedrine	Immediate	1	4–6	ADHD Narcolepsy	C, T, A: 5–40 C, T, A: 5–60	bid–tid bid–tid
	Dexedrine Spansule	Bimodal—immediate and delayed	1	6–10	ADHD Narcolepsy	C, T, A: 5–40 C, T, A: 5–60	qam qam
Lisdexamfetamine	Vyvanse	Prodrug slowly metabolized to amphetamine	1.5–2	13–14	ADHD	C, T, A: 30–70 Capsule taken whole or contents dissolved in water	qam

TABLE 29–14. Selected psychostimulants (continued)

Generic name	Trade name	Release profile	Onset of action, h	Duration of action, h[a]	Indications	Usual dosage range, mg/day	Dosing interval[b]
Stimulants—amphetamine derivatives (continued)							
Dexmethylphenidate	Focalin	Immediate	1	4	ADHD	C, T, A: 5–20	bid
	Focalin XR	Bimodal—immediate and delayed	0.5	8–12	ADHD	C, T, A: 5–20 Capsule taken whole or sprinkled on applesauce; do not crush	qam
Stimulants—methylphenidate derivatives							
Methylphenidate	Concerta	Immediate and extended	1–2	8–12	ADHD	C, T: 18–54 A: 18–72 Tablet taken whole; do not crush	qam
	Daytrana	Transdermal continuous-release	2	8–12	ADHD	C, T, A: 10–30 mg/9-hour transdermal patch	qam
	Metadate CD	Bimodal—immediate and delayed	1.5	8	ADHD	C, T, A: 20–60 Capsule taken whole or sprinkled on applesauce; do not crush	qam
	Ritalin	Immediate	1	4	ADHD Narcolepsy	C, T, A: 10–60	bid–tid
	Ritalin SR	Delayed	1–2	6–8	ADHD Narcolepsy	C, T, A: 20–60 Tablet must be taken whole	qam–qam and q2pm

TABLE 29–14. Selected psychostimulants *(continued)*

Generic name	Trade name	Release profile	Onset of action, h	Duration of action, h[a]	Indications	Usual dosage range, mg/day	Dosing interval[b]
Stimulants—methylphenidate derivatives *(continued)*							
Methylphenidate *(continued)*	Ritalin LA	Bimodal—immediate and delayed	1–1.5	8–10	ADHD	C, T, A: 20–60 Capsule taken whole or sprinkled on applesauce; do not crush	qam
	Quillivant XR	Oral suspension (20% immediate, 80% extended release)		12	ADHD	C, T, A: 20–60 Vigorously shake for at least 10 seconds	qam
Nonstimulants							
Atomoxetine	Strattera		c	12	ADHD	C, T <70 kg: 0.5 mg/kg/day up to the lesser of 1.4 mg/kg/day or 100 mg C, T, A >70 kg: 40–100	qam–qam and q4pm qam–qam and q4pm
Clonidine	Kapvay	Extended release	c	12	ADHD	C, T: 0.1–0.4 Tablet taken whole; do not crush	bid (qam and qhs)
Guanfacine	Intuniv	Extended release	c	8–14	ADHD	C, T, A: 1–4 Tablet taken whole; do not crush	qam

TABLE 29–14. Selected psychostimulants *(continued)*

Generic name	Trade name	Release profile	Onset of action, h	Duration of action, h[a]	Indications	Usual dosage range, mg/day	Dosing interval[b]
Nonstimulants *(continued)*							
Armodafinil	Nuvigil		1	>8	Narcolepsy, OSA	A: 150–250	qam
					SWD	A: 150	1 hour before work
Modafinil	Alertec, Provigil		1	5	Narcolepsy, OSA	A: 200	qam
					SWD	A: 200	1 hour before work

Note. A=adult; ADHD=attention-deficit/hyperactivity disorder; bid=twice per day; C=child; CD=extended release; LA=extended release; OSA=obstructive sleep apnea; q2pm=at 2 P.M.; q4pm=at 4 P.M.; qam=every morning; qhs=every night at bedtime; SR=sustained release; SWD=shift work disorder; T=adolescent; tid=three times per day; XR=extended release.

[a] Approximate duration of single dose in ADHD.

[b] Unless otherwise noted, bid dosing is morning and noon; tid dosing is morning, noon, and 4 P.M.

[c] Therapeutic effect builds over several weeks of treatment.

Source. Product monographs. Lexicomp Online, Hudson, OH, Lexi-Comp, 2017; and U.S. National Library of Medicine: DailyMed (website). Available at: https://dailymed.nlm.nih.gov/dailymed. Accessed October 7, 2018.

Medication selection involves choice of both agent and drug-release profile. Although studies suggest that overall response is similar for methylphenidate and amphetamine-based stimulants, individual response may differ considerably between the two drug classes, and a switch to an agent in the other class may improve an inadequate response. Short-acting formulations have a limited duration of effect (only 4–6 hours), requiring twice- or thrice-daily dosing to maintain therapeutic effects over the school (or working) day. Repeat dosing not only is inconvenient but also increases the stigma of medication use, the chances for drug diversion, and the possibility of lapses in therapeutic coverage by impairing medication adherence in patients with organizational and attentional deficits. Long-acting formulations have been developed that use controlled drug release (delayed or bimodal [immediate and delayed]), transdermal absorption, and metabolic delivery of active drug from a prodrug. Delayed-release preparations provide an extended duration of therapeutic effect but have a slower onset of action. In this situation, the addition of an immediate-release preparation can hasten the onset of effect. Bimodal drug-release formulations provide an immediate initial dose for rapid onset of action, followed by delayed release of the remaining capsule contents for extended effects. Long-acting formulations with once-daily dosing provide greater convenience, more consistent blood levels and therapeutic effects, improved medication compliance, and a reduced potential for abuse. Methylphenidate is available in the United States as a long-acting transdermal patch that is worn for 9 hours but provides therapeutic effects through 12 hours, although the duration of effect can be modified by early removal of the patch.

Lisdexamfetamine is a prodrug that is slowly metabolized by enzymatic hydrolysis in the blood to dextroamphetamine. Because the drug must first undergo oral absorption and subsequent metabolism to dextroamphetamine, lisdexamfetamine has a slow onset of action (1.5–2 hours) but a long duration (13–14 hours) of effect.

Common adverse effects of stimulant agents include CNS (e.g., insomnia, headache, nervousness, social withdrawal) and gastrointestinal (e.g., stomachache, anorexia) symptoms. Adverse effects are generally mild and diminish with continued treatment, adjustment of dosage, or change in dose timing. Rebound ADHD symptoms (i.e., hyperactivity, irritability) may occur with falling blood levels after the last daily dose. Use of stimulants in children has been associated with weight loss and slowing of the growth rate.

Stimulants can cause elevated heart rate and blood pressure, palpitations, hypertension or hypotension, and cardiac arrhythmias when taken at higher dosages. However, large retrospective database studies have found no increased cardiac risk in children and adults taking prescribed stimulants (Cooper et al. 2011; Habel et al. 2011). Stimulants may exacerbate motor or phonic tics or psychotic symptoms. Adverse effects increase in incidence and severity with short-acting formulations and with increased dosages.

All stimulants may interact with sympathomimetics and MAOIs (including selegiline), resulting in headache, arrhythmias, hypertensive crisis, and hyperpyrexia. Stimulants should not be administered with MAOIs or within 14 days of MAOI discontinuation. Methylphenidate may interact pharmacodynamically with TCAs to cause increased anxiety, irritability, agitation, and aggression. Higher dosages of stimulants may also reduce the therapeutic effectiveness of antihypertensive medications.

When stimulants are used concurrently with β-blockers, the excessive α-adrenergic activity may cause hypertension, reflex bradycardia, and possible heart block.

Nonstimulants

Nonstimulant medications have a positive but less robust effect on ADHD symptoms than do stimulants. However, they generally have less abuse potential than stimulants.

Atomoxetine

Atomoxetine is a specific norepinephrine reuptake inhibitor indicated for the treatment of ADHD. Unlike the rapid response to stimulants (i.e., a few hours), the therapeutic effect of atomoxetine builds gradually over several weeks. Elimination of atomoxetine is reduced in patients with hepatic impairment.

Atomoxetine's side effects reported in clinical trials included nausea, decreased appetite, fatigue, abdominal pain, tachycardia, hypertension, insomnia, irritability, and urinary retention. Nausea is worse with once-daily versus twice-daily dosing. Symptoms of overdose include tachycardia, gastrointestinal symptoms, agitation, QT prolongation, hypertension, somnolence, dizziness, tremor, and dry mouth. Treatment is primarily supportive.

Similar to stimulants, atomoxetine may interact with sympathomimetics and MAOIs. It should not be administered with MAOIs or within 14 days of MAOI discontinuation. Atomoxetine is metabolized by CYP2D6 and is a mild inhibitor of CYP2D6. Potent CYP2D6 inhibitors (e.g., paroxetine, fluoxetine) may increase the plasma levels and toxicity of atomoxetine.

Clonidine and Guanfacine

Clonidine and guanfacine are α_2-adrenergic agonists available in extended-release formulations and are FDA approved for monotherapy or adjunctive treatment of ADHD. Immediate-release preparations of clonidine and guanfacine, and a clonidine weekly transdermal patch, are also available for the treatment of hypertension. In patients with suboptimal response to stimulant monotherapy, the combination of a stimulant and an α_2-adrenergic agonist is significantly more effective than a stimulant alone. Unlike the rapid response to stimulants (i.e., a few hours), the therapeutic effects of guanfacine and clonidine on ADHD symptoms builds gradually over several weeks. Tic symptoms appear to be responsive to guanfacine or clonidine, whereas they are often worsened by stimulants.

Guanfacine's adverse effects include dose-dependent somnolence, headache, fatigue, upper abdominal pain, hypotension, and dizziness. Clonidine's adverse effects include somnolence, upper respiratory tract infection, fatigue, irritability, insomnia, nightmares, hypotension, and emotional dysregulation. Caution is warranted for patients receiving other antihypertensive agents or drugs known to affect sinus node function or atrioventricular node conduction, such as digitalis, calcium channel blockers, and β-blockers. Blood pressure and heart rate should be measured before and monitored during treatment.

Overdose of clonidine or guanfacine may cause initial hypertension followed by hypotension, bradycardia, respiratory depression, hypothermia, lethargy, and impaired consciousness. Large overdoses may cause reversible cardiac conduction defects or dysrhythmias, apnea, coma, and seizures. Treatment is primarily supportive.

Modafinil and Armodafinil

Modafinil and its *R*-enantiomer armodafinil are reported to inhibit the dopamine re-uptake transporter, but in a manner different from traditional stimulants, which may account for their milder activating effects. Modafinil and armodafinil are indicated for promotion of wakefulness in patients with narcolepsy, shift work disorder, or obstructive sleep apnea. The two agents have similar therapeutic and adverse effects, but armodafinil has a longer duration of action due to slower metabolism. Modafinil and armodafinil have a lower potential for abuse than do traditional stimulants.

Adverse effects include headache, nausea, anxiety, dizziness, insomnia, and rhinitis. Serious skin rash and possible Stevens-Johnson syndrome may occur. To date, there are no reports of fatal overdose with modafinil or armodafinil.

Modafinil and armodafinil are moderate inducers of CYP3A4 and moderate inhibitors of CYP2C19. Significant metabolic drug interactions are most likely to involve decreased levels of drugs that undergo significant CYP3A4-mediated first-pass metabolism, such as cyclosporine, ethinyl estradiol, and triazolam. Prazosin may reduce the wakefulness-inducing effects of modafinil. Caution is advised when prescribing MAOIs concurrently with modafinil or armodafinil.

Cognitive Enhancers

Cognitive enhancers may provide symptomatic improvement for cognitive (memory, visual-spatial function, motor skills) and functional (personality and behavior) symptoms of dementia. There is no evidence that they alter the course of the underlying disease process. Agents currently approved for the treatment of Alzheimer's disease include the cholinesterase inhibitors donepezil, galantamine, and rivastigmine and the N-methyl-D-aspartate (NMDA) receptor antagonist memantine (Table 29–15).

Cholinesterase Inhibitors

Cholinesterase inhibitors increase acetylcholine availability and enhance cholinergic neurotransmission by decreasing the cholinesterase-mediated degradation of acetylcholine in the synaptic cleft.

A meta-analysis of 10 randomized double-blind, placebo-controlled 6-month trials of donepezil, galantamine, or rivastigmine in patients with mild to severe Alzheimer's disease reported similar efficacy among the three agents in regard to improvement in cognitive function, global clinical state, performance of activities of daily living, and behavior compared with placebo (Birks 2006), with the improvements occurring only in a subset of the subjects. Similar results were observed in a meta-analysis of six randomized trials of cholinesterase inhibitors in patients with dementia associated with Parkinson's disease (Rolinski et al. 2012; refer to Table 29–15 for the FDA-approved indications of each agent). Updated guidelines for Alzheimer's disease and other dementias (Rabins et al. 2014) suggest that higher-dosage (23 mg/day) oral donepezil does not confer any meaningful benefit over lower-dosage treatment (10 mg/day), whereas higher-dosage (13.3 mg/24 hour) transdermal rivastigmine may have a greater benefit than lower-dosage treatment (4.6 mg/24 hour).

TABLE 29–15. Cognitive enhancers

Generic name	Trade name	Indications	Dosage forms	Usual dosage range, mg/day	Dosing interval
Cholinesterase inhibitors					
Donepezil	Aricept	AD—mild, moderate, severe	O, ODT	5–10 / Severe: 10–23	qhs / qhs
Galantamine	Razadyne / Razadyne ER, Reminyl ER	AD—mild, moderate / AD—mild, moderate	O, L / O	16–24 / 16–24	bid / qam
Rivastigmine	Exelon	AD—mild, moderate / PDD—mild, moderate	O, L	6–12	bid
	Exelon patch	AD—mild, moderate / PDD—mild, moderate	TD	9.5–13.3 mg/24 hours	daily
NMDA receptor antagonists					
Memantine	Namenda, Ebixa / Namenda XR	AD—moderate, severe / AD—moderate, severe	O / O	20 / 28	bid / daily
Combination products					
Memantine/donepezil	Namzaric	AD—moderate, severe	O	28/10	qpm

Note. AD=Alzheimer's disease; bid=twice per day; ER=extended release; L=oral liquid; NMDA=N-methyl-D-aspartate; O=oral tablet or capsule; ODT=oral dissolving tablet; PDD=Parkinson's disease dementia; qam=every morning; qhs=every night at bedtime; qpm=every evening; TD=transdermal patch; XR=extended release.

Patients with hepatic or renal impairment may require dosage reduction of galantamine and rivastigmine. Initial dosage titration should be slow and according to patient tolerability. Galantamine should not be prescribed in patients with severe hepatic or renal impairment, and galantamine dosages should not exceed 16 mg/day in those with moderate hepatic or renal impairment.

Most adverse effects of cholinesterase inhibitors are mild, dose-related, and gastrointestinal in nature (e.g., nausea, vomiting, diarrhea, reduced appetite, anorexia), as expected from procholinergic agents. Rivastigmine tends to cause the worst gastrointestinal side effects. Gastrointestinal side effects lessen over time and can be minimized by slow dosage titration and administration with food. Adequate hydration reduces nausea. A brief treatment-discontinuation period of a few to several days, with reinitiation at the same or a lower dosage, can reduce anorexia or gastrointestinal adverse effects. The procholinergic properties of cholinesterase inhibitors may also cause muscle cramps, urinary incontinence, insomnia, and vivid dreams and increase vagotonic (e.g., bradycardia) and bronchoconstrictor effects. Cholinesterase inhibitors should be used with caution in patients with cardiac conduction abnormalities or a history of asthma or obstructive pulmonary disease. Procholinergic agents may promote seizures. Newer long-term evidence has focused on the safety concerns of cholinesterase inhibitors, which include anorexia, weight loss, falls, hip fractures, syncope, bradycardia, and potential increases in the need for cardiac pacemakers (Rabins et al. 2014).

Overdose of cholinesterase inhibitors can cause a potentially fatal cholinergic crisis, with bradycardia, hypotension, muscle weakness, nausea, vomiting, respiratory depression, sialorrhea, diaphoresis, and seizures.

Donepezil and galantamine are metabolized by CYP2D6 and CYP3A4 isozymes but are not associated with any clinically significant CYP-mediated pharmacokinetic interactions. Rivastigmine is unaffected by drugs that interact with CYP isozymes.

Cholinesterase inhibitors may exacerbate the effects of other cholinesterase inhibitors (e.g., physostigmine) or of cholinomimetic agents (e.g., bethanechol). Cholinesterase inhibitors should be discontinued several weeks before surgery. These agents prolong the duration of action of the depolarizing neuromuscular-blocking agent succinylcholine (suxamethonium) by inhibiting its metabolism. In contrast, a cholinesterase inhibitor–mediated increase in acetylcholine levels antagonizes the actions of nondepolarizing neuromuscular blockers (e.g., rocuronium).

Many psychotropics have anticholinergic properties that may antagonize the effects of cognitive enhancers. The use of anticholinergic agents in patients with compromised cognitive function should be minimized. A partial listing of drugs with significant CNS anticholinergic effects is presented in Table 29–16. Conversely, cholinesterase inhibitors may have a countertherapeutic effect in patients receiving anticholinergic medication for medical conditions such as asthma or chronic obstructive pulmonary disease.

N-Methyl-D-Aspartate Receptor Antagonists

Memantine is thought to reduce chronic neuronal excitotoxicity by acting as an NMDA receptor antagonist. Although memantine may provide symptomatic improvement for symptoms of Alzheimer's disease, there is no evidence that it prevents or slows neurodegeneration or alters the course of the underlying disease process.

TABLE 29–16. Commonly used drugs with significant anticholinergic effects

	Risk[a]		Risk[a]
Antidepressants		Antipsychotics	
Tertiary-amine TCAs	+++	Chlorpromazine	+++
Secondary-amine TCAs	++	Clozapine	+++
Paroxetine	++	Olanzapine	++
		Perphenazine	++
Antidiarrheals		Quetiapine	++
Loperamide	++	Thioridazine	+++
Antiemetics		Antispasmodics	
Prochlorperazine	++	Atropine	+++
Promethazine	+++	Clidinium	+++
		Dicyclomine	+++
Antihistamines		Flavoxate	++
Brompheniramine	+++	Glycopyrrolate	++
Chlorpheniramine	+++	Homatropine	+++
Cyproheptadine	+++	Hyoscine	+++
Dimenhydrinate	++	Hyoscyamine	+++
Diphenhydramine	++	Methscopolamine	+++
Hydroxyzine	+++	Oxybutynin	+++
Meclizine	+++	Propantheline	++
		Scopolamine	+++
Antiparkinsonian agents		Tolterodine	++
Amantadine	++		
Benztropine	+++	Skeletal muscle relaxants	
Orphenadrine	+++	Baclofen	++
Procyclidine	+++	Carisoprodol	+++
Trihexyphenidyl	+++	Chlorzoxazone	+++
		Cyclobenzaprine	+++
H$_2$ antagonists		Metaxalone	+++
Cimetidine	++	Methocarbamol	+++
		Tizanidine	+++

Note. TCAs=tricyclic antidepressants.
[a]Risk of anticholinergic adverse effects at therapeutic dosages: +++=high; ++=medium. Risk is increased in the elderly and with multiple agents with anticholinergic activity.
Source. Compiled from Cancelli et al. 2009; Chew et al. 2008; McEvoy 2017; Rudolph et al. 2008.

Because of the differing mechanisms of action of cholinesterase inhibitors and memantine, it has been suggested that use of the two classes in combination might provide synergistic benefit for patients with moderate to severe Alzheimer's disease (data do not support memantine's use in mild Alzheimer's disease). A systematic review of pooled data from three 6-month trials in patients with moderate to severe Alzheimer's disease receiving memantine plus a cholinesterase inhibitor (mainly donepezil) concluded that combination therapy resulted in small improvements in cognition, clinical global scores, and behavior but had no effect on functional performance in activities of daily living (Farrimond et al. 2012). Memantine has no effect on the pharmacokinetics of cholinesterase inhibitors and thus may be used in combination with these agents without dosage adjustment.

Memantine undergoes primarily renal elimination. Patients with severe renal impairment should not exceed a dosage of 5 mg twice daily with the immediate-release formulation or 14 mg/day with the extended-release formulation. Memantine has no significant CYP interactions with other drugs. Drugs that alkalinize urine may reduce memantine elimination by up to 80%, whereas urine acidifiers enhance memantine elimination.

Memantine has been shown to be well tolerated in Alzheimer's disease, with an adverse-effect profile similar to that of placebo. Memantine has no effect on respiration and is generally benign in patients with cardiovascular disease. Overdose has been reported, with symptoms of agitation, confusion, psychosis, bradycardia, and coma, followed by full recovery; no fatalities have occurred with memantine alone.

Psychotropic Drugs in Pregnancy

Management of any psychiatric disorder during pregnancy and lactation is complicated by the need to consider the effects of psychiatric medication on the fetus and newborn as well as the potential effects of maternal untreated illness on fetal development. In 2015, the FDA replaced the long-standing five-letter system of pregnancy risk categories (i.e., A, B, C, D, and X) with a new system for organizing and presenting safety and use information in prescription drug labeling. New medications approved after June 30, 2015, are required to use the revised FDA labeling, which provides information on pregnancy, lactation, and impact on both female and male reproductive potential. The labeling on older medications is gradually being updated. The intent is to give providers and patients detailed evidence on which to base their decisions, rather than relying on category designations. Information is continually evolving regarding risk versus benefit of treating mental illness during pregnancy. Updated reviews on reproductive toxicity of specific drugs are available online through the U.S. National Library of Medicine's Developmental and Reproductive Toxicology Database (www.nlm.nih.gov/pubs/factsheets/dartfs.html), Motherisk (www.motherisk.org), and MotherToBaby (mothertobaby.org).

Prospective studies found that 68% of pregnant women who discontinued antidepressant use because of pregnancy relapsed during the first or second trimester (Cohen et al. 2006), and 80% of women who discontinued mood stabilizers relapsed during pregnancy (Viguera et al. 2007). In women with severe psychiatric disorders, the decision of whether to continue mood-stabilizing or antidepressant treatment during the first trimester and throughout pregnancy should be carefully balanced against the risks of discontinuation and should be discussed with the patient, her psychiatrist, and her obstetrician. In women with mild mental illness and low relapse risk, the mood stabilizer or antidepressant may be tapered off or continued during efforts to conceive, and the patient can be monitored closely for relapse of mood symptoms. Compared with gradual tapering, abrupt cessation of mood stabilizers greatly increases the risk of relapse (50% within 2 weeks) (Viguera et al. 2007). Monitoring of maternal serum levels and dosage adjustment of medication is advised as pregnancy progresses and during the early postpartum period, because serum levels of lithium, TCAs, lamotrigine, and other psychotropics decrease with pregnancy-related increases in volume of distribution, metabolic capacity, and renal filtration. These changes reverse in the postpartum period, but timing is variable; therefore, monitoring is needed to guide dosage adjustments postpartum.

Antipsychotics

A large 10-year database review of Medicaid patients receiving an antipsychotic prescription during the first trimester concluded that antipsychotic use in early pregnancy did not cause a meaningful increase in risk of congenital malformations. The possible exception to this conclusion was risperidone, which was associated with a small increased risk for overall malformations (relative risk, 1.26; 95% confidence interval, 1.02–1.56; Huybrechts et al. 2016).

Exposure to SGAs during pregnancy can lead to greater maternal weight gain and greater risk of gestational diabetes (Kulkarni et al. 2015). A small study found that placental passage of antipsychotics was highest for olanzapine and haloperidol, followed by risperidone, with quetiapine having the least placental transfer (Kulkarni et al. 2015). Exposure to antipsychotics during the third trimester carries a risk of abnormal muscle movements, EPS, and withdrawal symptoms in the newborn. As stated previously, the risk of relapse should be balanced against the risk of antipsychotic exposure.

Mood Stabilizers

Use of lithium during pregnancy has been associated with an overall increase in rare fetal cardiac defects, most of which are correctable and many of which resolve spontaneously. Historically, the risk of Ebstein's anomaly with lithium exposure was described as increased 20-fold but still low (1 in 1,000 infants) (Giles and Bannigan 2006). A recent retrospective cohort study of more than 1 million pregnancies found an increased risk of Ebstein's anomaly in infants exposed to lithium, particularly at higher dosages; however, the comparative rate for exposed versus nonexposed infants (0.6% vs. 0.18%) was of much smaller magnitude than previous estimates (Patorno et al. 2017). With fetal exposure to lithium in the first trimester, ultrasonography or fetal echocardiography to assess fetal cardiac development is advised. In women with moderate illness and/or relapse risk who have previously shown a preferential response to lithium, one option is to slowly discontinue lithium before conception and then restart lithium at 12 weeks, after fetal cardiac structural development is complete.

Newborns exposed to lithium prior to delivery, especially at higher serum levels, may experience "floppy baby syndrome." Signs and symptoms include premature birth, cyanosis, muscle flaccidity, lethargy, and poor reflexes. If clinically feasible, consideration should be given to holding lithium 24–48 hours prior to delivery (Hogan and Freeman 2016).

Use of anticonvulsants during pregnancy has been studied mainly in women with epilepsy. Valproate exposure increases the incidence of any major congenital malformation to greater than 9% (compared with an incidence of approximately 3% in the U.S. general population), and therefore valproate is generally contraindicated in pregnancy (Hogan and Freeman 2016). Risk increases with higher dosages and combined anticonvulsant therapy. Valproate is associated with a significantly increased risk of incomplete neural tube closure (2%–5%), cardiac defects, craniofacial abnormalities, limb defects, and neurocognitive developmental deficits. Carbamazepine is also teratogenic, increasing the risk of neural tube defects (e.g., spina bifida), facial dysmorphism, and fingernail hypoplasia, but the risk of malformations is lower than with valproate. The risk of any major malformation at birth is 5.3%–7.7% with carbamazepine, notably at dosages higher than 1,000 mg/day (Hogan and Freeman 2016). Maternal folic acid supplementation during pregnancy may reduce the risk of neural tube defects in infants exposed to carbamazepine, although likely not in infants exposed to valproate. Overall, pregnancy registry data to date indicate no increased risk of congenital malformations with lamotrigine. Insufficient data are available to assess oxcarbazepine's teratogenicity.

Antidepressants

The risks of antidepressant exposure during pregnancy continue to be debated. SSRIs are not associated with an increased rate of stillbirths or major physical malformations (Wisner et al. 2009). Concerns regarding increased rates of cardiac defects in children born to women who took paroxetine during pregnancy, which prompted the FDA to issue a product warning, have not been confirmed (Einarson et al. 2009). Risk of cardiac malformations may be increased if SSRIs are combined with benzodiazepines (Oberlander et al. 2008; Wikner et al. 2007). Bupropion is infrequently prescribed during pregnancy. A systematic review found conflicting evidence regarding a small risk of cardiovascular defects with bupropion (Hendrick et al. 2017). A potentially increased rate of spontaneous abortion associated with first-trimester bupropion exposure was identified; however, the rates of miscarriage were not higher than rates reported for the general population (Hendrick et al. 2017). Mirtazapine has not been associated with any specific malformations (Smit et al. 2016). Although less formally studied compared with other antidepressant classes, TCAs do not seem to be associated with birth defects. Increased risks for premature birth, small-for-gestational-age birth, preeclampsia, and persistent pulmonary hypertension in the newborn have been reported in association with SSRI exposure during pregnancy; however, study results are conflicting, and the risk of one or more of these conditions occurring in association with SSRI exposure may be no worse than the risk of untreated depression in pregnancy (Altemus and Occhiogrosso 2017). A 2017 retrospective cohort study in Sweden found first-trimester antidepressant exposure to be associated with a small increase in preterm births; however, the study did not find any association between exposure and risk for small-for-gestational-age birth, autism spectrum disorder, or ADHD (Sujan et al. 2017).

A neonatal syndrome has been described with serotonergic antidepressant (e.g., SSRI) exposure in the third trimester. Symptoms include hypertonia, difficulty feeding, tremor, excessive crying, irritability, respiratory disturbances, tachypnea, and restless sleep. This syndrome most commonly is associated with paroxetine, venlafaxine, and fluoxetine. Reported rates range from no signs to up to 30% of exposed infants (Yang et al. 2017). Symptoms are similar to those seen in premature infants, although duration may differ.

In 2006, the FDA warned of a association between third-trimester exposure to SSRIs and persistent pulmonary hypertension of the newborn (PPHN), based on a single study; in 2011, the advisory was altered to state that the risk was unclear due to conflicting data (U.S. Food and Drug Administration 2011). Most recently, two large pregnancy databases in the United States (Medicaid, 46 states; Huybrechts et al. 2015) and Canada (Quebec; Bérard et al. 2017) reported that late-pregnancy exposure to SSRIs was associated with a small absolute increase in risk of PPHN. Huybrechts et al. (2015) reported higher rates of PPHN in infants exposed to SSRIs (31.5 per 10,000 births) and infants exposed to non-SSRI antidepressants (29.1 per 10,000 births) compared with rates in nonexposed infants (20.8 per 10,000 births). It is unclear whether SNRIs also carry this risk, given the lack of statistical power (Bérard et al. 2017).

Anxiolytics and Sedative-Hypnotics

Retrospective case–control studies, which are prone to recall bias, observed a threefold increased risk of oral cleft associated with use of benzodiazepines during pregnancy (Dolovich et al. 1998). Subsequent studies have not found evidence of teratogenic risk when benzodiazepines are used as monotherapy during pregnancy (Bellantuono et al. 2013). Recent studies have found some increased obstetrical or neonatal risks with benzodiazepines during pregnancy (Freeman et al. 2018; Yonkers et al. 2017), but confounding by co-medication, psychiatric and medical comorbidity, and socioeconomic differences may account for the increased risks (Askaa et al. 2014). If benzodiazepines are used late in pregnancy, infants should be closely monitored for neonatal adverse effects, including irritability, tremor, withdrawal seizures, floppy baby syndrome, and apnea and other respiratory difficulties.

Psychostimulants

Insufficient human data are available to fully evaluate the teratogenic effects of amphetamines, methylphenidate, atomoxetine, clonidine, guanfacine, modafinil, and armodafinil during pregnancy (Besag 2014). Stimulant medications should generally be avoided during pregnancy, with emphasis placed on nonpharmacological approaches for treating ADHD and sleep–wake disorders.

Conclusion

In this chapter we have attempted to provide a clinical overview of the major psychotropic drug classes and their uses. We hope that the reader has gained an understanding of the strengths and liabilities of the available armamentarium. As research into the biological mechanisms of psychiatric disorders progresses, inevitably our medication treatments will be further refined to target these specific derangements, resulting in increased efficacy, reduced adverse effects, and improved patient outcomes.

Key Clinical Points

- The use of psychopharmacological agents for a given psychiatric disorder should be based on the best available clinical evidence.

- When appropriate, psychopharmacology should be combined with evidence-based psychosocial and psychotherapeutic modalities so as to enhance medication adherence, reduce symptom burden and risk of relapse, and improve patient functioning.

- The choice of psychopharmacological agent is based on multiple factors, including evidence for efficacy, side effects, desirable secondary pharmacodynamic effects, routes of administration, drug–drug interactions, medical and psychiatric comorbidities, and personal and family history of medication response.

- There is tremendous inter- and intraindividual variation in response to psychotropics.

- If a patient does not respond to one drug in a given class, that does not necessarily mean that the patient will not respond to another drug from the same class.

- In general, drugs that are approved for specific disorders are equally efficacious and differ primarily in terms of pharmacokinetics, adverse-effect profiles, and drug–drug interactions. The most notable exception to this rule is clozapine, which has unique efficacy for treatment-refractory schizophrenia.

- Because it increases the risk of medication toxicity and drug–drug interactions, polypharmacy should be minimized where possible.

References

Altemus M, Occhiogrosso M: Obstetrics and gynecology, in Clinical Manual of Psychopharmacology in the Medically Ill, 2nd Edition. Edited by Levenson JL, Ferrando SJ. Washington, DC, American Psychiatric Publishing, 2017, pp 429–470

American Diabetes Association, American Psychiatric Association, American Association of Clinical Endocrinologists, et al: Consensus development conference on antipsychotic drugs and obesity and diabetes. Diabetes Care 27(2):596–601, 2004 14747245

Askaa B, Jimenez-Solem E, Enghusen Poulsen H, Traerup Andersen J: Maternal characteristics of women exposed to hypnotic benzodiazepine receptor agonist during pregnancy. Obstet Gynecol Int 2014:945621, 2014 24817891

Beach SR, Celano CM, Noseworthy PA, et al: QTc prolongation, torsades de pointes, and psychotropic medications. Psychosomatics 54(1):1–13, 2013 23295003

Bellantuono C, Tofani S, Di Sciascio G, Santone G: Benzodiazepine exposure in pregnancy and risk of major malformations: a critical overview. Gen Hosp Psychiatry 35(1):3–8, 2013 23044244

Bérard A, Sheehy O, Zhao JP, et al: SSRI and SNRI use during pregnancy and the risk of persistent pulmonary hypertension of the newborn. Br J Clin Pharmacol 83(5):1126–1133, 2017 27874994

Besag FMC: ADHD treatment and pregnancy. Drug Saf 37(6):397–408, 2014 24794209

Bilo L, Meo R: Polycystic ovary syndrome in women using valproate: a review. Gynecol Endocrinol 24(10):562–570, 2008 19012099

Birks J: Cholinesterase inhibitors for Alzheimer's disease. Cochrane Database Syst Rev (1):CD005593, 2006 16437532

Boyer EW, Shannon M: The serotonin syndrome. N Engl J Med 352(11):1112–1120, 2005 15784664

Bunchorntavakul C, Reddy KR: Drug hepatotoxicity newer agents. Clin Liver Dis 21(1):115–134, 2017 27842767

Cancelli I, Beltrame M, Gigli GL, et al: Drugs with anticholinergic properties: cognitive and neuropsychiatric side-effects in elderly patients. Neurol Sci 30(2):87–92, 2009 19229475

Caroff SN: Hyperthermia associated with other neuropsychiatric drugs, in Neuroleptic Malignant Syndrome and Related Conditions, 2nd Edition. Edited by Mann SC, Caroff SN, Keck PE Jr, et al. Washington, DC, American Psychiatric Publishing, 2003a, pp 93–120

Caroff SN: Neuroleptic malignant syndrome, in Neuroleptic Malignant Syndrome and Related Conditions, 2nd Edition. Edited by Mann SC, Caroff SN, Keck PE Jr, et al. Washington, DC, American Psychiatric Publishing, 2003b, pp 1–44

Chew ML, Mulsant BH, Pollock BG, et al: Anticholinergic activity of 107 medications commonly used by older adults. J Am Geriatr Soc 56(7):1333–1341, 2008 18510583

Cohen LS, Altshuler LL, Harlow BL, et al: Relapse of major depression during pregnancy in women who maintain or discontinue antidepressant treatment. JAMA 295(5):499–507, 2006 16449615

Cooper WO, Habel LA, Sox CM, et al: ADHD drugs and serious cardiovascular events in children and young adults. N Engl J Med 365(20):1896–1904, 2011 22043968

Cukor D, Levenson JL, Rosenthal-Asher D, Kimmel PL: Renal disease, in American Psychiatric Publishing Textbook of Psychosomatic Medicine and Consultation-Liaison Psychiatry, 3rd Edition. Edited by Levenson JL. Washington, D.C., American Psychiatric Association Publishing, 2019, pp 571–591

de Silva VA, Suraweera C, Ratnatunga SS, et al: Metformin in prevention and treatment of antipsychotic induced weight gain: a systematic review and meta-analysis. BMC Psychiatry 16(1):341, 2016 27716110

Detke MJ, Lu Y, Goldstein DJ, et al: Duloxetine 60 mg once daily dosing versus placebo in the acute treatment of major depression. J Psychiatr Res 36(6):383–390, 2002 12393307

Dolovich LR, Addis A, Vaillancourt JM, et al: Benzodiazepine use in pregnancy and major malformations or oral cleft: meta-analysis of cohort and case-control studies. BMJ 317(7162):839–843, 1998 9748174

Dunkley EJ, Isbister GK, Sibbritt D, et al: The Hunter Serotonin Toxicity Criteria: simple and accurate diagnostic decision rules for serotonin toxicity. QJM 96(9):635–642, 2003 12925718

Einarson A, Choi J, Einarson TR, Koren G: Incidence of major malformations in infants following antidepressant exposure in late pregnancy: results of a large prospective cohort study. Can J Psychiatry 54(4):242–246, 2009 19321030

Farrimond LE, Roberts E, McShane R: Memantine and cholinesterase inhibitor combination therapy for Alzheimer's disease: a systematic review. BMJ Open 2(3):2, 2012 22689908

Freeman MP, Góez-Mogollón L, McInerney KA, et al: Obstetrical and neonatal outcomes after benzodiazepine exposure during pregnancy: results from a prospective registry of women with psychiatric disorders. Gen Hosp Psychiatry 53:73–79, 2018 29958100

Giles JJ, Bannigan JG: Teratogenic and developmental effects of lithium. Curr Pharm Des 12(12):1531–1541, 2006 16611133

Gitlin M: Lithium side effects and toxicity: prevalence and management strategies. Int J Bipolar Disord 4(1):27, 2016 27900734

Grigg J, Worsley R, Thew C, et al: Antipsychotic-induced hyperprolactinemia: synthesis of world-wide guidelines and integrated recommendations for assessment, management and future research. Psychopharmacology (Berl) 234(22):3279–3297, 2017 28889207

Grundy SM, Cleeman JI, Daniels SR, et al: Diagnosis and management of the metabolic syndrome: an American Heart Association/National Heart, Lung, and Blood Institute Scientific Statement. Circulation 112(17):2735–2752, 2005 16157765

Habel LA, Cooper WO, Sox CM, et al: ADHD medications and risk of serious cardiovascular events in young and middle-aged adults. JAMA 306(24):2673–2683, 2011 22161946

Harden CL, Goldstein MA: Mood disorders in patients with epilepsy: epidemiology and management. CNS Drugs 16(5):291–302, 2002 11994019

Hendrick V, Suri R, Gitlin MJ, et al: Bupropion use during pregnancy: a systematic review. Prim Care Companion CNS Disord 19(5), 2017 28973846

Hogan CS, Freeman MP: Adverse effects in the pharmacologic management of bipolar disorder during pregnancy. Psychiatr Clin North Am 39(3):465–475, 2016 27514299

Huybrechts KF, Bateman BT, Palmsten K, et al: Antidepressant use late in pregnancy and risk of persistent pulmonary hypertension of the newborn. JAMA 313(21):2142–2151, 2015 26034955

Huybrechts KF, Hernandez-Diaz S, Patorno E, et al: Antipsychotic use in pregnancy and the risk for congenital malformations. JAMA Psychiatry 73(9):938–946, 2016 27540849

Keck PE Jr, McElroy SL, Tugrul KC, Bennett JA: Valproate oral loading in the treatment of acute mania. J Clin Psychiatry 54(8):305–308, 1993 8253698

Kuehn BM: FDA: Antipsychotics risky for elderly. JAMA 300(4):379–380, 2008 18647971

Kulkarni J, Storch A, Baraniuk A, et al: Antipsychotic use in pregnancy. Expert Opin Pharmacother 16(9):1335–1345, 2015 26001182

Lehman AF, Lieberman JA, Dixon LB, et al; American Psychiatric Association; Steering Committee on Practice Guidelines: Practice guideline for the treatment of patients with schizophrenia, second edition. Am J Psychiatry 161(2 suppl):1–56, 2004 15000267

Levenson JL, Ferrando SJ (eds): Clinical Manual of Psychopharmacology in the Medically Ill, 2nd Edition. Washington, DC, American Psychiatric Publishing, 2017

Lewis SW, Barnes TR, Davies L, et al: Randomized controlled trial of effect of prescription of clozapine versus other second-generation antipsychotic drugs in resistant schizophrenia. Schizophr Bull 32(4):715–723, 2006 16540702

Lieberman JA, Stroup TS, McEvoy JP, et al: Effectiveness of antipsychotic drugs in patients with chronic schizophrenia. Clinical Antipsychotic Trials of Intervention Effectiveness (CATIE) Investigators. N Engl J Med 353(12):1209–1223, 2005 16172203

McEvoy GE: American Hospital Formulary Service (AHFS) Drug Information 2017. Bethesda, MD, American Society of Health-System Pharmacists, 2017

Meyer JM, Proctor G, Cummings MA, et al: Ciprofloxacin and clozapine: a potentially fatal but underappreciated interaction. Case Rep Psychiatry 2016:5606098, 2016 27872784

Oberlander TF, Warburton W, Misri S, et al: Major congenital malformations following prenatal exposure to serotonin reuptake inhibitors and benzodiazepines using population-based health data. Birth Defects Res B Dev Reprod Toxicol 83(1):68–76, 2008 18293409

Patorno E, Huybrechts KF, Bateman BT, et al: Lithium use in pregnancy and the risk of cardiac malformations. N Engl J Med 376(23):2245–2254, 2017 28591541

Rabins PV, Rovner BW, Rummans T, et al: Guideline Watch (October 2014): Practice Guideline for the Treatment of Patients With Alzheimer's Disease and Other Dementias. Arlington, VA, American Psychiatric Association, 2014. Available at: http://psychiatryonline.org/pb/assets/raw/sitewide/practice_guidelines/guidelines/alzheimerwatch.pdf. Accessed November 12, 2018.

Raja M: Clozapine safety, 35 years later. Curr Drug Saf 6(3):164–184, 2011 22122392

Ray WA, Chung CP, Murray KT, et al: Atypical antipsychotic drugs and the risk of sudden cardiac death. N Engl J Med 360(3):225–235, 2009 19144938

Reis M, Källén B: Maternal use of antipsychotics in early pregnancy and delivery outcome. J Clin Psychopharmacol 28(3):279–288, 2008 18480684

Richardson T, Macaluso M: Clinically relevant treatment considerations regarding lithium use in bipolar disorder. Expert Opin Drug Metab Toxicol 13(11):1105–1113, 2017 28965429

Rolinski M, Fox C, Maidment I, et al: Cholinesterase inhibitors for dementia with Lewy bodies, Parkinson's disease dementia and cognitive impairment in Parkinson's disease. Cochrane Database Syst Rev (3):CD006504, 2012 22419314

Rosenstein DL, Nelson JC, Jacobs SC: Seizures associated with antidepressants: a review. J Clin Psychiatry 54(8):289–299, 1993 8253696

Rudolph JL, Salow MJ, Angelini MC, et al: The anticholinergic risk scale and anticholinergic adverse effects in older persons. Arch Intern Med 168(5):508–513, 2008 18332297

Salem H, Pigott T, Zhang XY, et al: Antipsychotic-induced tardive dyskinesia: from biological basis to clinical management. Expert Rev Neurother 17(9):883–894, 2017 28750568

Schatzberg AF, Nemeroff CB (eds): The American Psychiatric Publishing Textbook of Psychopharmacology, 5th Edition. Arlington, VA, American Psychiatric Publishing, 2017

Seo H, Chiesa A, Lee SJ, et al: Safety and tolerability of lamotrigine: results from 12 placebo-controlled clinical trials and clinical implications. Clin Neuropharmacol 34(1):39–47, 2011 21242744

Smit M, Dolman KM, Honig A: Mirtazapine in pregnancy and lactation—a systematic review. Eur Neuropsychopharmacol 26(1):126–135, 2016 26631373

Sternbach H: The serotonin syndrome. Am J Psychiatry 148(6):705–713, 1991 2035713

Stone M, Laughren T, Jones ML, et al: Risk of suicidality in clinical trials of antidepressants in adults: analysis of proprietary data submitted to US Food and Drug Administration. BMJ 339:b2880, 2009 19671933

Sujan AC, Rickert ME, Öberg AS, et al: Associations of maternal antidepressant use during the first trimester of pregnancy with preterm birth, small for gestational age, autism spectrum disorder, and attention-deficit/hyperactivity disorder in offspring. JAMA 317(15):1553–1562, 2017 28418479

Tsuda Y, Saruwatari J, Yasui-Furukori N: Meta-analysis: the effects of smoking on the disposition of two commonly used antipsychotic agents, olanzapine and clozapine. BMJ Open 4(3):e004216, 2014 24595134

U.S. Food and Drug Administration: FDA Drug Safety Communication: Selective serotonin reuptake inhibitor (SSRI) antidepressant use during pregnancy and reports of a rare heart and lung condition in newborn babies. December 14, 2011. Available at: https://www.fda.gov/Drugs/DrugSafety/ucm283375.htm. Accessed November 12, 2018.

U.S. Food and Drug Administration: FDA Drug Safety Communication: FDA approves new label changes and dosing for zolpidem products and a recommendation to avoid driving the day after using Ambien CR. U.S. Food and Drug Administration website, May 14, 2013. Available at: http://www.fda.gov/Drugs/DrugSafety/ucm352085.htm. Accessed February 10, 2018.

Vieweg WV, Hasnain M, Howland RH, et al: Citalopram, QTc interval prolongation, and torsade de pointes. How should we apply the recent FDA ruling? Am J Med 125(9):859–868, 2012 22748401

Viguera AC, Whitfield T, Baldessarini RJ, et al: Risk of recurrence in women with bipolar disorder during pregnancy: prospective study of mood stabilizer discontinuation. Am J Psychiatry 164(12):1817–1824, quiz 1923, 2007 18056236

Whyte IM, Dawson AH, Buckley NA: Relative toxicity of venlafaxine and selective serotonin reuptake inhibitors in overdose compared to tricyclic antidepressants. QJM 96(5):369–374, 2003 12702786

Wikner BN, Stiller CO, Bergman U, et al: Use of benzodiazepines and benzodiazepine receptor agonists during pregnancy: neonatal outcome and congenital malformations. Pharmacoepidemiol Drug Saf 16(11):1203–1210, 2007 17894421

Wisner K, Sit D, Hanusa B, et al: Major depression and antidepressant treatment: impact on pregnancy and neonatal outcomes. Am J Psychiatry 166(5):557–566, 2009 19289451

Wu CC, Pai TY, Hsiao FY, et al: The effect of different carbapenem antibiotics (ertapenem, imipenem/cilastatin, and meropenem) on serum valproic acid concentrations. Ther Drug Monit 38(5):587–592, 2016 27322166

Yang A, Ciolino JD, Pinheiro E, et al: Neonatal discontinuation syndrome in serotonergic antidepressant-exposed neonates. J Clin Psychiatry 78(5):605–611, 2017 28570796

Yonkers KA, Gilstad-Hayden K, Forray A, Lipkind HS: Association of panic disorder, generalized anxiety disorder, and benzodiazepine treatment during pregnancy with risk of adverse birth outcomes. JAMA Psychiatry 74(11):1145–1152, 2017 28903165

Zivin K, Pfeiffer PN, Bohnert AS, et al: Evaluation of the FDA warning against prescribing citalopram at doses exceeding 40 mg. Am J Psychiatry 170(6):642–650, 2013 23640689

Recommended Readings

Gardner DM, Murphy AL, O'Donnell H, et al: International consensus study of antipsychotic dosing. Am J Psychiatry 167(6):686–693, 2010 20360319

Kripalani M, Shawcross J, Reilly J, et al: Lithium and chronic kidney disease. BMJ 339:b2452, 2009. Available at: http://www.bmj.com/content/339/bmj.b2452. Accessed October 7, 2018.

Levenson JL, Ferrando SJ (eds): Clinical Manual of Psychopharmacology in the Medically Ill, 2nd Edition. Washington, DC, American Psychiatric Publishing, 2017

Schatzberg AF, Nemeroff CB (eds): The American Psychiatric Publishing Textbook of Psychopharmacology, 5th Edition. Washington, DC, American Psychiatric Publishing, 2017

Online Resources

Drug Interactions

Clozapine REMS Program: https://www.clozapinerems.com

DailyMed: https://dailymed.nlm.nih.gov/dailymed/

epocrates: https://online.epocrates.com/

HIV InSite: http://hivinsite.ucsf.edu/

Medline Plus: Serotonin syndrome. Bethesda, MD, U.S. National Library of Medicine, 2018. Available at: https://medlineplus.gov/ency/article/007272.htm. Accessed October 7, 2018.

MedScape Drug Interactions Checker: https://reference.medscape.com/drug-interactionchecker

Neuroleptic Malignant Syndrome Information Service (NMSIS) (part of the Malignant Hyperthermia Association of the United States [MHAUS]): https://www.mhaus.org/nmsis/about-us/what-is-nmsis/. Accessed October 7, 2018.

U.S. Food and Drug Administration: Postmarketing Information on Drug Safety for Patients and Providers. Silver Spring, MD, U.S. Food and Drug Administration, 2017. Available at: https://www.fda.gov/Drugs/DrugSafety/PostmarketDrugSafetyInformationforPatients andProviders/default.htm. Accessed October 7, 2018.

Utah Poison Control Center for Health Professionals: Serotonin syndrome. Utox Update 4(4), 2002. Available at: https://poisoncontrol.utah.edu/newsletters/pdfs/toxicology-today-archive/Vol4_No4.pdf. Accessed October 7, 2018.

Drugs in Pregnancy and Lactation

Armstrong C: ACOG guidelines on psychiatric medication use during pregnancy and lactation. Am Fam Physician 78(6):772–778, 2008. Available at: https://www.aafp.org/afp/2008/0915/p772.html. Accessed October 7, 2018.

Developmental and Reproductive Toxicology Database (DART) (A TOXNET Database): https://toxnet.nlm.nih.gov/newtoxnet/dart.htm

Drugs and Lactation Database (LactMed) (A TOXNET Database): https://toxnet.nlm.nih.gov/newtoxnet/lactmed.htm

Motherisk: http://www.motherisk.org

MotherToBaby (Organization of Teratology Information Specialists): http://mothertobaby.org

U.S. Food and Drug Administration: FDA Drug Safety Communication: Selective Serotonin Reuptake Inhibitor (SSRI) Antidepressant Use During Pregnancy and Reports of a Rare Heart and Lung Condition in Newborn Babies. Silver Spring, MD, U.S. Food and Drug Administration, 2018. Available at: https://www.fda.gov/Drugs/DrugSafety/ucm283375.htm. Accessed October 7, 2018.

CHAPTER 30

Brain Stimulation Therapies

Corey Keller, M.D., Ph.D.

Mahendra T. Bhati, M.D.

Jonathan Downar, M.D., Ph.D.

Amit Etkin, M.D., Ph.D.

The notion of applying an electrical current to the brain to modulate neural activity and treat patients has existed since the eighteenth century. Brain stimulation interventions, specifically electroconvulsive therapy (ECT), preceded the discovery of psychiatric medications and remain one of the most effective psychiatric treatments. Despite the tremendous benefit, for decades ECT remained the only brain stimulation treatment in psychiatry, and there remains little understanding of the mechanism underlying its treatment effects. However, in the past 20 years, brain stimulation therapies have undergone a revolution with the development of a number of novel brain stimulation interventions (Table 30–1). Many of these new therapies have emerged from progress in neuroimaging and brain stimulation technology, and some are entering routine clinical use. Brain stimulation interventions represent a novel and expanding approach to understanding and treating psychiatric disorders.

Over the past 20 years, older treatments have improved, and novel technologies have been developed. Older treatments such as ECT have become less fraught with side effects with the advent of new, modified procedures performed under generalized anesthesia. Vagus nerve stimulation (VNS) has anticonvulsant effects and is an effective device-based intervention for treatment-resistant depression despite its limited availability. Deep brain stimulation (DBS) has revolutionized the treatment of movement disorders, and in 2008, DBS for treatment-resistant obsessive-compulsive disorder (OCD) was approved by the U.S. Food and Drug Administration (FDA) under a humanitarian device exemption. There is great interest in DBS and related technologies, which are becoming more targeted with the help of electrophysiology and neuroimaging. Repetitive transcranial magnetic stimulation (rTMS) represents the first

TABLE 30–1.　Brain stimulation therapies

	Type of stimulation	Convulsive?	Preclinical use?	Therapeutic use?	FDA approved?	Examples (manufacturers)
Electromagnetic—noninvasive						
Electroconvulsive therapy (ECT)	Electrical (AC)	Yes	—	Yes	Yes (depression)	Mecta Spectrum, Thymatron
Focal electrically administered seizure therapy (FEAST)	Electrical (DC)	Yes	Yes	Yes	No	—
Magnetic seizure therapy (MST)	Magnetic	Yes	Yes	Yes	No	MagVenture
Repetitive or patterned transcranial magnetic stimulation (rTMS)	Magnetic	No	Yes	Yes	Yes (depression)	Neuronetics, Brainsway, MagVenture, Magstim, Neurosoft
Synchronized transcranial magnetic stimulation (sTMS)	Magnetic	No	Yes	Yes	No	NeoSync
Low-field magnetic stimulation (LFMS)	Magnetic	No	Yes	No	No	—
Electromagnetic—invasive						
Deep brain stimulation (DBS)	Electrical (AC)	No	Yes	Yes	Yes (OCD)	Medtronic
Vagus nerve stimulation (VNS)	Electrical (AC)	No	Yes	Yes	Yes (depression)	Cyberonics
Epidural cortical stimulation (ECS)	Electrical (AC)	No	Yes	Yes	No	—
Other—noninvasive						
Focused ultrasound (FUS)	Mechanical (acoustic)	No	Yes	No	No	Insightec
Sonomagnetic stimulation	Mechanical (acoustic), and magnetic	No	Yes	No	No	—

TABLE 30–1. **Brain stimulation therapies** *(continued)*

	Type of stimulation	Convulsive?	Preclinical use?	Therapeutic use?	FDA approved?	Examples (manufacturers)
Other—noninvasive *(continued)*						
Transcranial electrical stimulation (TES)						
Transcranial direct current stimulation (tDCS)	Electrical (DC)	No	Yes	Yes	No	APeX, TCT, Soterix, Thync, foc.us
Transcranial alternating current stimulation (tACS)	Electrical (AC)	No	Yes	No	No	—
Cranial electrical stimulation (CES)	Electrical (DC)	No	Yes	Yes	No	Fisher Wallace (Alpha-Stim)

Note. AC=alternating current; DC=direct current; FDA=U.S. Food and Drug Administration; OCD=obsessive-compulsive disorder.

widespread use of an office-based, noninvasive brain stimulation treatment modality targeting specific brain regions and functions. In combination with neuroimaging and electrophysiology, rTMS is now moving from a one-size-fits-all standard treatment to a more personalized approach targeting different brain circuits and using stimulation parameters specific to the patient's symptomatology in a method better described as "circuitology." Newer experimental tools involve the ability to noninvasively modulate neural activity in superficial brain regions with much-lower-powered stimulation (i.e., transcranial direct-current stimulation [tDCS] and low-field magnetic stimulation [LFMS]) or to target deep brain structures focally, using acoustic rather than electromagnetic energy (i.e., focused ultrasound [FUS]).

In this chapter, we provide a comprehensive overview of current theory, practice, and research in brain stimulation therapies in psychiatry. We first focus on noninvasive and FDA-approved treatment modalities that are commonly employed in medication-resistant depression (ECT, rTMS). We then discuss FDA-approved invasive modalities (DBS, VNS), and we conclude with a survey of novel investigational therapies (tDCS, focal electrically administered seizure therapy [FEAST], magnetic seizure therapy [MST], epidural cortical stimulation [ECS], responsive neurostimulation [RNS], FUS).

Noninvasive Modalities

Electroconvulsive Therapy

Overview

Convulsive therapies in psychiatry emerged from the observation that seizures were associated with improved symptoms in patients with severe psychiatric illness—particularly those with mood disorders and catatonia. In 1934, Ladislas Meduna was the first psychiatrist to report on the benefit of chemically induced (via pentylenetetrazol) seizures for treatment of schizophrenia (Fink 1984). However, chemical induction of seizures with compounds proved unreliable, and two Italian psychiatrists, Ugo Cerletti and Lucio Bini, first used electrical stimulation in 1938 to successfully treat a patient with catatonic schizophrenia (Bini 1995). ECT quickly became widely adopted throughout the world as the first bona fide treatment in modern psychiatry and saved the lives of numerous patients during a time when there were no effective treatments for psychiatric disorders. ECT remains one of the most effective and rapidly acting treatments in psychiatry, yet it is vastly underutilized, due in part to stigma and the need for a specialized treatment setting involving anesthesia and physiological monitoring.

Indications

ECT is currently indicated for the treatment of unipolar depression, bipolar depression, catatonia, schizophreniform disorder, schizophrenia, and schizoaffective disorder (McDonald et al. 2016). Indications for use of ECT for unipolar depression include 1) illness refractory to other antidepressant therapy; 2) situations involving a need for rapid treatment, such as acute psychiatric illness during pregnancy, food refusal leading to nutritional compromise, or persistent suicidal intent; 3) presence of psychotic features; 4) medical comorbidity preventing use of antidepressant medications; and 5) catatonia. ECT has particular benefit for treatment of geriatric depression and is a treatment option that, if needed, can be safely used in critically ill, catatonic, pediatric, or pregnant patients. The legal and regulatory (FDA) requirements surrounding the use of ECT necessitate obtaining specific types of consent, which vary state by state. Some states (e.g., Texas, California) have strict requirements, which have the unfortunate effect of limiting access to ECT despite its being a safe and potentially lifesaving intervention. In these states, a court order is necessary to provide ECT in cases in which patients are severely ill, cannot consent, and need ECT.

Treatment Parameters

Modern ECT is typically delivered in a hospital setting and requires patients to undergo preparation similar to that required for an outpatient surgical procedure. Immediately prior to receiving ECT, patients typically receive an intravenous anesthetic such as methohexital, etomidate, or propofol, followed by administration of a muscle relaxant, usually succinylcholine. A tourniquet is commonly used to isolate an extremity (e.g., foot, arm) from the muscle relaxant to facilitate monitoring of the motor response to an induced seizure. General anesthesia induces unconsciousness, analgesia, and paralysis—all necessary elements to ensure the safety and tolerability of ECT. Anesthesia is brief (several minutes), and during this time patients are hydrated and oxygenated, with vital sign monitoring, electrocardiography (ECG), and encephalography (EEG), before receiving a brief alternating-current (AC; between 20–120 Hz) electrical stimulus for approximately 5 seconds to deliver an approximate 100–500 mC charge and induce a therapeutic seizure. A bite block is used to prevent oral injuries as a result of direct electrical stimulation of the masseter muscles and jaw clenching. The goal of ECT is to achieve a therapeutic effect via induction of a robust generalized seizure lasting approximately 30 seconds. Some practitioners use electromyography (EMG) to monitor motor seizure duration. During the seizure, transient increases in intracranial pressure and acute cerebrovascular changes occur secondary to changes in parasympathetic and sympathetic tone from the stimulation and seizure.

Stimulation is delivered to the brain via the scalp by placement of electrodes in a unilateral or bilateral fashion (Figure 30–1). Unilateral ECT is associated with fewer cognitive side effects compared with bilateral ECT but is thought to be less effective. Despite this perception of its lower efficacy, high-dose unilateral ECT of the nondominant hemisphere (typically the right) appears to be equivalent in antidepressant effect to medium-dose bilateral ECT. Because sinusoidal AC stimulation results in excessive electrical stimulation (thought to be associated with more severe cognitive side effects), the AC stimulus is delivered in the form of brief square-wave pulses.

Although use of ECT remains relatively unchanged since its invention, advances have been made in the type of stimulation used to induce a seizure with maximum treatment effects and minimum side effects. Induction of a seizure of optimal quality is achieved by utilizing ultrabrief-pulse stimulation (<0.5 ms per pulse) and high-dose unilateral ECT (Sackeim et al. 2008). For ECT to be effective, a robust generalized seizure needs to be generated, and research has shown that use of high-dose, ultrabrief, unilateral ECT is similar in effectiveness to bilateral ECT. Furthermore, ultrabrief-pulse ECT exposes the brain to less electrical current than does standard brief-pulse stimulation and therefore also results in fewer cognitive side effects. Changes to stimulus delivery have made ECT more tolerable, yet many patients continue to require standard bilateral ECT to induce a seizure and get a treatment effect, which can

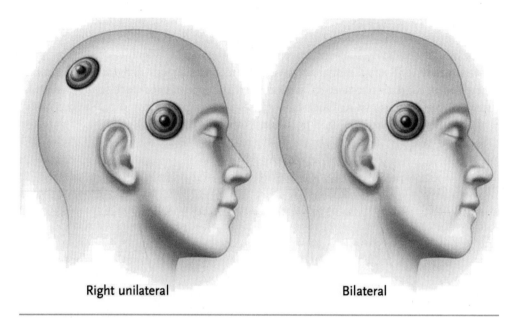

Right unilateral   Bilateral

FIGURE 30–1.   ECT electrode placement.

Right unilateral ECT uses electrodes placed on the one side of the head and positioned to the right of the vertex and right frontotemporal position. Bilateral electrode placement uses electrodes placed on both left and right frontotemporal positions.

Source.   Reprinted from Figure 1 (p. 1942) in: Lisanby SH: "Electroconvulsive Therapy for Depression." *New England Journal of Medicine* 357(19):1939–1945, 2007. Copyright 2007, Massachusetts Medical Society. Used with permission.

make ECT a less favorable treatment option. Ultimately, if one can induce a robust generalized seizure with the minimal necessary electrical stimulation and rapid recovery, one can minimize cognitive side effects while maximizing clinical response.

Concurrent Medications

Noradrenergic agents such as tricyclic antidepressants and serotonin-norepinephrine reuptake inhibitors (Sackeim et al. 2009), lithium, and antipsychotics (particularly clozapine) may be used to augment the therapeutic effects of ECT. Despite its clear benefit, lithium should be used with caution in combination with ECT because it may increase the risk of delirium and cognitive side effects during ECT. These potential side effects can usually be avoided by reducing or holding doses of lithium. As a general rule, anticonvulsants are to be avoided with ECT, because their use will directly interfere with the ability to induce a seizure, thereby disrupting the therapeutic effects of ECT (Sienaert and Peuskens 2007). Benzodiazepines should likewise be avoided, but if they are necessary, short-acting benzodiazepines are recommended, which are less likely to interfere with the induction of a therapeutic seizure. If use of benzodiazepines interferes with the ability to induce a seizure, use of pre-ECT flumazenil can be used to reverse the anticonvulsant effects of benzodiazepines (Krystal et al. 1998). Most nonanticonvulsant medications can be safely coadministered with ECT except for theophylline, which is rarely used. Use of theophylline during ECT can lead to prolonged seizures and result in status epilepticus (Rasmussen and Zorumski 1993).

Treatment Outcomes

Multiple meta-analyses show the lasting and robust antidepressant effect of ECT over pharmacotherapy for unipolar and bipolar depression. ECT remains the most effective antidepressant available and has been shown to reduce mortality and decrease hospital readmission. Evidence and experience support the effectiveness of ECT for the treatment of a range of conditions, including bipolar depression, catatonia, neuroleptic malignant syndrome, schizophrenia, and schizoaffective disorder. When used to treat depression, ECT has an overall response rate of 50%–90%. When used in patients with treatment-resistant depression that has failed to respond to multiple antidepressant medications, ECT has a lower response rate, of 50%–70%. Remission rates after ECT for treatment-resistant depression are typically reported between 50% and 80%. However, because the therapeutic effect is highly dependent on technique, including electrode placement and dosage, remission rates can range from 20% to 80% (Lisanby 2007). Response and remission rates are higher for patients with the psychotic subtype of depression, where ECT is more effective than antidepressants alone (Petrides et al. 2001). Response rates are also higher in elderly individuals (O'Connor et al. 2001). In conditions such as Parkinson's disease and epilepsy, in which comorbid depression is common, ECT can be used to treat the motor and seizure symptoms in addition to depression. The presence of comorbid anxiety reduces the effectiveness of ECT, and ECT has not shown benefit for treatment of primary anxiety or OCD. Remission rates are lower for certain populations, including persons with borderline personality disorder (~20%).

A typical course of ECT involves administration of 2–3 treatments per week. Most patients experience remission after 6–12 ECT treatments, with a mean number of 7 treatments required to achieve remission (Kellner et al. 2006). However, some patients may need as many as 20 treatments to achieve a full response. More frequent administration of ECT is associated with greater cognitive side effects, yet there may be rare conditions such as a malignant catatonia where more frequent and aggressive ECT is needed. If ECT induces cognitive side effects and complicates treatment, reducing the frequency of treatments often decreases this side effect.

Case: Catatonia Treated With Electroconvulsive Therapy

A 30-year-old pregnant female in the third trimester with a history of schizophrenia was admitted to a labor unit after several weeks of declining health with decreased oral intake and concerns for the viability of her fetus. After an extensive medical workup identified no specific medical cause of her symptoms, psychiatrists were asked to see this patient and determined a diagnosis of catatonia based on signs of stupor, catalepsy, and mutism. She did not respond to antipsychotics or to high doses of benzodiazepines, and a court order was obtained to perform emergency ECT. The patient underwent six bilateral treatments and had rapid resolution of her catatonia. After 2 weeks of treatment, she was nearly back to her normal function and soon thereafter had a successful and uncomplicated delivery.

Risks and Adverse Effects

Contrary to popular belief, ECT is a safe and highly effective treatment. ECT is considered one of the safest procedures performed under general anesthesia and has a mortality rate of two to four deaths per 100,000 treatments. *Generalized anesthesia* and *physiological monitoring* are two modifications to ECT that have greatly increased its safety profile. Mortality during ECT is most often related to cardiopulmonary events. Today, patients receiving ECT undergo a modified version of the procedure that includes use of general anesthesia and muscle relaxants. General anesthesia prevents the patient from experiencing the painful electrical stimulation and discomfort during a convulsion. Muscle relaxants limit tonic-clonic motor movements during a seizure and eliminate the risk of physical injury and bone fracture. Use of modified ECT procedures and anesthesia has increased the safety and reduced the risks; the most common adverse effects associated with ECT are aspiration, dental and tongue injuries, headache, nausea, and cognitive impairment.

Fifty percent to 80% of patients report cognitive side effects during and after a course of ECT (Rose et al. 2003). These side effects include acute confusion, anterograde amnesia, and retrograde amnesia. Type and degree of cognitive impairment depend on underlying cognitive status, medications, ECT electrode placement, type of stimulation, frequency of stimulation, anesthesia, and postictal effects from therapeutically induced seizures. Objective neuropsychological testing indicates that cognitive side effects are generally short lived (Semkovska and McLoughlin 2010), with retrograde amnesia being the most persistent. Despite the incidence of cognitive side effects, patients with cognitive impairment due to psychiatric illness may show improved cognition after a successful course of ECT.

Contraindications

There is no absolute contraindication to performing ECT. However, it is recommended that the clinician obtain a medical evaluation with appropriate laboratory workup for the patient prior to performing ECT to identify potential conditions or factors that may complicate treatment, such as ischemic heart disease, cardiac arrhythmias, uncontrolled hypertension, severe respiratory disease, apnea, dental problems, epilepsy, intracranial mass, skull defects, and prior adverse reactions to anesthesia.

Relapse Prevention and Maintenance Treatment

ECT can also be effective when used more sparingly as a continuation and maintenance treatment to prevent relapse of symptoms. *Continuation ECT* is defined as treatments administered with decreased frequency within 6 months after completion of an acute course of treatment. Continuation treatment is administered less frequently than the two or three times per week typical of an acute course of ECT. More than 50% of patients who achieve remission after an acute course of ECT but do not move to continuation treatment will experience a relapse (Prudic et al. 2004), a finding that emphasizes the importance of continuation treatment. If a patient who responds to ECT remains in remission for 6 months, his or her chances of sustained remission and recovery increase, especially in the context of pharmacotherapy with periodic maintenance ECT treatments. *Maintenance ECT* is typically administered every 4–6 weeks but varies depending on the patient's response to previous ECT treatments. Maintenance ECT is often performed in the context of pharmacological treatment, because evidence suggests that the combined use of pharmacotherapy and ECT is more effective than pharmacotherapy alone (Kellner et al. 2016; Navarro et al. 2008).

Mechanisms of Action

The therapeutic mechanism underlying ECT's effects is unknown; however, the effects are thought to be the direct result of the induced seizure. Numerous changes occur during a seizure, including alterations in brain metabolism, changes to sympathetic and parasympathetic nervous system tone, and the release of neurotransmitters including monoamines, glutamate, and γ-aminobutyric acid (GABA). Seizures specifically involve brain excitation followed by inhibition, during which there are alterations in corticothalamic connectivity and function. Several features of the EEG during ECT influence treatment response: 1) seizure quality, 2) seizure duration, and 3) degree of postictal EEG suppression after the seizure. Quantitative EEG studies suggest that ECT results in increased slow (delta) wave activity in the prefrontal cortex, which is associated with clinical response (Sackeim et al. 1996). Neuroimaging studies reveal gray matter volume changes in the hippocampus, amygdala, and temporal lobes after ECT. Other work suggests that ECT may result in an antidepressant effect by reducing functional connectivity in the dorsolateral prefrontal cortex (DLPFC; Perrin et al. 2012) and increasing connectivity with the hippocampus (Abbott et al. 2014) and frontolimbic circuits (Lyden et al. 2014). Positron emission tomography (PET) studies demonstrate decreased metabolic activity in the frontal and cingulate cortex after ECT (Nobler et al. 2001). Finally, the antidepressant effects of ECT might also be the result of hypothalamic and pituitary hormone release or increased production of brain-derived neurotrophic factor. In summary, ECT has numerous effects on brain function that lead to complex therapeutic as well as disruptive effects.

Conclusion and Future Directions

Despite the continued effectiveness and safety of ECT, it remains a vastly underutilized treatment in psychiatry. This underuse is primarily due to stigma, and secondarily due to limited knowledge of the procedure, limited numbers of facilities providing the procedure, regulatory and legal barriers, a lack of trained ECT practitioners, patients' difficulty accessing the treatment, the need for repeated rounds of general anesthesia, and cognitive side effects. Attempts to reduce ECT-related cognitive side effects have led to the development and research of novel convulsive techniques, such as focal electrically administered seizure therapy (FEAST) and magnetic seizure therapy (MST) (see "Investigational Modalities" section later in this chapter), which may further improve the utility and tolerability of convulsive therapies.

Repetitive Transcranial Magnetic Stimulation

rTMS is a noninvasive brain stimulation technique using powerful (1–2 T), focused magnetic field pulses to induce electrical currents in neural tissue. These pulses are generated via an electromagnetic inductor coil placed against the scalp (Figure 30–2). Single pulses can induce action potentials in a target brain region. For example, stimulation of the region of motor cortex controlling the hand can elicit muscle contractions in the digits or wrist. A session of repeated trains of pulses can cause a more durable excitation or inhibition of the stimulated neural circuit via the mechanisms of neuroplasticity. A course of repeated sessions, administered over several days, can exert still more durable effects lasting weeks to months.

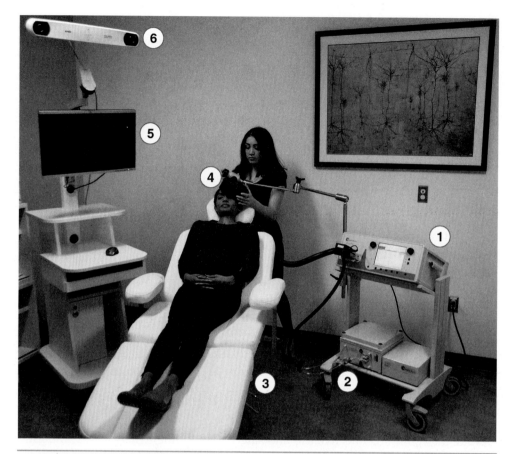

FIGURE 30–2. Components of a therapeutic rTMS treatment suite.

During rTMS sessions, the patient is awake and seated while the treatment technician positions the coil, enters the stimulation parameters, and activates the device to deliver the pulses of stimulation according to the intended protocol. Equipment includes the stimulator device **(1),** which generates the pulse sequence according to the set protocol; the stimulation coil **(2),** an electromagnetic inductor coil connected to the stimulator device and positioned over the target region on the scalp; and the treatment chair **(3),** upon which the patient is seated and stabilized in position during treatment. Some devices also include a cooling device to avoid overheating of the inductor coil during treatment **(4),** Some suites also incorporate a frameless stereotactic neuronavigation system **(5)** to localize the coil over the brain during treatment, using a previously acquired magnetic resonance imaging scan. Such devices employ a high-accuracy stereotactic camera system **(6),** similar to those used in neurosurgery, which can monitor in real time the positions of tracking markers attached to the patient's head and the coil in order to calculate the position of the coil with reference to the head, and thus the brain itself. Note that in this depiction, the patient is undergoing stimulation of the right dorsolateral prefrontal cortex (DLPFC) rather than the left DLPFC (which is more common).

Source. Reprinted with adaptations from Figure 1 (p. 1176) in: Downar J, Blumberger DM, Daskalakis ZJ: "Repetitive Transcranial Magnetic Stimulation: an Emerging Treatment for Medication-Resistant Depression." *Canadian Medical Association Journal* 188(16):1175–1177, 2016. Copyright 2016, Canadian Medical Association. Used with permission.

The rTMS technique was first introduced in 1985 by the engineer Anthony Barker at the University of Sheffield as a means of studying the neurophysiology of the motor cortex. Subsequent research demonstrated that trains of pulses could strengthen or weaken the elicited motor evoked potentials (reviewed in Ziemann et al. 2008). These observations led to proposals that rTMS, targeting the prefrontal regions implicated in depression in the early neuroimaging literature, might be used therapeutically as a less-invasive, more-tolerable alternative to ECT in the treatment of medication-resistant depression.

The first successful randomized controlled studies of rTMS in depression took place in the mid-1990s. Over the following two decades, more than 100 sham-controlled randomized controlled trials enrolling thousands of patients have demonstrated efficacy for rTMS in depression resistant to medications (Berlim et al. 2014; Kedzior et al. 2015). In 2008, following a key multisite study in 2007 (O'Reardon et al. 2007), the first rTMS device (manufactured by Neuronetics) received FDA approval for acute treatment of depression. Subsequently, devices from several other manufacturers (MagVenture, Magstim, Brainsway) have also received FDA clearance for this indication.

rTMS is now available in hundreds of clinics in most major U.S. cities and is covered by public and private insurance plans in most regions. Internationally, rTMS is also available in Europe, Canada, Australia and New Zealand, Israel, China, Japan, and a growing number of other countries. Published clinical guidelines on rTMS treatment are available in the United States (2018) as well as Europe (Lefaucheur et al. 2014) and Canada (Milev et al. 2016).

Indications

The major FDA-approved indication (and by far the most common use) for therapeutic rTMS is in the treatment of major depressive disorder (MDD) that has been resistant to at least one adequate medication trial. As previously mentioned, the initial approval for rTMS was in 2008, and since then, multiple TMS devices have gained approval. However, a wide variety of investigational uses are encountered in the literature. To date, published meta-analyses provide supportive evidence for the efficacy of rTMS in bipolar disorder, posttraumatic stress disorder (PTSD), OCD, alcohol and nicotine dependence, and schizophrenia. In 2018, rTMS received FDA approval for the treatment of OCD. Other uses remain off-label at present. Some neurological applications of rTMS (e.g., certain pain disorders, tinnitus) also have meta-analytic support, and an FDA-approved single-pulse TMS device is available for migraine. TMS is also approved for the presurgical mapping of eloquent cortex (i.e., motor, language cortical areas). Other less-well-studied applications in psychiatry include eating disorders (e.g., bulimia nervosa), dissociative disorders, conversion disorder, and borderline personality disorder.

Treatment Parameters

The effects of rTMS are critically dependent on the precise parameters of treatment, which include the target of stimulation, the pattern (frequency) of stimulation, the intensity of stimulation, the number of sessions, the interval between sessions, and the type of electromagnetic coil being used. Different coil geometries generate different magnetic fields, and conventional handheld coils ("figure 8–shaped" or "butterfly" coils) provide focal stimulation of target regions 1–4 cm deep to the scalp. Helmet-shaped "deep" rTMS coils employ larger windings with more complex geometry to allow stimulation of regions up to 5–8 cm deep to the scalp. However, all coils are subject to a trade-off between depth and focality (the deeper the stimulation, the less the focality). Thus, selective focal stimulation of deep structures such as the amygdala or nucleus accumbens is beyond the capability of any currently approved rTMS device (although indirect stimulation of such structures may be achieved via their connections to more superficial regions of the brain (Wang et al. 2014).

Different patterns of stimulation exert different effects on plasticity (Figure 30–3). Classically, low-frequency stimulation (1–5 Hz) has been considered "inhibitory," whereas high-frequency stimulation (5–30 Hz) is considered "excitatory," although these mechanisms are not well characterized in the prefrontal cortex and are likely oversimplistic. Conventional rTMS protocols deliver high- or low-frequency stimulation in 2- to 10-second trains of pulses at 4- to 60-second intervals over sessions lasting 20–60 minutes. However, newer protocols such as theta-burst stimulation (TBS) also exist and require just 1–3 minutes of stimulation. TBS comes in two forms: intermittent TBS (iTBS), which is considered excitatory, and continuous TBS (cTBS), which is considered inhibitory. TBS protocols mimic the brain's endogenous theta rhythms, which are thought to be more potent for inducing neuroplasticity. In preclinical and clinical studies to date (Di Lazzaro et al. 2011; Li et al. 2014), cTBS and iTBS do appear to match or exceed the potency of conventional protocols despite requiring much less time to administer. Recently, a large randomized trial found that 3 minutes of left DLPFC iTBS achieved outcomes that were noninferior to those of the conventional 10 Hz protocol requiring 37.5 minutes (Blumberger et al. 2018). The 3-minute iTBS treatments subsequently received FDA approval for clinical use.

Variability of effect is a current challenge for all rTMS protocols (see Figure 30–3). It is now recognized that a substantial proportion of people (20%–40%) can show neutral or paradoxical opposite-direction effects on plasticity for a given type of stimulation. This variability applies to both conventional rTMS and newer TBS protocols. To date, there is no known rTMS protocol with a consistent direction of effect across all people, and this variability may account for a substantial proportion of nonresponse to rTMS.

The therapeutic effects of rTMS sessions are cumulative, and the optimal number and frequency of sessions is a topic of active investigation. Clinical trials and naturalistic studies (McClintock et al. 2018) suggest that in depression, 26–28 rTMS sessions are needed for maximal effect, and some individuals may continue to improve with even longer courses (40 sessions or more). Standard treatment protocols deliver rTMS once daily, 5 days per week, on weekdays. Protocols delivering rTMS 3 days per week have been reported to be effective, although a longer period of time is required to complete the full course. Some protocols use an acute course of 20 daily sessions followed by a tapering course of twice-weekly and/or once-weekly sessions to sustain the effect. Among individuals who respond, the trajectory of improvement appears to be similar over time, session by session, regardless of the pattern of stimulation used (e.g., high frequency, low frequency, TBS).

The optimal intensity of stimulation is still under investigation. Stimulation intensity is conventionally determined on the basis of the individual's resting motor threshold (RMT), defined as the minimum intensity required to elicit muscle twitches in relaxed upper or lower extremities, by visual inspection or electromyography. The most commonly used intensity in rTMS studies to date is 110% RMT, and intensities of 110%–120% may achieve outcomes that are superior to those achieved by lower-intensity stimulation (McClintock et al. 2018). TBS is more commonly delivered at lower intensities, although it has also been found to be safe at 120% RMT (McClintock et al. 2018). Stimulation intensities above 120% RMT for any protocol fall outside current treatment guidelines (see "Risks and Adverse Events").

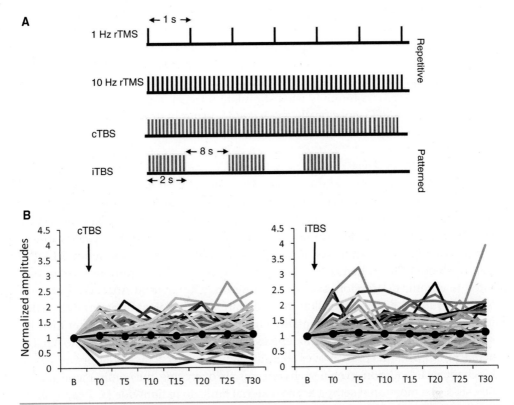

FIGURE 30–3. Stimulation protocols in common use for therapeutic repetitive transcranial magnetic stimulation (rTMS).

(A) Conventional stimulation protocols apply trains of stimulation at specific frequencies. Low frequency, 1-Hz stimulation is widely used in clinical settings as an inhibitory protocol to reduce activity/connectivity in the target brain circuit. High-frequency stimulation, commonly at 10 Hz (but also at 5 Hz or 20 Hz) is widely used as an excitatory protocol to increase activity/connectivity in the target circuit. Stimulation sessions of 10–40 minutes' duration are common for conventional rTMS protocols. More recently, theta-burst stimulation (TBS) protocols have entered clinical use. These protocols use triplet bursts at 30–50 Hz applied five or six times per second to induce plasticity more rapidly and with fewer pulses than conventional protocols. Continuous TBS (cTBS) involves application of a single train of 600 pulses over 40 seconds and is used for inhibitory stimulation. Intermittent TBS (iTBS) involves application of twenty 2-second trains of theta-burst stimulation with an 8-second interval (totaling 600 pulses) over approximately 3 minutes and is used for excitatory stimulation. The potency of TBS protocols matches or exceeds that of conventional protocols.

(B) Variability of effect across individuals is a current problem for all rTMS protocols, conventional or otherwise. Here, the amplitude of motor evoked potentials is plotted separately for many different individuals, measured over a 30-minute period after application of either cTBS *(left)* or iTBS *(right)* to motor cortex. Although cTBS is considered inhibitory, note that many individuals show motor excitation (amplitude >1) rather than inhibition; likewise, although iTBS is usually considered excitatory, many individuals show motor inhibition (<1) rather than facilitation (excitation). The same interindividual variability of effect is also observed with conventional 1-Hz, 10-Hz, and 20-Hz protocols.

Source. **Image A:** Adapted from Figure 2A in Dayan E, Censor N, Buch ER, et al: "Noninvasive Brain Stimulation: From Physiology to Network Dynamics and Back." *Nature Neuroscience* 16(7):838–844, 2013. **Image B:** Reprinted from Figure 4 (A & B) in Hamada M, Murase N, Hasan A, et al.: "The Role of Interneuron Networks in Driving Human Motor Cortical Plasticity." *Cerebral Cortex* 23(7):1593–1605, 2013. Copyright 2013, Oxford University Press. Used with permission.

Finally, the site of stimulation is a critical parameter for rTMS. rTMS may exert effects on diverse brain functions, such as motor function, visual or auditory perception, working memory, impulse control, theory of mind tasks (i.e., mentalizing), or emotion regulation, depending on the site of stimulation. Different rTMS targets have been studied for different indications (e.g., OCD, PTSD, substance dependence). In MDD, by far the most commonly used stimulation target (as per the FDA-approved protocol) is the DLPFC, specifically the left side, using high-frequency stimulation, usually at 10 Hz (Figure 30–4).

Treatment Outcomes

For context in interpreting treatment outcomes for rTMS, it is worth reviewing outcomes for other types of interventions in treatment-resistant depression (usually defined as failure of two or more medication trials of adequate dosage and duration). After two failed trials, remission rates for subsequent medication trials are as low as 10%–15% in published studies of sequential treatment, such as the landmark STAR*D trial (Rush et al. 2006). Remission rates for intensive psychotherapy programs dedicated to chronic depression, such as the Cognitive Behavioral Analysis System of Psychotherapy (CBASP; McCullough 2010), fare little better, at approximately 20%. Response rates for ECT are substantially higher, at 50%–90%; however, fewer than 1% of patients with treatment-resistant depression receive ECT, due to a variety of factors including stigma and concern over cognitive adverse effects (as noted previously in this chapter). In addition, even if such concerns are overcome, the requirements for anesthesia and a monitored setting act as material limits to nationwide ECT capacity, so that the likelihood of being able to offer ECT to a 10- or 20-fold larger number of patients with treatment-resistant depression is low. As a result, there is a need for treatments that surpass the 15%–20% remission rates of medication trials or psychotherapy in treatment-resistant depression while at the same time offering better patient acceptability and access than ECT. This is the treatment niche that rTMS addresses.

Regarding efficacy, early rTMS studies in MDD were directed at demonstrating efficacy of active versus sham stimulation at a time when the optimal number of sessions was unknown; as a result, many studies applied as few as 5–10 sessions compared with the current typical course length of 20–30 sessions. Many meta-analyses incorporating early studies accordingly have a low average course length of as few as 10–15 sessions among studies included—a course length that is sufficient to address the question of efficacy for active versus sham stimulation but that may not provide an accurate estimate of outcomes for full courses of 30 or more sessions. The issue of course length adequacy thus needs to be considered in interpreting the literature to date.

High-frequency (most often, 10 Hz) left DLPFC rTMS is the most widely used and widely studied protocol in depression, with efficacy supported by several meta-analyses and more than 100 studies to date. The most widely cited meta-analysis of rTMS in medication-resistant depression surveyed 29 trials enrolling 1,371 patients and found superiority for active over sham stimulation (Berlim et al. 2014). With an average course length of 12.9 sessions, response and remission rates averaged only 29% and 19%, respectively. Another meta-analysis of individual outcomes from 11 trials enrolling 1,132 patients, typically treating with 4–6 weeks of treatment, achieved substantially better outcomes, at 46% response and 31% remission (Fitzgerald et al. 2016). These outcomes are more in line with those in the most recent trials using optimized

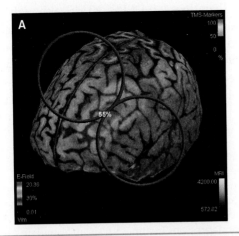
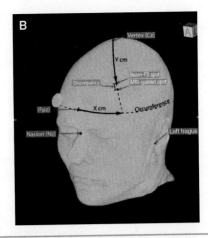

FIGURE 30–4. Techniques for localizing the stimulation site during repetitive transcranial magnetic stimulation (rTMS) treatment.

(A) Magnetic resonance imaging (MRI)–guided neuronavigation employs frameless stereotactic equipment, tracking devices attached to the coil and the patient's head, and an MRI of the patient to localize the focus of stimulation with accuracies of less than 4 mm under ideal conditions. The operator can monitor the position of the rTMS coil in real time in order to position it over the target site. Here, the left dorsolateral prefrontal cortex (DLPFC) is targeted, and the predicted electrical field of the coil during stimulation is superimposed on the patient's MRI.

(B) An alternative to MRI-guided neuronavigation in routine therapeutic rTMS involves the use of scalp landmarks to localize the target of stimulation. One commonly used method, known as BeamF3 (Beam et al. 2009), employs the standard electroencephalography (EEG) sensor site "F3" (in the international 10–20 EEG system) as a proxy for the scalp site corresponding to the left DLPFC. The procedure for locating the F3 site is based on three cardinal scalp measurements: 1) nasion–inion distance from anterior to posterior, 2) tragus–tragus distance from left to right ear, and 3) head circumference.

To view this figure in color, see Plate 10 in Color Gallery in middle of book.

Source. **Image A:** From the lab of Jonathan Downar, M.D., Ph.D. Used with permission.
Image B: Reprinted from Figure 1C (p. 967) in Mir-Moghtadaei A, Caballero R, Fried P, et al.: "Concordance Between BeamF3 and MRI-Neuronavigated Target Sites for Repetitive Transcranial Magnetic Stimulation of the Left Dorsolateral Prefrontal Cortex." *Brain Stimulation* 8(5):965–973, 2015. Copyright 2015, Elsevier.

stimulation parameters and adequate (20–30 sessions) course lengths, which report response in 45%–55% and remission in 30%–40% of medication-resistant depression patients (Blumberger et al. 2018; Levkovitz et al. 2015). Similar outcomes are reported in naturalistic case series in the community (Carpenter et al. 2012).

Right DLPFC rTMS using low-frequency (1 Hz) stimulation also has a large evidence base of meta-analyses and studies and appears to achieve outcomes similar to those of left DLPFC rTMS. The most recent meta-analysis (Berlim et al. 2013) found response and remission rates of 38% and 35%, respectively, for right DLPFC rTMS, despite an average course length of just 12.6 sessions in the analyzed studies. Studies directly comparing outcomes for right versus left DLPFC rTMS have found similar trajectories of outcome for both types of treatment (Cao et al. 2018). Tolerability and safety may be superior for 1 Hz rTMS, because low-frequency stimulation does not appear to carry the same seizure risk, and the lower number and frequency of pulses may result in less scalp discomfort.

Bilateral DLPFC rTMS (high-frequency left and low-frequency right) is also widely used, although evidence of superiority over unilateral left or right DLPFC rTMS is not clear. Community practitioners commonly report that right DLPFC rTMS often achieves better effects on comorbid anxiety than does left DLPFC rTMS, although to date no systematic investigation of left versus right DLPFC rTMS effects on mood versus anxiety has been performed. On a related note, however, a recent study (Weissman et al. 2018) found that bilateral rTMS achieved 40% remission from suicidal ideation, versus 13% for left DLPFC rTMS alone. Specific anxiolytic and antisuicidal effects of right DLPFC rTMS may be an important topic for future study.

Case: Depression Treated With rTMS

A 55-year-old female who had experienced recurrent MDD for more than 10 years had failed to respond to therapeutic dosages of sertraline and duloxetine. Although she had considered ECT, she had concerns about its potential cognitive effects and was worried about undergoing general anesthesia. Her primary psychiatrist referred her to a TMS provider, who thought she was a good candidate for the treatment based on the moderate severity of her depressive episodes, antidepressant treatment resistance, and absence of a history of seizures or implanted metal in her head. She underwent 6 weeks of daily high-frequency (10 Hz) left-sided rTMS over the DLPFC and achieved remission of her depression symptoms. She experienced few side effects other than mild scalp discomfort, and she remained well after tapering off rTMS.

Risks and Adverse Effects

Safety and tolerability are relative advantages of rTMS over pharmacotherapy. Reviews and large trials (Berlim et al. 2014; Blumberger et al. 2018) have reported an all-cause discontinuation rate of 5%–10% for rTMS, which compares favorably to the antidepressant discontinuation rate of approximately 25%. The most common adverse effect of rTMS treatment is a static electricity–like *painful sensation* at the site of stimulation as a result of contraction of scalp muscles during TMS. Pain may also be reported in other areas of the face, such as the eye, nose, sinuses, or teeth. The majority of patients report painful yet tolerable sensations of this type during treatment. Habituation does occur over time, with one study (Borckart et al. 2013) reporting that average pain ratings improved on a visual analogue scale (from 6/10 to 3/10) over the course of treatment. Transient *headache* or *fatigue* may occur after stimulation sessions (25%–30%); these symptoms also diminish over time and typically respond well to over-the-counter analgesia. Some patients receiving deep TMS will experience uncomfortable involuntary movements as a result of stimulation over wider areas of the brain extending to motor regions. About 2%–4% of patients discontinue treatment due to pain.

The most serious adverse event with rTMS is induction of a *generalized tonic-clonic seizure* during stimulation. The overall seizure risk is estimated at approximately 1 per 30,000 treatment sessions or 1 per 1,000 patients treated (0.1%; Rossi et al. 2009). For comparison, the seizure incidence associated with use of antidepressant medications is estimated at 0.1%–0.6%. All reported rTMS-associated seizures to date have been self-limited, have occurred during rather than after the treatment session, and have not progressed to epilepsy in any patient. Patients suffering a seizure during rTMS normally should not undergo further rTMS treatment.

Other adverse events that occur include *mania or hypomania, vasovagal syncope,* and short-term *hearing loss.* rTMS-induced mania or hypomania is a rare adverse event, with an estimated incidence of less than 1% in patients receiving rTMS for treatment-resistant depression, compared with an incidence of 3.4% per year for emergent mania or hypomania in patients diagnosed with MDD and treated with antidepressant medication (Rossi et al. 2009). A more common adverse event during treatment (reported by ~1% of patients) is vasovagal syncope, particularly during the initial sessions of treatment (Rossi et al. 2009). Patients experiencing syncopal episodes may proceed with treatment after recovery and reassurance. Video recordings of treatment sessions may aid in distinguishing syncope from seizure. Tinnitus or short-term hearing loss is a rare adverse event caused by the TMS click during discharge of each magnetic pulse. To avoid this adverse effect, patients and technicians should wear hearing protection (e.g., earplugs) during treatment sessions; such measures have been shown to be effective in preventing hearing problems associated with rTMS (Rossi et al. 2009). Whereas cognitive adverse effects are a common concern for ECT, rTMS's effects on cognition appear benign. Meta-analyses and reviews have found no evidence of significant cognitive adverse effects for rTMS across a wide variety of domains, including episodic memory, working memory, or executive function.

Contraindications

There are relatively few absolute contraindications to rTMS. High-frequency (>5 Hz) rTMS is generally contraindicated in patients with a history of previous seizures. Low-frequency (~1 Hz) rTMS has been performed safely in patients with epilepsy as an investigational treatment for seizures and does not appear to cause seizures in this setting; for this reason, some practitioners will consider use of low-frequency rTMS, after a discussion of risks and benefits, in MDD patients who have a possible seizure history. Patients who have a history of febrile seizures, medication- or electrolyte-induced seizures, substance use, or substance withdrawal may be considered for rTMS by some practitioners.

rTMS is also contraindicated in patients with intracranial ferromagnetic material, foreign metal bodies, or implanted devices such as DBS electrodes. For patients with implanted medication pumps, cardiac defibrillators or pacemakers, vagal nerve stimulators, or cochlear implants, TMS is generally considered safe.

Relapse Prevention and Maintenance Treatment

As in ECT, relapse is common after a successful course of rTMS that is not followed by maintenance treatment. There is substantial variability in time to symptom recurrence, which can range from as little as 2–3 months in some patients to more than 1 year in particularly strong responders.

Repeated rTMS treatments do appear to be successful in most patients who have previously responded to rTMS. For full relapse, a repeated full course of stimulation may be administered. Alternatively, a maintenance course of treatment consisting of fewer than the usual five sessions per week may be offered. There is currently no single standard protocol for maintenance treatment, perhaps because of the variability among patients in time to relapse and propensity to relapse. Commonly encountered maintenance schedules in clinical practice vary from once-weekly or biweekly sessions to once-monthly sessions; other approaches use "clustered" maintenance sessions, such as five sessions administered over 3 days once a month. Such maintenance protocols do appear to extend the time to relapse, in comparison with no maintenance (Milev et al. 2016).

So far there is insufficient evidence to recommend any particular rTMS maintenance schedule over another. In clinical practice, maintenance sessions are often scheduled as a compromise between the burden of disability associated with relapse and the logistical burdens of commuting to the clinic and arranging for time away from work or other responsibilities. In addition, U.S. insurance companies currently do not routinely pay for maintenance treatments. The optimal maintenance schedule may therefore reflect clinical, financial, and lifestyle factors for a given patient.

Mechanisms of Action

The therapeutic mechanisms of action for rTMS are still incompletely understood. At the synaptic level, rTMS is thought to act via the mechanisms of neuroplasticity, including long-term potentiation (LTP) and long-term depression (LTD). The mechanisms of LTP allow pre- and postsynaptic neurons that are simultaneously activated ("fire together") to increase the efficiency of their synaptic connection ("wire together"), either by adding more receptors or by growing new connections such as dendritic spines. As an analogous inhibitory process, LTD allows synaptic connections that are activated asynchronously to weaken in strength.

LTP and LTD are thought to rely upon a complex cascade of cellular mechanisms, including glutamatergic signaling via the N-methyl-D-aspartate (NMDA) receptor, dopaminergic signaling via the D_1 and D_2 receptors, intracellular calcium signaling, gene expression, and protein synthesis, all of which are subject to pharmacological manipulation. For example, NMDA antagonists such as memantine can block the neuroplastic effects of rTMS. Conversely, the dopamine agonist L-dopa (which activates D_1–D_5 receptors) can enhance the neuroplastic potency of both low- and high-frequency rTMS. However, pramipexole (an agonist at D_2, D_3, and D_4 receptors) does *not* appear to enhance rTMS-induced plasticity, suggesting that D_1 receptor mechanisms may be particularly important for both low- and high-frequency rTMS. The D_2 antagonist amisulpride blocked rTMS-induced plasticity in a preclinical study (Monte-Silva et al. 2011), raising the question of whether patients taking antipsychotics might have poorer rTMS outcomes. However, a subsequent study (Schulze et al. 2017) found that patients taking antipsychotics did not have poorer rTMS outcomes but instead trended nonsignificantly toward better outcomes.

At the circuit level, the mechanisms of rTMS may involve changes in both cortico-cortical and corticostriatal connections to the site of stimulation. For example, studies using resting-state functional magnetic resonance imaging (fMRI) have demonstrated that a single session of rTMS delivered to one node of a resting-state network such as the "default mode network" (DMN) can cause changes in resting-state functional connectivity (i.e., correlation of ongoing activity) to the other nodes of that network (Eldaief et al. 2011). The direction of effect may depend on the pattern of stimulation, with different effects ensuing from high- versus low-frequency stimulation (Eldaief et al. 2011).

Ligand studies using PET (Strafella et al. 2003) have found that a single rTMS session targeting a given region of the frontal lobe (e.g., motor cortex or DLPFC) causes a tightly localized increase in D_2 receptor occupancy in the associated region of the striatum. These observations suggest that rTMS may induce dopamine release (with associated effects on plasticity) in whichever corticostriatal loop circuit is targeted by the stimulation. These corticostriatal effects may be critical to the therapeutic effects of rTMS; several studies using resting-state fMRI have found that cortico-striatal-thalamo-cortical (CSTC) connectivity through the stimulation target is both a predictor and a correlate of response to rTMS (reviewed in Peters et al. 2016).

If rTMS selectively affects the specific corticocortical and cortico-striatal-thalamic networks connected to whichever brain region is being stimulated, then the therapeutic mechanisms of rTMS for psychiatric illnesses may also depend critically on which network is chosen for targeting. For this reason, there is currently much active research focused on identifying the optimal target networks for stimulation and localizing their nodes in individual patients, often using resting-state fMRI. As an example, one influential study found that across 14 neurological and psychiatric disorders, effective targets for DBS (discussed later) belonged to the same resting-state fMRI network as effective targets for rTMS (Fox et al. 2014). A related study found that for DLPFC rTMS, the optimal target site could be localized by finding the point that on resting-state fMRI was most negatively correlated with the subcallosal cingulate cortex—a target for DBS in MDD (Fox et al. 2012).

A related framework suggests that rTMS acts by targeting specific resting-state brain networks that are abnormally active across multiple types of psychiatric illness. One such network, the *salience network,* includes the DLPFC as well as the anterior cingulate and anterior insular regions and maps fairly well onto the effective target sites of rTMS. The salience network shows both volumetric and functional abnormalities across many psychiatric disorders (Goodkind et al. 2015). In healthy individuals, the salience network is critical for cognitive control (i.e., self-regulation of thoughts, behaviors, and emotions). By targeting this network, DLPFC rTMS may act, not specifically as an antidepressant per se, but rather more fundamentally as an enhancer of cognitive control. Because cognitive control deficits are a transdiagnostic feature of many psychiatric and personality disorders, this framework would predict the success of rTMS across populations with multiple types of illness as well as its failure among individuals with relatively preserved cognitive control.

The DMN may also play an important role in depression and the ability of rTMS to elicit clinical improvement. The DMN, which comprises multiple brain networks that are active in the absence of external stimuli, is involved in self-reflective thought, episodic memory, and theory of mind tasks (i.e., mentalizing). In a study using resting-state fMRI, the DMN was hyperconnected in patients with MDD prior to rTMS treatment and to become normalized following rTMS (Liston et al. 2014), suggesting that normalization of DMN connectivity may be an important part of the therapeutic action of rTMS.

In summary, an emerging if incomplete picture suggests that the mechanism of action of rTMS has multiple layers. The neurochemical mechanisms of synaptic plasticity may provide a generic mechanism for rewiring connections to the stimulation target. The choice of target may determine which corticocortical and corticostriatal networks are rewired. A few specific networks may play transdiagnostic roles in psychiatric pathology, and strengthening or inhibiting those networks may allow rTMS to address the specific deficits driving pathology in individual patients.

Future Directions

Brief protocols.   Conventional stimulation sessions are lengthy: 20–40 minutes for FDA-approved left DLPFC rTMS and as long as 60 minutes for bilateral stimulation.

Long protocols limit the number of patients who can be treated per device per day, thereby reducing clinic capacity and accessibility and increasing per-session costs. In preclinical studies, newer protocols such as theta-burst stimulation (TBS) require only 1–3 minutes to achieve the same or stronger effects on plasticity produced by conventional-length protocols. Recent randomized controlled studies (Li et al. 2014) suggest that TBS protocols show superiority over sham stimulation, with outcomes comparable to those of conventional rTMS stimulation. A recently published large trial that directly compared 3-minute iTBS against conventional 37.5-minute 10-Hz rTMS found equivalent, noninferior outcomes and trajectories of improvement (Blumberger et al. 2018). Another large trial (Brunelin et al. 2014) found that an 8-minute 1-Hz rTMS protocol targeting the right DLPFC was also effective, suggesting that brief protocols may be viable even without TBS. Brief protocols have the potential to improve the cost and clinic capacity for rTMS severalfold, which could allow rTMS to make meaningful reductions in the current 2% population prevalence of treatment-resistant depression.

Accelerated courses.   Conventional rTMS is delivered in once-daily sessions. Because 20, 30, or even 40 sessions of rTMS may be required for full effect, this limitation on sessions imposes a high logistical burden on patients commuting to the clinic over 4–8 weeks; such regimens are also too lengthy to be practical for most inpatient stays. Recent studies have begun to investigate "accelerated" rTMS courses that deliver multiple sessions per day to achieve full effects more rapidly. Studies delivering up to 10 sessions per day suggest that at least some patients may be able to achieve full remission in 2–10 days via such regimens. A recent study (Modirrousta et al. 2018) directly compared a course of conventional once-daily rTMS treatment for 20 days against a course of three-times-daily treatment over 6 half-days. Outcomes were the same in both groups, and patients greatly preferred the accelerated regimens. Some studies have also used TBS in accelerated regimens, thereby combining gains in clinic capacity with gains in course length (Duprat et al. 2016). Although accelerated rTMS regimens appear promising, the optimal number of sessions per day and the minimum necessary interval between sessions are still unknown.

New stimulation targets.   Conventional rTMS for depression targets the left and/or right DLPFC. However, not all patients respond to this target. Converging evidence from lesion, stimulation, neuroimaging, and connectivity studies suggests that several other rTMS-accessible regions may also be important in MDD, including the dorsomedial prefrontal cortex, the orbitofrontal cortex, and the frontopolar cortex (Downar and Daskalakis 2013). These alternative targets are now being studied in MDD. The dorsomedial prefrontal cortex appears promising in some studies (Bakker et al. 2015), and the orbitofrontal cortex likewise shows early indications of effectiveness in MDD (Feffer et al. 2018). Notably, patients not responding to stimulation at one target have been found to achieve remission with stimulation at another target. The potential may therefore exist to achieve cumulative remission rates of greater than 50% by pursuing treatment of alternative targets in nonresponders to standard DLPFC rTMS. However, given the fairly embryonic evidence base to date, these new targets will require further study under randomized conditions.

Invasive Modalities

Vagus Nerve Stimulation

VNS involves neurosurgical implantation of a device outside the brain to chronically stimulate the left vagus nerve, which contains predominantly afferent nerve fibers. VNS has significant effects on brain function and is an FDA-approved treatment for epilepsy and treatment-resistant unipolar and bipolar depression. VNS was first used as an anticonvulsant treatment; the observation that depressed patients with epilepsy who received VNS often had improved mood led to investigation of VNS for the treatment of depression. In VNS, an electrode—attached to the left vagus nerve extending through the neck and connected to a pulse generator implanted in the chest—delivers preset trains of chronic electrical stimulation at varying pulse widths, frequencies, currents, voltages, and cycles (Figure 30–5). Side effects of VNS are most often the result of direct stimulation of the vagus nerve and include hoarseness, throat pain, coughing, shortness of breath, tingling, and muscle pain. Although VNS can potentially alter cardiac function, studies have found no clinically relevant effects of VNS on cardiac function (Frei and Osorio 2001). Most side effects observed with VNS resolve with adjustment of stimulation parameters.

A 10-week sham-controlled VNS study in patients with treatment-resistant unipolar and bipolar depression failed to show an antidepressant effect after several weeks (Rush et al. 2005), but long-term, open-label trials have demonstrated long-term antidepressant effects (Nahas et al. 2005). These findings led to FDA approval of VNS in 2005 for use in treatment-resistant depression. However, despite having received approval for this indication, VNS is not generally available to patients in the United States because insurers have determined that it is not a cost-effective intervention for treatment-resistant depression.

Although its mechanism of action is unknown, VNS is theorized to act by indirectly modulating brain activity via bottom-up stimulation of monoaminergic cell bodies and brain regions involved in seizures and mood. VNS can be safely used with ECT to provide a combined anticonvulsive and convulsive treatment. VNS can also be safely used with TMS to provide a bottom-up and top-down approach to modulating brain networks involved in the pathophysiology of depression. Newer VNS devices attempt to noninvasively stimulate the vagus nerve through use of an external transcutaneous device that targets the auricular branch of the vagus nerve (Stefan et al. 2012). VNS will continue to evolve and may eventually become a more widely used antidepressant treatment in psychiatry.

Deep Brain Stimulation

Attempts to treat severe psychiatric disorders through invasive neurosurgery began well before the widespread use of pharmacotherapy and noninvasive brain stimulation techniques. Early neurosurgical interventions were often crude and were usually lesion based, and thus irreversible. However, the advent of modern stereotactic neuro-

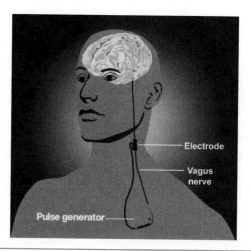

FIGURE 30–5. Vagus nerve stimulation (VNS) with electrode connecting left vagus nerve with an implanted pulse generator.

Source. Reprinted from National Institute of Mental Health: Brain Stimulation Therapies (web page), revised June 2016. Available at: https://www.nimh.nih.gov/health/topics/brain-stimulation-therapies/brain-stimulation-therapies.shtml#part_152878. Accessed August 20, 2018.

surgery and technological advances in brain stimulation brought the more recent technique of DBS. DBS is an invasive but reversible form of brain stimulation in which neurosurgically implanted deep brain electrodes connected to pulse generators implanted in the chest target and electrically stimulate white and gray matter areas deep inside the brain in a focal manner (Figure 30–6). Stimulator electrodes contain multiple contacts along their length and can stimulate brain circuits in a variety of ways, using stimulation patterns that differ in polarity, duration/times of stimulation, pulse width, frequency, and current. DBS is typically delivered in an open-loop fashion because it is preset and administered in a constant and chronic manner. However, new technologies are combining electrophysiological recording with stimulation to provide responsive closed-loop stimulation (see "Investigational Modalities" section later in chapter).

DBS was first developed to modulate basal ganglia circuitry in movement disorders and has been demonstrated to alleviate the motor symptoms of Parkinson's disease and tremor (DeLong and Benabid 2014). It revolutionized the treatment of movement disorders and has gained significant interest in psychiatry. The FDA approved DBS for humanitarian use in treatment-resistant OCD in 2008, and despite its invasive nature, DBS is relatively safe, adjustable, and reversible in comparison with other ablative neurosurgical methods used in OCD, such as capsulotomy. DBS carries a small risk of hardware infection as well as the potential for intracranial hemorrhage, seizure, stroke, confusion, and headache. DBS can cause hypomania in patients with or without a history of bipolar disorder. Successful use of DBS requires long-term maintenance of battery-powered devices, which can lead to significant burden for patients and providers. Multiple targets for DBS have been explored for treatment of a range of psychiatric disorders. The FDA-approved target for use in OCD is the ventral capsule/ventral striatum. Ventral capsule/ventral striatum DBS is thought to target dysfunctional CSTC circuits specific to OCD that connect the orbitofrontal cortex, medial

Brain Stimulation Therapies 883

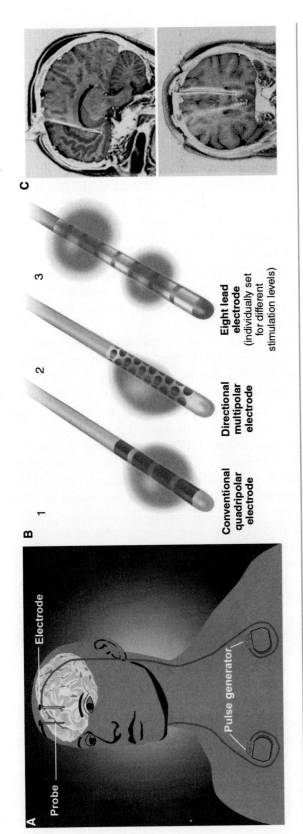

FIGURE 30–6. Deep brain stimulation (DBS).

(A) DBS with bilateral electrodes connected to bilateral implanted pulse generators. (B) Various types of DBS electrodes. (C) Magnetic resonance imaging scans showing sagittal and coronal views of DBS electrodes implanted in the subcallosal cingulate region in a patient with major depressive disorder.

Source. **Image A:** Reprinted from National Institute of Mental Health: Brain Stimulation Therapies (web page), Last Revised: June 2016. Available at: https://www.nimh.nih.gov/health/topics/brain-stimulation-therapies/brain-stimulation-therapies.shtml#part_152878. Accessed August 20, 2018.
Image B: Reprinted from Figure 3 in: Hickey P, Stacy M: "Deep Brain Stimulation: A Paradigm Shifting Approach to Treat Parkinson's Disease." *Frontiers in Neuroscience* 10:173, 2016. Copyright 2016, Frontiers Media SA.
Image C: From the lab of Jonathan Downar, M.D., Ph.D. Used with permission.

prefrontal cortex, basal ganglia, and thalamus (Greenberg et al. 2010b). The mechanism underlying the therapeutic effects of DBS is unknown. However, it is posited that continuous application of high-frequency (>100 Hz) stimulation inhibits local neuronal activity and disrupts abnormal downstream activity in the CSTC regions connected to the stimulation site. DBS is thought to disrupt this CSTC circuit, thus leading to its therapeutic effect.

Multiple randomized trials and meta-analyses suggest therapeutic benefits from DBS for OCD. Two randomized trials (Denys et al. 2010; Mallet et al. 2008) demonstrated significant reductions in OCD symptoms (as assessed with the Yale-Brown Obsessive-Compulsive Scale [Y-BOCS]) from DBS compared with sham DBS. In addition, there was significant improvement on DSM-IV Global Assessment of Functioning (GAF) scale scores (Mallet et al. 2008). After years of experience with DBS, it has become apparent that many patients benefit from this intervention. Studies suggest that patients show symptom reductions averaging about 45% on the Y-BOCS (Alonso et al. 2015). Patients who undergo DBS often show changes in mood, and the most common side effect seen from DBS in OCD is transient hypomania (Greenberg et al. 2010a). These observations have partly led to an interest in using DBS for treatment of mood disorders, specifically depression.

Therapeutic use of DBS for depression has been widely explored and informed by neuroimaging studies as well as by neurosurgical interventions such as cingulotomy. Multiple DBS targets have been investigated for depression, including the subcallosal cingulate, the nucleus accumbens, the ventral capsule/ventral striatum, the thalamus, the globus pallidus, the anterior limb of the internal capsule, the habenula, and the medial forebrain bundle. Neuroimaging findings in depression implicate overactivation of the subcallosal cingulate (Mayberg et al. 1999), and this region typically normalizes following antidepressant therapy, regardless of treatment modality (Goldapple et al. 2004; Mayberg et al. 2000). Initial open-label studies targeting DBS to the subcallosal cingulate white matter for treatment-resistant depression showed promise, with reported response and remission rates of approximately 50% or greater (Holtzheimer et al. 2012; Lozano et al. 2012). However, a randomized double-blind, sham-controlled study failed to achieve separation from placebo after 6 months (Holtzheimer et al. 2017). In an effort to replicate the antidepressant effects observed in OCD, the ventral capsule/ventral striatum was targeted for depression in a sham-controlled trial. Antidepressant effects of DBS at the ventral capsule/ventral striatum failed to separate from those of sham stimulation after 16 weeks (Dougherty et al. 2015). Multiple reasons have been proposed for these failures, including 1) biased patient selection and lack of physiological phenotyping, 2) suboptimal anatomic targeting, and 3) the short duration of these studies. Interestingly, many of these patients continued to improve months after randomization during open-label long-term DBS. Although DBS remains a promising tool for deep, targeted brain stimulation, it does not show a clear and consistent benefit in depression. Future research in DBS should include studies focused on optimizing treatment sites and targeting and refining treatment parameters to potentially enhance response. Ongoing studies are investigating the use of DBS in substance use disorders, PTSD, eating disorders, Alzheimer's disease, and other conditions.

Investigational Modalities

Cranial Electrical Stimulation

Cranial electrical stimulation (CES) involves transdermal application of low-energy alternating current to the scalp. The mechanism of effect of CES is unknown. Given the safety, availability, and low cost of these low-power devices, consumers are allowed to purchase and use such brain stimulation devices under existing FDA approvals extending back to the early 1990s. Despite the number and availability of these CES devices, there is limited evidence of clear benefit from CES when used to treat a number of psychiatric conditions, including depression (Kavirajan et al. 2014), anxiety, insomnia, pain, and drug withdrawal.

Transcranial Direct Current Stimulation

tDCS is a newer form of neurostimulation involving application of low-intensity direct current (in contrast to ECT, which uses high-intensity alternating current) to modulate neuronal activity. In contrast to TMS, ECT, or DBS, which alter neural activity enough to elicit action potentials, tDCS is thought to change the resting membrane potential of neurons in a subthreshold manner strong enough to alter excitability but not strong enough to elicit action potentials. tDCS is not FDA approved for depression but is readily available for purchase and administration. tDCS has minimal side effects, which include headache and pruritus at the site of stimulation. Due to the low cost and mobility of the device, tDCS has gained much interest as a potential treatment for depression and other psychiatric disorders. Use of tDCS has been shown to potentially improve cognition (Dedoncker et al. 2016). However, a double-blind noninferiority antidepressant trial demonstrated that whereas tDCS and escitalopram were each superior to placebo, tDCS did not show noninferiority to escitalopram and was associated with more adverse events (Brunoni et al. 2017). Although more studies are needed, to date tDCS has shown minimal clinical utility in depression and other psychiatric disorders, and therefore it is still investigational at this time.

Focal Electrically Administered Seizure Therapy

FEAST is a modified approach to ECT that employs monophasic rather than biphasic stimulation pulses and uses a nonstandard montage (i.e., specific electrode placement) consisting of a small electrode over the frontal pole and a larger electrode over the right parietal region. These modifications are intended to maximize effective stimulation of regions implicated in depression (e.g., subcallosal cingulate) while minimizing stimulation of nontarget areas associated with cognitive side effects (e.g., the anterior hippocampus). However, there is currently insufficient information on how FEAST compares with conventional ECT in regard to either efficacy or cognitive tolerability, and at present, FEAST remains an investigational technique.

Magnetic Seizure Therapy

MST is an experimental convulsive therapy using a higher-powered rTMS device to deliberately induce therapeutic seizures. In comparison with ECT, the electromagnetic fields of MST are thought to be more focal, avoiding stimulation of nontarget regions associated with cognitive side effects. Early clinical studies suggested that MST has relatively few cognitive adverse effects. However, large studies comparing MST and ECT for efficacy and tolerability are currently lacking, and MST remains an investigational technique.

Synchronized Transcranial Magnetic Stimulation

Synchronized TMS involves application of rTMS at a personalized frequency based on an individual's EEG alpha (8–12 Hz) peak frequency. Preliminary studies showed that a low-field form of this stimulation was safe, associated with few to no side effects, and potentially easier to provide to patients for treatment of symptoms of schizophrenia and depression (Leuchter et al. 2015). However, more studies are needed before synchronized TMS can be offered as a clinical treatment.

Epidural Cortical Stimulation

Epidural cortical stimulation (ECS) involves neurosurgical implantation of epidural electrodes. Unlike DBS, ECS electrodes do not penetrate the dura, and are thus somewhat less invasive than DBS electrodes. Although restricted to superficial brain regions, ECS electrodes offer the theoretical advantage of being suitable for implantation by a much wider range of neurosurgical centers, because the specialized expertise and equipment needed for stereotactic implantation of DBS electrodes are not required and the electrodes are simply positioned by the surgeon on the dura overlying the target region. ECS was initially investigated as a potential treatment for stroke patients but failed to show benefit. Early case series studying the effect of dorsolateral prefrontal ECS in depressed patients suggested an antidepressant effect (Williams et al. 2016). The technique remains investigational at present.

Focused Ultrasound

Focused ultrasound (FUS) is a noninvasive, nonionizing technology that delivers acoustic rather than electromagnetic pulses to target brain regions. When applied focally at high intensities and frequencies, FUS can create discrete thermal lesions capable of ablating brain tissue without a craniotomy and without damaging overlying tissues. Thus, this technique may be used in situations where radiofrequency ablation of brain tissue has previously been successful; the advantage is that the procedure is "closed-head," with no craniotomy required.

FUS can be applied in a variety of ways to target cortical circuits and potentially treat neuropsychiatric disorders. High-frequency magnetic resonance–guided FUS (MRgFUS) targeting the thalamus is an FDA-approved treatment for essential tremor in Parkinson's disease (Magara et al. 2014; Figure 30–7). An open-label case study of MRgFUS capsulotomies in four patients with OCD suggested beneficial effects from the treatment (Jung et al. 2015).

Aside from its use as a noninvasive lesion technique, FUS is being combined with ultrasound-sensitive, drug-filled nanoparticles to investigate the effects of focal deliv-

A

B 2 days post-FUS

3 months post-FUS

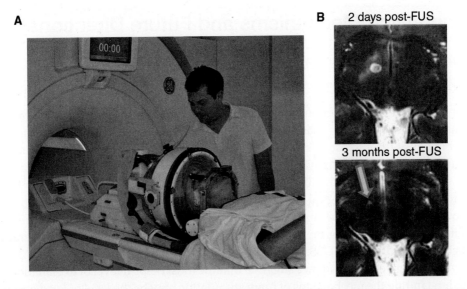

FIGURE 30–7. Magnetic resonance imaging (MRI)–guided focused ultrasound (FUS).

(A) An MRI-guided focused ultrasound device consists of a hemispheric array of ultrasonic transducers positioned very precisely using a stereotactic frame mounted on the patient's head, with the procedure taking place within the bore of an MRI scanner.

(B) MRI images 2 days after *(top)* and 3 months after *(bottom)* delivery of an ultrasonic ablation. Note the extremely focal nature of the lesions created by the ultrasonic intervention.

Source. Reprinted (with adaptations) from Figures 1 and 5 in: Magara A, Bühler R, Moser D, et al: "First Experience With MR-Guided Focused Ultrasound in the Treatment of Parkinson's Disease." *Journal of Therapeutic Ultrasound* 2:11, 2014. Copyright 2014, BMC Springer.

ery of pharmacological agents to specific areas of the body and brain, potentially reducing side effects from the relatively nonspecific nature of standard medication treatments. Finally, FUS at lower intensities can elicit action potentials without damage to neurons and may represent a potential method to specifically, reversibly, and focally modulate deep-brain activity.

Responsive Neurostimulation

Neurosurgically implanted RNS was the first closed-loop treatment FDA approved for use in epilepsy. It provides a personalized platform for detecting seizures and stimulating specific areas involved in seizures. It involves the use of implanted cortical or depth recording and stimulating electrodes connected to a device implanted in the skull to record, monitor, detect, and responsively stimulate the brain to prevent seizures. Unlike DBS, RNS does not deliver chronic and continuous stimulation in a preset manner. Rather, it delivers periodic bursts of individualized stimulation in response to a predefined electrophysiological signal. Given the episodic nature of pathological mental states in many psychiatric disorders, a closed-loop RNS system may provide a novel brain stimulation technology to individualize and enhance psychiatric treatments.

Underlying Mechanisms and Future Directions

What Is the Optimal Explanatory Level for Brain Stimulation Treatments?

For any given intervention in psychiatry, the underlying mechanism often has an optimal "explanatory level" that lies somewhere on a spectrum extending from molecular biology at the microscopic end to broad societal factors at the macroscopic end. For example, antipsychotics may be best understood in terms of their effects on D_2 receptor signaling, whereas cognitive-behavioral therapy may be best understood in terms of its effects on psychological mechanisms such as cognitive distortions and automatic thoughts. If we extend this approach, it is worth asking which explanatory level is best suited for understanding the therapeutic mechanisms of brain stimulation therapies such as ECT, rTMS, and DBS.

A growing body of evidence suggests that the most helpful level of explanation for understanding the mechanisms of brain stimulation may be the level of *functional networks* of brain regions. A key discovery emerging from neuroimaging studies since the 1990s is that brain regions are organized into functional networks whose activity is correlated over time, whether during task performance or at rest. These networks have a consistent anatomy across individuals, such that surveys of large samples of healthy individuals ($N=1,000$) can reliably identify at least seven discrete functional networks (Figure 30–8).

Some of these functional networks—for example, visual networks in the occipital cortex or primary somatosensory and motor networks bordering the central sulcus—perform low-level sensory or motor functions. Other networks perform higher-level integrative functions. The best-known of these higher-level networks is the DMN, which is active during resting, introspective activities such as self-reflection, recollection of past events, and imagining future scenarios. Other examples of higher-level networks are the dorsal and ventral frontoparietal networks associated with attention or working memory. Importantly, each network of correlated regions also has a corresponding "antinetwork" of regions whose activity shows an opposed negative or *anticorrelation* in activity. Thus, every brain region, whether at rest or during task performance, is associated with both a functional network and a functional *antinetwork.*

Association of Functional Networks With Transdiagnostic Dimensions of Pathology in Psychiatric Illness

Converging evidence from neuroimaging, stimulation, and lesion studies has identified three functional networks as playing particularly important, transdiagnostic roles across a variety of psychiatric illnesses (Figure 30–9). One of these is the *salience network*, whose core nodes include the dorsal anterior cingulate cortex (dACC) and the anterior insula, along with regions in the DLPFC and the inferior parietal lobule. The salience network is active during a variety of tasks requiring cognitive control or response inhibition/selection: the Stroop task, Flanker task, and go/no-go task are examples. Notably, a meta-analysis of 193 structural neuroimaging studies in more than 7,000 patients across a variety of psychiatric disorders (MDD, bipolar disorder, schizo-

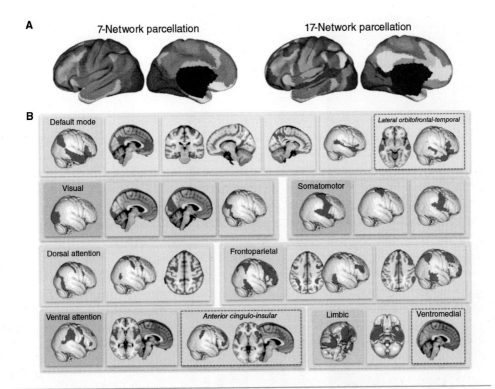

FIGURE 30–8. Networks of coherent functional activity in the resting human brain.

(A) The intrinsic, ongoing activity of the brain at rest or during tasks can be separated into at least seven distinct functional networks, appearing consistently across large datasets of up to 1,000 individuals. These networks can also be further subdivided into subnetworks. A 17-network parcellation has been identified as being stable across individuals (Yeo et al. 2011).

(B) The 17 resting-state networks identified by Yeo et al. (2011) included low-level visual and somatosensory cortical areas, higher-level networks involving premotor and sensory association areas, and larger fronto-parietal networks involved in attention, cognition, and executive control. However, three networks (highlighted in *dashed red lines*) are of particular interest as neural substrates for psychiatric endophenotypes: a ventromedial prefrontal "incentive" network corresponding to the classical reward circuit, a "nonreward" lateral orbitofrontal-temporal network (LOFTN) involved in emotional reappraisal and hypothetical reward valuation, and an anterior cinguloinsular "salience" network (aCIN) involved in cognitive control and response inhibition.

To view this figure in color, see Plate 11 in Color Gallery in middle of book.

Source. Reprinted from Figure 1 (A & B) in: Dunlop K, Hanlon CA, Downar J: "Noninvasive Brain Stimulation Treatments for Addiction and Major Depression." *Annals of the New York Academy of Sciences* 1394(1):31–54, 2017. Copyright 2017, John Wiley & Sons Inc.

phrenia, OCD, anxiety disorders, and substance use disorders) found that the most consistent sites of gray matter loss were in core salience network nodes in the dACC and anterior insula (Goodkind et al. 2015). Deficits in cognitive control, reflected in hypofunctioning of the salience network, have thus been proposed as a central and transdiagnostic dimension of pathology across a variety of psychiatric disorders.

Another key network is the limbic or *incentive network* associated with reward, motivation, and incentive salience. This network centers on the ventral striatum and includes its projection sites in the ventromedial prefrontal cortex as well as its inputs in the temporopolar cortex. Again, this network shows patterns of abnormal activation in a variety of psychiatric disorders, indicating pathological incentives/motivations.

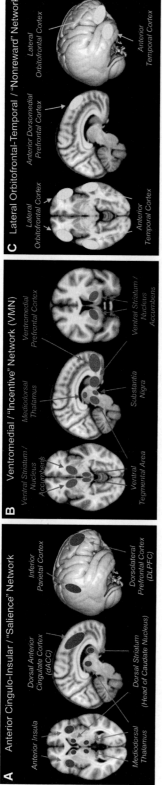

FIGURE 30–9.   Functional networks associated with transdiagnostic dimensions of pathology in psychiatric illness.

(A) The *salience network* has core nodes in the dorsal anterior cingulate and anterior insular cortex, with additional nodes in the dorsolateral prefrontal cortex and lateral parietal cortex, along with their striatal and thalamic counterparts. Closely linked to the Research Domain Criteria (RDoC) domain of *cognitive control*, the salience network is hypoactive transdiagnostically across multiple psychiatric disorders.

(B) The ventromedial *incentive network* corresponds closely to the classical *reward circuit* projecting from midbrain dopaminergic regions to the ventral striatum and ventromedial prefrontal cortex. Closely linked to the RDoC domain of *positive valence systems*, the incentive network is also abnormally active transdiagnostically across multiple psychiatric disorders. It is observed to be anticorrelated to the salience network in its activity.

(C) The lateral orbitofrontal-temporal network is sometimes linked to *nonreward functions* and the RDoC domain of *negative valence systems*. It centers on lateral orbitofrontal regions and their input regions in the lateral temporal cortex. Involved in emotional reappraisal, these regions are also abnormally overactive or underactive during tasks requiring cognitive control or response inhibition across a variety of psychiatric disorders.

To view this figure in color, see Plate 12 in Color Gallery in middle of book.

Source.   From the lab of Jonathan Downar, M.D., Ph.D. Used with permission.

The best-known of these patterns would be drug cues in substance use disorders; however, analogous patterns of abnormal activation can be observed in OCD, MDD, bulimia nervosa, and schizophrenia, among other disorders. Of note, the activity of the limbic network at rest is anticorrelated to the salience network, and tasks that involve the exercise of cognitive control (e.g., desisting from loss-chasing among pathological gamblers) reveal both activation of the salience network and suppression of the incentive network.

A third network, sometimes known as the *nonreward network*, is active during negative stimuli, missed rewards, or other worse-than-expected outcomes. This network centers on the ventrolateral prefrontal cortex and the adjacent lateral orbitofrontal cortex, particularly on the right hemisphere. It also has nodes in the lateral temporal lobe and includes ventral striatal circuits that may be distinct from circuits of the "reward" pathways. This nonreward region is active during (negative) reappraisal of emotional stimuli and has been identified as a nexus of activity in patients with MDD. Indeed, a recently proposed *nonreward attractor theory of depression* suggests that reactivating and self-perpetuating processes in this network may underlie core symptoms of negative affect, anhedonia, and rumination in depression (Rolls 2016).

Formulating Psychiatric Illness in Terms of Dimensions of Pathology and Associated Functional Networks

Although these three networks do not appear to map well onto categorical DSM diagnoses such as MDD or OCD, they do appear to map well onto *dimensions* or *domains* of pathology that cut across conventional disorders. Furthermore, these domains appear to correspond fairly well to the more biologically grounded Research Domain Criteria (RDoC) proposed by the National Institutes of Health (Insel et al. 2010) for formulating psychiatric illnesses for research purposes. Three of the five major domains in the RDoC matrix are cognitive control, positive valence systems, and negative valence systems. In the RDoC approach, patients would receive a dimensional diagnostic formulation on these three domains, with symptoms understood in terms of abnormalities in cognitive control, aberrant incentives, and aberrant disincentives.

This approach to formulation only becomes truly clinically useful, however, if it can be used to plan an approach to treatment. Here, the biological grounding of the domains may prove helpful. Tasks that engage cognitive control, positive valence systems (incentives), and negative valence systems (disincentives) tend to engage the salience network, limbic/incentive network, and lateral orbitofrontal/nonreward network, respectively. Thus, a "neuroanatomic" approach to formulation in psychiatry would assess each patient in terms of the relative contributions of deficient cognitive control, pathological/compulsive incentives, or pathological/compulsive disincentives. This diagnostic approach would identify neuroanatomically well-defined networks of pathology to be targeted for therapeutic intervention in each patient. Treatment would require a suite of neuroanatomically precise interventions capable of targeting these networks precisely and specifically and of modulating or normalizing their aberrant activity.

Brain Stimulation Treatments Modulate the Activity of Functional Networks

Mounting evidence suggests that currently available brain stimulation treatments (e.g., ECT, rTMS, DBS) do indeed affect not only the directly stimulated brain region but also the rest of its network of functionally connected regions. For example, during DBS of the subgenual cingulate cortex for depression, changes in metabolic activity are seen not only in the implanted region itself but also in a wide variety of other regions that belong to its functional network (e.g., the ventromedial prefrontal cortex) as well as its antinetwork. During ECT, changes in metabolic activity are seen not only under the stimulation electrodes but also in a widespread network of other cortical and subcortical regions throughout the brain. During rTMS, activations are seen not only in the region under the focus of the rTMS coil but also in other cortical and subcortical regions throughout the brain that belong to that region's network and antinetwork.

In addition to being a reliable observation across different techniques, these changes in network activity also appear to be central to the therapeutic effects of the techniques. For example, rTMS of the DLPFC and of the dorsomedial prefrontal cortex have both been found to modulate the integrity of the salience network, and patients showing such effects seem to have the best clinical response. Similarly, ECT leads to specific changes in network activity among the patients who show the strongest response to treatment. Along similar lines, it may be possible to predict treatment outcome for ECT or for rTMS based on the network activity of multiple brain regions, with treatment responders and nonresponders characterized by distinctly different patterns of activity in salience, limbic, or default mode networks prior to undergoing treatment. Multiple functional brain networks may therefore prove useful both as predictors and as correlates of successful treatment outcome.

One final but important finding is that the brain's functional networks may provide a common therapeutic mechanism for both invasive and noninvasive brain stimulation techniques. Fox et al. (2014) reviewed 14 different types of neurological or psychiatric illnesses (including MDD, OCD, Parkinson's disease, Tourette's disorder, and addiction) for which both DBS and rTMS had shown benefit in the literature. Taking the target location of the DBS electrode for each illness, these investigators mapped that region's functional network and antinetwork. The successful rTMS targets for each illness were located in the same network/antinetwork as the successful DBS targets. Furthermore, polarity seemed to matter: performing the wrong type of rTMS (high frequency to the antinetwork, or low frequency to the network) seemed to make symptoms worse rather than better.

Conclusion

It is worth noting that a key feature distinguishing brain stimulation therapies from other types of psychiatric interventions is that they are more anatomically specific in their effects. An rTMS stimulator, or a DBS electrode, can exert a wide range of very different effects on the brain, depending on whether it is used to target motor regions, visual regions, or other higher-level networks. Because the brain is arranged as a set of interconnected functional networks, stimulating any given brain region also exerts an effect on the other nodes of that region's network and antinetwork. Thus, the best level of explanation for understanding the mechanisms of brain stimulation treatments may be that of functional brain networks rather than individual brain regions or specific molecules or receptors.

Similarly, when planning a treatment strategy that uses brain stimulation, the best approach to diagnostic formulation may be one that considers pathology in terms of the underlying brain networks. This neuroanatomic approach to formulation is still in its infancy, but early indications suggest that certain well-characterized brain networks may underlie specific domains or dimensions of illness: for example, the salience network and the capacity for cognitive control. As we become more proficient in understanding psychiatric illnesses as "circuitopathies," our suite of brain stimulation treatments will steadily become more useful and may ultimately provide a more reliable pathway to remission for the many patients who do not improve with conventional treatments.

Key Clinical Points

- Brain stimulation preceded the use of medications and therapy in psychiatry.

- Interventional psychiatry involves the use of brain stimulation treatments.

- Brain stimulation can be convulsive or nonconvulsive and invasive or noninvasive.

- Electroconvulsive therapy (ECT) is the oldest, most rapidly acting, and most effective treatment for depression and catatonia.

- Transcranial magnetic stimulation (TMS) is a nonconvulsive treatment for medication-resistant depression.

- Vagus nerve stimulation (VNS) is approved but not currently reimbursed for treatment-resistant depression.

- Deep brain stimulation (DBS) has received a humanitarian exemption approval from the FDA for use in severe obsessive-compulsive disorder that is unresponsive to other treatments.

- New stimulation technologies are providing novel ways to understand and treat psychiatric disorders.

- Brain stimulation may provide a personalized, circuit-based approach to treating brain disorders.

- Brain stimulation may potentially be used to augment treatment with medications and psychotherapy.

References

Abbott CC, Jones T, Lemke NT, et al: Hippocampal structural and functional changes associated with electroconvulsive therapy response. Transl Psychiatry 4:e483, 2014 25405780

Alonso P, Cuadras D, Gabriëls L, et al: Deep brain stimulation for obsessive-compulsive disorder: a meta-analysis of treatment outcome and predictors of response. PLoS One 10(7):e0133591, 2015 26208305

Bakker N, Shahab S, Giacobbe P, et al: rTMS of the dorsomedial prefrontal cortex for major depression: safety, tolerability, effectiveness, and outcome predictors for 10 Hz versus intermittent theta-burst stimulation. Brain Stimul 8(2):208–215, 2015 25465290

Beam W, Borckardt JJ, Reeves ST, et al: An efficient and accurate new method for locating the F3 position for prefrontal TMS applications. Brain Stimulat 2(1):50–54, 2009 20539835

Berlim MT, Van den Eynde F, Daskalakis ZJ: Clinically meaningful efficacy and acceptability of low-frequency repetitive transcranial magnetic stimulation (rTMS) for treating primary major depression: a meta-analysis of randomized, double-blind and sham-controlled trials. Neuropsychopharmacology 38(4):543–551, 2013 23249815

Berlim MT, van den Eynde F, Tovar-Perdomo S, et al: Response, remission and drop-out rates following high-frequency repetitive transcranial magnetic stimulation (rTMS) for treating major depression: a systematic review and meta-analysis of randomized, double-blind and sham-controlled trials. Psychol Med 44(2):225–239, 2014 23507264

Bini L: Professor Bini's notes on the first electro-shock experiment. Convuls Ther 11(4):260–261, 1995 8919577

Blumberger DM, Vila-Rodriguez F, Thorpe K, et al: Effectiveness of theta burst versus high-frequency repetitive transcranial magnetic stimulation in patients with depression (THREE-D): a randomised non-inferiority trial. Lancet 391(10131):1683–1692, 2018 [Erratum in: Lancet 391(10139):e24, 2018] 29726344

Borckardt JJ, Nahas ZH, Teal J, et al: The painfulness of active, but not sham, transcranial magnetic stimulation decreases rapidly over time: results from the double-blind phase of the OPT-TMS Trial. Brain Stimul 6(6):925–928, 2013 23769413

Brunelin J, Jalenques I, Trojak B, et al: The efficacy and safety of low frequency repetitive transcranial magnetic stimulation for treatment-resistant depression: the results from a large multicenter French RCT. Brain Stimul 7(6):855–863, 2014 25192980

Brunoni AR, Moffa AH, Sampaio-Junior B, et al: Trial of electrical direct-current therapy versus escitalopram for depression. N Engl J Med 376(26):2523–2533, 2017 28657871

Cao X, Deng C, Su X, Guo Y: Response and remission rates following high-frequency vs. low-frequency repetitive transcranial magnetic stimulation (RTMS) over right DLPFC for treating major depressive disorder (MDD): a meta-analysis of randomized, double-blind trials. Front Psychiatry 9:413, 2018 30245641

Carpenter LL, Janicak PG, Aaronson ST, et al: Transcranial magnetic stimulation (TMS) for major depression: a multisite, naturalistic, observational study of acute treatment outcomes in clinical practice. Depress Anxiety 29(7):587–596, 2012 22689344

Dedoncker J, Brunoni AR, Baeken C, Vanderhasselt MA: A systematic review and meta-analysis of the effects of transcranial direct current stimulation (tDCS) over the dorsolateral prefrontal cortex in healthy and neuropsychiatric samples: influence of stimulation parameters. Brain Stimul 9(4):501–517, 2016 27160468

DeLong MR, Benabid AL: Discovery of high-frequency deep brain stimulation for treatment of Parkinson disease: 2014 Lasker Award. JAMA 312(11):1093–1094, 2014 25198255

Denys D, Mantione M, Figee M, et al: Deep brain stimulation of the nucleus accumbens for treatment-refractory obsessive-compulsive disorder. Arch Gen Psychiatry 67(10):1061–1068, 2010 20921122

Di Lazzaro V, Dileone M, Pilato F, et al: Modulation of motor cortex neuronal networks by rTMS: comparison of local and remote effects of six different protocols of stimulation. J Neurophysiol 105(5):2150–2156, 2011 21346213

Dougherty DD, Rezai AR, Carpenter LL, et al: A randomized sham-controlled trial of deep brain stimulation of the ventral capsule/ventral striatum for chronic treatment-resistant depression. Biol Psychiatry 78(4):240–248, 2015 25726497

Downar J, Daskalakis ZJ: New targets for rTMS in depression: a review of convergent evidence. Brain Stimulat 6(3):231–240, 2013 22975030

Duprat R, Desmyter S, Rudi de R, et al: Accelerated intermittent theta burst stimulation treatment in medication-resistant major depression: a fast road to remission? J Affect Disord 200:6–14, 2016 27107779

Eldaief MC, Halko MA, Buckner RL, et al: Transcranial magnetic stimulation modulates the brain's intrinsic activity in a frequency-dependent manner. Proc Natl Acad Sci U S A 108(52):21229–21234, 2011 22160708

Feffer K, Fettes P, Giacobbe P, et al: 1Hz rTMS of the right orbitofrontal cortex for major depression: safety, tolerability and clinical outcomes. Eur Neuropsychopharmacol 28(1):109–117, 2018 29153927

Fink M: Meduna and the origins of convulsive therapy. Am J Psychiatry 141(9):1034–1041, 1984 6147103

Fitzgerald PB, Hoy KE, Anderson RJ, et al: A study of the pattern of response to rTMS treatment in depression. Depress Anxiety 33(8):746–753, 2016 27059158

Fox MD, Buckner RL, White MP, et al: Efficacy of transcranial magnetic stimulation targets for depression is related to intrinsic functional connectivity with the subgenual cingulate. Biol Psychiatry 72(7):595–603, 2012 22658708

Fox MD, Buckner RL, Liu H, et al: Resting-state networks link invasive and noninvasive brain stimulation across diverse psychiatric and neurological diseases. Proc Natl Acad Sci U S A 111(41):E4367–E4375, 2014 25267639

Frei MG, Osorio I: Left vagus nerve stimulation with the neurocybernetic prosthesis has complex effects on heart rate and on its variability in humans. Epilepsia 42(8):1007–1016, 2001 11554886

Goldapple K, Segal Z, Garson C, et al: Modulation of cortical-limbic pathways in major depression: treatment-specific effects of cognitive behavior therapy. Arch Gen Psychiatry 61(1):34–41, 2004 14706942

Goodkind M, Eickhoff SB, Oathes DJ, et al: Identification of a common neurobiological substrate for mental illness. JAMA Psychiatry 72(4):305–315, 2015 25651064

Greenberg BD, Gabriels LA, Malone DA Jr, et al: Deep brain stimulation of the ventral internal capsule/ventral striatum for obsessive-compulsive disorder: worldwide experience. Mol Psychiatry 15(1):64–79, 2010a 18490925

Greenberg BD, Rauch SL, Haber SN: Invasive circuitry-based neurotherapeutics: stereotactic ablation and deep brain stimulation for OCD. Neuropsychopharmacology 35(1):317–336, 2010b 19759530

Holtzheimer PE, Kelley ME, Gross RE, et al: Subcallosal cingulate deep brain stimulation for treatment-resistant unipolar and bipolar depression. Arch Gen Psychiatry 69(2):150–158, 2012 22213770

Holtzheimer PE, Husain MM, Lisanby SH, et al: Subcallosal cingulate deep brain stimulation for treatment-resistant depression: a multisite, randomised, sham-controlled trial. Lancet Psychiatry 4(11):839–849, 2017 28988904

Insel T, Cuthbert B, Garvey M, et al: Research domain criteria (RDoC): toward a new classification framework for research on mental disorders. Am J Psychiatry 167(7):748–751, 2010 20595427

Jung HH, Kim SJ, Roh D, et al: Bilateral thermal capsulotomy with MR-guided focused ultrasound for patients with treatment-refractory obsessive-compulsive disorder: a proof-of-concept study. Mol Psychiatry 20(10):1205–1211, 2015 25421403

Kavirajan HC, Lueck K, Chuang K: Alternating current cranial electrotherapy stimulation (CES) for depression. Cochrane Database Syst Rev (7):CD010521, 2014 25000907

Kedzior KK, Reitz SK, Azorina V, et al: Durability of the antidepressant effect of the high-frequency repetitive transcranial magnetic stimulation (rTMS) In the absence of maintenance treatment in major depression: a systematic review and meta-analysis of 16 double-blind, randomized, sham-controlled trials. Depress Anxiety 32(3):193–203, 2015 25683231

Kellner CH, Knapp RG, Petrides G, et al: Continuation electroconvulsive therapy vs pharmacotherapy for relapse prevention in major depression: a multisite study from the Consortium for Research in Electroconvulsive Therapy (CORE). Arch Gen Psychiatry 63(12):1337–1344, 2006 17146008

Kellner CH, Husain MM, Knapp RG, et al: A novel strategy for continuation ECT in geriatric depression: phase 2 of the PRIDE study. Am J Psychiatry 173(11):1110–1118, 2016 27418381

Krystal AD, Watts BV, Weiner RD, et al: The use of flumazenil in the anxious and benzodiazepine-dependent ECT patient. J ECT 14(1):5–14, 1998 9661088

Lefaucheur JP, André-Obadia N, Antal A, et al: Evidence-based guidelines on the therapeutic use of repetitive transcranial magnetic stimulation (rTMS). Clin Neurophysiol 125(11):2150–2206, 2014 25034472

Leuchter AF, Cook IA, Feifel D, et al: Efficacy and safety of low-field synchronized transcranial magnetic stimulation (sTMS) for treatment of major depression. Brain Stimulat 8(4):787–794, 2015 26143022

Levkovitz Y, Isserles M, Padberg F, et al: Efficacy and safety of deep transcranial magnetic stimulation for major depression: a prospective multicenter randomized controlled trial. World Psychiatry 14(1):64–73, 2015 25655160

Li CT, Chen MH, Juan CH, et al: Efficacy of prefrontal theta-burst stimulation in refractory depression: a randomized sham-controlled study. Brain 137(pt 7):2088–2098, 2014 24817188

Lisanby SH: Electroconvulsive therapy for depression. N Engl J Med 357(19):1939–1945, 2007 17989386

Liston C, Chen AC, Zebley BD, et al: Default mode network mechanisms of transcranial magnetic stimulation in depression. Biol Psychiatry 76(7):517–526, 2014 24629537

Lozano AM, Giacobbe P, Hamani C, et al: A multicenter pilot study of subcallosal cingulate area deep brain stimulation for treatment-resistant depression. J Neurosurg 116(2):315–322, 2012 22098195

Lyden H, Espinoza RT, Pirnia T, et al: Electroconvulsive therapy mediates neuroplasticity of white matter microstructure in major depression. Transl Psychiatry 4:e380, 2014 24713861

Magara A, Bühler R, Moser D, et al: First experience with MR-guided focused ultrasound in the treatment of Parkinson's disease. J Ther Ultrasound 2:11, 2014 25512869

Mallet L, Polosan M, Jaafari N, et al; STOC Study Group: Subthalamic nucleus stimulation in severe obsessive-compulsive disorder. N Engl J Med 359(20):2121–2134, 2008 [Erratum in: N Engl J Med 361(10):1027, 2009] 19005196

Mayberg HS, Liotti M, Brannan SK, et al: Reciprocal limbic-cortical function and negative mood: converging PET findings in depression and normal sadness. Am J Psychiatry 156(5):675–682, 1999 10327898

Mayberg HS, Brannan SK, Tekell JL, et al: Regional metabolic effects of fluoxetine in major depression: serial changes and relationship to clinical response. Biol Psychiatry 48(8):830–843, 2000 11063978

McClintock SM, Reti IM, Carpenter LL, et al: Consensus recommendations for the clinical application of repetitive transcranial magnetic stimulation (rTMS) in the treatment of depression. J Clin Psychiatry 79(1), 2018 28541649

McCullough JP: CBASP, the third wave and the treatment of chronic depression. European Psychotherapy 9(1):169–190, 2010. Available at: https://cip-medien.com/wp-content/uploads/10.-CBASP-McCullough.pdf. Accessed February 6, 2019.

McDonald WM, Weiner RD, Fochtmann LJ, et al: The FDA and ECT. J ECT 32(2):75–77, 2016 27191123

Milev RV, Giacobbe P, Kennedy SH, et al: Canadian Network for Mood and Anxiety Treatments (CANMAT) 2016 clinical guidelines for the management of adults with major depressive disorder, section 4: neurostimulation treatments. Can J Psychiatry 61(9):561–575, 2016 27486154

Modirrousta M, Meek BP, Wikstrom SL: Efficacy of twice-daily vs once-daily sessions of repetitive transcranial magnetic stimulation in the treatment of major depressive disorder: a retrospective study. Neuropsychiatr Dis Treat 14:309–316, 2018 29398915

Monte-Silva K, Ruge D, Teo JT, et al: D2 receptor block abolishes theta burst stimulation-induced neuroplasticity in the human motor cortex. Neuropsychopharmacology 36(10):2097–2102, 2011 21697824

Nahas Z, Marangell LB, Husain MM, et al: Two-year outcome of vagus nerve stimulation (VNS) for treatment of major depressive episodes. J Clin Psychiatry 66(9):1097–1104, 2005 16187765

Navarro V, Gastó C, Torres X, et al: Continuation/maintenance treatment with nortriptyline versus combined nortriptyline and ECT in late-life psychotic depression: a two-year randomized study. Am J Geriatr Psychiatry 16(6):498–505, 2008 18515694

Nobler MS, Oquendo MA, Kegeles LS, et al: Decreased regional brain metabolism after ECT. Am J Psychiatry 158(2):305–308, 2001 11156816

O'Connor MK, Knapp R, Husain M, et al: The influence of age on the response of major depression to electroconvulsive therapy: a C.O.R.E. Report. Am J Geriatr Psychiatry 9(4):382–390, 2001 11739064

O'Reardon JP, Solvason HB, Janicak PG, et al: Efficacy and safety of transcranial magnetic stimulation in the acute treatment of major depression: a multisite randomized controlled trial. Biol Psychiatry 62(11):1208–1216, 2007 17573044

Perrin JS, Merz S, Bennett DM, et al: Electroconvulsive therapy reduces frontal cortical connectivity in severe depressive disorder. Proc Natl Acad Sci U S A 109(14):5464–5468, 2012 22431642

Peters SK, Dunlop K, Downar J: Cortico-striatal-thalamic loop circuits of the salience network: a central pathway in psychiatric disease and treatment. Front Syst Neurosci 10:104, 2016 28082874

Petrides G, Fink M, Husain MM, et al: ECT remission rates in psychotic versus nonpsychotic depressed patients: a report from CORE. J ECT 17(4):244–253, 2001 11731725

Prudic J, Olfson M, Marcus SC, et al: Effectiveness of electroconvulsive therapy in community settings. Biol Psychiatry 55(3):301–312, 2004 14744473

Rasmussen KG, Zorumski CF: Electroconvulsive therapy in patients taking theophylline. J Clin Psychiatry 54(11):427–431, 1993 8270586

Rolls ET: A non-reward attractor theory of depression. Neurosci Biobehav Rev 68:47–58, 2016 27181908

Rose D, Fleischmann P, Wykes T, et al: Patients' perspectives on electroconvulsive therapy: systematic review. BMJ 326(7403):1363, 2003 12816822

Rossi S, Hallett M, Rossini PM, et al: Safety, ethical considerations, and application guidelines for the use of transcranial magnetic stimulation in clinical practice and research. Clin Neurophysiol 120(12):2008–2039, 2009 19833552

Rush AJ, Marangell LB, Sackeim HA, et al: Vagus nerve stimulation for treatment-resistant depression: a randomized, controlled acute phase trial. Biol Psychiatry 58(5):347–354, 2005 16139580

Rush AJ, Trivedi MH, Wisniewski SR, et al; STAR*D Study Team: Bupropion-SR, sertraline, or venlafaxine-XR after failure of SSRIs for depression. N Engl J Med 354(12):1231–1242, 2006 16554525

Sackeim HA, Luber B, Katzman GP, et al: The effects of electroconvulsive therapy on quantitative electroencephalograms. Relationship to clinical outcome. Arch Gen Psychiatry 53(9):814–824, 1996 8792758

Sackeim HA, Prudic J, Nobler MS, et al: Effects of pulse width and electrode placement on the efficacy and cognitive effects of electroconvulsive therapy. Brain Stimulat 1(2):71–83, 2008 19756236

Sackeim HA, Dillingham EM, Prudic J, et al: Effect of concomitant pharmacotherapy on electroconvulsive therapy outcomes: short-term efficacy and adverse effects. Arch Gen Psychiatry 66(7):729–737, 2009 19581564

Schulze L, Remington G, Giacobbe P, et al: Effect of antipsychotic pharmacotherapy on clinical outcomes of intermittent theta-burst stimulation for refractory depression. J Psychopharmacol 31(3):312–319, 2017 27852961

Semkovska M, McLoughlin DM: Objective cognitive performance associated with electroconvulsive therapy for depression: a systematic review and meta-analysis. Biol Psychiatry
68(6):568–577, 2010 20673880

Sienaert P, Peuskens J: Anticonvulsants during electroconvulsive therapy: review and recommendations. J ECT 23(2):120–123, 2007 17548985

Stefan H, Kreiselmeyer G, Kerling F, et al: Transcutaneous vagus nerve stimulation (t-VNS) in
pharmacoresistant epilepsies: a proof of concept trial. Epilepsia 53(7):e115–e118, 2012
22554199

Strafella AP, Paus T, Fraraccio M, Dagher A: Striatal dopamine release induced by repetitive
transcranial magnetic stimulation of the human motor cortex. Brain 126(pt 12):2609–2615,
2003 12937078

Wang JX, Rogers LM, Gross EZ, et al: Targeted enhancement of cortical-hippocampal brain networks and associative memory. Science 345(6200):1054–1057, 2014 25170153

Weissman CR, Blumberger DM, Brown PE, et al: Bilateral repetitive transcranial magnetic stimulation decreases suicidal ideation in depression. J Clin Psychiatry 79(3), 2018 29701939

Williams NR, Short EB, Hopkins T, et al: Five-year follow-up of bilateral epidural prefrontal
cortical stimulation for treatment-resistant depression. Brain Stimulat 9(6):897–904, 2016
27443912

Yeo BT, Krienen FM, Sepulcre J, et al: The organization of the human cerebral cortex estimated
by intrinsic functional connectivity. J Neurophysiol 106(3):1125–1165, 2011 21653723

Ziemann U, Paulus W, Nitsche MA, et al: Consensus: motor cortex plasticity protocols. Brain
Stimulat 1(3):164–182, 2008 20633383

Recommended Readings

American Psychiatric Association: The Practice of Electroconvulsive Therapy: Recommendations for Treatment, Training, and Privileging: A Task Force Report of the American Psychiatric Association, 2nd Edition. Washington DC, American Psychiatric Press, 2001

McClintock SM, Reti IM, Carpenter LL, et al: Consensus recommendations for the clinical application of repetitive transcranial magnetic stimulation (rTMS) in the treatment of depression. J Clin Psychiatry 79(1), 2018 28541649

Milev RV, Giacobbe P, Kennedy SH, et al; CANMAT Depression Work Group: Canadian Network for Mood and Anxiety Treatments (CANMAT) 2016 Clinical Guidelines for the Management of Adults with Major Depressive Disorder, Section 4: Neurostimulation Treatments. Can J Psychiatry 61(9):561–575, 2016 27486154

CHAPTER 31

Brief Psychotherapies

Mantosh J. Dewan, M.D.

Brett N. Steenbarger, Ph.D.

Roger P. Greenberg, Ph.D.

Brief psychotherapy refers to a class of treatments that seek to accelerate change through the active, focused interventions of therapists and enhanced patient involvement. Treatment is designed to be brief and is limited from the start to less than 6 months or fewer than 24 sessions. In the past several decades, various brief approaches to therapy have evolved, ranging from single-session treatments and several sessions of strategic interventions to short-term psychodynamic modalities that frequently exceed 20 sessions. At the same time, rigorously performed outcome studies of brief therapy have matched patients and presenting concerns likely to benefit from specific approaches. This has also led to the application of brief therapies to a wider range of patients, including targeted interventions for severe conditions, including schizophrenia. The overarching message from this research is that the value of short-term work is significant but also highly dependent on the characteristics of patients and their therapists.

Brief Therapy: A Short Background

Surprisingly, Freud's own cases showed that psychoanalytic therapy was frequently of brief duration. For example, in *Studies on Hysteria* (Breuer and Freud 1955), Freud described three of his patients as having treatments that lasted for 9 weeks (Lucie R.), 7 weeks (Emmy Von N.), and one session (Katharina)! However, this brevity was not by design, and he tended not to focus on treatment outcome in his writing. Instead, he emphasized that having a neutral therapist who was not overly involved in how treatment would turn out could lead to important discoveries about the development of psychopathology (Fisher and Greenberg 1985).

Brief therapy arguably dates back to the publication of Alexander and French's (1946) classic work *Psychoanalytic Therapy: Principles and Applications*. They were the first to formally place the therapist in the active role of promoting patient health. Change, they argued, was not primarily a function of insight but of experience. Therefore, the therapist's role was to foster "corrective emotional experiences." These are replays of previous conflicted situations that end more positively within the helping relationship. This reformulation took therapists out of their historic role as "blank screens" and cast them as active treatment agents who could use their relationships with patients to catalyze needed developmental experiences. Research has since supported the usefulness of this more active approach. Lengthy treatments, which associated therapeutic gains primarily with the attainment of patient insights, have not turned out to be as central to change as many psychoanalysts assumed (Fisher and Greenberg 1996). With the writings of Peter Sifneos, James Mann, David Malan, and Habib Davanloo, brevity has become an accepted part of the psychoanalytic lexicon (Dewan et al. 2018).

The rise of behavior therapies contributed significantly to the prominence of brief work. Behavioral treatments cast the therapist in the role of teacher. No longer was therapy about self-exploration. Rather, it was intended to teach coping skills and alter learned action patterns. This permitted therapy to be highly circumscribed, emphasizing directive teaching and structured homework assignments between sessions. Behavior therapy found its first formal exposition in the writings of Skinner in the 1950s, along with the influential *Psychotherapy by Reciprocal Inhibition* (Wolpe 1958). By the 1970s, behavior therapy had become part of the therapeutic mainstream (Dewan et al. 2018).

Albert Ellis applied the learning paradigm to cognition with rational-emotive therapy in the 1950s. This blended the psychodynamic interest in the patient's inner life with hands-on behavioral methods. The cognitive method of teaching patients to unlearn dysfunctional thought patterns and acquire new, constructive ones continued with Aaron Beck's writings in the 1960s and the influential *Cognitive Therapy and the Emotional Disorders* (Beck 1976). The combination of a tight treatment focus and structured patient involvement between sessions ensured that cognitive therapy, like its behavioral sibling, possessed core ingredients of brevity.

Yet a third type of brief therapy emerged with the writings of Jay Haley, whose *Strategies of Psychotherapy* and *Problem-Solving Therapy* drew heavily on the clinical practices of Milton Erickson (Dewan et al. 2011). Erickson viewed the presenting concerns of patients as failed efforts to solve normal life problems. These lead to cycles in which attempted solutions reinforce initial problems, much as an insomniac patient's active efforts to sleep sustain wakefulness. The role of the therapist, Erickson held, is neither as significant other (as in brief psychodynamic work) nor as cognitive-behavioral teacher. Rather, the therapist is a problem solver who interrupts and redirects these self-reinforcing cycles. This frequently could be accomplished in a matter of several sessions through the prescription of directed tasks. With the publication of Watzlawick et al.'s (1974) classic work on change processes, the strategic approach became a therapeutic staple, notably in the family therapy literature.

In the 1980s, rising health care costs led to managed care, and brief therapy found an economic and a practice rationale (Dewan et al. 2011). Budman and Gurman (1988) found that therapy could be conducted in a time-effective manner. Research suggesting that brief modalities were effective for a variety of patients and problems supported the adoption of short-term work. The movement toward evidence-based medicine spurred the development of manualized psychotherapeutic treatments, which, by their very nature, are highly structured and limited in duration. With such popularity, however, also emerged concerns about the limitations of such treatments, especially for severe and persistent emotional disorders and conditions with high relapse rates. These concerns are being systematically addressed, and brief therapies have been devised for personality disorders and psychotic disorders (Beck et al. 2004; Linehan 2014; Wright et al. 2010). It is fair to say that by the twenty-first century brief therapies had become the practice rule rather than the exception among psychotherapists.

Current Models

Although "common factors" are essential and form the base of all successful therapies (Greenberg 2018), the various brief therapies make different assumptions about the causes of presenting problems and the specific procedures necessary to alter them. These approaches cluster within three broad models: relational, learning, and contextual (Steenbarger 2002). Because of their distinctive assumptions and practice patterns, each of these models defines *brevity* differently. We describe the key elements of each model and suggest that the reader enrich the text by referring to detailed illustrative cases and video clips provided for each therapy in *The Art and Science of Brief Psychotherapies: An Illustrated Guide*, 3rd Edition (Dewan et al. 2018).

Relational Therapies

Relational modalities include short-term psychodynamic treatments and interpersonal therapy (IPT). The key assumption of these approaches is that the presenting problems of patients reflect difficulties in significant relationships. Several important differences are evident between short-term dynamic therapies and IPT, chief among them being the focus on the therapeutic relationship as a vehicle for change.

Psychodynamic Therapy

Psychodynamic brief therapies share the premise of all psychodynamic therapies that the presenting problems of patients result from an internalization of conflicts from earlier significant relationships. The anxiety from these conflicts is controlled through defenses that aid short-term coping but forestall the conscious assimilation and working through of core relational issues. As a result, these issues resurface in future relationships whenever similar anxiety and conflict are experienced, triggering old patterns of defense. These coping efforts are no longer appropriate to present-day relationship contexts, yielding secondary conflict and the consequences that typically bring people to therapy. Thus, the psychodynamic therapist views presenting problems as more than symptoms of an underlying disorder. They are the result of outmoded, currently maladaptive (defensive) efforts in the face of repeated interpersonal conflict.

Traditional psychodynamic therapy works backward from presenting complaints to underlying core conflicts. The chief therapeutic strategy in this process is interpretation, as therapists promote insight into outmoded defenses and repeated interpersonal struggles. The therapeutic relationship becomes the locus for such insight as those struggles are reenacted in the transference relationship. As patients replay their maladaptive defensive patterns and interpersonal struggles within sessions, the dynamically oriented therapist engages the real relationship—the mature alliance between the self-observing patient and the therapist—to help the patient become aware of what is happening and why. With this insight into repetitive patterns and their consequences, patients can then attempt to rework the ways in which they handle interpersonal threats within the safe confines of the helping relationship.

Because traditional long-term psychodynamic work requires an unfolding of historical patterns within the therapeutic relationship, it cannot be an abbreviated treatment. The focus on interpretation as a chief therapeutic tool and insight as a goal—with in-session work and an exhaustive exploration of the past as the primary context for change efforts—ensures that such therapy spans months, if not years, of analysis.

Several features of short-term psychodynamic therapy enable it to accelerate this change curve:

- *Circumscribed, here-and-now focus*—Brief dynamic work focuses on "core conflictual relationship themes" (Luborsky and Mark 1991) that represent "cyclical maladaptive patterns" (Binder and Strupp 1991) linking current, past, and therapeutic relationships. Although an understanding of the role of the past in the genesis of these themes is relevant, it is not the primary focus of short-term dynamic therapy. Rather, brief dynamic work actively focuses on highly salient present-day manifestations of the cyclical patterns (Binder 2010; Levenson 2017).
- *Patient selection criteria*—Most short-term psychodynamic practitioners acknowledge that brief treatment is not appropriate for all patients and disorders. By limiting such work to patients who are experiencing emotional discomfort, able to readily form a trusting relationship, and open to viewing problems in an interpersonal context, therapists help ensure that treatment will progress efficiently (Levenson 2018). Levenson (2017) observed that inclusion criteria can be broad as long as patients are capable of working within the framework of cyclical patterns.
- *Active provision of positive relationship experiences within the therapy*—Following Alexander and French's (1946) early formulations, brief dynamic therapists do not rely primarily on interpretation as a source of change. Rather, change is catalyzed by the involvement of the therapist in the core relationship patterns, breaking the cycles of repetition by providing responses different from those anticipated by patients (Levenson 2017). Moreover, countertransference is not viewed merely as something for the therapist to guard against but as an inevitable and potentially useful experience that allows therapists to detect and counteract the emotional pulls of their patients.
- *Creation of heightened emotional contexts for change*—The work of Sifneos (1972) and Davanloo (1980) suggested that change can be accelerated by fostering an enhanced state of experiencing among patients. Such anxiety-provoking therapies seek to challenge and break through patterns of defense and resistance rather than relying solely on interpretation (Dewan et al. 2018). Levenson (2018) noted that in brief dynamic work, emotion can be used to change emotion by drawing upon powerful emotional experiences. Under conditions of heightened emotion, patients can more readily gain access to memories, impulses, and feelings associated with core conflictual patterns, facilitating an accelerated working through of these experiences within therapy.

In short, brief dynamic therapists, unlike their traditional counterparts, take an active role in the helping process, fostering and sustaining a treatment focus and initiating interventions within this focus to challenge maladaptive defensive patterns and provide new, corrective relationship experiences (Table 31–1). Although such short-term work may not be brief by insurance company standards, often extending to 20 or more sessions, it significantly abbreviates the traditional treatment course of psychoanalytically oriented psychotherapy. There is good evidence that brief dynamic therapy is effective for a wide range of patients (Dewan et al. 2018). Furthermore, studies have found that both in brief therapy and in traditional psychoanalysis, the strength of the relationship, persuasion, suggestion, catharsis, and the therapist as a model are much more pivotal to the change process than was previously recognized (Fisher and Greenberg 1996; Wallerstein 1989).

Interpersonal Therapy

Like dynamic therapy, IPT sustains a focus on relationship issues and also on interpersonal communication. However, it is distinct from dynamic therapy in that the primary focus of IPT is on the patients' relationships and communication patterns with others who are *currently* important in their lives; the IPT therapist does not seek to understand how past events and relationships may have influenced current relationships and therefore does not work on transference relationships with patients or reenactments of past interpersonal patterns. As a result, IPT tends to be briefer than most short-term psychodynamic therapies, often 8–20 sessions (Stuart 2018). Indeed, unlike short-term psychodynamic therapy, IPT began in 1984 as a brief manualized treatment that has been successfully applied to a variety of presenting problems and interpersonal concerns. In general, IPT has been found to be particularly efficacious for patients with mood and anxiety disorders (Stuart 2018).

IPT is based on the biopsychosocial diathesis–stress model. An acute interpersonal crisis (stress), particularly in the absence of sufficient social support, will cause distress and symptoms in the area in which the person is vulnerable (diathesis). The first one or two sessions are used for a comprehensive assessment. The patient's family history and health status are elicited. What is their attachment style: secure, anxious/preoccupied, dismissive, or fearful/avoidant? An *interpersonal inventory* consists of a succinct account of the important people in a patient's life. How effectively does the patient offer and ask for support? These threads are woven into an *interpersonal formulation*. IPT targets three problem areas (Stuart 2018):

- *Grief and loss* may be related to death, divorce, or loss of health or a job. The therapist helps the patient create a multidimensional picture of him- or herself to ease the grieving process and encourages the patient to develop new relationships and strengthen existing ones in order to decrease isolation and increase support.
- *Interpersonal disputes* require an understanding of the patient's communication pattern and how this may contribute to the problem. A fresh incident can be examined in detail and the communication analyzed. The patient considers ways to communicate more effectively to get what he or she needs. Role playing or bringing in the partner is often helpful. IPT also emphasizes altering expectations within relationships.

TABLE 31–1.　Differences between short-term and traditional psychodynamic therapies

	Short-term dynamic therapies	Traditional dynamic therapies
Therapeutic focus	Focal relationship patterns	Personality change
Therapist role	Active significant other	Blank screen
Emphasized change mechanism	Corrective relationship experiences	Insight
Mechanism for dealing with resistances	Challenge and confrontation	Interpretation

- *Role transitions* include social transitions such as marriage, divorce, change in job status, and retirement as well as natural transitions such as childbirth and aging. Transitions, even when they are eagerly anticipated, such as retirement, require an adjustment to the loss of the familiar and possibly shrinkage of the social circle and finances as well. IPT therapists encourage grieving this loss after a realistic appraisal of the old role and assist the patient in strengthening social supports.

In IPT, the therapist takes an active role in treatment, sustaining the focus on these issues. After assessment and establishment of a focus, the rationale and goals of treatment are made explicit and a therapeutic contract executed. Current interpersonal concerns are then explored, and patient and therapist brainstorm ways of handling them (Table 31–2). These potential solutions form the basis for between-session efforts (homework) by patients, securing their active involvement in treatment. Subsequent sessions review and refine these efforts, casting the therapist in the role of collaborative problem solver. Resistance to change is dealt with in a straightforward manner by the therapist, not as pattern reenactments to be interpreted and worked through. The goal of therapy is to promote independent functioning on the part of the patient, as well as symptom relief. As Stuart (2018) emphasized, IPT, unlike other therapies, does not presume a complete termination of therapy at the end of treatment. Rather, therapists assume that future sessions may be necessary to maintain gains and prevent relapse. IPT is also welcoming of the concomitant use of medications, which is consistent with IPT's biopsychosocial diathesis–stress model.

Current Models: Comparison and Summary

In summary, the relational model of therapy achieves brevity by creating a circumscribed focus on the patient's interpersonal patterns and by limiting treatment to patient groups able to sustain this focus. Whereas the role of the therapist is different in short-term dynamic therapy (a significant other) compared with IPT (a collaborative problem solver), the ultimate goal is similar: altering problem patterns by generating new, constructive relational experiences.

Learning Therapies

The learning model of treatment, which includes a wide range of cognitive-behavioral therapies, starts from a different set of premises from those in the relational

TABLE 31–2. **Differences between interpersonal therapy and short-term psychodynamic therapy**

	Interpersonal therapy	Short-term psychodynamic therapy
Therapeutic focus	Current patterns in interpersonal communications and attachments	Patterns repeated in past, present, and therapeutic relationships
Therapist role	Problem solver	Transference object
Emphasized change mechanism	Attempting new patterns of communication and altered expectations in extratherapeutic relationships	Corrective relationship experiences within therapy
Structure	Brief; manualized	Time-effective; open-ended

model. The presenting concerns of patients are viewed as learned maladaptive patterns that can be unlearned. Moreover, patients are seen as capable of acquiring new, adaptive patterns of thought and action through skill development. As a result, the learning therapies feature the therapist in an active, directive teaching mode and the patient as a student. This structuring of the helping relationship lends itself to active skill rehearsal within sessions and directed homework between meetings. The combination of a tight learning focus and active practice of techniques ensures that most learning therapies are short term by their very nature.

For purposes of exposition, it is helpful to distinguish between primarily *behavioral treatments* that emphasize exposure as a central therapeutic ingredient and *cognitive approaches* that more broadly target dysfunctional patterns of information processing for restructuring. Although these approaches have elements that overlap (e.g., patients exposed to traumatic cues may rehearse thoughts that emphasize self-control), the relative degree of emphasis is different, which affects the conduct and brevity of treatment.

Behavior Therapy

Learning therapies that use *exposure* as a core therapeutic ingredient include the work of Edna Foa and colleagues (Gallagher et al. 2018) in the treatment of posttraumatic stress disorder (PTSD) and obsessive-compulsive disorder (OCD) and David Barlow's work on panic disorder and unified protocols for the treatment of emotion-driven behaviors (Barlow 2002; Barlow and Farchione 2017). Gallagher et al. (2018) distinguished between 1) exposure and response prevention (ERP), which is designed to treat OCD in a 17-session protocol, and 2) prolonged exposure, which is designed to treat PTSD in 8–15 sessions. In both models, treatment begins with two sessions of assessment and psychosocial education. During this time, patients may keep detailed logs that track the appearance of symptoms and the circumstances surrounding them. Examination of these logs during the early sessions helps to generate a focus on the specific triggers for symptom appearance. Concurrently, therapists educate patients about the learning model, explaining how and why symptoms appear. This can be highly reassuring for patients who may be bewildered by their symptoms. The goal is to make patients experts in their own care so that they will be empowered to sustain change processes.

Also early in treatment, exposure-based learning therapies introduce specific skills designed to help control symptoms. These skills can include efforts at relaxation, thought stopping, self-reassurance, and seeking social support. The skills are typically introduced one at a time, explained in detail as part of the aforementioned psychosocial education, modeled in session by the therapist, and rehearsed in session by patients. Only after patients understand and master skills in session do they rehearse the skills as part of their between-session homework.

An important component of the brevity of these therapies stems from the subsequent employment of these skills. Once triggers for presenting symptoms have been identified, they are deliberately introduced into therapy sessions via imagery and in vivo exercises. Patients are thus required to actively use their coping skills while they are exposed to the very stimuli that have provoked symptoms. For example, a patient with PTSD secondary to assault is treated with prolonged imaginal exposure—that is, she is asked to reexperience aspects of the assault in as vivid detail as possible. This produces high anxiety, so support and relaxation techniques are used to help the patient habituate to these memories. This is repeated several times in each session, and the patient repeatedly listens to a tape of this retelling at home. Once this imagined assault loses its power to traumatize her, the patient is encouraged to gradually confront the attack in reality (in vivo), such as by a visit to the scene (presuming it is normally a safe place), first with a friend and then by herself. A patient with a handwashing compulsion might be exposed to dirt and then prevented from washing his hands (i.e., ERP). A patient experiencing panic might simulate panic experiences by spinning in a chair (interoceptive exposure) and then using cognitive and relaxation skills to maintain composure.

Such in-vivo exposure provides patients with firsthand emotional experiences of mastery that appear to accelerate the pace of symptom resolution. Once initial gains are achieved, efforts at generalization commence, and the skills are used across a variety of symptom-related cues (Table 31–3). Variations in technique—and the specific needs of patients—dictate whether the exposure is attempted in a gradual way or in a more rapid, intensive fashion. As Shapiro's (2001) work suggested, exposure appears to be effective because of the opportunity it affords patients to reprocess cues associated with distress. Exposure work activates fear structures and provides new information and experiences incompatible with fear, allowing for reprocessing and mastery (Gallagher et al. 2018).

Cognitive Therapy

Whereas the exposure therapies have found their greatest application in the treatment of anxiety disorders, *cognitive reprocessing therapies* have been applied to depression, anxiety, eating disorders, and child and adolescent disorders (Hollon and Beck 2004), and more recently to personality disorders, eating disorders, bipolar disorder, and schizophrenia (Barlow and Farchione 2017; Beck and Hindman 2018; Beck et al. 2004; Wright et al. 2010). Symptoms, according to this approach, can be traced to automatic thought patterns that distort information processing and produce negative thoughts about self, others, and the future (cognitive triad). The goal of therapy is to identify these thought patterns, challenge them, and replace them with more constructive alternatives (Beck 2011). The combination of in-session rehearsal and out-of-

TABLE 31–3.   **Comparison of learning and relational models of brief therapy**

	Learning models	Relational models
View of presenting problems	Learned maladaptive patterns of behavior and thought	Internalized relationship conflicts and patterns
Goal of therapy	Unlearning old dysfunctional patterns; acquiring new, constructive ones	Novel interpersonal experiences that can be internalized
Therapist role	Directive teacher	Facilitator of exploration
Emphasized change mechanism	Rehearsal of skills and experiences of mastery during problematic situations	Changing interpersonal patterns in current relationships
Structure	Brief, often manualized or highly structured	Sometimes brief and manualized (interpersonal therapy); sometimes not (short-term dynamic)

session homework targeting core patterns of automatic thought ensures that the cognitive work is time-efficient.

Like the exposure-based learning therapies, cognitive restructuring treatments begin with a period of assessment and psychosocial education. The education in the cognitive model helps patients understand the relation between thoughts and feelings and the ways in which automatic thought patterns can sustain unwanted patterns of emotion and action. Beck and Hindman (2018) presented a common example: a patient returns from work and sees disarray in her apartment (situation) and thinks, "I'm a total basket case. I'll never get my act together" (automatic thoughts), which makes her feel sad (emotion) and heavy in her body (physiological reaction), leading to her lying down with her coat on (behavior). Throughout cognitive therapy, therapists engage patients in a highly collaborative manner, minimizing resistance and sustaining the helping alliance.

This collaboration continues with the maintenance of a dysfunctional thought record in which patients track events, reactions to those events, and mediating beliefs. Most of these core beliefs pertain to the sense of being helpless (e.g., "I am incompetent," "I am trapped," "I am inferior") or unlovable (e.g., "I am ugly," "I am worthless," "I will be rejected") (Beck and Hindman 2018); patients then form schemas around these core beliefs that filter and color future perception, which creates cognitive distortions. The dysfunctional thought record enables therapists to create cognitive conceptualizations of patients, linking core beliefs to automatic thoughts, emotions, and behaviors. The record also helps patients observe their distortions as they are occurring and realize their role in maintaining presenting symptoms. From the observations of patients and therapists, a focus for intervention emerges that targets specific cognitive distortions.

Central to the cognitive restructuring therapies is a Socratic process of guided discovery between therapist and patient that questions these distortions and encourages a consideration of alternative explanations. What is the evidence for and against this idea? Is there an alternate explanation? What is the worst or best that could happen? How would you cope with the worst? What is the most realistic outcome? What is the effect of believing the automatic thought? What could be the effect of changing it? (Beck and Hindman 2018). This process also occurs between sessions because therapists encourage patients to use thought records to evaluate their own degree of belief in the distortions. Each dysfunctional thought pattern is viewed by therapist and patient as a hypothesis to be questioned and tested. Behavioral experiments devised during sessions are carried out between meetings to provide direct experiential tests of patient assumptions. The goal of this "collaborative empiricism" (Beck 2011) is to create vivid experiences of disconfirmation for patients that aid the building of new, accurate schemas (Table 31–4).

Learning Therapies: Comparison and Summary

Whereas the exposure therapies target specific conditioned responses for extinction, the cognitive restructuring therapies entail a comprehensive collaborative relationship between therapist and patient that evaluates and restructures a range of cognitive patterns. For this reason, as well as the differences between the therapies in the range of problems that they typically address, the exposure treatments can be briefer (fewer than 10 sessions) than the restructuring therapies (10–20 visits). Despite the differences in their specific methods, many similarities link these learning therapies. They are highly structured and focused, with active assignments during and between sessions. They seek to directly challenge and undercut the patterns that bring patients to therapy, achieving brevity by replacing verbal exploration with experiences of mastery and a reprocessing of emotional cues.

Contextual Therapies

The aforementioned relational and learning therapies begin with a common premise— that the presenting concerns of patients are acquired over the life span as the result of problematic experiences: faulty relationships or faulty learning. Both therapies, in that sense, place the locus of problems within the patient. Contextual brief therapies, on the other hand, do not view problems as intrinsic to patients. Rather, problems are seen as artifacts of person–situation interactions that, once identified, can be rapidly modified. Short-term couples therapies, for instance, view problem patterns as sustained by the reciprocal contributions of each partner (Baucom et al. 2012). Because difficulties are seen as situational, targeted problem-solving interventions to alter these situations make the contextual therapies among the briefest of therapies.

Strategic Therapy

Strategic therapies, including single-session treatments, view presenting concerns as the result of attempts at solutions that unwittingly reinforce the very problems patients are attempting to address. A person concerned about rejection in relationships, for instance, might interact in guarded ways, leading others to avoid future interaction. The problem, from the vantage point of the strategic therapist, is a function of the patient's construal of the situation and the ways in which that construal is reinforced through social interaction (Quick 2008). It can be resolved through skillful reframing that opens the door to new action alternatives (Watzlawick et al. 2011) and the creation of directed tasks (Levy and Shelton 1990) that disconfirm existing understandings. The goal of treatment is to catalyze initial change that patients can then

TABLE 31–4. **Differences between exposure and cognitive restructuring brief therapies**

	Exposure therapies	**Cognitive restructuring therapies**
View of presenting problems	Conditioned patterns of emotion and behavior triggered by internal and environmental cues	The result of information processing distortions arising from dysfunctional schemas
Goal of therapy	Deconditioning of patterns through skill enactment during exposure to symptom triggers	Challenging and replacing cognitive distortions with realistic, constructive alternatives
Therapist role	Directive teacher	Collaborative empiricist
Emphasized change mechanism	Firsthand experiences of mastery	Altered cognitive schemas
Structure	Brief, with circumscribed symptom focus; often manualized or highly structured	More extended, with broader focus; often manualized or highly structured

sustain on their own, not to effect fundamental changes of personality. For this reason, strategic therapies are intentionally brief.

The initial interview of strategic therapy is designed to identify current complaints of patients and their attempts at resolution. The therapist's conceptualization is neither a diagnosis nor a formulation of personality but a description of the current situational factors that help to maintain the patient's presenting concerns (Watzlawick et al. 2011). This description includes the people involved in the patient's concerns and the roles they take, the patient's view of the situation, the sequence of behaviors that result in the patient's complaints, and the specific contexts in which these complaints arise (Rosenbaum 1990). From this conceptualization, therapists gain an appreciation of the ways in which patients feel stuck in their attempts at resolution and can begin to generate ways of becoming unstuck.

As Rosenbaum (1990) emphasized, the goal of the therapy is not to find a solution for a patient's problem but to create a situation that lends itself to spontaneous goal attainment. Many times, fresh construals and solutions will result simply when old patterns are disrupted and patients behave in new and unpredictable ways (Quick 2008). The patient who is afraid of social interaction, for instance, will not interact with others if rejection is anticipated. That same patient, however, may view him- or herself to be a kind, sensitive person and will initiate interactions to help others. Such interactions offer the possibility of positive feedback and fresh incentives to seek out further social contact. By changing the patient's context—from being stuck in a pattern to enacting a strength—the therapist allows naturally occurring growth processes to take their own course. In that sense, strategic therapy is a process for removing barriers to change and not a self-contained change process in itself (Table 31–5).

Solution-Focused Therapy

An offshoot of strategic therapy, solution-focused brief therapy provides a somewhat different contextual approach to short-term change. Solution-focused brief therapists

TABLE 31–5.	Contextual models of brief therapy

Presenting complaints are the result of self-reinforcing problem–solution cycles.

Problems are a function of patients and their context, not internal to patients.

Goal of therapy is initiating change, not seeing it to completion.

Role of therapist is to structure experiences that undermine the stuck behavior of patients.

Therapy is highly abbreviated.

start from the premise that people are changing all the time, enacting solution patterns as well as problem ones (Ratner et al. 2012). Indeed, there is an important sense in this therapy in which problems do not exist at all. When patients cannot reach their goals, they at some point identify that they have a problem. This reification becomes self-fulfilling: the more patients focus on their problems, the more troubled they feel and act. Equally important, such a problem focus blinds patients to the occasions in which they do, in fact, reach their goals.

The aim of solution-focused brief therapy is to break this self-fulfilling conceptualization. The therapist accomplishes this by focusing on solution patterns rather than on problems. Thus, in the initial assessment therapists ask patients to identify positive pre-session changes and occasions during which problems either do not occur or occur less often or less intensely (Walter and Peller 1992). Enacting these exceptions to problem patterns—doing more of what is already working (O'Hanlon and Weiner-Davis 1989)—is the focus of therapy, not an analysis of core conflicts or a teaching of skills to remediate deficits. Because the therapy is not initiating new behavior and thought patterns but instead is building on existing ones, it tends to be highly targeted, lasting several sessions on average (Steenbarger 2018). A manualized version has demonstrated effectiveness across a variety of populations and presenting concerns (Franklin et al. 2011).

Several other factors contribute to the brevity of solution-focused therapy, including working within patient goals to minimize resistance, maintaining a tight solution focus, involving patients in between-session efforts to enact solution patterns, and having a high degree of therapist activity (Steenbarger 2018). The emphasis on patient strengths undercuts the cycle of problem-based thinking and stuck emotion and behavior. The focus on constructive change also paves the way for therapists and patients to frame goals in positive action terms that can be supported by directed homework tasks extending the solution patterns. Such goals can be formulated with minimal historical exploration, which further contributes to brevity.

Gingerich and Eisengart (2000) listed the specific techniques that facilitate solution-focused brief therapy:

- *A search for pre-session change:* This asks for patients to look out for changes that occur between the time of the initial phone call (usually their worst point) and the first session and zooms in on positive solutions that were used by the patient to make things a bit better.
- *Goal setting:* Goals come from the patient and are stated in a positive, active, here-and-now, specific, and attainable form ("I will reach out to others when I am depressed and will call two friends today").

- *Use of the miracle question:* "Suppose that one night, while you were asleep, there was a miracle, and this problem was solved. How would you know? What would be different? How would your husband know without your saying a word to him about it?" (de Shazer 1988, p. 5).
- *Use of scaling questions:* "On a scale from 1 to 10, where 1 is 'constantly arguing' and 10 is 'getting along perfectly,' on average, how would you rate your relationship over the past month?" (Steenbarger 2018).
- *A search for exceptions:* "No one argues every hour of the day. Tell me, what are you doing differently when you are not arguing or maybe even getting along?"
- *A message including compliments and a task:* Sessions end with the therapist providing a summary, praising the positive steps taken, and giving a specific task to be completed before the next session.

Steenbarger (2018) noted that a key assumption of solution-focused brief therapy is that exceptions to presented problem patterns often contain the kernel to solutions. For this reason, this therapy modality is closely aligned with positive psychology and approaches to helping that focus on the building of strengths. Because those kernels to solutions are present in all people, those seeking help are viewed as experts in their own care.

Contextual Therapies: Comparison and Summary

One way that solution-focused brief therapy differs from strategic brief therapies is that it lends itself to manualization. Such manuals (de Shazer 1988; Franklin et al. 2011; Ratner et al. 2012; Walter and Peller 1992) view therapy as a series of steps involving the identification of pre-session change, the formulation of solution-based goals, the use of the miracle question and scaling questions to elicit exceptions to patient complaints, the provision of feedback to support change, and the assignment of tasks to extend solution patterns (Table 31–6). Like strategic therapies, solution-focused therapy relies less on verbal exploration and more on direct experience to break circular patterns that interfere with the achievement of patient goals. The goal of both therapies is not so much to resolve a problem as it is to help patients see that what they thought was a problem was in fact a function of their punctuation of experience—their ways of construing themselves and the world.

Differences and Similarities Among the Brief Therapies

The foregoing discussion has focused on describing the major schools of brief therapy and highlighted the differences among these models. Therapists approaching patients from relational, learning, and contextual vantage points differ in their conceptualization of presenting problems and the procedures necessary to address these. These therapeutic modalities differ in other ways as well:

- *Scope*—Some of the brief therapies define a relatively wide set of goals; others are much more targeted. Short-term dynamic therapies, for instance, tackle broader relationship goals than does IPT; exposure therapies and the contextual variants

TABLE 31–6.   Differences between strategic and solution-focused brief therapies

	Strategic therapies	Solution-focused therapies
View of presenting problems	Attempted solutions to problems further reinforce those problems	De-emphasis of problems and emphasis on exceptions to problem patterns
Goal of therapy	Interruption of problem cycles and attempts to initiate new action patterns	Creating solution patterns out of exceptions to problem patterns
Therapist role	Facilitator of change through structured tasks and experiences	Facilitator of change through construction of solution patterns
Emphasized change mechanism	Reframing of problems and direct experiences of novel action patterns	Undermining of problem focus through enactment of solutions
Structure	Highly abbreviated but not highly structured	Highly abbreviated; often manualized or highly structured

are more tightly focused than are cognitive restructuring therapies. As might be expected, the treatments that are most narrowly gauged tend to be the briefest; the broader therapies tend to be of longer duration.

- *Degree of structure*—A subset of the brief therapies, including short-term dynamic therapy and strategic therapy, stress in-session experience as central to change. These therapies tend to feature deft use of the helping relationship and are difficult to capture in therapy manuals. Other short-term treatments, such as exposure work, cognitive restructuring therapy, and solution-focused brief therapy, rely heavily on between-session tasks as change elements. These tasks are relatively easy to standardize and codify in manuals.
- *Use of time in treatment*—A few of the brief treatments, such as IPT and the contextual therapies, are very explicitly brief and are frequently conducted in a time-limited mode, setting limits on the number of sessions at the outset. Other brief therapies, such as short-term psychodynamic work and cognitive restructuring, are time effective (Budman and Gurman 1988) but do not typically set upward bounds on the number of available sessions.
- *Nature of therapist activity*—Exposure therapy and the contextual therapies make extensive use of assigned tasks, placing the therapist in a directive role. The relational therapies feature a relative emphasis on exploration between therapist and patient, with less use of structured homework assignments.

Because of the described differences, we can conceptualize the brief therapies along a continuum, ranging from highly abbreviated and highly structured contextual therapies to more exploratory relational treatments. The briefest treatments emphasize that the patient's presenting complaints are artifacts of self-construal and can be addressed in the here and now through experiences that undermine those construals. These highly abbreviated therapies view patients as capable of growth and change and seek only to catalyze these naturally occurring processes. The more ex-

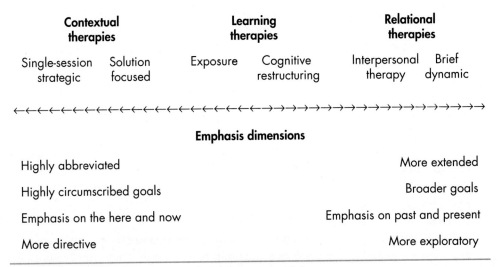

FIGURE 31–1. Differences among brief therapy models.

tended short-term therapies place presenting problems into a historical context and stress insight and corrective emotional experiences in a developed relationship as essential to change. Patients are viewed as caught in maladaptive relational patterns that are replayed across a variety of situations and thus need more than a change catalyst. Between these extremes, the learning therapies emphasize here-and-now unlearning of overlearned dysfunctional patterns and the acquisition of constructive alternatives through structured learning experiences (Figure 31–1).

Despite these evident differences, many underlying similarities among the brief therapies help to account for their brevity. It is not surprising that the brief therapies embody common ingredients (Greenberg 2018); a wealth of research (Lambert 2013; Wampold and Imel 2015) has found that factors shared by the various psychotherapies account for a significant proportion of the variance in patient change. A list of common factors across all psychotherapy models (both brief and longer term) typically would include the creation of a strong therapist-patient alliance, opportunities to confront and face problems, the development of patient mastery experiences, and the facilitation of patient hope and positive expectations about the future. Specific ingredients found across the short-term treatments include the following:

- *Brevity by design*—As Budman and Gurman (1988) first noted, brief therapies are brief by design, not by default. Time is an integral part of the treatment plan, regardless of whether the therapies are explicitly time limited or simply efficient in their use of time. Increasingly, this brevity by design is accomplished through the creation and use of treatment manuals that standardize helping approaches.
- *Creation and maintenance of a therapeutic focus*—Some of the short-term modalities are briefer than others, but all of them target focal patient patterns rather than attempting broader personality reconstruction. A major role of the therapist is to maintain this focus from session to session by guiding discussion and facilitating between-session efforts.
- *Selectivity*—To achieve brevity, therapists need to establish a rapid rapport with patients, which means that they must work with patients capable of forming a

quick alliance. Most brief therapies incorporate inclusion and exclusion criteria because patients with chronic and severe problem patterns frequently need more ongoing support than can be provided in short-term treatment.

- *Avoidance of resistance*—Many of the brief therapies include procedures designed to elicit the understanding and cooperation of patients, such as explicit efforts at education, the use of the patient's own language in framing goals, and the collaborative formulation of treatment goals. They aim to minimize resistance to change and sustain favorable expectations for outcome.
- *Activity*—Across the brief therapies, therapists take responsibility for initiating change efforts by providing new relationship experiences, teaching skills, and fostering contexts for new patterns of behavior. Patients in brief therapy are expected to explore problem patterns but also to tackle these actively through in-session experiences and between-session tasks and homework.
- *Enhanced patient experiencing*—The brief therapies emphasize the provision of new experiences, in and out of session, as facilitators of change. They supplement verbal explorations of presenting concerns with emotionally charged interventions.

Steenbarger (2002) suggested that the brief therapies have structural similarities characterized by a series of change stages (Table 31–7). Treatment begins with a period of engagement in which patient and therapist forge a working alliance that engages the patient's desire for change and mutually creates targets for change efforts. Central to the formation of this alliance is a translation of patients' presenting complaints into the language of a particular therapeutic approach, enabling patients to perceive their problems in a new light and fashion fresh possibilities for change. Therapy then draws on the procedures of the particular approach to create discrepant experiences that challenge old patterns of thought and behavior, facilitating new understandings and action patterns. The final phase of therapy seeks to consolidate these new understandings and skills by generalizing them to a variety of situations, thus cementing an internalization of new patterns and helping to prevent relapse. The brief therapies, from this vantage point, may be viewed as devices for generating novel experiences in the context of enhanced experiencing (Steenbarger 2006), accelerating learning processes that occur in all short-term modalities.

Research Pertaining to Brief Therapy and Its Effectiveness

An impressive body of research documents the effectiveness of psychotherapy across a variety of presenting problems (Lambert 2013; Roth and Fonagy 2006) and the importance of psychosocial factors even in psychopharmacological treatment (Greenberg 2016). This is relevant to brief therapy because most treatments that have been tested for efficacy—including the manualized therapies commonly used in controlled, double-blind outcome studies—are short term. Indeed, it would not be an exaggeration to say that most of the studies on psychotherapy outcomes are investigations of the effectiveness of short-term therapies. This is partly because cognitive and behavioral therapies dominate the outcome literature (Roth and Fonagy 2006), al-

TABLE 31–7.   **Structural elements common to the brief therapies**

Engagement

  Rapid formation of a therapeutic alliance and translation of presenting problems into focal goals

Discrepancy

  Provision of novel skills, insights, and experiences that challenge patient patterns and facilitate new understandings and actions

Consolidation

  Rehearsal of new patterns in varied contexts, accompanied by feedback, to ensure internalization and relapse prevention

though a sizable body of studies does support the effectiveness of short-term dynamic therapy, IPT, and solution-focused brief therapy (Dewan et al. 2018).

Research on Time and Outcome in Psychotherapy

A review of duration and outcome in therapy (Lambert 2013; Steenbarger 1994) observed that this relation is complicated by several factors:

- *The patient population*—If we plotted change in psychotherapy as a function of time, the curve would look different for patients with personality disorders and chronic, severe presenting problems than for those with more recent and less severe Axis I concerns (Howard et al. 1986). In general, outcomes are more slowly achieved among patients with significant psychiatric disorders than among less impaired individuals (Lambert 2013).
- *The outcome measures used*—Measures of patient well-being and symptom relief typically show change before measures of functional improvement do (Steenbarger 1994); as Lambert (2013) observed in his review, the dosage of therapy needed to reach a level of success depends on the success criterion chosen. It is quite possible that brief therapies differ in their time/outcome curves simply as a function of selecting different targets for change. The relational therapies, in particular, tend to focus on functional change as a criterion of improvement, whereas behavioral therapies are more likely to emphasize symptom change.
- *The time at which change is measured*—The goal of psychotherapy, brief and otherwise, is to foster lasting change, not just improvement from the beginning of treatment to the end. The duration/outcome equation looks far more favorable for all therapies when outcomes are measured at termination rather than at longer-term follow-up periods. This is particularly the case for disorders that have high known rates of relapse, such as major depressive disorder and substance use disorders (Roth and Fonagy 2006). Although several studies support the long-term effectiveness of IPT and cognitive-behavioral therapies (Lambert 2013), data also suggest that highly abbreviated treatments may run an enhanced risk of patient relapse (Steenbarger 1994) and that ongoing maintenance sessions can be effective in reducing relapse rates (Lambert 2013) and improving long-term outcome.

Early investigations of the dose–effect relation in psychotherapy found that approximately 50% of patients experience significant improvement within 8 sessions of therapy; 75% reach such improvement within 26 sessions (Howard et al. 1986). More recent research reviewed by Castonguay et al. (2013) found that clinically significant change occurs in half of all patients within 11–18 sessions. Similarly, Lambert's (2013) review noted that limiting sessions to fewer than 20 would mean that 50% of patients would not achieve significant gains from treatment. Clearly, many patients, but far from all, benefit from brevity. Indeed, it appears that both patients and therapists are sensitive to good-enough levels of change, such that therapy lasts as long as needed to achieve initial aims (Lambert 2013). This suggests that no single dose–effect curve describes the relation between time and change across all patients. It is safe to say, however, that if the goal of treatment is sustained functional change, most individuals meeting DSM diagnostic criteria would require more time for change than is typically afforded by the briefest treatment models.

Patient Selection Criteria

These findings highlight the importance of patient selection in the conduct of brief therapy. The dose–effect research suggests some of the following inclusion criteria:

- *Duration of presenting problems*—Chronic emotional and behavioral patterns are likely to have been overlearned and thus are more likely to require ongoing intervention than are problems of more recent origin (Steenbarger 2002).
- *Interpersonal functioning*—Given the importance of the therapeutic alliance to change across all psychotherapies (Crits-Christoph et al. 2013; Lambert and Barley 2002), it is unlikely that patients with poor interpersonal functioning and difficulties sustaining relationships will benefit from brief intervention. Indeed, they may need many sessions before they can even forge a trusting relationship.
- *Severity of presenting problems*—As noted earlier, most patients with severe presenting concerns and characterological and interpersonal problems (Lambert 2013) do not achieve clinically significant outcomes in a brief time frame. This is particularly the case when the severity of presenting symptoms prevents patients from actively engaging in within-session and between-session change efforts. When presenting problems are not overwhelming, patients are more likely to be able to tolerate the added discomfort of change efforts.
- *Complexity of presenting problems*—Some problems brought to therapy, such as phobias, are relatively simple, manifesting in limited ways in limited situations. Other problems, such as eating disorders, are highly complex, with manifestations cutting across mood, interpersonal functioning, and self-concept. A perusal of the outcome literature (Roth and Fonagy 2006) suggests that therapeutic outcomes are more favorable for less complex concerns, probably because targets for treatment can be more narrowly circumscribed. Many complex concerns, such as eating and substance use disorders, have high relapse rates that, in themselves, might require ongoing maintenance therapy and other extensions of treatment duration.
- *Understanding of the need for change*—Prochaska and Norcross (2002) found that the course of therapy is different for patients who have a clear understanding and acceptance of their problems and the need for change than for patients who lack

TABLE 31–8.	Patient selection criteria predictive of success in brief therapy (DISCUS)

Duration of presenting problems: Brief

Interpersonal functioning: Good, able to quickly form a trusting relationship

Severity of presenting problems: Mild to moderate

Complexity of presenting problems: Limited, circumscribed, with low relapse potential

Understanding of the need for change: Ready to take action

Social supports: Strong and easily accessible

such understanding. Patients in an action phase of readiness for change are much more likely to embrace the change techniques of brief treatment than are patients in precontemplative or contemplative modes. These latter groups, in fact, may require numerous sessions of problem exploration before they even acknowledge a need for change, and then targeted goals for treatment can be formulated.

- *Social supports*—When patients have weak or nonexistent social supports, they may look to therapy for support as well as for targeted change. In those cases, they are unlikely to embrace time limits on treatment. Brief therapy is most likely to proceed smoothly and without resistance if it is conducted with patients whose goals include rapid and targeted change.

These listed criteria, which form the acronym *DISCUS* (Table 31–8), can be useful during initial interviews in determining the likelihood that treatment changes will be achieved within a brief time frame. This can be helpful in settings such as community mental health centers, managed health care plans, and college and university counseling centers, which must rationally allocate scarce treatment resources to the treatment needs of a population. The criteria also suggest that firm, brief time limits on treatment for all patients are likely to prove ineffective for a significant proportion of the population. Patients with chronic, severe, and complex presenting concerns are much more likely to require extended intervention than are patients with recent, nonsevere, and simple presentations. Similarly, brief treatments are likely to be most relevant to patients with a high readiness for change and problems with low rates of relapse.

Nevertheless, brief therapy techniques may still prove useful in the conduct of ongoing psychotherapy. Cummings and Sayama (1995) made a compelling case for intermittent brief therapy throughout the life cycle, so that the benefits of focused change are blended with the benefits of longer-term assistance. Marsha Linehan's dialectical behavior therapy (Wilks and Linehan 2018), which uses sequential short-term cognitive-behavioral interventions in the treatment of personality disorders, illustrates one way in which brevity may be compatible with longer-term assistance. Indeed, a close investigation of dialectical behavior therapy (Wilks and Linehan 2018) found that patients could benefit from distinct skill-building modules in areas such as mindfulness, interpersonal effectiveness, and emotion regulation. More research is needed to determine the promise and limits of sequential short-term interventions in the treatment of pervasive psychiatric disorders, particularly in light of findings that outcomes for many disorders are enhanced by the combination of brief therapies with psychopharmacological intervention (Dewan 2018; Thase and Jindal 2004).

What Works in Brief Therapy?

As mentioned earlier, a large body of research suggests that the ingredients common to the psychotherapies are more important than their specific interventions in generating clinical outcomes (Greenberg 2018; Wampold and Imel 2015). These common effective ingredients include the quality of the therapeutic relationship (Crits-Christoph et al. 2013; Lambert and Barley 2002); patient expectations, readiness for change, and capacity for attachment (Clarkin and Levy 2004; Greenberg et al. 2006); and therapist ability to engage patients in a constructive manner (Beutler et al. 2004). Bateman and Fonagy (2018) made a strong case for mentalizing as an overarching common factor among psychotherapies, as each modality helps patients represent and differentiate the mind states of self and others. From this perspective, the brief therapies represent active interventions in which the therapeutic relationship provides a fresh opportunity for attachment, through which mentalizing can develop. A vexing finding in the psychotherapy literature is that researchers who champion specific treatment approaches consistently report more favorable results from their approaches than do researchers who do not champion specific approaches (Wampold and Imel 2015). This allegiance effect likely speaks to the role of the therapist's, as well as the patient's, expectations in generating outcomes. Indeed, when outcome studies have sought to eliminate allegiance as an outcome factor and limit outcome variance to specific treatment effects by requiring strict adherence to therapy manuals, the benefits of psychotherapy have been attenuated (Wampold and Imel 2015).

Given these findings, the brief therapies likely achieve their results by 1) intensifying the change ingredients found among all therapies, including longer-term ones (Steenbarger 2002), and 2) limiting application of short-term methods to patient populations most likely to benefit from psychosocial interventions. Lambert and Archer (2006) reported that patients who benefited from the initial sessions of therapy were most likely to have favorable outcomes by the end of treatment and at follow-up periods. This is significant because it suggests that the course and outcome are determined before most of the procedures that distinguish the various therapeutic schools have been initiated.

Among the brief therapies, therapists' skill factors—their ability to facilitate and sustain a treatment focus and their ability to provide novel experiences for patients—may be more important than the specific methods they use (Baldwin and Imel 2013). Lambert and Archer (2006) observed that therapists who are given feedback about the progress of their poor-prognosis patients early in treatment have more favorable outcomes than do therapists who are not given feedback. This points to skill factors among therapists as potential mediators of outcome. A detailed analysis by Wampold and Imel (2015) indicated that therapist competence accounts for greater treatment variance than do specific treatments themselves. Indeed, when outcome studies have assigned therapists to multiple treatments, competent therapists tended to have significantly better outcomes than did less competent ones, regardless of the treatment modality.

Finally, this research suggests that the factors that make therapy efficient are not entirely separable from those that make therapy effective. It may not be far wrong to assert that therapy is most likely to be brief when it is performed skillfully with patients most open to, and likely to benefit from, psychosocial intervention. The skills that make for successful treatment—the ability to foster novel experiences of self and others in an emotionally charged context via the medium of a supportive alliance—appear to be equally essential to brevity.

Recent Advances in Brief Therapy

Steenbarger (1993) described tensions that exist between brief therapy models and multicultural approaches to therapy that require a delving into the meaning systems of patients. He described a multicontextual approach to helping that delineates change targets and approaches those in time-effective ways. Aggarwal and Lewis-Fernandez (2018) extended this integration and showed how a cultural formulation interview can deepen our understanding of patients and contribute toward a stronger alliance. Indeed, their review found significantly better outcomes among culturally trained therapies over their nonadapted counterparts, leading them to emphasize the role of the patient as an expert in his or her treatment. This is particularly notable in solution-focused brief therapy, which looks to build upon the unique strengths of patients. In fostering a superior alliance and avoiding potential sources of resistance, cultural awareness appears to contribute to both the efficacy and the efficiency of psychotherapy. This is a promising area of future research, practice, and training.

The tremendous expansion of the online medium has led to the development of new models of delivery for brief psychotherapies. Yellowlees (2018) reported positive brief therapy outcomes via telepsychiatry, where visits occur via videoconferencing. The online medium has proven user friendly, convenient, and safe for patients, thereby enhancing the therapeutic alliance. Hybrid approaches, combining in-person and online contacts, help maintain the continuity of therapy, maximizing total contact even within a brief number of face-to-face sessions. Andersson and Carlbring (2018) reviewed promising developments in Internet-based therapy, in which treatment manuals are available online for self-directed treatment. Weekly contact with a therapist enhances compliance and outcome, but those contacts can be delivered in a number of ways, from chat and video to in-person meetings. The authors noted that Internet-based treatments tend to be focused and time limited, lending themselves well to brief formats, such as cognitive-behavioral therapies. A major advantage of such self-directed therapies is their availability 24/7 and the ability to access treatment from any geographic locale. The combination of manualized, evidence-based, self-directed therapies with ongoing online and in-person contact in a therapeutic relationship represents a fresh development in time-effective treatment.

Finally, ongoing work in the area of motivational interviewing (Paris and Martino 2018) is extending brief interventions to populations not yet in an action state of readiness for change. As in the case of dialectical behavior therapy applied to borderline personality disorder (Wilks and Linehan 2018), motivational interviewing applies sequential short-term interventions in the area of addictions to facilitate ongoing contact and progress. The use of sequential, highly structured brief therapies for the ongoing treatment of conditions not traditionally considered appropriate for short-term intervention is yet another promising development.

Conclusion

Seeking to make psychotherapy treatment more efficient, innovative psychoanalysts originally presented the key components of brief therapy. They stressed narrowed patient inclusion criteria, narrowed treatment focus, an active therapist, a limit on time and/or number of sessions, and facilitation of corrective emotional experiences. Building on dynamic tradition, behaviorists, cognitive therapists, and strategic therapists went on to develop three broad models of brief therapy based on their understanding about the causes of presenting problems and the techniques necessary to alter them. *Relational therapies,* which assume that presenting symptoms are a result of problems with significant relationships, include brief psychodynamic therapies and interpersonal therapy. *Learning therapies,* such as behavior therapies and cognitive therapy, view symptoms as arising from maladaptive learned behavior patterns that can be unlearned. *Contextual therapies* place the emphasis on ways in which presenting problems are situated within—and sustained by—their psychosocial contexts. Strategic therapies and solution-focused therapy are major models of contextual therapy.

Studies find that therapy is often brief by default due to patient dropout, restricted coverage, therapeutic rupture, and so on. This chapter provides guidelines for therapies that are brief by design. Brief therapies vary from single-session approaches and very brief strategic treatments to dynamic interventions that often exceed 20 sessions. Behavioral and cognitive therapies are of intermediate duration. Manuals developed by several treatment schools have made it easier to practice these techniques with fidelity and to conduct research. Indeed, most psychotherapy research is focused on brief therapy and clearly supports the efficacy of brief therapy approaches for a broad range of patients. As a result of the growth of brief therapy models, manuals, and research evidence, in association with fiscal constraints and demonstrated positive patient outcomes, brief therapy has become the norm for the majority of today's patients. New models of service delivery, focused on integrating the online medium, building upon cultural training to further the alliance, and integrating multiple short-term therapies in the treatment of more severe and complex conditions, promise further advances in brief therapy.

Key Clinical Points

- Brief therapy consists of a group of approaches to psychotherapy that include short-term psychodynamic, interpersonal, behavioral, cognitive, strategic, and solution-focused modalities.

- The various brief therapies differ in their average treatment duration (generally defined as fewer than 24 sessions or less than 6 months), their targets for change, and their assumptions regarding change processes.

- Several common ingredients link the brief therapies, including a circumscribed treatment focus, increased therapist and patient activity, an emphasis on generating novel experiences, and restricted patient inclusion criteria.

- Brief therapies overall are effective but are most likely to benefit patients who are ready for change and who present concerns that are recent, nonsevere, and simple. Patients with severe, chronic disorders benefit from specific, targeted treatments.

- Although a sizable proportion of patients can benefit from short-term treatment, the relation between time and change is complex, mediated by the nature of the outcomes measured, the time at which progress is assessed, and the degree of patient impairment.

- Brief therapies appear to be effective to the degree that they intensify the common factors that account for change across all therapies.

- Brief therapies can also be provided effectively via televideo and more autonomously over the Internet.

References

Aggarwal NK, Lewis-Fernandez R: Integrating culture and psychotherapy through the DSM-5 Cultural Formulation Interview, in The Art and Science of Brief Psychotherapies: An Illustrated Guide, 3rd Edition. Edited by Dewan MJ, Steenbarger BN, Greenberg RP. Washington, DC, American Psychiatric Association Publishing, 2018, pp 39–56

Alexander F, French TM: Psychoanalytic Therapy: Principles and Application. Oxford, UK, Ronald Press, 1946

Andersson G, Carlbring P: Internet-based brief therapies, in The Art and Science of Brief Psychotherapies: An Illustrated Guide, 3rd Edition. Edited by Dewan MJ, Steenbarger BN, Greenberg RP. Washington, DC, American Psychiatric Association Publishing, 2018, pp 315–326

Baldwin SA, Imel ZE: Therapist effects: findings and methods, in Bergin and Garfield's Handbook of Psychotherapy and Behavior Change, 6th Edition. Edited by Lambert MJ. Hoboken, NJ, Wiley, 2013, pp 258–297

Barlow D: Anxiety and Its Disorders: The Nature and Treatment of Anxiety and Panic, 2nd Edition. New York, Guilford, 2002

Barlow D, Farchione TJ (eds): Applications of the Unified Protocol for Transdiagnostic Treatment of Emotional Disorders. New York, Oxford University Press, 2017

Bateman AW, Fonagy P: Mentalizing as a common factor in psychotherapy, in The Art and Science of Brief Psychotherapies: An Illustrated Guide, 3rd Edition. Edited by Dewan MI, Steenbarger BN, Greenberg RP. Washington, DC, American Psychiatric Association Publishing, 2018, pp 29–38

Baucom DH, Epstein NB, Sullivan LJ: Brief couple therapy, in The Art and Science of Brief Psychotherapies: An Illustrated Guide, 2nd Edition. Edited by Dewan MJ, Steenbarger BN, Greenberg RP. Washington, DC, American Psychiatric Publishing, 2012, pp 239–276

Beck AT: Cognitive Therapy and the Emotional Disorders. New York, International Universities Press, 1976

Beck AT, Freedman A, Davis D, et al: Cognitive Therapy of Personality Disorders, 2nd Edition. New York, Guilford, 2004

Beck JS: Cognitive Therapy: Basics and Beyond, 2nd Edition. New York, Guilford, 2011

Beck JS, Hindman R: Cognitive therapy, in The Art and Science of Brief Psychotherapies: An Illustrated Guide, 3rd Edition. Edited by Dewan MJ, Steenbarger BN, Greenberg RP. Washington, DC, American Psychiatric Association Publishing, 2018, pp 97–134

Beutler LE, Malik M, Alimohamed S, et al: Therapist variables, in Bergin and Garfield's Handbook of Psychotherapy and Behavior Change, 5th Edition. Edited by Lambert MJ. New York, Wiley, 2004, pp 227–306

Binder JL: Key Competencies in Brief Dynamic Psychotherapy: Clinical Practice Beyond the Manual. New York, Guilford, 2010

Binder JL, Strupp HH: The Vanderbilt approach to time-limited dynamic psychotherapy, in Handbook of Short-Term Dynamic Psychotherapy. Edited by Crits-Christoph P, Barber JP. New York, Basic Books, 1991, pp 137–165

Breuer J, Freud S: Studies in hysteria (1893–1895), in The Standard Edition of the Complete Psychological Works of Sigmund Freud, Vol 2. Translated and edited by Strachey J (in collaboration with Freud A). London, Hogarth Press, 1955, pp 1–311

Budman SH, Gurman AS: Theory and Practice of Brief Therapy. New York, Guilford, 1988

Castonguay L, Barkham M, Lutz N, et al: Practice oriented research, in Handbook of Psychotherapy and Behavior Change, 6th Edition. Edited by Lambert M. New York, Wiley, 2013, pp 85–133

Clarkin JF, Levy KN: The influence of client variables on psychotherapy, in Bergin and Garfield's Handbook of Psychotherapy and Behavior Change, 5th Edition. Edited by Lambert MJ. New York, Wiley, 2004, pp 194–226

Crits-Christoph P, Gibbons MBC, Mukherjee D: Psychotherapy process-outcome research, in Bergin and Garfield's Handbook of Psychotherapy and Behavior Change, 6th Edition. Edited by Lambert MJ. Hoboken, NJ, Wiley, 2013, pp 298–340

Cummings N, Sayama M: Focused Psychotherapy: A Casebook of Brief, Intermittent Psychotherapy Throughout the Life Cycle. New York, Brunner/Mazel, 1995

Davanloo H: Short-Term Dynamic Psychotherapy. New York, Jason Aronson, 1980

de Shazer S: Clues: Investigating Solutions in Brief Therapy. New York, WW Norton, 1988

Dewan MJ: Combining brief psychotherapy and medications, in The Art and Science of Brief Psychotherapies: An Illustrated Guide, 3rd Edition. Edited by Dewan MJ, Steenbarger BN, Greenberg RP. Washington, DC, American Psychiatric Association Publishing, 2018, pp 57–66

Dewan MJ, Steenbarger BN, Greenberg RP: Brief psychotherapies, in Essentials of Psychiatry, 3rd Edition. Edited by Hales RE, Yudofsky SC, Gabbard GO. Washington, DC, American Psychiatric Publishing, 2011, pp 525–539

Dewan MJ, Steenbarger BN, Greenberg RP (eds): The Art and Science of Brief Psychotherapies: An Illustrated Guide, 3rd Edition. Washington, DC, American Psychiatric Publishing, 2018

Fisher S, Greenberg RP: The Scientific Credibility of Freud's Theories and Therapy. New York, Columbia University Press, 1985

Fisher S, Greenberg RP: Freud Scientifically Reappraised: Testing the Theories and Therapy. New York, Wiley, 1996

Franklin C, Trepper TS, McCollum EE, et al (eds): Solution-Focused Brief Therapy: A Handbook of Evidence-Based Practice. New York, Oxford University Press, 2011

Gallagher T, Hembree EA, Gillihan SJ, et al: Exposure therapy for anxiety disorders, OCD, and PTSD, in The Art and Science of Brief Psychotherapies: An Illustrated Guide, 3rd Edition. Edited by Dewan MJ, Steenbarger BN, Greenberg RP. Washington, DC, American Psychiatric Association Publishing, 2018, pp 135–172

Gingerich WJ, Eisengart S: Solution-focused brief therapy: a review of the outcome research. Fam Process 39(4):477–498, 2000 11143600

Greenberg RP: The rebirth of psychosocial importance in a drug-filled world. Am Psychol 71(8):781–791, 2016 27977264

Greenberg RP: Essential ingredients for successful psychotherapy: effect of common factors, in The Art and Science of Brief Psychotherapies: An Illustrated Guide, 3rd Edition. Edited by Dewan MJ, Steenbarger BN, Greenberg RP. Washington, DC, American Psychiatric Association Publishing, 2018, pp 17–28

Greenberg RP, Constantino MJ, Bruce N: Are patient expectations still relevant for psychotherapy process and outcome? Clin Psychol Rev 26(6):657–678, 2006 15908088

Hollon SD, Beck AT: Cognitive and cognitive-behavioral therapies, in Bergin and Garfield's Handbook of Psychotherapy and Behavior Change, 5th Edition. Edited by Lambert MJ. New York, Wiley, 2004, pp 447–492

Howard KI, Kopta SM, Krause MS, et al: The dose-effect relationship in psychotherapy. Am Psychol 41(2):159–164, 1986 3516036

Lambert MJ: The efficacy and effectiveness of psychotherapy, in Bergin and Garfield's Handbook of Psychotherapy and Behavior Change, 6th Edition. Edited by Lambert MJ. Hoboken, NJ, Wiley, 2013, pp 169–218

Lambert MJ, Archer A: Research findings on the effects of psychotherapy and their implications for practice, in Evidence-Based Psychotherapy: Where Practice and Research Meet. Edited by Goodheart CD, Kazdin AE, Sternberg RJ. Washington, DC, American Psychological Association, 2006, pp 111–130

Lambert MJ, Barley DE: Research summary on the therapeutic relationship and psychotherapy outcome, in Psychotherapy Relationships That Work: Therapist Contributions and Responsiveness to Patients. Edited by Norcross JC. New York, Oxford University Press, 2002, pp 17–36

Levenson H: Time-limited dynamic psychotherapy: an integrative perspective, in The Art and Science of Brief Psychotherapies: An Illustrated Guide, 3rd Edition. Edited by Dewan MJ, Steenbarger BN, Greenberg RP. Washington, DC, American Psychiatric Publishing, 2018, pp 259–300

Levenson H: Brief Dynamic Therapy, 2nd Edition. Washington, DC, American Psychological Association, 2017

Levy RL, Shelton JL: Tasks in brief therapy, in Handbook of Brief Therapies. Edited by Wells RA, Giannetti VJ. New York, Plenum, 1990, pp 145–164

Linehan MM: DBT Skills Training Manual, 2nd Edition. New York, Guilford, 2014

Luborsky L, Mark D: Short-term supportive-expressive psychoanalytic psychotherapy, in Handbook of Short-Term Dynamic Psychotherapy. Edited by Crits-Christoph P, Barber JP. New York, Basic Books, 1991, pp 110–136

O'Hanlon W, Weiner-Davis J: In Search of Solution: A New Direction in Psychotherapy. New York, WW Norton, 1989

Paris M, Martino S: Motivational interviewing, in The Art and Science of Brief Psychotherapies: An Illustrated Guide, 3rd Edition. Edited by Dewan MJ, Steenbarger BN, Greenberg RP. Washington, DC, American Psychiatric Association Publishing, 2018, pp 69–96

Prochaska JO, Norcross JC: Stages of change, in Psychotherapy Relationships That Work: Therapist Contributions and Responsiveness to Patients. Edited by Norcross JC. New York, Oxford University Press, 2002, pp 303–314

Quick EK: Doing What Works in Brief Psychotherapy, 2nd Edition. Burlington, MA, Elsevier, 2008

Ratner H, George E, Iveson C: Solution Focused Brief Therapy: 100 Key Points and Techniques. New York, Routledge, 2012

Rosenbaum R: Strategic psychotherapy, in Handbook of the Brief Psychotherapies. Edited by Wells RA, Giannetti VJ. New York, Plenum, 1990, pp 351–404

Roth A, Fonagy P: What Works for Whom? A Critical Review of Psychotherapy Research, 2nd Edition. New York, Guilford, 2006

Shapiro F: Eye Movement Desensitization and Reprocessing: Basic Principles, Protocols, and Procedures, 2nd Edition. New York, Guilford, 2001

Sifneos PE: Short-Term Psychotherapy and Emotional Crisis. Cambridge, MA, Harvard University Press, 1972

Steenbarger BN: A multicontextual model of counseling: bridging brevity and diversity. Journal of Counseling and Development 72(1):8–15, 1993

Steenbarger BN: Duration and outcome in psychotherapy: an integrative review. Professional Psychology: Research and Practice 25(2):111–119, 1994

Steenbarger BN: Brief therapy, in Encyclopedia of Psychotherapy, Vol 1. Edited by Hersen M, Sledge W. New York, Elsevier, 2002, pp 349–358

Steenbarger BN: The importance of novelty in psychotherapy, in Clinical Strategies for Becoming a Master Psychotherapist. Edited by O'Donohue W, Cummings NA, Cummings JL. New York, Academic Press, 2006, pp 278–293

Steenbarger BN: Solution-focused brief therapy: building strengths, achieving goals, in The Art and Science of Brief Psychotherapies: An Illustrated Guide, 3rd Edition. Edited by Dewan MJ, Steenbarger BN, Greenberg RP. Washington, DC, American Psychiatric Association Publishing, 2018, pp 199–218

Stuart S: Interpersonal psychotherapy, in The Art and Science of Brief Psychotherapies: An Illustrated Guide, 3rd Edition. Edited by Dewan MJ, Steenbarger BN, Greenberg RP. Washington, DC, American Psychiatric Publishing, 2018, pp 219–258

Thase ME, Jindal RD: Combining psychotherapy and psychopharmacology for treatment of mental disorders, in Bergin and Garfield's Handbook of Psychotherapy and Behavior Change, 5th Edition. Edited by Lambert MJ. New York, Wiley, 2004, pp 743–766

Wallerstein RS: The psychotherapy research project of the Menninger Foundation: an overview. J Consult Clin Psychol 57(2):195–205, 1989 2708605

Walter JL, Peller JE: Becoming Solution-Focused in Brief Therapy. New York, Brunner/Mazel, 1992

Wampold BE, Imel ZE: The Great Psychotherapy Debate: The Evidence for What Makes Psychotherapy Work, 2nd Edition. New York, Routledge, 2015

Watzlawick P, Weakland H, Fisch R: Change: Principles of Problem Formation and Problem Resolution. New York, WW Norton, 1974

Watzlawick P, Weakland H, Fisch R: Change: Principles of Problem Formation and Problem Resolution, Reprint Edition. New York, WW Norton, 2011

Wilks CR, Linehan MM: Application and techniques of dialectical behavior therapy, in The Art and Science of Brief Psychotherapies: An Illustrated Guide, 3rd Edition. Edited by Dewan MJ, Steenbarger BN, Greenberg RP. Washington, DC, American Psychiatric Association Publishing, 2018, pp 173–198

Wolpe J: Psychotherapy by Reciprocal Inhibition. Stanford, CA, Stanford University Press, 1958

Wright J, Sudak D, Turkington D, et al: High-Yield Cognitive-Behavior Therapy for Brief Sessions. Washington, DC, American Psychiatric Publishing, 2010

Yellowlees P: Telepsychiatry, in The Art and Science of Brief Psychotherapies: An Illustrated Guide, 3rd Edition. Edited by Dewan MJ, Steenbarger BN, Greenberg RP. Washington, DC, American Psychiatric Association Publishing, 2018, pp 303–314

Recommended Readings

Barlow DH: Clinical Handbook of Psychological Disorders, 3rd Edition. New York, Guilford, 2001

Beck JS: Cognitive Behavior Therapy: Basics and Beyond, 2nd Edition. New York, Guilford, 2011

Dewan MJ, Steenbarger BN, Greenberg RP: The Art and Science of Brief Psychotherapies: An Illustrated Guide, 3rd Edition. Washington, DC, American Psychiatric Association Publishing, 2018

Levenson H: Brief Dynamic Therapy, 2nd Edition. Washington, DC, American Psychological Association, 2017

Stuart S: Interpersonal Psychotherapy: A Clinician's Guide, 3rd Edition. London, Taylor and Francis, 2017

Walter JL, Peller JE: Becoming Solution-Focused in Brief Therapy. New York, Brunner/Mazel, 1992

Online Resources

Academy of Cognitive Therapy: www.academyofct.org
Association of Advancement of Behavior Therapy/Association for Behavioral and Cognitive Therapies: www.abct.org
International Society for Interpersonal Psychotherapy: www.interpersonalpsychotherapy.org
Society for Psychotherapy Research: www.psychotherapyresearch.org
Solution Focused Brief Therapy Association: www.sfbta.org

CHAPTER 32

Psychodynamic Psychotherapy

Eve Caligor, M.D.

John F. Clarkin, Ph.D.

Frank E. Yeomans, M.D., Ph.D.

Otto F. Kernberg, M.D.

Psychodynamic psychotherapy refers not to a single treatment, but rather—like cognitive-behavioral therapy (CBT)—to a family of therapies embedded in a shared model of mental functioning. Psychodynamics offer clinicians an approach to psychiatric disorders that focuses on the complex interplay of mental processes within each individual patient; psychodynamic approaches view the mind as in flux and as capable of changing. Different forms of psychodynamic therapy have different goals, ranging from ameliorating symptoms (e.g., depression or anxiety) to enhancing adaptation in a focal area of functioning (e.g., improving interpersonal functioning, reducing passivity) to improving overall personality functioning (e.g., resolution of borderline personality disorder). As a group, psychodynamic treatments aim to enhance the patient's awareness of the thoughts, feelings, and behaviors underlying the difficulties that bring the patient to treatment.

In an effort to define psychodynamic treatment, Blagys and Hilsenroth (2000) compared the interventions of psychodynamic therapists with those of therapists providing CBT. The psychodynamic treatments were distinguished on the basis of 1) a focus on affect and emotional expression; 2) identification of recurring patterns of behavior, feelings, experiences, and relationships; 3) a focus on interpersonal relationships; 4) exploration of the therapeutic relationship; 5) exploration of the patient's tendency to defend against and avoid certain issues; and 6) exploration of wishes, dreams, and fantasies.

Although other forms of psychotherapy may make use of some of these interventions, and not all psychodynamic treatments focus equally on all of these techniques, in concert, this constellation distinguishes psychodynamic treatments as a group from other treatment approaches. With time and the gathering of empirical evidence, there is a trend toward gradual convergence among different psychotherapeutic approaches (Wachtel 2008) as different forms of treatment incorporate aspects of clinical intervention that prove effective across treatments. As a result, even though we emphasize distinguishing features of psychodynamic treatments in this chapter, much is shared with other psychotherapeutic approaches—for example, focusing on developing a therapeutic alliance, striving to understand the patient's view and perspective, and helping the patient to confront his or her difficulties (so-called common factors).

Description of *psychodynamic psychotherapy* is complicated by the many different forms of this approach, including short-term, long-term, individual, couples, and group treatments for adults and those for children and adolescents. Furthermore, dynamic treatments are delivered in a variety of settings, including outpatient mental health clinics and private practice offices, psychiatric inpatient or day hospital units, and medical inpatient units. Psychodynamic treatments are often combined with other therapeutic modalities, including pharmacotherapy, self-help groups, and certain CBT-informed interventions (e.g., harm reduction). Given constraints of space, we focus in this chapter on individual, or dyadic, psychodynamic treatments for adults and as much as possible on those treatment approaches supported by an evidence base.

Dimensions along which different individual psychodynamic approaches can be characterized include 1) focus of treatment (symptom relief, improvement in a focal area of functioning, personality change), 2) treatment frame (duration of treatment, which can range from several sessions to several years; frequency of sessions, typically once or twice weekly; whether treatment is time limited, with total number of sessions specified before treatment begins, or open ended), 3) relative emphasis placed on supportive in contrast to exploratory interventions, and 4) management of the therapeutic relationship, including the therapist's stance and use of transference.

Basic Assumptions of the Psychodynamic Model

Every form of psychotherapy is embedded within a specific model of psychological functioning. Basic concepts and theoretical perspectives shared by psychodynamic therapies include

- *Treatment of the patient as a unique individual:* Presenting complaints are assessed and understood in the context of the whole person. The psychodynamic therapist seeks to understand each patient as an individual, with attention to personal strengths and vulnerabilities, in the context of the patient's social and interpersonal milieu, biological predispositions, personality organization, and internalized relationship patterns.
- *Recognition of complexity:* Symptoms and maladaptive personality functioning that bring the patient to treatment are understood as emerging from a complex interplay of psychological, biological, and social factors that may shift in relative influence over time and in different contexts.
- *Psychological causation and focus on the internal world:* Clinical problems can be understood in terms of the individual's conscious and unconscious beliefs, fears,

thoughts, and feelings, which are seen as playing a significant role in organizing and perpetuating presenting difficulties.

- *Unconscious motivation and intentionality:* In addition to conscious beliefs, fears, and motivations, factors outside of conscious awareness play a significant role in mental functioning and in organizing and perpetuating symptoms and maladaptive personality functioning; to fully understand conscious experience and individual subjectivity requires reference to psychological factors outside of full awareness.

- *Defensive operations:* Defenses, psychological strategies involuntarily used to minimize psychological discomfort in the face of internal conflicts and external stressors, are a universal feature of psychological functioning. Defenses operate by in some way altering aspects of experience that would generate discomfort if experienced without modification. Different defenses can be more or less adaptive, introducing a lesser or greater degree of distortion and rigidity into psychological functioning; lower-level defenses are highly maladaptive and are associated with personality pathology, whereas higher-level defenses are relatively adaptive, more flexible, and associated with normal[1] and neurotic personality functioning.[2]

- *Internal representations and internalized relationship patterns:* Early significant relationships are internalized to form mental representations of self in relation to other (e.g., an attentive parent in relation to a well-taken-care-of self associated with feelings of security), sometimes referred to as internal object relations. Within a psychodynamic frame of reference, internalized relationship patterns need not correspond in a one-to-one fashion to the individual's actual developmental experiences; rather, these patterns reflect a combination of actual early experience, wished-for experience, and defense. These internal patterns of relating organize interpersonal functioning—both expectations and experiences of the self in relation to others. In areas of psychological conflict, patterns of relating tend to be enacted in an especially repetitive, predictable, and rigid fashion. When internal relationship patterns are activated in relation to the therapist, we use the term *transference*.

- *Structural perspective:* Presenting complaints, including symptoms, maladaptive behaviors, and painful subjective states, can be understood as the observable expressions of underlying constellations of mental processes, referred to as psychological *structures*. For example, internal relationship patterns, defensive operations, identity, motivational systems, and psychological conflicts are psychological structures central to psychological functioning and psychopathology. Psychodynamic treatments attempt to modify the structures underlying and organizing presenting complaints, shifting them toward higher levels of integration and greater flexibility, with the expectation that these structural changes will result in symptomatic improvement.

- *Centrality of self and other functioning:* Psychodynamic perspectives on personality emphasize the centrality of self and other functioning. Central to self and other

---

[1] As used in this chapter, *normal* personality functioning refers to flexible and adaptive self and interpersonal functioning in conjunction with the predominance of higher-level defenses (see Table 32–3).

[2] The term *neurotic* may be widely used but is often loosely defined. It is used here to describe a group of relatively high-functioning individuals who use predominantly higher-level defenses (see Table 32–3).

functioning is the construct of *identity,* the psychological structure that organizes the individual's sense of self and sense of significant others. It may be useful to consider a patient as falling on a continuum of identity formation. Normal identity formation, or identity consolidation, is marked by relative consistency in values, interests, and pursuits; in contrast, pathology of identity formation, or identity diffusion, is marked by inconsistencies in values and interests, with radical or abrupt changes or failures of investment in work or relationships. The normal and neurotic personalities are characterized by normal identity formation; personality disorders are characterized by pathology of identity formation.

- *Developmental perspective:* Current personality functioning, dysfunction, and symptoms are understood in the context of the individual's developmental history. An individual's early history affects the formation and organization of psychological structures underlying current functioning, and the persistence of these structures represents the influence of the past in the present. Childhood adversity, including trauma, abuse, neglect, and inadequate attachment experiences as they interact with temperamental factors, plays an especially powerful role in pathogenesis.
- *Continuity between normal and disrupted personality development:* Pathology in particular domains of personality functioning is conceptualized as falling on a continuous spectrum of severity, spanning from the most severe pathology to healthy personality functioning. Psychodynamic treatments aim to move the patient toward the healthy end of the continuum, focusing on specific domains of functioning. For example, treatment may promote a shift from defensive operations that are rigid and maladaptive toward defenses that are more consistent with flexible and adaptive functioning.

Techniques of Psychodynamic Therapy and the Supportive–Expressive Continuum

Within the general framework that we have outlined, the dynamic therapist makes use of a range of techniques. Interventions used in dynamic therapies can be visualized as falling along a *supportive–expressive continuum* (Figure 32–1). All psychodynamic treatments use a combination of expressive and supportive interventions. The use of expressive interventions—also referred to as *exploratory* interventions—distinguishes dynamic therapies from other forms of treatment. There is a fair amount of variability across psychodynamic treatments with regard to use of supportive techniques.

As a group, expressive interventions help the patient explore his or her internal experience, emotions, behavior, and experience of others. Exploratory interventions aim to "open things up"—to bring to the patient's awareness aspects of himself or herself that are defended against and therefore lie outside full awareness, and ultimately to help the patient make sense of these parts of the self and to take responsibility for them. The techniques used by the psychodynamic therapist that fall at the most expressive end of the continuum are referred to as *interpretive interventions.*

The process of interpretation can be conceptualized as using three kinds of techniques. The most basic is clarification, followed by confrontation and interpretation proper (Table 32–1). In serial progression, these interventions gradually broaden the

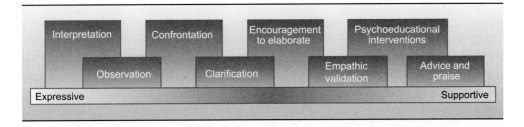

FIGURE 32–1. An expressive–supportive continuum of interventions.

Source. Reprinted from Gabbard GO: *Long-Term Psychodynamic Psychotherapy: A Basic Text,* 3rd Edition. Arlington, VA, American Psychiatric Association Publishing, 2017, p. 79. Copyright 2017, American Psychiatric Association. Used with permission.

TABLE 32–1. Techniques used in the interpretive process

Clarification—Asking for explanation of consciously experienced and described material that is vague or unclear

Confrontation—Calling attention to contradictions or omissions not fully in the patient's awareness, often denied or rationalized, in material that has been clarified

Interpretation proper—Offering a hypothesis about why the patient may be experiencing or doing things as he or she is, making sense of manifestly irrational elements in confronted material by invoking unconscious motivations, anxieties, and personal meanings in the here and now that are driving defensive operations

patient's level of self-awareness and self-understanding to include aspects of experience and behavior that have been defended against. In psychodynamic psychotherapy, interpretive interventions focus on exploring psychological conflicts linked to the patient's symptoms and presenting difficulties.

Supportive interventions include a heterogeneous group of techniques used in many different forms of psychotherapy. Whereas expressive interventions tend to place the therapist in the position of an observer, helping the patient to reflect on his or her behavior and emotional states, supportive interventions can be seen as placing the therapist in a more active role. In some supportive interventions, the therapist is directive, suggesting certain behaviors, whereas in others, the therapist focuses more on supporting the patient emotionally—alleviating distress, reducing confusion, and providing an experience of being cared for. Supportive interventions routinely used in dynamic therapy include psychoeducation; empathic validation; directing the patient's attention to particular aspects of his or her thoughts, feelings, and behaviors that appear to be relevant to issues currently active in the therapy; and requests for elaboration or clarification.

Additional techniques further along the supportive continuum (see Figure 32–1) that may be used in some forms of psychodynamic therapy include providing direct, concrete advice or guidance; teaching coping skills; and offering reassurance or praise. Finally, specialized psychodynamic treatments developed for the treatment of personality disorders often make use of supportive interventions to help the patient control destructive and disruptive behaviors—for example, contracting or setting limits in relation to self-harm or requiring ongoing consultation with a nutritionist or participation in a 12-step program as a necessary condition for continuing treatment.

Although we make distinctions between expressive and supportive interventions, in psychodynamic therapy, expressive and supportive interventions often work synergistically to promote change. For example, a supportive intervention such as empathic validation may support an alliance or provide affective containment, creating a setting in which the patient is better able to reflect and explore—to be more open; to experience potentially threatening aspects of internal experience; and to communicate private thoughts, feelings, and fantasies. Similarly, expressive interventions, such as the therapist's formulation of a particular anxiety in words for the patient to consider, often serve supportive and expressive functions—for example, by helping the patient contain anxiety or by communicating empathy and concern.

Clinical Assessment and Consultation

Patients seen in psychiatric consultation present with a wide range of problems and often with several different problems in combination. Most commonly, patients present with depression and/or anxiety, cognitive disturbances, or maladaptive behaviors such as substance misuse, eating disorders, or chronic self-injury. On evaluation, many patients can be seen to have difficulty regulating their emotions, leading to symptoms such as affective instability or inappropriate expressions of anger, or to be experiencing painful or dysphoric subjective states, such as constant self-criticism, feelings of emptiness, chronic boredom, global lack of satisfaction, or an inability to identify meaningful goals. Furthermore, patients presenting with a wide variety of complaints may additionally be experiencing difficulty in establishing or maintaining intimate relationships or in functioning or succeeding at work.

Psychodynamic therapies offer a unique perspective on treatment of a broad range of symptoms and personality pathology, by maintaining a focus on self and other functioning as organizing principles of mental health and psychopathology.[3] For example, on close inspection, many instances of anxiety are closely related to self-evaluation and interactions with others; similarly, depressive affects often arise in relation to self-appraisal and interpersonal stressors. Some clinical problems can be seen as direct expressions of pathology of self and interpersonal functioning or personality pathology (e.g., feelings of emptiness or chronic dysphoria, self-injurious behavior, difficulty identifying meaningful goals), whereas many other complaints are best conceptualized as co-occurring with and expressed in the context of the patient's personality and social milieu (e.g., substance misuse, major depressive disorder).

Diagnostic Assessment

Clinical assessment for psychodynamic therapy begins with the assumption that the *person*, within his or her unique environment, is the context for development and expression of symptoms and maladaptive personality functioning (Lingiardi and McWilliams 2017). Diagnostic assessment will always involve assessment of both symptoms

---

[3] The growing awareness of domains of dysfunction that extend across diagnostic boundaries has led to a recent shift in interest toward the development of transdiagnostic treatments, both for symptoms such as anxiety (Barlow et al. 2017) and for the personality disorders (Caligor et al. 2018).

and personality functioning or dysfunction, and both are conceptualized as being embedded in a particular *personality organization* (Caligor and Clarkin 2010). Our emphasis on evaluation of *both* symptoms and personality reflects the clinical reality that many individuals who present for treatment of symptoms have some level of personality dysfunction, and many with diagnosable personality pathology have symptom conditions. The presence of personality pathology will greatly affect clinical prognosis and the clinical approach to symptoms; conversely, the presence of symptoms invariably becomes a focus of clinical attention in the treatment of personality pathology.

Assessment focuses on domains most relevant to treatment planning and enables the clinician to tailor treatment to the needs of the individual patient based on severity of presenting symptoms, personality traits, and level of personality organization. Thorough assessment will guide the selection of treatment structure, focus, and level of care. By the end of the assessment process, the clinician will have acquired a clear understanding of the patient's 1) presenting problems, 2) DSM-5 or ICD-10 diagnoses (American Psychiatric Association 2013; World Health Organization 1992), 3) personality functioning, 4) level of personality organization, and 5) personal goals for treatment. Throughout assessment, the psychodynamic clinician attends to the burgeoning treatment relationship, promoting the development of an early therapeutic alliance while noting patterns beginning to emerge in the treatment relationship (i.e., transference dispositions). Content domains and a suggested outline for a comprehensive assessment interview are summarized in Table 32–2.

Presenting Symptoms, Pathological Personality Traits, and Psychiatric History

Patient assessment begins with identification and characterization of the symptoms and pathological personality traits that brought the patient to treatment, followed by a thorough and systematic evaluation of all symptoms and areas of dysfunction, beginning with current areas of difficulty and incorporating a review of the psychiatric history. This portion of the consultation involves data collection that would be part of any general psychiatric assessment. If the patient has a history of treatment, medication use, or hospitalization, this information is reviewed in depth, as are the patient's medical history, history of substance misuse, and family history of psychiatric illness and substance use. In addition, clinicians should inquire specifically about any history of physical or sexual abuse, neglect, or other trauma.

A thorough review of previous treatments, including any difficulties that emerged in the course of treatment, how the treatment ended, and the patient's view of each previous treatment experience (i.e., what felt helpful and what did not), is especially useful for treatment planning; such a review aids in anticipating difficulties likely to emerge during the consultation as well as during any treatment that may follow. The interviewer will follow up on this line of inquiry by contacting previous treaters to obtain a complete history of treatments.

Personality Functioning and Level of Organization

Having characterized the patient's difficulties, the consultant turns next to exploring the patient's personality, focusing on the degree to which symptoms and pathological personality traits interfere with personality functioning, as well as on the level of personality organization. The interviewer will explore the nature of the patient's inter-

TABLE 32–2.   **Content domains of assessment interview for psychodynamic therapy**

Presenting symptoms, pathological personality traits, and psychiatric history

Symptoms and pathological personality traits that brought the patient to treatment

Thorough and systematic evaluation of all symptoms and difficulties, beginning with current areas of difficulty and reviewing history

History of psychiatric treatment, medication, and hospitalization

Medical history, history of substance misuse, family history of psychiatric illness, and history of physical or sexual abuse or neglect or other trauma

Complete psychiatric review of symptoms, including those of affects, anxiety, psychosis, eating disorders, learning disorders, substance misuse, self-destructive behaviors, and history of violence or illegal activity

Review of previous treatments, including difficulties that emerged in the course of treatment, how the treatment ended, and patient's view of each previous treatment experience

Personality functioning in relationships, work, and leisure time

Degree to which symptoms and pathological personality traits interfere with personality functioning

Interpersonal functioning

Work functioning, current and past

Personal interests and use of free time

Assessment of structural features of personality: dimensional assessment of personality organization and structural diagnosis

Identity formation (sense of self, sense of others, and capacity to invest in and pursue longer-term goals)

Quality of object relations (both interpersonal functioning and the individual's understanding of relationships in terms of mutuality vs. need fulfillment)

Defensive style (predominantly flexible-adaptive, repression-based, or splitting-based)

Management of aggression (well-modulated and adaptive expression of aggression vs. inhibited expression or maladaptive aggressive behavior directed toward self or others)

Moral functioning (internalized values and ideals guiding behavior vs. a failure of internal values and ideals leading to unethical or antisocial behavior)

Overall dimensional appraisal of health vs. severity of pathology, taking into account assessment of each of these five domains

Personal/developmental history

Developmental history (history of trauma, antisocial behavior, positive relationships)

personal functioning, intimate relationships, current functioning at work and work history, finances, and use of leisure time (see Table 32–2). This portion of the consultation is a more comprehensive and detailed version of the social history taken as part of the standard psychiatric interview. The assessor will note whether difficulties are focused predominantly in a single domain (e.g., interpersonal functioning) or represent more global forms of dysfunction presenting across multiple domains (work and interpersonal functioning).

Assessment of personality functioning naturally leads to characterization of personality organization. Level of personality organization—which can be classified as (from healthiest to most pathological) normal personality organization, neurotic personality organization, high-level borderline personality organization, mid-level borderline personality organization, or low-level borderline personality organization[4])—is based on assessment of key psychological structures and reflects severity of personality pathology versus healthy personality functioning. Assessment of personality organization focuses on 1) identity formation (sense of self, sense of others, and capacity to invest in and pursue longer-term goals), 2) quality of object relations (interpersonal functioning and the individual's internal working models of relationships), 3) defensive style (predominantly flexible–adaptive, repression-based, or splitting-based), 4) management of aggression (well-modulated, adaptive expression of aggression versus inhibited expression or maladaptive aggressive behavior directed toward self or others), and 5) moral functioning (internalized values and ideals that guide behavior versus a failure of internal values and ideals leading to unethical or antisocial behavior).

This model of psychodynamic assessment and classification was first articulated by Kernberg and Caligor (2005). Although based on psychodynamic object relations theory, the model corresponds closely with the Alternative DSM-5 Model for Personality Disorders (AMPD) in DSM-5 Section III. Prototypes for different levels of personality organization, provided in Table 32–3, can be seen to overlap with the five levels of personality functioning outlined in the Level of Personality Functioning Scale in the AMPD.

Determination of level of personality organization is essential to guiding differential treatment planning. Psychodynamic intervention with individuals who present with high-level personality functioning (normal and neurotic personality organization) is constructed differently from intervention with patients with a borderline level of organization (Caligor et al. 2018) (Table 32–4). Individuals with a normal or neurotic level of personality organization have a very favorable prognosis and can benefit from relatively unstructured treatments and a variety of treatment approaches. These patients typically do not have difficulty establishing and maintaining a therapeutic alliance, and transferences tend to be slowly developing, consistent, relatively realistic, and subtle. In contrast, individuals organized at a borderline level, particularly those in the mid- and low-borderline range, require a highly structured treatment setting. These individuals have great difficulty establishing and maintaining a therapeutic alliance; transferences develop rapidly and are grossly distorted, highly affectively charged, and extreme, often leading to disruption of the treatment.

Process of Assessment

A major decision for the clinical assessor is whether to use a clinically guided interview or a semistructured interview with predetermined areas of inquiry. The former is the time-honored approach (MacKinnon et al. 2009) and has the advantage of favoring the experienced clinician's freedom. The latter type of interview ensures standard coverage of crucial areas and allows clinicians to compare their assessments

---

[4] We wish to clarify the distinction between DSM-5 borderline personality disorder and the borderline level of personality organization. Borderline personality disorder is a specific personality disorder diagnosed on the basis of a constellation of descriptive features. Borderline personality organization is a much broader category based on structural features—in particular, pathology of identity formation. The organization diagnosis subsumes DSM-5 borderline personality disorder as well as all the severe personality disorders.

TABLE 32–3. Structural approach to classification of personality pathology reflecting severity across five dimensions

Level of personality organization	Identity	Predominant defensive functioning	Quality of object relations	Aggression	Moral values
Normal	Consolidated; coherent conception of self and others	Higher-level defenses; mature	Deep, mutual	Modulated	Present; flexible
Neurotic (subsyndromal)		Higher-level defenses; repression	Deep, mutual with some conflicts	Modulated; inhibition	Present; rigid
High-level borderline (mild PD)	Mild identity pathology	Higher-level and splitting-based defenses	Some dependent relations	Varying degrees of aggression	Variable; combination of rigidity and some deficits
Middle-level borderline (severe PD)	Lack of coherent conception of self and others	Splitting-based defenses	Relations based on need fulfillment	Aggression toward self and others	Significant deficits but variable
Low-level borderline (most severe PD)			Relations based on exploitation; sadism		Severe pathology; callous disregard for others

Note. PD=personality disorder.

TABLE 32–4. Personality organization and prognosis for dynamic treatment of personality pathology and co-occurring disorders

Neurotic personality organization

Mild pathology; excellent overall prognosis

Treatment need not be highly structured

Patients can do well in a variety of treatments

Pathology best characterized as "maladaptive personality rigidity" rather than "personality disorder," given relatively mild severity of impairment and typically high level of functioning

More focal pathology (i.e., limited predominantly to a particular domain of functioning vs. globally affecting all domains of functioning) and less severe rigidity have better prognosis

Obsessive-compulsive, depressive, and hysterical personalities

High-level borderline personality organization

Least severe personality disorders within borderline personality organization spectrum; positive prognosis but less consistently so than for neurotic personality organization group

Patients do poorly in unstructured treatments

Patients do well in structured forms of dynamic therapy

Relative absence of significant pathology of moral functioning and capacity to form dependent relationships characterize this group and are positive prognostic features in dynamic therapy

Histrionic, dependent, and avoidant personality disorders, as well as healthier narcissistic patients

Mid-level borderline personality organization

Severe personality disorders; moderate prognosis with high rate of treatment dropout

Despite severity, many patients can benefit from a variety of specialized treatments

Require structured frame and contract; early phases of treatment often characterized by acting out

More severe impairment of moral functioning and object relations brings more guarded prognosis

Borderline, paranoid, and schizoid personality disorders

Personal/developmental history

Extremely guarded prognosis; treatments carry a high risk of destructive acting out

Contracting must be extensive and involve participation of third parties

Narcissistic personality disorder with significant antisocial features (often comorbid with borderline personality disorder), malignant narcissistic personality disorder, and antisocial personality disorder

Antisocial personality disorder is a contraindication for dynamic therapy

with those of others. On balance, we recommend using the clinical interview as the primary assessment tool for routine clinical practice because it allows the clinician to elicit information in ways that foster the alliance and engage the patient in treatment.

The clinical diagnostic interview can be complemented and is often enhanced by the introduction of structured assessment instruments in the form of self-report questionnaires inquiring about symptoms and maladaptive traits. For assessment of personality organization, the Structured Interview of Personality Organization–Revised (STIPO-R; J.F. Clarkin, E. Caligor, B.L. Stern, et al: "Structured Interview for Personality Organization–Revised [STIPO-R]," unpublished manuscript, Weill Cornell Medical College,

2015) can be integrated into the assessment process. The STIPO-R is a semistructured interview that facilitates clinical assessment of personality organization, focusing on the domains of identity formation, defenses, object relations, aggression, and moral functioning. The STIPO-R may be particularly helpful to clinicians who are inexperienced in assessment of personality organization.

During assessment, the balance between a focus on current functioning and a focus on past developmental history presents the assessor with another decision point. Within the dictates of time, we recommend a thorough evaluation of the current functioning with relatively less attention to the past, except when it has direct implications for current functioning; information about past difficulties in development, traumatic experiences, and the history of current ways of relating to others is most relevant. More complete information about the past will emerge during the course of treatment but in general is not needed for diagnostic assessment and treatment planning.

Enhancement of the Treatment Alliance Through Assessment

The quality of the early therapeutic alliance is associated with the rate of premature dropout from treatment as well as with long-term outcome (a higher-quality alliance is associated with lower dropout and better outcome). For this reason, alliance-building techniques should be used throughout the clinical assessment (Hilsenroth and Cromer 2007). Specifically, the developing alliance is supported by a longer and collaborative in-depth assessment that allows ample opportunity for the patient to voice concerns. Rapport is increased by avoiding the use of jargon or technical terms and instead using clear, concrete, and experience-near language (i.e., language that the patient can readily relate to his or her experience). Detailed exploration of the patient's immediate concerns emerging during the interview fosters the alliance and helps patients commit to treatment.

Sharing of Diagnostic Impressions

After completing the assessment process, the clinician will share his or her diagnostic impressions with the patient, explaining the rationale for diagnoses, providing psychoeducation, and leaving time to answer any questions the patient may have. This process naturally leads to discussion of treatment options.

Principles of Psychodynamic Therapy

In the same way that psychodynamic therapies are united by a shared model of psychological functioning, the family of psychodynamic therapies shares a general clinical framework. We focus here on principles of treatment essential for and specific to the psychodynamic therapy approach.

- *Treatment frame:* Treatment begins with the therapist introducing the treatment frame. This process establishes frequency and duration of sessions, handling of intersession contact, payment, cancellations and emergencies, the respective roles of patient and therapist, and how they will work together in the treatment.
- *Free and open communication:* Sessions are not structured, and the therapist does not set an agenda. Patients are encouraged to speak as openly and freely as possible

while the therapist attends closely to the patient's communications, making use of three channels of communication (Caligor et al. 2018)—the patient's verbal communications, the patient's nonverbal communications, and the feelings stimulated in the therapist by the patient's verbal and nonverbal communications.

- *Identification of a focus:* The therapist identifies a dominant issue in each session, which becomes a focus for intervention. To identify a dominant issue, the therapist attends to the three channels of communication, listening in particular for expressions of affect, descriptions of repetitive relationship patterns, communications about the therapist or about treatment, and evidence of activation of defenses— for example, contradictions, inconsistencies, vagueness, or omissions evident in the patient's communications. The dominant issue is understood to be an expression of conflict and defense currently active in the session. As the therapist works to identify a focus, he or she remains mindful of the treatment goals.

- *Requests for elaboration:* Having identified a dominant issue, the therapist asks for elaboration, inviting the patient to clarify his or her communications and to observe his or her own thoughts, feelings, and behavior in relation to the dominant issue.

- *Exploration:* The therapist works with the patient to gradually broaden the patient's awareness and understanding of his or her experience and behavior in the identified area of conflict and defense and to tolerate the anxieties associated with doing so. Interventions highlight how the patient's defenses and repetitively activated internal relationship patterns affect the patient's experience and behavior. Over time, anxieties defended against are identified and elaborated, followed by interpretation of underlying conflicts (the process of exploration is illustrated in the "Strategies of Psychodynamic Treatment: Promoting Structural Change Through Exploration" section later in this chapter).

Goals of Psychodynamic Treatment: What Changes in Psychodynamic Therapy?

Historically, some forms of psychodynamic treatment have not focused on specific treatment goals. However, empirical studies support the benefits of establishing clear goals for treatment, which may enhance both alliance and outcome (see, e.g., Goldman et al. 2013), and we believe that identifying specific and explicit goals with the patient before beginning treatment is essential. Typical goals for psychodynamic therapy include improved interpersonal functioning and capacity to sustain satisfying intimate and sexual relationships, improved occupational functioning or capacity to derive satisfaction from work, enhanced self-definition or improved self-esteem, enhanced ability to pursue long-term goals, better management of aggression (e.g., temper outbursts or inappropriate expressions of hostility, passivity, or failure of assertiveness), and amelioration of symptoms of anxiety and depression. Throughout treatment, the therapist remains mindful of the treatment goals. Identified goals orient the therapist during the course of treatment, focusing his or her thinking and interventions, and goals make it possible for therapist and patient to assess progress in treatment over time.

In addition to descriptive treatment goals, which reflect the patient's concerns and the specific difficulties that brought the patient to treatment, the dynamic therapist has in mind a set of structural goals for the treatment, with the expectation that structural changes will lead to symptomatic improvement. Barber et al. (2013) suggested five unique, empirically supported ways in which dynamic therapy seeks to help patients: 1) fostering insight into unconscious conflict, 2) increasing the use of adaptive psychological defenses, 3) decreasing rigidity in interpersonal perceptions and behavior, 4) improving the quality of the patient's mental representations of relationships (i.e., improving the quality of object relations), and 5) increasing the patient's comprehension of his or her own and others' mental states (i.e., improving the capacity for mentalization).

Each of these developments represents a form of structural change—a shift in specific functions, processes, or capacities within the patient toward higher levels of integration and flexibility. These changes can be considered mediators of outcome, where outcome is measured in terms of resolution of presenting symptoms or maladaptive behaviors; these changes also could be considered in and of themselves as outcomes of dynamic therapy (Barber et al. 2013).

Strategies of Psychodynamic Treatment: Promoting Structural Change Through Exploration

The overarching strategies organizing psychodynamic therapies can be understood from the perspective of promoting the kinds of structural changes outlined by Barber et al. (2013). To illustrate this approach, consider the patient who presents with marital problems. The patient complains about his wife in session; from the patient's perspective, his wife is once again criticizing him. As the patient complains, it becomes clear that he and his wife are stuck in a repetitive cycle that leaves him feeling victimized, frustrated, and angry.

In this patient's treatment, the basic strategy adopted by the dynamic therapist would be to help the patient develop more complete awareness and better understanding of his experience and behavior during exchanges with his wife, with the expectation that over time, enhanced self-awareness, reflectiveness, and self-understanding would lead him to feel and behave differently in interactions with his wife. The primary focus of clinical attention would be on the patient: his moment-to-moment experience and behavior with his wife and significant others, and perhaps with the therapist as well. As part of this process, the dynamic therapist would also help the patient more fully consider his understanding of his wife's experience of their interactions.

The dynamic therapist might begin by asking the patient for further details about his experience and behavior, as well as those of his wife, during their exchanges (this sort of intervention—asking for elaboration—is an example of the technique of *clarification*). This line of inquiry would lead to elaboration and articulation of the relationship pattern playing out between the patient and his wife, calling attention to the repetitive nature of the patient's behavior in these interactions. This kind of intervention promotes self-observation and self-awareness on the part of the patient (the patient's experience and behavior are to be examined; it seems he keeps having the same experience over and over again; he has the same experience perhaps not only with his wife but also in other relationships—and perhaps, although not necessarily, even with the therapist) while simultaneously communicating empathy ("I am listening"; "I understand what you are feeling").

The next strategy is to help the patient gradually expand his awareness to include aspects of the situation of which he is less fully aware, particularly those aspects in which he seems to be denying or ignoring elements of his communications, behavior, or experience that seem inconsistent or contradictory. This sort of intervention involves the therapist's offering the patient a bid for reflection; it is an example of the technique of *confrontation*. This strategy invites the patient to entertain an alternative perspective on repetitive thoughts, feelings, and behaviors. In our example, the therapist might invite the patient to consider that at the same time that he feels chronically criticized, underappreciated, and frustrated in relation to his wife, his reflexive and unreflective behavior during their exchanges might leave her feeling similarly; this may be the case when, for example, the patient responds to his wife's complaints either by insisting that she is entirely unreasonable or by giving her the silent treatment, refusing to acknowledge her concerns, or responding with a litany of complaints about her inadequacies as a partner.

Here the therapist is calling the patient's attention to aspects of his own behavior and experience that he is not attending to (his withholding and frustrating behavior and attitude, his hostility and critical attitude) and to his playing out of a rigid internal relationship pattern (his wife is critical and demanding, and he responds by withholding and rejecting; they are both angry). At the same time, the therapist is encouraging the patient to reflect, both on his own experience and behavior and on his wife's, implicitly encouraging greater empathy with her situation.

In summary, the therapist's strategy is to target processes (i.e., psychological structures) within the patient that are organizing chronic problems in the marriage: the *repetitive relationship pattern* that the patient finds himself unable to end, the effect of maladaptive *defenses* on his experience and behavior, his failure to *reflect on internal states* (either his own or his wife's), and the way he comes to *see his wife as an enemy* and fails to maintain an *empathic perspective in relation to her experience* during their arguments. With these objectives in mind, the therapist intervenes to promote self-observation and self-awareness on the patient's part, to support his ability to reflect on his own internal state and his wife's, and to encourage him to step out of familiar patterns to entertain alternative perspectives. These new perspectives involve acquiring greater awareness of and assuming responsibility for aspects of his behavior and internal experience previously defended against, as well as greater empathy for his wife—all of which leave him less vulnerable to feeling angry and victimized and more likely to challenge himself to try new, more constructive ways of interacting.

Psychodynamic strategies rely on repetition; rarely does a single intervention or exchange lead to change. Rather, it is repetitive implementation of basic treatment strategies applied in a variety of contexts across time (a process described as *working through*) that facilitates structural shifts within the patient—movement away from rigid interpersonal patterns to greater flexibility, a shift toward higher-level defenses that enable him to behave in a more flexible and adaptive manner, modification of his representations of himself in interaction with his wife so that they involve less distortion, and an ability to sustain a more mindful and empathic appraisal of her experience. These structural changes will correspond with achieving the overall treatment goal of improved marital relations.

Insight

Historically, insight into unconscious conflict was the sine qua non of psychodynamic treatments. Patients were thought to benefit from making the unconscious conscious and from receiving explanations of presenting difficulties based on an elaboration of unconscious meanings linked to the patient's developmental past. These assumptions were largely derived from early psychoanalytical models of change in which uncovering repressed motivations and conflicts was considered the major mechanism of therapeutic action. Many patients coming for dynamic treatment today continue to have the expectation that this is what treatment entails.

Contemporary views offer a broader understanding of what constitutes insight. Today's definition of insight need not necessarily involve an in-depth understanding of an unconscious conflict or necessarily include a link to the developmental past; instead, we might view insight in a more general sense: as the acquisition of an emotional and cognitive understanding of an aspect of self-functioning that has been defensively kept from awareness, in the setting of concern regarding what is newly understood. For example, our unhappily married patient's more complete awareness of his behavior in the marriage, of the hostility he covertly and overtly expresses, and of how his behavior affects his wife could be described as a form of insight, to the extent that he feels concern about this aspect of himself or motivated to try to behave differently. This essential "insight" need not necessarily be linked to an understanding of unconscious conflict or to the past.

Interpretation of Unconscious Conflict

What would insight into unconscious conflict look like for our patient complaining about his wife? Within a classic psychodynamic frame of reference, *insight* would refer to the patient's understanding of psychological conflicts organizing and driving his experience and behavior with his wife. For example, his marital difficulties could be seen to reflect, at least in part, conflicts in relation to his own hostile motivations and affects, aspects of himself that are conflictual (i.e., from his perspective unacceptable) and therefore defended against. Rather than being fully aware of these aspects of his internal experience and behavior and managing them consciously, flexibly, and adaptively (e.g., thoughtfully sharing with his wife that her criticism angers him and suggesting alternative ways that they might communicate, or taking personal responsibility for more hostile and rejecting aspects of himself that he disavows by apologizing to his wife for aspects of his behavior that are withholding or dismissive), he avoids taking responsibility for hostile motivations and related behaviors by using a combination of defenses that leave him feeling that it is not he who is critical, hostile, or at fault—rather, it is his wife who is all of these things; to the extent that he appears angry, his anger is reactive and justified.

To convey such a formulation to the patient, the therapist might begin by pointing out: "It is as if—in the heat of those exchanges with your wife—you are experiencing her almost as an enemy, as if in those moments you entirely lose sight of the woman you love." The therapist might go on to offer a possible explanation for this observation, in the form of an interpretation (see Table 32–1): "I wonder if seeing her as an enemy doesn't protect you in some way…perhaps from the pain you might feel if you were aware that your wishes to withhold from her, or even to hurt her, are directed toward someone whom you love." Here the therapist has suggested a hypothesis about why the patient might defensively distort his own image of his wife, suggesting that he does so, automatically and involuntarily, to protect himself from pain and guilt associated with expression of hostility directed toward a loved one. Within a classic psychodynamic framework, this interpretation might be further elaborated by drawing a link between the patient's conflicts in relation to expression of hostility and his developmental past—for example, by elaborating a connection between the patient's current conflicts with his wife and the patient's conflicts in relation to his father dating back to childhood and adolescence.[5]

Many contemporary psychodynamic therapists might expect to help this patient develop a similar understanding of his current difficulties with his wife at some point in the treatment and in the process to help the patient gain a more complete understanding of himself. However, rather than viewing the elaboration of an "explanation" of this kind (referred to as an *interpretation*) as the only, or even the major, mutative element in treatment, we can see it as one of many elements of change. Rather than assuming that an insight of this kind will lead directly to structural change, we might see this understanding as a way to help the patient more flexibly manage hostile aspects of his self-experience that are conflictual and to take responsibility for them—a step toward more adaptive and flexible self and interpersonal functioning and enhanced capacity for intimacy.

The Therapeutic Relationship

All psychotherapies are deeply embedded in the patient–therapist relationship, and it is generally agreed that this relationship serves not simply as a context for the techniques of treatment but also as a central vehicle of change. In psychodynamic therapy, the ongoing interactions between patient and therapist lie at the very core of the treatment. The relationship established between patient and dynamic therapist is highly specialized, characterized by clear professional boundaries and a singular focus on the needs of the patient. In this relationship, the role of the patient is to communicate his or her inner needs, thoughts, and feelings as fully as possible while the therapist refrains from doing so; the role of the therapist is to use his or her expertise to support self-awareness and self-exploration on the part of the patient.

The psychotherapeutic relationship is established at the beginning of treatment and evolves throughout its course. Therapeutic alliance, therapist stance, transference, and countertransference are all embedded within the matrix of ongoing interactions between patient and therapist.

---

[5] Making links to the patient's past, sometimes referred to as making a *genetic interpretation*, is not without risk. Premature genetic interpretation can lead to intellectualized or even counterproductive treatment developments; for example, the patient could use such a formulation to continue to "blame" his wife and his father rather than to develop the capacity to take responsibility for his own hostile and rejecting behaviors.

Therapist's Attitude and Stance

In his or her attitude toward the patient, the dynamic therapist sets the emotional tone of the treatment. The therapist's objective is to establish a relationship in which the patient feels as free as possible to openly explore and share his or her experience and behavior. Toward this end, the dynamic therapist is active, collaborative, warm, and respectful. In interacting with the patient, the therapist's stance is professional—emotionally responsive but restrained. The therapist does not try to hide his or her personality, but does refrain from speaking at length about his or her personal life, keeping the focus on the patient and the patient's difficulties.

In response to what the patient says and does, the dynamic therapist strives to be empathic, flexible, tolerant, and nonjudgmental. The therapist communicates openness to all aspects of the patient's internal situation, including those that the patient himself or herself rejects. Thus, the therapist is positioned as an observer in relation to the patient's communications and behavior. In assuming this "neutral"[6] stance (Auchincloss and Samberg 2012), the therapist makes an effort not to take sides in the patient's conflicts or to support one part of the patient in relation to another. Rather, the dynamic therapist strives to be open to all sides of the patient's conflicts, and the therapist attempts to frame interventions from the perspective of helping the patient do the same.

To facilitate self-observation and reflection on the patient's part, the dynamic therapist often refrains from providing advice or actively intervening in the patient's life (e.g., making suggestions to the patient in our vignette about how to better manage his wife, or perhaps suggesting that the patient leave the marriage). At the same time, the therapist is pragmatic and will choose to be more directive based on clinical circumstances. For example, patients with significant functional deficits who are receiving psychodynamic therapy may at times require or derive significant benefit from advice and guidance from the therapist. It also goes without saying that in response to a patient's engaging in frankly self-destructive or dangerous behaviors or becoming acutely suicidal, depressed, manic, or psychotic, the psychodynamic therapist will adopt an active, directive stance, making use of standard psychiatric management strategies to set limits on destructive behaviors, arrange for emergency management, and contact third parties as needed. In summary, the dynamic therapist favors exploration, but the therapist's focus is first and foremost on the immediate clinical and practical needs of the individual patient.

In dynamic therapies that fall at the more expressive end of the supportive–expressive continuum, therapists maintain a more consistently neutral stance, protecting their role as that of an observer who promotes reflection; in treatments at the more supportive end of the continuum, therapists freely make use of supportive interventions that require a more active or directive stance—in contrast to an observing one—in relation to the patient's conflicts.

To illustrate what is meant by the therapist's initiating a process of exploration while maintaining the position of a neutral observer in relation to the patient's conflicts, we can return to our patient complaining about his wife. In her interventions,

[6] We make a conceptual distinction between the therapist's emotionally supportive attitude toward *the patient as a person* and the therapist's relatively neutral stance in relation to *the patient's conflicts* (as communicated in the patient's thoughts, feelings, and behavior in session).

the therapist avoided joining with the patient in his criticism of his wife—for example, by commiserating with him about what he had to put up with. The therapist also abstained from siding with the wife in her criticism of the patient's passivity—for example, by encouraging him to be more assertive. Instead, the therapist made an effort to step back, to observe neutrally in her mind the interaction between patient and wife, and to encourage the patient to do so as well.

Therapeutic Alliance

The *therapeutic alliance* is an important component of the psychotherapeutic relationship (Bender 2005). In a psychodynamic framework, the alliance is understood as the working relationship established between the self-observing (healthier) part of the patient that wants and is able to make use of help and the therapist in the role of helpful expert (Auchincloss and Samberg 2012). Operationally, the therapeutic alliance reflects, on the one hand, the patient's realistic expectations and experience of the therapist as having something to offer on the basis of training, expertise, and concern and, on the other hand, the therapist's commitment to helping the patient by making use of this expertise and developing understanding of the patient.

The alliance requires the participation of both therapist and patient; it is jointly established between them. Establishing a therapeutic alliance is a central task of the opening phase of dynamic therapy, and monitoring and managing the alliance remains a task for the therapist throughout the course of the therapy.

Much of the psychotherapy outcome literature has focused on three related components of the alliance: shared goals, clearly defined tasks, and the patient–therapist bond (Bordin 1979). In this literature, the alliance has been found to be a relatively strong predictor of outcome in various forms of psychotherapy, predicting approximately 15% of variance in outcome (Horvath et al. 2011). The development of the bond between patient and dynamic therapist is facilitated by the therapist's nonjudgmental and accepting attitude, his or her attentiveness and interest, warmth and concern, and communication of empathy. In psychodynamic therapy, exploration of negative feelings about the treatment and the therapist is used to support the development and stabilization of an alliance and can help to repair the alliance when it is breached. In treatments at the supportive end of the supportive–expressive continuum, supportive interventions, such as offering the patient reassurance or praise, are also routinely used to support the alliance.

The patient's level of personality organization often predicts the ease with which the patient is able to form an alliance with the therapist. Patients with higher-level personality organization are for the most part able to establish a relatively stable alliance in the early phases of therapy (Bender 2005); initial difficulties or ruptures of the alliance that may arise over the course of treatment are relatively easily resolved and, once worked through, often serve to deepen the patient's self-understanding while further solidifying the working relationship between therapist and patient (Caligor et al. 2007; Safran et al. 2011).

In contrast, patients with more significant personality pathology often have difficulty establishing a therapeutic alliance, and the quality of the alliance is susceptible to wide fluctuation across sessions and even moment-to-moment within a session (Wnuk et al. 2013; Yeomans et al. 2015). Ruptures are common and inevitable; they may be accompanied by strong emotional reactions on the part of the patient. Not uncommonly, these reactions may include hostility, accusations, and even paranoia. Exploration of ruptures as they occur throughout the treatment is central to the psychotherapeutic process in this setting, especially in the treatment of severe personality disorders. In the successful treatment of patients with such disorders, we see the gradual consolidation of a stable therapeutic alliance over the course of the treatment.

Transference

Attention to transference and countertransference is a defining feature of dynamic therapy. The construct of transference has been a cornerstone of dynamic treatments since Freud's development of psychoanalytic technique in the early twentieth century (see Auchincloss and Samberg 2012 and Høglend 2014 for excellent reviews and citations). Views of countertransference have developed in tandem. Contemporary perspectives view transference–countertransference as a complex intersubjective field, molded in an ongoing fashion by the therapist's interactions with the patient. This matrix provides a unique opportunity to explore the patient's internal world.

A basic assumption of psychodynamic models is that early, significant, and emotionally charged interactions, colored by genetic and temperamental factors and dynamically and developmentally based distortions, come to be organized in the mind in the form of memory structures or internalized relationship patterns. These psychological structures, organized as neural networks, function as latent schemas—ways in which the individual can potentially organize his or her experience—that will be activated in particular contexts (Kernberg and Caligor 2005). Once activated, these relationship patterns will color the individual's expectations of interpersonal interactions and will lead the individual to act and feel in ways that correspond with these expectations.

The term *transference* is most commonly used to refer to enactment of these schemas or relationship patterns in relation to the therapist. However, it is widely accepted that transference to the therapist is but one example of a more general process wherein internal patterns of relating and associated representations and affects tend to be activated and enacted in one's interpersonal life and tend to organize one's experience of self in relation to others (Høglend 2014). Thus, transference constitutes a specific example of the routine ebb and flow of day-to-day experience. Transference manifestations differ according to the nature of the patient's psychopathology and, in particular, according to the patient's level of personality organization (Table 32–5). Furthermore, any given patient will have many different transference dispositions, and the quality and content of a patient's transferences will shift over the course of treatment. In dynamic therapy, relationship patterns enacted in relation to the therapist can become a jumping-off point for exploration of the patient's internal world; the patient's relationship with the therapist can offer a special opportunity for patient and therapist to explore, in their immediate here-and-now interactions, the patient's internal structures and interpersonal patterns of relating.

Classical dynamic approaches to transference focused on "reliving" the past in the present, and considerable attention was directed toward exploring the relationship between childhood experience and current relational patterns (Auchincloss and Samberg 2012). More contemporary models of transference focus not on the past as relived in the present but rather on information processing in the here and now. Dynamic therapists

TABLE 32–5. Transference and countertransference at different levels of personality functioning

Higher-level personality (neurotic and normal organization)	Personality disorder (borderline personality organization)
Transference	
Transference often not affectively dominant	Transference often affectively dominant
Transference often not conscious	Transference often conscious
Transference is subtle and gradually developing; may be ego-syntonic	Transference is affectively charged, rapidly developing, and ego-dystonic
Transference often conveyed in verbal communication	Transference often conveyed in nonverbal communication and countertransference
Excessive attention to transference can tax therapeutic alliance	Attention to transference can support therapeutic alliance
Transference analysis not preferentially associated with positive outcome	Transference analysis preferentially associated with positive outcome
Transference analysis may not be major source of insight	Transference analysis often major source of insight
Focus on transference may come across as peculiar, forced, or divorced from patient's concerns	Focus on transference directs clinical attention to dominant issues in the treatment and in the patient's life
Transference analysis may not be a major vehicle of change	Transference analysis seen as a major vehicle of change
Treatment not consistently transference-focused	Treatment often transference-focused
Countertransference	
Countertransference typically not dominant channel of communication relative to verbal	Countertransference dominant and often primary channel of communication
Countertransference relatively subtle and easy to overlook	Countertransference often extreme, intrusive, and affectively charged
Countertransference can be contained within mind of therapist with reflection	Countertransference induces pressure on the therapist to act and may be difficult to contain
Countertransference reflects interaction of patient's transference and therapist's transferences to patient	Countertransference often reflects largely patient's transference; says more about patient than about therapist
Use of countertransference need not be central to clinical technique	Use and containment of countertransference are central to clinical technique

are interested primarily in elaborating how the patient's current psychological organization affects his or her current subjectivity and behavior. This approach is compatible with that of Høglend (2014), who defines transference as "the patient's patterns of feelings, thoughts, perceptions, and behavior that emerge within the therapeutic relationship and reflect aspects of the patient's personality functioning (regardless of the developmental origin of these patterns)" (p. 1057).

Different forms of dynamic therapy focus to a greater or lesser degree on exploration of transference versus exploration focusing on the patient's self states and subjective experience and behavior in his or her interpersonal life. Historically, it has been thought that patients who do not have significant personality pathology benefit preferentially from transference work, whereas patients with personality disorders are less able to benefit. However, more recent perspectives suggest that in psychodynamic therapy for relatively healthy patients, transference work need not play a central role (Caligor et al. 2018), and that these patients may do equally well in dynamic treatments that focus on transference and those that do not (Høglend et al. 2006). In practice, patients in this group often experience an excessive focus on transference as unhelpful—as somehow peculiar, forced, or divorced from the patient's dominant concerns. In contrast, patients with more severe pathology may preferentially benefit from transference work. With this population, transferences tend to be affectively dominant and are often negative and intrusive (see Table 32–5)—both demanding of clinical attention and providing a central vehicle for exploration and change.

Countertransference

A defining feature of the therapeutic relationship in all forms of dynamic therapy is the therapist's ongoing attention to his or her emotional reactions to the patient. The dynamic therapist's ability to monitor and contain these reactions enables him or her to maintain an attitude of authentic warmth and concern toward the patient in the face of clinical challenges that may arise, while sustaining an observing stance in relation to the patient's conflicts.

Countertransference is the umbrella concept for the therapist's emotional reactions to the patient within a psychodynamic frame of reference (Auchincloss and Samberg 2012). Awareness of countertransference can help focus the therapist's attention as he or she attends to the patient's verbal—and especially nonverbal—communications and will inform the therapist's understanding of the internal relationship patterns organizing the patient's experience and behavior. At the same time, countertransference can cause blind spots in the therapist and can make it difficult for the therapist to understand and empathize with particular aspects of the patient's conscious and dissociated or unconscious experience.

Some countertransferences emerge largely from within the therapist, reflecting the therapist's conflicts and personal needs. For example, a middle-aged therapist finds that a particular patient reminds him of his adolescent daughter and realizes that this has hampered his ability to more fully explore the patient's sexual history. Another therapist who is having financial difficulties finds herself feeling envious of her wealthy patients. Countertransferences of this kind tell us more about the therapist than they do about the patient.

Other countertransferences may originate largely within the patient. For example, a well-known television personality relied heavily on narcissistic defenses to bolster his own sense of superiority by covertly diminishing others and leaving them feeling inadequate and inferior. This patient's highly accomplished therapist noticed that he often found himself feeling diminished and inadequate, questioning his ability to be of help, when meeting with this patient. This countertransference reaction may have more to do with the patient's conflicts and defenses than with the therapist's.

The first form of countertransference, the therapist-centered one, tells us how different therapists might respond differently to the same patient, whereas the second, patient-centered countertransference, reflects how different therapists might respond similarly to the same patient.

As the dynamic therapist monitors his or her internal reactions to the patient, he or she maintains an open attitude toward exploring their sources. The therapist will reflect on the extent to which personal reactions to the patient provide information about the patient's internal world and to what degree the therapist's reactions say more about the therapist's current needs and conflicts than they do about the patient's.

As a general rule, as personality pathology becomes more severe, attending to countertransference becomes increasingly central to clinical work. In the treatment of patients with personality disorders, countertransference reactions tend to be more powerful than those stimulated by healthier patients and often create a strong sense of pressure within the therapist to act on them (see Table 32–5); for example, the therapist of the television personality might feel powerfully tempted in the countertransference to tell his patient about an influential lecture he had recently delivered. This pressure to act on one's countertransference reactions is experienced regardless of whether the treatment is directed toward personality pathology per se or toward co-occurring problems such as depression, anxiety, eating disorder, or substance misuse.

Treatment Selection

Few empirical studies provide information about the relative effectiveness of psychodynamic treatments compared with other psychotherapeutic approaches. When two active treatments are compared, the most common finding is no difference in outcome (the "dodo bird verdict"[7]), and when differences are reported, these differences often seem to reflect allegiance effects on the part of the "home team" therapists. In light of general empirical support for both psychodynamic and cognitive-behavioral therapies, with little clear empirical guidance with regard to superiority of one treatment over another for most disorders (Steinert et al. 2017), practitioners must rely on their clinical judgment when recommending a particular treatment approach. In this setting, the patient's goals and treatment preferences, resources, motivation for change, social support, ability to attach to a therapist, and capacity to reflect on personal experience can guide differential treatment planning.

As the clinician provides psychoeducation, reviews treatment options, and recommends a particular form of treatment, he or she initiates a process of obtaining informed consent. This process entails sharing sufficient information to enable the patient to make a reasoned decision about whether to start a particular treatment, and weighing relative risks and benefits, as well as potential risks and benefits of not pursuing treatment.

In choosing between cognitive-behavioral and psychodynamic approaches, a helpful rule of thumb is that CBT tends to focus more specifically than psychodynamic therapy on the chief complaint and symptom constellation—for example, reduction of depression, alleviation of anxiety, or improved management of parasuicidal behavior. In comparison, psychodynamic treatments tend to have a broader treatment focus,

---

[7] The "dodo bird verdict" (its name taken from the *Alice's Adventures in Wonderland* story) argues that "all [psychotherapies] have won and all must have prizes" (Wampold and Imel 2015).

placing greater emphasis on modifying domains of personality functioning related to presenting symptoms. For example, psychodynamic therapy for panic disorder (Busch et al. 2011) seeks to enhance the patient's capacity for conscious processing of and reflection on anxieties in relation to dependency, seen to precipitate panic. These changes likely will lead to a reduction in symptoms as well as enhanced interpersonal functioning. Similarly, dynamic treatment approaches to borderline personality disorder—both transference-focused psychotherapy (Yeomans et al. 2015) and mentalization-based treatment (Bateman and Fonagy 2006)—focus on helping the patient expand his or her ability to examine interpersonal experience during momentary affective arousal and place it into a meaningful context. This capacity decreases impulsivity while enhancing mentalization and improving interpersonal functioning.

When choosing among psychodynamic treatments—for example, deciding whether to recommend longer- or shorter-term therapy or to recommend a treatment focusing primarily on symptom reduction or a more ambitious treatment focused on modifying underlying personality structure—the intersection of treatment goals and level of personality organization provides one general guideline for differential treatment planning (see Table 32–4). Another useful rule of thumb is that the more general the patient's complaints and symptoms, and the more global and severe the personality pathology, the longer the duration of treatment likely to be needed will be, and the more likely it is that in-depth attention to personality functioning will be of benefit for the motivated patient. For more focal pathology or more symptom-focused complaints, shorter-term, less-intensive, and more symptom-focused treatments are often adequate.

Evidence Base and Indications

Guidelines for evaluating and comparing different forms of psychotherapy place primary value on the randomized clinical trial, a study design in which patients with a shared disorder are randomly assigned to one of two or more manualized forms of treatment. The trial design emphasizes internal validity by enrolling a carefully selected, relatively homogeneous group of patients (shared diagnosis, typically limited comorbidities) who receive treatment by specifically trained and highly motivated therapists who use a treatment manual.

Although randomized clinical trials remain the gold standard for establishing empirically supported psychotherapeutic treatments, with time and experience, the need for studies that complement efficacy studies is increasingly recognized, particularly 1) process studies designed to identify modifiers and mediators of outcome—that is, studies addressing the questions of "What treatments work for whom, and by what mechanisms?"; and 2) naturalistic outcome (effectiveness) studies that are more practically relevant to ordinary clinical practice (i.e., more generalizable to a wider variety of patients and therapists).

Efficacy Studies

The empirical evidence for the efficacy of psychodynamic treatments has expanded dramatically in the past decade (see Leichsenring et al. 2015 for an updated and thorough review). There is support for the efficacy of manualized psychodynamic treatments for a broad range of common symptom disorders, including major depressive disorder, dysthymia, pathological grief, panic disorder, social anxiety disorder, generalized anxiety disorder, somatic symptom and related disorders, and anorexia nervosa. The efficacy of psychodynamic therapy in the treatment of personality disorders is established for borderline personality disorder, Cluster C personality disorders, and complex mental disorders (defined by Leichsenring and Rabung [2012] as personality disorders, chronic mental disorders, or multiple mental disorders). A comprehensive analysis by Steinert et al. (2017), which reviewed the outcome literature, concluded that existing evidence supports the general equivalence of psychodynamic psychotherapy to other forms of psychotherapy of established efficacy (largely CBT).

The psychodynamic treatments examined in the randomized clinical trials included in reviews and meta-analyses are heterogeneous with regard to duration, frequency of sessions, and technique to some degree. Manualized treatments for symptom disorders are typically 8–30 sessions long, whereas treatments for personality disorders are longer term, usually ranging from a minimum of 30 sessions for less severe personality pathology to weekly or twice-weekly sessions over the course of several years for more severe pathology.

Process Studies

The growing body of efficacy research on psychodynamic treatment raises the important question "How do these treatments work?" Do psychodynamic treatments work through common factors—those factors shared with other forms of effective therapy—or do psychodynamic techniques and treatment models have specific therapeutic benefits not fully shared by other forms of treatment?

Process studies focusing on the specific nature of therapeutic intervention during treatment (which interventions are used, how frequently, how skillfully) and their effect on the patient can help to answer these questions. Understanding how a treatment works is the first step in understanding how the treatment can be improved or how more effective treatments can be developed. In approaching these questions, it is helpful to distinguish between *change processes* introduced by the therapist and the treatment model (e.g., use of particular interventions, therapist competence in delivering the interventions) and *change mechanisms* taking place within the patient (e.g., patient self-understanding, reflective functioning) (Crits-Christoph et al. 2013). Both should be linked to positive outcome.

Common and Specific Factors

Discussion of change mechanisms in psychotherapy immediately leads to the controversial question of the extent to which a given treatment approach provides therapeutic benefit through implementation of specific techniques as opposed to common factors. *Common factors* are treatment elements that are provided by diverse forms of therapy—for example, therapeutic alliance, therapist empathy, use of a coherent and consistent clinical approach, patient expectation of change, and encouragement to face personal difficulties—and that overlap considerably with supportive interventions; in contrast, *specific factors* are more or less unique to an individual treatment—for example, focusing on emotions or enhancing self-understanding in psychodynamic therapies or assigning homework or questioning negative cognitions in CBT.

Given constraints of space, in this chapter we have chosen to focus on specific aspects of psychodynamic treatment and technique thought to contribute uniquely to therapeutic change. For an up-to-date review and discussion of common factors in psychotherapy outcome, we refer the reader to Laska et al. (2014). Although debate is ongoing and active in regard to the relative impacts of common and specific factors on psychotherapy outcome, it is widely accepted that common factors play a role in therapeutic outcome in psychodynamic treatments (Barber et al. 2013). It is also clear that, at least in some settings, specific factors play a significant role in outcome (see, e.g., Diener et al. 2007; Høglend 2014; Johansson et al. 2010; Slavin-Mulford et al. 2011).

Change Processes

Conceptually, in studying how psychodynamic therapy brings about change, one would want to show empirically that the use of specific expressive techniques is associated with better outcome; that is, that the use of expressive techniques constitutes a change process in psychodynamic therapy. However, a review of published studies examining the average use of expressive interventions as a group in relation to positive outcome in psychodynamic therapy reported inconsistent and contradictory findings (positive relation, no relation, and occasionally negative relation) (Barber et al. 2013).[8] One interpretation of this finding in light of the demonstrated efficacy of psychodynamic treatments is that major change processes in psychodynamic therapy are the use of supportive techniques and common factors, in contrast to the use of expressive techniques. Another, and in our minds more likely, interpretation is that expressive techniques do contribute to change but that looking at the average use of different techniques is insufficient from both a methodological perspective (e.g., lumping together effective and ineffective interventions and averaging out to no effect) and a clinical perspective.

From a clinical perspective, our interpretation of these data is that in dynamic therapy, selection among expressive techniques and their subsequent implementation must be done competently to be effective; to function as change processes, expressive techniques must be used at an appropriate frequency and depth, taking into account severity of the pathology, status of the therapeutic alliance, phase of treatment, and skill of the therapist. To illustrate, a review of the literature on transference interpretations suggested that 1) the optimal "dose" of interpretations with regard to change process appears to be a *low* frequency of interventions (from one to several interventions per session), 2) use of *high-frequency* interpretations has been found to be associated with *poorer* outcome, and 3) the positive relation of low-frequency interpretations with outcome varies with severity of symptoms (Høglend 2014).

In contrast to studies examining the overall use of expressive interventions, those examining the relation between positive outcome and specific kinds of interventions in psychodynamic therapy have yielded more consistent and clinically useful findings that support the specific effects of dynamic interventions. Notably, the therapist's exploration of affect has been consistently linked to more positive outcomes (Diener et al. 2007), as has the therapist's focus on interpersonal themes (Slavin-Mulford et al. 2011).

---

[8] Interestingly, studies investigating the effect of supportive interventions measured in aggregate have found no correlation with outcome (Barber et al. 2013).

In addition, studies have found a strong positive correlation between accuracy of interpretation and outcome (Barber et al. 2013). In summary, the relation between the use of technique and outcome in dynamic psychotherapy is complex. Interpersonal and affective exploration and the sparing use of accurate interpretations appear to be generally helpful.

Change Mechanisms

Studies of change mechanisms in dynamic psychotherapy have provided empirical support for the role of both patients' self-understanding and patients' reflective functioning. Across a variety of studies and patient samples, changes in patients' self-understanding of interpersonal patterns have been found to be predictive of change in symptoms and may be a specific effect of dynamic therapy (see Barber et al. 2013).

A particularly powerful illustration of the potential value of research focused on process in psychotherapy was provided in the First Experimental Study of Transference conducted by Høglend et al. (2006), which examined the effect of "transference work" on clinical outcome in a mixed outpatient sample receiving a 50-session weekly dynamic therapy. This study used a randomized dismantling design in which patients were randomly assigned to one of two treatments, which were identical except that one employed low-frequency, transference-based interventions and the other avoided transference work. The investigators found that *on average,* use of transference work had no significant effect on outcome.

However, when the investigators performed a moderator analysis, they found that transference work was significantly associated with superior outcome in patients with a poor quality of object relations and more severe personality pathology, whereas for those with better personality functioning, transference work did not significantly contribute to outcome (Høglend et al. 2006). Further (mediator) analysis (Johansson et al. 2010) led the authors to conclude that in the group with more severe pathology, transference work led to insight or self-understanding, which functioned as a mediator of transference work on outcome (i.e., when the effect of transference work on insight was statistically removed from the equation, the preferential effect of transference work on outcome dropped out). In the healthier group of patients, transference work did not contribute to insight. This study suggested that in psychodynamic therapy for patients with more severe personality pathology, transference work is a change process, and insight as a result of working in the transference is a change mechanism.

Although recent advances in psychodynamic therapy process and outcome studies are impressive, their limitations point to areas requiring greater research efforts. There is an urgent need for studies that can shed further light on the mechanisms whereby treatments lead to change, as well as clarify which patients benefit most from which forms of treatment. Efficacy studies have focused largely on short-term psychodynamic treatments (with the exception of longer-term treatments for borderline personality disorder), but in actuality, many patients require treatments lasting longer than 16–20 weeks. Finally, because the effects of psychodynamic treatments go beyond symptom relief, there is a need to develop assessment instruments that are capable of capturing the subtlety of psychodynamic outcomes (e.g., improved reflective functioning, shift in defensive style) without being excessively labor intensive.

Conclusion

Psychodynamic theory and related treatments have an extensive clinical history and accumulated experience. In recent decades, there has been an explosion of research efforts to investigate the effect of psychodynamic treatments on symptom and personality disorders. At present, psychodynamic approaches to the assessment and treatment of a wide range of psychiatric conditions provide an empirically supported approach for practicing clinicians. The psychodynamic model provides a coherent approach to conceptualizing patients' presenting problems, identifying assessment foci, and organizing clinical intervention.

Key Clinical Points

- Psychodynamic psychotherapy refers to a family of treatments that are embedded in a shared model of mental functioning with the goal of reducing symptoms and improving adaptation through enhancing patient awareness of thoughts, feelings, and behaviors.

- Basic assumptions of the psychodynamic model include a person-oriented perspective with a focus on psychological causation and the internal world of the patient.

- The techniques of psychodynamic treatment fall on a continuum of supportive–expressive interventions.

- With a focus on self-functioning and functioning in relation to others, psychodynamic treatment is relevant for many symptom and relationship difficulties.

- Clinical assessment in the psychodynamic model enables the clinician to tailor treatment to the needs of the individual patient, on the basis of severity of presenting symptoms and problems, personality traits, and level of structural pathology.

- The level of personality organization (i.e., neurotic; high-, mid-, or low-level borderline) is crucial to the prognosis, therapeutic alliance, and nature of transferences that will arise in the treatment.

- The goals of psychodynamic treatment include symptom change but extend to improved satisfaction and engagement in friendships, intimate relationships, and work and professional functioning.

- The relationship between therapist and patient in psychodynamic therapy is at the core of treatment, with the therapeutic objective being to create an atmosphere in which the patient feels as free as possible to openly explore and share his or her experiences with an empathic and nonjudgmental other.

- The construct of transference, which refers to the patient's enactment of internal relationship patterns with the therapist, is a manifestation of a more general process in which internal patterns of relating are enacted in daily life.

- The empirical evidence for the efficacy and effectiveness of psychodynamic treatments across symptom disorders and personality disorders has expanded dramatically in the past decade.

References

American Psychiatric Association: Diagnostic and Statistical Manual of Mental Disorders, 5th Edition. Arlington, VA, American Psychiatric Association, 2013

Auchincloss AL, Samberg E (eds): Psychoanalytic Terms and Concepts. New Haven, CT, Yale University Press, 2012

Barber JP, Muran C, McCarthy KS, et al: Research on dynamic therapies, in Bergin and Garfiend's Handbook of Psychotherapy and Behavior Change, 6th Edition. Edited by Lambert MJ. Hoboken, NJ, Wiley, 2013, pp 443–494

Barlow DH, Farchione TJ, Bullis JR, et al: The unified protocol for transdiagnostic treatment of emotional disorders compared with diagnosis-specific protocols for anxiety disorders: a randomized clinical trial. JAMA Psychiatry 74(9):875–884, 2017 28768327

Bateman A, Fonagy P: Mentalization-Based Treatment for Borderline Personality Disorder. Oxford, UK, Oxford University Press, 2006

Bender DS: The therapeutic alliance in the treatment of personality disorders. J Psychiatr Pract 11(2):73–87, 2005 15803042

Blagys M, Hilsenroth M: Distinctive features of short-term psychodynamic-interpersonal psychotherapy: an empirical review of the comparative psychotherapy process literature. Clinical Psychology Science and Practice 7(2):167–188, 2000

Bordin ES: The generalizability of the psychoanalytic concept of the working alliance. Psychotherapy 16(3):252–260, 1979

Busch FN, Milrod BS, Singer MB, et al: Manual of Panic-Focused Psychodynamic Psychotherapy—Extended Range, 2nd Edition. New York, Routledge, 2011

Caligor E, Clarkin JF: An object relations model of personality and personality pathology, in Psychodynamic Psychotherapy for Personality Disorders: A Clinical Handbook. Edited by Clarkin JF, Fonagy P, Gabbard G. Washington, DC, American Psychiatric Publishing, 2010, pp 3–36

Caligor E, Kernberg OF, Clarkin JF: Handbook of Dynamic Psychotherapy for Higher Level Personality Pathology. Washington, DC, American Psychiatric Publishing, 2007

Caligor E, Kernberg OF, Clarkin JF, et al: Psychodynamic Therapy for Personality Pathology: Treating Self and Interpersonal Functioning. Arlington, VA, American Psychiatric Association Publishing, 2018

Crits-Christoph P, Connolly Gibbons M, Mukherjee D: Psychotherapy process-outcome research, in Bergin and Garfield's Handbook of Psychotherapy and Behavior Change, 6th Edition. Edited by Lambert MJ. Hoboken, NJ, Wiley, 2013, pp 298–340

Diener MJ, Hilsenroth MJ, Weinberger J: Therapist affect focus and patient outcomes in psychodynamic psychotherapy: a meta-analysis. Am J Psychiatry 164(6):936–941, 2007 17541054

Gabbard G: Long-Term Psychodynamic Psychotherapy: A Basic Text, 2nd Edition. Washington, DC, American Psychiatric Publishing, 2010

Goldman RE, Hilsenroth MJ, Owen JJ, et al: Psychotherapy integration and alliance: use of cognitive-behavioral techniques within a short-term psychodynamic treatment model. Journal of Psychotherapy Integration 23(4):373–385, 2013

Hilsenroth MJ, Cromer TD: Clinical interventions related to alliance during the initial interview and psychological assessment. Psychotherapy (Chic) 44(2):205–218, 2007 22122211

Høglend P: Exploration of the patient-therapist relationship in psychotherapy. Am J Psychiatry 171(10):1056–1066, 2014 25017093

Høglend P, Amlo S, Marble A, et al: Analysis of the patient-therapist relationship in dynamic psychotherapy: an experimental study of transference interpretations. Am J Psychiatry 163(10):1739–1746, 2006 17012684

Horvath AO, Del Re AC, Flückiger C, et al: Alliance in individual psychotherapy. Psychotherapy (Chic) 48(1):9–16, 2011 21401269

Johansson P, Høglend P, Ulberg R, et al: The mediating role of insight for long-term improvements in psychodynamic therapy. J Consult Clin Psychol 78(3):438–448, 2010 20515219

Kernberg OF, Caligor E: A psychoanalytic theory of personality disorders, in Major Theories of Personality Disorder, 2nd Edition. Edited by Lenzenweger ML, Clarkin JF. New York, Guilford, 2005, pp 114–156

Laska KM, Gurman AS, Wampold BE: Expanding the lens of evidence-based practice in psychotherapy: a common factors perspective. Psychotherapy (Chic) 51(4):467–481, 2014 24377408

Leichsenring F, Rabung S: Long-term psychodynamic psychotherapy in complex mental disorders: update of a meta-analysis. Br J Psychiatry 199(1):15–22, 2011 [Erratum in: Br J Psychiatry 200(5):430, 2012] 21719877

Leichsenring F, Kruse J, Rabung S: Efficacy of psychodynamic psychotherapy in specific disorders: an update, in Handbook of Psychodynamic Approaches to Psychopathology. Edited by Luyten P, Mayes LC, Fonagy P, et al. New York, Guilford, 2015, pp 485–511

Lingiardi V, McWilliams N (eds): Psychodynamic Diagnostic Manual, 2nd Edition (PDM-2). New York, Guilford, 2017

MacKinnon RA, Michels R, Buckley PJ: The Psychiatric Interview in Clinical Practice, 2nd Edition. Washington, DC, American Psychiatric Publishing, 2009

Safran JD, Muran JC, Eubanks-Carter C: Repairing alliance ruptures, in Psychotherapy Relationships That Work: Evidence-Based Responsiveness. Edited by Norcross JC. New York, Oxford University Press, 2011, pp 224–238

Slavin-Mulford J, Hilsenroth M, Weinberger J, et al: Therapeutic interventions related to outcome in psychodynamic psychotherapy for anxiety disorder patients. J Nerv Ment Dis 199(4):214–221, 2011 21451344

Steinert C, Munder T, Rabung S, et al: Psychodynamic therapy: as efficacious as other empirically supported treatments? A meta-analysis testing equivalence of outcomes. Am J Psychiatry 174(10):943–953, 2017 28541091

Wachtel PL: Relational Theory and the Practice of Psychotherapy. New York, Guilford, 2008

Wampold BE, Imel ZE: The Great Psychotherapy Debate: The Evidence for What Makes Psychotherapy Work, 2nd Edition. New York, NY, Routledge, 2015

Wnuk S, McMain S, Links PS, et al: Factors related to dropout from treatment in two outpatient treatments for borderline personality disorder. J Pers Disord 27(6):716–726, 2013 23718760

World Health Organization: International Statistical Classification of Diseases and Related Health Problems, 10th Revision. Geneva, World Health Organization, 1992

Yeomans F, Clarkin JF, Kernberg OF: Transference-Focused Psychotherapy for Borderline Personality Disorder: A Clinical Guide. Arlington, VA, American Psychiatric Publishing, 2015

Recommended Readings

Caligor E, Diamond D, Yeomans FE, et al: The interpretive process in the psychoanalytic psychotherapy of borderline personality disorder. J Am Psychoanal Assn 57:271–301, 2009

Høglend P: Exploration of the patient-therapist relationship in psychotherapy. Am J Psychiatry 171:1056–1066, 2014

Kernberg OF: The basic components of psychoanalytic technique and derived psychoanalytic psychotherapies. World Psychiatry 15:287–288, 2016

Steinert C, Munder T, Rabung S, et al: Psychodynamic therapy: as efficacious as other empirically supported treatments? A meta-analysis testing equivalence of outcomes. Am J Psychiatry 174(10):943–953, 2017

Trachsel M, Grosse Holtforth M, Biller-Andorno N, et al: Informed consent for psychotherapy: still not routine. Lancet Psychiatry 2(9):775–777, 2015

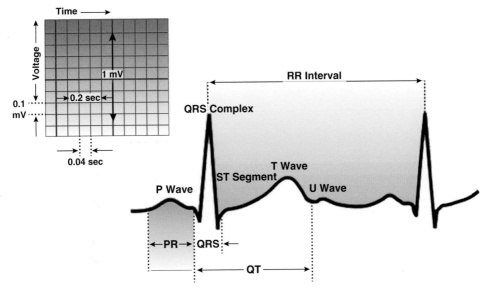

PLATE 1. *(Figure 5–1)* Electrocardiogram waves and intervals.

The P wave represents atrial activation; the PR interval is the time from onset of atrial activation to onset of ventricular activation. The QRS complex represents ventricular activation; the QRS duration is the duration of ventricular activation. The ST–T wave represents ventricular repolarization. The QT interval is the duration of ventricular activation and recovery. The U wave probably represents "afterdepolarizations" in the ventricles.

Source. Reprinted from the ECG Learning Center (https://ecg.utah.edu/), a webpage created by the Spencer S. Eccles Health Sciences Library, University of Utah, and available under a Creative Commons CC-BY license. Content copyright ©1997, Frank G. Yanowitz, M.D., Professor of Medicine (Retired), University of Utah School of Medicine, Salt Lake City.

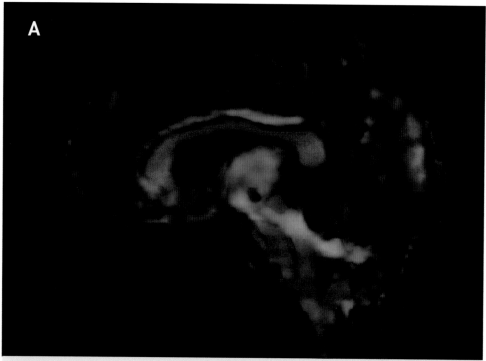

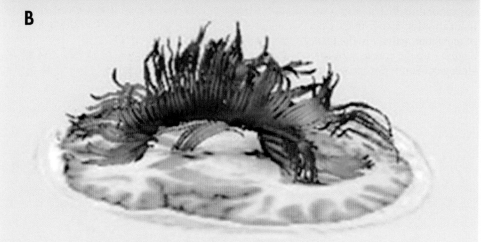

PLATE 2. *(Figure 5–6)* Diffusion tensor imaging (DTI).

(A) Fractional anisotropy color map derived from DTI in the sagittal plane. *Red* indicates white matter fibers coursing in a right–left direction, *blue* indicates fibers running in a superior–inferior direction, and *green* reflects fibers oriented in an anterior–posterior direction. **(B)** Fiber tracking using DTI of the total corpus callosum overlaid on a T1-weighted inversion recovery image from the same brain.

Source. Images courtesy of Elisabeth A. Wilde, Ph.D., Department of Neurology, University of Utah, Salt Lake City, Utah.

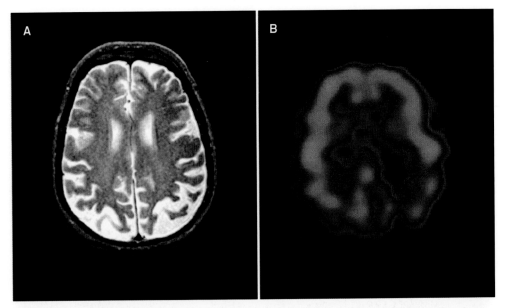

PLATE 3. *(Figure 5–7)* Side-by-side comparison of structural and functional neuroimaging: magnetic resonance imaging (MRI) and positron emission tomography (PET).

(A) Axial view of brain MRI (fluid attenuated inversion recovery [FLAIR] sequence) and **(B)** corresponding PET scan of a patient with Alzheimer's disease. The MRI scan **(A)** shows prominent atrophic change in the posterior regions of the brain, consistent with the striking reduction of metabolic activity in the posterior parietal lobes on PET imaging **(B)**.

Source. Image courtesy of Ziad Nahas, M.D., M.S.C.R., Department of Psychiatry, Medical College of South Carolina, Charleston, South Carolina.

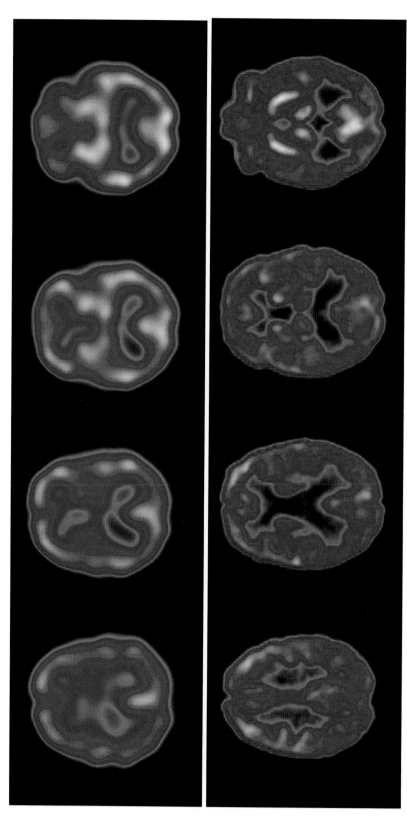

PLATE 4. *(Figure 5–8)* Comparison of single-photon emission computed tomography (SPECT) and positron emission tomography (PET).

SPECT (*top row*) and PET (*bottom row*) images from two patients with clinically similar degrees of mild cognitive impairment. The PET scan shows parietal abnormalities, suggesting that this patient may be at risk of developing Alzheimer's disease. The PET scan also shows superior resolution compared with the SPECT scan.

Source. Images courtesy of Paul E. Schulz, M.D., Department of Neurology, University of Texas Health Science Center at Houston (UTHealth), Houston, Texas.

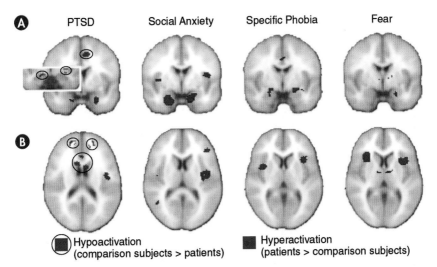

PLATE 5. *(Figure 13–1)* Clusters in which significant hyperactivation or hypoactivation was found in patients with posttraumatic stress disorder (PTSD), social anxiety disorder, or specific phobia relative to comparison subjects and in healthy subjects undergoing fear conditioning.

Results are shown for **(A)** amygdalae and **(B)** insular cortices. Note that within the left amygdala there were two distinct clusters for PTSD, a ventral anterior hyperactivation cluster and a dorsal posterior hypoactivation cluster. The right side of the image corresponds to the right side of the brain.

Source. Reprinted from Etkin A, Wager TD: "Functional Neuroimaging of Anxiety: A Meta-analysis of Emotional Processing in PTSD, Social Anxiety Disorder, and Specific Phobia." *American Journal of Psychiatry* 164(10):1476–1488, 2007. Copyright 2007, American Psychiatric Association. Used with permission.

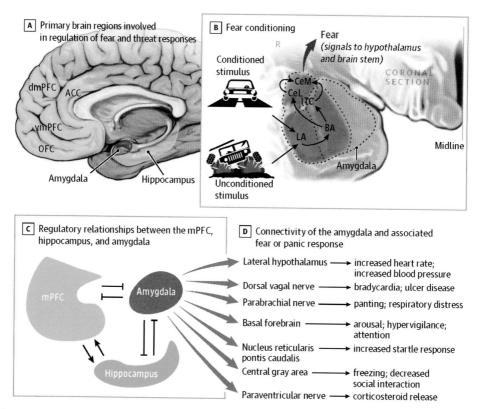

PLATE 6. *(Figure 15–1)* Schematic diagram of neural circuitry involved in fear conditioning and posttraumatic stress disorder.

(A) Primary brain regions involved in regulating fear and threat responses are the amygdala, the hippocampus, and the medial prefrontal cortex (mPFC), which consists of the dorsal (dmPFC) and ventral (vmPFC) subdivisions, the orbitofrontal cortex (OFC), and the anterior cingulate cortex (ACC).

(B) Shown are the amygdala-specific circuits involved in fear conditioning. The sensory information representing the *conditioned stimulus* (e.g., previously neutral stimulus such as driving a car) is integrated within the amygdala with the *unconditioned stimulus* information (e.g., a traumatic event such as an explosion in a car). The amygdala is central in the neural circuit involved in regulating fear conditioning. In general, input to the lateral nucleus (LA) of the amygdala leads to learning about fear, whereas the central amygdala (lateral [CeL] and medial [CeM] subdivisions) is responsible for sending output signals about fear to the hypothalamus and brain stem structures. The intercalated cell masses (ITC) are thought to regulate inhibition of information flow between the basal nucleus (BA) and the central amygdala.

(C and D) Interactions between components of the mPFC and the hippocampus constantly regulate the amygdala's output to subcortical brain regions activating the fear reflex. The mPFC (in particular, the vmPFC) is classically thought to inhibit amygdala activity and reduce subjective distress, while the hippocampus plays a role both in the coding of fear memories and in the regulation of the amygdala. The hippocampus and the mPFC also interact in regulating context and fear modulation.

Source. Reprinted from Figure 1 in Ross DA, Arbuckle MR, Travis MJ, et al.: "An Integrated Neuroscience Perspective on Formulation and Treatment Planning for Posttraumatic Stress Disorder: An Educational Review." JAMA Psychiatry 74(4):407–415, 2017. Copyright 2017, American Medical Association. Used with permission. Panels C and D adapted from Parsons and Ressler 2013.

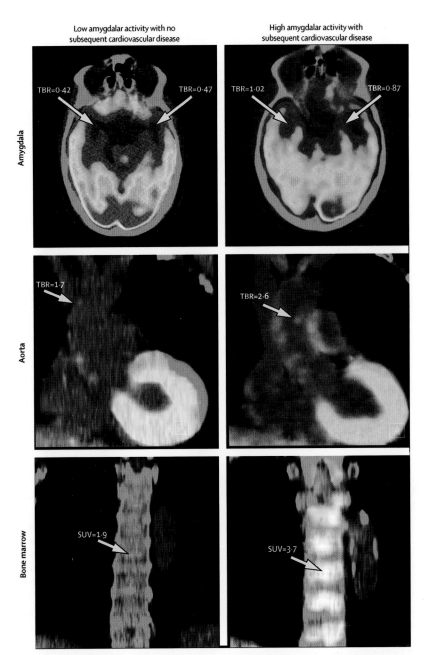

PLATE 7. *(Figure 15–2)* Pathogenic pathway linking stress to increased risk of cardiovascular disease: amygdalar, arterial, and bone-marrow uptake of ^{18}F-FDG in individuals with and without subsequent cardiovascular disease events.

Axial views of amygdala (**top,** *left and right*), coronal views of aorta (**middle,** *left and right*), and coronal views of bone marrow (**bottom,** *left and right*) are shown. ^{18}F-FDG uptake was increased in the amygdala, bone marrow, and arterial wall (aorta) in a patient who experienced an ischemic stroke during the follow-up period *(right)* compared with a patient who did not *(left)*. ^{18}F-FDG=[18]F fluorodeoxyglucose; SUV=standardized uptake value; TBR=target-to-background ratio.

Source.   Reprinted from Figure 1 in Tawakol A, Ishai A, Takx RA, et al.: "Relation Between Resting Amygdalar Activity and Cardiovascular Events: A Longitudinal and Cohort Study." *Lancet* 389(10071):834–845, 2017. Copyright 2017, Elsevier Inc.

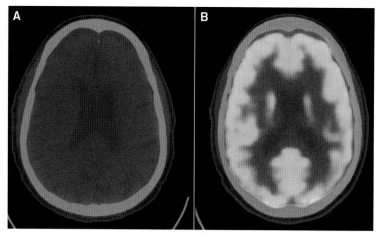

PLATE 8. *(Figure 25–1)* Florbetapir F 18 (^{18}F-AV-45) positron emission tomography scans for β-amyloid in two patients with a diagnosis of dementia.

The negative scan **(A)** suggests an underlying pathology other than Alzheimer's disease, whereas the positive scan **(B)** suggests that Alzheimer's pathology is the cause of cognitive decline.

Source.   Images courtesy of Steven Z. Chao, M.D., Ph.D.

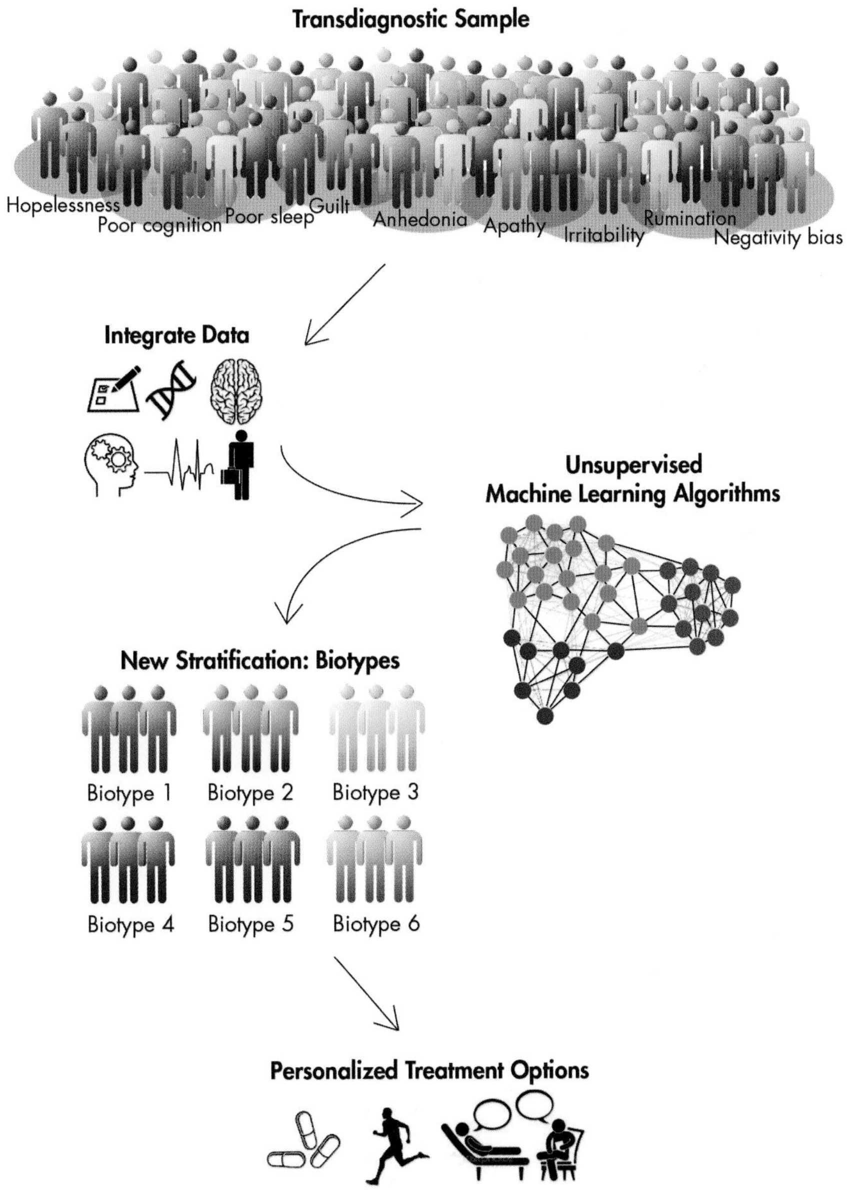

PLATE 9. *(Figure 28–1)* One path toward closing the clinical translational gap between research insights and clinical practice.

This flow diagram illustrates a proposed framework for escalating progress toward a clinically applicable precision psychiatry model of mental disorders: **(1) Transdiagnostic Sample**—Use standardized protocols and assessments that apply across multidiagnostic clinical samples and normative samples, allowing for a focus on features that are common to individuals across as well as within diagnoses; **(2) Integrate Data**—Gather and integrate data across clinical, genomic, imaging, cognitive behavior, physiological, and life history domains; **(3) Unsupervised Machine Learning Algorithms**—Harness new computational approaches to learn from the integrated data; **(4) New Stratification: Biotypes**—Identify coherent relations between clinical features and integrated domains of data that define new ways to stratify patients that may cut across some traditional diagnostic boundaries; for example, the term *biotype* is used to refer to coherent relations between profiles of brain function assessed by neuroimaging and profiles of symptoms and behavior; **(5) Personalized Treatment Options**—Use these data-derived stratification approaches in prospective and target-driven trials to optimize the choice of existing interventions and develop.

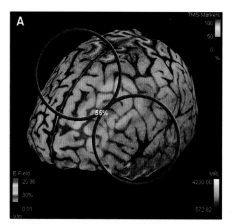
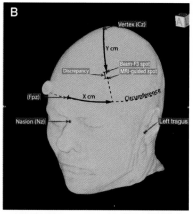

PLATE 10. *(Figure 30–4)* Techniques for localizing the stimulation site during repetitive transcranial magnetic stimulation (rTMS) treatment.

(A) Magnetic resonance imaging (MRI)–guided neuronavigation employs frameless stereotactic equipment, tracking devices attached to the coil and the patient's head, and an MRI of the patient to localize the focus of stimulation with accuracies of less than 4 mm under ideal conditions. The operator can monitor the position of the rTMS coil in real time in order to position it over the target site. Here, the left dorsolateral prefrontal cortex (DLPFC) is targeted, and the predicted electrical field of the coil during stimulation is superimposed on the patient's MRI.

(B) An alternative to MRI-guided neuronavigation in routine therapeutic rTMS involves the use of scalp landmarks to localize the target of stimulation. One commonly used method, known as BeamF3 (Beam et al. 2009), employs the standard electroencephalography (EEG) sensor site "F3" (in the international 10–20 EEG system) as a proxy for the scalp site corresponding to the left DLPFC. The procedure for locating the F3 site is based on three cardinal scalp measurements: 1) nasion–inion distance from anterior to posterior, 2) tragus–tragus distance from left to right ear, and 3) head circumference.

Source.   **Image A:** From the lab of Jonathan Downar, M.D., Ph.D. Used with permission.

Image B: Reprinted from Figure 1C (p. 967) in Mir-Moghtadaei A, Caballero R, Fried P, et al.: "Concordance Between BeamF3 and MRI-Neuronavigated Target Sites for Repetitive Transcranial Magnetic Stimulation of the Left Dorsolateral Prefrontal Cortex." *Brain Stimulation* 8(5):965–973, 2015. Copyright 2015, Elsevier.

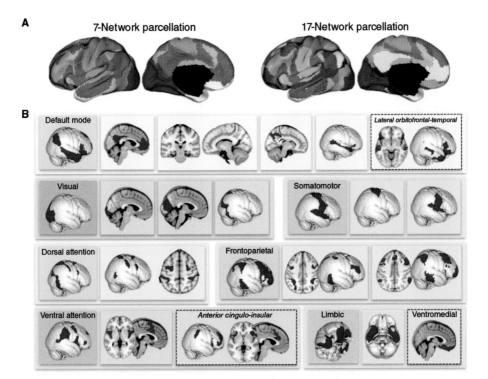

PLATE 11. *(Figure 30–8)* Networks of coherent functional activity in the resting human brain.

(A) The intrinsic, ongoing activity of the brain at rest or during tasks can be separated into at least seven distinct functional networks, appearing consistently across large datasets of up to 1,000 individuals. These networks can also be further subdivided into subnetworks. A 17-network parcellation has been identified as being stable across individuals (Yeo et al. 2011).

(B) The 17 resting-state networks identified by Yeo et al. (2011) included low-level visual and somatosensory cortical areas, higher-level networks involving premotor and sensory association areas, and larger frontoparietal networks involved in attention, cognition, and executive control. However, three networks (highlighted in *dashed red lines*) are of particular interest as neural substrates for psychiatric endophenotypes: a ventromedial prefrontal "incentive" network corresponding to the classical reward circuit, a "nonreward" lateral orbitofrontal-temporal network (LOFTN) involved in emotional reappraisal and hypothetical reward valuation, and an anterior cinguloinsular "salience" network (aCIN) involved in cognitive control and response inhibition.

Source. Reprinted from Figure 1 (A & B) in: Dunlop K, Hanlon CA, Downar J: "Noninvasive Brain Stimulation Treatments for Addiction and Major Depression." *Annals of the New York Academy of Sciences* 1394(1):31–54, 2017. Copyright 2017, John Wiley & Sons Inc.

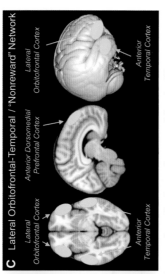

A Anterior Cingulo-Insular / "Salience" Network

Anterior Insula

Dorsal Anterior Cingulate Cortex (dACC)

Inferior Parietal Cortex

Mediodorsal Thalamus

Dorsal Striatum (Head of Caudate Nucleus)

Dorsolateral Prefrontal Cortex (DLPFC)

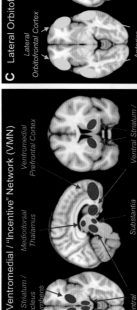

B Ventromedial / "Incentive" Network (VMN)

Ventral Striatum / Nucleus Accumbens

Mediodorsal Thalamus

Ventromedial Prefrontal Cortex

Ventral Tegmental Area

Substantia Nigra

Ventral Striatum / Nucleus Accumbens

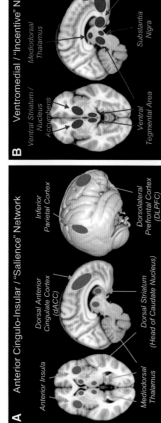

C Lateral Orbitofrontal-Temporal / "Nonreward" Network

Lateral Orbitofrontal Cortex

Anterior Dorsomedial Prefrontal Cortex

Lateral Orbitofrontal Cortex

Anterior Temporal Cortex

PLATE 12. *(Figure 30–9)* Functional networks associated with transdiagnostic dimensions of pathology in psychiatric illness.

(A) The *salience network* has core nodes in the dorsal anterior cingulate and anterior insular cortex, with additional nodes in the dorsolateral prefrontal cortex and lateral parietal cortex, along with their striatal and thalamic counterparts. Closely linked to the Research Domain Criteria (RDoC) domain of *cognitive control*, the salience network is hypoactive transdiagnostically across multiple psychiatric disorders.

(B) The ventromedial *incentive network* corresponds closely to the classical *reward circuit* projecting from midbrain dopaminergic regions to the ventral striatum and ventromedial prefrontal cortex. Closely linked to the RDoC domain of *positive valence systems*, the incentive network is also abnormally active transdiagnostically across multiple psychiatric disorders. It is observed to be anticorrelated to the salience network in its activity.

(C) The lateral orbitofrontal-temporal network is sometimes linked to *nonreward functions* and the RDoC domain of *negative valence systems*. It centers on lateral orbitofrontal regions and their input regions in the lateral temporal cortex. Involved in emotional reappraisal, these regions are also abnormally overactive or underactive during tasks requiring cognitive control or response inhibition across a variety of psychiatric disorders.

Source. From the lab of Jonathan Downar, M.D., Ph.D. Used with permission.

CHAPTER 33

Cognitive-Behavioral Therapy

Jesse H. Wright, M.D., Ph.D.

Michael E. Thase, M.D.

Aaron T. Beck, M.D.

Cognitive-behavioral therapy (CBT) is a system of psychotherapy based on theories of pathological information processing in mental disorders. Treatment is directed primarily at modifying distorted or maladaptive cognitions and related behavioral dysfunction. Therapeutic interventions are usually focused and problem oriented. Although the use of specific techniques is a major feature of this approach, there can be considerable flexibility and creativity in the clinical application of CBT.

In this chapter, we trace the historical origins of CBT, explain basic theories, and detail commonly used CBT techniques. The main focus is on the treatment of depression and anxiety disorders in adults; CBT procedures for psychosis, bipolar disorder, personality disorders, and other psychiatric conditions are briefly described. The extensive research on the effectiveness of CBT is summarized. Methods have been developed for using CBT with children and adolescents, but these applications are not discussed in this chapter. Readers who wish to learn about CBT for younger persons are referred to the excellent books on this topic, including those by Friedberg and McClure (2015), Szigethy (2012), and Reinecke et al. (2003).

The authors have provided statements describing relevant financial and nonfinancial affiliations (see "Disclosure of Interests" section at the beginning of the textbook).

Historical Background

The CBT approach to depression was first proposed by Beck in the early 1960s (Beck 1963, 1964). He had begun to study depression from a psychoanalytical perspective several years earlier but had been struck by incongruities between the "retroflexed hostility" concept of psychoanalysis and his observations that depressed individuals usually hold negatively biased constructions of themselves and their environment (Beck 1963, 1964). Subsequently, a comprehensive CBT method for depression was articulated, and the treatment model was extended to a variety of other conditions, including anxiety disorders. CBT was described in a fully developed form in *Cognitive Therapy of Depression* (Beck et al. 1979).

CBT is linked philosophically to the concepts of the Greek stoic philosophers and Eastern schools of thought such as Taoism and Buddhism (Beck et al. 1979). The writing of Epictetus in the *Enchiridion* ("Men are disturbed not by things which happen, but by the opinions about the things") captures the essence of the perspective that our ideas or thoughts are a controlling factor in our emotional lives. The existential phenomenological approach to philosophy, as exemplified in the writings of Kant, Jaspers, Frankl, and others, has also been linked to the basic concepts of CBT (Clark et al. 1999). A number of developments in the field of psychotherapy during the twentieth century contributed to the formulation of the CBT approach. The neo-Freudians, such as Adler, Horney, Alexander, and Sullivan, focused on the importance of perceptions of the self and on the salience of conscious experience. Other contributions came from the field of developmental psychology and from Kelly's theory of personal constructs (Clark et al. 1999). These writers stressed the significance of schemas (cognitive templates) in perceiving, assimilating, and acting on information from the environment.

CBT also incorporates theories and treatment methods of behavior therapy (Meichenbaum 1977). Procedures such as activity scheduling, graded task assignment, exposure, and social skills training play a fundamental role in CBT (Beck et al. 1979; Wright et al. 2017).

In the half-century since Beck introduced CBT concepts and methods, a very large research effort has documented the efficacy of this approach (for comprehensive reviews of the early research literature, see Gaffan et al. 1995; Robinson et al. 1990), and CBT methods have been studied for a broad range of problems, including depression, anxiety disorders, psychosis, eating disorders, substance abuse, and personality disorders. Related therapies such as mindfulness-based CBT (Williams et al. 2007), well-being therapy (Fava 2016), and dialectical behavior therapy (DBT; Linehan 1993) also have been developed (Wright et al. 2017), and computer-assisted delivery methods (Eells et al. 2015) are now available to improve efficiency and increase access to CBT.

Basic Concepts

The Cognitive Model

The cognitive model for psychotherapy is grounded on the theory that there are characteristic errors in information processing in psychiatric disorders and that these alterations in thought processes are closely linked to emotional reactions and dysfunctional behavior patterns (Alford and Beck 1997; Beck 1976; Clark et al. 1999; Dobson et al. 2018). For example, Beck and coworkers (Beck 1976) have proposed that people with depression are prone to cognitive distortions in three major areas—self, world/environment, and future (i.e., the "negative cognitive triad")—and that people with anxiety disorders habitually overestimate the danger or risk in situations. Cognitive distortions such as misperceptions, errors in logic, and misattributions are thought to lead to dysphoric moods and maladaptive behavior. Furthermore, a vicious cycle is perpetuated when the behavioral response confirms and amplifies negatively distorted cognitions:

> Mr. S is a 45-year-old recently divorced, depressed man. After being rebuffed on his first attempt to ask a woman for a date, Mr. S had a series of dysfunctional cognitions such as, "You should have known better; you're a loser.... There's no use trying." His subsequent behavioral pattern was consistent with these cognitions—he made no further social contacts and became more lonely and isolated. The negative behavior led to additional maladaptive cognitions (e.g., "No one will want me; I'll be alone the rest of my life.... What's the use of going on?").

The CBT perspective can be summarized in a working model (Figure 33–1) that expands on the well-known stimulus–response paradigm (Wright et al. 2017). Cognitive mediation is given a central role in this model. However, an interactive relationship between environmental influences, cognition, emotion, and behavior is also recognized. It should be emphasized that this working model does not presume that cognitive pathology is the cause of specific syndromes or that other factors such as genetic predisposition, biochemical alterations, or interpersonal conflicts are not involved in the etiology of psychiatric illnesses. Instead, the model is used as a guide for the actions of the cognitive therapist in clinical practice. It is assumed that most forms of psychopathology have complex etiologies involving cognitive, biological, social, and interpersonal influences and that there are multiple potentially useful approaches to treatment. In addition, it is assumed that cognitive changes are accomplished through biological processes and that psychopharmacological treatments can alter cognitions. This position is consistent with outcome research on CBT and pharmacotherapy (Blackburn et al. 1986) and with other studies that have documented neurobiological changes associated with conditioning in animals (Kandel and Schwartz 1982) and psychotherapy in humans (Fonzo et al. 2017; Goldapple et al. 2004).

The model in Figure 33–1 posits a close relationship between cognition and emotion. The general thrust of CBT is that emotional responses are largely dependent on cognitive appraisals of the significance of environmental cues. For example, sadness is likely when a person perceives an event (or memory of an event) in a negative way (e.g., as a loss, a defeat, or a rejection), and anger is common when a person judges that there are threats to oneself or one's loved ones. The cognitive model also incorporates the effects of emotion on cognitive processing. Heightened emotion can stimulate and intensify cognitive distortions. Therapeutic procedures in CBT involve interventions at all points in the model diagrammed in Figure 33–1. However, most of the effort is directed at stimulating either cognitive or behavioral change.

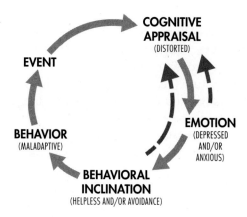

FIGURE 33–1.   Basic cognitive-behavioral model.

Source.   Reprinted from Wright JH, Brown GK, Thase ME, Basco MR: *Learning Cognitive-Behavior Therapy: An Illustrated Guide,* 2nd Edition (Core Competencies in Psychotherapy Series; Glen O. Gabbard, series ed). Arlington, VA, American Psychiatric Association Publishing, 2017, p. 4. Copyright © 2017, American Psychiatric Association Publishing. Used with permission.

Levels of Dysfunctional Cognitions

Beck and colleagues (Beck 1976; Beck et al. 1979) have suggested that there are two major levels of dysfunctional information processing: 1) automatic thoughts and 2) basic beliefs incorporated in schemas. *Automatic thoughts* are the cognitions that occur rapidly while a person is in a situation (or recalling an event). These automatic thoughts usually are not subjected to rational analysis and often are based on erroneous logic. Although the individual may be only subliminally aware of these cognitions, automatic thoughts are accessible through questioning techniques used in CBT (Beck et al. 1979; Wright et al. 2017). The different types of faulty logic in automatic thinking have been termed *cognitive errors* (Beck et al. 1979). Descriptions of typical cognitive errors are provided in Table 33–1.

   Schemas, or core beliefs, are deeper cognitive structures that contain the basic rules for screening, filtering, and coding information from the environment (Beck et al. 1979; Clark et al. 1999). These organizing constructs are developed through early childhood experiences and subsequent formative influences. Schemas can play a highly adaptive role in allowing rapid assimilation of data and appropriate decision making. However, in psychiatric disorders, there are clusters of maladaptive schemas that perpetuate dysphoric mood and ineffective or self-defeating behavior (Beck 1976; Beck and Freeman 1990).

   Although some authors (e.g., Dobson et al. 2018) divide the schema level of cognitive processing into core beliefs and underlying assumptions (conditional propositions such as "if–then" statements), we prefer the parsimonious method of describing all underlying basic cognitive constructs as schemas. In this chapter, we use the terms *schemas* and *core beliefs* interchangeably. Examples of adaptive and maladaptive schemas are presented in Table 33–2.

   One of the basic tenets of CBT is that maladaptive schemas often lie dormant until they are triggered by stressful life events (Beck et al. 1979; Clark et al. 1999; Dobson et al. 2018). The newly emerged schema then influences the more superficial level of

TABLE 33–1. Cognitive errors

Selective abstraction (sometimes termed *mental filter*)	Drawing a conclusion based on only a small portion of the available data
Arbitrary inference	Coming to a conclusion without adequate supporting evidence or despite contradictory evidence
Absolutistic thinking ("all-or-none" thinking)	Categorizing oneself or one's personal experiences into rigid dichotomies (e.g., all good or all bad, perfect or completely flawed, success or total failure)
Magnification or minimization	Over- or undervaluing the significance of a personal attribute, a life event, or a future possibility
Personalization	Linking external occurrences to oneself (e.g., taking blame, assuming responsibility, criticizing oneself) when there is little or no basis for making these associations
Catastrophic thinking	Predicting the worst possible outcome while ignoring more likely eventualities

Source. Adapted from Wright et al. 2017.

TABLE 33–2. Adaptive and maladaptive schemas

Adaptive	Maladaptive
If I work at something, I can master it.	If I choose to do something, I must succeed.
I'm a survivor.	I'm a fake.
Others can trust me.	Without a woman [man], I'm nothing.
I'm lovable.	I'm stupid.
People respect me.	No matter what I do, I won't succeed.
I can figure things out.	Others can't be trusted.
If I prepare, I usually do better.	I can never be comfortable around others.
I like to be challenged.	If I make one mistake, I'll lose everything.
There's not much that can scare me.	The world is too frightening for me.
No matter what happens, I can manage—somehow.	I must be perfect to be accepted.

cognitive processing so that automatic thoughts are consistent with the rules of the schema. This theory applies primarily to episodic disorders such as depression. In chronic conditions (e.g., personality disturbances, eating disorders), schemas that pertain to the self may be present consistently and may be more resistant to change than in depression or anxiety disorders (Beck et al. 2015).

> Mrs. C, a 39-year-old schoolteacher who was married for the second time, was functioning well until her husband made an unwise financial investment. When the family's economic situation changed, Mrs. C became depressed and started to have crying spells in her classroom. During the course of CBT, several important schemas were uncovered. One of these was the maladaptive belief "You'll fail no matter how hard you try." This schema was associated with a host of negative automatic thoughts (e.g., "We messed up again; we'll lose everything. It's not worth the effort."). Although there had

been a significant financial loss, and the marriage was stressed because of the situation, the emergence of Mrs. C's underlying schema led to an overgeneralization of the significance of the problem and a perpetuation of dysfunctional automatic thoughts.

Cognitive Pathology in Depression and Anxiety Disorders

The role of cognitive functioning in depression and anxiety disorders has been studied extensively. Information processing also has been examined in eating disorders, characterological problems, and other psychiatric conditions. In general, the results of this investigative effort have confirmed Beck's hypotheses (Beck 1963, 1964, 1976; Beck et al. 1979; Clark et al. 1999; Dobson et al. 2018). A full review of this research is not attempted here. However, we provide a synthesis of results of significant studies on depression and anxiety. These findings have played an important role in both confirming and shaping the treatment procedures used in CBT. Cognitive pathology in eating disturbances, personality disorders, and psychoses is described in the section "Cognitive-Behavioral Therapy Applications" later in this chapter.

Reviews of the voluminous research on cognitive processes in depression have found strong evidence for a negative cognitive bias in this disorder (Clark et al. 1999; Dobson et al. 2018). For example, distorted automatic thoughts and cognitive errors have been found to be much more frequent in depressed persons than in control subjects (Blackburn et al. 1986; Dobson et al. 2018).

Substantial evidence also has been collected to support the concept of the negative cognitive triad of self, world/environment, and future (Clark et al. 1999; Dobson et al. 2018), and a large group of investigations has established that one of the elements of this triad, a view of the future as hopeless, is highly associated with suicide risk. For example, Beck et al. (1985) found that hopelessness was the strongest predictor of eventual suicide in a sample of depressed inpatients followed up 10 years after discharge. CBT has been shown to be an effective treatment approach for reducing hopelessness and suicide attempts (Brown et al. 2005).

Studies of information processing in anxiety disorders have provided additional confirmation for the cognitive model of psychopathology (Clark 2018; Clark and Beck 2011). Anxious patients have been found to have an attentional bias in responding to potentially threatening stimuli (Clark and Beck 2011). Individuals with significant levels of anxiety are more likely than nonanxious persons to have a facilitated intake of information about potential threat; furthermore, those with anxiety disorders are prone to interpret environmental situations as being unrealistically dangerous or risky and to underestimate their ability to cope with these situations (Clark 2018; Clark and Beck 2011). Anxious patients also have been shown to have an enhanced recall for memories associated with threatening situations or past anxiety states and misinterpretations of bodily stimuli (Clark 2018; Clark and Beck 2011). Thus, dysfunctional thinking in anxiety disorders spans several phases of information processing, including attention, elaboration and inference, and retrieval from memory.

Comparisons of depressed and anxious patients have identified differences between the two groups and common features of the disorders. Findings of studies on cognitive pathology in depression and anxiety disorders are summarized in Table 33–3.

TABLE 33–3.   Pathological information processing in depression and anxiety disorders

Predominant in depression	Predominant in anxiety disorders	Common to both depression and anxiety disorders
Hopelessness	Fears of harm or danger	Demoralization
Low self-esteem	High sensitivity to information about potential threat	Self-absorption
Negative view of environment	Automatic thoughts associated with danger, risk, uncontrollability, incapacity	Heightened automatic information processing
Automatic thoughts with negative themes	Overestimates of risk in situations	Maladaptive schemas
Misattributions	Enhanced recall of memories for threatening situations	Reduced cognitive capacity for problem solving
Overestimates of negative feedback		
Enhanced recall of negative memories		
Impaired performance on cognitive tasks requiring effort, abstract thinking		

Therapeutic Principles

General Procedures

CBT is usually a short-term treatment, lasting from 5 to 20 sessions. In some instances, very brief treatment courses are used for patients with mild or circumscribed problems, or longer series of CBT sessions are used for those with chronic or especially severe conditions. However, the typical patient with major depressive disorder or an anxiety disorder can be treated successfully within the short-term format. Research studies on CBT for depression and anxiety disorders typically have used traditional "50-minute hours" to deliver treatment, and the book *Learning Cognitive-Behavior Therapy: An Illustrated Guide,* 2nd Edition (Wright et al. 2017), focuses on the use of 50-minute sessions. However, psychiatrists have developed methods for combining CBT and medication in briefer sessions for some patients (Wright et al. 2010). In this chapter, we describe traditional CBT delivered in 50-minute sessions. Readers interested in methods of adapting CBT for briefer sessions can find guidelines in *High-Yield Cognitive-Behavior Therapy for Brief Sessions: An Illustrated Guide* (Wright et al. 2010).

After acute-phase treatment with CBT is completed, booster sessions may be useful in some cases, particularly for individuals with a history of recurrent illness or incomplete remission. Booster sessions can help maintain gains, solidify what has been learned in CBT, and decrease the chances of relapse. Also, longer-term CBT can be woven into the ongoing psychiatric treatment of bipolar disorder, schizophrenia, and other conditions that are managed by psychiatrists over many years (Wright et al. 2010).

Although CBT is primarily directed at the here and now, knowledge of the patient's family background, developmental experiences, social network, and medical history helps guide the course of therapy. Collecting a thorough history is an essential component of the early phase of treatment. The therapist can augment the history taking in CBT by asking the patient to write a brief "autobiography" as one of the early homework assignments. This material is then reviewed during subsequent therapy session.

The bulk of the therapeutic effort in CBT is devoted to working on specific problems or issues in the patient's current life. The problem-oriented approach is emphasized for several reasons. First, directing the patient's attention to current problems stimulates the development of action plans that can help reverse helplessness, hopelessness, avoidance, or other dysfunctional symptoms. Second, data on cognitive responses to recent life events are more readily accessible and verifiable than are those for events that happened years in the past. Third, practical work on current problems helps to prevent the development of excessive dependency or regression in the therapeutic relationship. Finally, current problems usually provide ample opportunity to understand and explore the effect of past experiences.

The Therapeutic Relationship

The therapeutic relationship in CBT is characterized by a high degree of collaboration between patient and therapist and an empirical tone to the work of therapy. The therapist and patient function much like an investigative team. They develop hypotheses about the validity of automatic thoughts and schemas, and about the effectiveness of patterns of behavior. A series of exercises or experiments is then designed to test the validity of the hypotheses and, subsequently, to modify cognitions or behavior. Beck et al. (1979) termed this form of therapeutic relationship *collaborative empiricism*. Methods of building a collaborative and empirical relationship are listed in Table 33–4.

The development of a collaborative working relationship is dependent on a number of therapist and patient characteristics. The "nonspecific" therapist variables that are important components of all effective psychotherapies (Wright et al. 2017) are equally significant in CBT (see Table 33–4). Professionals who are kind and understanding and can convey appropriate empathy make good cognitive-behavioral therapists. Other factors of significance are the ability of the therapist to generate trust, to demonstrate a high level of competence, and to show equanimity under pressure.

The therapist usually is more active in CBT than in most other psychotherapies. The degree of therapist activity varies with the stage of treatment and the severity of the illness. Generally, a more directive and structured approach is emphasized early in treatment, when symptoms are severe. For example, a markedly depressed patient who is beginning treatment may benefit from considerable direction and structure because of symptoms such as helplessness, hopelessness, low energy, and impaired concentration. As the patient improves and understands more about the methods of CBT, the therapist can become somewhat less active. By the end of treatment, the patient should be able to use self-monitoring and self-help techniques with little reinforcement from the therapist.

Collaborative empiricism is fostered throughout the therapy, even when directive work is required. Although the therapist may suggest specific strategies or give homework assignments designed to combat severe depression or anxiety, the patient's input is always solicited, and the self-help component of CBT is emphasized from the outset of treatment. Also, it is made clear that CBT is not an attempt to convert all negative thoughts to positive ones. Bad things do occur to people, and some individuals have behaviors that are ineffective or self-defeating. It is emphasized that in CBT one seeks to obtain an accurate assessment of 1) the validity of cognitions and 2) the adaptive versus maladaptive nature of behavior. If cognitive distortions have occurred, the patient and therapist will work together to develop a more rational perspective. On the other hand, if actual negative experiences or characteristics are identified, the patient and therapist will attempt to find ways of coping or changing.

Additional procedures that cognitive therapists use to encourage collaborative empiricism are 1) providing feedback throughout sessions, 2) recognizing and managing transference, 3) customizing therapy interventions, and 4) using gentle humor. The therapist gives feedback to keep the therapeutic relationship anchored in the here and now and to reinforce the working aspect of the therapy process. Comments are made frequently throughout the session to summarize major points, give direction, and keep the session on target. Also, the therapist asks questions at several intervals in each session to determine how well the patient has understood a concept or has grasped the essence of a therapeutic intervention. Because CBT is highly psychoeducational, the therapist functions to some degree as a teacher. Thus, discreet positive feedback is given to help stimulate and reward the patient's efforts to learn. On a cautionary note, however, the cognitive therapist needs to avoid overzealous coaching or providing inaccurate or overdone positive feedback. Such actions will usually undermine the development of a good collaborative relationship.

TABLE 33–4.   Methods of enhancing collaborative empiricism

Work together as an investigative team.

Adjust therapist activity level to match the severity of illness and phase of treatment.

Encourage self-monitoring and self-help.

Obtain an accurate assessment of the validity of cognitions and efficacy of behavior patterns.

Develop coping strategies for real losses and actual deficits.

Promote essential "nonspecific" therapist variables (e.g., kindness, empathy, equanimity, positive general attitude).

Provide and request feedback on a regular basis.

Recognize and manage transference.

Customize therapy interventions.

Use gentle humor.

Patients also are encouraged to give feedback throughout the sessions. In the beginning of treatment, patients are told that the therapist will want to hear from them regularly about how the sessions are going. What are the patient's reactions to the therapist? What things are going well? What would the patient like to change? What points are clear and make sense? What seems confusing?

A collaborative therapeutic relationship with frequent opportunities for two-way feedback generally discourages the formation of a transference neurosis. CBT methodology and the short-term nature of treatment promote pragmatic working relationships as opposed to recapitulations of dysfunctional early relationships. Nevertheless, significant transference reactions can occur. These are more likely with patients who have personality disorders or other chronic illnesses that require longer-term treatment. The formation of negative or problematic transference reactions is rare in conventional short-term CBT for persons with uncomplicated depression or anxiety disorders. When transference reactions occur, the cognitive therapist applies CBT procedures to understand the phenomenon and to intervene. Typically, automatic thoughts and schemas that pertain to the therapeutic relationship are identified, explored, and modified if possible.

Another feature of CBT that increases the collaborative nature of the therapeutic relationship is the customization of therapy interventions to meet the level of the patient's cognitive and social functioning. A profoundly depressed or anxious individual with concentration difficulties may require a primarily behavioral approach, with limited efforts at understanding concepts such as automatic thoughts and schemas, especially in the beginning of treatment. Conversely, a less symptomatic patient with the ability to grasp abstract concepts may be able to profit from schema assessment early in therapy. If treatment procedures are pitched at a proper level, the patient is more likely to understand the material of therapy and to form a collaborative relationship with the therapist who is directing the treatment.

The therapeutic relationship also can be enhanced by using appropriate humor during CBT sessions. For example, the therapist may encourage the patient's sense of humor by providing opportunities to laugh together at some improbable situation or humorously distorted cognition. On occasion, the therapist may use hyperbole in a discreet manner to point out an inconsistency or an illogical conclusion. Humor needs to be injected carefully into the therapeutic relationship. Although some patients respond quite well to humor, others may be limited in their ability to use this feature of therapy. However, humor can strengthen the therapeutic relationship in CBT if patient and therapist are able to laugh with each other and to use humor to deflate exaggerated or distorted cognitions.

See Videos 1 and 2 accompanying the book *Learning Cognitive-Behavior Therapy: An Illustrated Guide,* 2nd Edition (Wright et al. 2017), for examples showing that a cognitive-behavioral therapist can be quite active in sessions, structuring therapy to focus on coping with specific problems while conveying considerable empathy and understanding.

Assessment and Case Conceptualization

Assessment for CBT begins with completion of a standard history and mental status examination. Although special attention is paid to cognitive and behavioral elements, a full biopsychosocial evaluation is completed and used in formulating the treatment plan. The Academy of Cognitive Therapy (www.academyofct.org), a certifying organization for cognitive therapists, has outlined a method for assessment and case conceptualization that involves consideration of developmental influences, family history, social and interpersonal issues, genetic and biological contributions, and strengths and assets in addition to key automatic thoughts, schemas, and behavioral patterns (Figure 33–2). *Learning Cognitive-Behavior Therapy: An Illustrated Guide,* 2nd Edition (Wright et al. 2017), provides detailed methods, worksheets, and examples of use of the Academy of Cognitive Therapy formulation methods. Worksheets from this book can be downloaded from the American Psychiatric Association Publishing web site (https://www.appi.org/wright). Also, the Academy of Cognitive Therapy web site supplies illustrations of how to complete case conceptualizations.

The key elements of the case conceptualization (Table 33–5) are 1) an outline of the most salient aspects of the history and mental status examination; 2) detailing of at least three examples from the patient's life of the relationship between events, automatic thoughts, emotions, and behaviors (specific illustrations of the cognitive model as it pertains to this patient); 3) identification of important schemas; 4) listing of strengths; 5) a working hypothesis that weaves together all of the information in numbers 1–4 with the cognitive and behavioral theories that most closely fit the patient's diagnosis and symptoms; and 6) a treatment plan (including choices for specific CBT methods) that is based on the working hypothesis. The conceptualization is continually developed throughout therapy and may be augmented or revised as new information is collected and treatment methods are tested.

One of the common myths about CBT is that it is a "manualized" therapy that follows a "cookbook" approach. Although it is true that CBT has been distinguished by clear descriptions of theory and methods, this treatment is guided by an individualized case conceptualization. Experienced therapists typically use considerable creativity in matching CBT interventions to the unique attributes, cultural background, life stresses, and strengths of each patient (see Table 33–5).

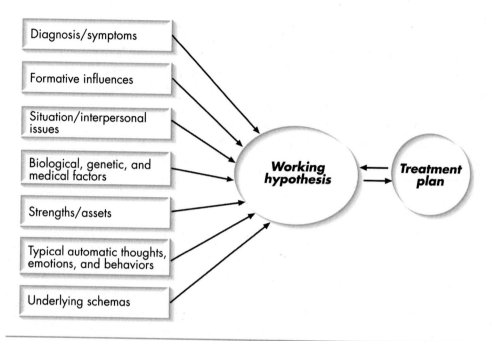

FIGURE 33–2. Case conceptualization flowchart.

Source. Reprinted from Wright JH, Brown GK, Thase ME, Basco MR: *Learning Cognitive-Behavior Therapy: An Illustrated Guide,* 2nd Edition (Core Competencies in Psychotherapy Series, Glen O. Gabbard, series ed). Arlington, VA, American Psychiatric Association Publishing, 2017, p. 50. Copyright © 2017, American Psychiatric Association Publishing. Used with permission.

TABLE 33–5. Key elements of cognitive-behavioral therapy case conceptualization

History and mental status examination

Examples of cognitive-behavioral model from patient's life

Identification of major schemas

List of strengths

Working hypothesis

Treatment plan

Structuring Therapy

Several of the structuring procedures commonly used in CBT are listed in Table 33–6. One of the most important techniques for CBT is the use of a therapy agenda. At the beginning of each session, the therapist and patient work together to derive a short list of topics, usually consisting of two to four items. Generally, it is advisable to shape an agenda that 1) can be managed within the time frame of an individual session, 2) follows up on material from earlier sessions, 3) reviews any homework from the previous session and provides an opportunity for new homework assignments, and 4) contains specific items that are highly relevant to the patient but are not too global or abstract.

Agenda setting helps to counteract hopelessness and helplessness by reducing seemingly overwhelming problems into workable segments. The agenda-setting pro-

TABLE 33–6. Structuring procedures for cognitive-behavioral therapy
Set agenda for therapy sessions.
Give constructive feedback to direct the course of therapy.
Use common cognitive-behavioral therapy techniques on a regular basis.
Assign homework to link sessions together.

cess also encourages patients to take a problem-oriented approach to their difficulties. Simply articulating a problem in a specific manner often can initiate the process of change. In addition, the agenda keeps the patient focused on salient issues and encourages efficient use of the therapy time.

The agenda is set in a collaborative manner, and decisions to depart from the agenda are made jointly between therapist and patient. When work on an agenda item generates important information on a topic that was not foreseen at the beginning of the session, the therapist and patient discuss the merits of diverting or modifying the agenda. An excessively rigid approach to using a therapy agenda is not advocated. There must be sufficient flexibility to investigate promising new leads or to allow the patient to express significant thoughts or feelings that were unexpected at the beginning of the session. However, an overall commitment to setting and following the therapy agenda gives needed structure to patients who are unable to define problems clearly or think of ways to cope with them.

Feedback procedures described earlier are also used in structuring CBT sessions. For example, the therapist may observe that the patient is drifting from the established agenda or is spending time discussing a topic of questionable relevance. In situations such as these, constructive feedback is given to direct the patient back to a more profitable area of inquiry. Commonly used CBT techniques add an additional structural element to the therapy. Examples include activity scheduling, thought recording, and graded task assignments. These interventions, and others of a similar nature, provide a clear and understandable method for reducing symptoms. Repeated use of procedures such as recording, labeling, and modifying automatic thoughts helps to link sessions together, especially if the concepts and strategies that are introduced in therapy are then assigned as homework.

Psychoeducation

Psychoeducational procedures are a routine component of CBT. One of the major goals of the treatment approach is to teach patients a new way of thinking and behaving that can be applied in resolving their current symptoms and in managing problems that will be encountered in the future. The psychoeducational effort usually begins with the process of socializing the patient to therapy. In the opening phase of treatment, the therapist explains the basic concepts of CBT and introduces the patient to the format of CBT sessions. The therapist also devotes time early in treatment to discussing the therapeutic relationship in CBT and the expectations for both patient and therapist. Psychoeducational work during a course of CBT often involves brief explanations or illustrations coupled with homework assignments. These activities are woven into treatment sessions in a manner that emphasizes a collaborative, active learning approach. Some cognitive-behavioral therapists have described the use of "mini-lectures," but a heavily didactic approach is generally avoided.

Psychoeducation can be facilitated with reading assignments and computer programs that reinforce learning, deepen the patient's understanding of CBT principles, and promote the use of self-help methods. Table 33–7 contains a list of useful psychoeducational tools, including books and computer programs, that teach the CBT model and encourage self-help. Most cognitive-behavioral therapists liberally use psychoeducational tools as a basic part of the therapy process.

Cognitive Techniques

Identifying Automatic Thoughts

Much of the work of CBT is devoted to recognizing and then modifying negatively distorted or illogical automatic thoughts (Table 33–8). The most powerful way of introducing the patient to the effects of automatic thoughts is to find an in vivo example of how automatic thoughts can influence emotional responses. Mood shifts during the therapy session are almost always good places to pause to identify automatic thoughts. The therapist observes that a strong emotion such as sadness, anxiety, or anger has appeared and then asks the patient to describe the thoughts that "went through your head" just prior to the mood shift. This technique is illustrated in the example of Mr. B, a 50-year-old depressed man who had suffered several recent losses and had developed extremely low self-esteem.

> Therapist: How did you react to your wife's criticism?
> Mr. B: (Suddenly appears much more sad and anxious) It was just too much to take.
> Therapist: I can see that this really upsets you. Can you think back to what went through your mind right after I asked you the last question? Just try to tell me all the thoughts that popped into your head.
> Mr. B: (Pauses, then recounts) I'm always making mistakes. I can't do anything right. There's no way to please her. I might as well give up.
> Therapist: I can see why you felt so sad. When these kinds of thoughts just automatically pop into your mind, you don't stop to think if they are accurate or not. That's why we call them automatic thoughts.
> Mr. B: I guess you're right. I hardly realized I was having those thoughts until you asked me to say them out loud.
> Therapist: Recognizing that you're having automatic thoughts is one of the first steps in therapy. Now let's see what we can do to help you with your thinking and with the situation with your wife.

Beck (1989) has described emotion as the "royal road to cognition." The patient usually is most accessible during periods of affective arousal, and cognitions such as automatic thoughts and schemas generally are more potent when they are associated with strong emotional responses. Hence, the cognitive therapist capitalizes on spontaneously occurring affective states during the interview and also pursues lines of questioning that are likely to stimulate emotion. One of the misconceptions about CBT is that it is an overly intellectualized form of therapy. In fact, CBT, as formulated by Beck et al. (1979), involves efforts to increase affect and to use emotional responses as a core ingredient of therapy.

TABLE 33–7.	Psychoeducational materials and programs for cognitive-behavioral therapy	
Authors	**Title**	**Description**
Barlow and Craske 2007	*Mastery of Your Anxiety and Panic*	Self-help for anxiety
Burns 1980, 1999	*Feeling Good*	Book with self-help program
Foa and Wilson 2001	*Stop Obsessing! How to Overcome Your Obsessions and Compulsions*	Self-help for obsessive-compulsive disorder
Greenberger and Padesky 1995	*Mind Over Mood*	Self-help workbook
Proudfoot et al. 2003	*Beating the Blues*	Computer-assisted therapy and self-help program
Wright and McCray 2012	*Breaking Free From Depression: Pathways to Wellness*	Book with self-help program; integrates cognitive-behavioral therapy and biological approaches
Wright et al. 2005, 2012	*Good Days Ahead: The Multimedia Program for Cognitive Therapy*	Computer-assisted therapy and self-help program

TABLE 33–8.	Methods for identifying and modifying automatic thoughts

Socratic questioning (guided discovery)

Use of mood shifts to demonstrate automatic thoughts in vivo

Imagery exercises

Role-play

Thought recording

Generating alternatives

Examining the evidence

Decatastrophizing

Reattribution

Cognitive rehearsal

One of the most frequently used procedures in CBT is Socratic questioning. There is no set format or protocol for this technique. Instead, the therapist must rely on his or her experience and ingenuity to formulate questions that will help patients move from having a "closed mind" to a state of inquisitiveness and curiosity. Socratic questioning stimulates recognition of dysfunctional cognitions and development of a sense of dissonance about the validity of strongly held assumptions.

Socratic questioning usually involves a series of inductive questions that are likely to reveal dysfunctional thought patterns. The use of this technique to identify automatic thoughts is illustrated in the case of Ms. W, a 42-year-old woman with an anxiety disorder.

Therapist: What things seem to trigger your anxiety?

Ms. W: Everything. It seems like no matter what I do, I'm nervous all the time.

Therapist: I suppose that "everything" could trigger your anxiety and that you have no control over it. But let's stop for a moment and see if there are any other possibilities. Is that okay?

Ms. W: Sure.

Therapist: Then try to think of a situation where your anxiety is very high and one where it's much lower.

Ms. W: Well, a high-anxiety time would be whenever I try to go out in public, like to go shopping or to a party. And a low-anxiety time would be sitting at home watching TV.

Therapist: So there's some variation depending on what you are doing at the time.

Ms. W: I guess that's right.

Therapist: Would you like to find out what's behind the variation?

Ms. W: I guess. But I suppose it's just because being out with people makes me nervous and being at home feels safe.

Therapist: That's one explanation. I wonder if there might be any others—ones that would give you some clues on how to get over the problem.

Ms. W: I'm willing to look.

Therapist: Well then, let's try to find out something about the different thoughts that you have about these two situations. When you think of going out to a party, what comes to mind?

Ms. W: I'll be embarrassed. I won't have any idea what to say or do. I'll probably panic and run out the door.

This example depicts the typical use of Socratic questions early in the therapy process. Further questioning would be required to help the patient fully understand how dysfunctional cognitions are involved in her anxiety responses and how changing these cognitions could dampen her anxiety and promote a higher level of functioning.

Imagery and role-play are used as alternative methods of uncovering cognitions when direct questions are unsuccessful in generating suspected automatic thinking. These techniques also are selected when only a limited number of automatic thoughts can be brought out through Socratic questioning, and the therapist expects that more important automatic thoughts are present. Some patients may be able to use imagery procedures with few prompts or directions. In this case, the clinician may only need to ask the patient to imagine himself or herself back in a particularly troubling or emotion-provoking situation and then to describe the thoughts that occurred. However, most patients, particularly in the early phases of therapy, can benefit from "setting the scene" for the use of imagery. The patient is asked to describe the details of the setting. When and where did it take place? What happened immediately before the incident? How did the characters in the scene appear? What were the main physical features of the setting? Questions such as these help bring the scene alive in the patient's mind and facilitate recall of cognitive responses to the situation.

Role-play is a related technique for evoking automatic thoughts. When this procedure is used, the therapist first asks a series of questions to try to understand a vignette involving an interpersonal relationship or other social interchange that is likely to stimulate dysfunctional automatic thinking. Then, with the permission of the patient, the therapist briefly steps into the role of the individual in the scene and facilitates the playing out of a typical response set. Role-play is used less frequently than Socratic questioning or imagery and is best suited to therapeutic situations in which there is an excellent collaborative relationship and the patient is unlikely to respond to the role-play exercise with a negative or distorted transference reaction.

Thought recording is one of the most frequently used CBT procedures for identifying automatic thoughts (Wright et al. 2017). Patients can be asked to log their thoughts in several different ways. The simplest method is the two-column technique—a procedure that often is used when the patient is just beginning to learn how to recognize automatic thoughts. The two-column technique is illustrated in Table 33–9. In this case, the patient was asked to write down automatic thoughts that occurred in stressful or upsetting situations. Alternatively, the patient could try to identify emotional reactions in one column and automatic thoughts in the other. A three-column exercise could include a description of the situation, a list of automatic thoughts, and a notation of the emotional response. Thought recording helps the patient to recognize the effects of underlying automatic thoughts and to understand how the basic cognitive model (i.e., relationship between situations, thoughts, feelings, and behaviors) applies to his or her own experiences. This procedure also initiates the process of modifying dysfunctional cognitions.

Modifying Automatic Thoughts

There usually is no sharp division in CBT between the phases of eliciting and modifying automatic thoughts. In fact, the processes involved in identifying automatic thoughts often are enough to initiate substantive change. As the patient begins to rec-

TABLE 33–9. Two-column thought recording	
Situation	Automatic thoughts
Call from boss to submit a report	I can't do this. I don't know what to do. It won't be acceptable.
My wife asks me to help more around the house	Nothing I do is ever enough. She thinks I don't try.
Car won't start	I was stupid to buy this car. Nothing works right anymore. This is the last straw.

ognize the nature of his or her dysfunctional thinking, there typically is an increased degree of skepticism regarding the validity of automatic thoughts. Although patients can start to revise their cognitive distortions without specific additional therapeutic interventions, modification of automatic thoughts can be accelerated if the therapist applies Socratic questioning and other basic CBT procedures to the change process (see Table 33–8).

Techniques used for revising automatic thoughts include 1) generating alternatives, 2) examining the evidence, 3) thought recording, 4) reattribution, and 5) cognitive rehearsal. Socratic questioning is used in all of these procedures. *Generating alternatives* is illustrated in the case of Ms. D, a 32-year-old woman with major depressive disorder. The therapist's questions were pointed toward helping Ms. D to see a broader range of possibilities than she had originally considered.

Ms. D: Every time I think of going back to school, I panic.
Therapist: And when you start to think of going to school, what thoughts come to mind?
Ms. D: I'll botch it up. I won't be able to make it. I'll feel so ashamed when I have to drop out.
Therapist: What else could happen? Anything even worse, or are there any better possibilities?
Ms. D: Well, it couldn't get much worse unless I never even tried at all.
Therapist: How would that be so bad?
Ms. D: Then I'd just be the same—stuck in a rut, not going anywhere.
Therapist: We can take a look at that conclusion later—that not going to school would mean that you would stay in a rut. But for now, let's look at the other possibilities if you do try to go to school again.
Ms. D: Okay. I guess there's some chance that it would go pretty well, but it'll be hard for me to manage school, the house, and all my family responsibilities.
Therapist: When you try to step back from the situation and not listen to your automatic thoughts, what's the most likely outcome of your going back to school?
Ms. D: It will be a difficult adjustment, but it's something I want to do. I have the intelligence to do it if I apply myself.

Examining the evidence is a major component of the collaborative empirical experience in CBT. Specific automatic thoughts or clusters of related automatic thoughts are set forth as hypotheses, and the patient and therapist then search for evidence both for and against each hypothesis. In the case of Ms. D, the thought "If I don't go to school, I'd just be the same—stuck in a rut, not going anywhere" was selected for an exercise in examining the evidence. The therapist believed that returning to school was probably an adaptive action for the patient to take. However, the therapist also thought that seeing further education as the only route to change would excessively load this activity with a "make or break" mentality and would promote a disregard for other modifications that might increase self-esteem and self-efficacy.

Five-column thought change records (TCRs) (Beck et al. 1979; Table 33–10) or other similar devices for *thought recording* are standard tools used in modification of automatic thoughts. The five-column TCR is used to encourage both identification of and change in dysfunctional cognitions. Two additional columns (rational response and outcome) are added to the three-column thought record (situation, automatic thoughts, and emotions) typically used to identify automatic thoughts. The patient is instructed to use this form to capture and change automatic thoughts. Either a stressful event or a memory of an event or situation is noted in the first column. Automatic thoughts are recorded in the second column and are rated for degree of belief (how much the patient believes them to be true at the moment they occur) on a 0–100 scale. The third column is used to observe the emotional response to the automatic thoughts. The intensity of emotion is rated on a 1–100 scale. The fourth column, rational response, is the most critical part of the TCR. The patient is asked to stand back from the automatic thoughts, assess their validity, and then write out a more rational or realistic set of cognitions. A wide variety of procedures can be used to facilitate the development of rational thoughts for the TCR.

Most patients can learn about cognitive errors and can start to label specific instances of erroneous logic in their automatic thoughts. This is often the first step in generating a more rational pattern of cognitive responses to life events. Previously described techniques such as generating alternatives and examining the evidence also are used by the patient in a self-help format when the TCR is assigned for homework. In addition, the therapist often is able to help the patient refine or add to the list of rational thoughts when the TCR is reviewed at a subsequent therapy session. Repeated attention to generating rational thoughts on the TCR is usually quite helpful in breaking maladaptive patterns of automatic and negatively distorted thinking.

The fifth column of the TCR, outcome, is used to record any changes that have occurred as a result of modifying automatic thoughts. Although use of the TCR usually will lead to development of a more adaptive set of cognitions and reduction in painful emotions, on some occasions the initial automatic thoughts will prove to be accurate. In such situations, the therapist helps the patient take a problem-solving approach, including the development of an action plan, to manage the stressful or upsetting event.

The use of *reattribution techniques* is based on findings of studies on the attributional process in depression. Depressed individuals have been found to have negatively biased attributions in three dimensions: global versus specific, internal versus external, and fixed versus variable (Abramson et al. 1978). Several different types of reattribution procedures are used, including psychoeducation about the attributional process, Socratic questioning to stimulate reattribution, written exercises to recognize and reinforce alternative attributions, and homework assignments to test the accuracy of attributions.

Cognitive rehearsal is used to help uncover potential negative automatic thoughts in advance and to coach the patient in ways of developing more adaptive cognitions. First, the patient is asked to use imagery or role-play to identify possible distorted cognitions that could occur in a stressful situation. Second, the patient and therapist

TABLE 33–10. Thought change record—an example

Situation	Automatic thought(s)	Emotion(s)	Rational response	Outcome
Describe	a. Write automatic thought(s) that preceded emotion(s).	a. Specify sad, anxious, angry, etc.	a. Identify cognitive errors.	a. Once again, rate belief in automatic thought(s), 0%–100%.
a. Actual event leading to unpleasant emotion; or	b. Rate belief in automatic thought(s), 0%–100%.	b. Rate degree of emotion, 1%–100%.	b. Write rational response to automatic thought(s).	b. Specify and rate subsequent emotion(s), 0%–100%.
b. Stream of thoughts, daydream, or recollection leading to unpleasant emotion; or			c. Rate belief in rational response, 0%–100%.	
c. Unpleasant physiological sensations				
Date: 3/15/13				
I wake up and I'm immediately troubled. I start to worry about work.	1. I can't face another day. (90%)	Sad: 90% Anxious: 80%	1. Magnification. Even though it has been rough, I have been able to get to work every day. Get a shower and make breakfast—that will get things started. (80%)	Sad: 30% Anxious: 40%
	2. The big project is due in 2 weeks; I'll never get it done. (100%)		2. Catastrophizing, all-or-none thinking. Don't panic. About half of the work is done. Break it down into pieces. Taking one step at a time helps. (95%)	
	3. Everybody knows I'm ready to fall apart. (90%)		3. Overgeneralization, magnification. Some people know I've been in trouble, but they haven't gotten down on me. I'm the one who puts me down. (95%)	
	4. It's hopeless. (85%)		4. Magnification. I know my job well and have a good track record. If I stick with this, I can probably make it. (90%)	

work together to modify the dysfunctional cognitions. Third, imagery or role-play is used again, this time to practice the more adaptive pattern of thinking. Finally, for a homework assignment, the patient is asked to try out the newly acquired cognitive patterns in vivo.

See Videos 2 and 8 accompanying the book *Learning Cognitive-Behavior Therapy: An Illustrated Guide*, 2nd Edition (Wright et al. 2017), for examples of CBT methods for helping patients revise negative automatic thoughts.

Identifying and Modifying Schemas

The process of identifying and modifying schemas is somewhat more difficult than changing negative automatic thoughts, because these core beliefs are more deeply embedded and usually have been reinforced through years of life experience. However, many of the same techniques described for automatic thoughts are used successfully in therapeutic work at the schema level. Procedures such as Socratic questioning, imagery, role-play, and thought recording are used to uncover maladaptive schemas (Table 33–11).

As the patient gains experience in recognizing automatic thoughts, repetitive patterns begin to emerge that may suggest the presence of underlying schemas. Therapists have several options at this point. A psychoeducational approach can be used to explain the concept of schemas (which may be alternatively termed *core beliefs*) and their linkage to more superficial automatic thoughts. Patients may then start to recognize schemas on their own. However, when the patient first starts to learn about core beliefs, the therapist may need to suggest that certain schemas might be operative and then engage the patient in collaborative exercises that test these hypotheses.

Modification of schemas may require repeated attention, both in and out of therapy sessions. One commonly used procedure is to ask the patient to list in a therapy notebook all the schemas that have been identified to date. The schema list can be reviewed before each session. This technique promotes a high level of awareness of schemas and usually encourages the patient to place issues pertaining to schemas on the agenda for therapy.

CBT interventions that are particularly helpful in modifying schemas include examining the evidence, listing advantages and disadvantages, generating alternatives, and using cognitive rehearsal. After a schema has been identified, the therapist may ask the patient to do a pro/con analysis (examining the evidence) using a double-column procedure. This technique usually induces the patient to doubt the validity of the schema and to start to think of alternative explanations.

> Ms. R is a 24-year-old woman with depression and bulimia. During the course of her CBT, Ms. R identified an important schema that was affecting both the depression and the eating disorder ("I must be perfect to be accepted."). By examining the evidence, she was able to see that her core belief was based at least in part on faulty logic (Table 33–12).

Ms. R also used the technique of listing advantages and disadvantages as part of the strategy to modify this maladaptive schema (Table 33–13). Some schemas appear to have few, if any, advantages (e.g., "I'm stupid"; "I'll always lose in the end"), but many core beliefs have both positive and negative features (e.g., "If I decide to do something, I must succeed"; "I always have to work harder than others or I'll fail").

TABLE 33–11. Methods for identifying and modifying schemas
Socratic questioning
Imagery and role-play
Thought recording
Identifying repetitive patterns of automatic thoughts
Psychoeducation
Listing schemas in therapy notebook
Examining the evidence
Listing advantages and disadvantages
Generating alternatives
Cognitive rehearsal

TABLE 33–12. Schema modification through examining the evidence

Schema: "I must be perfect to be accepted."

Evidence for	Evidence against
The better I do, the more people seem to like me.	Others who aren't "perfect" seem to be loved and accepted. Why should I be different?
Women who have a perfect figure are most attractive to men.	You don't have to have a perfect figure. Hardly anybody has one—just the models on television.
My parents have the highest standards; they are always pushing me to do better.	My parents want me to do well. But they'll probably accept me as long as I try to do my best, even if I don't meet all of their expectations. This statement is absolute and sets me up for failure, because no one can be perfect all the time.

The latter group of schemas may be maintained even in the face of their dysfunctional aspects because they encourage hard work, perseverance, or other behaviors that are adaptive. Yet the absolute and demanding nature of the beliefs ultimately leads to excessive stress, failed expectations, low self-esteem, or other deleterious results. Listing advantages and disadvantages helps the patient to examine the full range of effects of the schema and often encourages modifications that can make the schema both more adaptive and less damaging. In Ms. R's case, this exercise set the stage for another step of schema modification, generating alternatives (Table 33–14).

The list of alternative schemas usually includes several different options, ranging from rather minor adjustments to extensive revisions in the schema. The therapist uses Socratic questioning and other CBT techniques such as imagery and role-play to help the patient recognize potential alternative schemas. A "brainstorming" attitude is encouraged. Instead of trying to be sure that a revised schema is entirely accurate at first glance, the therapist usually suggests trying to generate a variety of modified schemas without initially considering their validity or practicality. This stimulates creativity and gives the patient further encouragement to step aside from long-standing rigid schemas.

After alternatives are generated and discussed, the therapy turns toward examining the potential consequences of changing basic attitudes. Cognitive rehearsal can be

TABLE 33–13. **Schema modification through listing advantages and disadvantages**

Schema: "I must be perfect to be accepted."

Advantages	Disadvantages
I've tried very hard to be the best.	I never really feel accepted because I've never reached perfection.
I've received top marks in school.	I'm always down on myself. I've developed bulimia. I'm obsessed with my body size.
I'm in lots of activities, and I've won dancing competitions.	I have trouble accepting my successes. I drive myself too hard and can't enjoy ordinary things.

TABLE 33–14. **Schema modification through generating alternatives**

Schema: "I must be perfect to be accepted."

Possible alternatives

People who are successful are more likely to be accepted.

If I try to do my best (even if it's not perfect), others are likely to accept me.

I would like to be perfect, but that's an impossible goal. I'll choose certain areas to try to excel (school, work, and career) and not demand perfection everywhere.

You don't need to be perfect to be accepted.

I'm worthy of love and acceptance without trying to be perfect.

used in the therapy session to test a schema modification. This may be followed by a homework assignment to try out the revised schema in vivo. Therapist and patient work together to choose the most reasonable modifications for underlying schemas and to reinforce learning these new constructs through multiple practice sessions in therapy sessions and in real-life experiences.

Behavioral Procedures

Behavioral interventions are used in CBT to 1) change dysfunctional patterns of behavior (e.g., helplessness, isolation, phobic avoidance, inertia, bingeing and purging); 2) reduce troubling symptoms (e.g., tension, somatic and psychic anxiety, intrusive thoughts); and 3) assist in identifying and modifying maladaptive cognitions. Table 33–15 presents a list of behavioral techniques. As discussed earlier in this chapter, the basic cognitive-behavioral model (see Figure 33–1) suggests that there is an interactive relationship between cognition and behavior. Thus, behavioral initiatives should influence cognition, and cognitive interventions should have an effect on behavior.

The Socratic questions used in cognitively oriented procedures have a direct parallel when the emphasis is on behavioral change. The therapist asks a series of questions that help differentiate actual behavioral deficits from negatively distorted accounts of behavior. Depressed and anxious patients usually overreport their symptomatic distress or the difficulties they have in managing situations. Often, well-framed questions can identify cognitive distortions and also stimulate change as the patient considers the negative effect of dysfunctional behavior. We explain four spe-

---

TABLE 33–15.   Behavioral procedures used in cognitive-behavioral therapy

Questioning to identify behavioral patterns

Activity scheduling with mastery and pleasure recording

Self-monitoring

Graded task assignments

Behavioral rehearsal

Exposure and response prevention

Coping cards

Distraction

Relaxation exercises

Respiratory control

Assertiveness training

Modeling

Social skills training

---

cific behavioral techniques—activity scheduling, graded task assignments, exposure, and coping cards—in the following discussion. A more detailed description of behavioral methods is available in Wright et al. (2017) or Meichenbaum (1977).

Activity scheduling is a structured method of learning about the patient's behavioral patterns, encouraging self-monitoring, increasing positive mood, and designing strategies for change. The patient is asked to record what he or she does during each hour of the day in a daily or weekly activity log and then to rate each activity for mastery and pleasure on a 0–10 scale. When the activity record is first introduced, the therapist usually asks the patient to make a record of baseline activities without attempting to make any changes. The data are then reviewed in the next therapy session. Almost invariably, the patient rates some activities higher than others for mastery and pleasure.

> Mr. G, a 48-year-old depressed man who had told his therapist that "I don't enjoy anything anymore," described several activities on his daily activity log that contradicted this statement. Reading while sitting alone was rated as a 6 on mastery and 8 on pleasure, and attending his son's choir concert was rated as 7 on mastery and 10 on pleasure. Conversely, attempting to work in his home office was rated as a 1 on mastery and a 0 on pleasure. Discussion of the activity scheduling assignment with Mr. G helped him to see that he was still capable of performing reasonably well in certain activities and also that he was able to derive considerable enjoyment from some of his actions. In addition, the schedule was used to target problem areas (e.g., working in his home office) that would require further work in therapy. Finally, the activity schedule provided data that could be used in adjusting Mr. G's daily routine to promote a heightened sense of mastery and greater enjoyment.

Another behavioral procedure, the *graded task assignment*, can be used when the patient is facing a situation that seems excessively difficult or overwhelming. A challenging behavioral goal is broken down into small steps that can be taken one at a time. The graded task assignment is somewhat similar to the systematic desensitization protocols that are used in traditional behavior therapy; however, a cognitive component is added to the methodology. An added emphasis is placed on improving self-esteem and self-efficacy, countering hopelessness and helplessness, and using the graded task assignment to disprove maladaptive thoughts and schemas. With depressed individuals, the graded task assignment typically is used as a problem-solving technique. This stepwise approach, coupled with cognitive techniques such as Socratic questioning and thought recording, can reactivate the patient and help him or her to focus in a productive manner. For example, a graded task assignment was used in the case of Mr. G, the 48-year-old man introduced in the previous case study.

> One of the particularly troublesome items uncovered with activity scheduling was Mr. G's difficulty in getting to work at his home office. Socratic questioning revealed that Mr. G had been unable to work in his home office for more than 6 weeks. Mail, bills, and e-mail were piled up to the point that he saw the situation as impossible. Cognitions related to this problem included automatic thoughts such as "It's too much; I've procrastinated too long this time; I'm totally swamped; I can't handle it."
>
> The therapist and patient constructed a series of steps that encouraged Mr. G to approach the task and eventually master the problem. The graded task assignment included the following steps: 1) walk into the office and sit down at the desk for at least 15 minutes; 2) spend at least 20 minutes sorting letter mail into categories; 3) open and discard any junk mail; 4) open and stack all bills; 5) clean the office; 6) open e-mail, delete all messages that don't require a response, and answer messages that do; 7) balance the checkbook; and 8) pay all current or overdue bills. Reasonable goals for specific time intervals were discussed, and the therapist used coaching, Socratic questioning, and other cognitive techniques to help Mr. G accomplish the task.

Videos 12, 13, 14, and 15 accompanying the book *Learning Cognitive-Behavior Therapy: An Illustrated Guide,* 2nd Edition (Wright et al. 2017), show examples of behavioral methods for helping depressed patients reactivate and restore a sense of enjoyment in daily activities.

Exposure techniques are a central part of cognitive-behavioral approaches to anxiety disorders. For example, a phobia can be conceptualized as an unrealistic fear of an object or a situation coupled with a conditioned pattern of avoidance. Treatment can proceed along two complementary lines: 1) cognitive restructuring to modify the dysfunctional thoughts and 2) exposure therapy to break the pattern of avoidance. Typically, a hierarchy of feared stimuli is developed with the patient. The hierarchy should contain several different stimuli that cause varying degrees of distress. Usually the items are ranked by degree of distress. One commonly used system involves rating each item on a scale from 0 to 100, with 100 representing the maximum distress possible. After the hierarchy is established, the therapist and patient work collaboratively to set goals for gradual exposure, starting with the items that are ranked lower on the distress scale. Breathing training, relaxation exercises, and other behavioral methods (see Table 33–15) may be used to enhance the patient's ability to carry out the exposure protocol. Exposure can be done with imagery in treatment sessions or in vivo. Also, innovative virtual reality methods have been developed for exposure therapy (Rothbaum et al. 1995; Valmaggia et al. 2016). Clinician-administered exposure therapy is frequently used as part of the cognitive-behavioral approach to simple phobias, panic disorder with agoraphobia, and social phobia.

Coping cards are another commonly used method to achieve behavioral change. The therapist helps the patient identify specific actions that are likely to help him or her cope with an anticipated problem or put CBT skills into action. These ideas are then written down on a small card, which the patient carries as a reminder and as a tool to help in solving problems. Coping cards often contain both cognitive and behavioral interventions, as illustrated in Figure 33–3.

Other behavioral techniques used in CBT include behavior rehearsal (a procedure that is usually combined with cognitive rehearsal, described earlier in "Modifying Automatic Thoughts"), response prevention (a collaborative exercise in which the patient agrees to stop a dysfunctional behavior, such as prolonged crying spells, and to monitor cognitive responses), relaxation exercises, respiratory control, assertiveness training, modeling, and social skills training (Meichenbaum 1977; Wright et al. 2017).

Computer-Assisted Cognitive-Behavioral Therapy

Computer-assisted CBT (CCBT) offers significant potential for increasing the efficiency of cognitive-behavioral interventions and improving patient access to treatment (Richards and Richardson 2012). For example, Wright et al. (2005) and Thase et al. (2018) have developed a multimedia form of CCBT that is designed to be suitable for a wide range of patients, including those with no previous computer or keyboard experience. This online program, "Good Days Ahead," features large amounts of video, along with interactive self-help exercises such as thought change records, activity schedules, and coping cards. Randomized controlled trials of CCBT for drug-free patients with depression conducted with the Wright and colleagues program found that CCBT was equivalent to standard CBT, even though the total therapist time in CCBT was reduced to about half in one study (Wright et al. 2005) and two-thirds in another (Thase et al. 2018). Another multimedia CBT program, "Beating the Blues," was found to be effective in a controlled trial with primary care patients (Proudfoot et al. 2004); however, this program was not more effective than treatment as usual in another study in which the computer program was self-guided (Gilbody et al. 2015). Meta-analyses have concluded that the overall results of CCBT research support the effectiveness of this method for both depression and anxiety disorders (Adelman et al. 2014; Davies et al. 2014; Richards and Richardson 2012; Wright et al. [in press]). However, clinician-supported CCBT has typically performed better than self-directed CCBT.

Virtual reality methods for computer-assisted therapy have been directed primarily at phobias and other anxiety disorders. The virtual environment is used to simulate feared situations and to promote exposure therapy. Controlled research has supported the efficacy of virtual reality as part of a CBT treatment package for fear of flying, height phobia, and other phobias (Rothbaum et al. 2000; Valmaggia et al. 2016). This method is also showing promise in the treatment of social anxiety disorder and panic disorder with agoraphobia (Pull 2005) as well as posttraumatic stress disorder (PTSD). For these conditions, the virtual environment may include simulations of other people or places, such as crowded public spaces, public speaking experiences, and scenes from war zones.

Although typically not developed or studied as full treatment programs, several CBT-based apps for smartphones have been introduced. These apps have been used for self-monitoring, psychoeducation, and specific techniques such as relaxation or breathing training (Sucala et al. 2017; Van Ameringen et al. 2017; Wang et al. 2018). Systematic reviews of mobile apps for mental health have noted that few mobile apps have been empirically tested, and many apps have been developed by persons with-

Situation: My girlfriend comes in late or does something else that makes me think she doesn't care.

Coping strategies:

Spot my extreme thinking, especially when I use absolute words like never or always.

Stand back from the situation and check my thinking before I start yelling or screaming.

Think of the positive parts of our relationship—I think she does love me.

We've been together for 4 years, and I want to make it work.

Take a "time-out" if I start getting into a rage. Tell her that I need to take a break to calm down. Take a brief walk or go to another room.

FIGURE 33–3. Mr. W's coping card.

This example shows how Mr. W, a middle-aged man with bipolar disorder, developed an effective coping strategy for managing anger in situations with his girlfriend.

Source. Reprinted from Wright JH, Brown GK, Thase ME, Basco MR: *Learning Cognitive-Behavior Therapy: An Illustrated Guide,* 2nd Edition (Core Competencies in Psychotherapy Series, Glen O. Gabbard, series ed). Arlington, VA, American Psychiatric Association Publishing, 2017, p. 125. Copyright © 2017, American Psychiatric Association Publishing. Used with permission.

out clinical training. Also, these reviews suggest that security and privacy concerns should be considered when recommending that patients use mobile apps as part of their treatment. However, mobile apps have considerable appeal and may be a useful adjunct to CBT for some patients.

Selecting Patients for Cognitive-Behavioral Therapy

CBT procedures have been described for many diagnostic categories (Beck 1993; Wright et al. 2017). Although there are no contraindications to using this treatment approach, CBT is usually not attempted with patients who have severe memory disturbances. CBT can be considered a primary treatment for 1) disorders in which it has been proven to be effective in controlled research (e.g., unipolar depression [nonpsychotic], anxiety disorders, eating disorders, and psychophysiological disorders) and 2) other conditions for which a clearly detailed treatment method has been developed (e.g., personality disorders, substance abuse) and some evidence supports CBT's effectiveness. CBT should be considered as an adjunctive therapy for disorders such as major depressive disorder with psychotic features, bipolar disorder, and schizophrenia—disorders for which there is clear evidence for the effectiveness of pharmacotherapy but limited or no research examining the effectiveness of CBT alone compared with pharmacotherapy.

Chronicity and symptom severity have been associated with poorer response to CBT (e.g., Thase et al. 1993, 1994), although these findings may reflect the more negative prognostic effect of these variables. When CBT has been compared directly with pharmacotherapy, most studies have found little relation between severity or endogenous subtype and differential treatment outcome (e.g., DeRubeis et al. 1999).

Investigations of biological predictors have yielded suggestive results. Thase et al. (1996a) found that poorer response to an intensive inpatient CBT program was associated with high levels of urinary free cortisol levels. In a large ($N=90$) outpatient study, an abnormal sleep profile (defined by multiple disturbances of electroencephalographic sleep recordings) was associated with a lower recovery rate and higher risk for relapse (Thase et al. 1996b). A specific alteration in cortical activation (as measured by functional magnetic resonance imaging scanning) was strongly associated with more favorable short-term CBT response (Siegle et al. 2006, 2012). In another study, greater connectivity between the frontal cortex and the cingulate cortex was associated with higher rates of remission with CBT compared with medication in the treatment of major depressive disorder (Dunlop et al. 2017). Although these studies suggest that various biological markers of depression may be associated with response or nonresponse to CBT, research evidence to date does not justify the use of laboratory tests to select patients for CBT.

Clinical experience has suggested that those patients who do not have severe character pathology (especially borderline or antisocial features), who have previously formed trusting relationships with significant others, who believe in the importance of self-reliance, and who have a curious or inquisitive nature are especially suitable for CBT (Wright et al. 2017). Above-average intelligence is not associated with better outcome, and CBT procedures can be simplified for those with subnormal intellectual skills or impaired learning and memory functioning. A flexible approach can be used in which CBT procedures are customized to match the special characteristics of each patient's social background, intellectual level, personality structure, and clinical disorder (Wright et al. 2017).

Cognitive-Behavioral Therapy Applications

The basic procedures described in this chapter are used in all CBT applications. However, the targets for change, selection of techniques, and timing of interventions may vary depending on the condition being treated and the format for therapy. A full discussion of the multiple applications and formats for CBT is beyond the scope of this chapter. The reader is referred to comprehensive books on CBT for a more detailed accounting of the modifications of this treatment approach for different clinical disorders (see "Recommended Readings" at end of chapter). In this portion of the chapter, we briefly examine the distinctive features of CBT for six common psychiatric illnesses: depression, anxiety disorders, eating disorders, personality disorders, psychosis, and bipolar disorder.

Data on CBT effectiveness are presented in the later section "Effectiveness of Cognitive-Behavioral Therapy."

Depression

In the opening phase of treatment of depression, the cognitive-behavioral therapist focuses on establishing a collaborative relationship and introducing the patient to the CBT model. Agendas, feedback, and psychoeducational procedures are used to structure sessions. Early in therapy, a special effort may be placed on relieving hopelessness because of the close link between this element of the negative cognitive triad and suicide risk. Also, a reduction in hopelessness can be an important step in reactivating and reenergizing the depressed patient. The clinician carefully matches the therapeutic work to the patient's level of cognitive functioning so that learning is encouraged and the patient is not overwhelmed with the material of therapy. Behavioral techniques such as activity scheduling and graded task assignment often are a major component of the opening phase of CBT for depression.

The middle portion of treatment is usually devoted to eliciting and modifying negatively distorted automatic thoughts. Behavioral techniques continue to be used in most cases. By this point in the therapy, patients should understand the CBT model and be able to employ thought-monitoring techniques to reverse all three elements of the negative cognitive triad (self, world, and future). Typically, the patient is taught to identify cognitive errors (e.g., selective abstraction, overgeneralization, absolutistic thinking) and to use procedures such as generating alternatives and examining the evidence to alter negatively distorted thinking.

Work on eliciting and testing automatic thoughts continues during the latter portion of treatment. However, if there have been gains in functioning and the patient has grasped the basic principles of CBT, therapy can focus more heavily on identifying and altering maladaptive schemas. The concept of schemas usually has been introduced earlier in therapy, but the principal efforts at changing these underlying structures are typically reserved for the late phase of treatment, when the patient is more likely to grasp and retain complex therapeutic initiatives. Before therapy concludes, the therapist helps the patient review what has been learned during the course of treatment and also suggests thinking ahead to possible circumstances that could trigger a return of depression. The potential for relapse is recognized, and problem-solving strategies are developed that can be used in future stressful situations.

Anxiety Disorders

Although the techniques used in CBT for anxiety disorders are similar to those used in the treatment of depression, treatment efforts are directed toward altering four major types of dysfunctional anxiety-producing cognitions: 1) overestimates of the likelihood of a feared event, 2) exaggerated estimates of the severity of a feared event, 3) underestimation of personal coping abilities, and 4) unrealistically low estimates of the help that others can offer. Most authors have recommended that a mixture of cognitive and behavioral measures be used in working with patients who have anxiety disorders (Barlow and Cerney 1988; Clark and Beck 2011).

In panic disorder, the emphasis is on helping the patient recognize and change grossly exaggerated estimates of the significance of physiological responses or fears of imminent psychological disaster. For example, an individual with panic disorder may begin to perspire or breathe more rapidly, after which cognitions such as "I can't catch my breath; I'll pass out; I'll have a stroke" increase the intensity of the autonomic nervous system activity. The vicious cycle interaction between catastrophic cognitions and physiological arousal can be broken in two complementary ways: 1) altering the dysfunctional cognitions and 2) interrupting the cascading autonomic hyperactivity. Commonly used cognitive interventions include Socratic questioning, imagery, thought recording, generating alternatives, and examining the evidence. Behavioral measures such as relaxation training and respiratory control are used to dampen the physiological arousal associated with panic (Clark and Beck 2011; Clark et al. 1985). Also, when panic attacks are stimulated by specific situations (e.g., driving, public speaking, crowds), graded exposure may be particularly useful in helping patients to both master a feared task and overcome their panic symptoms.

CBT for phobic disorders centers on modifying unrealistic estimates of risk or danger in situations and engaging the patient in a series of graded exposure assignments. Generally, cognitive and behavioral procedures are used simultaneously. For example, a graded task assignment for an individual with agoraphobia might include a stepwise increase in experiences in a social setting accompanied by use of a TCR to record and revise maladaptive automatic thinking. Patients with generalized anxiety disorder usually have diffuse cognitive distortions about many circumstances in their lives (e.g., physical health, finances, loss of control, family issues) coupled with persistent autonomic arousal (Clark and Beck 2011). The CBT approach to generalized anxiety disorder is closely related to methods used for panic disorder and phobias. However, special attention is paid to defining the stimuli that are associated with increased anxiety. Breaking down the generalized state of anxiety into workable segments can help the patient gain mastery over what initially appears to be an uncontrollable situation.

Obsessive-Compulsive Disorder and Posttraumatic Stress Disorder

Behavioral techniques such as exposure and response prevention are used together with cognitive restructuring for patients with obsessive-compulsive disorder (OCD) (Clark and Beck 2011). Cognitive interventions include questioning the validity of obsessional thoughts, attempting to replace dysfunctional cognitions with positive self-statements, and modifying negative automatic thoughts. A combined approach of cognitive techniques to modify maladaptive thought patterns and behavioral interventions to counter patterns of avoidance is also used in CBT for PTSD (Clark and Beck 2011; Foa et al. 2005).

Eating Disorders

CBT is a well-established first-line treatment for bulimia nervosa and binge-eating disorder. CBT for both conditions was given a grade A rating by the United Kingdom's National Institute for Health and Care Excellence, indicating that CBT has strong support for efficacy from empirical trials (Brownley et al. 2016; Wilson and Shafran 2005). Considerably less research has been conducted on CBT for anorexia nervosa than for other eating disorders; however, cognitive and behavioral interventions can be included in comprehensive treatment programs for this difficult-to-treat condition.

Individuals with eating disorders may have many of the same cognitive distortions that are seen in depression. In addition, they have a cluster of cognitive biases about body image, eating behavior, and weight (Clark et al. 1989). Patients with eating disorders usually place inordinate value on body shape as a measure of self-worth and as a condition for acceptance (e.g., "I must be thin to be accepted"; "If I'm overweight, nobody will want me"; "Fat people are weak"). They also may believe that any variance from their excessive standards means a total loss of control.

CBT interventions are used to subject these maladaptive cognitions to empirical testing. Commonly used procedures include eliciting and testing automatic thoughts, examining the evidence, using reattribution, and giving in vivo homework assignments. Also, behavioral techniques are used to stimulate more adaptive eating behavior and to uncover significant cognitions related to eating. As in treatment of other disorders, the relative emphasis on cognitive procedures compared with behavioral measures is dictated by the severity of the illness and the phase of treatment. An individual with anorexia nervosa who is malnourished and has an electrolyte imbalance may require hospitalization with an emphasis on behavioral interventions during the initial part of treatment. Patients with this level of illness may have a significant impairment in learning and memory functioning and therefore have limited capacity to understand thought recording or other cognitive interventions. In contrast, a patient with uncomplicated bulimia nervosa may be able to benefit from relatively demanding cognitively oriented procedures early in treatment.

One of the critical factors in treating patients with eating disorders is the development of an effective working relationship. Compared with individuals with depression or anxiety disorders, those with eating disturbances often are reluctant to fully engage in therapy. Frequently, they have long-standing patterns of hiding their behavior from others and have developed elaborate methods of maintaining their dysfunctional approach to meals, body weight, and exercise. Thus, the patient with an eating disorder poses a special problem for the cognitive-behavioral therapist. A thorough psychoeducational effort and considerable patience are usually required for the formation of a collaborative empirical relationship. If the therapist focuses in the beginning on problem areas that the patient clearly wants to change (e.g., low self-esteem, hopelessness, loss of interest), struggles over control of eating disorders can be avoided until there have been successful experiences in working together in therapy.

Personality Disorders

Beck et al. (2015) articulated a CBT approach to personality disorders that is based on a cognitive conceptualization of characterological disturbances. They suggested that the different personality types have idiosyncratic cognitions in basic beliefs, view of self and others, and strategies for social interaction. For example, an individual with a narcissistic personality pathology might believe, "I'm special; I'm better than the rest; ordinary rules don't apply to me." This cognitive set leads to behavioral strategies such as manipulation, breaking rules, and exploiting others (Beck et al. 2015). In contrast, a person with a dependent personality disorder might have core beliefs such as, "I need others to survive; I can't manage on my own; I can't be happy if I'm alone." The interpersonal strategies associated with these beliefs would include efforts to cling to or entrap others (Beck et al. 2015).

CBT methods typically used in treatment of mood disorders may not be successful with characterological problems (Beck et al. 2015). Recommendations that have been made for modifying CBT for treatment of personality disorders are summarized in Table 33–16 (Beck et al. 2015). The problem-oriented, structured, and collaborative empirical characteristics of CBT are retained in therapeutic work with patients who have personality disturbances, but there is an added emphasis on the therapeutic relationship. Treatment of personality disorders with CBT may take considerably lon-

TABLE 33–16. **Modifications of cognitive-behavioral therapy for personality disorders**

Pay special attention to the therapeutic relationship.

Attend to one's own (the therapist's) cognitive responses and emotional reactions.

Develop an individualized case conceptualization (including an assessment of the effect of developmental experiences, significant traumas, and environmental stresses).

Place an initial focus on increasing self-efficacy.

Use behavioral techniques, such as rehearsal and social skills training, to reverse actual deficits in interpersonal functioning.

Set firm, reasonable limits.

Set realistic goals.

Anticipate adherence problems.

Review and repeat treatment interventions.

ger than therapy for more circumscribed problems such as depression or anxiety. Patients with personality disturbances have deeply ingrained schemas that are unlikely to change within the short-term format used for other disorders. When the course of therapy lengthens, the chance for development of transference and countertransference reactions is greater. In CBT, transference is viewed as a manifestation of underlying schemas. Therefore, transference phenomena are recognized as opportunities for examining and modifying core beliefs.

An individualized case conceptualization is used. This formulation includes hypotheses on the role of maladaptive schemas in symptom production. Consideration also is given to the influences of parent–child conflicts, traumatic experiences, and the current social network on cognitive and behavioral pathology. Patients with personality disorders often have significant real-life problems, including severely disturbed interpersonal relationships and pronounced social skills deficits.

Although an ultimate goal of treatment is to modify ineffective or maladaptive schemas, initial efforts (using procedures such as behavioral techniques or thought recording) may be directed at more readily accessible targets such as increasing self-efficacy or decreasing dysphoric mood. Self-monitoring, self-help exercises, and the structuring procedures used in CBT help prevent excessive dependency. However, patients with character disorders (especially those with borderline, narcissistic, or dependent personalities) are prone to have excessive expectations, to be overly demanding, or to exhibit manipulative behavior. Thus, the cognitive therapist needs to set firm but reasonable limits and to help the patient articulate realistic treatment goals (Beck et al. 2015).

Adherence to treatment recommendations can be another problem in CBT for personality disorders. The therapist can use procedures such as Socratic questioning or schema identification to uncover the reasons for nonadherence and help the patient follow through with homework assignments or other therapeutic work. Reviewing and repeating treatment interventions is another important component of CBT for personality disorders. Considerable patience and persistence are required from the therapist as efforts are made to help the patient reverse chronic, deeply embedded psychopathology.

DBT is a specialized form of CBT developed by Linehan (1993) and others for treatment of borderline personality disorder. DBT employs cognitive and behavioral methods in addition to mindfulness and acceptance strategies derived from Zen teaching and practice. Therapy with DBT is long-term and involves repeated behavioral analysis, behavioral skills instruction, contingency management, cognitive restructuring, exposure interventions to reduce avoidance and dysfunctional emotions, and mindfulness training. DBT has been used successfully in borderline patients with suicidal behavior and substance abuse (Linehan et al. 1991, 1999, 2006).

Psychosis

Although biological treatments are the accepted form of therapy for psychotic patients, randomized controlled trials have found that CBT can reduce both positive and negative symptoms in patients who have residual symptomatology after stabilization on medication. It also has been observed that cognitive psychotherapy can help psychotic individuals understand their disorders, adhere to treatment recommendations, and develop more effective psychosocial functioning (Wright et al. 2009).

In CBT for patients who have psychotic symptoms, the therapist conveys that maladaptive cognitions and reactions to life stress may interact with biological factors in the expression of the illness. Therefore, attempts to develop more adaptive cognitions or to learn how to cope better with environmental pressures can assist with efforts toward managing the disorder. During the early part of therapy with a psychotic patient, there is a strong emphasis on building a therapeutic alliance. The therapist tries to normalize and destigmatize the condition (Wright et al. 2009) and explains the rationale for antipsychotic medication in combination with CBT. Attempts may be made to stimulate hope by modifying a patient's intensely negative cognitions about the illness or its treatment (e.g., "I'm to blame; Nothing will help; Drugs don't work."). Usually, work on examining hallucinations or delusions directly is delayed until a solid therapeutic relationship has been established. However, efforts are made to reverse delusional self-destructive cognitions as early as possible in the treatment process.

Reality testing is performed in a gentle, nonconfrontational manner. Usually, delusions with the lowest level of conviction are targeted first. The therapist uses guided discovery as a major intervention but also may help the patient to record and change distorted automatic thoughts or perform examining the evidence exercises. Behavioral techniques such as activity scheduling, graded task assignment, and social skills training also are used with psychotic patients. These procedures can be used to provide needed structure or to teach adaptive behaviors. Negative symptoms are typically approached slowly in a manner that gives consideration to the difficulty of changing this manifestation of psychotic disorders. Other components of the CBT approach to psychotic disorders may include 1) use of CBT techniques that enhance medication adherence, 2) identification of potential triggers for symptom exacerbation, 3) development of cognitive and behavioral strategies to manage stressful life events, and 4) implementation of family and/or group therapy applications of CBT (Wright et al. 2009).

Bipolar Disorder

CBT methods for bipolar disorder focus primarily on attempts to help patients understand and cope with a disease that is thought to have strong genetic and biological influences. Basco and Rush (2005) recommended extensive psychoeducation, in addition to techniques such as mood graphing and symptom summary worksheets. The latter interventions are used to assist patients in recognizing early signs of a mood swing and then devising methods to reduce the risk of cycling into a full depression or mania. For example, a person who notes that decreased sleep typically heralds the onset of a manic episode might be coached on cognitive-behavioral strategies for improving sleep patterns, or a patient who recognizes that pressured activity and distractibility often progress to more severe symptoms of mania may practice cognitive-behavioral methods for slowing down and staying focused on productive task completion. Medication adherence is another important goal of CBT for bipolar disorder (Basco and Rush 2005). Dysfunctional cognitions about medication can be modified with CBT, and behavioral interventions, such as reminder systems and behavioral plans to overcome obstacles to adherence, can be used.

Treatment of depressive episodes in bipolar disorder uses many of the same interventions described for CBT for major depression. Typically, CBT is not used as a mainstay of treatment for severe mania when persons are markedly agitated or grossly psychotic. Instead, the CBT effort is greater when symptoms are less extreme and the patient can concentrate on the work of therapy. The overall goals of CBT for bipolar disorder are to lower symptoms of both depression and mania, improve psychosocial functioning, gain stress management skills, and reduce the risk for relapse.

Learning Cognitive-Behavioral Therapy

Psychiatry residents are now required to achieve competency in CBT before completing their training, and many other mental health disciplines are emphasizing CBT training in their educational programs. Also, clinicians who have previously completed their training without special emphasis on CBT may be interested in gaining expertise in this approach. Although there are many ways to receive training in CBT and to achieve competency, typical programs include at least 1 year of educational experiences with a series of didactic presentations, readings, video and role-play illustrations, and supervision.

The Beck Institute (www.beckinstitute.org) offers an extramural fellowship and online courses for clinicians who do not have CBT training available locally and wish to enter an intensive CBT educational program. Several other centers for CBT have been established throughout the world to provide clinical service and training. Workshops on CBT are offered at annual meetings of the American Psychiatric Association, the American Psychological Association, the Association for Behavioral and Cognitive Therapies, and others.

Basic textbooks used for training in CBT include *Learning Cognitive-Behavior Therapy: An Illustrated Guide,* 2nd Edition (Wright et al. 2017), which includes videos of CBT methods; *Cognitive Behavior Therapy: Basics and Beyond,* 2nd Edition (Beck 2011); and *Cognitive Behavioral Therapy for Clinicians* (Sudak 2006). Other recommended readings and web sites are provided at the end of this chapter. The Academy of Cognitive Therapy has an especially useful web site (www.academyofct.org) for those interested in learning CBT.

Effectiveness of Cognitive-Behavioral Therapy

CBT has been investigated in many carefully designed outcome trials that have documented the effectiveness of this treatment approach. The most intensive research has been directed at CBT for depression and anxiety disorders. There also has been a steady increase in investigations of CBT for OCD, PTSD, eating disorders, psychosis, bipolar disorder, and other conditions. The large amount of CBT research was summarized by Hofmann et al. (2012), who performed a review that identified 269 meta-analytic investigations. Our focus here is on providing a brief overview of outcome research.

Meta-analyses of numerous outcome studies of depression documented that CBT is, at the least, as effective as other proven treatments for depression, including antidepressant pharmacotherapy (Cuijpers et al. 2011, 2016; Driessen and Hollon 2010). A two-center trial conducted at the University of Pennsylvania and Vanderbilt University (DeRubeis et al. 2005) is particularly noteworthy because the study was limited to patients with moderate to severe depressive symptoms. DeRubeis et al. (2005) found CBT to be as effective as a two-drug sequential algorithm across 16 weeks of therapy. Although the weight of the evidence indicates that CBT and antidepressant pharmacotherapy are comparable in effectiveness to acute-phase therapies, results of several investigations indicate that CBT has more durable effects for at least 1 year after termination of acute-phase therapy (see Vittengl et al. 2007). This finding was fully replicated in the University of Pennsylvania–Vanderbilt University collaboration (Hollon et al. 2005), in which acute-phase CBT had sustained efficacy comparable to that of continuation pharmacotherapy.

CBT likewise has been found to be an effective therapy for anxiety disorders (Bandelow et al. 2015; Cuijpers et al. 2016). Especially strong evidence has been collected to support the utility of CBT and related therapies in treatment of panic disorder. Two major forms of therapy have been developed: panic control treatment—a combination of relaxation training, cognitive restructuring, and exposure (Barlow and Cerney 1988)—and focused cognitive therapy—a more cognitively oriented treatment that uses exposure but places less emphasis on behavioral interventions than does panic control treatment (Clark and Beck 2011). In one of the larger studies of Beck's model of cognitive therapy in panic disorder, the treatment was compared with relaxation training, imipramine, and a wait-list control condition (Clark et al. 1994). All three active treatments were superior to the control condition, but CBT led to greater reductions in anxiety levels, catastrophic cognitions, and frequency of panic attacks. CBT also has been found to be an effective option for helping patients with panic disorder to discontinue benzodiazepines and for helping those whose symptoms did not respond to antidepressant or anxiolytic medications (Heldt et al. 2006).

Other studies have demonstrated that CBT is an effective treatment for generalized anxiety disorder (Cuijpers et al. 2016) and social anxiety disorder (Clark et al. 2003; Cuijpers et al. 2016).

Exposure and response prevention, a treatment that is primarily behavioral in focus, is the best-established therapy for OCD, either alone or (more typically) combined with CBT in comprehensive treatment packages (Salkovskis and Westbrook 1989; Simpson et al. 2006). Similarly, PTSD also has been shown to be responsive to CBT (Foa et al. 2005; McDonagh et al. 2005).

Numerous experimental trials have found that CBT significantly improves the symptoms of bulimia nervosa, with complete remission observed in at least 50% of cases (e.g., Brownley et al. 2016; Wilson and Shafran 2005).

There has been a growing interest in studying the use of CBT for schizophrenia and related psychotic disorders (Grant et al. 2012; Jauhar et al. 2014; Mehl et al. 2015). Meta-analyses typically have found small to medium effect sizes for positive symptoms and small effect sizes for negative symptoms (Burns et al. 2014; Jauhar et al. 2014; Mehl et al. 2015; Velthorst et al. 2015). A notable individual study of recovery-oriented CBT in patients with schizophrenia found superior effects for CBT compared with treatment as usual, and these positive results were maintained at follow-up (Grant et al. 2012, 2017).

Although fewer studies have evaluated the efficacy of CBT in the longer-term treatment of bipolar disorder, studies have yielded both positive (e.g., Lam et al. 2003; Miklowitz et al. 2007) and failed (e.g., Scott et al. 2006) results. In the study by Scott et al. (2006), the effects of CBT were moderated by patients' past number of episodes, with a beneficial effect among the patients who had experienced fewer prior episodes. A recent meta-analysis of randomized controlled trials of CBT in patients with bipolar disorder (Chiang et al. 2017) found moderate effect sizes for relapse prevention and improvement of depression, mania, and psychosocial functioning.

A substantial amount of research has examined the utility of CBT for a wide range of other disorders. Although a review of studies is beyond the scope of this chapter, it is accurate to say that CBT has become a major treatment option for several conditions in behavioral medicine, including chronic pain (Richmond et al. 2015), insomnia (Trauer et al. 2015), irritable bowel syndrome (Laird et al. 2017), and chronic fatigue syndrome (Malouff et al. 2008). When viewed within a broader framework of CBT, relapse prevention strategies have been a cornerstone of psychosocial interventions for substance abuse disorders for more than a decade (Carroll and Onken 2005) and have now been augmented by mindfulness-based strategies (Witkiewitz et al. 2014). Similarly, DBT (Linehan 1993)—which draws heavily on mindfulness-based strategies—is one of the few empirically validated treatments for borderline personality disorder.

Conclusion

CBT is a system of psychotherapy that is linked philosophically with a long tradition of viewing cognition as a primary determinant of emotion and behavior. The theoretical constructs of CBT are supported by a large body of experimental findings regarding dysfunctional information processing and maladaptive behavior in psychiatric disorders. In clinical practice, CBT is usually short term, problem oriented, and highly collaborative. Therapists and patients work together in an empirical style, seeking to identify and modify maladaptive patterns of thinking. Behavioral techniques are used to uncover distorted cognitions and to promote more effective functioning. Also, psychoeducational procedures and homework assignments help reinforce concepts learned in therapy sessions. The goals of CBT include both immediate symptom relief and the acquisition of cognitive and behavioral skills that will decrease the risk for relapse.

The efficacy of CBT for depression, anxiety disorders, eating disorders, and other conditions has been established in a wide range of outcome studies. Detailed treatment manuals or other guidelines for therapy have been described for most psychiatric illnesses.

CBT has evolved into one of the major psychotherapeutic orientations in modern psychiatric treatment. Future challenges for this therapy model include study of the relative importance of treatment components, detailed examination of predictors for outcome, elucidation of the interface between biological and cognitive processes, and incorporation of new developments in computer-assisted learning. The empirical nature of CBT should promote further exploration of the potential uses for this treatment approach.

Key Clinical Points

- Studies of information processing in mental disorders have found characteristic patterns of cognitions that are linked with dysphoric emotions and maladaptive behavior.

- Treatment with cognitive-behavioral therapy (CBT) involves modification of dysfunctional cognitions and associated behaviors.

- CBT is an active treatment characterized by a highly collaborative therapeutic relationship.

- Structure, psychoeducation, and homework are important components of treatment.

- Cognitive-behavioral therapists help patients identify and change automatic thoughts and core beliefs (schemas).

- Behavioral methods are used to reverse helplessness, anhedonia, avoidance, and other core symptoms of mental disorders.

- CBT has been extensively researched. Strong empirical support exists for the efficacy of this treatment approach.

- CBT methods have been developed for many conditions, including mood and anxiety disorders, schizophrenia, eating disorders, substance abuse, and personality disorders.

References

Abramson LY, Seligman MEP, Teasdale JD: Learned helplessness in humans: critique and reformulation. J Abnorm Psychol 87(1):49–74, 1978 649856

Adelman CB, Panza KE, Bartley CA, et al: A meta-analysis of computerized cognitive-behavioral therapy for the treatment of DSM-5 anxiety disorders. J Clin Psychiatry 75(7):e695–e704, 2014 25093485

Aguileria A, Muench F: There's an app for that: information technology applications for cognitive behavioral therapy practitioners. Behav Ther (NY NY) 35(4):65–73, 2012 25530659

Alford BA, Beck AT: The Integrative Power of Cognitive Therapy. New York, Guilford, 1997

Bandelow B, Reitt M, Röver C, et al: Efficacy of treatments for anxiety disorders: a meta-analysis. Int Clin Psychopharmacol 30(4):183–192, 2015 25932596

Barlow DH, Cerney JA: Psychological Treatment of Panic. New York, Guilford, 1988

Barlow DH, Craske MG: Mastery of Your Anxiety and Panic, 4th Edition. New York, Oxford University Press, 2007

Basco MR, Rush AJ: Cognitive-Behavioral Therapy for Bipolar Disorder. New York, Guilford, 2005

Beck AT: Thinking and depression, I: idiosyncratic content and cognitive distortions. Arch Gen Psychiatry 9:324–333, 1963 14045261

Beck AT: Thinking and depression, II: theory and therapy. Arch Gen Psychiatry 10:561–571, 1964 14159256

Beck AT: Cognitive Therapy and the Emotional Disorders. New York, International Universities Press, 1976

Beck AT: Cognitive therapy and research: a 25-year retrospective. Presented at the World Congress of Cognitive-Behavior Therapy, Oxford, UK, June 1989

Beck AT: Cognitive therapy: past, present, and future. J Consult Clin Psychol 61(2):194–198, 1993 8473571

Beck AT, Freeman A: Cognitive Therapy of Personality Disorders. New York, Guilford, 1990

Beck AT, Rush AJ, Shaw BF, et al: Cognitive Therapy of Depression. New York, Guilford, 1979

Beck AT, Steer RA, Kovacs M, et al: Hopelessness and eventual suicide: a 10-year prospective study of patients hospitalized with suicidal ideation. Am J Psychiatry 142(5):559–563, 1985 3985195

Beck AT, Davis DD, Freeman A (eds): Cognitive Therapy of Personality Disorders, 3rd Edition, New York, Guilford, 2015

Beck JS: Cognitive Behavior Therapy: Basics and Beyond, 2nd Edition. New York, Guilford, 2011

Blackburn IM, Jones S, Lewin RJP: Cognitive style in depression. Br J Clin Psychol 25(Pt 4):241–251, 1986 3801730

Brown GK, Ten Have T, Henriques GR, et al: Cognitive therapy for the prevention of suicide attempts: a randomized controlled trial. JAMA 294(5):563–570, 2005 16077050

Brownley KA, Berkman ND, Peat CM, et al: Binge-eating disorder in adults: a systematic review and meta-analysis. Ann Intern Med 165(6):409–420, 2016 27367316

Burns AMN, Erickson DH, Brenner CA: Cognitive-behavioral therapy for medication-resistant psychosis: a meta-analytic review. Psychiatr Serv 65(7):874–880, 2014 24686725

Burns DD: Feeling Good. New York, William Morrow, 1980

Burns DD: Feeling Good: The New Mood Therapy. New York, HarperCollins, 1999

Carroll KM, Onken LS: Behavioral therapies for drug abuse. Am J Psychiatry 162(8):1452–1460, 2005 16055766

Chiang KJ, Tsai JC, Liu D, et al: Efficacy of cognitive-behavioral therapy in patients with bipolar disorder: a meta-analysis of randomized controlled trials. PLoS One 12(5):e0176849, 2017 28472082

Clark DA: Cognitive therapy for anxiety, in Science and Practice in Cognitive Therapy: Foundations, Mechanisms, and Applications. Edited by Leahy RL. New York, Guilford, 2018, pp 298–316

Clark DA, Beck AT: Cognitive Therapy of Anxiety Disorders. New York, Guilford, 2011

Clark DA, Feldman J, Channon S: Dysfunctional thinking in anorexia and bulimia nervosa. Cognitive Therapy and Research 13(4):377–387, 1989

Clark DA, Beck AT, Alford BA: Scientific Foundations of Cognitive Theory and Therapy of Depression. New York, Wiley, 1999

Clark DM, Salkovskis PM, Chalkley AJ: Respiratory control as a treatment for panic attacks. J Behav Ther Exp Psychiatry 16(1):23–30, 1985 3998171

Clark DM, Salkovskis PM, Hackmann A, et al: A comparison of cognitive therapy, applied relaxation and imipramine in the treatment of panic disorder. Br J Psychiatry 164(6):759–769, 1994 7952982

Clark DM, Ehlers A, McManus F, et al: Cognitive therapy versus fluoxetine in generalized social phobia: a randomized placebo-controlled trial. J Consult Clin Psychol 71(6):1058–1067, 2003 14622081

Cuijpers P, Andersson G, Donker T, et al: Psychological treatment of depression: results of a series of meta-analyses. Nord J Psychiatry 65(6):354–364, 2011 21770842

Cuijpers P, Cristea IA, Karyotaki E, et al: How effective are cognitive behavior therapies for major depression and anxiety disorders? A meta-analytic update of the evidence. World Psychiatry 15(3):245–258, 2016 27717254

Davies EB, Morriss R, Glazebrook C: Computer-delivered and web-based interventions to improve depression, anxiety, and psychological well-being of university students: a systematic review and meta-analysis. J Med Internet Res 16(5):e130, 2014 24836465

DeRubeis RJ, Gelfand LA, Tang TZ, et al: Medications versus cognitive behavior therapy for severely depressed outpatients: mega-analysis of four randomized comparisons. Am J Psychiatry 156(7):1007–1013, 1999 10401443

DeRubeis RJ, Hollon SD, Amsterdam JD, et al: Cognitive therapy vs. medications in the treatment of moderate to severe depression. Arch Gen Psychiatry 62(4):409–416, 2005 15809408

Dobson KS, Poole JC, Beck JS: The fundamental cognitive model, in Science and Practice in Cognitive Therapy: Foundations, Mechanisms, and Applications. Edited by Leahy RL. New York, Guilford, 2018, pp 29–47

Driessen E, Hollon SD: Cognitive behavioral therapy for mood disorders: efficacy, moderators and mediators. Psychiatr Clin North Am 33(3):537–555, 2010 20599132

Dunlop BW, Rajendra JK, Craighead WE, et al: Functional connectivity of the subcallosal cingulate cortex and differential outcomes to treatment with cognitive-behavioral therapy or antidepressant medication for major depressive disorder. Am J Psychiatry 174(6):533–545, 2017 28335622

Eells TD, Barrett MS, Wright JH, et al: Can cognitive therapy be conducted by computers? Curr Behav Neurosci Rep 2(4):209–215, 2015

Fava GA: Well-Being Therapy, Treatment Manual and Clinical Applications. New York, Karger, 2016

Foa E, Wilson R: Stop Obsessing! How to Overcome Your Obsessions and Compulsions, Revised Edition. New York, Bantam Books, 2001

Foa EB, Hembree EA, Cahill SP, et al: Randomized trial of prolonged exposure for posttraumatic stress disorder with and without cognitive restructuring: outcome at academic and community clinics. J Consult Clin Psychol 73(5):953–964, 2005 16287395

Fonzo GA, Goodkind MS, Oathes DJ, et al: Selective effects of psychotherapy on frontopolar cortical function in PTSD. Am J Psychiatry 174(12):1175–1184, 2017 28715907

Friedberg RD, McClure JM: Clinical Practice of Cognitive Therapy With Children and Adolescents: The Nuts and Bolts. New York, Guilford, 2015

Gaffan EA, Tsaousis I, Kemp-Wheeler SM: Researcher allegiance and meta-analysis: the case of cognitive therapy for depression. J Consult Clin Psychol 63(6):966–980, 1995 8543719

Gilbody S, Littlewood E, Hewitt C, et al; REEACT Team: Computerised cognitive behaviour therapy (cCBT) as treatment for depression in primary care (REEACT trial): large scale pragmatic randomised controlled trial. BMJ 351:h5627, 2015 [Erratum in: BMJ 352:i195, 2016] 26559241

Goldapple K, Segal Z, Garson C, et al: Modulation of cortical-limbic pathways in major depression: treatment-specific effects of cognitive behavior therapy. Arch Gen Psychiatry 61(1):34–41, 2004 14706942

Grant PM, Huh GA, Perivoliotis D, et al: Randomized trial to evaluate the efficacy of cognitive therapy for low-functioning patients with schizophrenia. Arch Gen Psychiatry 69(2):121–127, 2012 21969420

Grant PM, Bredemeier K, Beck AT: Six-month follow-up of recovery-oriented cognitive therapy for low-functioning individuals with schizophrenia. Psychiatr Serv 68(10):997–1002, 2017 28566022

Greenberger D, Padesky CA: Mind Over Mood. New York, Guilford, 1995

Heldt E, Gus Manfro G, Kipper L, et al: One-year follow-up of pharmacotherapy-resistant patients with panic disorder treated with cognitive-behavior therapy: outcome and predictors of remission. Behav Res Ther 44(5):657–665, 2006 16038874

Hofmann SG, Asnaani A, Vonk IJJ, et al: The efficacy of cognitive behavioral therapy: a review of meta-analyses. Cognit Ther Res 36(5):427–440, 2012 23459093

Hollon SD, DeRubeis RJ, Shelton RC, et al: Prevention of relapse following cognitive therapy vs. medications in moderate to severe depression. Arch Gen Psychiatry 62(4):417–422, 2005 15809409

Jauhar S, McKenna PJ, Radua J, et al: Cognitive-behavioural therapy for the symptoms of schizophrenia: systematic review and meta-analysis with examination of potential bias. Br J Psychiatry 204(1):20–29, 2014 24385461

Kandel ER, Schwartz JH: Molecular biology of learning: modulation of transmitter release. Science 218(4571):433–443, 1982 6289442

Laird KT, Tanner-Smith EE, Russell AC, et al: Comparative efficacy of psychological therapies for improving mental health and daily functioning in irritable bowel syndrome: a systematic review and meta-analysis. Clin Psychol Rev 51:142–152, 2017 27870997

Lam DH, Watkins ER, Hayward P, et al: A randomized controlled study of cognitive therapy for relapse prevention for bipolar affective disorder: outcome of the first year. Arch Gen Psychiatry 60(2):145–152, 2003 12578431

Linehan MM: Cognitive-Behavioral Treatment of Borderline Personality Disorder. New York, Guilford, 1993

Linehan MM, Armstrong HE, Suarez A, et al: Cognitive-behavioral treatment of chronically parasuicidal borderline patients. Arch Gen Psychiatry 48(12):1060–1064, 1991 1845222

Linehan MM, Schmidt H 3rd, Dimeff LA, et al: Dialectical behavior therapy for patients with borderline personality disorder and drug-dependence. Am J Addict 8(4):279–292, 1999 10598211

Linehan MM, Comtois KA, Murray AM, et al: Two-year randomized controlled trial and follow-up of dialectical behavior therapy vs. therapy by experts for suicidal behaviors and borderline personality disorder. Arch Gen Psychiatry 63(7):757–766, 2006 16818865

Malouff JM, Thorsteinsson EB, Rooke SE, et al: Efficacy of cognitive behavioral therapy for chronic fatigue syndrome: a meta-analysis. Clin Psychol Rev 28(5):736–745, 2008 18060672

McDonagh A, Friedman M, McHugo G, et al: Randomized trial of cognitive-behavioral therapy for chronic posttraumatic stress disorder in adult female survivors of childhood sexual abuse. J Consult Clin Psychol 73(3):515–524, 2005 15982149

Mehl S, Werner D, Lincoln TM: Does cognitive behavior therapy for psychosis (CBTp) show a sustainable effect on delusions? A meta-analysis. Front Psychol 6:1450, 2015 26500570

Meichenbaum DB: Cognitive-Behavior Modification: An Integrative Approach. New York, Plenum, 1977

Miklowitz DJ, Otto MW, Frank E, et al: Psychosocial treatments for bipolar depression: a 1-year randomized trial from the Systematic Treatment Enhancement Program. Arch Gen Psychiatry 64(4):419–426, 2007 17404119

Proudfoot J, Goldberg D, Mann A, et al: Computerized, interactive, multimedia cognitive-behavioural program for anxiety and depression in general practice. Psychol Med 33(2):217–227, 2003 12622301

Proudfoot J, Ryden C, Everitt B, et al: Clinical efficacy of computerised cognitive-behavioural therapy for anxiety and depression in primary care: randomised controlled trial. Br J Psychiatry 185:46–54, 2004 15231555

Pull CB: Current status of virtual reality exposure therapy in anxiety disorders. Curr Opin Psychiatry 18(1):7–14, 2005 16639177

Reinecke MA, Dattilio FM, Freeman A (eds): Cognitive Therapy With Children and Adolescents: A Casebook for Clinical Practice, 2nd Edition. New York, Guilford, 2003

Richards D, Richardson T: Computer-based psychological treatments for depression: a systematic review and meta-analysis. Clin Psychol Rev 32(4):329–342, 2012 22466510

Richmond H, Hall AM, Copsey B, et al: The effectiveness of cognitive behavioural treatment for non-specific low back pain: a systematic review and meta-analysis. PLoS One 10(8):e0134192, 2015 26244668

Robinson LA, Berman JS, Neimeyer RA: Psychotherapy for the treatment of depression: a comprehensive review of controlled outcome research. Psychol Bull 108(1):30–49, 1990 2200072

Rothbaum BO, Hodges LF, Kooper R, et al: Effectiveness of computer-generated (virtual reality) graded exposure in the treatment of acrophobia. Am J Psychiatry 152(4):626–628, 1995 7694917

Rothbaum BO, Hodges L, Smith S, et al: A controlled study of virtual reality exposure therapy for the fear of flying. J Consult Clin Psychol 68(6):1020–1026, 2000 11142535

Salkovskis PM, Westbrook D: Behaviour therapy and obsessional ruminations: can failure be turned into success? Behav Res Ther 27(2):149–160, 1989 2930440

Scott J, Paykel E, Morriss R, et al: Cognitive-behavioural therapy for severe and recurrent bipolar disorders: randomised controlled trial. Br J Psychiatry 188:313–320, 2006 16582056

Siegle GJ, Carter CS, Thase ME: Use of FMRI to predict recovery from unipolar depression with cognitive behavior therapy. Am J Psychiatry 163(4):735–738, 2006 16585452

Siegle GJ, Thompson WK, Collier A, et al: Toward clinically useful neuroimaging in depression treatment: prognostic utility of subgenual cingulate activity for determining depression outcome in cognitive therapy across studies, scanners, and patient characteristics. Arch Gen Psychiatry 69(9):913–924, 2012 22945620

Simpson HB, Huppert JD, Petkova E, et al: Response versus remission in obsessive-compulsive disorder. J Clin Psychiatry 67(2):269–276, 2006 16566623

Sucala M, Cuijpers P, Muench F, et al: Anxiety: there is an app for that. A systematic review of anxiety apps. Depress Anxiety 34(6):518–525, 2017 28504859

Sudak D: Cognitive Behavioral Therapy for Clinicians. Baltimore, MD, Lippincott Williams & Wilkins, 2006

Szigethy E (ed): Cognitive-Behavior Therapy for Children and Adolescents. Washington, DC, American Psychiatric Publishing, 2012

Thase ME, Simons AD, Reynolds CF 3rd: Psychobiological correlates of poor response to cognitive behavior therapy: potential indications for antidepressant pharmacotherapy. Psychopharmacol Bull 29(2):293–301, 1993 8290680

Thase ME, Reynolds CF 3rd, Frank E, et al: Response to cognitive-behavioral therapy in chronic depression. Journal of Psychotherapy Practice & Research 3(3):204–214, 1994

Thase ME, Dubé S, Bowler K, et al: Hypothalamic-pituitary-adrenocortical activity and response to cognitive behavior therapy in unmedicated, hospitalized depressed patients. Am J Psychiatry 153(7):886–891, 1996a 8659610

Thase ME, Simons AD, Reynolds CF 3rd: Abnormal electroencephalographic sleep profiles in major depression: association with response to cognitive behavior therapy. Arch Gen Psychiatry 53(2):99–108, 1996b 8629894

Thase ME, Wright JH, Eells TD, et al: Improving the efficiency of psychotherapy for depression: computer-assisted versus standard CBT. Am J Psychiatry 175(3):242–250, 2018 28969439

Trauer JM, Qian MY, Doyle JS, et al: Cognitive behavioral therapy for chronic insomnia: a systematic review and meta-analysis. Ann Intern Med 163(3):191–204, 2015 26054060

Valmaggia LR, Latif L, Kempton MJ, et al: Virtual reality in the psychological treatment for mental health problems: an systematic review of recent evidence. Psychiatry Res 236:189–195, 2016 26795129

Van Ameringen M, Turna J, Khalesi Z, et al: There is an app for that! The current state of mobile applications (apps) for DSM-5 obsessive-compulsive disorder, posttraumatic stress disorder, anxiety and mood disorders. Depress Anxiety 34(6):526–539, 2017 28569409

Velthorst E, Koeter M, van der Gaag M, et al: Adapted cognitive-behavioural therapy required for targeting negative symptoms in schizophrenia: meta-analysis and meta-regression. Psychol Med 45(3):453–465, 2015 24993642

Vittengl JR, Clark LA, Dunn TW, et al: Reducing relapse and recurrence in unipolar depression: a comparative meta-analysis of cognitive-behavioral therapy's effects. J Consult Clin Psychol 75(3):475–488, 2007 17563164

Wang K, Varma DS, Prosperi M: A systematic review of the effectiveness of mobile apps for monitoring and management of mental health symptoms or disorders. J Psychiatr Res 107:73–78, 2018 30347316

Williams JMG, Teasdale JD, Segal ZV, et al: The Mindful Way Through Depression: Freeing Yourself From Chronic Unhappiness. New York, Guilford, 2007

Wilson GT, Shafran R: Eating disorders guidelines from NICE. Lancet 365(9453):79–81, 2005 15639682

Witkiewitz K, Bowen S, Harrop EN, et al: Mindfulness-based treatment to prevent addictive behavior relapse: theoretical models and hypothesized mechanisms of change. Subst Use Misuse 49(5):513–524, 2014 24611847

Wright JH, McCray LW: Breaking Free From Depression: Pathways to Wellness. New York, Guilford, 2012

Wright JH, Wright AS, Albano AM, et al: Computer-assisted cognitive therapy for depression: maintaining efficacy while reducing therapist time. Am J Psychiatry 162(6):1158–1164, 2005 15930065

Wright JH, Turkington D, Kingdon D, et al: Cognitive-Behavior Therapy for Severe Mental Illness. Washington, DC, American Psychiatric Publishing, 2009

Wright JH, Sudak D, Turkington D, et al: High-Yield Cognitive-Behavior Therapy for Brief Sessions: An Illustrated Guide. Washington, DC, American Psychiatric Publishing, 2010

Wright JH, Wright AS, Beck AT: Good Days Ahead 3.0. San Francisco, CA, Empower Interactive, 2012

Wright JH, Brown GK, Thase ME, Basco MR: Learning Cognitive-Behavior Therapy: An Illustrated Guide, 2nd Edition (Core Competencies in Psychotherapy Series; Gabbard GO, series ed). Arlington, VA, American Psychiatric Association Publishing, 2017

Wright JH, Owen JJ, Eells TD, Richards D, Richardson T, Brown GK, Barrett M, Rasku MA, Polser G, Thase ME: Computer-assisted cognitive-behavior therapy for depression: a systematic review and meta-analysis. J Clin Psychiatry (in press)

Recommended Readings

Barlow DH, Cerney JA: Psychological Treatment of Panic. New York, Guilford, 1988

Basco MR, Rush AJ: Cognitive-Behavioral Therapy for Bipolar Disorder. New York, Guilford, 2005

Beck AT, Freeman A: Cognitive Therapy of Personality Disorders. New York, Guilford, 1990

Beck AT, Rush AJ, Shaw BF, et al: Cognitive Therapy of Depression. New York, Guilford, 1979

Beck AT, Wright FD, Newman CF, et al: Cognitive Therapy of Substance Abuse, Revised Edition. New York, Guilford, 2001

Beck AT, Emery GD, Greenberg RL: Anxiety Disorders and Phobias: A Cognitive Perspective, Deluxe Edition. New York, Basic Books, 2005

Beck AT, Davis DD, Freeman A: Cognitive Therapy of Personality Disorders. New York, Guilford, 2015

Beck JS: Cognitive Behavior Therapy: Basics and Beyond, 2nd Edition. New York, Guilford, 2011

Clark DA, Beck AT: Cognitive Therapy of Anxiety Disorders: Science and Practice. New York, Guilford, 2011

Clark DA, Beck AT, Alford BA: Scientific Foundations of Cognitive Theory and Therapy of Depression. New York, Wiley, 1999

Clark DM, Fairburn CG (eds): Science and Practice of Cognitive Behavior Therapy. New York, Oxford University Press, 1997

Fairburn C, Brownell K (eds): Eating Disorders and Obesity: A Comprehensive Handbook, 2nd Edition. New York, Guilford, 2002

Freeman A, Mahoney MJ, DeVito P: Cognition and Psychotherapy, 2nd Edition. New York, Spring Publishing, 2004

Friedberg RD, McClure JM: Clinical Practice of Cognitive Therapy With Children and Adolescents: The Nuts and Bolts. New York, Guilford, 2015

Kendall PC (ed): Child and Adolescent Therapy: Cognitive-Behavioral Procedures. New York, Guilford, 2012

Kingdon D, Turkington D: Cognitive Therapy for Schizophrenia. New York, Guilford, 2005

Leahy R (ed): Science and Practice in Cognitive Therapy. New York, Guilford, 2018

Linehan MM: Cognitive-Behavioral Treatment of Borderline Personality Disorder. New York, Guilford, 1993

Meichenbaum DB: Cognitive-Behavior Modification: An Integrative Approach. New York, Plenum, 1977

Reinecke MA, Dattilio FM, Freeman A (eds): Cognitive Therapy With Children and Adolescents: A Casebook for Clinical Practice, 2nd Edition. New York, Guilford, 2003

Salkovskis PM (ed): Frontiers of Cognitive Therapy. New York, Guilford, 1996

Sudak D: Cognitive Behavioral Therapy for Clinicians. Baltimore, MD, Lippincott Williams & Wilkins, 2006

Szigethy E (ed): Cognitive-Behavior Therapy for Children and Adolescents. Washington, DC, American Psychiatric Publishing, 2012

Wilkes TCR, Belsher G, Rush AJ, et al: Cognitive Therapy for Depressed Adolescents. New York, Guilford, 1994

Wright JH, Turkington D, Kingdon D, Basco MR: Cognitive-Behavior Therapy for Severe Mental Illness: An Illustrated Guide, 2nd Edition, Washington, DC, American Psychiatric Publishing, 2009

Wright JH, Sudak D, Turkington D, et al: High-Yield Cognitive-Behavior Therapy for Brief Sessions: An Illustrated Guide. Washington, DC, American Psychiatric Publishing, 2010

Wright JH, Brown GK, Thase ME, Basco MR: Learning Cognitive-Behavior Therapy: An Illustrated Guide, 2nd Edition (Core Competencies in Psychotherapy Series; Gabbard GO, series ed). Arlington, VA, American Psychiatric Association Publishing, 2017

Online Resources

Academy of Cognitive Therapy: https://www.academyofct.org

American Psychiatric Association Publishing (for downloading of worksheets from Learning Cognitive-Behavior Therapy: An Illustrated Guide, 2nd Edition, by Wright JH, Brown GK, Thase ME, Basco MR): https://www.appi.org/wright

Association for Behavioral and Cognitive Therapies: http://www.abct.org/Home

Beck Institute: https://beckinstitute.org

British Association for Behavioural and Cognitive Psychotherapies: http://www.babcp.com

Empower Interactive (for computer-assisted CBT software): http://www.empower-interactive.com

International Association for Cognitive Psychotherapy: https://www.the-iacp.com

CHAPTER 34

Supportive Psychotherapy

Arnold Winston, M.D.
Laura Weiss Roberts, M.D., M.A.

Supportive psychotherapy is an extensively practiced form of individual psychotherapy that focuses on ameliorating symptoms, improving self-esteem, fostering resilience, and strengthening adaptive skills. Supportive psychotherapy has value in the care of highly diverse conditions occurring across the age spectrum, and it is well received by patients who may not tolerate or be suited to other forms of psychotherapy. Especially in the context of a strong therapeutic alliance, supportive psychotherapy is as efficacious as other forms of treatment for several mental disorders (Arnow et al. 2013; Winston and Winston 2002).

Supportive psychotherapy involves approaches that are integrated intentionally and flexibly by the therapist into the care of individual patients. Supportive psychotherapy is not merely a supportive relationship between the therapist and the patient. Supportive psychotherapy is highly intentional therapeutic work that emphasizes relational and interpersonal issues and the self within the reality of the present everyday world as opposed to conflict and instinctual issues and a focus on the past. A supportive patient–therapist relationship affords the patient the safety to access and acknowledge painful experiences and beliefs. Supportive psychotherapy does not seek to change the patient's underlying personality structure; instead, supportive psychotherapy is oriented toward coping, adaptation, and well-being.

From a theoretical perspective, supportive psychotherapy has been conceptualized in three ways (Brenner 2012). First, it is a general approach that uses the core elements present in all psychotherapies—namely, the creation and sustenance of a therapeutic relationship along with empathy, compassion, genuineness, safety, and trust. Second, supportive psychotherapy has been viewed as an extension of psychoanalytic psychotherapy, with an emphasis on ego psychology and development, object relations theory, self psychology issues, interpersonal and relational approaches, and attachment theory. Third, supportive psychotherapy is seen as a therapeutic modality that includes specifically definable techniques or interventions that draw from across the fields of psychiatry and psychology.

A Continuum of Patient Impairment

Human beings are endowed with complex psychological structures and, as a group, function along a sickness–health continuum according to their level of need and impairment, adaptive capacity, self-concept, and ability to relate to others. This continuum is conceptualized as extending from the most impaired patients to the most intact, well-put-together individuals. Impairments consist of behaviors that interfere with an individual's ability to function in everyday life, form relationships, think clearly and realistically, and behave in a relatively adaptive and mature fashion. Individuals on the healthier side of the continuum tend to function well, have good relationships, and lead productive lives. They are able to enjoy a wide range of activities relatively free of conflict. The adaptation and behavior of individuals in the middle of the continuum are uneven. These individuals have significant problems in maintaining consistent functioning and stable relationships. An individual's position on the continuum can vary over time, depending on a few factors, including response to environmental stressors, physical illness, maturational growth, and psychotherapy and pharmacotherapy.

An individual's placement on the continuum is associated with the nature and severity of symptomatology or the presence of a mental disorder. For example, patients with a serious anxiety, developmental, mood, or psychotic disorder or a severe personality disorder generally experience greater impairment and fall on the more burdened and impaired side of the psychopathology continuum. Patients with better potential for healthy functioning may have conditions such as dysthymia, panic disorder, adjustment disorder, or traits of personality disorders. Substance abuse problems occur across the continuum. Although diagnosis can provide a general idea of where a person might reside on the continuum, the actual placement will depend on the individual's level of psychopathology and adaptation.

Matching the psychotherapeutic strategy to the patient's locus on the continuum is of crucial importance. Individual psychotherapies may be conceptualized as an array that extends from supportive psychotherapy to expressive or exploratory psychotherapy, as shown in Figure 34–1. Supportive psychotherapy uses a variety of interventions directed toward building psychological structure, stability, relationships, self-esteem, and a sense of self. Expressive psychotherapy explores relational and conflict issues, seeking personality change through analysis of the relationship between therapist and patient and through the development of insight into previously unrecognized feelings, thoughts, and needs.

Most individuals do not lie at either end of the psychopathology continuum but instead have both conflict and structural problems. Many patients will require work in both areas, generally beginning with relationship problems and structure building and then perhaps going on to address conflict issues. For these reasons, the psychotherapeutic approach often will be a combined supportive–expressive psychotherapy.

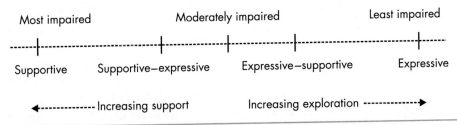

FIGURE 34–1. Attunement of psychotherapy to the patient's degree of impairment.

Indications

Supportive psychotherapy has value in the care of very impaired individuals, in the care of less impaired individuals in acute situational distress, in the care of medically ill patients, in the context of grief, and as an adjuvant strategy in the care of individuals living with addiction.

Supportive psychotherapy is helpful for the most impaired patients, who require direct interventions aimed at improving ego functions, day-to-day coping, and self-esteem. In caring for these more symptomatic individuals, the therapist focuses on the patient's daily activities, medications, and use of resources for recovery and well-being. These individuals may experience any of the following:

- *Poor reality testing and primitive defenses:* Individuals with severe and chronic illness use defenses such as projection and denial, which are often maladaptive. They have great difficulty in separating self from other and may have hallucinations, delusions, thought broadcasting, and other psychotic symptoms.
- *Impaired object relations and interpersonal relationships:* These individuals have less capacity for mutuality and reciprocity and are unable to maintain stable relationships or sustained levels of intimacy or trust. This inability can lead to major problems in the patient–therapist relationship. In addition, such individuals cannot engage in self-observation and exploration, which limits their ability to introspect and develop insight.
- *Inadequate affect regulation and poor impulse control:* These patients have great difficulty containing aggression and tend to engage in destructive behavior.
- *Overwhelming anxiety:* Issues of separation or individuation can lead to severe anxiety, rendering these individuals incapable of exploring their feelings.

Supportive psychotherapy may be of great value to patients with these experiences. Importantly, psychotherapy that is primarily expressive is contraindicated for this group of patients.

Interestingly, supportive psychotherapy is also helpful for patients who are otherwise relatively healthy but have become symptomatic as a result of a severe and often overwhelming traumatic event. Under other circumstances, persons in this group might be referred for expressive treatment, because they have good reality testing, high-level object and interpersonal relations with good social supports and an ability to form a working alliance, a capacity to tolerate and contain affects and impulses, and a capacity for introspection.

In such crisis situations, supportive psychotherapy is usually delivered in a time-sensitive or episode-of-care model. An acute crisis is not a diagnosis but rather a general syndromal description for patients whose customary coping skills and defenses have been overwhelmed by an often unexpected event, resulting in intense anxiety and other symptoms (Dewald 1994). Patients in this context may meet formal criteria for an adjustment disorder. Supportive psychotherapy can help these patients manage uncomfortable feeling states and can enhance their coping strategies. The focus of the treatment is to reassure the patient that symptoms are generally time limited, to ensure safety in real time, to reduce stress by clarifying and providing information about what the patient is having difficulty adjusting to, and to support novel coping and problem-solving methods, including environmental change.

For many medical conditions, supportive psychotherapy is the only psychotherapeutic treatment that should be recommended. An understanding of a patient's defensive, cognitive, and interpersonal styles enables the therapist to assist the patient in developing better coping strategies. Early studies showed that supportive psychotherapy could be successfully used in patients with breast cancer, in HIV-positive patients with depression, in patients with pancreatic cancer, in cancer patients with depression, in patients with chronic pain, in patients with HIV-related neuropathic pain, and in patients with somatization disorder (Winston et al. 2012).

In the care of patients with substance use disorders, supportive psychotherapy may play an invaluable adjuvant role, helping individuals to develop coping strategies to control or reduce substance use and diminish anxiety and dysphoria. The therapist focuses first on the development of a therapeutic alliance to enhance treatment retention and to create an environment within which the patient can begin cognitive and motivational work. The therapist must actively strive to maintain a positive therapeutic alliance so that the patient can remain in treatment and actively contribute to the work of therapy. Newer evidence-based strategies such as psychoeducation, relapse prevention (Marlatt and Gordon 1985), and motivational interviewing (Rollnick and Miller 1995) should be integrated into supportive psychotherapy, along with 12-Step programs and group psychotherapy.

Supportive psychotherapy is also helpful in caring for a person after an acute loss of a loved one. Acute bereavement can overwhelm coping skills and produce symptoms such as self-reproach, social withdrawal, an inability to mourn, and depression and anxiety. Supportive psychotherapy affords the patient an empathic holding environment in which the work of mourning can safely take place. In addition, healthy defenses are strengthened, concrete assistance for routine activities is offered when needed, and social withdrawal is prevented.

Supportive psychotherapy is contraindicated in very few circumstances. In other words, supportive psychotherapy is contraindicated only when psychotherapy itself is contraindicated, such as in patients with delirium, drug intoxication, late-stage dementia, or malingering, or when providing supportive psychotherapy would deprive the patient of a more appropriate form of care.

In considering whether supportive psychotherapy is appropriate, it is important to note that for some conditions, treatments other than supportive psychotherapy have been shown to be more effective. For example, panic disorder (Barlow and Craske 1989) and obsessive-compulsive disorder (Foa and Franklin 2002) have been shown to have better outcomes with cognitive-behavioral therapy (CBT) than with supportive psychotherapy. A recent meta-analysis failed to show better health outcomes for treatment as usual compared with supportive psychotherapy when evaluated across 24 studies of schizophrenia care (Buckley et al. 2015).

For individuals with severe impairments, such as patients with schizophrenia, a broader approach of social skills training (Benton and Schroeder 1990) and psychoeducation (Goldman and Quinn 1988) is indicated. Combining these approaches with supportive psychotherapy would include providing education about the illness, facilitating reality testing, promoting medication adherence, helping the patient with problem solving, and reinforcing adaptive behaviors with praise (Lamberti and Herz 1995). In addition, the therapist would use supportive techniques such as behavioral goal setting, encouragement, modeling, shaping, and praise to teach interpersonal skills. Studies have demonstrated the utility of these interventions in improving social competence (Heinssen et al. 2000).

Interestingly, in the care of chronic depression, empirical research comparing CBT and supportive psychotherapy suggested that the quality of the therapeutic alliance is of greater importance to health outcomes than the specific form of therapy (Arnow et al. 2013). Another small project (Yrondi et al. 2015) showed that patients with depression had a preference for supportive psychotherapy over psychodynamic therapy and CBT, a finding that has important implications when balancing modern-day patient-centered care practices and health outcomes. For these reasons, attunement between the therapist and the patient and the patient's preferences is important in the selection of supportive psychotherapy over other potential treatments.

Strategies

Supportive psychotherapy relies on direct methods rather than change induced by insight. A major tenet of traditional psychoanalytic psychotherapy is that unconscious conflict produces the symptom or personality problem. Once the conflict becomes conscious, is explored, and is worked through, the symptom or personality problem improves because it is no longer psychologically necessary. The working-through process involves exploring the patient's history, particularly early relationships, to understand the genesis of the problem. In supportive psychotherapy, the therapist should understand many of the patient's dynamic issues and unconscious conflicts, but these generally are not explored. Some patients may not be able to contain or explore feelings and impulses and may become overwhelmed by anxiety, particularly in a time-limited treatment context. Instead, conscious problems and conflicts in the patient's current life are addressed (Table 34–1) (Dewald 1971).

The five key strategies in supportive psychotherapy focus on the following:

1. *Defenses*—From the point of view of psychoanalytic theory, supportive psychotherapy supports the patient's defenses. When therapy is primarily expressive, defenses are challenged and explored so that underlying conflicts, wishes, and feelings that were being defended against become available for exploration and resolution. In supportive psychotherapy, defenses are questioned or confronted only when they are maladaptive and interfere with functioning. In practice, the

TABLE 34–1.	Strategies in supportive psychotherapy

Strengthening and supporting defenses

Maintaining and repairing the therapeutic relationship

Promoting patient self-esteem

Employing therapeutic self-disclosure and modeling

Working primarily in the present

clinician does not work directly with a defense, but rather works on the attitude or behavior it expresses.

2. *Therapeutic relationship*—The relationship between patient and therapist is a professional one, with the therapist providing a service that the patient needs. The therapist, as in all forms of psychotherapy, must maintain proper therapist–patient boundaries. The patient may need love or friendship, but the therapist does not become a lover or a friend. The therapist does not advise the patient about what to invest in, how to vote, or where to vacation. These are products of the therapist's private, not professional, opinion. With that said, however, the therapist providing supportive psychotherapy is active and conversational, takes positions, answers questions, and self-discloses. The relationship between patient and therapist is supportive, providing security and safety for the patient. The therapist serves more as a model of identification than as a transference figure. A positive patient–therapist relationship is always actively fostered by the therapist and is addressed and repaired when a misalliance develops (Winston and Winston 2002).

3. *Self-esteem*—Improvement in self-esteem is an important goal of supportive psychotherapy. The therapist's positive regard, approval, acceptance, interest, respect, and genuineness help to promote the patient's self-esteem. A patient who cannot form relationships with others finds in the therapist a person who is accepting and interested. The therapist communicates interest in the patient by making it evident that he or she remembers their conversations and is aware of the patient's likes, dislikes, attitudes, and general sensibility. Acceptance is communicated by the avoidance of arguing or criticizing verbal interactions and by the avoidance of defensiveness on the part of the therapist.

4. *Self-disclosure*—Intentional revelations by the therapist about himself or herself should have a therapeutic rationale—that is, they should be in the interest of the patient (Roberts 2016). Therapists' decisions about self-disclosure generally are related to modeling and educating, promoting the therapeutic alliance, validating reality, and fostering the patient's sense of autonomy. Straightforward answers to personal questions from the patient can be given within appropriate social conventions of privacy and reticence. Self-disclosure does have transference implications, and if self-disclosure is in the therapist's interest and takes the form of bragging, complaining, seductiveness, and so on, then it is a boundary violation and exploitative.

5. *Working in the present*—Supportive psychotherapy focuses on current coping and adaptation, with less attention paid to past issues. Change in underlying personality structure is not the objective of supportive psychotherapy; instead, improvements in the quality of everyday life are the goal of this form of therapeutic work.

Assessment and Case Formulation

The process of evaluation and case formulation is an essential element of all psychotherapeutic approaches. A central objective of the assessment process is to diagnose the patient's illness and characterize the patient's problems so that the patient can be treated appropriately. Another important objective of the evaluation process is to establish a therapeutic relationship that can further the patient's interest in and commitment to psychotherapy. A thorough evaluation should help the clinician select the appropriate treatment approach. The treatment approach should be individualized to meet the patient's needs and goals and should be based on the central issues identified in the assessment and case formulation.

The therapist generally does not know the extent of a patient's impairment, psychopathology, or strengths when they meet for the first time. Therefore, the therapist should begin the initial interview by attempting to understand why the patient has come for treatment. Every patient should have a thorough evaluation of current problems and history. At the end of the evaluation, the therapist should understand the patient's problems, interpersonal relationships, everyday functioning, and psychological or executive structure.

The evaluation should not be a simple series of questions and answers but more of an exploration of the patient's life. The evaluation should be therapeutic and should help to motivate the patient for treatment while promoting the therapeutic alliance. The evaluation should promote the objectives of supportive psychotherapy: to ameliorate symptoms and to maintain, restore, or improve self-esteem, adaptive skills, and ego or psychological functions (Pinsker 1997). In a supportive approach, a therapeutic evaluation generally involves the use of supportive psychotherapy interventions such as praise, reassurance, encouragement, clarification, and confrontation.

The case formulation is an explanation of the patient's symptoms and psychosocial functioning and depends on an accurate and thorough assessment of the patient. The therapist's formulation governs his or her choice of interventions as well as which issues in the patient's life he or she will focus on. Having a sense of the patient's underlying issues at the start of treatment enhances the therapist's ability to respond empathically. At the same time, having empathy for the patient helps the therapist to guide and plan therapy effectively. The initial formulation must be modified over the course of psychotherapy as more is learned about the patient. The DSM diagnosis is one important part of case formulation, but it does not illuminate an individual's adaptive or maladaptive characteristics or explain his or her unique life history.

There are many approaches to case formulation, which include what Winston et al. (2012) have defined as structural, genetic, dynamic, and cognitive-behavioral elements.

- A *structural* case formulation attempts to capture the relatively fixed characteristics of an individual's personality, which are understood within a functional context. The structural approach is also an assessment of psychopathology and enables the clinician to place the patient on the psychopathology continuum with some degree of accuracy. The major components of the structural approach are relation to reality, object relations, affect, impulse control, defenses, thought processes, and autonomous functions (i.e., perception, intention, intelligence, language, and motor development) and synthetic functions (i.e., ability to form a cohesive whole), as well as conscience, morals, and ideals.

- The *genetic* approach to case formulation involves exploration of early development and life events that may help to explain an individual's current situation. Life presents many challenges, conflicts, and crises. These challenges can be traumatic, depending on their severity, the developmental stage during which they occurred, and the quality of an individual's support system. An example of a persistent difficulty or traumatic situation is a young child growing up with a violent alcoholic father who is demeaning and at times physically abusive.

- The *dynamic* approach concerns mental and emotional tensions that may be conscious or unconscious. The approach focuses on conflicting wishes, needs, or feelings and on their meanings. The genetic approach is concerned with a person's childhood traumas and conflicts, whereas the dynamic approach focuses on current conflicts.

- The *cognitive-behavioral* approach addresses an individual's underlying psychological structure and the content of his or her thoughts. The cognitive-behavioral case formulation model has been described by Tomkins (1996) as encompassing several components, including the problem list, core beliefs, origins, precipitants, and predicted obstacles to treatment.

Overall, the structural and cognitive-behavioral formulations are the most important in supportive psychotherapy, because mapping out current areas of difficulty and ameliorating them are more important than understanding the genetic basis or dynamic cause of the difficulty.

A well-thought-out and comprehensive treatment plan should emerge from the case formulation. Generally, this plan will include treatment goals, the types of interventions to be used, and the frequency of sessions. In supportive psychotherapy, the frequency of visits should be flexible, depending on the patient's needs. Patients in crisis situations may be seen frequently, whereas more stable patients may be seen less often. Setting a specific repeated time to meet tends to reduce anxiety, which is an important objective of supportive psychotherapy.

Overall Goals

For patients requiring supportive psychotherapy, organizing goals, as stated by most authors, are the amelioration of symptoms and the improvement and enhancement of adaptation, self-esteem, and overall functioning (Table 34–2).

In the past, it had been assumed that long-term changes in symptoms, self-esteem, conflicts, and adaptation could not occur in supportive psychotherapy, because this type of therapy focuses on well-being, resilience, and effectiveness in everyday life and does not aim at changing personality or ego structure. Studies have suggested, however, that supportive psychotherapy can produce personality change in patients on the healthier side of the sickness–health continuum (Winston et al. 2001).

Both therapist and patient must agree on the treatment goals in psychotherapy. The goals that are set within the first few sessions should be viewed as preliminary and open to change. Both immediate objectives for each session and ultimate goals for treat-

TABLE 34–2.	Goals of supportive psychotherapy

Ameliorate symptoms

Improve adaptation

Enhance self-esteem

Improve functioning

ment should be considered. For example, an immediate goal for a patient who has temporarily left work would be to return to work within a week or so. An ultimate goal would be to promote job stability and improve relationships with coworkers.

Clearly outlined goals help to motivate patients and promote the therapeutic alliance as patient and therapist work toward a common end. The goals of therapy should be realistic and generally should be based on the patient's needs. In the event of disagreement, the therapist should enter into an exploration of the problem. For example, many patients with chronic psychiatric illness discontinue their medications. In such cases, a major goal of treatment is to help patients continue taking medications. Exploring the reasons for discontinuation and educating patients about the risks of discontinuing are therefore in order.

Treatment goals should never be regarded as fixed and unchangeable. If a patient improves, then goals can be expanded or changed.

Goals in the Context of Crisis Intervention

Parad and Parad (1990) defined *crisis* as an "upset in a steady state, a turning point leading to better or worse, a disruption or breakdown in a person's or family's normal or usual pattern of functioning" (pp. 3–4). A crisis occurs when an individual encounters a situation that leads to a breakdown in functioning, creating disequilibrium. Generally, a crisis is precipitated by a traumatic event or stressor, such as a catastrophe or disaster (e.g., earthquake, fire, war, terrorist act), a relationship rupture or loss, rape, or abuse. A crisis also may result from a series of difficult events or mishaps rather than from one major occurrence.

During crises, individuals perceive their lives, needs, security, relationships, and sense of well-being to be at risk. An individual's reaction to stress is the result of numerous factors, including age, health, personality issues, experience with stressful events, support and belief systems, and underlying biological or genetic vulnerability. Individuals in crisis may become impulsive. Crises tend to be time limited, generally lasting no more than a few months; the duration depends on the stressor and on the individual's perception of and response to the stressor.

Crisis intervention is a therapeutic process aimed at restoring homeostatic balance and diminishing vulnerability to the stressor (Parad and Parad 1990; Winston et al. 2004, 2012). Restoring homeostasis is accomplished by helping to mobilize the individual's abilities and social network and by promoting adaptive coping mechanisms. Crisis intervention is a short-term approach that focuses on solving the immediate problem and includes the entire therapeutic repertoire for helping patients deal with the challenges and threats of overwhelming stress (Table 34–3).

TABLE 34–3.   **Terminology**

Crisis—a situation that can lead to a breakdown in functioning, creating disequilibrium

Crisis intervention—a brief therapeutic process aimed at restoring homeostatic balance and promoting adaptive coping mechanisms

The distinction between crisis intervention and psychotherapy is often blurred, because the two approaches may overlap with regard to technique and length of treatment. Crisis intervention is generally expected to involve one to three sessions, whereas the duration of brief psychotherapy can extend from a few visits to 20 or more sessions. Brief psychotherapy, a more comprehensive form of crisis therapy, is based on several different treatments, including supportive–expressive, cognitive–behavioral, humanistic, family, and systems approaches, as well as the use of medication when indicated (Winston et al. 2012). Systems approaches can be broad and can encompass actions such as working with and referral to social service agencies, mobile crisis units, suicide hotlines, and law enforcement agencies. An additional focus of crisis intervention has been emergency management and prevention through the use of various forms of debriefing (Everly and Mitchell 1999).

Thoroughly evaluating a patient in crisis is critical. The individual's capacity to deal with stress, maintain ego structure and equilibrium, and deal with reality should be assessed, as well as the individual's problem-solving and coping abilities. The evaluation session should be therapeutic and diagnostic, because the patient is in crisis and is seeking relief from suffering. (See Vignette 5 on the evaluation process in crisis intervention in *Learning Supportive Psychotherapy: An Illustrated Guide* by Winston et al. 2012.)

Suicidal thoughts and behaviors are common in patients in crisis. It is essential to ask patients about suicidal ideas and attempts. A careful and thorough assessment of the suicidal patient is critical to determine the diagnosis and the proper treatment approach. Crisis intervention approaches, generally accompanied by the use of medication, often play an important role in the treatment of suicidal individuals (Winston et al. 2012).

Therapeutic Interventions

Supportive psychotherapy depends on clearly defined techniques designed to achieve the goals of maintaining or improving the patient's self-esteem, functioning, and adaptation to the environment. In supportive treatment, important objectives include reduction of anxiety, promotion of stability, and relief of symptoms. These goals are accomplished by working in the here and now rather than in the past. The therapeutic relationship becomes a focus in a real as opposed to a transferential manner. Generally, resistance is not addressed, and adaptive defenses are strengthened and supported (Winston and Winston 2002).

In current practice, supportive psychotherapy uses many ideas and techniques derived from CBT and learning theory. Cognitive-behavioral techniques are an indispensable part of supportive psychotherapy and can be used for targeted problems such as panic, depression, phobias, obsessive-compulsive symptoms, and dysfunctional thinking. Many psychotherapies of different types—including mindfulness, interpersonal, and acceptance and commitment therapies—can be considered a form of carefully orchestrated learning (Etkin et al. 2005) through the acquisition of a combination of skills and knowledge. In general, *learning* is the cognitive process of acquiring skill or knowledge. *Memory* is the retention of learned information. Learning does not take place as a simple recording process. Learning requires active processing during psychotherapy sessions through an interpretive process in which new information is stored by relating it to what an individual already knows. From this perspective, it is important for the therapist to facilitate effective processing during psychotherapy sessions with the techniques of interpretation, elaboration, generation, and critical reflection. Table 34–4 presents a list of interventions used in supportive psychotherapy.

The *style of communication* in supportive psychotherapy tends to be more conversational than in expressive psychotherapy. Silences are avoided because they can raise the individual's level of anxiety. There is a give-and-take exchange, and challenging questions are not asked. Questions beginning with "Why" are avoided because they can increase anxiety and threaten self-esteem.

Praise, reassurance, and encouragement are considered useful techniques for promoting patient self-esteem, especially if the therapist is genuine when using these techniques. Patients quickly pick up on comments that are patronizing or gratuitous and may feel misunderstood. Praise, when offered, tends to be reality based and tends to support more adaptive behaviors. Examples of praise include, "It's good that you can be so considerate of other people" and "It's terrific that you got yourself to go to that lecture."

Words spoken in an attempt to reassure a patient must not be empty or without basis. The patient must believe that the reassurance is based on an understanding of his or her unique situation. Furthermore, the therapist must limit reassurance to areas in which he or she has expert knowledge or dependable common information (Winston et al. 2004). Many patients ask their therapist if they will get better. A response of "Yes, you will get better" may be misleading and false. A more appropriate response would be "Most people with your condition improve."

Encouragement has a major role in general medicine and rehabilitation. Patients living with chronic illnesses may become inactive, mentally and physically. The psychiatrist encourages the patient to maintain hygiene, to get exercise, to interact with other people, sometimes to be more independent, and sometimes to accept the care and concern of others. It is useful to think about encouragement as a form of coaching to help patients engage in different behaviors and activities (Pinsker 1997). For example, a patient complained that she was inept because she was unable to write a cover letter for a job application. The therapist said, "You just need to get started. Let's see what we can do now to help you get started."

Advice is an important tactic in supportive psychotherapy and should be based on the therapist's knowledge and expertise in the field of psychiatry. In contrast to the more abstinent therapeutic stance used in expressive psychotherapy, the therapist conducting supportive psychotherapy can be direct and take an active role with patients. The therapist gives advice and teaches about the supportive psychotherapy objectives of improving ego functions and adaptive skills. When a therapist is telephoned by a patient who becomes disorganized in response to minimal stress, for example, the therapist tells her to get dressed, have breakfast, and then straighten up

TABLE 34–4.	Therapeutic interventions used in supportive psychotherapy

Conversational style of communication

Praise, reassurance, and encouragement

Advice

Rationalizing and reframing

Rehearsal or anticipatory guidance

Empathic confrontation, clarification, and interpretation

Processing, elaborative processing, generation, interleaving, and critical reflection

the house; here, the therapist is not giving advice but rather providing help with routine, predictability, and structure.

Rationalizing and reframing are important CBT techniques that provide the patient with an alternative way of looking at an event that was previously perceived as painful or negative. The challenge in using rationalization and reframing is to avoid sounding fatuous or arguing with and contradicting a patient. For example, a young mother complained that her toddler had started to run away from her, and expressed her belief that the child was losing interest in her. The therapist might reframe this painful and negative perception by saying, "She feels secure enough with you that she's free to explore the world."

Rehearsal or *anticipatory guidance* is a technique that is as useful in supportive psychotherapy as it is in CBT. Anticipatory guidance is a useful technique for helping patients prepare for future encounters with situations perceived as potentially problematic. Preparation for a difficult event can be likened to studying for an examination or rehearsing for a performance. The objective is to consider in advance what the obstacles might be to a proposed course of action and then to prepare strategies for dealing with each potential obstacle. Gaining mastery over an anticipated situation diminishes anxiety and enhances self-esteem. An example of anticipatory guidance would be taking a patient through an initial telephone call to a prospective employer. The patient expects a cold reception and rejection. Rehearsal provides the patient with various scenarios and responses so that he or she will be equipped to cope with the anxiety engendered by making the telephone call and will have a repertoire of responses ready.

Empathic confrontation addresses a patient's defensive behavior by bringing to the patient's attention a pattern of behaviors, ideas, or feelings he or she has not recognized or has avoided. In supportive psychotherapy, confrontations are generally framed with gentleness and empathy and are used to address maladaptive defenses; adaptive defenses are encouraged. Confrontation in a supportive mode is illustrated in the following dialogue:

Patient: I went to my parents' home to speak with them about borrowing some money to pay for several unexpected bills, but I got into a silly argument with them and never had a chance to ask them.

Therapist: We know that it's hard for you to ask them for anything, so could it be that you got into the argument with them to avoid asking them for money?

Clarification is summarizing, paraphrasing, or organizing without elaboration or inference. It is central to the style of communication between patient and therapist and is the most frequently used intervention in supportive–expressive psychotherapies. It demonstrates that the therapist is attentive and is processing what he or she hears. Clarification frames communication so that both parties agree on what is being discussed. Summarizing and restating help organize the patient's thinking and provide structure. In the following example, the therapist clarifies through summarizing:

> Patient: I can't seem to concentrate on anything. My house is costing too much, so I have to sell it, but I have to fix some things in it first.... I can't seem to get started. Collection agencies are after me, and my ex-wife keeps calling about child support— and now my car got hit, so I can't use it.
> Therapist: It sounds like a lot of things are troubling you and you are experiencing being overwhelmed. Let's examine these things one at a time and see what we can come up with.

An *interpretation* is an explanation that brings meaning to the patient's behavior or thinking. Generally, it makes the individual aware of something that was not previously conscious. An interpretation can link thoughts, feelings, and behaviors toward people in the patient's current life to people from the past and/or to the therapist. In supportive psychotherapy, interpretation is generally more limited in scope. Present rather than past relationships are emphasized.

A major approach to facilitate learning is effective processing (deWinstanley and Bjork 2002), which includes interpretation, elaboration, generation, and interleaving. *Processing* involves interpretation that is focused and accurate, accompanied by thorough elaboration. Information that can be interpreted (linked) through associations with preexisting knowledge will be easier to learn than information that is not interpreted. It is important to note that interpretation as a technique of learning theory is not the same as the classic technique of interpretation in dynamic psychotherapy; instead, it is more of a linkage to preexisting knowledge. *Elaborative processing* involves thinking about new information in different ways and connecting it with other previously known information. *Generation* (Richland et al. 2005) is the production of information during learning rather than the presentation of information by a teacher or therapist. *Interleaving* (Richland et al. 2005) involves the learning of two or more sets of information in which instruction and focus continually alternate between the two sets (as opposed to focusing on each set separately until it is mastered). In supportive psychotherapy, the therapist promotes the use of these processing techniques by asking questions designed to help the patient think about his or her problems in several different ways without supplying the answers. The patient is encouraged to process information in collaboration with the therapist.

Critical reflection (Mezirow 1998) is an important technique of learning theory. It is the process by which a person questions and then replaces or reframes an assumption. It is the process through which alternative perspectives are formed on ideas, actions, and forms of reasoning previously taken for granted. Supportive psychotherapy and other psychotherapy approaches use reframing and critical reflection to attempt to provide patients with alternative ways of thinking about the world, relating to others, and solving problems.

Therapeutic Relationship

Historically, the components of the therapeutic relationship have been considered to be the transference–countertransference configuration, the real relationship, and the therapeutic alliance (Greenson 1967). Although these three components are intimately related and form a cohesive whole, discussing each of these components separately provides more clarity. Transference and real relationship issues play a role in every transaction within the therapeutic relationship. At certain times, transference aspects may be more important, whereas at other times, real relationship issues may predominate. From this point of view, a continuum exists between transference issues and real issues that corresponds to the supportive–expressive psychotherapy continuum. Expressive therapy places more emphasis on the transference, whereas supportive psychotherapy focuses more on the real relationship.

Pinsker (1997) and others (e.g., Misch 2000) have described general principles that address the relationship of supportive psychotherapy and the therapeutic relationship. These principles are listed in Table 34–5.

Transference and the Real Relationship

Classically, *transference* has been described as a special type of object relationship consisting of behaviors, thoughts, feelings, wishes, and attitudes directed at the therapist that are related to important people in the patient's past. Essentially, the past is revived in the present.

The real relationship underlies all psychotherapy. It exists in the here and now of the therapeutic interaction between patient and therapist, encompassing a genuine mutual liking for each other that is authentic, trusting, and realistic, without the distortions that are characteristic of transference (Greenson 1967). The real relationship includes the patient's hopes and aspirations for help, care, understanding, and love, as well as the everyday interactions that take place on a social level between individuals.

At the supportive end of the psychotherapy continuum, transference can be used to guide therapeutic interventions. However, transference generally is not discussed unless negative transference threatens to disrupt treatment. Positive transference reactions generally are not explored but rather are simply accepted. Negative reactions always must be investigated, however, because they may compromise treatment (Winston and Winston 2002). The real relationship is paramount and is based on overt mutuality in the conduct of therapy.

In expressive psychotherapy, however, both positive and negative transference phenomena are of pivotal importance for identifying intrapsychic conflict; therapeutic gain is ascribed to the emotional working-through of these relationships. Transference clarification and interpretation are important interventions. The real relationship serves as more of a backdrop, and the emphasis is on the transference.

Therefore, transference is increasingly worked with as one moves across the psychotherapy continuum from supportive to expressive psychotherapy. The emphasis on the real relationship increases as one moves from expressive to supportive psychotherapy. In the middle of the continuum, where most psychotherapy takes place, a mixture of supportive and expressive approaches to transference takes place. In supportive psychotherapy, the therapist clarifies often, confronts at intervals, and inter-

TABLE 34–5. The patient–therapist relationship in supportive psychotherapy

Positive feelings and thoughts about the therapist generally are not focused on in order to maintain the therapeutic alliance.

The therapist is alert to distancing and negative patient behaviors, so as to anticipate and avoid a disruption in treatment.

When a patient–therapist problem is not resolved through practical discussion, the therapist moves to discussion of the therapeutic relationship.

The therapist attempts to modify the patient's distorted perceptions using clarification and confrontation but usually not interpretation.

If indirect means fail to address negative transference or therapeutic impasses, explicit discussion about the therapeutic relationship may be warranted.

The therapist uses only the amount of expressive technique necessary to address negative issues in the patient–therapist relationship.

A positive therapeutic alliance may allow the patient to listen to the therapist present material that the patient would not accept from anyone else.

When making a statement that the patient might experience as criticism, the therapist may have to frame the statement in a supportive, empathic manner or first offer anticipatory guidance.

prets infrequently. The therapist's interventions help the patient to recognize and address maladaptive behavior and cognitive problems that are reflected in behavior with the therapist and are illustrative of the patient's behavior with others. The goal of these interventions is in keeping with the goals of supportive psychotherapy: to increase self-esteem and adaptive functioning.

The following example illustrates some of the strategies used to address positive transference reactions.

> Mr. A, age 54 years, tells his therapist how much his relationship with his wife has improved since he started therapy. He attributes this improvement to the therapist's interest in him. In supportive psychotherapy, the therapist would not explore this compliment but would simply accept it, conceptualizing Mr. A's statement as a reflection of the real relationship, and might say, "I'm glad to be of help to you." The opportunity also might be used to bolster Mr. A's self-esteem by adding, "Our work has been a joint effort, so you have to take some of the credit, too."

Countertransference

Classically, *countertransference* is the therapist's transference to the patient (Greenson 1967). It includes behaviors, thoughts, wishes, attitudes, and conflicts derived from the therapist's past and displaced onto the patient. A broader definition includes the real relationship, consisting of reactions most people would have to the patient, determined by moment-to-moment interactions in the therapeutic relationship, which is a transactional construct affected by what the therapist brings to the situation as well as by what the patient projects (Gabbard 2001; Winston and Winston 2002).

The therapist's countertransference reactions can lead to misunderstanding of the patient and can result in inappropriate behavior toward the patient. Countertransference reactions also can be a powerful tool for understanding and empathizing with the patient (Gabbard 2001). The therapist must monitor his or her own feelings toward the patient to help gain access to the patient's inner world and unconscious.

The use of empathy is important in facilitating, impeding, or distorting counter-transference awareness. *Empathy* can be defined as "feeling oneself into" something or someone (Wolf 1983). Empathy thus becomes a method of gathering data about the mental life of another person. The ability to empathize by accurately sensing and understanding what a person is experiencing will enable the therapist to attend to countertransference reactions in the care of the patient. The following is an example of the use of countertransference in supportive psychotherapy:

> Mr. B, a middle-aged man, began to describe how people at work tended to avoid him, even when he thought he was being friendly. The therapist responded empathically by remarking, "That must be hard for you." Mr. B reacted in an angry manner. The therapist responded by saying, "I'm finding my temperature rising because of your criticisms of me, and I can't help wondering if you get your coworkers feeling the same way. However, I won't act on my feelings the way they do. I'll continue to sit and talk with you; I won't make excuses and leave."

In supportive psychotherapy approaches, it is safer, more respectful, and more protective of the therapeutic alliance to say "I'm finding my temperature rising" than to say "I'm very angry with you." The therapist's modulated expression of countertransference not only offers disconfirmation of the patient's maladaptive construal style but also models adult restraint and containment, not denial of affect. The therapist who responds to the patient's hostility in a complementarily hostile manner is arguing. Arguing not only is poor technique but also is predictive of poor therapeutic outcome (Henry et al. 1990).

Therapeutic Alliance

The therapeutic alliance is a component of the real relationship and forms an essential part of the foundation on which all psychotherapy stands. Zetzel (1956) first used the term *therapeutic alliance* for the "unobjectionable positive transference" that was seen as an essential element in the success of psychotherapy. She believed that the capacity to form an alliance is based on an individual's early experiences with the primary caregiver. In the absence of this capacity, the task of the therapist in early treatment is to provide a supportive relationship to foster the development of a therapeutic alliance. Greenson (1967) emphasized the collaborative nature of the alliance, in which the patient and therapist work together to promote therapeutic change. Bordin (1979) operationalized the therapeutic alliance concept as the degree of agreement between patient and therapist concerning the tasks and goals of psychotherapy and the quality of the bond between them. He conceptualized the alliance as evolving and changing as the result of a dynamic interactive process occurring between patient and therapist.

Outcome research in psychotherapy supports the idea that the quality of the therapeutic alliance is the best predictor of treatment outcome (Horvath and Symonds 1991). Research evidence indicates that in brief supportive and supportive–expressive psychotherapies, an early and strong therapeutic alliance is predictive of positive outcome (Arnow et al. 2013; Hellerstein et al. 1998; Luborsky 1984).

Alliance Ruptures

The stability of the therapeutic alliance appears to be related to the psychotherapy continuum. The alliance tends to be more stable on the supportive psychotherapy side of the continuum because it is not threatened by challenging confrontations or interpretations that may heighten patient anxiety (Hellerstein et al. 1998).

Patients vary in their capacity to establish a positive alliance with a therapist. Those on the impaired side of the psychopathology continuum, who have structural deficits, especially in object relations, may have problems developing a positive relationship with the therapist. The inability to establish "basic trust" (Erikson 1950) interferes with the establishment of a therapeutic bond. With these patients, a major therapeutic task, especially early in treatment, is building a trusting relationship.

Breaks in the therapeutic alliance are not unusual. In fact, misunderstandings between therapist and patient occur for many reasons. Over the course of psychotherapy, the patient may at various times experience the therapist as critical, insensitive, distant, withholding, untrustworthy, intrusive, unempathic, and so on, any of which can contribute to a misalliance.

In supportive psychotherapy, ample opportunity and breadth of strategy exist for the therapist to intervene effectively when problems in the alliance occur. Less constraint is placed on the therapist about communicating his or her sincere regret at having unwittingly impugned or patronized the patient or having raised a subject that the patient found intrusive, anxiety provoking, or simply unpalatable. Generally, when the therapist anticipates or notices a misalliance, supportive techniques are used as the first line of repair (Bond et al. 1998). The therapist attempts to address the problem in a practical manner, staying within the current situation before moving to symbolic or transference issues.

Educational Preparation

It is essential for clinical psychiatrists to have a working knowledge of supportive psychotherapy, because it is the most commonly used psychotherapy. In all forms of psychiatric practice—outpatient, inpatient, consultation–liaison, medication management, and so on—the strategies and techniques of supportive psychotherapy are invaluable. Every psychiatrist should be able to perform a thorough patient evaluation and diagnostic interview and to formulate a comprehensive treatment plan, which can encompass many possible approaches, including psychopharmacological and psychosocial treatments. In addition, psychiatrists should have an understanding of the therapeutic relationship and how to establish a therapeutic alliance. Concepts such as transference and countertransference, defenses, adaptive styles, and self-esteem issues all need to be understood and worked with in an effective manner.

Unfortunately, supportive psychotherapy has not been taught in any kind of systematic fashion in residency training programs. The requirements of the Residency Review Committee for Psychiatry have mandated since 2007 that psychiatry residents demonstrate competence in three types of psychotherapy, one of which is supportive psychotherapy (Accreditation Council for Graduate Medical Education 2017). These requirements may help to foster the teaching and supervision of supportive psychotherapy in residency training programs.

Conclusion

Supportive psychotherapy is a broad-based treatment that is effective for many different types of patients and psychiatric disorders. Despite being the most widely used psychotherapy, it remains undervalued and is rarely taught in a systematic fashion. However, this situation appears to be changing as a result of the requirements for the teaching of supportive psychotherapy in residency training programs. It is clear that more research in supportive psychotherapy is needed to help define and distinguish which strategies and techniques are useful with what type of patient. In addition, the field needs to develop a better understanding of the mechanism of change and a more comprehensive and integrated theoretical foundation for supportive psychotherapy.

Key Clinical Points

- *Supportive psychotherapy* can be defined as a treatment that uses direct measures to ameliorate symptoms and to maintain, restore, or improve self-esteem, ego functions, and adaptive skills.

- Matching the psychotherapy technique to the patient's locus on the psychopathology continuum is of crucial importance.

- There are few absolute contraindications to supportive psychotherapy. In general, supportive psychotherapy is contraindicated only when psychotherapy itself is contraindicated.

- Major supportive psychotherapy strategies include strengthening defenses, maintaining and repairing the therapeutic alliance, enhancing self-esteem, and using therapeutic modeling and self-disclosure.

- Major supportive psychotherapy interventions include use of a conversational communication style, praise, reassurance, encouragement, advice, rationalizing, reframing, rehearsal, clarification, confrontation, and interpretation.

- Supportive psychotherapy focuses more on the real relationship and less on transference.

- Supportive psychotherapy involves much more than provision of a supportive relationship.

References

Accreditation Council for Graduate Medical Education: ACGME Program Requirements for Graduate Medical Education in Psychiatry. Chicago, IL, Accreditation Council for Graduate Medical Education, July 2017. Available at: http://www.acgme.org/Portals/0/PFAssets/ProgramRequirements/400_psychiatry_2017-07-01.pdf?ver=2017-05-25-083803-023.pdf. Accessed December 20, 2017.

Arnow BA, Steidtmann D, Blasey C, et al: The relationship between the therapeutic alliance and treatment outcome in two distinct psychotherapies for chronic depression. J Consult Clin Psychol 81(4):627–638, 2013 23339536

Barlow D, Craske M: Mastery of Your Anxiety and Panic. Albany, Center for Stress and Anxiety Disorders, State University of New York, 1989

Benton MK, Schroeder HE: Social skills training with schizophrenics: a meta-analytic evaluation. J Consult Clin Psychol 58(6):741–747, 1990 2149858

Bond M, Banon E, Grenier M: Differential effects of interventions on the therapeutic alliance with patients with personality disorders. J Psychother Pract Res 7(4):301–318, 1998 9752641

Bordin ES: The generalizability of the psychoanalytic concept of the working alliance. Psychotherapy: Theory, Research and Practice 16(3):252–260, 1979

Brenner AM: Teaching supportive psychotherapy in the twenty-first century. Harv Rev Psychiatry 20(5):259–267, 2012 23030214

Buckley LA, Maayan N, Soares-Weiser K, et al: Supportive therapy for schizophrenia. Cochrane Database Syst Rev (4):CD004716, 2015 25871462

Dewald PA: Psychotherapy: A Dynamic Approach (1964). New York, Basic Books, 1971

Dewald PA: Principles of supportive psychotherapy. Am J Psychother 48(4):505–518, 1994 7872414

deWinstanley PA, Bjork RA: Successful lecturing: presenting information in ways that engage effective processing, in Applying the Science of Learning to University Teaching and Beyond (New Directions for Teaching and Learning, No 89). Edited by Halpern DF, Hakel MD. San Francisco, CA, Jossey-Bass, 2002, pp 19–31

Erikson EH: Childhood and Society. New York, WW Norton, 1950

Etkin A, Pittenger C, Polan HJ, et al: Toward a neurobiology of psychotherapy: basic science and clinical applications. J Neuropsychiatry Clin Neurosci 17(2):145–158, 2005 15939967

Everly GS Jr, Mitchell JT: Critical Incident Stress Management (CISM): A New Era and Standard of Care in Crisis Intervention, 2nd Edition. Ellicott City, MD, Chevron, 1999

Foa EB, Franklin ME: Psychotherapies for obsessive compulsive disorder: a review, in Obsessive Compulsive Disorder, 2nd Edition. Edited by Maj M, Sartorius N, Okasha A, et al. Chichester, UK, Wiley, 2002, pp 93–115

Gabbard GO: A contemporary psychoanalytic model of countertransference. J Clin Psychol 57(8):983–991, 2001 11449380

Goldman CR, Quinn FL: Effects of a patient education program in the treatment of schizophrenia. Hosp Community Psychiatry 39(3):282–286, 1988 3356434

Greenson RR: The Technique and Practice of Psychoanalysis. New York, International Universities Press, 1967

Heinssen RK, Liberman RP, Kopelowicz A: Psychosocial skills training for schizophrenia: lessons from the laboratory. Schizophr Bull 26(1):21–46, 2000 10755668

Hellerstein DJ, Rosenthal RN, Pinsker H, et al: A randomized prospective study comparing supportive and dynamic therapies: outcome and alliance. J Psychother Pract Res 7(4):261–271, 1998 9752637

Henry WP, Schacht TE, Strupp HH: Patient and therapist introject, interpersonal process, and differential psychotherapy outcome. J Consult Clin Psychol 58(6):768–774, 1990 2292626

Horvath AO, Symonds BD: Relation between working alliance and outcome in psychotherapy: a meta-analysis. Journal of Counseling Psychology 38(2):139–149, 1991

Lamberti JS, Herz MI: Psychotherapy, social skills training, and vocational rehabilitation in schizophrenia, in Contemporary Issues in the Treatment of Schizophrenia. Edited by Shriqui CL, Nasrallah HA. Washington, DC, American Psychiatric Press, 1995, pp 713–734

Luborsky L: Principles of Psychoanalytic Psychotherapy: A Manual for Supportive-Expressive Treatment. New York, Basic Books, 1984

Marlatt GA, Gordon JR: Relapse Prevention: Maintenance Strategies in the Treatment of Addictive Behaviors. New York, Guilford, 1985

Mezirow J: On critical reflection. Adult Education Quarterly 48:185–198, 1998

Misch DA: Basic strategies of dynamic supportive therapy. J Psychother Pract Res 9(4):173–189, 2000 11069130

Parad HJ, Parad LG: Crisis Intervention, Book 2: The Practitioner's Sourcebook for Brief Therapy. Milwaukee, WI, Family Service America, 1990

Pinsker H: A Primer of Supportive Psychotherapy. Hillsdale, NJ, Analytic Press, 1997

Richland LE, Bjork RA, Finley JR, et al: Linking cognitive science to education: generation and interleaving effects, in Proceedings of the 27th Annual Conference of the Cognitive Science Society. Mahwah, NJ, Erlbaum, 2005, pp 1850–1855

Roberts LW: A Clinical Guide to Psychiatric Ethics. Arlington, VA, American Psychiatric Association Publishing, 2016

Rollnick S, Miller WR: What is motivational interviewing? Behav Cogn Psychother 23(4):325–334, 1995

Tomkins MA: Cognitive-behavioral case formulation: the case of Jim. Journal of Psychotherapy Integration 6(2):97–105, 1996

Winston A, Winston B: Handbook of Integrated Short-Term Psychotherapy. Washington, DC, American Psychiatric Publishing, 2002

Winston A, Rosenthal RN, Muran JC: Supportive psychotherapy, in Handbook of Personality Disorders: Theory, Research, and Treatment. Edited by Livesley WJ. New York, Guilford, 2001, pp 344–358

Winston A, Rosenthal RN, Pinsker H: Introduction to Supportive Psychotherapy. Washington, DC, American Psychiatric Publishing, 2004

Winston A, Rosenthal RN, Pinsker H: Learning Supportive Psychotherapy: An Illustrated Guide. Washington, DC, American Psychiatric Publishing, 2012

Wolf ES: Empathy and countertransference, in The Future of Psychoanalysis. Edited by Goldberg A. New York, International Universities Press, 1983, pp 309–326

Yrondi A, Rieu J, Massip C, et al: Depressed patients' preferences for type of psychotherapy: a preliminary study. Patient Prefer Adherence 9:1371–1374, 2015 26491265

Zetzel E: Current concepts of transference. Int J Psychoanal 37(4–5):369–375, 1956 13366506

Recommended Readings

Bhola P, Kapur M: The development and role of the therapeutic alliance in supportive psychotherapy with adolescents. Psychol Stud 58:207–215, 2013

Dewald PA: Principles of supportive psychotherapy. Am J Psychother 48:505–518, 1994

Ehlers A, Hackmann A, Grey N, et al: A randomized controlled trial of 7-day intensive and standard weekly cognitive therapy for PTSD and emotion-focused supportive therapy. Am J Psychiatry 171:294–304, 2014

Harder S, Koester A, Valbak K, et al: Five-year follow-up of supportive psychodynamic psychotherapy in first-episode psychosis: long-term outcome in social functioning. Psychiatry 77:155–168, 2014

Jorgensen CR, Freund C, Boye R, et al: Outcome of mentalization-based and supportive psychotherapy in borderline personality disorder: a randomized trial. Acta Psychiatr Scand 127:305–317, 2013

Markowitz JC: What is supportive psychotherapy? FOCUS 12:285–289, 2014

Misch DA: Basic strategies of dynamic supportive therapy. J Psychother Pract Res 9(4):173–189, 2000

Pinsker H: A Primer of Supportive Psychotherapy. Hillsdale, NJ, Analytic Press, 1997

Winston A, Winston B: Handbook of Integrated Short-Term Psychotherapy. Washington, DC, American Psychiatric Publishing, 2002

Winston A, Rosenthal RN, Pinsker H: Learning Supportive Psychotherapy: An Illustrated Guide. Washington, DC, American Psychiatric Publishing, 2012 (Contains a DVD with six clinical vignettes illustrating supportive psychotherapy process)

CHAPTER 35

Mentalizing in Psychotherapy

Jon G. Allen, Ph.D.
Peter Fonagy, Ph.D., F.B.A., F.Med.Sci., FAcSS

We define *mentalizing* as the natural human imaginative capacity to perceive and interpret behavior in self and others as conjoined with intentional mental states, such as desires, motives, feelings, and beliefs. In plain language, we characterize mentalizing as attentiveness to thinking and feeling in self and others—or, in shorthand, as holding mind in mind.

Although it does not appear in many current dictionaries, *mentalizing* has been in the lexicon for two centuries and in the *Oxford English Dictionary* for the past century. French psychoanalysts introduced the concept into the professional literature in the second half of the twentieth century (Lecours and Bouchard 1997), and mentalizing came into English-language professional literature on the brink of the final decade: Morton (1989) construed enduring impairments of mentalizing as the core deficit in autism, and Fonagy (1989) proposed that more transient impairments of mentalizing associated with profound insecurity in attachment relationships play a key role in the developmental psychopathology that contributes to borderline personality disorder (BPD). This proposal was the wellspring for the development of mentalization-based treatment (MBT) (Bateman and Fonagy 2016).

This chapter is not intended to promote a brand of psychotherapy but rather to acquaint clinicians with the value of considering mentalizing in understanding psychopathology and conducting psychotherapy, regardless of their theoretical approach or preferred treatment modalities. We begin with an explication of mentalizing, its various dimensions, and overlapping concepts. Then we review the development of mentalizing in attachment relationships, including developmental failures contributing to later psychopathology. We advance the thesis that effective psychotherapy entails a natural pedagogical process that rekindles the patient's openness to interpersonal influence and thus unblocks obstacles to social learning that stem from a history of social adversity. With this developmental frame, we describe MBT for BPD and summarize the results of controlled research on its effectiveness. Given the developmental thesis we articulate regarding the pedagogical process of psychotherapy, BPD was a natural domain for the development of a mentalization-based approach to treatment. Yet given the pervasive influence of social adversity on the development of psychopathology, along with the cardinal importance of social learning in its amelioration, we have expanded our purview beyond BPD. Accordingly, we articulate our view that mentalizing plays a crucial role as a common therapeutic factor in diverse psychotherapies as applied to a broad range of psychiatric disorders. In covering such a wide territory, we are hitting the highlights; we intend this chapter merely to be a gateway into the burgeoning literature on mentalizing and related developments in attachment theory and research.

Facets of Mentalizing and Related Concepts

Mentalizing is an umbrella term that encompasses many facets (Allen et al. 2008), outlined in Table 35–1. Therapists must attend to the multifaceted nature of mentalizing, because individuals' mentalizing capacity varies along several dimensions, and significant individual differences in the nature of this variability relate to psychopathology. Linking different conceptual dimensions of mentalizing to activation in somewhat distinct brain regions contributes to the accurate parsing of these dimensions (Fonagy and Luyten 2016).

Most fundamentally, we distinguish mentalizing in relation to self and others. Plainly, some individuals are more adept at interpreting others' mental states than their own, whereas others can be more attuned to their own mental states and relatively indifferent or oblivious to those of other people. Learning to differentiate mental states of self and others is a complex developmental achievement, and this differentiation can break down in the context of interpersonal stress. As research on mirror neurons attests (Iacoboni 2008), brain regions that respond similarly to observing, acting, and feeling equip a person for emotional resonance and contagion; this capacity for resonance develops into true empathy only in conjunction with inhibitory processes in more advanced brain regions that permit perspective taking and reflection on the differences between self and other. As we explain to patients in educational groups, individuals must project their own experience when mentalizing in relation to others, but they also must recognize their projections as such and attend to differences in experience and perspectives.

We also distinguish between explicit and implicit mentalizing. *Explicit* mentalizing is relatively controlled, predominantly taking the form of narrative; people routinely tell stories to others and themselves about their mental states, the reasons for them, and their history. These stories are more or less elaborate, ranging from simply putting feelings into words to creating more complex autobiographical narratives. Explicit mentalizing, like consciousness more generally, permits mental time travel: people mentalize not only about the present (e.g., exploring reasons for current feelings) but also about the past (e.g., reconstructing the basis for a previous interpersonal conflict or impulsive action) and the future (e.g., anticipating the best way to address a relationship challenge). Thus, as in psychotherapy, individuals use explicit

TABLE 35–1.   **Facets of mentalizing**

Awareness of mental states in *self* vs. awareness of mental states in *others*

Explicit mentalizing (controlled, deliberate, conscious) vs. *implicit* mentalizing (automatic, intuitive, procedural)

Focus on *external* behavior (directly observable) vs. *internal* mental states (inferred)

Focus on *cognition* (thoughts and beliefs) vs. *affect* (emotional feelings)

Source.   Adapted from Allen JG: *Restoring Mentalizing in Attachment Relationships: Treating Trauma With Plain Old Therapy.* Washington, DC, American Psychiatric Publishing, 2013, p. 29. Used with permission.

mentalizing to learn from past mistakes in the service of interacting more effectively in the future.

In contrast, *implicit* mentalizing is relatively automatic, procedural, and nonconscious, such as in turn-taking in conversation, adapting voice tone and posture to others' emotional states, and taking others' knowledge into account automatically (e.g., not referring to "Jane" when the other person has no idea who Jane is). In general, people rely on implicit mentalizing when all goes smoothly in interactions, whereas explicit mentalizing exemplifies the function of consciousness and deliberation more generally. Individuals mentalize explicitly when they encounter novel or inexplicable behavior (in self or others) and when deliberately addressing and resolving intrapsychic or interpersonal conflicts.

We also distinguish cognitive and affective mentalizing, in relation to which individual differences are plainly evident. Extreme imbalance in either direction poses challenges for psychotherapy. For example, relying on cognition, obsessive and intellectualizing patients might be adept at generating explicit reasons for their own or others' behavior, but such insight—devoid of any real emotional meaning—does not promote change. Conversely, patients who are more prone to being flooded with affect (e.g., as in BPD) are using implicit processes conducive to emotional contagion and impaired self–other differentiation. For patients at both ends of this spectrum, mentalizing emotion—thinking and feeling about thinking and feeling—is a crucial therapeutic goal.

Finally, we distinguish between external and internal mentalizing. *External* mentalizing entails responsiveness to external, observable aspects of behavior—most prominently facial expressions but also voice tone and posture. In contrast, *internal* mentalizing requires inference and imagination in the service of understanding the mental states conjoined with external behavior (i.e., desires, feelings, beliefs, and relationship proclivities). As evident in the context of BPD (see section "Mentalization-Based Treatment" later in this chapter), implicit, affective, and external mentalizing can lead to problematic interpersonal behavior—for example, a patient may respond to the therapist's momentary frown of puzzlement as an indication of hostile rejection and be convinced that the therapist is eager to terminate the therapy. Such implicit responses call for therapeutic explication in which the therapist's perspective can be brought to bear on the patient's experience.

Implicit in the foregoing discussion are individual differences in mentalizing capacity or skill. Our psychotherapeutic efforts are directed toward identifying areas of mentalizing deficits and improving mentalizing skills in these domains. To a great degree, skillful mentalizing (as highlighted in Table 35–2) entails flexible integration of

TABLE 35–2.   **Hallmarks of skillful mentalizing**

Engaging in mentalizing when indicated (vs. indifference or avoidance of mentalizing)

Mentalizing with reasonable accuracy (vs. distorted mentalizing or excessively elaborate or obsessive mentalizing—i.e., hypermentalizing)

Mentalizing with awareness of the possibility of inaccuracy (vs. certainty in one's perceptions and interpretations)

Mentalizing with benevolent intent (vs. misusing mentalizing for the purpose of manipulation or exploitation)

Flexibly integrating the multiple facets of mentalizing (vs. limiting mentalizing to specific facets)

Grounding mentalizing in authentic emotion (vs. pseudomentalizing, as evident in intellectualization, use of clichés, or "psychobabble")

the multiple facets of mentalizing that we have just delineated: balancing focus on self and others; integrating cognitive and affective mentalizing; being able to link external behavior with internal mental states; and relying on implicit and intuitive mentalizing while engaging explicit and reflective mentalizing when confronting problems or engaging in more complex interactions (e.g., in challenging negotiations or psychotherapy).

Given that mentalizing is fundamental to human relationships—relating to oneself as well as relating to others—it is little wonder that mentalizing overlaps in various ways with many cognate concepts, including empathy, psychological mindedness, observing ego, insight, theory of mind, mind reading, social cognition, metacognition, social intelligence, and emotional intelligence. The term *reflective functioning* bears especially close kinship to mentalizing in being a well-established measure of mentalizing capacity, based on assessments of the arena in which mentalizing is most challenging—namely, narratives regarding childhood attachment relationships, a common component of psychotherapeutic discourse.

The distinction between mentalizing and mindfulness bears particular attention because the two concepts are easily confused and conflated. Moreover, mindfulness has become extremely popular and is likely to be far more familiar to clinicians and patients who question the difference when they hear about mentalizing. Our view of the relations between these two concepts is summarized in Table 35–3. Most simply, mindfulness refers to present-centered attention, which can include attention to mental states in self or others—mindfulness of mind. In contrast, mentalizing also includes reflection and interpretation, typically in the form of narrative. In our view, mindful attentiveness to mental states is a necessary condition for skillful mentalizing. Mindfulness and mentalizing overlap in two key respects: 1) both emphasize the need to distinguish between mental states and the reality they represent, and 2) both advocate a nonjudgmental, open-minded attitude of curiosity and inquisitiveness about mental states in oneself and others, which we call the *mentalizing stance.*

Readers might wonder, with all these cognate concepts, what is the justification for adding another, and an unusual word to boot—mentalizing. None of these concepts has an exact synonym, and they spring from diverse clinical and research traditions. As discussed in the next section, mentalizing has the distinct advantage of being embedded in attachment theory and research, which anchors it in developmental psycho-

TABLE 35–3.	Mentalizing and mindfulness

Mentalizing

Constructing biographical and autobiographical narrative

Reflecting on the meaning of mental states

Making inferences about mental states

Overlapping aspects of mentalizing and mindfulness

Awareness of mental states as representational

Nonjudgmental attitude of acceptance, compassion, curiosity

Mindfulness

Attentiveness to mental states in self and others

Present-centered bare attention

TABLE 35–4.	Prementalizing modes of experience

Psychic equivalence: Mental contents are equated with reality (e.g., as in dreams, posttraumatic flashbacks, and paranoid delusions); the failure to distinguish mental representations from the external reality they represent is associated with loss of tentativeness in perceptions and interpretations.

Pretend mode: Mental states are too divorced from reality, taking on a feeling of unreality, often relating to a lack of anchoring in emotion or sense of self (e.g., dissociative states, discourse devoid of emotional meaning).

Teleological mode: Mental states are expressed in goal-directed action rather than articulated in narrative communication (e.g., anger expressed in nonsuicidal self-injury or demand that caring be expressed through physical contact).

Source. Adapted from Allen JG, Fonagy P, Bateman AW: *Mentalizing in Clinical Practice.* Washington, DC, American Psychiatric Publishing, 2008, p. 91. Used with permission.

pathology. In addition, stemming from *mentalization,* mentalizing has the advantage of a verb form; we advocate to patients—and therapists—that mentalizing is something they must *do*—more consistently and skillfully.

The theory of mentalizing is also distinct from other related concepts in that it proposes a developmentally and neuroscientifically based conceptualization of the processes that are activated when mentalizing fails. These processes are called *prementalizing,* or *nonmentalizing,* modes of experience (Table 35–4), and they are associated with the interpersonal or intrasubjective dysfunction most commonly associated with personality disorder but also with many experiences of mental disorder.

Development of Mentalizing in Attachment Relationships

Our thinking about mentalizing is heavily steeped in attachment theory; in particular, our original developmental work on the emergence of mentalizing in infancy and early childhood was strongly shaped by attachment paradigms. In this section we briefly explain the relationship between mentalizing and attachment theory, and provide an update on how our thinking has more recently evolved to consider the broader social-cognitive processes at work in the relationship between the social environment and developmental psychopathology (Fonagy et al. 2017).

The far more refined account of the relationship between attachment and mentalization provided by Gergely and Unoka (2008) can be condensed as follows: Infants begin to develop a sense of self (and self-awareness) through a complex process of emotional mirroring. The mother, for example, mentalizes her infant's emotion and expresses this emotion in her face and demeanor, in effect representing (i.e., re-presenting) the emotion to the infant in such a way that the infant gradually links his or her internal experience to his or her mother's representation of it. The mentalizing mother responding to her infant's frustration, for instance, does not express her own frustration *with* the infant but rather expresses the infant's frustration *for* him or her to see in her face, hear in her voice, and feel in her touch (e.g., intermingling an expression of frustration with an element of caring and concern). Later, in mentalizing interactions, the mother puts the child's emotions (and her own) into words. Ultimately, through mentalizing narratives, the relational contexts for emotional feelings are explicated.

Research on the intergenerational transmission of attachment patterns and the capacities for mentalizing (or nonmentalizing) embedded in these patterns provided a developmental foundation for a mentalizing approach to psychotherapy. Fonagy et al. (1991) used the Reflective Functioning Scale to assess the quality of mentalizing in mothers pregnant with their first child, who were also interviewed about their attachment relationships with their own parents in childhood with the Adult Attachment Interview. To examine the relationship between parental mentalizing in the Adult Attachment Interview and subsequent infant attachment security, Fonagy et al. (1991) used Ainsworth's Strange Situation, which entails moderately stressful parent–child separations and reunions in a playroom. In short, securely attached infants are more or less distressed by the separation; regardless, at the point of reunion, they seek contact and comfort from their mother, and then, reassured, they return to play. Mothers' mentalizing capacity in relation to their own attachment history predicted their infants' attachment security in relation to them.

At the opposite extreme, trauma in attachment relationships contributes to the intergenerational transmission of impaired mentalizing capacities. The most profound form of parental insecurity in the Adult Attachment Interview regarding parents' childhood attachment, classified as unresolved–disorganized, is evident prototypically in lapses of coherence of discourse associated with the intrusion of unresolved traumatic childhood experiences. Infants of parents classified as unresolved–disorganized are at higher risk for showing the most severe form of insecure attachment in the Strange Situation—namely, disorganized attachment. Infant disorganized attachment behavior is anomalous in showing extreme conflict (e.g., screaming in protest when the parent leaves the room and then running away when the parent returns) as well as manifesting frankly confused or disoriented behavior (e.g., wandering around the room as if lost, or entering into a dissociative, trancelike state). Liable to have their own traumatic attachment history evoked in response to their infant's attachment needs or distress, profoundly insecure parents become frightening or frightened and unable to mentalize; in turn, their infants are liable to feel frightened and unable to seek solace in the relationship.

Disorganized attachment in infants, related to unresolved trauma in parents, was first found to occur in relation to frank maltreatment (Main and Solomon 1990). Subsequent research has identified more subtle disturbances in parents' attachment discourse and parent–child interactions that are associated with disorganized attachment. That is, infant disorganization relates not only to parents' trauma-related lapses (including dissociative states) in attachment interviews but also to more pervasive indications of hostile or helpless states of mind throughout the interviews (Melnick et al. 2008). In addition, infant disorganization is associated both with frank maltreatment—abuse and neglect—and with more pervasive disturbances of emotional communication in parent–infant interactions (Lyons-Ruth and Jacobvitz 2016) and a more generally disabled caregiving system (George and Solomon 2011). More fundamentally, Tronick's (2007) demonstrably stressful still-face procedure (i.e., the mother adopting an expressionless and unresponsive demeanor, which invariably distresses her infant) is the prototype of emotional neglect, which can be traumatic in the form of chronic unresponsiveness.

We construe the crux of attachment trauma as being left psychologically alone in unbearable emotional states. Such experience precludes the development of mentalizing when it is most urgently needed, resulting in a threefold cascade of developmental liabilities, as highlighted in Table 35–5. Fonagy and Target (1997) initially articulated the adverse consequences of attachment trauma in proposing a *dual liability:* such trauma 1) evokes extreme distress and 2) undermines the development of the capacity to regulate distress—namely, the capacity to develop secure attachments, which requires mentalizing. We now propose that attachment trauma creates a further and most profound liability in its potential to disrupt the individual's capacity for *epistemic trust* (by which we mean openness to the reception of social communication that is of personal relevance and of generalizable significance; i.e., social and cultural information about one's world and how best to function within it). One particularly pernicious consequence of social trauma may be the destruction of this trust in social knowledge of all kinds.

In adding this third component to our thinking about atypical attachment experiences, we are in effect recalibrating the nature of the role of attachment in generating vulnerability to psychological disorder and distress in later childhood and adulthood. The theory of epistemic trust in relation to developmental psychopathology starts with the evolutionarily informed idea that the human infant is adapted to be open to receiving social communication from primary caregivers. The acceptance of implicit and explicit knowledge as being personally relevant and generally applicable enables the human infant to absorb a wealth of cultural understanding about the social milieu that the infant and his or her caregivers share. Gergely and Csibra (2005) proposed the term *pedagogic stance* to designate the uniquely human predispositions to teach and learn new and relevant cultural information in an efficient way, as summarized in Table 35–6. In contrast, for example, to the arduous process of trial-and-error learning, cultural knowledge—no matter how painstakingly acquired by our species, groups, or individuals—can be transmitted rapidly through pedagogy. To navigate the social world, we must be open to learning about new objects, expected behaviors, and social contexts. Concomitantly, we must be able to correct our ideas, beliefs, expectations, and fantasies in light of communications from others as well as to learn from the situations we create and find ourselves in. This kind of adaptation

TABLE 35–5.	Threefold liability associated with attachment trauma
1.	Evokes unbearable emotional states
2.	Undermines the development of mentalizing and thereby the capacity to regulate emotion
3.	Promotes epistemic mistrust and thereby undermines the capacity to benefit from interpersonal influence, hampering social learning and the refinement of social cognition

TABLE 35–6.	Overview of natural pedagogy
	Facilitates rapid transmission of cultural knowledge through teaching and learning
	Includes knowledge about psychological and interpersonal functioning essential to social cognition
	Permits correction of misunderstandings and of distorted perceptions and interpretations regarding mental states in oneself and others
	Is triggered by ostensive cues signaling intent to impart information (e.g., establishing eye contact, addressing recipient by name)
	Requires epistemic trust, which is essential for openness to social influence and learning

is essential in infancy, and it is part and parcel of the developmental progression throughout life, including specific developmental phases, such as early childhood and adolescence, that require particularly intensive instruction and learning from caregivers and others. In short, we all benefit from inheriting an evolutionarily selected interpersonal channel for acquiring information about the world that we can trust—in effect, a biologically designed epistemic superhighway for the rapid and efficient transmission of socially maintained information that is essential for survival and adaptation in a human community.

In infancy, special cues trigger the pedagogic stance of learning from caregivers in the role of teachers. These cues signal to the child that the information that the caregiver is about to transmit is trustworthy and generalizable beyond the current situation (Gergely 2007). These ostensive communicative cues in infancy include making eye contact, raising the eyebrows, addressing the recipient by name, and using a special voice tone (motherese). These different cues are all ways of marking the interaction as special by signaling that the caregiver is paying attention to the infant's subjectivity in the context of intention to communicate (Fonagy et al. 2007).

This pedagogical template for social learning continues to hold beyond infancy. That is, we continue to require special triggers to open our minds so that we can take in new information about the world. If we are to learn from them, others who seek to communicate with us first must establish their credentials as trustworthy social pedagogues by showing us that they are interested in our minds. Only then does the epistemic superhighway open up. Our feeling that these persons can see the world from our perspective (i.e., when they mentalize us) is the basis for epistemic trust and opens up our wish to learn about the world. Hence, epistemic trust is a precondition for learning about the social world through the pedagogical route. In our view, the attachment system serves the evolutionary function of establishing general epistemic trust in the social world by producing an expectation that others will respond to us in a sensitively responsive and psychologically attuned way—that is, enabling us to feel that we are known. A well-established body of evidence shows that securely attached children are more cognitively open and flexible than those who are insecurely attached, and this cognitive capacity is reflected in superior academic performance (Thompson 2008). Concomitantly, as Bowlby (1988) also asserted in the context of psychotherapy, security in attachment relationships is conducive to exploring one's own and others' mental states. In summary, the experience of feeling thought about promotes the sense of safety needed to think and learn about the social world in interactions with others throughout life. Most pertinent to our concerns in this chapter, epistemic trust, established on the basis of the clinician's mentalizing effort, is a precondition for effective psychotherapy, which promotes openness to social influence.

Human infants therefore are instinctively inclined to epistemic openness to caregivers. However, one must be able to exercise some vigilance in relation to other people's social communication: whether through malign intent or unreliability, or both, other people can feed us misleading or incorrect information. In the case of an infant whose caregiver can be hostile, abusive, neglectful, or pathologically inconsistent and unreliable, it may be adaptive for the infant to adopt a position of epistemic vigilance, or outright mistrust, toward social communications. Once epistemic trust is disrupted and the mind is closed to processing new information, the behavioral repertoire of traumatized individuals becomes rigid and inaccessible to change through the mere presentation of fresh information. Although this rigidity makes it more difficult for the individual to adapt and survive, in the context of social adversity it must be understood as self-protective. Yet without a capacity to develop epistemic trust through entertaining a feeling of being understood, the capacity to learn from experience comes to exclude many forms of learning through human communication. We suggest that the destruction of epistemic trust can constitute one of the most damaging and chronic consequences of trauma in the context of early caregiver relationships. The role of attachment, according to this thinking, is as a powerful form of social communication about the nature of the social environment that the infant inhabits. Secure attachment is a powerful cue that stimulates the opening of epistemic trust. Attachment therefore remains highly significant in this developmental model, but it is also a model that locates attachment as both a reflection and a mediator of wider social learning about the prevailing environment (Fonagy et al. 2017). This allows us to account for some of the complexity of findings cumulatively emerging from contemporary attachment research—that the relationship between infant attachment style and later outcomes is not as straightforward as early studies suggested, and that the influence of infant attachment fluctuates across the life span (for a review, see Fonagy et al. 2017).

The cognitive-dynamic model we have advanced has far-reaching clinical implications. In effect, the human brain has evolved to be prepared for knowledge transfer by communication (now including the century-old invention of psychological therapy); we are ready to learn from others about ourselves, just as we are ready to learn from them about the social world. To the extent that we find the meaning of our own subjective experience within the social world (i.e., within the other) and not simply in self-reflection, we are eager to learn about our own opaque mental world from those around us through mentalizing dialogue. Reaching out to a trusted confidant to make sense of puzzlingly intense distress about an interaction is a commonplace example of such mentalizing dialogue. The epistemic mistrust that follows trauma entailing intense social adversity, maltreatment, or abuse impinges on this natural disposition to learn through such dialogue. Persons with a history of extreme social adversity are difficult to reach by means of ordinary communication, posing enormous challenges for psychotherapy, the goal of which is enduring change in the capacity for social understanding.

To work effectively with traumatized individuals in psychotherapy, therapists must consider not only the "what" but also the "how" of learning. Before learning can begin, negative expectations about the trustworthiness or value of human communication must be radically shifted. Benevolence is necessary but not sufficient; epistemic trust rests on competence and credibility—first and foremost on the patient feeling understood and his or her agency being recognized. Toward this end, the psychotherapist must create a social situation that aims largely to open patients' minds by establishing a relationship in which they feel that their subjective experience is being thought about empathically so that they can begin to trust the social world again. If a secure attachment relationship is the marker of trust and trustworthiness, then the establishment of such a relationship with the patient is a critical precondition for change. Psychotherapists' sensitivity and psychological attunement are paramount, not because they enable therapists to delineate the specific content of the patient's mind with pinpoint accuracy, but rather because these capacities generate epistemic trust. Such trust opens up the patient not only to therapeutic influence but also— more importantly—to the influence of the wider social network, to the extent that this experience of being known and open to new learning generalizes to other relationships. Thus, it is not what is taught in psychotherapy that brings change; rather, effective psychotherapy rekindles the evolutionary capacity for learning from others, which is crucial to the lifelong development and refinement of social cognition.

Mentalization-Based Treatment

As noted in this chapter's introduction, MBT was originally developed for the treatment of BPD. The core symptoms of BPD—emotional dysregulation, impulsivity, self-destructive behavior, and unstable relationships—are embedded in highly insecure (i.e., preoccupied and disorganized) attachment relationships and severe mentalizing impairments. More specifically, patients with BPD show marked impairments in the explicit, internal, and cognitive facets of mentalizing: they are reactive to external behavioral cues (e.g., a grimace or a yawn), they have difficulty linking such cues appropriately to internal mental states, and they are subject to implicit mentalizing and emotional contagion concomitant with impaired capacity for explicit, reflective thinking (Fonagy and Luyten 2009). The following vignette illustrates such nonmentalizing reactivity and the therapist's efforts to reestablish mentalizing.

> Ms. A sought psychotherapy in her late 20s for depression embedded in turbulent relationships with her parents and boyfriends since her early adolescence. She had started and quit psychotherapy twice previously, stating that it had been a waste of time and that therapists only wanted her money.
> Despite her apparent cynicism about psychotherapy, Ms. A seemed reasonably engaged in the first two sessions, showing some awareness of her pattern of moving quickly into romantic relationships, becoming infatuated and then increasingly frustrated and disillusioned with her partner's flagging attentiveness. She began the third

session stating that she was in a particularly "foul mood," and she attributed this mood to the therapy, which she said amounted to only a rehashing of all her "messed up" relationships, rubbing her nose in her failures. The therapist frowned, leaned back, paused to think, looked at her intently, and then said, "That sounds grim." Ms. A bristled, protesting, "You've given up on me! This therapy is going nowhere, and the way you're glaring at me tells me that you're going to blame it all on me."

The therapist leaned forward and said, "Sorry, I've learned that I seem to stare when I'm thinking, and that can be off-putting." Ms. A responded, "You got that right!" The therapist continued, "I wasn't aware of glaring at you. It's interesting that you thought I intended to blame you, because when I paused, I was thinking that I'm not giving you enough help and starting to wonder what we might do differently." Ms. A's tone softened a bit, but she replied, "That doesn't change the fact that you've concluded I'm beyond help." The therapist responded, "I wonder if you're equating my feelings with yours—maybe you feel like giving up and interpreted my comment about this 'grim' situation as indicating that I see you the way you see yourself." Ms. A responded, "Sometimes I'm convinced I'm beyond help—I've even thought about killing myself. Why wouldn't you believe therapy is pointless?" The therapist responded, "I don't know how successful we will be, but I'm encouraged that you're speaking up about your frustrations with this process, and you're also willing to listen to me. So maybe you won't quit before we figure out what might be of help."

In instances such as these, when mentalizing collapses, patients' behavior is governed by prementalizing modes (see Table 35–4). In the psychic equivalence mode, as Ms. A's response exemplifies, patients feel complete conviction in their perceptions and interpretations, unable to consider multiple perspectives or to adopt the as-if mode of thought. Alternatively, in the pretend mode, patients' experience becomes dissociated from reality and, losing grounding in reality, their perceptions can be highly distorted. Finally, in the teleological mode, action takes the place of thought, as patients' anger is expressed in self-destructive action, and caring must be conveyed in touch rather than gaze, demeanor, and words.

It is easier for therapists to empathize with the apparent inaccessibility of patients with BPD to social influence (including psychotherapy) if they respect patients' inability to detect and respond to ostensive cues signaling the therapists' interest in the patients' subjective experiences and the therapists' perspectives on them. Such cues would normally generate epistemic trust and open the individual to learning from trusted others. What appears as rigidity in persons with BPD is instead a failure of a key reflective (i.e., mentalizing) capacity coupled with an inability to respond openly to—and to learn from—human communication.

Although there are multiple developmental pathways to BPD, a nonmentalizing family environment makes an important contribution. Family relationships marked by impaired emotional communication are not conducive to coherent discourse regarding feelings, thoughts, needs, motives, and different perspectives. Such interactions also do not exemplify the mentalizing stance of empathic and mindful concern and may help set the stage for a developmental cascade that results in BPD. To summarize:

> One developmental path to impairments in mentalizing in BPD is a combination of early neglect, which might undermine the infant's developing capacity for affect regulation, with later maltreatment or other environmental circumstances, including adult experience of verbal, emotional, physical and sexual abuse, that are likely to activate the attachment system chronically. (Fonagy and Luyten 2009, p. 1366)

Bateman and Fonagy developed MBT to provide a comparatively mentalizing-rich and trustworthy interpersonal environment in which these core deficits in social cognition can be rectified. In its original iteration (Bateman and Fonagy 1999), MBT was developed in the context of a day-hospital (partial hospitalization) program centered on individual and group psychotherapy but also including expressive therapies (e.g., involving artwork and writing). Patients attended the program 5 days a week, and the maximum length of stay ranged from 18 to 24 months. Subsequently, Bateman and Fonagy (2009) established an 18-month intensive outpatient program consisting of once-weekly 50-minute individual psychotherapy sessions coupled with once-weekly 90-minute group psychotherapy sessions. In both programs, the individual psychotherapist is separate from the group therapist. Both programs were designed with common features of effective treatments for BPD in mind (Table 35–7).

The overall aims of MBT, a highly straightforward treatment approach, can be summarized simply:

> It is a therapy to enhance capacities of mentalization and to make them more stable and robust so that the individual is better able to solve problems and to manage emotional states (particularly within interpersonal relationships), or at least to feel more confident in doing so. Our intention with the patient is to promote a mentalizing attitude to relationships and problems, to instill doubt where there is certainty, and to enable the patient to become increasingly curious about his or her own mental states and those of others. (Bateman and Fonagy 2012, p. 274)

The mentalizing focus is guided by the most prominent mentalizing impairments in patients with BPD: interventions are aimed at slowing down the patient in the face of emotional reactivity by encouraging explicit thinking about internal mental states, while shifting fluidly to maintain a balance of mentalizing in relation to self and others. Although MBT has substantial roots in psychoanalysis, the mentalizing approach does not specify the content of the treatment process; rather, the content is guided by the patient's concerns, albeit with a focus on interpersonal problems and attachment relationships in particular. Importantly, consistent with our developmental thesis regarding the natural pedagogical process, the treatment does not focus on acquiring insight but rather on enhancing openness to influence and mentalizing skills for the sake of effectiveness in interpersonal and intrapersonal problem solving.

Our developmental thesis is consistent with the fact that different therapeutic approaches are effective in the treatment of BPD, as is also true for many other psychiatric disorders. Feeling reliably understood, perhaps for the first time, the patient is ready to hear the therapist's message and to engage in a process of learning and change. However, we should entertain the possibility that it may not be the therapist's specific observations and suggestions that are of greatest potential in the therapeutic process. Given the research evidence that many theoretical approaches and therapeutic modalities are effective for this group of patients, it is highly likely that change comes about through the mere fact of establishing trust and interpersonal understanding in the consulting room that serves to clear barriers on the epistemic superhighway. Patients leave the consulting room with a mind that is able to learn—that is, to absorb new information and integrate it into their current and past patterns of thought. With the benefit of effective psychotherapy, they are able to continue the process of psychological exploration and learning with partners, parents, friends, and

TABLE 35–7.	Common features of effective treatments for borderline personality disorder

Clear treatment structure

Efforts to enhance treatment adherence

Focus on self-injurious and problematic interpersonal behavior

Supportive therapeutic relationships

High level of therapist activity and engagement

Long duration of treatment

Integration with other health care services and community resources

colleagues. The information to which they are exposed may not necessarily be new; rather, previously imparted information from these various sources was mistrusted, because the biological cue for internalization—epistemic trust—could not be triggered without the ability to feel understood by others.

In the interest of establishing trust and promoting interpersonal learning, MBT includes significant attention to transference and countertransference in a qualified sense: along with other relationships, the patient–therapist relationship is addressed in the service of improving mentalizing. As DeFife et al. (2015) also advocated in promoting therapeutic immediacy, patients and therapists think together about their relationship, comparing and contrasting their perspectives. Continuous and perfect alignment of perspectives would not promote learning; therapy invariably entails a fluid process of alignment, misalignment, and realignment of perspectives. The therapist must grasp the patient's experience with reasonable accuracy much of the time while also challenging the patient's perspective by bringing in another point of view. Moreover, the therapist also must exemplify openness and flexibility by responsiveness to the patient's point of view, for example, when inevitably the therapist's comments are off the mark. This approach requires a high degree of transparency on the part of the therapist, which serves as a model of transparency for the patient—being able to speak directly and forthrightly about the experience of the relationship: "The patient has to find himself in the mind of the clinician and, equally, the clinician has to understand him-/herself in the mind of the patient if the two together are to develop a mentalizing process. *Both have to experience a mind being changed by a mind*" (Bateman and Fonagy 2016, p. 182; emphasis added).

The following clinical vignette illustrates the process of mentalizing the transference and of minds influencing minds.

Dr. B, a physician in her mid-40s, was hospitalized on an emergency basis after a 6-month spiral into depression that was precipitated by a contentious marital separation, compounded by increasingly confrontational disputes with a partner in her group practice—all exacerbated by binge drinking that culminated in an overdose. After she was stabilized, she was transferred to specialized inpatient treatment during which she received psychotherapy.

Dr. B denied that her overdose was a suicide attempt; rather, she said that she merely wanted to knock herself out for a time to escape from the pain of feeling continually berated and left alone to fend for herself. Despite disavowing suicide, she acknowledged that when she took the overdose, she would not have minded if she had died. By the time she was stabilized and was provided with respite from relentless stress, she was

horrified that she could have died, especially because of the potential effect of her suicide on her two children and the implications of her self-destructive behavior for a
brewing custody battle. Accordingly, Dr. B agreed that her safety after discharge from
the hospital should be a prominent focus for the psychotherapy.

Dr. B's long history of self-defeating behavior was a focus for psychotherapy and
came to the fore in the context of impending discharge when she faltered in developing
a concrete safety plan that included identifying individuals from whom she might seek
help in a crisis. In the context of a generally collaborative relationship, the therapist
evoked a rift in the alliance when he pointed out that Dr. B was repeating her "self-
defeating" pattern in "procrastinating" regarding planning for her safety when she left
the hospital. Dr. B took umbrage and protested angrily, "I've been working my ass off
in treatment!" She added that she was afraid she would not have the support she
needed when she left the hospital, and she maintained that she was not being "self-
defeating" but rather being "brutally realistic" in raising doubts about her safety, given
her "poor track record" in safeguarding her welfare over the course of her lifetime. Expressing her puzzlement forthrightly, Dr. B said that she could not understand where
the therapist was coming from.

Taken aback by Dr. B's challenge of an observation that seemed self-evident to him,
the therapist responded to her request to explain himself. He stated that he was responding to what seemed to be Dr. B's "balking" at working on a plan and that now he
was aware that his frustration was a reflection of his anxiety about her safety going forward—anxiety that the two of them obviously shared. He then said that—whether or
not Dr. B was being self-defeating—*he* was feeling defeated. This led to a mutual recognition of how he was resonating with Dr. B's struggle with her own feeling of being defeated by her recurrent depression and alcohol abuse, as well as her relentless self-
criticism. Responding to the therapist's feeling of defeat, she acknowledged that others—including her husband and partner—repeatedly had felt defeated by her behavior.
In the course of this reflection, Dr. B and the therapist shared the experience of minds
being influenced by minds, and they were freed up to explore the barriers to Dr. B's being able to identify durable sources of support.

Broadly, the ideal outcome of MBT is for the patient to internalize the mentalizing
stance from the therapeutic process, the crux of which is an enduring inclination to
explore and understand mental states with an open-minded attitude of curiosity. In
other words, epistemic trust must be (re)established so that patients can be open to
learning about their own and others' mental states. Of course, once established, such
mentalizing will flourish only in the context of reciprocity and mutuality. In patient
education groups conducted in a therapeutic milieu that cultivates this stance, patients commonly say something like, "You've got me trying to mentalize. Now tell me
how to get my spouse to do it!" We would reply that trying to force another person to
mentalize, ironically, is nonmentalizing. We adhere to the developmental principle
that mentalizing begets mentalizing, but this does not mean that it is possible to mentalize "at" someone. Indeed, when an individual is nonmentalizing, when affect is
raised in the context of interpersonal stressors, an overtly mentalizing approach may
appear heavy-handed and inappropriate. This may be the case, for example, when
patients are in the grip of psychic equivalence, making it impossible for them to imagine that the current reality is anything other than what they are experiencing; that no
matter how persecutory the situation may be, it is unalterable and utterly fixed. In
such a situation, the initial approach of a mentalization-based therapist would be to
attempt to see the position through the eyes of the patient, which may include seeing
him-/herself that way. This sounds straightforward but requires humility, discipline,
and imagination, as (naturally) one wants to hold on to the way one sees oneself. Ex-

periencing empathy in this way is a critical first step in learning about other ways of seeing the world: once the patient has had the experience of feeling understood and recognized, the therapist might be able to introduce alternative perspectives that might involve a shift in view. Developing an individual's capacity for mentalizing is analogous to physiotherapy to strengthen muscles after being in a cast—strength needs to be built up gradually, with careful consideration of areas of weakness and vulnerability to further injury, through gradual challenge.

Bateman and Fonagy have examined the effectiveness of MBT for treating BPD in a series of randomized controlled trials, with patients receiving treatment as usual in the community serving as comparison groups. The day-hospital program was investigated in a series of outcome studies, culminating in an 8-year follow-up study (Bateman and Fonagy 2008), the longest follow-up of treatment for BPD conducted to date. In comparison with treatment as usual, MBT was associated with decreased suicide attempts, emergency department visits, inpatient admissions, medication and outpatient treatment use, and impulsivity. Far fewer patients in the MBT group than in the comparison group met criteria for BPD at follow-up (13% vs. 87%). Moreover, in addition to symptomatic improvement, patients in the MBT group showed greater improvement in interpersonal and occupational functioning. Similarly, the intensive outpatient program proved more effective than structured clinical management for BPD at the end of the 18-month treatment period (Bateman and Fonagy 2009), particularly for patients with more than two personality disorder diagnoses (Bateman and Fonagy 2013). Compared with treatment as usual, the outpatient treatment resulted in lowered rates of suicidal behavior and nonsuicidal self-injury as well as fewer hospitalizations; in addition, the MBT group showed improved social adjustment coupled with diminished depression, symptom distress, and interpersonal distress. A randomized controlled trial of an adaptation of MBT for adolescents (MBT-A) found that in the treatment of young people who self-harm, MBT-A was more effective than treatment as usual in reducing both self-harm and depression (Rossouw and Fonagy 2012).

Another randomized controlled trial compared MBT for eating disorders (MBT-ED) with specialist supportive clinical management for patients with eating disorders and symptoms of BPD. The high dropout rate in this study (only 15 of the 68 participants eligible for randomization—22%—completed the 18-month follow-up) made results difficult to interpret; nonetheless, MBT-ED was associated with greater reductions in shape concern and weight concern on the Eating Disorder Examination (Robinson et al. 2016). Another recent randomized controlled trial of the effectiveness of MBT for comorbid antisocial personality disorder and BPD found that MBT was effective in the reduction of anger, hostility, paranoia, and frequency of self-harm and suicide attempts as well as in the improvement of negative mood, general psychiatric symptoms, interpersonal problems, and social adjustment (Bateman et al. 2016).

Mentalizing as a Common Factor in Psychotherapy

Decades of psychotherapy research have shown a consistent finding: compared with control conditions, many brands of psychotherapy are demonstrably effective, but it is difficult to show consistently that any particular brand is more effective than any other (Wampold and Imel 2015). Whereas differences among brands generally carry limited weight, extensive evidence attests to the substantial effect of the quality of the patient–therapist relationship on outcomes (Norcross 2011). Most notably, consistent evidence attests to the importance of the therapeutic alliance (Horvath et al. 2011) and the capacity to repair ruptures in the alliance (Safran et al. 2011). Our approach is entirely consistent with this emphasis on the therapeutic relationship, for which we use the language of mentalizing in the context of a secure attachment relationship. Bowlby (1988) summarized this approach elegantly in construing the therapist's role as providing "the patient with a secure base from which he can explore the various unhappy and painful aspects of his life, past and present, many of which he finds it difficult or perhaps impossible to think about and reconsider without a trusted companion to provide support, encouragement, sympathy, and, on occasion, guidance" (p. 138). When one of us (J.G.A.) made the observation in a trauma-education group that "the mind can be a scary place," a patient replied, "Yes, and you wouldn't want to go in there alone!" Bowlby might have applauded.

We have proposed immodestly that mentalizing is *"the most fundamental common factor* among psychotherapeutic treatments" (Allen et al. 2008, p. 1). With countervailing humility, we also have asserted the corollary: "mentalization-based treatment is the *least novel* therapeutic approach imaginable" (Allen and Fonagy 2006, p. xix; emphasis added). In our view, mentalizing is what psychotherapists do—with Oldham's (2008) caveat: when they are doing their job. Thankfully, one need not know about the concept in order to mentalize, although we believe that understanding the concept facilitates doing so by focusing attention to the crucial process. How could one conduct psychoanalysis, psychodynamic psychotherapy, interpersonal psychotherapy, cognitive therapy—or even behavior therapy—without mentalizing? And how could a therapist conduct any of these treatments without inviting the patient to mentalize? The behavior therapist must know the patient's view of the problem, and changing behavior can promote mentalizing (e.g., exposure to feared interpersonal situations can alter appraisals of their dangerousness and increase understanding and acceptance of one's emotional reactions).

Accordingly, in addition to being the fulcrum for a structured approach to the treatment of BPD, the mentalizing approach can be viewed as a distinctive *style* of psychotherapy as might be practiced by many generalists, as contrasted with the more specialized, disorder-centered treatments. Our experience in conducting workshops for psychotherapists in diverse clinical settings and in varied parts of the world suggests that this mentalizing style of psychotherapy has wide appeal. In part, this appeal stems from the commonsensical quality of the approach; once one gets past the esoteric word *mentalizing,* there is nothing unusual about it. We use one basic technique: mentalizing conversation. We explicitly encourage therapists to be ordinary and natural. We relieve them of the need to be the expert on the patient's mind. We commend a not-knowing stance, consistent with our understanding of the opacity of mental states, including one's own mental states.

If our experience is any guide, this approach to psychotherapy sounds easy—until one tries to do it consistently. As is true for patients, mentalizing is easily derailed for therapists, and for the same reasons: attachment insecurity, intense affect, defensiveness, and aversion to awareness. Moreover, although the mentalizing approach is not tied to a particular body of theory regarding personality and psychopathology, conducting psychotherapy—especially with patients who have severe and chronic psychiatric disorders—requires a great deal of professional knowledge. Given the close developmental ties of mentalizing to attachment relationships, knowledge of attachment theory and research is especially valuable, and this literature is vast. Moreover, although the mentalizing approach is neither highly structured nor prescriptive, it is not freewheeling: sound treatment must be based on an explicit formulation that guides the treatment—ideally, a written formulation provided to the patient based on a collaborative process of understanding (Allen et al. 2008). The following clinical example illustrates the potential value of such a formulation.

> Mr. C, a second-year medical student, was referred for inpatient treatment after being placed on medical leave. With his prospective career seriously threatened, he believed that he had "nowhere to go," and he was hospitalized after he plummeted into suicidal despair.
>
> Mr. C said that he had derived no benefit from previous therapy but thought that he would give it another try "in sheer desperation." He stated adamantly that he had been plagued with anxiety as long as he could remember and that he had "thought about every imaginable strategy for coping" for years. He stated flatly that in light of his long experience in trying to "outwit" his anxiety, the best any therapist might do is "scramble to catch up" with his thinking, while invariably remaining behind. In effect, he had nothing to learn and was impervious to influence.
>
> Despite his forthright skepticism and pessimism about the process, Mr. C discussed the childhood development of his anxiety forthrightly and poignantly. Mr. C's anxiety was all too conspicuous, and he said that his father had adopted a "drill-sergeant" approach to curing him of it. For example, Mr. C was afraid of the dark, and even through adolescence, he slept with a light on. His father would go into his room at night after he was asleep to turn off the light, leaving Mr. C to awaken in terror. Mr. C learned to "stuff" his feelings in his family, a pattern that continued into his adulthood. His friends were more like acquaintances, he dated only sporadically, and he had no emotional confiding relationships.
>
> The therapist quickly adopted Mr. C's pessimism about being able to outthink him, and after a few initial sessions, he made a serious blunder. Although Mr. C had revealed a great deal about himself, he continued to express frustration and disappointment about the failure of the therapy to relieve his anxiety. Intending to address the relationship implications of Mr. C's insistence that the best any therapist could do was aspire to catch up with Mr. C's understanding (but never improve on it), the therapist acknowledged feeling "inadequate" in the process. Mr. C immediately responded with marked despair, stating, "Right now I feel more hopeless than ever before in my life! You're telling me you can't help me." The therapist, feeling discouraged and guilty, with his own mentalizing capacity compromised, was unable to engage Mr. C in any productive reflection about the interaction throughout the rest of the session. His only effective intervention was urging strongly that Mr. C come back for another session, which Mr. C said he was willing to do.
>
> In the interim between sessions, the therapist wrote a two-page, single-spaced narrative formulation in an effort to rescue the process. The formulation began by stating the therapist's intention to address the "impasse" in their work so as to find a way to move forward. The formulation acknowledged the therapist's feeling of inadequacy and raised the possibility that the therapist was "resonating" with Mr. C's feeling of inadequacy in coping with his anxiety.
>
> The formulation summarized what the therapist had learned about the developmental origins of Mr. C's anxiety. It delineated the psychological and relationship factors contributing to Mr. C's suicide attempt, emphasizing how Mr. C had come to feel utterly alone in his despair. The formulation agreed with the futility of trying to "outthink" Mr. C or, indeed, of any aspiration to help Mr. C "think his way out" of the anxiety. Instead, the formulation raised the possibility that Mr. C's emotional pain might be

alleviated somewhat if he were to feel less alone with it. It made the point that, his aversion to closeness notwithstanding, Mr. C had confided openly and emotionally in the therapist about the problems that culminated in his suicidal state. It noted also that Mr. C had made initial efforts to confide in some of his peers in the hospital and had commented that merely knowing that others struggled in similar ways had been somewhat reassuring to him. Moreover, with the help of his social worker, he had begun to "open a dialogue" with his parents, who—to his surprise—had responded helpfully to his plight. In effect, the formulation pointed to the importance of attachment relationships in ameliorating his anxiety as well as the value of feeling and expressing his emotions as a potential way forward.

At the beginning of the next session, the therapist apologized straightforwardly to Mr. C for the "clumsy" and "hurtful" way he had approached the "challenges" of psychotherapy and their work together. He stated that he wanted to get the therapy "back on track" and that he thought it might be helpful for him to summarize his thinking about the therapy in writing. He invited Mr. C to read the formulation, and Mr. C did so with great concentration—underlining different passages as he went. When he finished, he looked up and declared, "That's about right." Specifically, having experienced glimmers of benefit from the therapeutic milieu in the hospital, he agreed with the broad point that the treatment as a whole would have a better outcome if it focused on feelings and relationships rather than on thinking. He commented that the formulation had offered what he had been wanting—that is, a different perspective on managing his anxiety.

We have introduced potential confusion in proposing mentalizing as both a specialized brand of therapy (i.e., MBT for BPD) and a common factor in psychotherapy. In the latter context, mentalizing is an integrative approach to psychotherapy—transtheoretical, transdiagnostic, and applicable to multiple treatment modalities. In this regard, mentalizing is consistent with the expansive applications of other therapeutic approaches—psychoanalysis, interpersonal psychotherapy, cognitive therapy, and mindfulness practice. In our view, MBT and related attachment research has provided the context of discovery in which we have refined our understanding of the psychotherapeutic potential of a fundamental psychological and interpersonal process—indeed, the process by which humans establish and maintain relationships as well as understand themselves. As was discovered more than two decades ago in the context of BPD (Fonagy 1989), mentalizing provides a unique window into the realm of developmental psychopathology. This window is continually opening wider.

In collaboration with colleagues, one of us (J.G.A.) began to explore the broader applicability of mentalizing in clinical work with patients at The Menninger Clinic, which specializes in intensive, multidisciplinary inpatient services for patients with complex, treatment-resistant psychopathology—a treatment approach that can be essential to interrupting entrenched treatment stalemates, as Mr. C's vignette exemplified. A history of attachment trauma is ubiquitous in this patient population. As is characteristic of the field of psychiatry more generally, the treatment is eclectic and uses several therapeutic modalities (i.e., individual, group, and family therapy, along with psychoeducation) and theoretical frameworks (i.e., ranging from psychodynamic to cognitive-behavioral). To bring conceptual coherence to this diverse practice, patients and staff members are educated about mentalizing in the context of attachment relationships as an overarching goal of treatment.

Concomitant with the appreciation of its generic role in psychotherapy, the wider applications of mentalizing are becoming increasingly systematic and formalized. For example, the mentalizing approach is being extended in diverse clinical settings nationally and internationally to the treatment of depression, substance abuse, eating disorders, trauma, and antisocial personality disorder (Bateman and Fonagy 2019). In addition, beyond its applications to individual and group therapy, mentalizing is being applied to family therapy as well as parent–infant and parent–child interventions. This burgeoning interest in diverse applications is consistent with our view of mentalizing as a common factor in psychopathology and in psychotherapy.

Key Clinical Points

- *Mentalizing is multifaceted:* Although we advocate a broad focus on mentalizing in psychotherapy, clinicians must attend at any given moment to particular facets that are impaired; primary distinctions are self versus others, implicit versus explicit, internal versus external, and cognitive versus affective.

- *Mentalizing begets mentalizing:* Psychotherapeutic practice builds on the finding that parental mentalizing in relation to the parent's attachment history as well as to the child's is conducive to the child's developing secure attachment and enhanced mentalizing capacity in what can be construed as a natural pedagogical process.

- *Mentalization-based treatment (MBT) is effective:* Long-term follow-up research on the treatment of borderline personality disorder (BPD) shows that MBT reduces an array of core symptoms and treatment use while improving interpersonal and occupational functioning.

- *Mentalizing is a common psychotherapeutic factor:* Core principles developed in MBT to promote mentalizing can be applied within diverse theoretical frameworks and for different treatment modalities; promoting mentalizing in the context of attachment constitutes a refinement of therapeutic practice based on research showing the prominent contribution of the patient–therapist relationship to treatment outcomes. The final common pathway that effective treatments share is the stimulation of epistemic trust, which is developed through the experience of being sensitively mentalized. Most important, such trust optimizes the patient's capacity for social learning, which fosters social adaptation where it matters most—beyond the consulting room.

- *Mentalizing applies to diverse psychopathology:* Although mentalizing-focused treatment was developed to ameliorate deficits in social cognition commonly associated with BPD, such deficits are evident in an array of psychiatric disorders for which mentalizing approaches are being developed, including substance abuse, eating disorders, depression, trauma, and other personality disorders.

References

Allen JG, Fonagy P: Preface, in Handbook of Mentalization-Based Treatment. Edited by Allen JG, Fonagy P. Chichester, UK, Wiley, 2006, pp ix–xxi

Allen JG, Fonagy P, Bateman A: Mentalizing in Clinical Practice. Washington, DC, American Psychiatric Publishing, 2008

Bateman A, Fonagy P: Effectiveness of partial hospitalization in the treatment of borderline personality disorder: a randomized controlled trial. Am J Psychiatry 156(10):1563–1569, 1999 10518167

Bateman A, Fonagy P: 8-Year follow-up of patients treated for borderline personality disorder: mentalization-based treatment versus treatment as usual. Am J Psychiatry 165(5):631–638, 2008 18347003

Bateman A, Fonagy P: Randomized controlled trial of outpatient mentalization-based treatment versus structured clinical management for borderline personality disorder. Am J Psychiatry 166(12):1355–1364, 2009 19833787

Bateman A, Fonagy P: Borderline personality disorder, in Handbook of Mentalizing in Mental Health Practice. Edited by Bateman A, Fonagy P. Washington, DC, American Psychiatric Publishing, 2012, pp 273–288

Bateman A, Fonagy P: Impact of clinical severity on outcomes of mentalisation-based treatment for borderline personality disorder. Br J Psychiatry 203(3):221–227, 2013 23887998

Bateman A, Fonagy P: Mentalization-Based Treatment for Personality Disorders: A Practical Guide. New York, Oxford University Press, 2016

Bateman A, Fonagy P (eds): Handbook of Mentalizing in Mental Health Practice, 2nd Edition. Washington, DC, American Psychiatric Association Publishing, 2019

Bateman A, O'Connell J, Lorenzini N, et al: A randomised controlled trial of mentalization-based treatment versus structured clinical management for patients with comorbid borderline personality disorder and antisocial personality disorder. BMC Psychiatry 16:304, 2016 27577562

Bowlby J: A Secure Base: Parent-Child Attachment and Healthy Human Development. New York, Basic Books, 1988

DeFife J, Hilsenroth MJ, Kuutmann K: Beyond transference: fostering growth through therapeutic immediacy, in Handbook of Psychodynamic Approaches to Psychopathology. Edited by Luyten P, Mayes LC, Fonagy P, et al. New York, Guilford, 2015, pp 512–528

Fonagy P: A child's understanding of others. Bulletin of the Anna Freud Centre 12:91–115, 1989

Fonagy P, Luyten P: A developmental, mentalization-based approach to the understanding and treatment of borderline personality disorder. Dev Psychopathol 21(4):1355–1381, 2009 19825272

Fonagy P, Luyten P: A multilevel perspective on the development of borderline personality disorder, in Developmental Psychopathology, Vol 3: Risk, Disorder, and Adaptation. Edited by Cicchetti D. New York, Guilford, 2016, pp 726–792

Fonagy P, Target M: Attachment and reflective function: their role in self-organization. Dev Psychopathol 9(4):679–700, 1997 9449001

Fonagy P, Steele H, Steele M: Maternal representations of attachment during pregnancy predict the organization of infant-mother attachment at one year of age. Child Dev 62(5):891–905, 1991 1756665

Fonagy P, Gergely G, Target M: The parent-infant dyad and the construction of the subjective self. J Child Psychol Psychiatry 48(3–4):288–328, 2007 17355400

Fonagy P, Luyten P, Allison E, Campbell C: What we have changed our minds about, part 2: borderline personality disorder, epistemic trust and the developmental significance of social communication. Borderline Personal Disord Emot Dysregul 4:9, 2017 28405338

George C, Solomon J: Caregiving helplessness: the development of a screening measure for disorganized maternal caregiving, in Disorganized Attachment and Caregiving. Edited by Solomon J, George C. New York, Guilford, 2011, pp 133–166

Gergely G: The social construction of the subjective self: the role of affect-mirroring, markedness, and ostensive communication in self development, in Developmental Science and Psychoanalysis. Edited by Mayes L, Fonagy P, Target M. London, Karnac, 2007, pp 45–82

Gergely G, Csibra G: The social construction of the cultural mind: imitative learning as a mechanism of human pedagogy. Interact Stud 6(3):463–481, 2005

Gergely G, Unoka Z: Attachment and mentalization in humans: the development of the affective self, in Mind to Mind: Infant Research, Neuroscience, and Psychoanalysis. Edited by Jurist EL, Slade A, Bergner S. New York, Other Press, 2008, pp 50–87

Horvath AO, Del Re AC, Fluckiger C, et al: Alliance in individual psychotherapy, in Psychotherapy Relationships That Work: Evidence-Based Responsiveness, 2nd Edition. Edited by Norcross JC. New York, Oxford University Press, 2011, pp 25–69

Iacoboni M: Mirroring People: The New Science of How We Connect With Others. New York, Farrar, Straus & Giroux, 2008

Lecours S, Bouchard MA: Dimensions of mentalisation: outlining levels of psychic transformation. Int J Psychoanal 78(Pt 5):855–875, 1997 9459091

Lyons-Ruth K, Jacobvitz D: Attachment disorganization from infancy to adulthood: neurobiological correlates, parenting contexts, and pathways to disorder, in Handbook of Attachment: Theory, Research, and Clinical Applications, 3rd Edition. Edited by Cassidy J, Shaver PR. New York, Guilford, 2016, pp 667–695

Main M, Solomon J: Procedures for identifying infants as disorganized/disoriented during the Ainsworth Strange Situation, in Attachment in the Preschool Years: Theory, Research, and Intervention. Edited by Greenberg MT, Cicchetti D, Cummings EM. Chicago, IL, University of Chicago Press, 1990, pp 121–160

Melnick S, Finger B, Hans S, et al: Hostile-helpless states of mind in the AAI: a proposed additional AAI category with implications for identifying disorganized infant attachment in high-risk samples, in Clinical Applications of the Adult Attachment Interview. Edited by Steele H, Steele M. New York, Guilford, 2008, pp 399–423

Morton J: The origins of autism. New Sci 1694:44–47, 1989

Norcross JC (ed): Psychotherapy Relationships That Work: Evidence-Based Responsiveness, 2nd Edition. New York, Oxford University Press, 2011

Oldham JM: Epilogue, in Mentalizing in Clinical Practice. Edited by Allen JG, Fonagy P. Washington, DC, American Psychiatric Publishing, 2008, pp 341–346

Robinson P, Hellier J, Barrett B, et al: The NOURISHED randomised controlled trial comparing mentalisation-based treatment for eating disorders (MBT-ED) with specialist supportive clinical management (SSCM-ED) for patients with eating disorders and symptoms of borderline personality disorder. Trials 17(1):549, 2016 27855714

Rossouw TI, Fonagy P: Mentalization-based treatment for self-harm in adolescents: a randomized controlled trial. J Am Acad Child Adolesc Psychiatry 51(12):1304–1313.e3, 2012 23200287

Safran JD, Muran JC, Eubanks-Carter C: Repairing alliance ruptures, in Psychotherapy Relationships That Work: Evidence-Based Responsiveness, 2nd Edition. Edited by Norcross JC. New York, Oxford University Press, 2011, pp 224–238

Thompson RA: Early attachment and later development: familiar questions, new answers, in Handbook of Attachment: Theory, Research, and Clinical Applications, 2nd Edition. Edited by Cassidy J, Shaver PR. New York, Guilford, 2008, pp 348–365

Tronick E: The Neurobehavioral and Social-Emotional Development of Infants and Children. New York, WW Norton, 2007

Wampold BE, Imel ZE: The Great Psychotherapy Debate: The Evidence for What Makes Psychotherapy Work, 2nd Edition. New York, Routledge, 2015

Recommended Readings

Allen JG: Mentalizing in the Development and Treatment of Attachment Trauma. London, Karnac, 2013

Allen JG: Restoring Mentalizing in Attachment Relationships: Treating Trauma With Plain Old Therapy. Washington, DC, American Psychiatric Publishing, 2013

Allen JG, Fonagy P, Bateman A: Mentalizing in Clinical Practice. Washington, DC, American Psychiatric Publishing, 2008

Bateman A, Fonagy P (eds): Handbook of Mentalizing in Mental Health Practice, 2nd Edition. Washington, DC, American Psychiatric Association Publishing, 2019

Bateman A, Fonagy P: Mentalization-Based Treatment for Personality Disorders: A Practical Guide. New York, Oxford University Press, 2016

Fonagy P: Attachment Theory and Psychoanalysis. New York, Other Press, 2001

Fonagy P, Gergely G, Jurist EL, et al: Affect Regulation, Mentalization, and the Development of the Self. New York, Other Press, 2002

Holmes J: Exploring in Security: Towards an Attachment-Informed Psychoanalytic Psychotherapy. New York, Routledge, 2010

Jurist EL, Slade A, Bergner S (eds): Mind to Mind: Infant Research, Neuroscience, and Psychoanalysis. New York, Other Press, 2008

CHAPTER 36

Hybrid Practitioners and Digital Treatments

Peter Yellowlees, M.B.B.S., M.D.

Jay Shore, M.D., M.P.H.

Technological changes—digital, nano, genomic, and cloud based, or some combination of these—are one of several trends currently transforming the U.S. health care environment (Yellowlees and Shore 2017), and as such are already affecting psychiatrists and the way that many psychiatric treatments are performed.

For many years, the introduction of technologies, sometimes even the telephone, into psychiatric care has been viewed with some suspicion, and a philosophical set of beliefs emerged during the late twentieth century that supported the use of, for instance, videoconferencing, only if and when in-person care was unavailable. Hence *telepsychiatry*—a term often used synonymously with *videoconferencing*—was frequently viewed as being a second-class approach to treatment (noting that before 2007, picture quality usually was poor) that had to be proven to be "no worse" than conventional in-person approaches to care. Over the past decade, high-definition videoconferencing and numerous other technologies have emerged and have become available for psychiatrists to use, especially in the mobile and monitoring sphere. With the simultaneous emergence of the millennial generation of physicians, who as "digital natives" have never known life without the Internet, psychiatrists now commonly practice as hybrid practitioners. This type of care involves patients being treated both in person and online in a much more flexible manner than was previously possible, at times and places that are mutually convenient and in a physician–patient relationship that is potentially 24/7. As psychiatrists change the way that they practice and deliver their therapies and therapeutic approaches, it is inevitable that there will be some potentially important unintended effects, which will need to be addressed by developing a set of rules or guidelines for this new form of more open practice with less solid boundaries.

The scientific literature and formal research studies are unable to keep up with this rapidly changing field. Although several influential reviews of the use of technology in mental health care have been published, traditionally validated randomized controlled trials are lacking in most areas of technology practice, with the only exception being some areas involving videoconferencing. The two most recent peer-reviewed publications of importance were by Bashshur et al. (2016) and Hilty et al. (2013). Others of importance are a book edited by Yellowlees and Shore (2017) covering all areas of telepsychiatry and a report from the National Academy of Sciences (2017) on veteran health care that includes a comprehensive review of technology-assisted mental health care; in addition, Shore (2013) has written an excellent one-stop-shop article for psychiatrists who want to start using videoconferencing. Among the organizations that publish guidelines and best practice documents in this area, the American Telemedicine Association has been the most prolific, having produced three guidelines for clinical telemental health and psychiatry within the past decade: adult telepsychiatry (Yellowlees et al. 2010), web-based videoconferencing (Turvey et al. 2013), and child and adolescent telemental health (Myers et al. 2017). In 2018, these various guidelines were updated and consolidated into a single "best practices" document endorsed by both the American Telemedicine Association and the American Psychiatric Association (Shore et al. 2018).

What Types of Technologies Are Currently Being Used for Psychiatric Treatment?

Yellowlees and Shore (2017) suggested that technologies can be divided into those that have already become a standard part of daily practice and those that are currently not yet in widespread use or deployment but are likely to become so over the next decade.

The base technologies currently being used for clinical purposes are as follows:

1. *Telephony:* Telephony has long been used with patients, especially to deal with emergent issues, although all practitioners will be aware of the pains involved in playing "phone tag" with patients. Interactive voice response systems have been used for several years to collect information and to monitor patients, and the increasing combination of traditional telephony approaches with those possible on smart devices is radically changing the way that telephony is thought about.

2. *E-mail or secure messaging:* E-mail or secure messaging occurs either in real time (synchronous) or in delayed time (asynchronous) and is especially useful for communication between or after sessions and for monitoring treatment. With the use of enterprise electronic medical record (EMR) systems, psychiatrists will increasingly communicate with their patients via secure messaging within the EMRs, and e-mail communication with patients will also be carried out via smartphones and similar devices. E-mail has already been transforming administrative communications around patient care for decades.

3. *Videoconferencing:* Live interactive videoconferencing has rapidly developed as a field over the past three decades. The American Telemedicine Association has reported that more than a million individual patients were treated with telepsychiatry in the United States in 2016 (Yellowlees and Shore 2017), with the Department

of Veterans Affairs being the biggest national provider of such services (National Academy of Sciences 2017). Videoconferencing has moved past a tipping point of use and is now commonly used by psychiatrists around the United States, with many commercial virtual telepsychiatry companies emerging and patients routinely asking their psychiatrists if they can be seen at home on video. Several articles have been published identifying areas where treatment with videoconferencing seems to be more effective than in-person treatment, such as in children with attention-deficit/hyperactivity disorder (Myers et al. 2015) and in patients with posttraumatic stress disorder (PTSD) (Azarang et al. 2018).

4. *Web-based applications:* Web-based applications are currently being widely deployed for clinical purposes, with a focus on psychoeducation and patient support, as well as monitoring and data collection. Many web sites incorporate synchronous and asynchronous communication capacities, allowing them to be used as an adjunct to treatment, taking the place of, for instance, paper charts or tools, or as the portal through which treatment occurs, such as with online cognitive-behavioral programs, which are becoming increasingly common, with an emerging evidence base confirming their utility. A review of YouTube.com will rapidly show how much psychiatric educational material is available for patients.

5. *Mobile devices:* Mobile telephones are arguably the mental health technology platform of the twenty-first century and encompass all of the time-honored uses of telephone systems along with texting and applications (apps) with monitoring, recording, and note-taking capacities. The typical smartphone is equipped with accelerometers to detect the position of the smartphone and estimate the activity of the user; with Wi-Fi and Global Positioning System to locate the user; and with software that can capture the user's interactions. Mobile devices not only provide an audiovisual medium for mobile telepsychiatry but also may serve as intelligent information-gathering devices for a range of biological, functional, and environmental data, leading the way for the development of a range of innovative future approaches to treatment.

Literally thousands of smartphone apps are currently available to assist patients and providers with everything from screening for disorders to maintaining lists of activities in a cognitive-behavioral treatment program and practicing mindfulness when anxious. Dulin et al. (2013) have described how smartphone apps can even intervene to help a patient with a substance use disorder at risk of relapse (e.g., by sending an alert when the patient approaches a liquor store or by coaching the patient through difficult social situations where alcohol is readily available, such as at weddings). The common theme of these applications is digitization and automation of much of the health care provider's therapies, so that they are available to patients in between telepsychiatry sessions with the therapist, or perhaps are supplemented by contact with an "avatar therapist" (artificial intelligence–supported patient technology) between sessions. Yellowlees et al. (2012) have even described a potential future in which the human therapist is replaced entirely with a technology-based avatar that is trained to respond therapeutically to movements and language.

Studies have shown how much patients like using mobile devices as a "therapist in the pocket," and increasing numbers of psychiatrists are incorporating device- or app-supported therapeutic techniques as part of their routine practice. The problem with all apps is the difficulty in judging the quality and validity of the app itself, but some good reviews have described how to do this (Torous et al. 2016). For clinicians who are concerned about the quality of apps, it is worthwhile to commence with any of the current batch of more than a dozen apps created by the Department of Veterans Affairs Palo Alto Health Care System group, all of which are excellent and can be downloaded free from the App Store.

6. *Electronic medical records:* EMRs are now used routinely by psychiatrists working in academic and health system settings, as well as by an increasing number of psychiatrists in private practice. Within a decade, all clinicians will routinely use EMRs. Most personal health records are now tethered (i.e., patients and physicians share the same EMR information, with patient access through a patient portal), as opposed to untethered (i.e., patient records are available only to providers). Adapting to the use of EMRs has been a significant stressor for many psychiatrists and other physicians and has commonly led to symptoms of burnout or, in some cases, to premature retirement, but the profession is adapting, driven by the increasing diffusion of EMR systems for clinical, administrative, and reimbursement purposes. Most EMRs already incorporate access to a range of educational and decision making support materials. In the future, "precision medicine" will likely automatically combine phenomic and genomic information about patients, allowing more precise prescribing of medications tailored to the individual. Videoconferencing and instant-messaging capacities are currently being introduced by some companies (e.g., Epic, Cerner) and will make these EMRs "one-stop shops" for clinical treatment of patients both in person and online in the near future. Technology platform and business integration currently remain significant but not insurmountable challenges.

Emergent technologies are those that are not yet in widespread and consistent use in the practice of psychiatry but are currently being pilot-tested in limited settings. Given the rapidly changing nature of technology, it is challenging to predict which of these technologies will ultimately attain widespread use. The scientific evidence base for these technologies ranges from sparse to nonexistent, although evidence is not necessarily the primary driver of widespread diffusion and adoption. Below, we briefly describe some of the more promising emergent technologies.

1. *Virtual reality:* Virtual reality involves the use of virtual gaming systems that use technology (wraparound three-dimensional goggles; body location sensors to direct movement, touch, smell, and other sensory components) to immerse the user in a computer-generated environment. For more than a decade, virtual reality has been used in exposure therapies (PTSD, phobia) and pain management, with more sophisticated applications under development.

2. *Virtual worlds:* Virtual worlds are massive online multiplayer systems (e.g., *Second Life*) that allow individuals to interact with both virtual environments and other individuals for psychoeducation and treatment purposes. The "Virtual Hallucinations" environment—created by the University of California–Davis (UCD) team and available on YouTube (https://www.youtube.com/watch?v=qHGa7dQtKiI)—has already been viewed by more than 200,000 people; this environment allows an individual to experience simulated psychotic symptoms, building understanding and empathy for those afflicted with these symptoms (Godwin et al. 2017).

3. *Spatial tracking systems:* As previously described, these tracking systems are used in mobile phones but are now also being used with physiological monitors (e.g., Fitbit), giving providers a wide range of information on patient activity (e.g., actigraphy).

4. *Social networking:* Both individual practitioners and health care organizations are exploring methods to leverage social networking apps for engaging and educating patients as well as for potentially monitoring (both actively and passively) patients' activities to assess location, social engagement, and so forth. This area is particularly fraught with ethical and legal issues, including patient–psychiatrist boundaries.

All of these and other technologies will probably find roles in clinical practice in the future.

What Types of Online or Hybrid Therapies or Treatment Strategies Are Emerging?

Yellowlees and Shore (2017) have described in detail a full range of online and hybrid therapies and treatment strategies. We examine several core issues here.

Integration of Psychiatric Care Into Primary Care Systems

A crucial step in expanding mental health care services to where patients are, which is mainly in the primary care setting, is to improve the flow of clinical work across primary care and specialty care settings. This workflow objective is best achieved by implementing efficient, provider-compatible, administratively simple electronic synchronous and asynchronous solutions to integrate behavioral health care into the primary care setting via a stepped-care model, delivering the right level of triage and treatment based on patients' needs.

Integrated behavioral health care is a comprehensive approach to care that involves a team of primary care and behavioral health clinicians working together with patients and families. It uses a systematic and cost-effective approach to provide patient-centered care for a defined population through an integrated primary care medical home (ICPMH; Katon and Unützer 2011).

Before the development of such systems, the main option for a primary care provider who wanted to have a patient psychiatrically assessed was to refer the patient for an in-person psychiatric consultation. The only alternative to this direct consultation was to telephone, or speak in person to, a psychiatric colleague and obtain a "curbside" consultation. Mental health care services in primary care are changing substantially with the implementation of integrated care models, and the following services are now becoming routine:

- *Evidence-based clinical reviews:* A multidisciplinary (including psychiatrists) team reviews panels of patients, or individual patients, often involving routine screening of patients with tools such as the Patient Health Questionnaire–9, Generalized Anxiety Disorder–7, and Alcohol Use Disorders Identification Test (AUDIT). Feedback and treatment planning suggestions are then returned to the patients' primary care physicians electronically through EMRs, messaging, or similar electronic systems (Raney et al. 2014).

- *Patient registries:* Registries of patients with specific disorders, such as depression or bipolar disorder, are reviewed by psychiatrists with expertise in those disorders to make sure that best practices are being followed—for instance, by checking that all patients taking lithium are receiving annual renal and thyroid function tests, or that all patients with depression are being offered therapeutic dosages of antidepressants and appropriate psychotherapies. When reviewers identify a patient who is an outlier or who seems not to be receiving guideline-based care, they are able to contact the primary care provider and local treatment team to reinforce whatever is missing and suggest alternatives.
- *Online provider to online provider (electronic):* E-consultations and responding to primary provider questions via EMR messaging are becoming increasingly common, and essentially represent an enhanced form of curbside consultations. In these communications, the psychiatrist receives a formal referral or set of questions from a primary care provider, perhaps with some algorithmically developed questions; ideally reviews the patient's notes in a shared EMR; and then responds with an opinion and treatment suggestions for the provider to consider.

These types of asynchronous clinical services provide the foundations that support the ICPMH model of care delivery. Technologies such as EMRs, e-mail, telephony, and secure electronic messaging through patient portals have created a series of electronically supported consultation choices for patients and providers. When primary care physicians are able to combine direct care with synchronous and asynchronous consultation options using videoconferencing or telephony, a multitude of care delivery approaches become possible, producing a more flexible and stepped-care structure in the ICPMH. Stepped models of care use less intensive and less expensive interventions at the outset and gradually add more intensive services if patients fail to improve (Hilty et al. 2013).

The Individual Psychiatrist Practicing in a Hybrid Manner

Yellowlees and Shore (2017) have described hybrid providers as "clinicians who interact with patients both in person and online, so that their doctor–patient relationships cross both environments. The addition of interactions via videoconferencing, e-mail, text messaging, and telephony leads to improved access and interactions at times and places not possible when care is restricted to the in-person venue" (p. 254).

This hybrid practice is rapidly becoming the preferred model of care for many psychiatrists who use the technologies described earlier to complement in-person care, depending on the psychiatrist's and patient's preferences (Yellowlees et al. 2015). The photograph in Figure 36–1 shows the setup of P. Y.'s office, where he sees patients both online and in person. Note that he has three screens on his desk for both online and in-person work and at all times can have the patient's EMR on one screen; digital communications software, such as e-mail or messaging, or educational web sites on another screen; and videoconferencing or video educational material on the third screen.

It also can be helpful to examine the current process of the psychiatrist–patient relationship, whether in-person or virtual, using an informatics perspective (Figure 36–2).

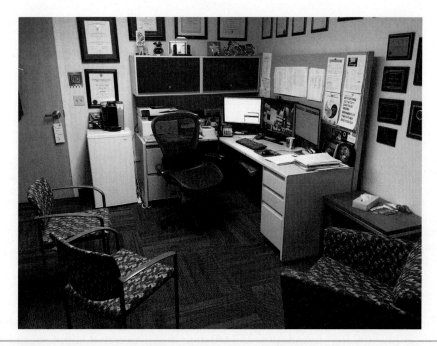

FIGURE 36–1. Office setup for both in-person and virtual care.
Source. Photograph courtesy of Peter Yellowlees, M.B.B.S., M.D. Used with permission.

Yellowlees et al. (2015) have described three core components of any physician–patient interaction:

1. History, physical examination, and information gathering; in informatics terms, this component is known as *data collection.*
2. Formulation of a diagnosis from this information; in the informatics field, this component is known as *data analysis.*
3. Creation of a treatment plan; in informatics, this component is known as *project implementation.*

The separation of these three components is a long-standing tradition in several medical specialties, such as radiology and pathology, in which actual data collection (e.g., via X ray or phlebotomy) is done by other personnel, with radiologists or pathologists subsequently reviewing the findings. Such separation of data collection from data analysis and treatment planning is now possible in psychiatry with the use of novel technologies (as discussed earlier). For instance, in asynchronous telepsychiatry, a nonphysician may conduct a recorded patient interview on one day and the psychiatrist may analyze the recorded interview and develop a treatment plan a few days later, with the primary care provider eventually implementing the psychiatrist's plan. Thus, the evolution of more mobile, team facilitated, and asynchronous environments will enable further separation of the components of the traditional in-person psychiatric consultation to allow more highly trained and paid psychiatrists to focus on the more difficult analytic and planning components of patient care.

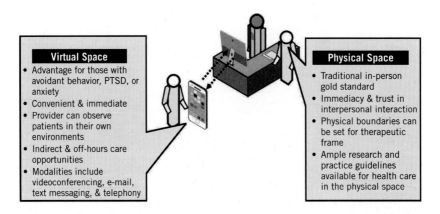

FIGURE 36–2. Elements of virtual and in-person care in a hybrid psychiatrist–patient relationship.

Note. PTSD=posttraumatic stress disorder.
Source. Created by and used with permission of Steven Chan, M.D.

The hybrid physician–patient relationship of the future undoubtedly will be based on the "gold standard" foundation of a trusting interaction that supports and promotes healing. How this key relationship is successfully sustained across multiple formats and team members will have an enormous impact on treatment outcomes. The weight of history supports the importance and power of the patient–physician relationship in managing treatment and disease. Technology can be used both to enhance and to create distance in interpersonal relationships. Used deftly, technology allows healing relationships to be built and maintained in multiple online interactions, which can be more strongly patient-focused and provide more frequent and convenient access to care—potentially anytime, anywhere. Careful attention to the patient–psychiatrist relationship—and to how that relationship is affected by different modes of communication—will become the responsibility and focus of all psychiatrists moving forward. Additionally, as psychiatrists increasingly become involved in settings providing team-based care, active management of interteam dynamics and team–patient interaction will also become essential in building the needed trust and rapport in the relationships that contain a patient's treatment. Potential downsides to these new models of care are the "always on" hybrid relationship, as well as the challenges of maintaining optimal physician–patient boundaries and navigating issues surrounding technology literacy. In this style of practice, psychiatrists need to ensure that appropriate professional boundaries—ethical, physical, technical, and time related—are maintained, as discussed by Yellowlees and Shore (2017); these authors have suggested that psychiatrists should design their practices to establish simple "rules" of communication and engagement with patients so that both parties have the same expectations about the relationship and respect each other's privacy.

The effect of the transition to providing hybrid care is also significant for the systems and providers that psychiatrists interact with. For example, as previously discussed (see "Integration of Psychiatric Care Into Primary Care Systems"), primary care physicians traditionally, when referring a patient to a psychiatrist, had only three options:

1. Arrange an in-person office consultation at a specialist psychiatry clinic.
2. Telephone for a curbside consultation.
3. Instruct the patient to go to the emergency department.

In a hybrid practice environment, many more options are available. For example, when a UCD primary provider wishes to obtain psychiatric advice, or to attend regular educational sessions offered by UCD psychiatrists, he or she may use the following additional options:

4. Schedule a psychiatric review through the care coordination team.
5. Submit an e-consultation request via the EMR.
6. Arrange an asynchronous telepsychiatry consultation for clinic or home.
7. Arrange a synchronous telepsychiatry consultation for clinic or home.
8. Arrange for a patient to be seen by a psychiatrist in the primary care clinic.

Unfortunately, although the potential menu of stepped-care choices available has expanded substantially, what is possible for an individual patient still ultimately depends on that patient's health insurance status. This stark reality speaks to the impact of our administrative and organizational systems in health care, which can have real effects on the provider–patient relationship—and, in terms of allowing access to care, can even control whether such a relationship is allowed to exist.

Online Psychotherapy

The published literature on online psychotherapy was recently reviewed by Kocsis and Yellowlees (2018). Historically, the major concerns documented have related to boundaries; technical impediments to communication, confidentiality, and privacy; and legal liability (Morland et al. 2015). The advantages documented have primarily involved reduced costs of treatment, improved access for underserved patient populations, and maintenance of continuity of psychotherapeutic relationships after one of the participants has relocated. Studies have documented that cognitive-behavioral therapy (Hedman et al. 2012) and psychodynamic psychotherapy (Johansson et al. 2013; Saeed and Anand 2015; Scharff 2013), when delivered online, are no less effective than when delivered in person.

Kocsis and Yellowlees (2018) have described some distinct advantages of online therapy:

1. *Reduction in patient anxiety and a shift toward more egalitarian power dynamics:* Telepsychotherapy can be less anxiety provoking, because patients have the option to be "seen" from their homes or other familiar settings. Similarly, therapists have the option of seeing patients from a setting that is more comfortable for them— such as from home. Kocsis and Yellowlees (2018) noted that this geographic relocation may help both parties to feel more relaxed or "settled" and could foster the development of psychotherapeutic intimacy.
2. *Increase in safety in the virtual space in which the consultation occurs:* Telepsychotherapy tends to result in more eye contact compared with in-person psychotherapy. However, the literal distance between patient and therapist also may create a type of psychological distance similar to that experienced through the use of an ana-

lytic couch. Kocsis and Yellowlees (2018) have discussed the concept of a "virtual space" in telepsychotherapy (see Figure 36–2), representing a combination of the increased physical and psychological distance that arises by virtue of the teleconferencing medium, which provides more safety to allow an increased sharing of intimacy. These authors further noted that in telepsychotherapy, the patient may be able to be more honest and to speak about important topics more candidly because of the "protection" afforded by the virtual space, all the while still maintaining intimacy-fostering eye contact (Kocsis and Yellowlees (2018).

3. *Improvement in the patient's sense of control:* In telepsychotherapy, the patient experiences a greater sense of physical and psychological control of the session; simultaneously, the therapist is less likely to be successful with a paternalistic approach (Kocsis and Yellowlees 2018). Although the experience is likely rare, the patient also can literally "switch off" the therapist by turning off the computer or video device.

4. *Option for use of a hybrid model:* Several groups of patients struggle to access and remain engaged with psychotherapeutic care. For patients with high levels of anxiety or hypervigilance, such as phobic patients, patients on the autism spectrum, and traumatized patients, leaving the home environment to seek therapy may feel tremendously difficult. These groups may more readily engage in telepsychotherapy than in traditional in-person psychotherapy, and Kocsis and Yellowlees (2018) have proposed that gradual integration of in-person sessions, after formation of an initial psychotherapeutic rapport from the "safety" of online sessions, may be a novel approach to exposure therapy.

What Types of Patients May Be Treated More Effectively With Online Technologies or Hybrid Care?

After years of telemedicine use by many psychiatrists in their practices, the consensus is clear that any type of patient with a psychiatric disorder may be seen via videoconferencing (Bashshur et al. 2016), and that this is likely to be the case with most of the technologies discussed here. The only absolute contraindications to a psychiatric interview or intervention via telepsychiatry are when a patient refuses to attend, as some do, or when a patient is actively acting out and engaging in behavior dangerous to him- or herself or others at the time of the interview.

Patients Receiving Hybrid Care or Being Treated in the Primary Care Setting

Patients routinely report that they value having multiple forms of contact with their psychiatrist, and the numbers of patients who report using e-mail or secure EMR-based messaging systems to communicate with their practitioners have grown dramatically. Yellowlees and Shore (2017) have emphasized the efficiency of hybrid care, in which psychiatrists can potentially provide care for many more patients if they work both in-person and online, doing a combination of synchronous and asynchronous electronic consultations (using e-mail, messaging, videoconferencing, and telephony), while also remaining in closer and more regular contact with patients. Most psychiatrists, driven by patient demands, will likely work in a hybrid manner in the future. Even when the clinician has no direct contact with the patient, such as during asynchronous telepsychiatry consultations (Yellowlees et al. 2017), we have had patients who recorded their thanks for the recommendations of these unknown psychiatrists when followed up for repeat consultations.

Psychotic Patients

By virtue of their illness, psychotic patients often seem to feel very unsafe, and despite some having paranoid thoughts about televisions and radios, these patients seem to feel more at ease when the provider is not in the room. The increased physical and psychological distance afforded with videoconferencing may reduce anxiety in this population (Sharp et al. 2011). For especially paranoid individuals, Kocsis and Yellowlees (2018) have noted that temporarily pointing the camera away from the patient (so that the provider has only audio information, but the patient can still both see and hear the provider) may allow enough distance for the patient to feel safe. Therapists also may feel safer with the removal of the threat of physical harm by psychotic patients who are potentially assaultive, as has been reported by clinicians who work with correctional populations.

Highly Anxious Patients

Psychotherapy via video may be particularly helpful for anxious patients who have difficulty leaving their homes (Morland et al. 2015). With a video-based modality, patients who might otherwise delay or forgo treatment can access a therapeutic relationship in a way that feels safe for them, as Fortney et al. (2015) have demonstrated. If a cognitive-behavioral therapy model is used for treatment, having the patient eventually come to the therapist's office could be set as a goal for therapy or could be one of the steps in a set of gradually escalating exposures.

Patients on the Autism Spectrum

Many higher-functioning patients on the autism spectrum enjoy using computers and find a sense of community online, such that they may feel more comfortable with this modality for receiving psychiatric care (Boada and Parellada 2017). Studies using online virtual reality systems designed to teach social skills to autistic children have shown early success (Georgescu et al. 2014).

Children and Teenagers

Pakyurek et al. (2010) have described how child therapists may obtain a more accurate picture of children's everyday behavior from the less intrusive vantage point of telepsychotherapy. Hilty and Yellowlees (2015) have suggested that for children with attention-deficit/hyperactivity disorder, multimodal online and in-person treatment should become the new standard of care. Teenagers are already completely accustomed to being online, and they may feel that this means of obtaining care offers both improved privacy and greater convenience (because they would not need their parents to drive them to appointments).

Traumatized Patients

Patients with significant childhood or adult abuse histories may have an especially difficult time feeling safe around the "authority figure" of the doctor or therapist in a closed office setting, and an online approach may help to build the important initial rapport and sense of safety.

Regarding treatment of PTSD, Morland et al. (2014) have conducted several studies examining the use of teleconferencing for delivery of cognitive processing therapy (both individual and group) and cognitive-behavioral therapy and have concluded that video delivery was noninferior to in-person delivery of these modalities.

Future Therapeutic Approaches and Directions

The numbers of different approaches to technology-enabled psychiatric care will increase rapidly in the future. Directions that appear most likely include the following:

- Increased use of mobile care, with more virtual consultations and monitoring that are bi- or multidirectional and continuously evaluated for quality and outcomes.
- Increased use of virtual reality, and the development of avatar-driven therapists directing and coordinating care, especially with cognitive-behavioral techniques, and improving patient engagement and adherence to care plans.
- Increased algorithmic screening of patients, using facial and voice recognition technologies, combined with use of open and closed social networks and substantially increased active (the patient inputs data deliberately) and passive (data are uploaded automatically without patient involvement) monitoring.
- Combination of multiple data sources and predictive assessments facilitated by changes in capacity to conduct "big data" analytics on the fly with potentially massive data sets of both genomic and phenomic data to customize treatments to an individual level.
- Creation of fully interoperable wireless cloud-based and patient-owned health histories that are accessible continuously, anytime and anywhere.

Management of Digital Treatments and Hybrid Relationships: Recommendations for Psychiatrists

As they navigate this new and constantly evolving environment, psychiatrists are encouraged to consider the following maxims:

- Stay abreast of base technologies (those in widespread use) and their important regulatory and administrative aspects.
- When trying out or adapting emergent technologies in clinical practice, become familiar with the evidence base supporting the technology and with the guidelines and procedures, and consider obtaining formal training if available.

- Remain mindful of how the choice of communication medium impacts the patient–psychiatrist relationship.
    - Determine whether the patient's technology literacy and the clinical setting are appropriately matched with the technologies being used.
    - In team-based settings, ascertain who is monitoring patient engagement and rapport.
    - Check in with patients at regular intervals to ascertain the frequency and quality of their interactions across platforms.
    - Consider creation of a formal written educational policy or handout for patients.

Key Clinical Points

- Hybrid psychiatrist–patient relationships are becoming routine and enable much better mutual communication as long as boundaries are well defined, especially when mobile devices are used.

- Patients enjoy using technologies to connect with their clinicians, and studies of telepsychiatry show very high patient satisfaction.

- Numerous studies have found that telepsychiatry clinical assessments are just as accurate as in-person assessments and that most psychotherapies can be carried out successfully via videoconferencing.

- Guidelines for both adult and child telepsychiatry are available and should be used by all mental health clinicians.

- Mental health care services in primary care are changing substantially with the implementation of technology-enabled integrated-care models that allow a wider range of patients to be treated.

- Some patients may be better treated virtually than purely in person, especially children and individuals with posttraumatic stress disorder.

- The only absolute clinical exclusions to the use of telepsychiatry are active violence or dangerousness during the call.

References

Azarang A, Pakyurek M, Giroux C, et al: Information technologies: an augmentation to posttraumatic stress disorder treatment among trauma survivors. Telemed J E Health July 13, 2018 [Epub ahead of print] 30004318

Bashshur RL, Shannon GW, Bashshur N, et al: The empirical evidence for telemedicine interventions in mental disorders. Telemed J E Health 22(2):87–113, 2016 26624248

Boada L, Parellada M: Seeing the doctor without fear: www.doctortea.org for the desensitization for medical visits in autism spectrum disorders. Rev Psiquiatr Salud Ment 10(1):28–32, 2017 27964853

Dulin PL, Gonzalez VM, King DK, et al: Smartphone-based, self-administered intervention system for alcohol use disorders: theory and empirical evidence basis. Alcohol Treat Q 31(3), 2013 24347811

Fortney JC, Pyne JM, Kimbrell TA, et al: Telemedicine-based collaborative care for posttraumatic stress disorder: a randomized clinical trial. JAMA Psychiatry 72(1):58–67, 2015 25409287

Georgescu AL, Kuzmanovic B, Roth D, et al: The use of virtual characters to assess and train non-verbal communication in high-functioning autism. Front Hum Neurosci 8:807, 2014 25360098

Godwin HT, Khan M, Yellowlees P: The educational potential of YouTube. Acad Psychiatry 41(6):823–827, 2017 28924869

Hedman E, Ljótsson B, Lindefors N: Cognitive behavior therapy via the Internet: a systematic review of applications, clinical efficacy and cost-effectiveness. Expert Rev Pharmacoecon Outcomes Res 12(6):745–764, 2012 23252357

Hilty DM, Yellowlees PM: Collaborative mental health services using multiple technologies: the new way to practice and a new standard of practice? J Am Acad Child Adolesc Psychiatry 54(4):245–246, 2015 25791139

Hilty DM, Ferrer DC, Parish MB, et al: The effectiveness of telemental health: a 2013 review. Telemed J E Health 19(6):444–454, 2013 23697504

Johansson R, Frederick RJ, Andersson G: Using the internet to provide psychodynamic psychotherapy. Psychodyn Psychiatry 41(4):513–540, 2013 24283446

Katon W, Unützer J: Consultation psychiatry in the medical home and accountable care organizations: achieving the triple aim. Gen Hosp Psychiatry 33(4):305–310, 2011 21762825

Kocsis BJ, Yellowlees P: Telepsychotherapy and the therapeutic relationship: principles, advantages, and case examples. Telemed J E Health 24(5):329–334, 2018 28836902

Morland LA, Mackintosh MA, Greene CJ, et al: Cognitive processing therapy for posttraumatic stress disorder delivered to rural veterans via telemental health: a randomized noninferiority clinical trial. J Clin Psychiatry 75(5):470–476, 2014 24922484

Morland LA, Poizner JM, Williams KE, et al: Home-based clinical video teleconferencing care: clinical considerations and future directions. Int Rev Psychiatry 27(6):504–512, 2015 26619273

Myers K, Vander Stoep A, Zhou C, et al: Effectiveness of a telehealth service delivery model for treating attention-deficit/hyperactivity disorder: a community-based randomized controlled trial. J Am Acad Child Adolesc Psychiatry 54(4):263–274, 2015 25791143

Myers K, Nelson E, Hilty DM, et al: American Telemental Association practice guidelines for telemental health with children and adolescents. Telemed J Health 23(10):779–804, 2017 28930496

National Academy of Sciences: Evaluation of the Department of Veterans Affairs Mental Health Services. Washington, DC, National Academies Press, 2017

Pakyurek M, Yellowlees P, Hilty D: The child and adolescent telepsychiatry consultation: can it be a more effective clinical process for certain patients than conventional practice? Telemed J E Health 16(3):289–292, 2010 20406115

Raney L, Pollack D, Parks J, et al: The American Psychiatric Association response to the "joint principles: integrating behavioral health care into the patient-centered medical home." Fam Syst Health 32(2):147–148, 2014 24955687

Saeed SA, Anand V: Use of telepsychiatry in psychodynamic psychiatry. Psychodyn Psychiatry 43(4):569–583, 2015 26583441

Scharff JS (ed): Psychoanalysis Online: Mental Health, Teletherapy, and Training (Library of Technology and Mental Health, Scharff JS, series editor). London, Karnac Books, 2013

Sharp IR, Kobak KA, Osman DA: The use of videoconferencing with patients with psychosis: a review of the literature. Ann Gen Psychiatry 10(1):14, 2011 21501496

Shore JH: Telepsychiatry: videoconferencing in the delivery of psychiatric care. Am J Psychiatry 170(3):256–262, 2013 23450286

Shore J, Yellowlees P, Caudill R, et al: Best practices in videoconferencing-based telemental health—April 2018. Telemed J E Health 24(11):827–832, 2018 30358514

Torous JB, Chan SR, Yellowlees PM, et al: To use or not? Evaluating ASPECTS of smartphone apps and mobile technology for clinical care in psychiatry. J Clin Psychiatry 77(6):e734–e738, 2016 27136691

Turvey C, Coleman M, Dennison O, et al: ATA practice guidelines for video-based online mental health services. Telemed J E Health 19(9):722–730, 2013 23909884

Yellowlees PM, Shore J (eds): Telepsychiatry and Health Technologies: A Guide for Mental Health Professionals. Arlington, VA, American Psychiatric Association Publishing, 2017

Yellowlees P, Shore J, Roberts L, et al: Practice guidelines for videoconferencing-based telemental health—October 2009. Telemed J E Health 16(10):1074–1089, 2010 21186991

Yellowlees PM, Holloway KM, Parish MB: Therapy in virtual environments—clinical and ethical issues. Telemed J E Health 18(7):558–564, 2012 22823138

Yellowlees P, Chan RS, Burke Parish M: The hybrid doctor-patient relationship in the age of technology—telepsychiatry consultations and the use of virtual space. Int Rev Psychiatry 27(6):476–489, 2015 26493089

Yellowlees PM, Shafqat S, Myers K: Indirect consultation and hybrid care (chapter 8), in Telepsychiatry and Health Technologies: A Guide for Mental Health Professionals. Edited by Yellowlees PM, Shore J. Arlington, VA, American Psychiatric Association Publishing, 2017, pp 251–287

Recommended Readings

Bashshur RL, Shannon GW, Bashshur N, et al: The empirical evidence for telemedicine interventions in mental disorders. Telemed J E Health 22(2):87–113, 2015

Hilty DM, Ferrer DC, Parish MB, et al: The effectiveness of telemental health: a 2013 review. Telemed J E Health 19(6):444–454, 2013

Myers K, Nelson E, Hilty DM, et al: American Telemental Association practice guidelines for telemental health with children and adolescents. Telemed J Health 23(10):779–804, 2017

Shore JH: Telepsychiatry: videoconferencing in the delivery of psychiatric care. Am J Psychiatry 170(3):256–262, 2013

Turvey C, Coleman M, Dennison O, et al: ATA practice guidelines for video-based online mental health services. Telemed J E Health 19(9):722–730, 2013

Yellowlees PM, Shore J (eds): Telepsychiatry and Health Technologies: A Guide for Mental Health Professionals. Arlington, VA, American Psychiatric Association Publishing, 2017

Yellowlees P, Shore J, Roberts L; American Telemedicine Association: Practice guidelines for videoconferencing-based telemental health—October 2009. Telemed J E Health 16(10):1074–1089, 2010

Yellowlees P, Richard Chan S, Burke Parish M: The hybrid doctor-patient relationship in the age of technology—telepsychiatry consultations and the use of virtual space. Int Rev Psychiatry 27(6):476–489, 2015

CHAPTER 37

Complementary and Integrative Psychiatry

Lila Massoumi, M.D., ABOIHM

Patricia L. Gerbarg, M.D.

Philip R. Muskin, M.D., M.A.

Uma Naidoo, M.D.

Conventional medicine is the practice of medicine taught in medical schools and treatments that meet the requirements of the generally accepted standard of care in a particular country. Nonmainstream treatments have been called *complementary and alternative medicine,* or CAM (Massoumi 2017a). *Integrative medicine,* the more current concept, is the integration of conventional medicine with complementary treatments that have an evidence base. A nationwide government survey released in February 2015 reported that approximately 33% of U.S. adults ages 18 years and older use some form of CAM (Clarke et al. 2015). In 2007, 83 million adults spent $33.9 billion out of pocket on CAM in the United States (National Center for Complementary and Integrative Health 2018).

Historically, CAM has been criticized for lacking evidence for efficacy and safety. The relatively smaller body of research is due in part to the high cost of clinical trials, which cannot be recovered in sales because most natural substances cannot be patented. The absence of a large evidence base for CAM treatments may not accurately reflect their potential therapeutic value. Additional concerns about CAM include supplement–drug interactions, purity, and potency (Gerbarg and Brown 2013). Physicians who choose to recommend CAM treatments may have concerns about liability risks when deviating from conventional care. Obtaining continuing medical education in nonmainstream therapies, consulting with experienced integrative physicians, obtaining board certification in integrative medicine (American Board of Physician Specialties), and implementing good informed consent practices can help reduce such risks. Physicians are advised to document informed consent in the medical record, including the discussion with the patient about both conventional and non-mainstream treatment options and the expected benefits and potential short- and long-term risks for each treatment.

In this chapter, we provide a brief overview of nutrients, phytomedicines, hormones, mind–body practices, and electromagnetic treatments commonly used in CAM. Readers interested in delving deeper into this topic are referred to the American Psychiatric Association Publishing textbook *Complementary and Integrative Treatments in Psychiatric Practice* (Gerberg et al. 2017).

Nutrients

Folic Acid and Vitamin B_{12}

Folate (vitamin B_9) is a vitamin required for the synthesis of methionine and *S*-adenosylmethionine (SAMe). It is best known for its role in preventing neural tube defects in infants. Folic acid supplements come in three forms: folate, folic acid (synthetic form), and L-methylfolate (the main biologically active form). Adjunctive L-methylfolate at 15 mg/day may be an effective treatment strategy for patients with major depressive disorder (MDD) who have a partial response or no response to selective serotonin reuptake inhibitors (SSRIs) (Bottiglieri 2013). L-Methylfolate may be more effective than folate for treatment-refractory depression (Sarris et al. 2016).

Vitamin B_{12} (cyanocobalamin, cobalamin, methylcobalamin, adenosylcobalamin, hydroxocobalamin) is required for the synthesis of succinyl–coenzyme A (an intermediate of the citric acid cycle) and the synthesis of methionine from homocysteine. The rates of folate and B_{12} deficiencies appear to be greater in depressed persons than in nondepressed control subjects (Bottiglieri 2013). Studies do not support the use of folate or B_{12} as monotherapies for MDD. Evidence that supplementation with folate or B_{12} can beneficially augment antidepressant treatment is stronger for patients with insufficiencies of these vitamins (Almeida et al. 2015). For example, up to 30% of elderly persons may have difficulty absorbing B_{12} from food because of low levels of stomach acid (from weakening of the stomach lining or the use of antacids), which may contribute to the vitamin insufficiency. Vitamin B_{12} supplementation also may help preserve cognitive function in geriatric patients. For patients with a serum vitamin B_{12} level less than 200 pg/mL, a vitamin B_{12} supplement of 0.5–2 mg (500–2,000 µg) per day should be recommended. No adverse effects or safe upper limit of B_{12} dose or level has been identified.

Vitamin D

Vitamin D is found in fish and eggs or added artificially to dairy products. In the presence of ultraviolet B light from the sun, the body produces vitamin D from cholesterol. Low vitamin D levels are associated with an increase in all-cause mortality in the general population independent of gender or race (Akhondzadeh et al. 2013). Two systematic reviews found that studies on vitamin D for MDD were inconclusive (Li et al. 2014; Shaffer et al. 2014). Although current evidence does not support a role for vitamin D in the treatment or prevention of depression, supplementation can be justified for "general health" in patients with confirmed vitamin D insufficiency, a common finding. In a population of 544 adult psychiatric patients in Chicago, Illinois, a chart review found that 75% had vitamin D insufficiency (<30 ng/mL), with a mean level of 22 ng/mL (Rylander and Verhulst 2013). Risk factors for insufficiency include low sunlight exposure (northern climes, winter months, indoor work, dark skin tone, bedridden status), obesity, advanced age, and chronic illness. Evidence indicates that supplementation with D_3 may be more efficient than D_2 for raising 25-hydroxyvitamin D levels (Tripkovic et al. 2012). For patients with 25-hydroxyvitamin D levels lower than 50 ng/mL, repletion can be accomplished with vitamin D_3 600–4,000 IU/day (Christakos et al. 2013). Vitamin D toxicity is extremely rare and generally occurs only after ingestion of large doses of vitamin D (>10,000 IU/day) for prolonged periods in patients with normal gut absorption (Kennel et al. 2010).

S-Adenosylmethionine

SAMe is an amino acid–derived metabolite that serves as the body's most avid methyl (CH_3) donor (Figure 37–1). In several European countries, SAMe is a well-established conventional treatment for depression, arthritis, and cholestasis of pregnancy.

More than 50 clinical trials of SAMe for depression have been conducted. A meta-analysis by the U.S. Department of Health and Human Services Agency for Healthcare Research and Quality (AHRQ), which included 28 double-blind, randomized controlled trials (RCTs), concluded that SAMe monotherapy was more effective than placebo and as effective as conventional antidepressants for treating MDD (overall effect size: 0.65; 95% confidence interval: –1.05 to –0.25) (see Sharma et al. 2017). It also concluded from 12 studies (total N >23,000) that SAMe 800–1,200 mg/day had analgesic and anti-inflammatory effects in patients with osteoarthritis, and in 7 of those studies SAMe had benefits equal to those of nonsteroidal anti-inflammatory drugs but fewer side effects. The AHRQ study also noted that SAMe may be safe for use in pregnancy, because SAMe treatment for cholestasis in pregnancy caused no adverse effects on neonates in the studies reviewed, including one study with follow-up to age 1 year. Because healthy infants have higher cerebrospinal fluid levels of SAMe than do adults, and because SAMe has been shown to improve myelination in children with genetic errors of methyl-transfer pathways, there are reasons to think that SAMe—as a natural metabolite supporting healthy neuronal function—would be less likely to cause adverse effects during pregnancy and breast feeding compared with conventional antidepressant medications.

SAMe has been shown to augment antidepressant effects of prescription antidepressants (Sharma et al. 2017). SAMe can be used in the treatment of hepatic disease and to protect the liver from hepatotoxic effects of alcohol and medication. Hepatoprotection occurs, in part, by increasing synthesis of the major antioxidant glutathione.

SAMe has few adverse effects. Common side effects include mild nausea, abdominal discomfort, and loose stools; less often, nausea or vomiting occurs. SAMe can be stimulating and may initially exacerbate anxiety. In patients with bipolar disorder, SAMe can induce hypomanic or manic symptoms.

SAMe should be taken in the morning on an empty stomach (at least 30 minutes before food) to maximize absorption. If nausea occurs, the first dose can be taken with a little food. Second doses can be taken in the early afternoon at least 30 minutes before or 2 hours after lunch. Because SAMe is an activating antidepressant, it should not be

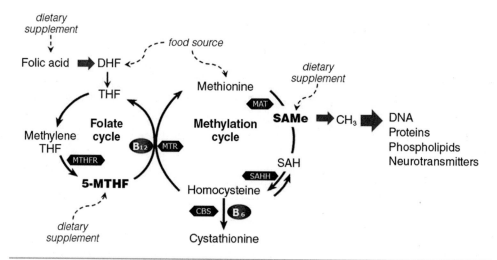

FIGURE 37–1.   Relationship between folate, vitamin B$_{12}$, and methylation.

Note.   5-MTHF=5-methyltetrahydrofolate; CBS=cystathionine β-synthase; DHF=dihydrofolate; MAT=
methionine adenosyltransferase; MTHFR=methyltetrahydrofolate reductase; MTR=methionine synthase;
SAH=*S*-adenosylhomocysteine; SAHH=*S*-adenosylhomocysteine hydrolase; SAMe=*S*-adenosylmethi-
onine; THF=tetrahydrofolate.

Source.   Reprinted from Figure 1 in Bottiglieri T: "Folate, Vitamin B$_{12}$, and *S*-Adenosylmethionine." *Psychiatric Clinics of North America* 36(1):3, 2013. Copyright 2013, Elsevier. Used with permission.

taken late in the afternoon or in the evening, because it may interfere with sleep. The
usual starting dose of SAMe is 400 mg, which can be increased in 400-mg increments
every 3–7 days as tolerated. The typical dosing range for mild to moderate depression
or for antidepressant augmentation is 800–1,200 mg/day; for moderate to severe depression, 1,600 mg/day; and for patients with treatment-resistant illness, up to 2,400
mg/day as tolerated. For elderly, debilitated, or medication-sensitive patients, dosing
may start at 200 mg/day, with slow upward titration.

The quality of SAMe products is critical, because low-quality products can lose up
to 50% of their potency while sitting on shelves. Because SAMe oxidizes on exposure
to air, tablets must be carefully manufactured, enteric coated, and protected in individual blister packs. SAMe tablets should *not* be refrigerated, because condensation
inside blister packs can degrade the product. High-quality, pharmaceutical-grade 1,4-
butanedisulfonate SAMe is manufactured in Europe (ademetionine) and in the
United States (Azendus). Many patients respond well to less-expensive brands containing toluenate or tosylate SAMe; however, for patients who do not, a trial of 1,4-
butanedisulfonate SAMe is indicated.

N-Acetylcysteine

N-Acetylcysteine (NAC) is an acetylated form of the amino acid cysteine, the rate-
limiting precursor to the major antioxidant glutathione. NAC is associated with reduced inflammatory cytokines and has neuroplastic properties. NAC is approved by
the U.S. Food and Drug Administration (FDA) as an antidote for acetaminophen
overdose (Heard 2008). It is also used as a mucolytic in chronic obstructive pulmonary disease, a renal protectant, and a therapeutic agent for HIV. Limited data sup-

port the use of adjunctive NAC for MDD and for depression in the maintenance phase of bipolar disorder (Wang and Pae 2017). Three double-blind RCTs in children with autism spectrum disorder showed greater improvement with NAC than with placebo (Ghanizadeh and Moghimi-Sarani 2013; Hardan et al. 2012; Nikoo et al. 2015). Two double-blind RCTs of patients with schizophrenia showed significantly greater improvement on Positive and Negative Syndrome Scale scores in NAC-treated patients compared with placebo-treated control subjects (Berk et al. 2008; Farokhnia et al. 2013). In one of the studies (Berk et al. 2008), the use of NAC was associated with decreased akathisia ($P=0.022$). A 24-week double-blind RCT in 43 elderly subjects with probable Alzheimer's disease reported that NAC improved performance in some cognitive domains compared with placebo (Adair et al. 2001). Studies of NAC have shown mixed results for trichotillomania, nail-biting disorder, and substance use disorder. Daily dosages greater than 2 g (e.g., 1,200 mg twice a day) are usually needed for effectiveness, and response may take 16 weeks or longer (possibly consistent with slow effects on neuroplasticity and neurogenesis) (Bloch et al. 2013; Ghanizadeh et al. 2013; Grant et al. 2009). Overall, NAC is well tolerated, with no significant differences in adverse events compared with placebo.

Acetyl-L-Carnitine

Acetyl-L-carnitine (ALC), a short-chain ester of carnitine, has been studied in depression, mild cognitive impairment (MCI), and Alzheimer's disease (Wang and Pae 2017). Out of nine double-blind RCTs of ALC for depression, three found ALC monotherapy to be more effective than placebo in MDD (Garzya et al. 1990; Gecele et al. 1991; Villardita et al. 1983), and two found ALC monotherapy to be better than placebo in dysthymia (Bella et al. 1990; Bersani et al. 2013). One showed ALC augmentation to be more effective than placebo in geriatric depression (Nasca et al. 1989), and two observed it to be as effective as fluoxetine (Bersani et al. 2013) or amisulpride (Zanardi and Smeraldi 2006) in this population. ALC had fewer significant side effects (experienced by 6/41 subjects) than fluoxetine (18/39 subjects) (Bersani et al. 2013). A meta-analysis of 21 double-blind RCTs identified significant advantages of ALC compared with placebo in MCI and Alzheimer's disease, with small effect sizes (0.20–0.32) (Montgomery et al. 2003). These RCTs suggest that ALC is generally safe and well tolerated. The most common side effects are diarrhea, foul-smelling urine, constipation, and dyspepsia. Dosages used in studies were 1–3 g.

Omega-3 Fatty Acids

Over the past century in Western societies, dietary consumption of omega-3 fatty acids has decreased dramatically, whereas consumption of omega-6 fatty acids from processed foods (high in vegetable oil) has increased (Mischoulon and Freeman 2013). This dietary shift has led to a lower physiological ratio of omega-3 to omega-6 fatty acids. A 1:1 ratio of omega-3 to omega-6 may be optimal for general health. The omega-3 fatty acids best utilized by the body are eicosapentaenoic acid (EPA; 20:5) and docosahexaenoic acid (DHA; 22:6). The primary dietary sources of omega-3 fatty acids are fish consumption and fish oil supplementation. Flaxseed and hemp oils contain the omega-3 fatty acid α-linoleic acid (ALA), which the body must convert to EPA or DHA. In approximately 15% of people, this conversion is impaired.

More than 30 controlled trials and meta-analyses support the efficacy of omega-3 fatty acids in depression. EPA rather than DHA appears to have the main antidepressant effect, because most of the significant positive studies in depression used at least 60% EPA. For mood disorders, a ratio of EPA to DHA of 3:2 or higher is recommended. Daily dosages of 1–3 g (EPA+DHA) are safe without physician supervision. Dosages greater than 3 g/day may affect platelet function and increase bleeding times. Physicians should check serum international normalized ratios in patients who have bleeding disorders or who are taking anticoagulants such as warfarin or aspirin. Most complaints of side effects, such as gastrointestinal upset and fishy aftertaste ("fish burps" or "seal burps"), can be avoided by freezing capsules before consuming or by ingesting them with food.

Phytomedicines

Phytomedicines (herbs) can contain many bioactive compounds with synergistic and polyvalent effects. Growing evidence supports the beneficial effects of herbal extracts on oxidative stress, mitochondrial energy production, cellular repair, neurotransmission, central nervous system activation or inhibition, neuroendocrine systems, and gene expression (Gerbarg and Brown 2013). Herbs can be used alone or in combination with other herbs, nutrients, and psychotropic medications. Few herbs relevant to psychiatric practice have clinically significant medication interactions. Herbal effects on cytochrome P450 (CYP) isoenzymes in vitro and in many animal studies do not necessarily occur in human studies. Digestion and metabolism convert herbal constituents to secondary metabolites whose effects on these isozymes are often negligible or even the opposite of the effects of the same herbal extracts in vitro. Caution is required when combining herbs that interact with drugs having a narrow therapeutic window (i.e., a small difference between therapeutic and toxic levels or between therapeutic and subtherapeutic levels) or with drugs having the potential to cause serious adverse effects at levels outside the therapeutic range, such as warfarin, cyclosporine, or digoxin. The risks of herb–drug interactions can be minimized by monitoring side effects and obtaining serum levels of medications that have a narrow therapeutic window. Among herbs used in psychiatric practice, most have no clinically significant interactions with drugs when used at therapeutic doses. The exceptions are St. John's wort (*Hypericum perforatum*) and kava.

As with all herbal preparations, the concentrations of bioactives within a species can vary between batches as a result of genetic variations, environmental conditions, parts of the plant used, adulterations, and processing and storage techniques. It is not surprising that clinical trials sometimes yield inconsistent outcomes for the same herb. Some manufacturers produce standardized products similar to pharmaceutical quality. When recommending phytomedicines, clinicians are encouraged to guide patients to brands or trademarked herbs that have been tested in clinical trials.

Adaptogenic Herbs

The term *adaptogen* denotes substances that "increase the ability of an organism to adapt to environmental stressors and prevent damage to the organism by such stressors" (Panossian 2013, p. 49). Starting in 1948, extensive research in the former Soviet Union found that adaptogens enhanced physical and mental performance under stress. Although many of these studies would be rated as low quality by modern standards, they still provide useful information. Over the past 25 years, better-quality studies have confirmed and extended earlier findings. Adaptogens increase energy and alertness, but unlike prescription stimulants, they do not cause addiction or withdrawal. They have demonstrated abilities to protect living organisms from oxidative stress, toxic chemicals, infection, neoplasms, heat, cold, radiation, hypoxia, physical exertion, and psychological stress. (For a review of molecular mechanisms, see Panossian 2013.) The dose–response curve of adaptogens is bell shaped, so excessively high doses are not more effective.

Rhodiola rosea (Arctic Root)

For more than 60 years, clinical and biochemical studies of *Rhodiola rosea* have increased our understanding of how this adaptogen exerts many of its therapeutic effects. Rosavins, salidroside (rhodioloside), and tyrosol have been used as active marker compounds in standardized extracts (e.g., SHR-5). In 1969, the Pharmacologic Committee of the U.S.S.R. Ministry of Health recommended the use of *R. rosea* for patients with asthenia neuroses and schizophrenia, as well as for healthy individuals doing intensive work requiring mental or physical exertion (Panossian and Amsterdam 2017). Numerous systematic reviews concluded that *R. rosea* standardized extract SHR-5 is significantly beneficial in stress-induced fatigue. A 6-week double-blind RCT of *R. rosea* (SHR-5) in mild to moderate depression showed significant antidepressant effects compared with placebo (Darbinyan et al. 2007). In patients with a variety of depressive conditions being treated with tricyclic antidepressants (TCAs), adjunctive *R. rosea* increased intellectual and physical activity and productivity, decreased TCA-induced side effects, and reduced time spent in the hospital (Brichenko et al. 1986). In patients with schizophrenia who had pronounced neuroleptic-induced extrapyramidal symptoms, *R. rosea* was reported to notably decrease extrapyramidal symptoms and fatigue after 1–1.5 months (Saratikov and Krasnov 1987).

   R. rosea is best absorbed when taken on an empty stomach 20 minutes or more before breakfast and/or lunch. If taken in the late afternoon or evening, its stimulating effects can disturb sleep. *R. rosea* can be taken continuously long-term or as needed before and during a stressful period. It is considered safe, and adverse effects are rare. Sensitive individuals, who may experience excessive stimulation such as anxiety, irritability, or insomnia, should start with lower dosages. The stimulatory effect can exacerbate agitation and irritability in bipolar disorder. Vivid dreams may occur during the first 2 weeks of use, but this effect usually abates. *R. rosea* can increase libido but rarely causes hypersexuality. Some patients may respond to small dosages (100 mg), but others may require dosages of 300 mg twice a day. For treatment-resistant depression, attention-deficit/hyperactivity disorder (ADHD), or cognitive impairment, dosages up to 900 mg daily may be necessary. At higher dosages, patients should be monitored for easy bruising and advised to avoid aspirin-containing products.

Schisandra chinensis (Schizandra)

In studies of *Schisandra* for schizophrenia, several trials reported remission of catatonic stupor, decreased hallucinations, and increased sociability (Panossian and Amsterdam 2017). Older studies with less rigorous methodology suggested that *Schisandra* may have a place in the treatment of schizophrenia for amelioration of catatonia, negative symptoms, fatigue, and side effects of first-generation antipsychotics and other sedating medications. In patients with bipolar disorder, *Schisandra* decreased depressive (but not hypomanic) symptoms. When used as adjunctive therapy with amitriptyline in patients with borderline states of exogenous–organic origin, *Schisandra* ameliorated side effects of headaches, dizziness, xerostomia, and bowel and urinary disorders in comparison with placebo (Sudakov et al. 1986). Dosages in studies were in tincture form, and thus optimal dosages cannot be extrapolated.

Eleutherococcus senticosus (Acanthopanax senticosus, Siberian Ginseng)

Eleutherococcus senticosus is widely used in Russia and China to increase physical and mental performance and quality of life. Studies of extracts from *E. senticosus* roots showed antistress, antiulcer, anti-irradiation, anticancer, anti-inflammatory, and hepatoprotective activity (Panossian and Amsterdam 2017). *E. senticosus* is usually well tolerated; however, safety during pregnancy or breast feeding has not been established. The standard dosage for *E. senticosus* is 300–1,200 mg/day.

Adaptogen Combination (ADAPT-232)

ADAPT-232 (Chisan, now called Adapt Life), a fixed combination of *R. rosea*, *E. senticosus*, and *S. chinensis*, has been used in Scandinavia since 1979 to treat decreased performance, fatigue, and weakness (Panossian 2013). Beneficial effects on cognitive function, attention, and memory have been reported in humans.

Panax ginseng (Asian Ginseng, Korean Ginseng, True Ginseng)

Panax ginseng has been used in traditional Chinese medicine for thousands of years to increase resistance to physical or mental stress, illness, and aging. Literally translated, *P. ginseng* means "all-healing man root" (Massoumi 2017b). A 2009 Cochrane review of ginseng for cognition in healthy adults and those with MCI or dementia concluded that clinical and preclinical studies suggested that a single 200- to 400-mg dose of *P. ginseng* improved at least one cognitive domain (e.g., quality of memory, secondary memory, speed of attention), although no single aspect of cognition improved consistently across studies (Geng et al. 2010).

American Ginseng (Panax quinquefolius, Xi Yang Shen)

American ginseng grows mainly in North America. Wild American ginseng is so extensively sought that it has been declared an endangered species in some states in the United States (Massoumi 2017b). Compared with *P. ginseng*, American ginseng is gentler, less stimulating, and less likely to cause agitation or headaches. As with *P. ginseng*, a single 100–400 mg dose of American ginseng may improve cognition. American ginseng has few side effects. Some animal and in vitro studies suggest that ginseng may have estrogenic activity, but the clinical significance of such activity in humans is unclear. American ginseng decreases international normalized ratios (INR) and reduces the effectiveness of warfarin.

Withania somnifera (Ashwagandha)

Compared with other adaptogens, *Withania somnifera* is more calming, possibly by improving γ-aminobutyric acid (GABA)-ergic signaling dysfunctions such as occur in anxiety disorders and insomnia. Four clinical studies have described *W. somnifera* as a safe and effective adaptogen for treating anxiety, and two studies indicated its effectiveness in bipolar disorder (Panossian and Amsterdam 2017). Dosing of *W. somnifera* as KSM-66 is 300 mg/day and as Sensoril is 500 mg nightly or twice per day. Doses should be decreased in cases of excessive daytime sedation. Doses are best absorbed on an empty stomach. If heartburn develops, the dose can be taken with a little food. *W. somnifera* is contraindicated in pregnancy because it may precipitate miscarriage.

Maca (*Lepidium meyenii*)

Maca is a Peruvian herb that grows at high altitudes in the Andes and is used to enhance sexual function, fertility, energy, alertness, mental focus, mood, and physical resilience (Gerbarg and Brown 2013). Research on maca consists primarily of animal studies and a small number of methodologically limited human trials, which suggest improvements in sexual desire and function without increasing serum testosterone, prolactin, or estradiol in men. A double-blind, randomized pilot study found that maca (3 g/day) significantly reduced SSRI-induced sexual dysfunction (Dording et al. 2008). Animal studies show no teratogenic or carcinogenic effects (Gonzales 2012). At recommended doses, maca causes minimal side effects; excess doses may cause overactivation. In clinical practice, maca can be a useful adjunctive treatment for asthenia, sexual dysfunction, or infertility (Gerbarg and Brown 2013).

Medicinal Herbs

St. John's Wort (*Hypericum perforatum*)

Research on St. John's wort supports its use for the treatment of mild to moderate depression and somatic symptom disorder (Sarris 2017b). A Cochrane review and meta-analysis reported that in 18 double-blind RCTs, St. John's wort showed a significantly greater response rate ratio (i.e., proportion of responders in treatment group divided by proportion of responders in control group) of 1.48 compared with placebo and an effect size equivalent to that of SSRIs (Linde et al. 2008). St. John's wort can augment response to TCAs and other antidepressants, including bupropion, venlafaxine, and SAMe, but should not be combined with monoamine oxidase inhibitors (MAOIs). Combining high-dose St. John's wort and serotonergic prescription antidepressants (SSRIs, serotonin–norepinephrine reuptake inhibitors) increases the risk of serotonin syndrome. A clear temporal association exists between St. John's wort use and induction of hypomania or mania. As with conventional antidepressants, caution is advised in people with a personal or family history of bipolar disorder. The average daily dosage of St. John's wort is between 900 mg and 1,800 mg (standardized to contain 0.3% hypericin and/or 1%–5% hyperforin) given in two or three doses. The most common adverse effects are reversible dermatological (phototoxic rash) and gastrointestinal symptoms (nausea, heartburn, loose stools). At higher dosages, St. John's wort may cause side effects similar to, but milder than, those of SSRIs, including sexual dysfunction, bruxism (teeth clenching), and restless legs syndrome. In humans, significant interactions have been reported between St. John's wort and oral contraceptives, antiretroviral medications, and immunosuppressants via induction of CYP3A4. The safety of St. John's wort in pregnancy and lactation has not been established.

Ginkgo Biloba

Sufficient evidence supports ginkgo as an adjunctive treatment for cognitive and neuropsychiatric symptoms associated with Alzheimer's disease, vascular dementia, cerebrovascular insufficiency, normal aging, and tinnitus (Diamond and Mondragon 2017). Ginkgo can be a primary treatment for dementia when acetylcholinesterase inhibitors are ineffective or contraindicated. Mechanisms of action include increasing cerebral blood flow, antioxidant effects, and anti-inflammatory effects. Pharmaceutical-grade ginkgo extracts are standardized to 24% ginkgo-flavone glycosides and 6% terpenoids. Most double-blind RCTs use Ginkgo biloba special extract EGb 761 (marketed as Indena, Tebonin, and Tanakan). Ginkgold, Vitanica VI3, Ginkgoforte (Blackmore), and Lichtwer's Li370 extract also contain standardized flavone glycoside and terpenoids. Products containing one of the scientifically tested standardized forms of ginkgo are more likely to be effective. A meta-analysis of 75 clinical trials totaling 7,115 patients with various psychiatric and medical issues found that EGb 761 at a dosage of 60–1,000 mg/day used for 2 days or up to 2 years was well tolerated, with no adverse events (Ihl et al. 2011). Inhibition of platelet activating factor by ginkgolide B suggests that ginkgo can have additive effects with drugs that affect platelet function and/or coagulation, such as nonsteroidal anti-inflammatory drugs (e.g., aspirin, ibuprofen, selective cyclooxygenase 2 [COX-2] inhibitors) and anticoagulants (e.g., warfarin). Doses of ginkgo between 120 and 240 mg taken two or three times per day are considered optimal in most cases. Overall, studies indicate that 4–6 weeks are needed for positive effects on memory (Gauthier and Schlaefke 2014).

Saffron (*Crocus sativus*)

Saffron has a long history of use extending back to the Persian Empire. The therapeutic dosage of saffron as a psychotropic agent is much higher than the amounts used in cooking. Seven RCTs documented benefits of saffron in mild to moderate depression (Akhondzadeh and Kashani 2017). Constituents of saffron show neuroprotective properties in animal models of ischemic, oxidative, traumatic, and inflammatory brain injury. Saffron's neuroprotective effects are probably a result of enhanced glutathione synthesis. In a 22-week double-blind RCT, saffron 30 mg/day was as effective as donepezil 10 mg/day for mild to moderate Alzheimer's disease, and the frequencies of adverse effects were similar between the two agents, with the exception of vomiting, which occurred significantly less frequently with saffron (Akhondzadeh et al. 2010). The same researchers found that 1 year of daily saffron given to patients with moderate to severe Alzheimer's disease was comparable to memantine in reducing cognitive decline (Farokhnia et al. 2014). For all of these studies, the tolerability of saffron 15–20 mg twice daily was similar to that of placebo. Because the cost of high-dosage saffron as a spice would be prohibitive, taking optimized saffron in capsule form is more affordable. A short-term (7-day) study of saffron 200 and 400 mg/day versus placebo showed that saffron slightly decreased some hematological parameters, such as red blood cell, hemoglobin, hematocrit, and platelet counts, but these measurements remained within normal ranges and were not clinically significant (Modaghegh et al. 2008). Consumption of saffron up to 1.5 g/day has not been associated with any adverse effects; however, doses higher than 5 g are toxic and doses of 20 g are lethal (Javadi et al. 2013). Saffron doses greater than 10 g have been used to induce abortion (Winterhalter and Straubinger 2000); therefore, saffron's use in pregnancy is not recommended.

Kava (Kava-Kava, *Piper methysticum*)

In traditional cultures, kava is used only ceremonially (i.e., not chronically) (Sarris 2017a). Kava has been studied for treatment of anxiety. A 2003 Cochrane review found that kava was more effective than placebo for treating anxiety; however, no comparisons against traditional anxiolytics were made (Pittler and Ernst 2003). A meta-analysis contained in the Pittler and Ernst (2003) review reported that 7 of the 12 RCTs that met its inclusion criteria showed that kava produced reductions in anxiety (as measured by Hamilton Anxiety Scale score) that were significantly greater ($P=0.01$) than reductions with placebo, demonstrating a strong clinical effect. In a 6-week comparison of kava with placebo for generalized anxiety disorder, the kava group had significant reductions in anxiety with no indications of hepatic dysfunction (Sarris et al. 2013). Long-term heavy use of kava can lead to facial swelling, scaly rash, dyspnea, low albumin levels, increased γ-glutamyltransferase, decreased white blood cell and platelet counts, hematuria, and pulmonary hypertension. Reports of kava hepatotoxicity, including 11 possible cases of liver failure, led to U.S. Food and Drug Administration (2002) warnings of potential liver injury. However, investigations revealed improper storage and the presence of a toxic mold as the cause, not the kava itself. In Australia and New Zealand, quality control of kava requires batch testing. Taking kava with alcohol, benzodiazepines, or muscle relaxants can result in coma. The use of kava is not recommended until more information is available on safety, efficacy, and quality.

Cannabis sativa

Cannabis sativa contains at least 144 cannabinoids in addition to 1,100 other compounds (Englund et al. 2017). The most abundant cannabinoids are Δ-9-tetrahydrocannabinol (THC) and cannabidiol (CBD), which the plant produces in varying ratios. The use of cannabis has been reported in the treatment of nausea (including nausea related to cancer or its treatment), anorexia, headaches, neuropathic pain, glaucoma, seizures, and muscle spasms (in patients with multiple sclerosis). The main adverse effects associated with cannabis are dependence, cognitive impairment, and psychosis (Englund et al. 2017). Over the past four decades, cannabis potency (percentage of THC) has doubled worldwide, whereas CBD concentrations have remained low or absent in most preparations. Preliminary evidence suggests that CBD can reverse or protect against the harmful effects of THC. In a study of 48 volunteers, pretreatment with 600 mg oral CBD before administration of 1–5 mg intravenous THC significantly reduced paranoia, psychotic symptoms, and cognitive impairment (Englund et al. 2013). The relative dose of CBD required to offset the negative effects of a given dose of THC is unknown. Increasing the concentration of CBD does not appear to alter the pleasurable effects of THC (e.g., feeling "stoned") (Haney et al. 2016). This finding is important, because consumers would reject safer products containing higher levels of CBD if the pleasurable, rewarding effects were lost (Lopez-Quintero et al. 2011). In 2017, the National Academies of Sciences, Engineering, and Medicine released a report on cannabis, noting the legalization of medical and recreational cannabis use in several states. They concluded,

However, despite this changing landscape, evidence regarding the short- and long-term health effects of cannabis use remains elusive. While a myriad of studies have examined cannabis use in all its various forms, often these research conclusions are not appropriately synthesized, translated for, or communicated to policy makers, health care providers, state health officials, or other stakeholders who have been charged with influencing and enacting policies, procedures, and laws related to cannabis use. (National Academies of Sciences, Engineering, and Medicine 2017, p. 25)

Hormones

Melatonin

In addition to its benefits in sleep disorders, melatonin has antioxidant properties and can be modestly helpful for tardive dyskinesia (Modabbernia 2017). Doses for sleep range from 0.5 to 10 mg; doses for tardive dyskinesia are 6–10 mg at night.

Mind–Body Modalities

Polyvagal Theory

The nervous system continuously monitors risk and safety. The assessment of danger versus safety shifts our autonomic state. Traditionally, the autonomic state was seen as being influenced by two opposing systems: the sympathetic ("fight or flight") and the parasympathetic ("rest and digest"). Polyvagal theory provides a more nuanced understanding of the autonomic system as a three-level hierarchical model of behavior, emotion, and cognition in which evolutionarily newer circuits inhibit phylogenetically older, more defensive circuits (Porges and Carter 2017). The newest circuit—unique to mammals—orchestrates states of social engagement and communication (e.g., facial expression, vocalization, listening). The optimal healthy state, when the animal feels safe, is associated with increased heart rate variability (HRV) (see "Breathing Practices" subsection later in this section); flexibility and adaptiveness; and the ability to love, bond, connect, feel soothed, and be cooperative (Table 37–1).

Humans and other mammals have two functionally distinct vagal circuits. One vagal circuit is phylogenetically older and unmyelinated. It originates in a brain-stem area called the *dorsal motor nucleus of the vagus*. The other vagal circuit is uniquely mammalian and myelinated. It originates in the brain-stem area called the *nucleus ambiguus*. The phylogenetically older unmyelinated vagal motor pathways are present in most vertebrates and, when not recruited as a defense system, function to support health, growth, and restoration via neural regulation of the subdiaphragmatic (below the diaphragm) organs. The "newer" mammalian myelinated vagal motor pathways regulate the supradiaphragmatic organs (heart and lungs). This newer vagal circuit, which slows heart rate and supports states of calmness, mediates the physiological state necessary for mind–body treatments to have positive effects. Provided that the organism feels safe, the newer circuit of social engagement will shut down or inactivate the phylogenetically older defensive states. The next level down is the defensive state of fight or flight, attributed to activation of the sympathetic nervous system,

TABLE 37–1. Neuroception of environmental conditions

Safety	Danger	Life threat
Parasympathetic system—Myelinated vagus	Sympathetic system	Parasympathetic system—Unmyelinated vagus
↑ Heart rate variability	↓ Heart rate variability	↓ Heart rate variability
↑ Body awareness	↓ Body awareness	↓ Body awareness
↑ Social engagement	↓ Social engagement	↓ Social engagement
Immobilization without fear	Mobilization	Immobilization with fear
Flexible and adaptive	Approach or withdrawal	Death-feign, collapse
Bond, connect, love, intimacy, soothing, healing, cooperative	Emotion dysregulation	Disconnect
	Hypervigilance	Dissociate
	Overactivity	
↑ Oxytocin	↑ Central vasopressin	↑ Peripheral vasopressin

Note. The polyvagal theory postulates three levels of autonomic response to perceived environmental conditions (Porges and Carter 2017). ↑=increased; ↓=decreased.

which we share with most vertebrates. Should "fighting" or "fleeing" fail to resolve the perceived danger, the oldest defense level (shared with reptiles) may become uninhibited, leading to the next level down, the "freeze" state of immobilization (feigning death when escape is not possible; dissociation; vasovagal syncope; behavioral shutdown). The theory is called *polyvagal* to highlight the coexistence of three vagal systems corresponding to the three evolutionary levels of development.

Porges coined the term *neuroception* to refer to the innate unconscious process of risk assessment (Porges 2004). Neuroception uses data from our environment, others around us, and signals from our own body to assess safety. Neuroception relies heavily on the vagus nerve, which has both sensory and motor fibers connecting the viscera to the brain. Polyvagal theory emphasizes that communication between brain and viscera is bidirectional. For example, feeling safe activates the autonomic state of spontaneous social interaction. Conversely, intimate social interactions can induce feelings of safety. The bidirectional influence is related not only to emotions but also to body states. Breathing rapidly can be interpreted by the neuroceptive process as a signal of danger. Conversely, a neuroceptive assessment of danger will create anxiety, thereby causing us to breathe quickly. By emphasizing the bidirectional communication between brain and viscera, polyvagal theory helps explain how mind–body practices can be used to our advantage to shift the autonomic state to one of safety. The most potent method for actively encouraging the neuroception of safety is through voluntarily regulated breathing practices (Gerbarg and Brown 2015).

Meditation

Among the many meditation practices in use, two general forms are focused attention and open monitoring. In focused-attention meditation, attention is typically focused on an anchor, such as breathing, a mantra, or an object. In open-monitoring meditation, attention is on open awareness and observation of environmental stimuli, thoughts, emotions, and physical sensations as they arise and as they pass. Focused attention and open monitoring are often combined during a single meditation session. Meditation can be practiced while sitting, while lying down, or while moving (e.g., walking meditation, yoga). In focused-attention meditation practiced during movement, attention is anchored in physical sensations as they occur with each step or pose.

Mindfulness

Mindfulness is a mental state in which attention is consciously focused on the present moment: internal stimuli (thoughts, emotions, proprioception, pain, and interoception); external stimuli (auditory, olfactory, and visual stimuli, as well as general awareness of the environment); and current motor behaviors. In the nonmindful state, the mind shifts automatically (as in "mind-wandering" or "autopilot"), and thoughts often relate to the past or the future (Marchand 2017). The goal of a mindfulness practice is to become skilled at recognizing when the autopilot state occurs and to shift back into the present moment. For many people, the seemingly simple state of awareness of the present is difficult to achieve.

Mindfulness-based interventions have been shown to be beneficial in the treatment of various psychiatric and substance use disorders. Mindfulness-type therapies include mindfulness-based stress reduction, mindfulness-based cognitive therapy, and mindfulness-based relapse prevention. Acceptance and commitment therapy and dialectical behavior therapy are often referred to as mindfulness-based approaches. The mechanism of action of mindfulness may be that focusing on the present allows us to step back from and be less identified with automatic thoughts and emotions, thereby reducing their power. Mindfulness requires dedication to the practice and thus is most appropriate for people who are highly motivated to practice regularly. Patients with psychosis are not good candidates for meditation or mindfulness, because psychotic thoughts may emerge during unstructured meditation.

Breathing Practices

Imbalances of the autonomic nervous system underlie and exacerbate stress-related conditions. Restoring sympathovagal balance and resiliency is fundamental to treatment of most disorders seen in psychiatric, pediatric, and general medical practices. The most efficient way to balance the sympathetic and parasympathetic branches of the autonomic nervous system is through voluntarily regulated breathing practices (VRBPs) (Brown and Gerberg 2012; Gerberg and Brown 2017). Breath and emotion are bidirectional. Each emotional state is associated with a particular breathing pattern. Conversely, by consciously changing the pattern of breath, one can shift emotional states.

Information from the respiratory system provides an enormous amount of data from millions of receptors (e.g., each alveolus contains three types of stretch receptors); bronchial, laryngeal, pharyngeal, and nasal passages; baroreceptors; chemoreceptors (registering changes in PO_2 and PCO_2); and receptors in the diaphragm, thoracic cavity, and chest wall. Every millisecond, respiratory information streams up vagal pathways to brain-stem nuclei and from there to central nervous system networks regulating emotion, perception, cognitive processing, and behavior. Evidence shows that slow breathing practices (through vagal afferents) can reduce overactivity in the amygdala, increase underactivity in prefrontal emotion regulatory centers, modulate hypothalamic-pituitary-adrenal function, increase levels of the inhibitory neurotransmitter GABA, stimulate oxytocin release, and improve cognitive function (Brown et al. 2013; Streeter et al. 2012). Respiratory sinus arrhythmia and HRV are derived mathematically from the normal changes in the cardiac beat-to-beat interval between inspiration and expiration (Gerberg and Brown 2017). These changes reflect the flexibility of the cardiovascular system. High respiratory sinus arrhythmia and high HRV are associated with better health and longevity. Low respiratory sinus arrhythmia and low HRV are associated with chronic stress, anxiety, panic disorder, posttraumatic stress disorder (PTSD), depression, and aging. The effects of paced breathing on respiratory sinus arrhythmia and HRV have been well documented. For most adults, gentle breathing at 4.5–6 cycles per minute significantly increases HRV (as indicated by HRV high-frequency spectra activity), leading to a calm state.

Slow VRBPs are the most useful clinically, because they can rapidly reduce the sympathetic overdrive associated with states of stress and anxiety while increasing parasympathetic activity. Studies show that slow VRBPs are associated with reduction in perceived stress, anxiety, insomnia, depression, and symptoms of PTSD (Brown et al. 2013; Gerberg and Brown 2017).

Yoga

In Indian tradition, yoga was originally designed as a spiritual practice for self-realization (Varambally and Gangadhar 2012). In the United States, yoga is a mind–body practice that combines physical postures, breathing techniques, and meditation or relaxation. Yoga is growing in popularity; according to the 2017 National Health Interview Survey, the use of yoga by U.S. adults has increased significantly in the past 5 years (from 9.5% in 2012 to 14.3% in 2017) (Black et al. 2018). In psychiatric practice, preliminary evidence suggests that yoga may be a safe and effective therapy whether used alone or adjunctively for depression, dysthymia, anxiety disorders, schizophrenia, alcohol use disorder, and ADHD of childhood (Cabral et al. 2011). An acute session of yoga has been shown to increase brain levels of GABA in healthy subjects (Streeter et al. 2007). Regular practice has been shown to reduce serum levels of cortisol and adrenocorticotropic hormone and to increase oxytocin in patients with schizophrenia (Jayaram et al. 2013). Methodological issues in yoga research include difficulty in double-blinding and finding a suitable placebo control for yoga. No consensus currently exists on which yoga school or tradition would be most helpful for a given condition.

Qigong/Tai Chi

Qigong is an ancient Chinese practice traditionally thought to cultivate and circulate the body's life force energy—*qi* (or *chi*)—via a series of orchestrated body movements, breathing techniques, vocalizations, and visualizations. Tai chi is a subtype of qigong. Comparative studies suggest that participation in qigong or tai chi may be more effective than conventional exercise for reducing anxiety, increasing frontal electroencephalographic theta-wave activity (indicating increased relaxation and mental focus), and maintaining a stable clinical dementia rating over 5 months (Abbott et al. 2017). Putative mechanisms of action include reduction of sympathetic output and decrease of inflammation.

Given that tai chi and qigong are low-intensity exercises that carry a minimal risk of adverse events, clinicians may consider recommending tai chi or qigong to any elderly patient who is motivated to practice a mind–body intervention. The movements of these practices are gentle, as participants are not required to lie down or contort into difficult postures. Because tai chi and qigong are often taught in groups, participation can provide a socialization benefit. Based on the average effective practice duration (dose) in the literature, clinicians should encourage patients to practice for a minimum of 30 minutes per session, three times a week.

Electromagnetic Treatments

Cranial Electrotherapy Stimulation

Cranial electrotherapy stimulation (CES) is FDA cleared for the treatment of anxiety, insomnia, and pain (Kirsch and Nichols 2013). The devices are benign-looking handheld units with two wired electrodes applied to opposite sides of the head (e.g., temples, mastoid process, or earlobes via clips). A mild electrical stimulation is delivered at a patented stimulus frequency pattern between 0.5 and 15,000 Hz at an intensity of 50 μA to 4 mA (using two AA batteries). Treatment is usually self-administered once or twice per day for 20–60 minutes. Functional magnetic resonance imaging studies of participants using CES indicate cortical deactivation (Feusner et al. 2012) and reduced pain processing (Taylor et al. 2013). Electroencephalograms show increased alpha brain-wave activity (indicating a relaxed but alert mental state) (Kennerly 2004). Adverse effects are rare (approximately 1%), mild, and self-limited, consisting mainly of skin irritation under the electrodes and headaches (Electromedical Products International 2012). In the United States, an FDA-cleared CES device costs between $600 and $1,200 and requires a prescription from a health care practitioner. Use of CES is contraindicated in patients with a cardiac pacemaker or other implanted electrical devices. CES safety in pregnancy has not been established.

Neurofeedback (Neurotherapy)

In biofeedback, patients are trained to become aware of and to learn to control their own physiology to improve physical and psychological health. Neurofeedback, a subspecialization of biofeedback (also called electroencephalographic biofeedback), uses the patient's electroencephalogram as feedback to modify the brain's electrical activity (Larsen and Sherlin 2013). Neurofeedback has been used for attention-deficit disorder/ADHD, epilepsy, anxiety disorders, depressive disorders, traumatic brain injury, alcohol and other substance use disorders, insomnia, and pain, as well as for enhancement of performance (Simkin et al. 2014). Neurofeedback protocols include operant conditioning, quantitative electroencephalography guided, z-score training, low-energy neurofeedback system, slow cortical potentials training, and NeuroField (NeuroField Inc., Bishop, CA). Neurofeedback usually involves 10–40 treatment sessions lasting 30–40 minutes each (typically 1–3 weekly sessions for 3–5 months). Several studies have reported persistence of benefit for up to 6 months after treatment (Gevensleben et al. 2010; Kouijzer et al. 2009; Steiner et al. 2014). Some patients may need additional periodic follow-up treatments. Treatment is best administered by a qualified professional who has received training from one of the neurofeedback organizations—the Association for Applied Psychophysiology and Biofeedback (www.aapb.org), the Biofeedback Certification International Alliance (www.bcia.org), or the International Society for Neurofeedback and Research (www.isnr.org).

Key Clinical Points

- Many patients with psychiatric disorders use complementary and alternative medicine (CAM) without telling their physicians. It is important for clinicians to ask their patients about CAM use to prevent adverse interactions between patients' medications and the supplements they may be taking.

- Studies do not support the use of vitamins B_9 (folic acid), B_{12}, or D as monotherapies for major depressive disorder. However, evidence indicates that supplementation with these nutrients can beneficially augment antidepressant treatment in patients with insufficiencies of these vitamins.

- Clinicians should provide patients with information about high-quality supplement brands, particularly those that are pharmaceutical grade or that have been tested in clinical trials.

- *S*-adenosylmethionine (SAMe) is effective as a monotherapy or an adjunctive treatment for major depressive disorder. SAMe does not cause many of the adverse effects of conventional antidepressants, such as sexual dysfunction, weight gain, or elevation of hepatic enzymes.

- Adaptogens can increase resilience to physical and emotional stress and may mitigate medication side effects such as extrapyramidal symptoms.

- Most herbs used in psychiatric practice do not have clinically significant cytochrome P450 (CYP) effects; the exception is St. John's wort (*Hypericum perforatum*), which induces CYP3A4.

- Polyvagal theory correlates the organism's perception of environmental safety or threat with the activation of three evolutionary hierarchical autonomic systems: unmyelinated parasympathetic, sympathetic, and myelinated parasympathetic. Mind–body modalities such as breathing practices can be used to shift the autonomic state to one of perceived safety.

- Voluntarily regulated breathing practices (VRBPs) can reduce overactivity in the amygdala, increase underactivity in prefrontal emotion regulatory centers, and modulate hypothalamic-pituitary-adrenal function. Preliminary evidence indicates that VRBPs also may increase levels of the inhibitory neurotransmitter γ-aminobutyric acid, stimulate oxytocin release, and improve cognitive function.

- Cranial electrotherapy stimulation and neurofeedback are valuable treatment options for anxiety, depression, pain, attention-deficit/hyperactivity disorder, and other conditions.

References

Abbott R, Chang DD, Eyre H, et al: Mind-body practices tai chi and qigong in the treatment and prevention of psychiatric disorders, in Complementary and Integrative Treatments in Psychiatric Practice. Edited by Gerbarg PL, Muskin PR, Brown RP. Arlington, VA, American Psychiatric Association Publishing, 2017, pp 261–280

Adair JC, Knoefel JE, Morgan N: Controlled trial of N-acetylcysteine for patients with probable Alzheimer's disease. Neurology 57(8):1515–1517, 2001 11673605

Akhondzadeh S, Kashani L: Saffron, passionflower, valerian, and sage for mental health, in Complementary and Integrative Treatments in Psychiatric Practice. Edited by Gerbarg PL, Muskin PR, Brown RP. Arlington, VA, American Psychiatric Association Publishing, 2017, pp 175–184

Akhondzadeh S, Shafiee Sabet M, Harirchian MH, et al: A 22-week, multicenter, randomized, double-blind controlled trial of Crocus sativus in the treatment of mild-to-moderate Alzheimer's disease. Psychopharmacology (Berl) 207(4):637–643, 2010 19838862

Akhondzadeh S, Gerbarg PL, Brown RP: Nutrients for prevention and treatment of mental health disorders. Psychiatr Clin North Am 36(1):25–36, 2013 2353807

Almeida OP, Ford AH, Flicker L: Systematic review and meta-analysis of randomized placebo-controlled trials of folate and vitamin B12 for depression. Int Psychogeriatr 27(5):727–737, 2015 25644193

Bella R, Biondi R, Raffaele R, Pennisi G: Effect of acetyl-L-carnitine on geriatric patients suffering from dysthymic disorders. Int J Clin Pharmacol Res 10(6):355–360, 1990 2099360

Berk M, Copolov D, Dean O, et al: N-acetyl cysteine as a glutathione precursor for schizophrenia—a double-blind, randomized, placebo-controlled trial. Biol Psychiatry 64(5):361–368, 2008 18436195

Bersani G, Meco G, Denaro A, et al: L-Acetylcarnitine in dysthymic disorder in elderly patients: a double-blind, multicenter, controlled randomized study vs. fluoxetine. Eur Neuropsychopharmacol 23(10):1219–1225, 2013 23428336

Black LI, Barnes PM, Clarke TC, et al: Use of yoga, meditation, and chiropractors among U.S. children aged 4–17 years. NCHS Data Brief, No. 324. Hyattsville, MD, National Center for Health Statistics, November 2018. Available at: https://www.cdc.gov/nchs/data/databriefs/db324-h.pdf. Accessed January 18, 2019.

Bloch MH, Panza KE, Grant JE, et al: N-Acetylcysteine in the treatment of pediatric trichotillomania: a randomized, double-blind, placebo-controlled add-on trial. J Am Acad Child Adolesc Psychiatry 52(3):231–240, 2013 23452680

Bottiglieri T: Folate, vitamin B12, and S-adenosylmethionine. Psychiatr Clin North Am 36(1):1–3, 2013 23538072

Brichenko VS, Kupriyanova IE, Skorokhodova TF: The use of herbal adaptogens together with tricyclic antidepressants in patients with psychogenic depressions, in Modern Problems of Pharmacology and Search for New Medicines, Vol 2. Edited by Goldsberg ED. Tomsk, Russia, Tomsk State University Press, 1986, pp 58–60

Brown RP, Gerbarg PL: The Healing Power of the Breath. Boulder, CO, Shambhala Press, 2012

Brown RP, Gerbarg PL, Muench F: Breathing practices for treatment of psychiatric and stress-related medical conditions. Psychiatr Clin North Am 36(1):121–140, 2013 23538082

Cabral P, Meyer HB, Ames D: Effectiveness of yoga therapy as a complementary treatment for major psychiatric disorders: a meta-analysis. Prim Care Companion CNS Disord 13(4), 2011 22132353

Christakos S, Hewison M, Gardner DG, et al: Vitamin D: beyond bone. Ann N Y Acad Sci 1287:45–58, 2013 23682710

Clarke TC, Black LI, Stussman BJ, et al: Trends in the use of complementary health approaches among adults: United States, 2002–2012. Natl Health Stat Rep (79):1–16, 2015 25671660

Darbinyan V, Aslanyan G, Amroyan E, et al: Clinical trial of Rhodiola rosea L. extract SHR-5 in the treatment of mild to moderate depression. Nord J Psychiatry 61(5):343–348, 2007 [Erratum in: Nord J Psychiatry 61(6):503, 2007] 17990195

Diamond BJ, Mondragon A: Ginkgo biloba: psychiatric indications, mechanisms, and safety, in Complementary and Integrative Treatments in Psychiatric Practice. Edited by Gerbarg PL, Muskin PR, Brown RP. Arlington, VA, American Psychiatric Association Publishing, 2017, pp 149–156

Dording CM, Fisher L, Papakostas G, et al: A double-blind, randomized, pilot dose-finding study of maca root (L. meyenii) for the management of SSRI-induced sexual dysfunction. CNS Neurosci Ther 14(3):182–191, 2008 18801111

Electromedical Products International: Cranial electrotherapy stimulator (CES) safety data submitted to FDA Neurologic Devices Panel, February 10, 2012. Available at: https://www.pharmamedtechbi.com/~/media/Supporting%20Documents/The%20Gray%20Sheet/38/7/FDA_Executive_Summary.pdf. Accessed January 18, 2019.

Englund A, Morrison PD, Nottage J, et al: Cannabidiol inhibits THC-elicited paranoid symptoms and hippocampal-dependent memory impairment. J Psychopharmacol 27(1):19–27, 2013 23042808

Englund A, Freeman TP, Murray RM, et al: Can we make cannabis safer? Lancet Psychiatry 4(8):643–648, 2017 28259650

Farokhnia M, Azarkolah A, Adinehfar F, et al: N-acetylcysteine as an adjunct to risperidone for treatment of negative symptoms in patients with chronic schizophrenia: a randomized, double-blind, placebo-controlled study. Clin Neuropharmacol 36(6):185–192, 2013 24201233

Farokhnia M, Shafiee Sabet M, Iranpour N, et al: Comparing the efficacy and safety of Crocus sativus L. with memantine in patients with moderate to severe Alzheimer's disease: a double-blind randomized clinical trial. Hum Psychopharmacol 29(4):351–359, 2014 25163440

Feusner JD, Madsen S, Moody TD, et al: Effects of cranial electrotherapy stimulation on resting state brain activity. Brain Behav 2(3):211–220, 2012 22741094

Garzya G, Corallo D, Fiore A, et al: Evaluation of the effects of L-acetylcarnitine on senile patients suffering from depression. Drugs Exp Clin Res 16(2):101–106, 1990 2205455

Gauthier S, Schlaefke S: Efficacy and tolerability of Ginkgo biloba extract EGb 761 in dementia: a systematic review and meta-analysis of randomized placebo-controlled trials. Clin Interv Aging 9:2065–2077, 2014 25506211

Gecele M, Francesetti G, Meluzzi A: Acetyl-L-carnitine in aged subjects with major depression: clinical efficacy and effects on the circadian rhythm of cortisol. Dementia and Geriatric Cognitive Disorders 2(6):333–337, 1991

Geng J, Dong J, Ni H, et al: Ginseng for cognition. Cochrane Database Syst Rev (12):CD007769, 2010 21154383

Gerbarg PL, Brown RP: Phytomedicines for prevention and treatment of mental health disorders. Psychiatr Clin North Am 36(1):37–47, 2013 23538075

Gerbarg PL, Brown RP: Breathing practices for mental health and aging, in Complementary and Integrative Therapies for Mental Health and Aging. Edited by Lavretsky H, Sajatovic M, Reynolds III C. New York, Oxford University Press, 2015, pp 239–256

Gerbarg A, Brown R: Breathing techniques in psychiatric treatment, in Complementary and Integrative Treatments in Psychiatric Practice. Edited by Gerbarg PL, Muskin PR, Brown RP. Arlington, VA, American Psychiatric Association Publishing, 2017, pp 241–250

Gerbarg PL, Muskin PR, Brown RP (eds): Complementary and Integrative Treatments in Psychiatric Practice. Arlington, VA, American Psychiatric Association Publishing, 2017

Gevensleben H, Holl B, Albrecht B, et al: Neurofeedback training in children with ADHD: 6-month follow-up of a randomised controlled trial. Eur Child Adolesc Psychiatry 19(9):715–724, 2010 20499120

Ghanizadeh A, Moghimi-Sarani E: A randomized double blind placebo controlled clinical trial of N-acetylcysteine added to risperidone for treating autistic disorders. BMC Psychiatry 13:196, 2013 23886027

Ghanizadeh A, Derakhshan N, Berk M: N-acetylcysteine versus placebo for treating nail biting, a double blind randomized placebo controlled clinical trial. Antiinflamm Antiallergy Agents Med Chem 12(3):223–228, 2013 23651231

Gonzales GF: Ethnobiology and ethnopharmacology of Lepidium meyenii (Maca), a plant from the Peruvian highlands. Evid Based Complement Alternat Med 2012:193496, 2012 21977053

Grant JE, Odlaug BL, Kim SW: N-acetylcysteine, a glutamate modulator, in the treatment of trichotillomania: a double-blind, placebo-controlled study. Arch Gen Psychiatry 66(7):756–763, 2009 19581567

Haney M, Malcolm RJ, Babalonis S, et al: Oral cannabidiol does not alter the subjective, reinforcing or cardiovascular effects of smoked cannabis. Neuropsychopharmacology 41(8):1974–1982, 2016 26708108

Hardan AY, Fung LK, Libove RA, et al: A randomized controlled pilot trial of oral N-acetylcysteine in children with autism. Biol Psychiatry 71(11):956–961, 2012 22342106

Heard KJ: Acetylcysteine for acetaminophen poisoning. N Engl J Med 359(3):285–292, 2008 18635433

Ihl R, Bachinskaya N, Korczyn AD, et al; GOTADAY Study Group: Efficacy and safety of a once-daily formulation of Ginkgo biloba extract EGb 761 in dementia with neuropsychiatric features: a randomized controlled trial. Int J Geriatr Psychiatry 26(11):1186–1194, 2011 21140383

Javadi B, Sahebkar A, Emami SA: A survey on saffron in major Islamic traditional medicine books. Iran J Basic Med Sci 16(1):1–11, 2013 23638288

Jayaram N, Varambally S, Behere RV, et al: Effect of yoga therapy on plasma oxytocin and facial emotion recognition deficits in patients of schizophrenia. Indian J Psychiatry 55 (suppl 3):S409–S413, 2013 24049210

Kennel KA, Drake MT, Hurley DL: Vitamin D deficiency in adults: when to test and how to treat. Mayo Clin Proc 85(8):752–757; quiz 757–758, 2010 20675513

Kennerly R: QEEG analysis of cranial electrotherapy: a pilot study (Student Scholarship Presentation Abstract). Journal of Neurotherapy: Investigations in Neuromodulation, Neurofeedback and Applied Neuroscience 8(2):112, 2004. Available at: http://www.isnr-jnt.org/article/view/16964/10886. Accessed January 18, 2019.

Kirsch DL, Nichols F: Cranial electrotherapy stimulation for treatment of anxiety, depression, and insomnia. Psychiatr Clin North Am 36(1):169–176, 2013 23538086

Kouijzer ME, de Moor JM, Gerrits BJ, et al: Long-term effects of neurofeedback treatment in autism. Research in Autism Spectrum Disorders 3(2):496–501, 2009

Larsen S, Sherlin L: Neurofeedback: an emerging technology for treating central nervous system dysregulation. Psychiatr Clin North Am 36(1):163–168, 2013 23538085

Li G, Mbuagbaw L, Samaan Z, et al: Efficacy of vitamin D supplementation in depression in adults: a systematic review. J Clin Endocrinol Metab 99(3):757–767, 2014 24423304

Linde K, Berner MM, Kriston L: St John's wort for major depression. Cochrane Database Syst Rev (4):CD000448, 2008 18843608

Lopez-Quintero C, Pérez de los Cobos J, Hasin DS, et al: Probability and predictors of transition from first use to dependence on nicotine, alcohol, cannabis, and cocaine: results of the National Epidemiologic Survey on Alcohol and Related Conditions (NESARC). Drug Alcohol Depend 115(1–2):120–130, 2011 21145178

Marchand WR: Mindfulness and meditation in psychiatric practice, in Complementary and Integrative Treatments in Psychiatric Practice. Edited by Gerbarg PL, Muskin PR, Brown RP. Arlington, VA, American Psychiatric Association Publishing, 2017, pp 281–292

Massoumi L: The growth of complementary and integrative medicine in psychiatric practice, in Complementary and Integrative Treatments in Psychiatric Practice. Edited by Gerbarg PL, Muskin PR, Brown RP. Arlington, VA, American Psychiatric Association Publishing, 2017a, pp 3–8

Massoumi L: Panax ginseng and American ginseng in psychiatric practice, in Complementary and Integrative Treatments in Psychiatric Practice. Edited by Gerbarg PL, Muskin PR, Brown RP. Arlington, VA, American Psychiatric Association Publishing, 2017b, pp 163–168

Mischoulon D, Freeman MP: Omega-3 fatty acids in psychiatry. Psychiatr Clin North Am 36(1):15–23, 2013 23538073

Modabbernia A: Melatonin and melatonin analogues for psychiatric disorders, in Complementary and Integrative Treatments in Psychiatric Practice. Edited by Gerbarg PL, Muskin PR, Brown RP. Arlington, VA, American Psychiatric Association Publishing, 2017, pp 211–220

Modaghegh MH, Shahabian M, Esmaeili HA, et al: Safety evaluation of saffron (Crocus sativus) tablets in healthy volunteers. Phytomedicine 15(12):1032–1037, 2008 18693099

Montgomery SA, Thal LJ, Amrein R: Meta-analysis of double blind randomized controlled clinical trials of acetyl-L-carnitine versus placebo in the treatment of mild cognitive impairment and mild Alzheimer's disease. Int Clin Psychopharmacol 18(2):61–71, 2003 12598816

Nasca D, Zurria G, Aguglia E: Action of acetyl-L-carnitine in association with mianserine on depressed old people. New Trends in Clinical Neuropharmacology 3:225–230, 1989

National Academies of Sciences, Engineering, and Medicine: The Health Effects of Cannabis and Cannabinoids: The Current State of Evidence and Recommendations for Research. Washington, DC, National Academies Press, 2017

National Center for Complementary and Integrative Health: The Use of Complementary and Alternative Medicine in the United States: Cost Data. Hyattsville, MD, National Center for Complementary and Integrative Health, 2018. Available at: https://nccih.nih.gov/news/camstats/costs/costdatafs.htm. Accessed September 10, 2018.

Nikoo M, Radnia H, Farokhnia M, et al: N-acetylcysteine as an adjunctive therapy to risperidone for treatment of irritability in autism: a randomized, double-blind, placebo-controlled clinical trial of efficacy and safety. Clin Neuropharmacol 38(1):11–17, 2015 25580916

Panossian AG: Adaptogens in mental and behavioral disorders. Psychiatr Clin North Am 36(1):49–64, 2013 23538076

Panossian A, Amsterdam JD: Adaptogens in psychiatric practice, in Complementary and Integrative Treatments in Psychiatric Practice. Edited by Gerberg PL, Muskin PR, Brown RP. Arlington, VA, American Psychiatric Association Publishing, 2017, pp 113–134

Pittler MH, Ernst E: Kava extract for treating anxiety. Cochrane Database Syst Rev (1):CD003383, 2003 12535473

Porges SW: Neuroception: a subconscious system for detecting threats and safety. Zero to Three 24(5):19–24, 2004. Available at: https://eric.ed.gov/?id=EJ938225. Accessed January 18, 2019.

Porges SW, Carter CS: Polyvagal theory and the social engagement system, in Complementary and Integrative Treatments in Psychiatric Practice. Edited by Gerberg PL, Muskin PR, Brown RP. Arlington, VA, American Psychiatric Association Publishing, 2017, pp 221–240

Rylander M, Verhulst S: Vitamin D insufficiency in psychiatric inpatients. J Psychiatr Pract 19(4):296–300, 2013 23852104

Saratikov AS, Krasnov EA: Rhodiola Rosea Is a Valuable Medicinal Plant (Golden Root). Tomsk, Russia: Tomsk State University Press, 1987

Sarris J: Kava (Piper methysticum) in the treatment of anxiety, in Complementary and Integrative Treatments in Psychiatric Practice. Edited by Gerberg PL, Muskin PR, Brown RP. Arlington, VA, American Psychiatric Association Publishing, 2017a, pp 157–162

Sarris J: St. John's wort (Hypericum perforatum) in the treatment of depression, in Complementary and Integrative Treatments in Psychiatric Practice. Edited by Gerberg PL, Muskin PR, Brown RP. Arlington, VA, American Psychiatric Association Publishing, 2017b, pp 143–148

Sarris J, Stough C, Bousman CA, et al: Kava in the treatment of generalized anxiety disorder: a double-blind, randomized, placebo-controlled study. J Clin Psychopharmacol 33(5):643–648, 2013 23635869

Sarris J, Murphy J, Mischoulon D, et al: Adjunctive nutraceuticals for depression: a systematic review and meta-analyses. Am J Psychiatry 173(6):575–587, 2016 27113121

Shaffer JA, Edmondson D, Wasson LT, et al: Vitamin D supplementation for depressive symptoms: a systematic review and meta-analysis of randomized controlled trials. Psychosom Med 76(3):190–196, 2014 24632894

Sharma A, Gerberg P, Bottiglieri T, et al: S-Adenosylmethionine (SAMe) for neuropsychiatric disorders: a clinician-oriented review of research. J Clin Psychiatry 78(6):e656–e667, 2017 28682528

Simkin DR, Thatcher RW, Lubar J: Quantitative EEG and neurofeedback in children and adolescents: anxiety disorders, depressive disorders, comorbid addiction and attention-deficit/hyperactivity disorder, and brain injury. Child Adolesc Psychiatr Clin N Am 23(3):427–464, 2014 24975621

Steiner NJ, Frenette EC, Rene KM, et al: In-school neurofeedback training for ADHD: sustained improvements from a randomized control trial. Pediatrics 133(3):483–492, 2014 24534402

Streeter CC, Jensen JE, Perlmutter RM, et al: Yoga Asana sessions increase brain GABA levels: a pilot study. J Altern Complement Med 13(4):419–426, 2007 17532734

Streeter CC, Gerberg PL, Saper RB, et al: Effects of yoga on the autonomic nervous system, gamma-aminobutyric-acid, and allostasis in epilepsy, depression, and post-traumatic stress disorder. Med Hypotheses 78(5):571–579, 2012 22365651

Sudakov VN, Savinykh AB, Agapov YK: The role of adaptogens in the psychoprophylaxis of patients with borderline states of exogenous-organic genesis, in Modern Problems of Pharmacology and Search for New Medicines, Vol 2. Edited by Goldsberg ED. Tomsk, Russia, Tomsk State University Press, 1986, pp 298–330

Taylor AG, Anderson JG, Riedel SL, et al: A randomized, controlled, double-blind pilot study of the effects of cranial electrical stimulation on activity in brain pain processing regions in individuals with fibromyalgia. Explore (NY) 9(1):32–40, 2013 23294818

Tripkovic L, Lambert H, Hart K, et al: Comparison of vitamin D2 and vitamin D3 supplementation in raising serum 25-hydroxyvitamin D status: a systematic review and meta-analysis. Am J Clin Nutr 95(6):1357–1364, 2012 22552031

U.S. Food and Drug Administration: Letter to Health Care Professionals: FDA Issues Consumer Advisory That Kava Products May Be Associated With Severe Liver Injury. Rockville, MD, U.S. Food and Drug Administration, March 25, 2002

Varambally S, Gangadhar BN: Yoga: a spiritual practice with therapeutic value in psychiatry. Asian J Psychiatr 5(2):186–189, 2012 22813667

Villardita C, Smirni P, Vecchio I: Acetyl-L-carnitine in depressed geriatric patients. European Review for Medical and Pharmacological Sciences 6:1–2, 1983

Wang SM, Pae CU: Acetyl-L-carnitine, N-acetylcysteine, and inositol in the treatment of psychiatric and neuropsychiatric disorders, in Complementary and Integrative Treatments in Psychiatric Practice. Edited by Gerbarg PL, Muskin PR, Brown RP. Arlington, VA, American Psychiatric Association Publishing, 2017, pp 53–73

Winterhalter P, Straubinger M: Saffron—renewed interest in an ancient spice. Food Reviews International 16(1):39–59, 2000

Zanardi R, Smeraldi E: A double-blind, randomised, controlled clinical trial of acetyl-L-carnitine vs. amisulpride in the treatment of dysthymia. Eur Neuropsychopharmacol 16(4):281–287, 2006 16316746

Recommended Readings

Brown RP, Gerbarg PL: The Healing Power of the Breath. Boulder, CO, Shambhala Press, 2012

Brown RP, Gerbarg PL, Muskin PR: How to Use Herbs, Nutrients, and Yoga in Mental Health Care. New York, WW Norton, 2009

Gerbarg PL, Muskin PR, Brown RP (eds): Complementary and Integrative Treatments in Psychiatric Practice. Arlington, VA, American Psychiatric Association Publishing, 2017

Knotkova H, Rasche D: Textbook of Neuromodulation. New York, Springer-Verlag, 2016

Muskin PR, Gerbarg PL, Brown RP: Complementary and Integrative Therapies for Psychiatric Disorders, An Issue of Psychiatric Clinics, Vol 36–1. London, Elsevier Health Sciences, 2013

Online Resources

American Psychiatric Association Caucus on Complementary and Integrative Psychiatry: https://www.intpsychiatry.com

Information on supplement efficacy: https://examine.com

Information on supplement quality: https://www.consumerlab.com

National Center for Complementary and Integrative Health (NCCIH): https://nccih.nih.gov

CHAPTER 38

Integrated and Collaborative Care

Ramanpreet Toor, M.D.

Deborah S. Cowley, M.D.

Mental disorders are responsible for significant morbidity and mortality, accounting for about 25% of disability worldwide (Murray et al. 2012). However, in the United States, only 12% of people with psychiatric disorders see a psychiatrist, and only 21% see any mental health specialist (Wang et al. 2005). Most people do not seek any medical care, and of those who do, more than half are seen in general medical settings, which have a low rate of adequate mental health care (Unützer and Ratzliff 2015). Access to specialty mental health care is poor, and only about half of the patients referred from primary care to specialty mental health care follow through with the referral (Grembowski et al. 2002). At the same time, patients with chronic severe mental illness have shorter life spans and higher rates of chronic medical conditions, primarily as a result of socioeconomic factors, side effects of psychotropic medications, and limited access to effective primary and preventive health care (Druss et al. 2011). These gaps in access to and quality of care have led to efforts to integrate behavioral and general medical services so as to improve both mental health and medical outcomes for patients.

Integrated behavioral health care has been defined as "the care that results from a practice team of primary care and behavioral health clinicians, working together with patients and families, using a systematic and cost-effective approach to provide patient-centered care for a defined population" (Peek and The National Integration Academy Council 2013, p. 2). This approach to care "may address mental health and substance abuse conditions, health behaviors (including their contribution to chronic medical illnesses), life stressors and crises, stress-related physical symptoms, and ineffective patterns of health care utilization" (Peek and The National Integration Academy Council 2013, p. 2). Studies of integrated care have confirmed the effectiveness of this approach in addressing the triple aim of improving access to care, improving quality and outcomes of care, and reducing total health care costs (Katon and Unützer 2011). The alignment of integrated care with patient-centered medical homes, accountable care organizations, and the Affordable Care Act has led to increased focus on this model of care over the past decade, and the American Psychiatric Association (2017) has both advocated for training in integrated care for medical students, residents, and fellows (Summers et al. 2014) and implemented such training for practicing psychiatrists.

Given the evidence base for and large-scale implementation of integrated care, there are increasing opportunities and needs for psychiatrists to work in this area. In this chapter, we describe models of integrated care, focusing primarily on the collaborative care model, which is the integrated care model with the strongest evidence base. We outline the core principles of collaborative care, some of which are applicable to enhancing any type of psychiatric practice, and discuss the psychiatrist's role within integrated care and a collaborative care team.

Models of Integrated Care

Integrated care delivery has several models, including colocation of a psychiatrist within a general medical setting (colocated care), collaborative care, telepsychiatry, and provision of general medical services to psychiatric patients with chronic severe mental illnesses. The target population, personnel, methods, advantages, and limitations of these various models are summarized in Table 38–1.

In colocated care, the psychiatrist or other behavioral health care specialist spends time within a general medical clinic and provides on-site consultation and direct care to patients referred by clinic providers. This model increases access, patient satisfaction, and communication and interaction between providers and improves outcomes for individual patients (van der Feltz-Cornelis et al. 2010). However, patients referred may be those most obviously distressed rather than those who most need specialty mental health care services, and once the service is well established, the on-site psychiatrist or behavioral health specialist often has a long wait list and limited availability for new referrals or follow-up appointments.

In contrast, collaborative care is a population-based model that uses systematic mental health screening of the clinic or health system population to identify patients for further diagnostic evaluation and evidence-based treatment. The psychiatrist serves as a consultant to the primary care provider and a behavioral health care provider or care manager, tracking outcomes of the care manager's caseload and focusing on patients who are not improving with first-line treatments, making further treatment recommendations to "step up" care as indicated, and seeing the patient for a direct consultation only as needed. For example, in the Improving Mood-Promoting Access to Collaborative Treatment (IMPACT) study treating late-life depression, the largest study of collaborative care to date, psychiatrists provided direct consultation for diagnostic clarification or treatment-refractory symptoms for only 11% of the patients in the intervention group (Unützer et al. 2002).

Collaborative care is supported by a substantial evidence base. For example, a review of 79 randomized controlled trials of collaborative care for depression and anxiety found significantly greater improvement in short- and long-term outcomes as well as benefits in terms of medication use, mental health quality of life, and patient

TABLE 38–1. Models of integrated care

	Colocated care	Collaborative care	Telepsychiatry	Medical care for psychiatric patients
Target population	Patients referred by primary care providers	Clinic or health system patient population	Providers or patients at distant sites or unable to come in person	Psychiatric patients, especially in community mental health
Personnel	Consulting psychiatrist or behavioral health specialist	Team of patient, primary care provider, care manager, psychiatrist	Psychiatrist or other mental health specialist	General medical provider
Methods	Direct (in-person) consultation	Population-based screening; team provides patient-centered and evidence-based interventions, outcome measurement, stepped care	Direct or indirect consultation by telephone or videoconferencing	Preventive and primary medical care delivered within psychiatric treatment setting
Advantages	Improved access, patient satisfaction, provider interactions, outcomes for referred patients	Improved access, care quality, population outcomes, cost-effectiveness	Improved access for smaller/rural areas, patients who are unable to come to appointments	Improved access to medical care
Limitations	Limited capacity; treats only referred patients	Requires changes in practice; varying reimbursement	Requires specialized equipment; varying reimbursement	Need for medical providers in mental health setting or psychiatrists providing medical care

satisfaction (Archer et al. 2012). Collaborative care also has resulted in improved outcomes for patients with opioid and alcohol use disorders (Watkins et al. 2017) and has reduced health care disparities in engagement in and response to treatment for depression (Angstman et al. 2015). In addition, a form of collaborative care adapted for patients with depression and comorbid medical conditions (diabetes and coronary heart disease) produced reductions in depression scores, systolic blood pressure, cholesterol levels, and glycated hemoglobin levels, as well as improvements in quality of life and satisfaction with care, in comparison with usual care (Katon et al. 2010), and was cost-effective (Katon et al. 2012).

Telepsychiatry has particular advantages in increasing access to mental health care for patients and their providers in smaller or rural communities and for patients who have difficulty coming in person to see a psychiatrist because of agoraphobia, physical disability, or lack of transportation. Telepsychiatry, including telephone and videoconferencing methodologies, can be used to provide education and consultation to providers, directly evaluate patients, and implement collaborative care in small or remote primary care practices. For example, pediatric access lines (Straus and Sarvet 2014) and perinatal psychiatry consultation lines (Byatt et al. 2016) provide specialized telephone consultation and education to primary care providers in the areas of child and adolescent psychiatry and treatment of pregnant and postpartum women, and Fortney et al. (2013) showed that a telemedicine-based collaborative care intervention for depression was superior to collaborative care delivered by local on-site staff in five rural federally qualified health centers.

Finally, several models have been proposed for improving general medical care for psychiatric patients (Kern 2015). These include education of psychiatrists in screening for and first-line treatment of common medical conditions, inclusion of care managers within community mental health centers to coach patients on how to make and navigate primary care appointments, addressing health behaviors with psychiatric patients, and colocation of a general medical provider within a community mental health setting.

Principles of Collaborative Care

Because collaborative care is the integrated care model that to date has the strongest evidence supporting its effectiveness, it is the focus of the remainder of this chapter. In 2011, a national expert panel convened by the Advancing Integrated Mental Health Solutions (AIMS) Center at the University of Washington developed a consensus statement regarding five core principles, all of which are required for effective collaborative care (Unützer and Ratzliff 2015):

1. *Patient-centered collaboration:* Collaborative care teams work together to provide patient-centered care. The team includes the informed patient, who participates actively in his or her care; the primary care provider; the care manager; and a psychiatric consultant. Team providers support the patient in achieving a shared treatment goal. For the team to collaborate successfully in providing excellent care, each team member must have a very clear role. These roles are described in detail later in this chapter.

2. *Population-based care:* Traditional psychiatric practice, like other forms of medical practice, focuses on the patient who presents for care. In contrast, collaborative care is population based. In population-based care, the focus is on a defined population, such as all individuals served by a particular primary care clinic, medical center, or health care system. Patients within the defined population are screened, and those identified as having a psychiatric disorder are treated, tracked in a comprehensive database (referred to as a registry; Figure 38–1), and monitored for adherence to treatment and clinical outcomes. The registry includes patient information, each patient's initial and last score on relevant symptom rating scales such as the Patient Health Questionnaire–9 (PHQ-9) for depression (Kroenke et al. 2001) and the Generalized Anxiety Disorder 7-item (GAD-7) scale for anxiety (Spitzer et al. 2006), assessments by the care manager, and psychiatric consultation notes. The registry allows the care manager and psychiatric consultant to keep track of all patients in treatment and to rapidly identify those who are not doing well or who are not following up with appointments. The care manager has the primary responsibility of monitoring and updating the registry and reviews the list weekly with the psychiatric consultant so that timely treatment adjustments can be made for patients who are not improving. The care manager also reaches out to patients who are not following up.

3. *Evidence-based care:* Treatments delivered in collaborative care use the best available evidence. The psychiatric consultant provides evidence-based medication recommendations, whereas the care manager is trained in and delivers evidence-based brief psychotherapy interventions. These interventions include behavioral activation, cognitive-behavioral therapy, interpersonal therapy, motivational interviewing, and problem-solving treatment (a skills-building treatment for depression used in primary care and community settings).

4. *Measurement-based treatment to target:* Measurement-based treatment to target is an approach familiar to psychiatrists from the Sequenced Treatment Alternatives to Relieve Depression (STAR*D) trial (Rush 2007). The collaborative care team establishes a patient-centered treatment goal for each person who is identified as having a mental health condition. Patients are then systematically tracked with the help of outcome measures, such as symptom rating scales, and timely treatment adjustments are made until the predefined goal is achieved. For example, a common goal in the treatment of depression is a PHQ-9 score less than 10 or a 50% reduction in the PHQ-9 score. A depressed patient with this kind of goal would complete the PHQ-9 at every visit with the care manager. Some patients respond to initial first-line treatments, whereas others may require additional interventions to reach treatment goals. Collaborative care uses a stepped-care model, progressively increasing the intensity and number of treatments (e.g., increasing dosages, changing medications, adding augmentation agents and/or psychosocial interventions) as needed, depending on the patient's response.

5. *Accountability:* All of the other principles described here must be in place to support the core principle of accountability. *Accountability* refers to the fact that the psychiatric consultants within collaborative care teams take responsibility both for the treatment outcomes of patients in their identified population who are active in treatment and for continuous improvement in the overall quality of care provided by their team.

View Record	Treatment Status	Name	Date of Initial Assessment	Date of Most Recent Contact	Date Next Follow-up Due	Number of Follow-up Contacts	Weeks in Treatment	PHQ-9				GAD-7				Psychiatric Case Review	
								Initial PHQ-9 Score	Last Available PHQ-9 Score	% Change in PHQ-9 Score	Date of Last PHQ-9 Score	Initial GAD-7 Score	Last Available GAD-7 Score	% Change in GAD-7 Score	Date of Last GAD-7 Score	Flag	Most Recent Psychiatric Case Review Note
View	Active	Nancy Fake	5/29/2017	5/29/2017	6/12/2017	0	6	No Score	No Score			No Score	No Score				
View	RP	Betty Test	12/15/2016	5/15/2017	6/14/2017	10	30	12	1	-92%	5/15/2017	9	3	-67%	5/15/2017		
View	Active	Susan Test	11/20/2016	6/2/2017	6/16/2017	10	33	22	15	-32%	6/2/2017	18	14	-22%	6/2/2017	Flag for discussion & safety risk	9/15/2016
View	Active	Bob Dolittle	3/2/2017	7/1/2017	7/15/2017	3	19	22	19	-14%	7/1/2017	12	10	-17%	7/1/2017	Flag as safety risk	9/17/2016
View	Active	Joe Smith	4/1/2017	7/11/2017	7/25/2017	6	14	15	8	-47%	7/11/2017	11	4	-64%	7/11/2017		10/24/2016
View	Active	Albert Smith	3/5/2017	6/30/2017	7/28/2017	5	18	18	18	0%	6/30/2017	14	10	-29%	6/30/2017	Flag for discussion	

Treatment Status note: The most recent contact was over 1 month (30 days) ago. The next follow-up contact is past due.

PHQ-9 note: The last available PHQ-9 score is at target (<5 or 50% decrease from initial score). The last available PHQ-9 score is more than 30 days old.

GAD-7 note: The last available GAD-7 score is at target (<10 or 50% decrease from initial score). The last available GAD-7 score is more than 30 days old.

FIGURE 38–1.   Example of a collaborative care registry.

Note.   GAD-7=Generalized Anxiety Disorder 7-item scale; PHQ-9=Patient Health Questionnaire 9-item depression scale.

Source.   Reprinted from AIMS (Advancing Integrated Mental Health Solutions) Center web page "Patient Tracking Spreadsheet With Example Data" (available at: https://aims.uw.edu/resource-library/patient-tracking-spreadsheet-example-data; accessed October 7, 2018). Copyright 2018, University of Washington. Used with permission.

Collaborative Care Team

In the collaborative care model, mental health care providers work together with primary care providers and the patient as a team. A collaborative care team consists of the patient and at least a primary care provider, a care manager or behavioral health care provider, and a psychiatric consultant (Figure 38–2). Each team member has a clear role in order to coordinate care most effectively (Ratzliff et al. 2016):

- *Patient:* In collaborative care, the patient is an active team member who works with other members of the team to establish treatment goals, reports symptoms and side effects, asks questions and raises concerns, and engages in treatment.
- *Primary care provider:* The primary care provider, usually a family physician, internist, pediatrician, nurse practitioner, or physician assistant, has the most established relationship with and is the first contact for the patient. This provider retains the overall responsibility of overseeing all aspects of care provided to the patient. He or she has several important roles, including identifying patients who need behavioral health treatment, doing the initial assessment, starting appropriate first-line treatment, introducing the collaborative care model to the patient, and referring the patient to the care manager for further assessment and treatment. The primary care provider works with the rest of the team to develop shared treatment goals, monitor treatment response, and encourage the patient to engage in collaborative care. The primary care provider prescribes medications, orders laboratory tests, and adjusts treatment in consultation with the care manager and psychiatric consultant.
- *Care manager or behavioral health care provider:* Care managers are typically licensed social workers, registered nurses, or psychologists. They are usually located in the primary care clinic but may be off-site, especially in rural areas with fewer patients and staff (Fortney et al. 2013). They work closely with the primary care provider and psychiatric consultant to provide mental health care to patients.

  The care manager has two main roles. The first is care management, which includes engaging the patient in treatment, seeing the patient every 2 weeks, performing systematic initial and follow-up assessments, coordinating the care being provided to the patient, adding the patient to the registry, maintaining and updating the registry, tracking the treatment response of the patient with behavioral health measures, and regularly reviewing the caseload with the psychiatric consultant, usually on a weekly basis. The focus of these caseload reviews is on patients who are not improving, are diagnostically challenging, or are not coming to appointments. The second major function of the care manager is to provide brief, evidence-based psychotherapies, such as behavioral activation, problem-solving therapy, cognitive-behavioral therapy, interpersonal therapy, and motivational interviewing.

  Typically, patients are in active treatment for 3–6 months, after which two outcomes are possible: either the patient achieves remission or the patient needs referral to specialized mental health care services for longer-term, more intensive treatment. Once the patient improves and enters remission, the care manager moves him or her to the relapse prevention phase and follows up monthly for 3 months to make sure that the patient continues to be stable before handing the care back to the primary care provider. If a patient does not improve despite multiple treatment ad-

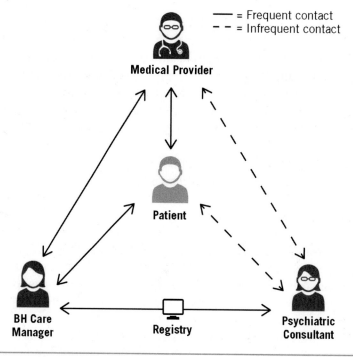

FIGURE 38–2.   Collaborative care team.

Note.   BH=behavioral health.

Source.   Reprinted from AIMS (Advancing Integrated Mental Health Solutions) Center web page "Collaborative Care Team Structure" (available at: https://aims.uw.edu/collaborative-care/team-structure; accessed October 7, 2018). Copyright 2017, University of Washington. Used with permission.

justments or requires a level of care that cannot be provided within the collaborative care model, the care manager facilitates referrals to specialty mental health care services and follows up until the patient has established care there.

- *Psychiatric consultant:* Almost all U.S. counties have unmet needs for psychiatric prescribers (Thomas et al. 2009). In the collaborative care model, a psychiatric provider can leverage his or her expertise in a more efficient way by working with a team and sharing the care of the patient instead of working alone. In this model, the psychiatric consultant performs primarily indirect consultation, reviewing care managers' caseloads and providing recommendations for additional assessment and treatment for patients whose symptoms are not improving. In a minority of cases, the psychiatric consultant sees the patient directly, either in person or by teleconferencing. In addition to this indirect and direct clinical consultation, the psychiatrist has several other important roles, including providing education and training for other team members, continuously working on improving the quality of care provided to the patients by the team, and taking on a leadership role to support the team and the collaborative care model (Raney 2015). The roles of the psychiatric consultant within integrated care and the collaborative care model are described in more detail in the following section.

The Psychiatrist's Role in Collaborative Care

As noted, the psychiatrist on a collaborative care team is not only a clinical consultant but also an educator and a leader. Having an actively engaged psychiatrist on the collaborative care team is associated with higher patient remission rates at 6 months (Whitebird et al. 2014).

Clinical Consultant

In other integrated care models, particularly colocated care and some telepsychiatry services, the psychiatrist provides direct consultation, seeing the patient in person or by teleconferencing, doing an assessment, and providing treatment recommendations to the primary care provider. In contrast, the psychiatric consultant in collaborative care spends most of his or her time providing indirect consultations. Indirect consultations include caseload reviews with the care manager and "curbside consults." For weekly caseload reviews, the psychiatric consultant reviews the registry (i.e., the comprehensive list of patients who are in active treatment) with the care manager and develops treatment recommendations without seeing the patient; this is done by gathering information from the care manager, from the assessment conducted by the primary care provider, and from behavioral health measures such as symptom rating scales. Patients are closely followed up by the care manager, usually twice a month, for brief evidence-based psychotherapy and assessment of symptoms with behavioral health measures. This frequent and systematic information gathered by the care manager gives the psychiatric consultant an opportunity to diagnose over time and also to make timely adjustments to the treatment plan until the patient reaches remission or the team's shared treatment goal. During caseload reviews, about 5–10 patients may be discussed in an hour, depending on the complexity of the patients' conditions. The psychiatric consultant documents recommendations in the registry and in the electronic health record, if he or she has access to it. The care manager has the responsibility of forwarding treatment recommendations to the primary care provider and the patient. In the collaborative care model, direct consultations are usually reserved for situations in which the psychiatric provider needs to see the patient to clarify the diagnosis or reassess the treatment approach in treatment-refractory cases.

In the collaborative care model, indirect consultation raises issues about the psychiatric provider's liability and billing (Raney 2015). The psychiatric provider remains a consultant to the primary care provider in these models and also should document the basis on which recommendations are made, the sources of information used, and whether he or she personally saw and evaluated the patient. Psychiatric providers should always have liability insurance coverage even if they do only indirect consultation. Although collaborative care is cost-effective in capitated health care systems, traditionally it has not been reimbursed by insurance companies or in fee-for-service settings. Increasingly, however, the indirect consultation provided by psychiatric providers in collaborative care is reimbursable.

Educator

The psychiatric consultant plays a key role in educating the collaborative care team, with the goal of improving team members' skills and building confidence to manage mental health disorders. Every consultation note or communication with the team provides an opportunity to educate. Because primary care providers and care managers are very busy, the most effective way to teach is to provide brief, concise teaching points. More formal and comprehensive education about specific topics can be provided by scheduling a time during lunch or a monthly provider meeting (Raney 2015).

Leader

Even if the psychiatric consultant is not in a formal leadership position, he or she plays a key role in supporting the functioning of the collaborative care team, clinically and at a systems level. In the early phase of implementation of the collaborative care model within a clinic or health care system, there can be confusion or disagreements about team member roles, treatment plans for patients, or how collaborative care fits into the clinic or system. It is important for the psychiatric consultant to be engaged and vigilant and to intervene when necessary to support the team. At times, there can be resistance at the provider, staff, or administrative level to making changes to accommodate this new model. In this situation, the psychiatric consultant's role is to make the case for collaborative care by providing education about the rationale, evidence base, health outcomes, and other benefits of this model. Once the collaborative care model is implemented, the psychiatric consultant has the responsibility to ensure adherence to the core principles of collaborative care, the best possible patient outcomes, and continuous quality improvement in the work of the team. The psychiatric consultant also can contribute to the workflow of the clinic by facilitating development of clinical protocols for different psychiatric disorders or situations, such as treatment algorithms, safety assessment protocols, procedures for managing psychiatric emergencies, and approaches to challenging patients and clinical situations (Ratzliff et al. 2015).

Preparing Psychiatrists for Careers in Integrated Care

Psychiatrists working in integrated care settings report overwhelmingly positive experiences and particularly value the patient-centered model of care, working with a team, the psychiatrist's role as an educator, and opportunities for growth and innovation (Norfleet et al. 2016). Increasingly, psychiatry residents and practicing psychiatrists have opportunities to learn about integrated care, and integrated care rotations are being developed and are encouraged during residency training (American Psychiatric Association 2017; Cowley et al. 2014; Summers et al. 2014). In addition to acquiring knowledge about integrated and collaborative care, some competencies and characteristics have been proposed as being particularly helpful in preparing psychiatrists to work in these settings (Cowley et al. 2014; Raney 2015; Ratzliff et al. 2015).

First, behavioral health care and primary care have very different "cultures," and integrating the two can present challenges. Primary care settings are usually fast-paced, with brief appointments of varying duration, flexible boundaries, double booking or "squeezing in" of patients, and frequent interruptions. Primary care providers often need to make decisions quickly and appreciate clear, specific, and succinct recommendations from consultants. Outpatient psychiatry settings are characterized by longer appointments of specified length and a firm treatment frame and boundaries. Psychiatrists working in primary care settings need to be flexible and able to adapt to and work effectively within a different model of practice. This includes being available and responsive; tolerating interruptions; providing brief recommendations without jargon; and outlining specific suggestions for medications, dosing, and titration.

Psychiatric providers working in integrated care may need to increase their knowledge base and seek consultation themselves so that they can help primary care providers and care managers who see patients and clinical situations outside of their usual practice, such as child and adolescent psychiatry, addictions, eating disorders, and cognitive disorders. To work in collaborative care, psychiatric providers need to learn skills in indirect consultation, reviewing caseloads, and providing recommendations without seeing the patient. Psychiatrists wanting to work in telepsychiatry or to offer first-line general or preventive medical care to patients will need to learn about relevant technology, primary care topics, and different modes of practice. The role of the psychiatric consultant also requires skills in educating other providers in the course of consultations and in working in and leading high-functioning teams. In a survey study, 52 psychiatrists working in integrated care identified the following educational priorities for their role: having knowledge of eating disorders, making pharmacological recommendations for children and adolescents, performing indirect consultations and caseload panel reviews, supervising care managers, advising teams about behavioral health issues, and supporting a clinic or an organization in building an effective integrated care team that fits their population and resources (Ratzliff et al. 2015). Clinicians best suited for working as psychiatric consultants in integrated care are flexible and team oriented, are willing to tolerate interruptions, and derive enjoyment and satisfaction from educating others (Raney 2015).

Conclusion

Integrated care, and especially collaborative care, offers an evidence-based care model to achieve the triple aim of mental health care: access, quality, and cost-effectiveness. It allows psychiatrists to leverage their time to help as many patients as possible and to focus their efforts on those patients who most need psychiatric expertise. In this chapter, we reviewed the rationale for and models of integrated care, as well as the core principles, team structure, and psychiatrist's role in collaborative care, the integrated care model with the strongest evidence base. Psychiatrists working in integrated care report finding this work rewarding, and opportunities for psychiatrists in this area will likely increase in the future.

Key Clinical Points

- Integrated care brings together mental health care and primary medical care to increase access to care and improve mental health and medical outcomes for patients in a cost-effective manner.

- Models of integrated care include colocation of a psychiatrist within a primary care setting, collaborative care, telepsychiatry, and delivery of preventive and general medical care to psychiatric patients.

- Collaborative care is the integrated care model with the strongest evidence base and has demonstrated effectiveness in improving mental health care quality, outcomes, and cost-effectiveness and reducing health care disparities in primary care settings.

- The five core principles of collaborative care are patient-centered collaboration, population-based care, evidence-based care, measurement-based treatment to target, and accountability.

- The collaborative care team consists of the patient, the primary care provider, the behavioral care manager, and the psychiatric consultant, with each team member having a clearly defined role.

- The psychiatric consultant in a collaborative care team provides indirect and direct consultation, education, and leadership.

- Psychiatrists working in integrated care benefit from knowledge about the care delivery model, consultation skills, appreciation of differences between primary care and psychiatric practice, flexibility, and enjoyment of working with a team.

References

American Psychiatric Association: Learn About Integrated Care. Arlington, VA, American Psychiatric Association Publishing, 2017. Available at: https://www.psychiatry.org/psychiatrists/practice/professional-interests/integrated-care/learn. Accessed August 31, 2017.

Angstman KB, Phelan S, Myszkowski MR, et al: Minority primary care patients with depression: outcome disparities improve with collaborative care management. Med Care 53(1):32–37, 2015 25464162

Archer J, Bower P, Gilbody S, et al: Collaborative care for depression and anxiety problems. Cochrane Database Syst Rev 10:CD006525, 2012 23076925

Byatt N, Biebel K, Moore Simas TA, et al: Improving perinatal depression care: the Massachusetts Child Psychiatry Access Project for Moms. Gen Hosp Psychiatry 40:12–17, 2016 27079616

Cowley D, Dunaway K, Forstein M, et al: Teaching psychiatry residents to work at the interface of mental health and primary care. Acad Psychiatry 38(4):398–404, 2014 24733538

Druss BG, Zhao L, Von Esenwein S, et al: Understanding excess mortality in persons with mental illness: 17-year follow up of a nationally representative US survey. Med Care 49(6):599–604, 2011 21577183

Fortney JC, Pyne JM, Mouden SB, et al: Practice-based versus telemedicine-based collaborative care for depression in rural federally qualified health centers: a pragmatic randomized comparative effectiveness trial. Am J Psychiatry 170(4):414–425, 2013 23429924

Grembowski DE, Martin D, Patrick DL, et al: Managed care, access to mental health specialists, and outcomes among primary care patients with depressive symptoms. J Gen Intern Med 17(4):258–269, 2002 11972722

Katon W, Unützer J: Consultation psychiatry in the medical home and accountable care organizations: achieving the triple aim. Gen Hosp Psychiatry 33(4):305–310, 2011 21762825

Katon WJ, Lin EH, Von Korff M, et al: Collaborative care for patients with depression and chronic illnesses. N Engl J Med 363(27):2611–2620, 2010 21190455

Katon W, Russo J, Lin EH, et al: Cost-effectiveness of a multicondition collaborative care intervention: a randomized controlled trial. Arch Gen Psychiatry 69(5):506–514, 2012 22566583

Kern JS: Providing primary care in behavioral health settings, in Integrated Care: Working at the Interface of Primary Care and Behavioral Health. Edited by Raney LE. Arlington, VA, American Psychiatric Association Publishing, 2015, pp 169–191

Kroenke K, Spitzer RL, Williams JB: The PHQ-9: validity of a brief depression severity measure. J Gen Intern Med 16(9):606–613, 2001 11556941

Murray CJL, Vos T, Lozano R, et al: Disability-adjusted life years (DALYs) for 291 diseases and injuries in 21 regions, 1990–2010: a systematic analysis for the Global Burden of Disease Study 2010. Lancet 380(9859):2197–2223, 2012 23245608

Norfleet KR, Ratzliff ADH, Chan Y-F, et al: The role of the integrated care psychiatrist in community settings: a survey of psychiatrists' perspectives. Psychiatr Serv 67(3):346–349, 2016 26695492

Peek CJ, The National Integration Academy Council: Lexicon for Behavioral Health and Primary Care Integration: Concepts and Definitions Developed by Expert Consensus (AHRQ Publ No 13-IP001-EF). Rockville, MD, Agency for Healthcare Research and Quality, 2013. Available at: http://integrationacademy.ahrq.gov/sites/default/files/Lexicon.pdf. Accessed September 3, 2017.

Raney LE: Integrating primary care and behavioral health: the role of the psychiatrist in the Collaborative Care Model. Am J Psychiatry 172(8):721–728, 2015 26234599

Ratzliff A, Norfleet K, Chan Y-F, et al: Perceived educational needs of the integrated care psychiatric consultant. Acad Psychiatry 39(4):448–456, 2015 26122347

Ratzliff A, Cerimele J, Katon W, et al: Working as a team to provide Collaborative Care, in Integrated Care: Creating Effective Mental and Primary Health Care Teams. Edited by Ratzliff A, Unützer J, Katon W, et al. Hoboken, NJ, Wiley, 2016, pp 1–23

Rush AJ: STAR*D: what have we learned? Am J Psychiatry 164(2):201–204, 2007 17267779

Spitzer RL, Kroenke K, Williams JB, et al: A brief measure for assessing generalized anxiety disorder: the GAD-7. Arch Intern Med 166(10):1092–1097, 2006 16717171

Straus JH, Sarvet B: Behavioral health care for children: the Massachusetts Child Psychiatry Access Project. Health Aff (Millwood) 33(12):2153–2161, 2014 25489033

Summers RF, Rapaport MH, Hunt JB, et al: Training psychiatrists for integrated behavioral health care: a report by the American Psychiatric Association Council on Medical Education and Lifelong Learning. Arlington, VA, American Psychiatric Association, 2014. Available at: https://www.med.upenn.edu/psychres/assets/user-content/documents/CMELL_ICReport_2232015%20(5).pdf. Accessed September 3, 2017.

Thomas KC, Ellis AR, Konrad TR, et al: County-level estimates of mental health professional shortage in the United States. Psychiatr Serv 60(10):1323–1328, 2009 19797371

Unützer J, Ratzliff AH: Evidence base and core principles, in Integrated Care: Working at the Interface of Primary Care and Behavioral Health. Edited by Raney LE. Arlington, VA, American Psychiatric Association Publishing, 2015, pp 3–16

Unützer J, Katon W, Callahan CM, et al: Collaborative care management of late-life depression in the primary care setting: a randomized controlled trial. JAMA 288(22):2836–2845, 2002 12472325

van der Feltz-Cornelis CM, Van Os TWDP, Van Marwijk HWJ, et al: Effect of psychiatric consultation models in primary care: a systematic review and meta-analysis of randomized clinical trials. J Psychosom Res 68(6):521–533, 2010 20488268

Wang PS, Lane M, Olfson M, et al: Twelve-month use of mental health services in the United States: results from the National Comorbidity Survey Replication. Arch Gen Psychiatry 62(6):629–640, 2005 15939840

Watkins KE, Ober AJ, Lamp K, et al: Collaborative care for opioid and alcohol use disorders in primary care: the SUMMIT randomized clinical trial. JAMA Intern Med 177(10):1480–1488, 2017 28846769

Whitebird RR, Solberg LI, Jaeckels NA, et al: Effective implementation of collaborative care for depression: what is needed? Am J Manag Care 20(9):699–707, 2014 25365745

Recommended Readings

Advancing Integrated Mental Health Solutions (AIMS) Center, University of Washington, web site: Available at: https://aims.uw.edu. Accessed August 28, 2017.

Bland DA, Lambert K, Raney L, et al: Resource document on risk management and liability issues in integrated care models. Am J Psychiatry 171 (5 suppl):1–7, 2014

McCarron RM, Xiong GL, Keenan CR, et al (eds): Preventive Medical Care in Psychiatry. Arlington, VA, American Psychiatric Association Publishing, 2015

Melek SP, Norris DT, Paulus J: Economic Impact of Integrated Medical-Behavioral Healthcare: Implications for Psychiatry. Milliman American Psychiatric Association Report. Denver, CO, Milliman, 2014. Available at: https://www.psychiatry.org/File%20Library/Psychiatrists/Practice/Professional-Topics/Integrated-Care/Milliman-Report-Economic-Impact-Integrated-Implications-Psychiatry.pdf. Accessed September 3, 2017.

National Institute of Mental Health: Integrated Care. Bethesda, MD, National Institute of Mental Health, 2017. Available at: https://www.nimh.nih.gov/health/topics/integrated-care/index.shtml. Accessed September 3, 2017.

Raney LE (ed): Integrated Care: Working at the Interface of Primary Care and Behavioral Health. Arlington, VA, American Psychiatric Association Publishing, 2015

Ratzliff A, Unützer J, Katon W, et al (eds): Integrated Care: Creating Effective Mental and Primary Health Care Teams. Hoboken, NJ, Wiley, 2016

CHAPTER 39

Standardized Assessment and Measurement-Based Care

Craig S. Rosen, Ph.D.

Steven N. Lindley, M.D., Ph.D.

Shannon Wiltsey Stirman, Ph.D.

The assessment process requires the clinician to make decisions by formulating, testing, and refining hypotheses based on clinical information that is often incomplete or inconsistent, often in the context of very brief clinical encounters. Evidence has been mounting for decades that in such contexts, subjective clinical judgment does not yield diagnoses that are as accurate or comprehensive as standardized diagnostic measures. Consequently, evidence-based assessment is now recognized as a key component of evidence-based care. The American Psychiatric Association guidelines recommend that "the initial psychiatric evaluation of a patient include quantitative measures of symptoms, level of functioning, and quality of life" (American Psychiatric Association Work Group on Psychiatric Evaluation 2016, p. 35). More recent research findings suggest that quantitative measures should be used not just at initial evaluation but also over the course of treatment to measure patient health and symptoms. Integrating the routine use of measurement within clinical care has been shown to result in faster improvement in client outcomes, including symptoms, interpersonal functioning, and quality of life, than routine care without ongoing assessment, particularly among patients at risk for deterioration (Bickman et al. 2011; Lambert et al. 2003). The Joint Commission (2017) has recognized the value of ongoing assessment, specifying that behavioral health care organizations should use standardized tools or instruments to monitor patient progress.

There has been a marked shift in the approach to psychological assessment over the past two decades in response to developments in research on assessment (Hunsely and Mash 2010). The field is deemphasizing use of projective tests and complex multidimensional instruments that require highly specialized training to administer and interpret. There is now a greater emphasis on brief, focused measures that can be administered in a range of treatment settings and readily interpreted by most clinicians. Advances in information technology also provide more tools for administering and interpreting mental health assessments and outcome measures (Hunsely and Mash 2010). Through these changes, standardized assessment is moving away from being a rare and highly specialized referral and toward becoming an integral part of routine care. In time, quantitative monitoring of psychiatric symptoms should become as routine as tracking blood pressure or white blood cell counts.

Why and When to Use Standardized Assessment Measures

Standardized assessment tools can improve care in a number of ways—by increasing accuracy and minimizing the likelihood of misdiagnosis, by demonstrating progress, or by flagging a lack of improvement that might require a change in treatment plan.

Screening

Mental disorders are often underdiagnosed in primary care settings and may be missed even in specialized settings. Several studies indicate that use of validated brief screening tools enables improved detection and more accurate diagnosis of mental disorders in primary care (Bufka and Campl 2010). Screening tools used in primary care or other settings are intended to identify people who may potentially have a psychiatric disorder who should be referred for further assessment. Because they are intended for routine use in all patients, screening tools are very short and easily interpreted without advanced training (Bufka and Campl 2010). Very brief (two- to four-item) screening measures are often not designed to make definitive diagnoses or to measure progress over time.

Case Formulation and Treatment Planning

Psychiatrists need to accurately determine diagnoses and level of severity prior to developing a treatment plan. Clinical judgment is subject to numerous cognitive biases (Hunsely and Mash 2010). Clinicians may attend to one salient detail and miss other parts of a patient's presentation or may be overly influenced by one recent case. Use of validated assessment measures can help clinicians to consider multiple domains of symptoms and functioning. They can help psychiatrists to more accurately assess severity of a given patient's symptoms by comparing the symptoms against established norms.

Monitoring Progress: Measurement-Based Care

Patients do not always get better. About one-third of patients will fail to respond to any given antidepressant, and others may have a more limited response, requiring a change of treatment approach (Kautzky et al. 2017). Unfortunately, clinical impressions alone are not very effective for assessing change, especially lack of change. Studies suggest that mental health providers' clinical judgment failed to detect most cases in which standardized assessments showed that patients' symptoms were failing to respond to treatment or were becoming worse (Fortney et al. 2017). If patients are appreciative, adherent to treatment, and gaining insight, it may not be immediately obvious if their symptoms and functioning are not improving.

In contrast, by using standardized symptom measures to assess change, psychiatrists could determine by the second week of treatment which patients with schizophrenia were likely to be nonresponsive to an antipsychotic (Samara et al. 2015). A similar study found that change scores on the nine-item depression scale of the Patient Health Questionnaire (PHQ-9) in the first 2 weeks of hospitalization predicted which patients were likely to eventually improve (Fowler et al. 2015).

Measurement-based care (MBC) refers to the ongoing administration of validated measures throughout the course of treatment to track patient progress, and the use of those data to inform clinicians' and patients' decisions about clinical interventions (Scott and Lewis 2015). Use of validated measures can provide a more objective indicator of client progress to inform treatment decisions. Research has indicated that routine outcome monitoring, accompanied by feedback on patient progress, may produce client outcomes that are superior to those found in usual care (Fortney et al. 2017; Gondek et al. 2016; Scott and Lewis 2015). In addition to demonstrated improved outcomes, MBC has several additional benefits. It can provide a way to measure and visualize progress. Measuring change can promote hope in patients, who may have difficulty in seeing the big picture of their progress toward recovery, and it provides a "jumping off point" for discussion about whether, and why, symptoms and functioning are or are not changing as desired. Use of routine outcome monitoring to inform treatment may therefore enhance communication between clients and providers and promote shared decision making (Scott and Lewis 2015). By repeatedly measuring the patient's clinical status, it is possible to identify problems before they become severe and to affirm progress as soon as it occurs (Fortney et al. 2017).

Types of Standardized Measures

Brief Self-Report Scales

Several different types of standardized measures can be used for psychological assessment. The most widely used standardized measures are self-report rating scales (Beidas et al. 2015; Bufka and Campl 2010). These can vary in length and complexity. Brief screening instruments can be as short as 2–6 items. Brief symptom measures used to track change typically are 7–50 items in length. A number of brief measures of symptoms and functioning that are freely available (together with their psychometric properties) have been identified for use in routine care (Beidas et al. 2015). One concern with self-report measures is that people can potentially exaggerate or minimize their symptoms. Several studies suggest that people are more likely to disclose stigmatizing problems such as substance use in an online survey or paper questionnaires than in a clinical interview (Del Boca and Darkes 2003).

Structured Interviews

A second type of standardized assessment is semistructured or structured clinical interviews such as the Mini International Neuropsychiatric Interview (Groth-Marnat and Wright 2016). Structured interviews require substantial training and often take a long time to administer, so they are used more often in research studies than in clinical practice. However, they can be extremely useful in informing treatment planning and differential diagnosis in complicated cases, and referral for formal assessment may be foundational to effective care in such cases.

Self-Report Measures for Personality Assessment and Differential Diagnosis

It may sometimes be useful to refer patients with particularly complex presentations to psychologists who specialize in assessment to be assessed with both structured interviews and self-report measures. These assessment referrals are typically for treatment planning, not for measuring treatment response. Assessments may include use of more extensive self-report questionnaires, such as the Minnesota Multiphasic Personality Inventory (MMPI), that assess personality disorders as well as other symptoms (Groth-Marnat and Wright 2016). These measures require specialized training to administer and score reliably. Clinical psychology training programs are placing increasing emphasis on use of validated self-report batteries rather than projective personality tests such as the Rorschach (Stedman et al. 2018).

Neuropsychiatric Assessment

Another type of standardized assessment involves tests of behavior, which assess people by rating their performance on standardized tasks (Groth-Marnat and Wright 2016). This is the approach used in neuropsychiatric assessment. Cognitive screening tests such as the Mini-Mental Status Exam (Folstein et al. 1975) can help identify individuals who may have cognitive impairment. Referral of those individuals for comprehensive neuropsychiatric assessment using standardized measures can enable detection of cognitive deficits and strengths that might not otherwise be immediately apparent (Roebuck-Spencer et al. 2017). Neuropsychiatric tests assess domains such as attention and concentration, memory, language, visuospatial abilities, and problem solving (Groth-Marnat and Wright 2016). Results of such assessments can inform recovery and treatment and can identify existing strengths that can be leveraged to improve functioning.

Psychometric Criteria

Standardized assessments of symptoms and functioning should be reliable, valid, and (if used to assess progress) sensitive to change. *Reliability* is the degree to which a measure yields consistent scores when administered to the same person under similar circumstances (Groth-Marnat and Wright 2016). A measure that has low reliability cannot be sensitive to change. Some ways of assessing reliability are test–retest reliability (administering the test on two different occasions and comparing results), internal consistency (comparing results from different items on the same scale), and interrater reliability (comparing results from two interviewers or observers assessing the same person) (Groth-Marnat and Wright 2016).

Validity is the extent to which a test measures the trait it is intended to measure (Groth-Marnat and Wright 2016; Tarescavage and Ben-Porath 2014). Content validity is how well items on the test appear to reflect the trait being measured. Construct validity is how well scores on a test match other measures of the same construct. For example, a good depression scale should be highly correlated with other measures of depression and weakly correlated with measures of other disorders. Criterion validity is how results of a test correspond with an established measure of the same construct. Two important indices of criterion validity for screening measures are sensitivity (how well it detects people who have the disorder) and specificity (how well it screens out people who do not have the disorder) (Groth-Marnat and Wright 2016).

Sensitivity to change is the extent to which scores on a test rise and fall in parallel with other measures of the same construct (Tarescavage and Ben-Porath 2014). Sensitivity to change is critical for monitoring patient outcomes. For example, the nine-item version of the PHQ (Beidas et al. 2015) is a depression measure with good sensitivity to change that is widely used in both research trials and clinical care. There is also a shorter, two-item version of the measure, the PHQ-2 (Kroenke et al. 2003), which is used for screening. The PHQ-2 has demonstrated validity in detecting which patients are likely to be depressed, but it is not nuanced enough to measure how patients' level of depression changes during treatment.

Benefits from using measures to assess progress and inform treatment planning—including more rapid and substantial improvements in symptoms, functioning, and quality of life, and greater engagement in treatment—have been demonstrated in several studies (Fortney et al. 2017; Gondek et al. 2016; Scott and Lewis 2015). However, in order to see these clinical benefits, measurement must occur frequently and providers must receive and examine the measure results at or near the time of treatment (Fortney et al. 2017). Use of MBC includes consideration of what measures to use, how to use them to guide treatment, and how to discuss them with patients, as well as the practical aspects of administration.

Selecting Measures

The measures used for initial treatment planning or monitoring progress should match the clinical purpose of the assessment and the clinical focus of the treatment (Table 39–1). One should avoid asking patients for information that will not be discussed with them. Patients must feel that the data being collected are relevant to their care and being used to actively guide the treatment plan. Although symptom severity is normally thought of as the primary target of MBC, outcome measures can encompass a wide range of domains, including medication side effects, social functioning, quality of life, and strength of the therapeutic alliance. The choice of outcome measure also can change over time as the goals of treatment shift. Many readily available brief questionnaires can be used to assess initial severity as well as to monitor change over time (Beidas et al. 2015; Tarescavage and Ben-Porath 2014). In addition to being brief to administer, outcome measures need to be able to be rapidly interpretable and quickly summarized by the provider to inform care decisions and discussions with a patient during the session.

Symptom Severity

Some symptom measures, such as the 45-item Outcome Questionnaire (OQ-45) and the Brief Symptom Inventory, assess a broad range of symptoms and presenting problems across disorders (Tarescavage and Ben-Porath 2014). Other measures, such as the PTSD Checklist for posttraumatic stress disorder, assess symptoms of a single disorder (Beidas et al. 2015). Still other symptom severity measures—such as the PHQ-9, which measures depressive symptoms, and the Generalized Anxiety Disorder seven-item scale (GAD-7), which measures anxiety—assess specific symptoms that may be present across several disorders (Beidas et al. 2015).

Functioning

Patients' goals for improvement often go beyond simple symptom reduction to include a return to their usual self, with an improvement in functioning and a heightened sense of well-being. Some validated assessment measures, such as the 32-item Behavior and Symptom Identification Scale (BASIS-32) and the Medical Outcomes Study 36-item Short Form (SF-36), assess overall functioning and quality of life (Tarescavage and Ben-Porath 2014). Patients may also identify very specific problem-focused goals, such as being able to enjoy life, having higher energy levels, being able to find work or succeed at work, improving relationships, having positive feelings about people, feeling connected to other people, engaging in positive activities, improving sleep quality or amount, or improving skills for coping with strong emotions or for handling conflict. Progress on such patient-specific goals can be assessed with measures tailored to the individual, using an approach such as goal attainment scaling (Kiresuk et al. 2014). Such "idiographic" or patient-specific measures may most closely reflect a given patient's goals; however, they do not have established validity and cannot be compared against norms. It is often helpful to use a mix of approaches, combining a patient-specific measure with other well-characterized measures that have psychometric validity.

Therapeutic Alliance

Although more the focus of psychotherapy treatment, the routine monitoring of the therapeutic alliance may be equally important for psychopharmacological treatment. Often providers are not aware that there is a problem. Routine monitoring of the therapeutic alliance along with symptom assessments has been shown to improve psychotherapy outcomes through early identification of problems that can then be openly discussed and addressed. Stronger therapeutic alliances have been associated with better adherence to antidepressant and antipsychotic treatment and with enhanced outcomes for both psychotherapy and pharmacotherapy in randomized clinical trials (Zilcha-Mano et al. 2014). Early detection of problems in the alliance is likely to improve patient engagement in and satisfaction with care. Several standardized, patient-reported brief measures of the therapeutic alliance are available, with the Working Alliance Inventory (Horvath and Greenberg 1989) being one of the more commonly used instruments.

TABLE 39–1. Purposes and uses of standardized measures

Type of measure	Purpose	Which patients	Who administers and interprets it	Examples
Screening tools	Identification of persons who should be referred for further assessment	Everyone	Primary care staff or mental health professionals	PHQ-2, AUDIT-C
Broad symptom measures	Treatment planning; assessment of progress	Patients in mental health treatment	Mental health professionals	OQ-45, Brief Symptom Inventory
Specific symptom measures	Treatment planning; assessment of progress	Patients in mental health treatment	Mental health professionals	PHQ-9, GAD-7
Scales of functioning or quality of life	Treatment planning; assessment of progress	Patients in mental health treatment	Mental health professionals	BASIS-24, SF-36
Ratings of quality of therapeutic alliance or patient satisfaction	Assessment of progress	Patients in mental health treatment	Mental health professionals	Working Alliance Inventory
Comprehensive self-report assessment batteries	Formulation of complex cases; personality assessment; differential diagnosis	Complex cases that pose assessment challenges	Assessment experts (typically psychologists)	MMPI, MCMI
Medication adherence and side effects	Assessment of medication compliance and physical side effects	Individuals using psychotropic medication	Psychiatrists	Morisky Medication Adherence Scale; UKU Side Effect Rating Scale
Neuropsychiatric assessments	Assessment of cognitive deficits and strengths relative to established norms	Individuals who may have cognitive impairment	Neuropsychologists	WAIS, Halstead-Reitan

Note. AUDIT-C = Alcohol Use Disorders Identification Test—Consumption; BASIS-24 = 24-item Behavior and Symptom Identification Scale; GAD-7 = Generalized Anxiety Disorder seven-item scale; MCMI = Millon Clinical Multiaxial Inventory; MMPI = Minnesota Multiphasic Personality Inventory; OQ-45 = 45-item Outcome Questionnaire; PHQ-2 = two-item Patient Health Questionnaire; PHQ-9 = nine-item Patient Health Questionnaire; SF-36 = Medical Outcomes Study 36-item Short Form; UKU = Udvalg fur Kliniske Undersøgelser; WAIS = Wechsler Adult Intelligence Scale.

Medication Adherence and Side Effects

Routine assessment of medication adherence and of presence and intensity of medication adverse effects can greatly improve the quality of care. Many side effects can go undetected unless patients are specifically queried about their presence, and undiscussed side effects can significantly impair adherence to treatment and impair the therapeutic alliance. If side effects are detected early, they can be openly discussed with patients. When combined with other outcome monitoring, routine assessment allows for a more informed, open discussion of the benefits versus burdens of psychopharmacological treatment to take place. As with other types of outcome monitoring, brevity is important for routine use in most settings, so questions cannot comprehensively cover all potential side effects. Instead, monitoring instruments can be tailored to particular classes of medication and designed to stimulate further investigation of potential side effects. Examples of standardized measures that can be used for medication monitoring include the Morisky Medication Adherence Scale (Morisky et al. 1986) and the patient-report version of the Udvalg for Kliniske Undersøgelser (UKU) Side Effect Rating Scale (Lindström et al. 2001).

Use and Interpretation of Measures in Routine Care

It is important to note that the data generated through MBC do not replace clinical judgment and collaboration; rather, they should *enhance* it. Quantitative measures with well-established norms can be used to compare a given patient with the larger patient population. For example, a patient's depression scores at intake can be compared with norms to determine whether the person has subthreshold, mild, moderate, or severe symptoms. This information can be used to weigh potential risks and benefits of medications with specific side-effect profiles. Several outcome measures, such as the OQ-45, are designed not just for assessing initial severity but also for benchmarking change over time (Gondek et al. 2016; Lyon et al. 2016). Such information enables clinicians to know whether a given patient's progress is in line with that of most patients in the clinic or in a national population, or whether a patient is showing slower-than-typical progress. This feedback loop can improve outcomes by cueing clinicians to assess further and to revise their treatment plans if patients are not responding as expected (Gondek et al. 2016). This use of benchmarks focuses on making decisions for an individual patient but allows clinicians to acknowledge legitimate reasons why a given patient might be having slower-than-usual improvement (e.g., emergence of new life stressors).

These same outcome norms can also inform efforts to improve quality of care at the clinician or program level, and MBC is consistent with recently introduced Joint Commission standards for behavioral health care (Joint Commission 2017). However, data on individual patients are often not designed for program evaluation and should be used with caution and with an understanding of the limitations. Comparing outcomes across clinicians or programs requires risk adjustment methods to statistically control for differences in the severity or acuity of clinicians' patient populations. Even with good risk adjustment models, too narrow a focus on achieving a particular measurement can divert attention from other aspects of care that are not being measured and could drive lower performers to make changes that are not necessarily the best care for particular patients or populations. Benchmarking for program improvement is best used as one part of a quality improvement process that is locally driven by front-line staff rather than a rigid top-down effort.

Use of Clinical Data to Inform Shared Decision Making

A key tenet of MBC is that patients should be involved in reviewing their progress and in making decisions regarding their care (Scott and Lewis 2015). The first step is to discuss the rationale for using MBC with patients. It is important that the discussion be linked to the patient's treatment goals. The patient should understand that symptoms are only *one* source of information about treatment effectiveness and that functioning, satisfaction, and other factors that are important to the patient (e.g., activity level) also inform treatment effectiveness. The discussion with the patient should include explanation of how the measurement will be used, along with the rationale for MBC. Using an analogy such as taking the temperature or blood pressure at every visit can help the patient understand how the information will be used—that is, it is one source of information that will be taken into account, along with other clinical information, to understand where the patient is in relation to his or her treatment goals and the progress that the patient is making. Furthermore, the provider can explain that MBC has a self-correcting function: clinical decision making is continually audited by the provider and patient for effectiveness, and based on this information, appropriate changes can be made to enhance the likelihood that the patient is achieving the treatment goals.

Once the patient understands the rationale, the measure can be given first to establish a baseline and then at every subsequent visit. Within each meeting, the feedback can be very brief and should be discussed in the context of both past visits and the patient's goals. The data should be presented in a way that is easily understandable by patients, with information discussed in terms of its implications for maintaining or altering the course of treatment. Categorizing results (e.g., recovered/asymptomatic, mild, moderate, severe) and discussing in terms of the degree of change and how results compare to expected outcomes can assist in these discussions. By providing data feedback to the patient, the clinician can elicit the patient's perspective on the clinical implications of the data and on contextual factors (e.g., recent life events) that may contribute to the observed outcomes. The information can be used as a backdrop to talk about treatment goals and barriers. It can also be used to explore whether there is a need to make changes, in terms of the treatment itself or of patient behaviors, to move closer to the treatment goals. The provider and the patient could consider potential relationships between variables that impact the patient's functioning. For example, they can reflect on whether the patient's mood seems to be better when he or she is taking medications as prescribed, drinking less, or engaging in more activities. Through such discussion, collaborative decisions about next steps, such as medication adjustments, behavioral changes, or adjunctive treatment, can be made.

Table 39–2 highlights some best practices for MBC. At times, clinicians or patients may feel some discomfort with the use of measurement, and clinicians have expressed concern that measurement feels impersonal or fails to reflect the patient's complexity

TABLE 39–2.	Best practices for measurement-based care

1. Introduce measurement-based care as a tool for increasing patients' control over their own treatment. People are individuals; no one treatment works for everyone. Monitoring progress helps patients and their providers judge what is working or identify things that need to be changed.

2. Select outcome measures that fit the patients' treatment goals, are reliable and valid, and are sensitive to change.

3. Standardized outcomes data should enhance clinical judgment and collaborative decision making, not replace it.

4. Provide some feedback every time patients complete an assessment to reinforce the idea that the assessment is a clinical tool to improve their care, not simply paperwork.

5. Elicit patients' reactions to their scores. What do they think about their progress? How do their symptoms align (or not) with other indicators of how they are doing? Reflect back the patients' comments and provide your own feedback.

6. Do not argue if a patient disagrees with what the measure is indicating. Explore the discrepancy with the patient's experience and validate his or her emotional reactions.

7. Emphasize that it is normal for the pace of change to be specific to the person, and for progress to be uneven.

8. If a patient is not responding, collaboratively explore possible nonadherence issues and/or whether there is some new stressor in the patient's life. Discuss whether to stay the course, change treatment intensity, or change the treatment approach.

and individuality. In such cases, it is important to emphasize that measures serve as a springboard to a larger discussion about treatment goals, adherence, and satisfaction, and that treatment planning remains a collaborative process, which is informed but not dictated by the measures. It is also helpful to examine not only the total score but also the patterns of response on items or subscales that might provide useful information for treatment planning. For example, if a patient's depressive symptoms are decreasing in all areas but somatic symptoms are increasing, this pattern may have implications for medication management. Finally, it is helpful to remember that when measures detect a lack of improvement, that finding should prompt the clinician to ask, "What am I missing?" It may be the case that further assessment is needed to better understand additional or underlying problems. There may be issues such as hopelessness about treatment or concerns about the current treatment plan that need to be discussed. Lack of improvement may also reflect a set of life circumstances or medical issues that can only be fully addressed through additional support and engagement of a multidisciplinary team. Lack of change can present an opportunity to work collaboratively with the patient or with peers, as appropriate, to broaden the focus of treatment or to identify previously undetected challenges to or facilitators of recovery.

Case Examples

Case 1

This first case demonstrates how intake assessment data can inform treatment selection.

Over a year after the death of his wife, an older man presented to see a psychiatrist. At 71 years of age, the patient was now retired and living alone at home for the first time in 40 years. He presented with many depressive symptoms, existential concerns, and questions regarding the value of life. Given the nature of his symptoms, the provider asked him to complete a Geriatric Depression Scale (GDS) form. The results of the survey were enlightening. Although the man noted feelings of emptiness, worthlessness, and lack of energy and happiness, his answers to other items indicated that he still had hope and did not feel helpless. The presence of hopefulness and personal agency as elucidated by the GDS led the psychiatrist to discuss psychotherapy as a first mode of treatment (rather than starting with an antidepressant). The patient was not started on medications at that initial visit but instead was referred for psychotherapy, and he began seeing a psychologist once weekly for several months. When the patient returned to the psychiatrist 2 months later, he reported marked improvement in his depressive symptoms. A follow-up GDS was performed that confirmed the patient's subjective report that he no longer felt worthless or empty and his energy levels had improved, indicating no need for psychiatric medication.

Case 2

This second case demonstrates how ongoing monitoring can help identify that a patient is failing to respond and may be at risk of giving up.

A 40-year-old veteran sought treatment for PTSD. He began cognitive processing therapy (CPT), a psychotherapy involving reassessment of his thoughts and feelings regarding an event during his military service about which he felt profoundly guilty. His symptoms were monitored weekly with the PTSD Checklist. At the start of the fifth session, the provider and patient reviewed his scores and noted that the man's PTSD symptoms had increased since the start of CPT. The patient said that these results showed that treatment could not help him, because what he had done was unforgivable. "I've prayed over this many times, and Jesus has not lifted this burden from me." This remark led to a discussion of the patient's spiritual beliefs about recovery. During that conversation, the patient affirmed that he believed that all sinners could be redeemed. The provider then explained that CPT involves working through long-suppressed memories and feelings, and that people sometimes feel a little worse before they get better. The clinician and patient decided to increase the frequency of sessions to twice a week, attend to his spiritual beliefs in the context of CPT, and continue assessing his symptoms. Soon thereafter, the patient had a breakthrough, and his PTSD symptoms dropped to a nonclinical level.

Integration of Measurement-Based Care Into Routine Practice

Despite the importance of routine MBC for achieving the highest quality of mental health care, putting MBC into routine practice can be a significant challenge. Barriers to and facilitators of MBC have been identified through research of MBC implementation efforts in a variety of settings (de Jong 2016; Ross et al. 2016). Some issues that need to be addressed in planning implementation include when and where the data will be collected, whether the measures will be administered by paper and pencil or by other means, and how reports of the results will be generated.

Timing and Location

Processes and procedures need to be individualized to best fit the work flow within the particular clinical setting (de Jong 2016). For example, outcome data can be collected prior to an appointment from home, in the waiting room before the appointment, or even at multiple data points between sessions. Selection of the best process for data collection depends on the size and staffing of the clinic. Whatever method of data collection is selected, it should not duplicate work for either providers or patients. Brevity is another important factor to consider, because the time burdens involved in collecting outcome measures are a commonly reported barrier (Ross et al. 2016). Collecting and reviewing measures takes time and can encroach on the limited time that the provider and patient have together. Evidence indicates that outcome measures need to be obtained frequently (usually every session) in order to jointly reassess progress and allow for timely adjustments in care (Fortney et al. 2017). In sessions that may be limited to 15–30 minutes, clinicians need to sacrifice thoroughness for practicality and sustainability. A way to achieve this compromise is by jointly defining treatment goals with patients in longer treatment-planning sessions and then targeting for assessment only those outcome measures that are most relevant to the goals of care. Typically, completion of measures would require 5 minutes or less and ideally would occur in the waiting room prior to the session. A plan can include collecting different types of data at different sessions to spread out the burden on patients and providers.

Method of Administration and Generation of Reports

Collecting outcome data by paper and pencil is simple and easy for the patient and can be done in settings that do not have an electronic medical record (EMR). However, staff then need a process for entering and scoring those data and for generating reports of the results. The full benefits of MBC are realized when interventions and outcomes are recorded in an EMR or an MBC platform in a manner that allows for easy extraction and analyses across a patient population. EMR-embedded MBC allows for progress to be tracked easily over time and to be graphically presented in a manner that facilitates patient–provider discussions. EMR embedding also expands the possibilities for collection of MBC data to include kiosks, mobile devices, and web-based applications, thereby decreasing the time spent in session to collect the data. Systems that use the outcomes to facilitate the creation of progress notes can improve standard work flows.

In addition to improving individual patient outcomes, EMR-embedded MBC has the potential to improve the overall quality of mental health care. Currently, quality assessment in mental health care is difficult, in part because we lack the capability to compare results across programs or treatment conditions. Well-designed mental health care EMR systems minimize the need for additional data entry and maintain ease of use. The ability to perform high-level tracking of care in a population of patients has the potential to improve not only individual patient outcomes but also the overall quality of mental health care.

If measures and graphical representations are not available in clinical records, a number of web-based platforms for outcomes monitoring are available for free or for a licensing fee (Lyon et al. 2016). Examples of such systems include the OQ analyst platform (www.oqmeasures.com/products); Willow (www.willow.technology), typically used for psychotherapy; PROMIS (www.healthmeasures.net/explore-measurement-systems/promis/obtain-administer-measures); and Outcome Tracker (www.outcometracker.org/indexProvider.php). Developers of these platforms typically comply with U.S. laws requiring privacy and confidentiality (e.g., Health Insurance Portability and Accountability Act [HIPAA] laws). These systems automate delivery of outcome tracking measures to and from patients, thereby allowing more time for therapeutic work during the patient's visit. A recent review (Lyon et al. 2016) of more than 40 currently available digital outcome tracking systems evaluated them in regard to the range of outcomes and care processes that they can monitor, their ability to generate provider alerts and automated feedback reports, and their comparison of patients' progress relative to established norms (Gondek et al. 2016). Several MBC software programs have graphical user interfaces that make the results rapidly accessible and understandable for shared decision making.

Potential Advances in Data Collection

Future advances in technology may greatly expand the type of outcome data that can be collected (Hallgren et al. 2017). Web-based and mobile technology can already be used by patients to record outcome data prior to appointments so that results are available at the time of their appointment. The same technologies allow for data to be collected by patients across multiple time points and in different settings. Patients can also use this type of data to monitor their own progress. Making this information easily interpretable and fitting it within a clinic's work flow will be imperative for routine use. As technologies enable ongoing assessment of patients in real time, clinics will need to develop processes for responding to data received between appointments. For example, ancillary staff, such as psychiatric technicians, might monitor outcomes to identify when changes in a patient's symptoms or side effects warrant a psychiatrist's attention.

In addition to patient-entered data, emerging technology allows for passive data collection from patients, if implemented with proper safeguards and patient consent (see Chapter 7, "Ethical Considerations in Clinical Psychiatry"). Voice analysis technology on mobile phones has the potential to monitor conversations and detect mood or psychosis episodes prior to patients' or providers' awareness of a pending episode. Actigraphy likewise can detect behavioral changes and disruptions in sleep that patients may not be aware of at the time. Natural language processing tools have the potential to detect changes in mood, thought processes, and suicidality from postings and other patient writings. As such data become available from large numbers of patients, improved "big data" analytics may help to identify markers of patients who can benefit from a change of intervention (Kautzky et al. 2017). Building a clinical infrastructure to address these multiple types of data will be a vital part of this transformation (Hallgren et al. 2017).

Conclusion

A growing body of evidence supports the value of MBC. Using standardized assessment measures to inform initial treatment planning and monitoring of progress can improve quality of care by enhancing case formulation, by reducing treatment failure, and by promoting shared decision making. Many brief, reliable, and valid measures are available; some are free. The process of integrating assessment into clinic work flows needs to be carefully thought out. When integration is done well, assessment becomes a routine part of care that enables both providers and patients to make better-informed decisions.

Key Clinical Points

- Use of validated standardized measures as part of initial assessment can facilitate accurate assessment and appropriate treatment planning.

- MBC (ongoing use of standardized measures to monitor progress and inform care decisions) can improve patient outcomes and reduce treatment failures.

- Standardized assessment measures should demonstrate *reliability* (consistency) and *validity* (measure what they claim to). Measures of progress over time must be *sensitive to change.*

- Many brief self-report questionnaires for screening and measuring patients' progress are readily available for use by psychiatrists and other staff. Several outcome-monitoring software packages are also available.

- Collecting outcome data is only the first step. What matters is how providers and patients use the results to inform their treatment decisions.

- Outcome results should be shared with patients in a way that elicits their input and promotes shared decision making.

References

American Psychiatric Association Work Group on Psychiatric Evaluation: Practice Guidelines for the Psychiatric Evaluation of Adults, 3rd Edition. Arlington, VA, American Psychiatric Association, 2016

Beidas RS, Stewart RE, Walsh L, et al: Free, brief, and validated: standardized instruments for low-resource mental health settings. Cognit Behav Pract 22(1):5–19, 2015 25642130

Bickman L, Kelley SD, Breda C, et al: Effects of routine feedback to clinicians on mental health outcomes of youths: results of a randomized trial. Psychiatr Serv 62(12):1423–1429, 2011 22193788

Bufka LF, Campl N: Brief measures for screening and measuring mental health outcomes, in Assessment and Treatment Planning for Psychological Disorders, 2nd Edition. Edited by Antony MM, Barlow DH. New York, Guilford, 2010, pp 62–94

de Jong K: Challenges in the implementation of measurement feedback systems. Adm Policy Ment Health 43(3):467–470, 2016 26518779

Del Boca FK, Darkes J: The validity of self-reports of alcohol consumption: state of the science and challenges for research. Addiction 98 (suppl 2):1–12, 2003 14984237

Folstein MF, Folstein SE, McHugh PR: "Mini-mental state." A practical method for grading the cognitive state of patients for the clinician. J Psychiatr Res 12(3):189–198, 1975 1202204

Fortney JC, Unützer J, Wrenn G, et al: A tipping point for measurement-based care. Psychiatr Serv 68(2):179–188, 2017 27582237

Fowler JC, Patriquin M, Madan A, et al: Early identification of treatment non-response utilizing the Patient Health Questionnaire (PHQ-9). J Psychiatr Res 68:114–119, 2015 26228409

Gondek D, Edbrooke-Childs J, Fink E, et al: Feedback from outcome measures and treatment effectiveness, treatment efficiency, and collaborative practice: a systematic review. Adm Policy Ment Health 43(3):325–343, 2016 26744316

Groth-Marnat G, Wright AJ: Handbook of Psychological Assessment, 6th Edition. Hoboken, NJ, John Wiley & Sons, 2016

Hallgren KA, Bauer AM, Atkins DC: Digital technology and clinical decision making in depression treatment: current findings and future opportunities. Depress Anxiety 34(6):494–501, 2017 28453916

Horvath AO, Greenberg LS: Development and validation of the Working Alliance Inventory. Journal of Counseling Psychology 36(2):223–233, 1989

Hunsely J, Mash EJ: The role of assessment in evidence-based practice, in Assessment and Treatment Planning for Psychological Disorders, 2nd Edition. Edited by Antony MM, Barlow DH. New York, Guilford, 2010, pp 3–22

Joint Commission: Comprehensive Accreditation Manual for Behavioral Health: The Official Handbook. Oak Brook, IL, Joint Commission Resources, 2017

Kautzky A, Baldinger-Melich P, Kranz GS, et al: A new prediction model for evaluating treatment-resistant depression. J Clin Psychiatry 78(2):215–222, 2017 28068461

Kiresuk TJ, Smith A, Cardillo JE: Goal Attainment Scaling: Applications, Theory, and Measurement. New York, Psychology Press, 2014

Kroenke K, Spitzer RL, Williams JB: The Patient Health Questionnaire-2: validity of a two-item depression screener. Med Care 41(11):1284–1292, 2003 14583691

Lambert MJ, Whipple JL, Hawkins EJ, et al: Is it time for clinicians to routinely track patient outcome? A meta-analysis. Clinical Psychology: Science and Practice 10(3):288–301, 2003. Available at: https://psycnet.apa.org/record/2003-07528-003. Accessed January 18, 2019.

Lindström E, Lewander T, Malm U, et al: Patient-rated versus clinician-rated side effects of drug treatment in schizophrenia. Clinical validation of a self-rating version of the UKU Side Effect Rating Scale (UKU-SERS-Pat). Nord J Psychiatry 55 (suppl 44):5–69, 2001 11860666

Lyon AR, Lewis CC, Boyd MR, et al: Capabilities and characteristics of digital measurement and feedback systems: results from a comprehensive review. Adm Policy Ment Health 43(3):441–466, 2016 26860952

Morisky DE, Green LW, Levine DM: Concurrent and predictive validity of a self-reported measure of medication adherence. Med Care 24(1):67–74, 1986 3945130

Roebuck-Spencer TM, Glen T, Puente AE, et al: Cognitive screening tests versus comprehensive neuropsychological test batteries: a national academy of neuropsychology education paper. Arch Clin Neuropsychol 32(4):491–498, 2017 28334244

Ross DF, Ionita G, Stirman SW: System-wide implementation of routine outcome monitoring and measurement feedback system in a national network of operational stress injury clinics. Adm Policy Ment Health 43(6):927–944, 2016 27444375

Samara MT, Leucht C, Leeflang MM, et al: Early improvement as a predictor of later response to antipsychotics in schizophrenia: a diagnostic test review. Am J Psychiatry 172(7):617–629, 2015 26046338

Scott K, Lewis CC: Using measurement-based care to enhance any treatment. Cognit Behav Pract 22(1):49–59, 2015 27330267

Stedman JM, McGeary CA, Essery J: Current patterns of training in personality assessment during internship. J Clin Psychol 74(3):398–406, 2018 28685823

Tarescavage AM, Ben-Porath YS: Psychotherapeutic outcomes measures: a critical review for practitioners. J Clin Psychol 70(9):808–830, 2014 24652811

Zilcha-Mano S, Dinger U, McCarthy KS, et al: Does alliance predict symptoms throughout treatment, or is it the other way around? J Consult Clin Psychol 82(6):931–935, 2014 24274627

Recommended Readings

Beidas RS, Stewart RE, Walsh L, et al: Free, brief, and validated: standardized instruments for low-resource mental health settings. Cogn Behav Pract 22(1):5–19, 2015

Bufka LF, Campl N: Brief measures for screening and measuring mental health outcomes, in Assessment and Treatment Planning for Psychological Disorders, 2nd Edition. Edited by Antony MM, Barlow DH. New York, Guilford, 2010, pp 62–94

Fortney JC, Unützer J, Wrenn G, et al: A tipping point for measurement-based care. Psychiatr Serv 68(2):179–188, 2017

Gondek D, Edbrooke-Childs J, Fink E, et al: Feedback from outcome measures and treatment effectiveness, treatment efficiency, and collaborative practice: a systematic review. Adm Policy Ment Health 43(3):325–343, 2016

Groth-Marnat G, Wright AJ: Handbook of Psychological Assessment, 6th Edition. Hoboken, NJ, John Wiley and Sons, 2016

Lyon AR, Lewis CC, Boyd MR, et al: Capabilities and characteristics of digital measurement and feedback systems: results from a comprehensive review. Adm Policy Ment Health 43(3):441–446, 2016

Scott K, Lewis CC: Using measurement-based care to enhance any treatment. Cogn Behav Pract 22(1):49–59, 2015

Tarescavage AM, Ben-Porath YS: Psychotherapeutic outcomes measures: a critical review for practitioners. J Clin Psychol 70(9):808–830, 2014

PART IV

Caring for Special Populations

CHAPTER 40

Women

Vivien K. Burt, M.D., Ph.D.

Sonya Rasminsky, M.D.

Erin Murphy-Barzilay, M.D.

Rita Suri, M.D.

Although men and women are at equal risk of developing a mental disorder in their lifetime, there are gender-specific differences in the prevalence, clinical course, and treatment of specific psychiatric illnesses (Table 40–1). Additionally, women are at particular risk of mood disorders at times of reproductive transition (e.g., menarche, pregnancy, perimenopause) or in response to exogenous hormones (e.g., contraceptives, menopausal hormone treatment, fertility medications) (Table 40–2).

The psychiatric evaluation of reproductive-age women should always include questions about sexual activity, use and form of birth control, history of unprotected intercourse, past pregnancies, and regularity of menstrual cycles. Because roughly 45% of pregnancies in the United States are unplanned, treatment decisions in women of reproductive age must account for the possibility of future pregnancy.

A variety of factors—including sex-specific differences in drug absorption, bioavailability, metabolism, and elimination—influence how women respond to psychotropic medications. Because women tend to have greater bioavailability and slower clearance of drugs, optimal dosages for men may be too high for women. Furthermore, women tend to take more medications than men and are more prone to side effects associated with drug–drug interactions.

Along with biological factors, multiple psychosocial issues directly affect women's mental health. In many cases, a woman's experience includes a history of childhood physical or sexual abuse, rape, or domestic violence. In addition, economic deprivation; wage inequality; lack of social, emotional, and financial support for raising children; and caring for aging parents are some of the many factors that disproportionately affect women and their mental health.

In addition to genetic loading, the risk for mood and anxiety disorders in women at and after puberty is increased by a history of childhood and adolescent trauma. Thus,

TABLE 40–1.   Gender differences in psychiatric disorders

Disorder	Ratio (female:male)	History, presentation, and course in women	Treatment issues in women
Schizophrenia	Incidence 1.0:1.4, but prevalence equal (Aleman et al. 2003)	Compared with men, women have a better premorbid history, are diagnosed later, and are more likely to have a family history of schizophrenia; have less substance abuse and are less likely to commit suicide; have more mood symptoms, more positive symptoms, and fewer negative symptoms; and have better language proficiency and better social functioning. 15% of women with schizophrenia have a midlife onset of disease.	Compared with men, women have a better treatment response but are at increased risk of antipsychotic-induced hyperprolactinemia. Women with schizophrenia require birth control counseling as well as behavioral therapy to avoid unwanted sexual advances.
Unipolar major depression	1.7:1.0 (Kessler et al. 1994)	Women have an increased risk of exacerbation at times of reproductive transition (i.e., premenstruum, postpartum, perimenopause).	Treatment of depression to remission is advisable in women of childbearing age to safeguard against relapse in pregnancy and postpartum depression. Careful risk–benefit analysis for both mother and fetus is important in cases of pregnancy for women with past or current depression.
Bipolar disorder	Overall, approximately equal (Hendrick et al. 2000; Smith et al. 2013)	Compared with men, women have more mixed states, more bipolar II disorder, and more comorbid PTSD. Women are at risk of premenstrual worsening.	Compared with men, women are at increased risk of lithium-induced hypothyroidism. Women have a possibly increased risk of PCOS (due to valproate effect, independent hypothalamic-pituitary-gonadal effect, or both) and a high risk of postpartum destabilization.

TABLE 40–1. Gender differences in psychiatric disorders *(continued)*

Disorder	Ratio (female:male)	History, presentation, and course in women	Treatment issues in women
Anxiety disorders	Panic disorder: 2.5:1.0 (Kessler et al. 1994) Generalized anxiety disorder: 1.8:1.0 (Kessler et al. 1994) OCD[a]: 1.5:1.0 (Karno et al. 1988) PTSD[b]: 2:1 (Kessler et al. 1994)	Women older than 45 years are at markedly increased risk of generalized anxiety disorder. Women have an increased risk for exacerbation at times of reproductive transition (i.e., premenstruum, postpartum, perimenopause, pregnancy [OCD]). Women with PTSD are at increased risk of PMDD.	Women are at increased risk of thyroid disorders, which may produce symptoms similar to those of an anxiety disorder. Clinician should assess for premenstrual anxious symptoms and differentiate PMS/PMDD from true anxiety disorder with premenstrual exacerbation. Clinician should assess for perimenopausal physical changes (e.g., vasomotor) that may mimic anxiety symptoms.

Note. OCD=obsessive-compulsive disorder; PCOS=polycystic ovary syndrome; PMDD=premenstrual dysphoric disorder; PMS=premenstrual syndrome; PTSD=posttraumatic stress disorder.

[a]In DSM-5, OCD is now classified with the Obsessive-Compulsive and Related Disorders.
[b]In DSM-5, PTSD is now classified with the Trauma- and Stressor-Related Disorders.

TABLE 40–2.   **Reproductive-related times and events of psychiatric consequence in women**

Age of menarche

Phase of menstrual cycle

Use of hormonal contraception

Pregnancy

Birth

Postpartum

Breastfeeding or weaning

Induced abortion

Miscarriage

Infertility treatment

Hysterectomy

Perimenopause

---

having a history of poor prepubertal attachments and exposure to domestic violence or sexual abuse and having experienced parental loss or absence (through death, divorce, or marital discord) are associated with negative self-image and an increase in early affective illness. Furthermore, repeated depressive episodes in childhood and adolescence increase the risk of recurrent depression throughout adulthood, and in women this risk is particularly high at times of reproductive transitions (e.g., premenstrually, perinatally, perimenopausally). For further details about adolescent mental health, the reader is referred to Chapter 41 in this volume, "Children and Adolescents."

Premenstrual Dysphoric Disorder

Premenstrual dysphoric disorder (PMDD) comprises recurrent physical and emotional symptoms that begin in the late luteal phase of the menstrual cycle and remit within several days following the onset of menstruation. In addition to experiencing physical symptoms (i.e., bloating, breast tenderness, cramping, and headaches), women with PMDD have emotional symptoms that may include depression, irritability, anxiety, and insomnia. With the publication of DSM-5 in 2013, the American Psychiatric Association moved PMDD from Appendix B in Section III to a formal categorical entity in Section II (American Psychiatric Association 2013). DSM-5 criteria state that symptoms must be present during the premenstrual week (rather than *most of the time* during the premenstrual week, as required in the DSM-IV [American Psychiatric Association 1994] research criteria) and place greater emphasis on mood lability, irritability, and anger. Because women with PMDD often are able to compensate and cope during their symptomatic days, the new criteria indicate that PMDD causes clinically significant distress *or* interferes with activities. The criteria also specify that the condition may co-occur with other disorders. Criterion G highlights the distinctiveness of PMDD from an ongoing medical condition or substance-induced condition.

Whereas most women of reproductive age experience premenstrual symptoms during at least some of their cycles, the 12-month prevalence of PMDD is 1.8%–5.8% of menstruating women (American Psychiatric Association 2013).

The pathophysiology of PMDD is thought to involve a complex interplay of genetic susceptibility, structural and functional brain heterogeneity, trauma, and stress as it relates to the hypothalamic, pituitary, and gonadal axes; inflammatory processes; the involvement of estrogen and serotonin; and the additional influence of the neuroactive hormones progesterone and allopregnanolone (Raffi and Freeman 2017). Women with PMDD have ovarian hormone levels indistinguishable from those of women without PMDD. Recent evidence supports the idea that mood symptoms in women with PMDD are uniquely triggered by changes in estradiol and progesterone rather than being the result of a steady-state level above a critical threshold (Schmidt et al. 2017). This abnormal sensitivity to changes in sex hormones has been associated with differences in the expression of a gene complex regulating epigenetic mechanisms for response to sex hormones and environmental stressors (Dubey et al. 2017).

Evaluation and Treatment

Evaluation for PMDD includes documentation of the course and nature of symptoms, possible precipitants, and prior treatment approaches and responses. The diagnosis is confirmed by prospective daily ratings over at least two menstrual cycles. Physical conditions that may cause symptoms in association with the premenstrual phase of the menstrual cycle (e.g., endometriosis, fibrocystic breast disease, migraine headaches) should be ruled out. Because premenstrual symptoms tend to be familial, assessment should include a family history of premenstrual symptoms and effective treatments. Over-the-counter and prescription medications should be noted, and possible psychiatric side effects of these substances should be considered. The use of caffeine, salt, alcohol, and nicotine should be ascertained, because these may cause symptoms that mimic those of PMDD (e.g., bloating, lethargy, irritability, breast tenderness). A good psychosocial history is important as well, because an association of PMDD with stressful life events and also with past sexual abuse has been noted.

Treatment for PMDD falls into four broad categories: 1) nonpharmacological treatments, 2) serotonin reuptake inhibitors, 3) hormonal treatments, and 4) complementary medicines.

Nonpharmacological Treatments

Mild premenstrual symptoms may be responsive to nonpharmacological interventions, such as sleep hygiene education, exercise, relaxation therapy, and cognitive-behavioral therapy. Dietary modifications, including reduction of salty foods, caffeine, red meat, and alcohol, along with increased consumption of fruits, legumes, whole grains, and water and consumption of smaller and more frequent meals high in carbohydrates, have been reported to improve tension and depression.

Serotonin Reuptake Inhibitors

The depression of PMDD is frequently as severe as that of major depressive disorder, and although PMDD symptoms occur solely during the luteal phase, the condition recurs monthly over years, often resulting in severe suffering and dysfunction. Fortunately, women with moderate to severe PMDD generally respond robustly to selective serotonin reuptake inhibitors (SSRIs) (Yonkers and Simoni 2018), and fluoxetine, sertraline, and paroxetine are approved by the U.S. Food and Drug Administration (FDA) for this indication. Both continuous and intermittent dosing are effective

(Lanza di Scalea and Pearlstein 2017). Continuous pharmacological treatment (i.e., throughout the month) is best for women who have comorbid depressive or anxiety disorders or for women who have difficulty with adherence to intermittent therapy. Luteal-phase treatment (i.e., during the 2 premenstrual weeks) works well for patients who have symptoms that are clearly localized to the premenstrual days and who may have side effects (e.g., sexual side effects) that dissipate on days when SSRIs are not used. Symptom-onset treatment (i.e., beginning with the start of symptoms and ending with the onset of menses) may also be effective and limits medication exposure significantly. Premenstrual anxiety and irritability may be treated with anxiolytics such as buspirone and alprazolam.

Hormonal Treatments

Oral contraceptives are frequently used in the treatment of PMDD, but evidence supporting their use is limited, and they should be considered primarily in women who also desire contraception. The best evidence is for medication containing the progesterone drospirenone: the combination of 3 mg of drospirenone and 20 µg of ethinyl estradiol (Yaz) is FDA approved for the treatment of PMDD. However, the FDA issued a warning in 2012 that drospirenone-containing pills may be associated with a higher risk of venous thromboembolism than pills containing other progestins, making individualized risk assessment essential (U.S. Food and Drug Administration 2012).

Gonadotropin-releasing hormone (GnRH) agonists such as leuprolide suppress ovulation and can lead to improvement in symptoms of PMDD. However, because the resulting hypoestrogenic state leads to bone loss, vaginal dryness, and other menopausal symptoms, GnRH agonists are considered a treatment of last resort (Lanza di Scalea and Pearlstein 2017; Yonkers and Simoni 2018).

Complementary Treatments

Many women choose to use herbal remedies to manage PMDD. Vitamin B_6 (pyridoxine) may be helpful at dosages up to 100 mg daily, but peripheral neuropathy can occur at dosages higher than 200 mg daily (Yonkers and Simoni 2018). *Vitex agnus-castus* extract (chasteberry) has shown benefit in comparison with placebo, pyridoxine, or magnesium. Calcium at dosages as low as 500 mg daily can improve symptoms. Because calcium (not exceeding 1,500 mg/day) and vitamin D may also reduce the risk of osteoporosis and have other health advantages, women should be encouraged to include these in their daily diets.

Psychiatric Disorders During Pregnancy

Pregnancy is not necessarily a time of emotional stability, particularly if the expectant mother has a prior history of psychiatric illness or has changed or discontinued a medication regimen that had kept her stable and functional (Cohen et al. 2006). Given the public health impact of perinatal mood disorders, in 2016 the U.S. Preventive Services Task Force (O'Connor et al. 2016) recommended universal screening for depression in pregnant and postpartum women, adding to the existing recommendations by the American College of Obstetricians and Gynecologists (2018) and the American Academy of Pediatrics (Earls et al. 2019). As of 2019, four states (New Jersey, Illinois, West

Virginia, and California) mandate screening for perinatal depression, and several others require education or have launched statewide awareness campaigns (Earls et al. 2019).

The ideal time for women with psychiatric histories to decide among possible treatment options during pregnancy is prior to becoming pregnant. In this way, a treatment plan can be formulated that considers safety and well-being for both patient and fetus. Although discontinuation of psychiatric medications should be considered when clinically feasible, nonpharmacological interventions may not be sufficient during pregnancy.

Psychiatric decompensation during pregnancy impacts both the mother and the fetus. A woman who is depressed, anxious, or psychotic may be unable to care for herself or to adhere to prenatal regimens. In addition, depression during pregnancy may be associated with obstetrical complications and adverse consequences for the fetus, such as preterm birth and low birth weight (Jarde et al. 2016). Antenatal psychiatric instability also increases the risk for illness during the postpartum period, when maternal responsibilities are new and particularly overwhelming. Patients should be advised that nicotine and alcohol are detrimental to the fetus and their own well-being, and strategies should be devised to ensure opportunities for adequate sleep and healthful nutrition. Psychotherapy, group support, and family and couples counseling may be helpful, because pregnancy is a stressful time and may be particularly challenging for psychiatrically ill women.

Although the FDA does not endorse the safety of any psychiatric medication during pregnancy, physicians may prescribe medications according to evidence-based knowledge and their own best clinical judgment. In 2015, the FDA replaced its pregnancy labeling categories of A, B, C, D, and X with the new "Pregnancy and Lactation Labeling Rule" (known as the "Final Rule"). The new labeling provides detailed information regarding a medication's use during pregnancy and lactation and in males and females of reproductive potential.

Before a psychotropic agent is administered to a pregnant patient, the risks and benefits to both the mother and the fetus should be evaluated and shared with the patient, her partner (whenever possible), and her obstetrician. Pregnancy counseling should emphasize that the goal is to weigh risks associated with psychotropic medications against risks of untreated disease for mother and baby, during both pregnancy and the postpartum period. Discussions should be documented, and the clinician should assess and note the patient's understanding and capacity to consent to the treatment plan.

Table 40–3 presents general guiding principles for the treatment of psychiatric illness during pregnancy.

Treatment of Depression During Pregnancy

Depression during pregnancy is common; depressive symptoms affect about 10% of pregnant women, with 5.1% having symptoms that meet criteria for probable major depressive disorder and 4.8% having symptoms that meet criteria for milder depression (Vigod et al. 2016). Nevertheless, depression may be overlooked during pregnancy because many of the neurovegetative symptoms of depression coincide with normal somatic complaints of pregnancy. The functional impairment that frequently occurs in association with depression is of particular concern during pregnancy because of its potential impact on the health of both the expectant mother and her fetus. Furthermore,

---

TABLE 40–3.   **Treatment of psychiatric illness in pregnancy**

The overall mental health of an expectant mother is an important determinant of the health of the fetus and neonate.

Psychiatric illness that compromises maternal function increases the risk of poor obstetrical outcomes.

Depression during pregnancy substantially increases the risk of postpartum depression.

Risks of maternal treatment with psychotropic medication should be weighed against known risks of untreated psychiatric disease for mother and baby.

Risk–benefit decisions during pregnancy should be made on a case-by-case basis by an informed patient in combination with her partner and doctors.

For mild to moderate psychiatric illness, nonpharmacological interventions should be tried first:

  Psychotherapy

  Couples counseling

  Stress-reduction strategies

  Mobilization of psychosocial supports

  Bright-light therapy (for depression)

For severe, disabling psychiatric illness, the risk of psychotropic medication to both mother and infant is generally less than the risk of symptomatic illness.

When a psychiatrically ill pregnant woman is being treated, regardless of whether treatment includes psychotropic medications, general maternal medical health indices, such as appetite, weight, and sleep patterns, should be carefully monitored to optimize maternal health and obstetrical outcomes.

---

depression during pregnancy significantly increases the risk of postpartum depression. For mild to moderate depression, nonpharmacological modalities such as individual or conjoint psychotherapy and stress-reduction counseling are good first options for treatment. However, for severe and treatment-resistant depression, particularly if symptoms jeopardize a patient's emotional stability and the viability of the pregnancy (e.g., if the woman is suicidal, psychotic, or not gaining weight or is reluctantly contemplating an abortion), psychopharmacological approaches to treatment are reasonable.

Because the use of antidepressants during pregnancy is not without some risk, nonpharmacological strategies, such as psychotherapy, should be tried first. Bright-light therapy is a noninvasive treatment option for antenatal depression. Transcranial magnetic stimulation appears to be an effective and safe treatment for depression during pregnancy. However, if a woman is experiencing severe, debilitating depression, or if she has a history of chronic depression with severe relapses following medication discontinuation, antidepressants should be considered. When antidepressants are used during pregnancy, dosages should be kept at the minimum necessary to promote ongoing mood stability and normal functioning. The major issues of concern when evaluating outcomes with any medications during pregnancy, and in this case with antidepressants, are the risks of congenital malformation, pregnancy loss, perinatal toxicity, shorter gestation length, and neurobehavioral sequelae to the fetus.

An enormous amount of controversy exists regarding the risks and benefits of antidepressants during pregnancy, largely because studies in pregnant women are notoriously difficult to do. Among the many problems that make conclusions extremely difficult are inadequate randomization, lack of adequate controls, failure to address confounders (e.g., the effect of depression, anxiety, or genetic loading on infant outcomes; the use of multiple medications; the use of illicit drugs and alcohol), lack of reliable data on the actual intake of medications, and lack of blinding to cases and controls. Because women often are undertreated during pregnancy because of concerns about fetal outcome, it may be that pregnant women who choose to remain on psychiatric medications have more severe illness. Thus, apparent associations between adverse infant outcomes and prenatal antidepressant exposure may be a function of variables related to maternal illness rather than a function of medication exposure (confounding by indication). Although absolute conclusions about risks during pregnancy for individual psychiatric medications are not possible, clinicians should carefully and critically analyze accruing data for individual medications and classes of agents in order to help women and their partners make informed decisions regarding the treatment of depression during pregnancy.

In the following subsections, which emphasize data from peer-reviewed studies, we review what is currently known about the use of antidepressants during pregnancy. Because serotonergic antidepressants (SSRIs and serotonin–norepinephrine reuptake inhibitors [SNRIs]) are the antidepressants most widely used to treat depression, and because of the large amount of conflicting and controversial data published on the subject of SSRI use during pregnancy, the discussion emphasizes the prenatal use of these agents.

Selective Serotonin Reuptake Inhibitors and Serotonin–Norepinephrine Reuptake Inhibitors

Teratogenicity. Although numerous peer-reviewed studies on the use of SSRIs during pregnancy have found no significantly increased risk of birth defects beyond the general population risk of 3% (Huybrechts et al. 2014; Margulis et al. 2013; Nordeng et al. 2012), several other studies have suggested possible teratogenicity with in utero exposure to SSRIs (Jimenez-Solem et al. 2012; Malm et al. 2011). Studies finding increased risks have been compromised by reliance on prescription data, lack of control for underlying psychiatric condition, low numbers of exposed subjects, low background absolute risk for uncommon defects, and inadequate control for substance and alcohol use or abuse. Although some studies have found that paroxetine may be associated with cardiac defects (especially right-ventricle defects) in 1–2 per 100 infants, a large-scale cohort study of close to 950,000 women found no significant association between cardiac malformations and first-trimester antidepressant use, including paroxetine (Huybrechts et al. 2014). Current consensus suggests that the risk of treatment discontinuation may outweigh the possible risks associated with antenatal antidepressant therapy (Ornoy and Koren 2017).

Neonatal adaptation syndrome. Third-trimester exposure to SSRIs is associated with an approximately 25% risk of perinatal symptoms—including irritability, jitteriness, poor muscle tone, weak or absent cry, respiratory distress, hypoglycemia, and seizures—that sometimes require admission to special care nurseries. If infants have these symptoms, they are usually mild, transient, and self-limited. It appears that neonatal symptoms do not differ between babies of women who discontinued SSRIs in the third trimester of pregnancy and babies of women who continued their antidepressant through delivery (Salisbury et al. 2016).

Persistent pulmonary hypertension of the newborn.   Late exposure to SSRIs has been reported to increase the risk of persistent pulmonary hypertension of the newborn (PPHN), a rare illness affecting fewer than 2 per 1,000 live births at baseline. Because data supporting the role of prenatal SSRIs in PPHN are confounded by other factors, in December 2011 the FDA issued a public safety announcement advising health care professionals not to alter their current clinical practice of treating depression during pregnancy, stating that "it is premature to reach any conclusion about a possible link between SSRI use during pregnancy and PPHN" (U.S. Food and Drug Administration 2011).

Gestation length, birth weight, and fetal growth.   While some studies have suggested that SSRIs may be associated with an increased risk of shorter gestation, small-for-gestational-age babies, and admission to special care nurseries, other studies, a large systematic review, and a meta-analysis of pregnancy and delivery outcomes after prenatal exposure to antidepressants (Ross et al. 2013) found statistically but not clinically significant decreases in length of gestation (3 fewer days), birth weight (75 grams lower), and Apgar scores (less than half a point on the 1- and 5-minute scores). Thus, although gestation length, birth weight, and fetal growth may be somewhat decreased with prenatal antidepressant exposure, the differences appear to be small, and Apgar scores, which measure the condition of neonates on delivery, are not clinically significantly different.

Neurobehavioral sequelae.   The long-term neurodevelopmental and behavioral outcomes of children exposed to antidepressants in utero is of significant interest. Numerous studies have found no adverse developmental outcomes in children exposed antenatally to SSRIs. A recent large population cohort study found that an increased risk of intellectual disability in the offspring of women who used antidepressants (both SSRIs and other antidepressants) during pregnancy was likely due to factors other than the antidepressants themselves (e.g., parental age, maternal psychiatric disorders) (Viktorin et al. 2017). Six recent meta-analyses reported an increased risk of autism spectrum disorder (ASD) in the children of women treated with antidepressants during pregnancy (Andalib et al. 2017; H.K. Brown et al. 2017; Kaplan et al. 2016, 2017; Kobayashi et al. 2016; Mezzacappa et al. 2017). Of importance, however, is the fact that the majority of these meta-analyses (H.K. Brown et al. 2017; Kaplan et al. 2016, 2017; Kobayashi et al. 2016; Mezzacappa et al. 2017) could not exclude maternal mental illness as a significant confounding factor that may have influenced the increased risk. In his comprehensive review of these meta-analyses, Andrade (2017a) stated that "the findings of these meta-analyses do not discourage the use of SSRIs during pregnancy if the condition being treated causes significant dysfunction, is associated with serious negative implications (e.g., suicidal risk), or is associated with negative behaviors that impact maternal or fetal well-being" (p. e1050). Among five recent observational studies examining the risk of ASD in children with prenatal antidepressant exposure, two studies did not find an increased risk (H.K. Brown et al. 2017; Sujan et al. 2017). The three studies that did suggest an association between in utero antidepressant exposure and ASD could also not exclude the influence of maternal mental illness or other factors, including environmental and genetic risks, on their findings (Liu et al. 2017; Rai et al. 2017; Viktorin et al. 2017). Thus, antidepressant use during pregnancy may be suggestive of more severe maternal mental illness, which in turn is likely to be related to adverse neurodevelopmental outcomes such as ASD in exposed offspring (Andrade 2017b). Because maternal depression and antidepressant exposure are so closely linked, and because antidepressant treatment itself may be indicative of the severity of depression during pregnancy, "evidence supporting an association between in utero exposure to antidepressant medications, especially selective serotonin reuptake inhibitors, and adverse long-term neurodevelopmental outcomes remains inconclusive" (Oberlander and Zwaigenbaum 2017, p. 1533). Of note, the large increase in ASD diagnoses over the past two decades does not appear to be connected to antenatal SSRI use. As always, the potential risk of medication exposure must be balanced against the risk to the mother or fetus of untreated mental illness.

Summary regarding use of SSRIs and SNRIs during pregnancy.   Because there are no rigorously controlled trials of the effect of prenatal antidepressants on infant outcomes, all such studies are necessarily limited by multiple real and potential confounds. In particular, a major limitation is of confounding by indication (i.e., confounding by presence and severity of maternal mental illness). Maternal depression is clearly a risk factor for mood disorders and other difficulties in offspring. Although there have been reports of small increased risks for certain rare congenital defects with various SSRIs, the absolute risks (if reports are true) are very small. Transient difficulties with neonatal adaptation must not be assumed to mean long-term difficulties, especially in the context of worsening maternal depression. The possibility of neurobehavioral and other long-term outcomes with in utero SSRI exposure and/or maternal depression and anxiety is currently a subject of study, and these studies, like those examining other adverse outcomes, are compromised by multiple confounders (especially the effect of postpartum mental illness on neurodevelopment in babies and children). What is apparent is that for women with impairing and disabling depression and anxiety, nontreatment during pregnancy is not a feasible option.

Other Antidepressant Classes

Table 40–4 presents major summary points about the antenatal use of SSRIs, SNRIs, and other antidepressant classes.

Treatment of Bipolar Disorder During Pregnancy

Pregnancy does not protect against bipolar mood instability when mood stabilizers are discontinued. Predictors of recurrence of mood episodes include treatment discontinuation, antidepressant use, younger age, early illness onset, prenatal mood episodes, and somatic complaints during pregnancy.

Table 40–5 lists basic principles of managing bipolar disorder during pregnancy. When long periods of interepisode euthymia have been demonstrated, an attempt may be made before conception to avoid mood stabilizers during the first trimester. Careful tapering may be attempted over a period of 2–4 weeks to reduce the likelihood of relapse. During pregnancy, gradual rather than rapid taper mitigates the risk of postpartum relapse. However, for women whose illness has historically required pharmacotherapy to remain stable, medication is best continued throughout pregnancy. Recurrence rates for pregnant women who discontinue mood stabilizers are

TABLE 40–4.   Use of antidepressants during pregnancy: summary points

Antidepressant class	Teratogenicity	Other adverse effects	Comments
Selective serotonin reuptake inhibitors (SSRIs)	As a group, SSRIs other than paroxetine do not appear to increase risk for major congenital malformations. Paroxetine may increase risk of congenital anomalies, particularly ventricular–septal defects.	Increased risk of poor neonatal adaptability Possible increased risk of persistent pulmonary hypertension of the newborn Increased risk for shorter gestational period and preterm birth (37 weeks' gestation) Increased risk of small-for-gestational-age birth (statistically but not clinically significant)	Paroxetine should be avoided if possible. Use of these agents is justified if history suggests that antenatal treatment is essential to keep a pregnant woman euthymic and functional. Targeted early second-trimester ultrasound should be considered for exposed fetuses. Clinician should Maintain awareness of possible neonatal side effects and observe exposed infants for several days beyond usual 1–2 days postpartum. Monitor maternal appetite, weight, and other indices of maternal health.
Tricyclic antidepressants (TCAs)	TCAs do not appear to increase risk for major congenital malformations.	Increased risk of poor neonatal adaptability Increased risk of shorter gestational period (37 weeks' gestation)	Use of these agents is justified if history suggests that antenatal treatment is essential to keep a seriously depressed pregnant woman euthymic and functional. Clinician should: Maintain awareness of possible neonatal side effects—observe exposed infants for several days beyond usual 1–2 days postpartum. Monitor maternal appetite, weight, and other indices of maternal health.

TABLE 40–4. Use of antidepressants during pregnancy: summary points *(continued)*

Antidepressant class	Teratogenicity	Other adverse effects	Comments
Other antidepressants: fluvoxamine, venlafaxine, bupropion, trazodone, nefazodone, duloxetine	Fewer cases have been published; more data are needed. Venlafaxine does not appear to increase risk for major congenital malformations (but more data are needed). Bupropion does not appear to increase the risk for major congenital malformations (but more data are needed). Mirtazapine does not appear to increase risk for congenital defects (more data are needed).	More data needed. Some suggestion that antidepressants may increase risk of shorter gestational period, preterm birth (37 weeks' gestation)	Use of these agents is justified only if history suggests that antenatal treatment is essential to keep a seriously depressed pregnant woman euthymic and functional. Clinician should: Maintain awareness of possible neonatal side effects—observe exposed infants for several days beyond usual 1–2 days postpartum. Monitor maternal appetite, weight, and other indices of maternal health.
Monoamine oxidase inhibitors (MAOIs)	Unknown (insufficient data)	Associated with blood pressure changes that are potentially detrimental to the fetus and that may compromise use of agents to prevent preterm labor and treat other obstetrical complications	MAOI antidepressants are best avoided during pregnancy.

TABLE 40-5.	Treatment of pregnant patients with bipolar disorder

For women with mild to moderate bipolar disorder, an attempt should be made to withhold mood stabilizers during the first trimester. (Caution: Careful psychiatric supervision is needed to monitor for early relapse.)

For women with moderate to severe bipolar disorder, mood stabilizers and other psychiatric medications should be continued as needed to maintain euthymia throughout pregnancy.

Because all mood stabilizers carry some teratogenic risk and potential for peripartum toxicity, choice of treatment should be made after a careful case-by-case analysis of the safest regimen to maintain maternal mood stability and fetal safety.

Lithium, despite its risk of cardiovascular teratogenicity, is probably a reasonable choice for the pregnant bipolar patient. Prenatal testing (nuchal lucency, level 2 ultrasound at week 18–20) and other guidelines of careful management should be followed.

high, and the risks of uncontrolled bipolar disorder during pregnancy must be weighed against the risks of pharmacological treatment. Lithium is preferable to carbamazepine and valproate because of its lower risk of teratogenicity.

Lithium

Maternal use of lithium during the first trimester is associated with an increased risk for cardiac malformations in general, although this risk is small (0.6%–4.1%) and may be dose dependent (Patorno et al. 2017). With first-trimester use of lithium, the risk for Ebstein's anomaly (a serious congenital defect in the formation of the tricuspid valve) has historically been estimated at about 1 in 1,000, compared with the background risk of 1 in 20,000. However, more recent data suggest that the risk of outflow-tract obstructions (which includes conditions related to Ebstein's anomaly, such as pulmonary atresia) is probably smaller than these previous estimates (Patorno et al. 2017). Additional potential adverse consequences to the neonate from maternal lithium use during pregnancy include rare transient perinatal effects. In utero lithium exposure does not incur adverse neurobehavioral effects.

If lithium is used during pregnancy, levels must be carefully monitored, and dosing may need to be adjusted as total body volume increases. Guidelines for managing lithium during pregnancy are presented in Table 40–6.

Anticonvulsants

Of the conventional mood stabilizers, valproate carries the highest risk for major malformations. In addition to an increased risk of spina bifida, valproate has been associated with significant developmental delay (Meador et al. 2013; Weston et al. 2016), atrial septal defect, cleft palate, hypospadias, polydactyly, craniosynostosis, and ASD. Cognitive deficits associated with valproate have been shown to persist up to 4.5 years (Meador et al. 2013). Given the significant adverse outcomes associated with antenatal valproate use, "delaying discussions of treatment risks until a pregnancy is considered will leave a substantial number of children at unnecessary risk. Women of childbearing potential should be informed of the potential risks of fetal valproate exposure before valproate is prescribed" (Meador and Loring 2013, p. 1731). If exposure has occurred, an amniotic α-fetoprotein analysis at week 16 and an ultrasound between weeks 18 and 22 should be obtained to assess for neural tube defects.

TABLE 40–6. **Guidelines for management of lithium in pregnant patients with bipolar disorder**

Maintain maternal target lithium concentrations at minimum clinically effective levels.

If possible, avoid situations that tend to increase lithium levels:

Use of agents that cause lithium concentrations to increase: nonsteroidal anti-inflammatory drugs (NSAIDs), diuretics, angiotensin-converting enzyme (ACE) inhibitors, calcium channel blockers

Sodium-restricted diet (e.g., to manage preeclampsia, edema) may result in increased maternal lithium serum concentration.

Maintain heightened awareness of possible maternal lithium toxicity in cases of the following:

Acute loss of fluids at delivery

Hyperemesis gravidarum

Preeclampsia

Monitor fetal development:

Nuchal translucency (12 weeks' gestation)

Level 2 structural ultrasound (at week 18–20)

Fetal echocardiogram

Dosing and levels:

Twice-daily dosing recommended

Check preconception lithium level to guide dosage during pregnancy and postpartum.

Monitor maternal lithium levels carefully:

Once every 3 weeks until 34 weeks' gestation

Weekly after 34 weeks until delivery

Labor and delivery:

Maintain fluids throughout labor and delivery; do not discontinue lithium.

Monitor lithium in mother twice per week during the first 2 weeks postpartum, with goal of achieving preconception lithium level.

Source. Adapted from Newport et al. 2005; Wesseloo et al. 2017.

The overall risk of major congenital malformations with carbamazepine has been estimated at 3.3%, similar to the background risk with no exposure. First-trimester exposure to carbamazepine is associated with an increased risk for spina bifida but not for other congenital malformations, and this risk is far less than that for valproate. In utero exposure to carbamazepine, unlike that to valproate, does not appear to have an adverse effect on IQ in exposed offspring (Meador et al. 2013).

Although the North American Antiepileptic Drug Pregnancy Registry suggested that lamotrigine monotherapy during the first trimester is associated with oral clefts, this finding was not substantiated by data derived from the EUROCAT (European Registration of Congenital Anomalies and Twins) congenital malformation registries, representing 10.1 million births (Dolk et al. 2016). Even if there is an association between antenatal lamotrigine exposure and oral clefts, the absolute risk of having a child with an oral cleft is about 0.7%, a risk that women whose condition is stable on lamotrigine may be willing to take when compared with adverse outcomes associated with relapse during pregnancy. Of note, maternal serum lamotrigine concentrations decline during pregnancy because of rising levels of estradiol. Levels should be monitored during pregnancy, and dosing may need to be adjusted. If the dosage is increased during pregnancy, it should be tapered back to the prepregnancy dosage over a 2-week period after delivery in order to prevent lamotrigine toxicity.

Because topiramate increases the risk of congenital malformations (especially oral clefts) and growth retardation in infants exposed in utero (Holmes and Hernandez-Diaz 2012), this medication should be avoided during pregnancy.

Combining valproate with either lamotrigine or carbamazepine significantly increases the risk of malformations among exposed infants.

Because of their higher risk for neural tube defects, pregnant women treated with anticonvulsants should take 4 mg of folic acid daily, beginning prior to conception.

Table 40–7 summarizes the risks of commonly used mood stabilizers in pregnancy.

Antipsychotics

Antipsychotics are sometimes used during pregnancy. Although low-potency phenothiazines may increase the risk of nonspecific congenital anomalies, high-potency antipsychotics have not been associated with major malformations. Atypical antipsychotics have not been shown to be teratogenic, with the possible exception of risperidone (Huybrechts et al. 2016), but more controlled studies are needed to establish that these agents are safe during pregnancy. Preliminary data from the prospectively derived National Pregnancy Registry for Psychiatric Medications, based at the Massachusetts General Hospital, are encouraging and suggest that atypical (i.e., second-generation) antipsychotics *as a group* do not appear to be teratogenic (Cohen et al. 2016). These data have been included by the FDA in its list of pregnancy exposure registries. Of concern during pregnancy is the risk of atypical antipsychotic–induced hyperglycemia and gestational diabetes, although this risk may be minimal for women who have used atypical antipsychotics without metabolic side effects prior to pregnancy (Panchaud et al. 2017).

Among infants exposed to first-generation antipsychotic agents in utero near the time of delivery, a transient syndrome of motor restlessness, tremor, hypertonia, and poor feeding has been noted. Antipsychotic exposure during pregnancy has been associated with lower scores on tests of neuromotor performance at age 6 months, although the extent of the relative contribution of underlying maternal mental illness is unclear, and it is not known whether these findings have any long-term clinical significance (Johnson et al. 2012).

Table 40–8 summarizes the risks associated with the use of antipsychotics during pregnancy.

Treatment of Schizophrenia During Pregnancy

Although some women with schizophrenia remain stable during pregnancy, others are at increased risk for poor prenatal care and adverse pregnancy outcomes. Patients should be assessed for substance misuse, psychosocial stressors, lack of housing and financial resources, and other factors that negatively affect parenting ability. Women with schizophrenia are more likely to have low dietary folate and obesity, factors that place them at increased risk of having a child with a neural tube defect. Psychosocial support should be maximized to enhance proper nourishment, adherence to prenatal

TABLE 40–7. Use of mood stabilizers during pregnancy

Medication	Teratogenicity	Potential perinatal effects
Lithium	Cardiac risk—including Ebstein's anomaly No long-term neurobehavioral sequelae	Hypotonia, poor feeding, cyanosis, neonatal goiter, diabetes insipidus
Valproate	Neural tube anomalies Craniofacial abnormalities Developmental delay Coagulopathy	Hypoglycemia Hepatic dysfunction Coagulopathy
Carbamazepine	Neural tube anomalies Possible association with craniofacial abnormalities, developmental delay, cardiovascular/coronary abnormalities, coagulopathy	Hypoglycemia Hepatic dysfunction
Lamotrigine	Possible oral cleft	None known

TABLE 40–8. Use of antipsychotics during pregnancy

Medication classes	Teratogenicity	Potential perinatal effects
Low-potency antipsychotic agents: phenothiazines	Nonspecific congenital anomalies	Behavioral irritability, restlessness Impaired feeding Jaundice
High-potency antipsychotic agents (e.g., haloperidol)	No known major congenital anomalies	Behavioral irritability, restlessness Impaired feeding
Atypical antipsychotics	Limited data reveal no major anomalies (olanzapine, quetiapine, clozapine); possible abnormalities with risperidone—more data needed	Behavioral irritability, restlessness, tremor Hyperreflexia Impaired feeding

instructions (including daily intake of vitamins and folate), preparation for the responsibilities of motherhood, location of appropriate housing, and access to social services.

Relapse of symptoms of schizophrenia places pregnant women and their offspring at significant risk for adverse outcomes; therefore, antipsychotic medications should be used during pregnancy when necessary. The limited yet growing data on these medications during pregnancy were detailed in the previous section on bipolar disorder and suggest that the atypical antipsychotics, with the possible exception of risperidone, do not appear to increase the risk of major congenital malformations (Huybrechts et al. 2016). The anticholinergic agents trihexyphenidyl and benztropine have been associated with minor congenital malformations and anticholinergic symptoms in the newborn, including functional bowel obstruction and urinary retention. Diphenhydramine does not appear to increase the risk of congenital malformations.

Treatment of Anxiety Disorders and Obsessive-Compulsive Disorder During Pregnancy

The course of panic disorder, generalized anxiety disorder, and obsessive-compulsive disorder (OCD) during pregnancy is variable. OCD in particular often presents for the first time during pregnancy or the postpartum period, and discontinuation of anxiolytic antidepressants and other medications at the onset of pregnancy can result in relapse. Stress and anxiety during pregnancy increase the risk for maternal self-neglect, postpartum exacerbation, and cognitive, behavioral, and emotional alterations in babies and children.

Nonpharmacological interventions for anxiety disorders include cognitive-behavioral therapy, elimination of caffeine, reduction of psychosocial stressors, and mindfulness-based therapy. Serotonin reuptake inhibitors are reasonable treatment options for severe symptoms that do not respond to those measures. For OCD, SSRI dosages generally are higher than those used for treatment of depression.

For severely anxious pregnant women, particularly as an SSRI begins to take effect, occasional small doses of benzodiazepines may be necessary. Intermittent use of low doses of benzodiazepines during pregnancy, particularly after the first trimester, does not appear to increase the risk of adverse neonatal sequelae. Nevertheless, the use of benzodiazepines during pregnancy is controversial, with some researchers noting a risk of oral clefts, particularly with diazepam and alprazolam. Although newer studies have not found an association with oral clefts or other major malformations (Bellantuono et al. 2013), an attempt should be made to avoid benzodiazepines during gestational weeks 5–9, because this is the period in which formation of the fetal palate occurs. Among the benzodiazepines, lorazepam is a reasonable choice, because it has no active metabolites and passes into the placenta to a lesser degree than do other benzodiazepines. Transient perinatal syndromes, including hypotonia, failure to feed, temperature dysregulation, apnea, and low Apgar scores, have been noted with third-trimester use of benzodiazepines. Near term, benzodiazepines should generally be kept at a minimum. Whenever possible, benzodiazepine dosage changes should be gradual to avoid precipitating in utero withdrawal. Recently, a large study demonstrated an association between long-term (but not occasional short-term) prenatal exposure to benzodiazepines during two or more trimesters and increased internalizing problems (anxiousness, emotional reactivity, somatic complaints) in children at 1.5 and 3 years of age (Brandlistuen et al. 2017). While this study demonstrated an association, the study groups were nonrandomized, and the effect size was small. Nonetheless, the reported association may represent another reason to limit benzodiazepine use to short-term treatment during pregnancy, in addition to the increased risk for tolerance and dependence with any long-term use of benzodiazepines.

Treatment of Other Psychiatric Disorders During Pregnancy

Attention-Deficit/Hyperactivity Disorder

As the prevalence of attention-deficit/hyperactivity disorder (ADHD) rises among adults, a large number of women enter their reproductive years taking stimulant medication. The data on stimulant use during pregnancy are limited, and much of the available information comes from women with large background differences, and who used these medications in other contexts, such as for weight management or substance abuse. Despite these limitations, stimulant medications do not appear to be major teratogens. A recent large, register-based cohort study of first-trimester exposure to methylphenidate and amphetamines found no overall increased risk of major congenital malformations in exposed infants (Huybrechts et al. 2018). That study also found that prenatal exposure to methylphenidate was associated with a 28% increased risk of cardiovascular malformations in exposed infants; no increased risk was found with prenatal amphetamine exposure. A critical analysis of this study has called into question the statistical and clinical significance of the risk with first-trimester methylphenidate exposure (Andrade 2018). At the same time, there continues to be some concern about the impact of stimulant exposure on fetal growth and neonatal outcomes (especially central nervous system–associated difficulties) (Norby et al. 2017). Given the need for further data, nonpharmacological alternatives are preferred. However, if a woman has significant functional impairment at work or school or while driving, decisions about prenatal use of stimulants should be made on a case-by-case basis.

Eating Disorders

As many as 25% of women may express weight and body shape concerns during early pregnancy, and as many as 7.5% may have symptoms that meet criteria for an eating disorder in the first trimester. Women with preexisting eating disorders may exhibit reduced symptomatology during pregnancy, and that pregnancy may represent a motivational time to discontinue harmful behaviors. Pregnancy may be a risk factor for new onset of disordered eating. Because of the high level of psychiatric comorbidity with eating disorders during pregnancy (particularly depression and anxiety), women with eating disorders should be closely monitored by mental health professionals during both pregnancy and the postnatal period (Easter et al. 2015).

Substance Use Disorders

Alcohol use during pregnancy can cause significant harm to both mother and fetus. In addition to causing premature labor, abruptio placentae, stillbirth, and other obstetrical complications, alcohol and its metabolite, acetaldehyde, are associated with teratogenic effects. Fetal alcohol syndrome, a lifelong disabling condition that results from in utero exposure to alcohol, occurs in as many as 1.5 in 1,000 live births in the United States. Isolated abnormalities (fetal alcohol effects) occur more often than the full syndrome. In utero exposure to alcohol increases the risk of fetal brain developmental deficits, microcephaly, abnormal facial features, and a number of psychiatric sequelae. No safe quantity of prenatal alcohol consumption has been established. Behavioral interventions are the cornerstone of treatment of alcohol use disorders during pregnancy (DeVido et al. 2015).

With the legalization of recreational marijuana in many states, the prevalence of marijuana use is increasing in pregnant women (Q.L. Brown et al. 2017). In the 2007–2012 National Survey on Drug Use and Health, 3.9% of pregnant women reported using marijuana in the past month, and 7% in the past 2–12 months (Ko et al. 2015). The effects of marijuana on the developing fetus are largely unknown but may include increased risk of stillbirth, fetal growth restriction, preterm birth, and adverse neurodevelopmental outcomes (Metz and Stickrath 2015). The American College of Obstetrics and Gynecology recommends avoiding marijuana during pregnancy (Committee on Obstetric Practice 2017).

Illicit drug use in pregnant women is a major public health concern. Commonly used illicit drugs include cocaine, heroin, stimulants (e.g., methamphetamine), and prescription analgesics, anxiolytics, and hypnotics. Antenatal cocaine use is associated with miscarriage, preterm labor, abruptio placentae, and other obstetrical complications secondary to cocaine's vasoconstrictive effects. Exposed neonates may experience a withdrawal syndrome lasting several months.

Over the past decade, prescription opioid abuse has become a national crisis, with the prevalence among pregnant women increasing dramatically. Pregnant women who are dependent on opioids tend to have inconsistent prenatal care, and antenatal opioid use has been associated with miscarriage, stillbirth, poor fetal growth, preterm labor, and sudden infant death syndrome. Exposed neonates are at risk for a neonatal abstinence syndrome characterized by irritability, poor feeding, respiratory difficulties, and tremulousness. For pregnant women addicted to opiates, the standard of care has been maintenance treatment with either methadone or buprenorphine, largely because of concerns that detoxification during pregnancy could lead to preterm labor, fetal distress, or stillbirth. However, more recent literature suggests that detoxification may be safer for the fetus than was previously thought (Guille et al. 2017). When women are treated for opioid dependence during pregnancy, significant attention should be paid to psychosocial interventions, including ongoing support with housing, transportation, and long-term mental health follow-up.

Use of Electroconvulsive Therapy During Pregnancy

Electroconvulsive therapy (ECT) is a feasible treatment option for pregnant patients with severe mood disorders because it appears to be safe and effective and exposes the developing fetus to a minimum of psychoactive medication. Special considerations in the administration of ECT to pregnant women include the need for a pelvic examination and uterine tocodynamometry to exclude uterine contractions and elevation of the right hip to ensure adequate placental perfusion. The muscle relaxant succinylcholine and the anticholinergic agent glycopyrrolate appear relatively safe for use during pregnancy. Propofol and methohexital sodium, the most frequently used anesthetic agents for ECT in the United States, are short acting and have not been associated with teratogenicity. Given the potential for fetal sedation, obstetric fetal monitoring during ECT is necessary. Following the procedure, maternal and fetal monitoring should continue, including use of cardiotocography and ultrasound between treatments (Leiknes et al. 2015). Treatment response rates among pregnant women with depression and schizophrenia have been found to be comparable to response rates among nonpregnant subjects, and ECT may be a reasonable option for pregnant women with severe symptoms, including psychotic catatonia or strong suicidality.

Postpartum Psychiatric Disorders

For many women, the period following delivery is a time of heightened risk for emotional instability. Conditions involving disordered mood following childbirth include postpartum blues, postpartum depression and anxiety, and postpartum psychosis (Table 40–9). Although no specific etiology has been found to explain the onset of psychiatric illness during the postpartum period, the causes probably reside in a combination of biological/endocrinological and psychosocial factors.

Postpartum Depression

The prevalence of postpartum depression varies widely across studies, depending on the population being studied, the definition used, and the mode of assessment employed (Norhayati et al. 2015). DSM considers postpartum depression not to be a stand-alone diagnosis but rather a specifier for major depressive episodes in the context of either major depressive disorder or bipolar disorder. With the publication of DSM-5, the "postpartum onset" specifier was changed to "peripartum onset," expanding the time frame of symptoms from 4 weeks postpartum to during pregnancy or within the first 4 weeks after childbirth. In clinical practice, however, the entire first postpartum year is considered a high-risk time for emergent mood disorders. The definition of postpartum depression is continually evolving and may have several distinct phenotypes (Postpartum Depression: Action Towards Causes and Treatment [PACT] Consortium 2015). Traditionally, the prevalence of postpartum depression is considered to be 15%, but it may be much higher if one includes women who have elevated scores on screening questionnaires such as the Edinburgh Postnatal Depression Scale (EPDS) or the 9-item depression scale of the Patient Health Questionnaire (PHQ-9).

Risk factors for postpartum depression include depression and anxiety during pregnancy, a personal history of depression, previous postpartum depression, a family history of postpartum depression, stressful life events, poor social and partner support, and low self-esteem. Additionally, endocrine risk factors, including elevated midpregnancy levels of placental corticotropin-releasing hormone, have been implicated as contributing to postpartum depression (Glynn and Sandman 2014), and neuroreceptor downregulation and plasticity during and following delivery may also contribute to the onset (Licheri et al. 2015). Thyroid function should always be evaluated in postpartum women with depression or anxiety, because the postpartum period is a time of increased risk for thyroid dysregulation. Once a woman has had one episode of postpartum depression, her risk of having another is significantly increased (Rasmussen et al. 2017).

It is important to screen for bipolar disorder in the context of postpartum depression, because postpartum depression is particularly common in women with bipolar disorder, and women who have experienced a postpartum psychiatric episode are at heightened risk of developing bipolar disorder in the future. Postpartum unipolar depression should be distinguished from postpartum bipolar depression in order to provide safe, appropriate, and effective psychopharmacological treatment.

Depressed mothers are more likely than nondepressed mothers to engage in negative parenting behaviors, and their children are at risk for behavioral problems and cognitive deficits from infancy to early childhood. Prompt and effective treatment of postpartum depression not only provides relief for new mothers but also reduces the likelihood of childhood behavior problems and patterns of insecure attachment that may have lasting effects throughout the life of affected offspring.

Postpartum depression is best treated comprehensively with individual and group psychotherapy, psychopharmacology, and psychoeducation. Interpersonal (both in-

TABLE 40–9. Postpartum psychiatric disorders

Disorder	Prevalence	Presentation	Treatment
Postpartum "blues"	Very common—up to 85%	Mood lability, emotional hypersensitivity, no dysfunction; resolves by week 2 in 80%, evolves to become postpartum depression in 20%	Provide support, reassurance, clinical monitoring (particularly for women with past histories of mood disorders or postpartum disorders). If severe, disabling, or lasting beyond 12 days, consider another diagnosis.
Postpartum depression	Approximately 15%, but estimates vary based on definition used	Major depressive episode, often with comorbid anxiety. Mother unable to sleep even when child care is provided for new baby. May be unipolar or bipolar depression (pure or mixed)	Provide individual psychotherapy (cognitive-behavioral or interpersonal), conjoint therapy to address interpersonal difficulties, group therapy for peer support, psychosocial assistance (child care, home care assistance). For unipolar postpartum depression, prescribe antidepressant, sometimes anxiolytic. For bipolar depression, administer mood stabilizer, with addition of augmenting agents if needed (e.g., anxiolytic). For psychotic or suicidal depression, hospitalize; consider use of antipsychotic or electroconvulsive therapy. Nursing mothers: educate regarding medications and breastfeeding; assess maternal and infant well-being.
Postpartum anxiety	8.5% overall Generalized anxiety disorder 3.6% Panic disorder 1.7% Obsessive-compulsive disorder[a] 2.5%	Excessive worry, intrusive ego-dystonic thoughts. Often underrecognized and underdiagnosed	Provide individual and/or group cognitive-behavioral therapy. Consider antidepressants and anxiolytics, which can be helpful.

TABLE 40–9. Postpartum psychiatric disorders *(continued)*

Disorder	Prevalence	Presentation	Treatment
Postpartum psychosis	<1/1,000, but higher with history of bipolar disorder or previous postpartum psychosis	Early onset, usually by day 2 or 3 postdelivery; often presenting as mixed/rapid cycling with psychotic features Mother unable to sleep Caution: risk of infanticide	Hospitalize patient, educate and reassure family, and emphasize medications and supportive care. Prescribe medications: mood stabilizer, antipsychotic, benzodiazepine. Consider electroconvulsive therapy if psychosis is refractory. In most cases, mothers with postpartum psychosis should not breastfeed.

[a]In DSM-5, obsessive-compulsive disorder is now classified with the Obsessive-Compulsive and Related Disorders.

dividual and group) and cognitive-behavioral therapies are helpful in treating post-partum depression. Standard antidepressants have been used successfully to treat postpartum unipolar depression. In cases of postpartum bipolar depression, treatment should include mood stabilizers; other augmenting agents are frequently required more acutely. Because antidepressants can precipitate mania in bipolar patients, caution should be exercised before treatment with an antidepressant. Decisions regarding medications should include consideration of whether the patient is breastfeeding (see subsection "Breastfeeding and Psychotropic Medications" later in this chapter).

Because women with a history of mood disorder are at higher risk of developing a postpartum episode, careful monitoring during and after pregnancy is essential. Pregnant women who develop mood symptoms during the third trimester are especially vulnerable to postpartum depression, with insomnia, suicidality, and poor functioning at work providing early warning signs (Suri et al. 2017). Lay advocacy groups (e.g., Postpartum Support International) and web-based education can be helpful for clinicians as well as for patients and their families. Assistance with household responsibilities and child care provides the patient with opportunities to reduce sleep deprivation.

The decision of whether or not to breastfeed should be discussed thoroughly, because breastfeeding may require a change in treatment modality or influence the choice of medication should pharmacotherapy be indicated. For patients whose depression is complicated by psychosis or suicidal thoughts, ECT is often the treatment of choice to provide rapid improvement.

Postpartum Psychosis

The most serious postpartum illness, postpartum psychosis, occurs in 0.25–0.6 of every 1,000 births. The condition is characterized by mood lability, agitation, confusion, thought disorganization, hallucinations, and disturbed sleep. Most cases of postpartum psychosis are thought to be manifestations of bipolar disorder. A family history of bipolar disorder heightens the risk of postpartum psychosis, and women who have their first psychotic episode during the postpartum period should be carefully monitored for subsequent mood episodes.

Because postpartum psychosis carries with it the risk of suicide, infant neglect, and infanticide, patients should be hospitalized. The initial evaluation includes a medical assessment to rule out pathophysiological causes such as postpartum thyroiditis, Sheehan's syndrome, pregnancy-related autoimmune disorders, N-methyl-D-aspartate-encephalitis, HIV-related infection, and intoxication or withdrawal states. Acute pharmacological treatment includes a benzodiazepine, an antipsychotic, and a mood stabilizer (with lithium as the preferred agent). Maintenance treatment for the patient whose postpartum psychosis was preceded by chronic recurrent mood episodes involves long-term treatment with a mood stabilizer. For patients with isolated postpartum psychosis, medications are often tapered and discontinued after 1 year of treatment, although these women should receive follow-up because of their high risk of subsequent mood episodes.

One-third of women with postpartum psychosis relapse during a subsequent pregnancy (Wesseloo et al. 2016). For women with bipolar disorder, the relapse risk is significantly decreased with medication during pregnancy (23% vs. 66%), so these women should be treated both prenatally and postnatally with a mood stabilizer (see subsection "Treatment of Bipolar Disorder During Pregnancy" earlier in this chapter).

Women with psychosis limited to the postpartum period can be placed on a prophylactic mood stabilizer immediately after delivery.

Breastfeeding and Psychotropic Medications

More than 80% of new mothers in the United States begin breastfeeding at birth, and 50% are still breastfeeding at 6 months (Centers for Disease Control and Prevention 2018). Breastfeeding can enhance mother–infant bonding and is an excellent source of nutrition for infants. For women who require pharmacological treatment for postpartum psychiatric disorders, the decision about whether to breastfeed can be difficult. Although no medication should be taken by a breastfeeding woman without careful assessment of risks and benefits for the nursing baby, it is also important to consider the possible harm to a mother that withholding a drug can cause. Table 40–10 lists issues that should be discussed when deciding whether or not to breastfeed.

All psychotropic medications are transmitted into the breast milk, but the quantity that a nursing infant ingests varies considerably, based on properties of individual medications, maternal dosage, infant age, and the frequency of feeding. The most up-to-date information about individual agents can be found in the National Institutes of Health LactMed database (https://toxnet.nlm.nih.gov/newtoxnet/lactmed.htm), a free resource for practicing clinicians. The American Academy of Pediatrics Committee on Drugs (2001), which previously classified the effects of psychotropic medications on nursing infants as "unknown but may be of concern," now recommends caution only with the small subset of medications for which the infant level is greater than 10% of the weight-adjusted maternal dosage (Sachs and Committee on Drugs 2013).

Infant hepatic drug clearance rises from about one-third of the mother's weight-adjusted clearance at birth to 100% at age 6 months. Thus, exposure to drugs through breast milk is greater in a neonate than in an older infant. Neonatologists should be consulted before premature infants are exposed to psychotropic medications through breast milk. Medications should be prescribed at the lowest dosage that achieves remission of psychiatric symptoms. Short-acting rather than long-acting medications are preferable, and supplementation of breast milk with formula reduces the infant's exposure to the drug. Because the clinical significance of any exposure to the baby of even small (and undetectable) doses of psychotropic agents is unknown, the baby's clinical status should be continually monitored.

Data on the use of SSRIs and tricyclic antidepressants during lactation are broadly reassuring (Burt et al. 2001). Because infants nursed by mothers taking SSRIs generally have extremely low serum levels of the medication, routine monitoring of serum concentrations is not necessary. Sertraline is considered the first-line choice for nursing mothers because of its low infant serum levels and limited adverse events; however, a different SSRI should be used if it is more effective for the mother. Data on SNRIs, bupropion, and mirtazapine in breastfeeding are limited. Monoamine oxidase inhibitors are best avoided, because they may cause hypertension in the infant.

Women with bipolar disorder require sleep to avoid postpartum relapse; breastfeeding is therefore to be undertaken with extreme caution. Lithium is associated with adverse effects, including cyanosis, poor muscle tone, and electrocardiogram changes, that have been noted in infants exposed to lithium through nursing. If a

TABLE 40–10.	Breastfeeding: issues to consider for postpartum women with psychiatric disorders

Breastfeeding provides the ideal form of nutrition for babies.

Breastfeeding fosters bonding between mother and infant.

Breastfeeding invariably results in sleep deprivation.

For many new mothers with psychiatric illness, the best way to ensure emotional stability is to avoid sleep deprivation. Consideration should therefore be given to ways in which to maximize sleep (e.g., formula feeding, supplementation of breastfeeding with formula).

All psychiatric medications are excreted into breast milk.

Amount of exposure via breast milk is invariably less than that through maternal–fetal circulation (during pregnancy).

Premature infants generally have immature cytochrome P450 enzymes and therefore may be at greater risk of side effects or toxicity when exposed to medications via breast milk.

The effect of neonatal medication exposure via breast milk on infant development is not known.

Appetite and weight should be monitored in breastfeeding women receiving psychiatric medications to ensure maternal well-being and to optimize the nutritional quality of breast milk.

woman does choose to breastfeed while taking lithium, her infant should be carefully monitored; lithium concentrations in infant serum contain about one-quarter the concentration of lithium in maternal serum. Although no significant clinical or behavioral effects have been noted in breastfed infants, exposed infants at least up to age 6 weeks should be carefully monitored clinically, and their sera should be evaluated for lithium, thyroid-stimulating hormone, blood urea nitrogen, and creatinine levels.

Valproate and carbamazepine are considered by the American Academy of Pediatrics Committee on Drugs (2001) to be compatible with breastfeeding; however, there have been rare reports of hepatic dysfunction and one possible case of transient seizure-like activity in infants exposed to carbamazepine via breast milk. Even though valproate accumulates in breast milk to a lesser extent than does carbamazepine, it should be used with caution in breastfeeding mothers because it has been associated with infant hepatotoxicity.

Lamotrigine is transmitted into the breast milk in relatively high concentrations; nursing infants whose mothers are taking lamotrigine have plasma levels averaging 30%–35% of maternal serum levels, and milk-to-plasma ratios are highly variable. Lamotrigine dosages are often increased during pregnancy, and as clearance returns to preconception levels over 2–3 weeks postpartum, maternal plasma and milk levels can rise dramatically if the dosage is not adjusted. In clinical practice, however, very few adverse events have been reported in infants exposed to lamotrigine via breast milk. Infants can have clinically insignificant thrombocytosis, and there has been one reported case of severe apnea in an exposed infant. If a woman chooses to breastfeed while taking lamotrigine, her infant should be carefully monitored, and breastfeeding should be discontinued if the infant develops a rash.

Data about atypical antipsychotics are limited but reassuring. While serious consideration should be given to the importance of sleep—and therefore forgoing breastfeeding—in the maintenance of psychiatric stability for a woman with psychosis, some women who require antipsychotic medication want to breastfeed. Most atypical antipsychotics appear to have a low milk/plasma ratio and low infant serum levels, and very few adverse events have been reported.

The American Academy of Pediatrics Committee on Drugs (2001) suggests that occasional use of short-acting benzodiazepines is compatible with breastfeeding. Infants breastfed by mothers taking a benzodiazepine in addition to another psychotropic medication did tend to be more sedated (Kelly et al. 2012). As a precaution, it is prudent to monitor benzodiazepine-exposed infants for sedation or other possible side effects.

Perimenopausal Depression and Anxiety

Menopause refers to the cessation of ovulation and menstrual cycling and usually occurs between ages 44 and 55 years (average age, 51.4 years). *Perimenopause* (climacteric) refers to the years before menopause during which ovarian function begins to decline. Numerous studies support the increased risk for depression and anxiety in women during the menopausal transition. Although perimenopausal depression cannot be fully explained by vasomotor discomfort, it is likely that hot flushes and adverse life events contribute to negative mood during the menopausal transition. Risk factors for perimenopausal depression include a history of depression (including postpartum and premenstrual), vasomotor symptoms, sleep difficulties, chronic health problems, loss of significant others, and psychosocial problems.

Treatment

Some studies have found that estrogen (e.g., transdermal 17β-estradiol) produces mood-elevating effects in perimenopausal and surgically menopausal women but not in postmenopausal women. At this time, estrogen alone is not accepted for long-term treatment of clinical depression. Whether estrogen may prime or augment standard antidepressants in perimenopausal depressed women is unclear.

For perimenopausal women with major depressive disorder, standard antidepressant treatment, often including psychotherapy, is considered first-line treatment. For perimenopausal women with severe hot flushes or night sweats who report subclinical depression and lethargy, hormone therapy may relieve the psychological symptoms as the vasomotor symptoms become less distressing. As women experience vasomotor symptom relief (usually within 2 weeks of beginning hormone replacement), depressive symptoms also should improve. Although paroxetine is the only nonhormonal therapy approved by the FDA for use in the treatment of menopausal vasomotor symptoms, the North American Menopause Society in its 2015 position statement noted that serotonergic antidepressants (SSRIs and SNRIs), gabapentin, and clonidine may be helpful for this indication (North American Menopause Society 2015). These nonhormonal treatments for vasomotor symptoms are best considered when the risk–benefit ratio for hormone therapy is unfavorable.

If, after resolution of vasomotor symptoms, depression persists or worsens, standard psychiatric treatment should be initiated. Psychosocial factors that may contribute to depressed mood also should be addressed, including stress related to caring for aging parents, new-onset health problems in the patient or her partner, financial difficulties, and changes in sexual functioning of the patient or her partner.

Menopausal Hormone Therapy

Menopausal hormone therapy incurs both benefits and risks, and the decision about whether to use hormone therapy can be complex and confusing. Hormone therapy is not generally recommended in women with a history of breast cancer, endometrial cancer, or thromboembolism. The Women's Health Initiative, a large prospective, randomized, placebo-controlled study initiated in the 1990s, evaluated the risks and benefits of hormone treatment and its effects on coronary events, stroke, pulmonary embolism, breast cancer, bone health, and cognition in 27,000 postmenopausal women. The estrogen-plus-progestin arm of the trial was stopped 3 years early (in 2002, after an average of 5.6 years) because of increases in breast cancer, coronary heart disease, stroke, and pulmonary embolism; the estrogen-only arm (for women with prior hysterectomy) was stopped 1 year early (in 2004, after an average of 7.2 years) because of an increase in stroke. A 2013 synthesis of 13 years of follow-up from the Women's Health Initiative found that overall, women taking hormone therapy had fewer fractures but more strokes, blood clots, gallbladder disease, and urinary incontinence. Estrogen plus progestin increased the risk for coronary heart disease, breast cancer, stroke, blood clots, and probable dementia; this regimen decreased the risk of hip fracture and colorectal cancer. In contrast, estrogen alone (for women posthysterectomy) increased the risk of stroke and blood clots but decreased the risk of coronary heart disease, breast cancer, and hip fracture; it did not impact the rate of colorectal cancer (Manson et al. 2013). Recently, an even longer-term follow-up (18 years) from the Women's Health Initiative found no increase in all-cause cardiovascular or cancer mortality in women exposed to hormone therapy (Manson et al. 2017).

The short-term use of estrogen for treatment of severe vasomotor symptoms and urogenital atrophy is acceptable for women up to age 59 years or within 10 years of menopause (Stuenkel et al. 2015). In perimenopausal and postmenopausal women who are at high risk of osteoporosis, estrogen therapy may be appropriate. However, hormone therapy as a primary long-term treatment to prevent heart disease and cognitive decline in postmenopausal women is not justified. As stated in the North American Menopause Society's 2017 statement on hormone therapy, prolongation of hormone therapy should be based on shared decision making and carefully documented indications, and the decision to continue hormone therapy should be regularly evaluated (The NAMS 2017 Hormone Therapy Position Statement Advisory Panel 2017). Topically applied low-dose estrogen therapy is effective and preferred for treatment of genitourinary symptoms. Both the North American Menopause Society and the American Congress of Obstetricians and Gynecologists recommend against the use of custom-compounded bio-identical hormones, given the lack of evidence regarding safety and efficacy as well as the lack of regulation of these products. More data are needed before short-term estrogen therapy can be considered a primary mode of treatment for depression in perimenopausal women.

Conclusion

When clinicians are assessing and treating women with psychiatric disorders, it is important that they recognize gender-specific issues that affect diagnosis and treatment.

In particular, reproductive-related transitions, including monthly menstrual cycles, pregnancy, the postpartum period, and perimenopause, present unique challenges for psychiatric care. Psychopharmacological and psychotherapeutic treatment modalities should address the special and changing needs of women over the course of their lives.

Key Clinical Points

- Although women and men are at equal lifetime risk of developing a psychiatric disorder, there are gender-specific differences in prevalence, clinical course, and treatment of specific psychiatric illnesses.

- Women are at particular risk for mood disorders at times of reproductive transition.

- For women, a comprehensive psychiatric evaluation should include an assessment of menstrual cycling, reproductive history, and birth control regimens.

- Premenstrual dysphoric disorder is diagnosed by prospective mood tracking and responds to luteal-phase or continuous dosing with selective serotonin reuptake inhibitors (SSRIs).

- The mental health of an expectant mother is an important determinant of the health and well-being of both the mother and her offspring.

- Decisions regarding the use of psychiatric medications during pregnancy are best made after weighing the risks of untreated mental illness against the risks of a particular medication.

- Depression and anxiety are common during both pregnancy and the postpartum period, and all women should be screened for these symptoms during and after pregnancy.

- Although data about antidepressant use during pregnancy is continually evolving, SSRIs are not considered to be teratogenic.

- In pregnant women with bipolar disorder, discontinuation of mood-stabilizing medication is associated with a high rate of relapse in both pregnancy and the postpartum period.

- In general, lithium remains the treatment of choice for pregnant women with bipolar disorder.

- Postpartum psychosis is a psychiatric emergency that requires hospitalization.

- Valproate incurs a relatively high risk for serious congenital and neurodevelopmental consequences in prenatally exposed offspring and should therefore be avoided in women who are pregnant or considering pregnancy.

- Women are at increased risk for depression as they move into and through perimenopause. That risk is particularly high for those with a past history of major depressive disorder.

References

Aleman A, Kahn RS, Selten JP: Sex differences in the risk of schizophrenia: evidence from meta-analysis. Arch Gen Psychiatry 60(6):565–571, 2003 12796219

American Academy of Pediatrics Committee on Drugs: The transfer of drugs and other chemicals into human milk. Pediatrics 108(3):776–789, 2001 11533352

American College of Obstetricians and Gynecologists: ACOG Committee Opinion No. 757: Screening for Perinatal Depression. Obstet Gynecol 132(5):e208–e212, 2018 30629567

American Psychiatric Association: Diagnostic and Statistical Manual of Mental Disorders, 4th Edition. Washington, DC, American Psychiatric Association, 1994

American Psychiatric Association: Diagnostic and Statistical Manual of Mental Disorders, 5th Edition. Arlington, VA, American Psychiatric Association, 2013

Andalib S, Emamhadi MR, Yousefzadeh-Chabok S, et al: Maternal SSRI exposure increases the risk of autistic offspring: a meta-analysis and systematic review. Eur Psychiatry 45:161–166, 2017 28917161

Andrade C: Antidepressant exposure during pregnancy and risk of autism in the offspring, 1: meta-review of meta-analyses. J Clin Psychiatry 78(8):e1047–e1051, 2017a 28994903

Andrade C: Antidepressant exposure during pregnancy and risk of autism in the offspring, 2: do the new studies add anything new? J Clin Psychiatry 78(8):e1052–e1056, 2017b 29099558

Andrade C: Risk of major congenital malformations associated with the use of methylphenidate or amphetamines in pregnancy. J Clin Psychiatry 79(1), 2018 29370484

Bellantuono C, Tofani S, Di Sciascio G, et al: Benzodiazepine exposure in pregnancy and risk of major malformations: a critical overview. Gen Hosp Psychiatry 35(1):3–8, 2013 23044244

Brandlistuen RE, Ystrom E, Hernandez-Diaz S, et al: Association of prenatal exposure to benzodiazepines and child internalizing problems: a sibling-controlled cohort study. PLoS One 12(7):e0181042, 2017 28746341

Brown HK, Ray JG, Wilton AS, et al: Association between serotonergic antidepressant use during pregnancy and autism spectrum disorder in children. JAMA 317(15):1544–1552, 2017 28418480

Brown QL, Sarvet AL, Shmulewitz D, et al: Trends in marijuana use among pregnant and nonpregnant reproductive-aged women, 2002–2014. JAMA 317(2):207–209, 2017 27992619

Burt VK, Suri R, Altshuler LL, et al: The use of psychotropic medications during breast-feeding. Am J Psychiatry 158(7):1001–1009, 2001 11431219

Centers for Disease Control and Prevention: Breastfeeding Report Card: United States, 2018. August 20, 2018. Available at: https://www.cdc.gov/breastfeeding/data/report-card.htm. Accessed January 9, 2019.

Cohen LS, Altshuler LL, Harlow BL, et al: Relapse of major depression during pregnancy in women who maintain or discontinue antidepressant treatment. JAMA 295(5):499–507, 2006 16449615

Cohen LS, Viguera AC, McInerney KA, et al: Reproductive safety of second-generation antipsychotics: current data from the Massachusetts General Hospital National Pregnancy Registry for Atypical Antipsychotics. Am J Psychiatry 173(3):263–270, 2016 26441156

Committee on Obstetric Practice: ACOG Committee Opinion no. 722: Marijuana use during pregnancy and lactation. Obstet Gynecol 130(4):e205–e209, 2017 28937574

DeVido J, Bogunovic O, Weiss RD: Alcohol use disorders in pregnancy. Harv Rev Psychiatry 23(2):112–121, 2015 25747924

Dolk H, Wang H, Loane M, et al: Lamotrigine use in pregnancy and risk of orofacial cleft and other congenital anomalies. Neurology 86(18):1716–1725, 2016 27053714

Dubey N, Hoffman JF, Schuebel K, et al: The ESC/E(Z) complex, an effector of response to ovarian steroids, manifests an intrinsic difference in cells from women with premenstrual dysphoric disorder. Mol Psychiatry 22(8):1172–1184, 2017 28044059

Earls MF, Yogman MW, Mattson G, Rafferty J; Committee on Psychosocial Aspects of Child and Family Health: Incorporating recognition and management of perinatal depression into pediatric practice. Pediatrics 143(1), 2019 30559120

Easter A, Solmi F, Bye A, et al: Antenatal and postnatal psychopathology among women with current and past eating disorders: longitudinal patterns. Eur Eat Disord Rev 23(1):19–27, 2015 25345371

Glynn LM, Sandman CA: Evaluation of the association between placental corticotrophin-releasing hormone and postpartum depressive symptoms. Psychosom Med 76(5):355–362, 2014 24915294

Guille C, Barth KS, Mateus J, et al: Treatment of prescription opioid use disorder in pregnant women. Am J Psychiatry 174(3):208–214, 2017 28245688

Hendrick V, Altshuler LL, Gitlin MJ, et al: Gender and bipolar illness. J Clin Psychiatry 61(5):393–396; quiz 397, 2000 10847318

Holmes LB, Hernandez-Diaz S: Newer anticonvulsants: lamotrigine, topiramate and gabapentin. Birth Defects Res A Clin Mol Teratol 94(8):599–606, 2012 22730257

Huybrechts KF, Palmsten K, Avorn J, et al: Antidepressant use in pregnancy and the risk of cardiac defects. N Engl J Med 370(25):2397–2407, 2014 24941178

Huybrechts KF, Hernández-Díaz S, Patorno E, et al: Antipsychotic use in pregnancy and the risk for congenital malformations. JAMA Psychiatry 73(9):938–946, 2016 27540849

Huybrechts KF, Bröms G, Christensen LB, et al: Association between methylphenidate and amphetamine use in pregnancy and risk of congenital malformations: a cohort study from the International Pregnancy Safety Study Consortium. JAMA Psychiatry 75(2):167–175, 2018 29238795

Jarde A, Morais M, Kingston D, et al: Neonatal outcomes in women with untreated antenatal depression compared with women without depression: a systematic review and meta-analysis. JAMA Psychiatry 73(8):826–837, 2016 27276520

Jimenez-Solem E, Andersen JT, Petersen M, et al: Exposure to selective serotonin reuptake inhibitors and the risk of congenital malformations: a nationwide cohort study. BMJ Open 2(3):e001148, 2012 22710132

Johnson KC, LaPrairie JL, Brennan PA, et al: Prenatal antipsychotic exposure and neuromotor performance during infancy. Arch Gen Psychiatry 69(8):787–794, 2012 22474072

Kaplan YC, Keskin-Arslan E, Acar S, et al: Prenatal selective serotonin reuptake inhibitor use and the risk of autism spectrum disorder in children: a systematic review and meta-analysis. Reprod Toxicol 66:31–43, 2016 27667009

Kaplan YC, Keskin-Arslan E, Acar S, et al: Maternal SSRI discontinuation, use, psychiatric disorder and the risk of autism in children: a meta-analysis of cohort studies. Br J Clin Pharmacol 83(12):2798–2806, 2017 28734011

Karno M, Golding JM, Sorenson SB, Burnam MA: The epidemiology of obsessive-compulsive disorder in five US communities. Arch Gen Psychiatry 45(12):1094–1099, 1988 3264144

Kelly LE, Poon S, Madadi P, Koren G: Neonatal benzodiazepine exposure during breastfeeding. J Pediatr 161(3):448–451, 2012 22504099

Kessler RC, McGonagle KA, Zhao S, et al: Lifetime and 12-month prevalence of DSM-III-R psychiatric disorders in the United States. Results from the National Comorbidity Survey. Arch Gen Psychiatry 51(1):8–19, 1994 8279933

Ko JY, Farr SL, Tong VT, et al: Prevalence and patterns of marijuana use among pregnant and nonpregnant women of reproductive age. Am J Obstet Gynecol 213(2):201.e1–201.e10, 2015 25772211

Kobayashi T, Matsuyama T, Takeuchi M, et al: Autism spectrum disorder and prenatal exposure to selective serotonin reuptake inhibitors: a systematic review and meta-analysis. Reprod Toxicol 65:170–178, 2016 27474253

Lanza di Scalea T, Pearlstein T: Premenstrual dysphoric disorder. Psychiatr Clin North Am 40(2):201–216, 2017 28477648

Leiknes KA, Cooke MJ, Jarosch-von Schweder L, et al: Electroconvulsive therapy during pregnancy: a systematic review of case studies. Arch Women Ment Health 18(1):1–39, 2015 24271084

Licheri V, Talani G, Gorule AA, et al: Plasticity of GABAA receptors during pregnancy and postpartum period: from gene to function. Neural Plast 2015:170435, 2015 26413323

Liu X, Agerbo E, Ingstrup KG, et al: Antidepressant use during pregnancy and psychiatric disorders in offspring: Danish nationwide register based cohort study. BMJ 358:j3668, 2017 28877907

Malm H, Artama M, Gissler M, et al: Selective serotonin reuptake inhibitors and risk for major congenital anomalies. Obstet Gynecol 118(1):111–120, 2011 21646927

Manson JE, Chlebowski RT, Stefanick ML, et al: Menopausal hormone therapy and health outcomes during the intervention and extended poststopping phases of the Women's Health Initiative randomized trials. JAMA 310(13):1353–1368, 2013 24084921

Manson JE, Aragaki AK, Rossouw JE, et al: Menopausal hormone therapy and long-term all-cause and cause-specific mortality: the Women's Health Initiative randomized trials. JAMA 318(10):927–938, 2017 28898378

Margulis AV, Abou-Ali A, Strazzeri MM, et al: Use of selective serotonin reuptake inhibitors in pregnancy and cardiac malformations: a propensity-score matched cohort in CPRD. Pharmacoepidemiol Drug Saf 22(9):942–951, 2013 23733623

Meador KJ, Loring DW: Risks of in utero exposure to valproate. JAMA 309(16):1730–1731, 2013 23613078

Meador KJ, Baker GA, Browning N, et al: Fetal antiepileptic drug exposure and cognitive outcomes at age 6 years (NEAD study): a prospective observational study. Lancet Neurol 12(3):244–252, 2013 23352199

Metz TD, Stickrath EH: Marijuana use in pregnancy and lactation: a review of the evidence. Am J Obstet Gynecol 213(6):761–778, 2015 25986032

Mezzacappa A, Lasica PA, Gianfagna F, et al: Risk for autism spectrum disorders according to period of prenatal antidepressant exposure: a systematic review and meta-analysis. JAMA Pediatr 171(6):555–563, 2017 28418571

The NAMS 2017 Hormone Therapy Position Statement Advisory Panel: The 2017 hormone therapy position statement of The North American Menopause Society. Menopause 24(7):728–753, 2017 28650869

Newport DJ, Viguera AL, Beach AJ, et al: Lithium placental passage and obstetrical outcome: implications for clinical management during late pregnancy. Am J Psychiatry 162(11):2162–2170, 2005 16263858

Norby U, Winbladh B, Kallen K: Perinatal outcomes after treatment with ADHD medication during pregnancy. Pediatrics 140(6), 2017 29127207

Nordeng H, van Gelder MM, Spigset O: Pregnancy outcome after exposure to antidepressants and the role of maternal depression: results from the Norwegian Mother and Child Cohort Study. J Clin Psychopharmacol 32(2):186–194, 2012 22367660

Norhayati MN, Hazlina NH, Asrenee AR, et al: Magnitude and risk factors for postpartum symptoms: a literature review. J Affect Disord 175:34–52, 2015 25590764

North American Menopause Society: Nonhormonal management of menopause-associated vasomotor symptoms: 2015 position statement of The North American Menopause Society. Menopause 22(11):1155–1172, quiz 1173–1174, 2015 26382310

Oberlander TF, Zwaigenbaum L: Disentangling maternal depression and antidepressant use during pregnancy as risks for autism in children. JAMA 317(15):1533–1534, 2017 28418464

O'Connor E, Rossom RC, Henninger M, et al: Primary care screening for and treatment of depression in pregnant and postpartum women: evidence report and systematic review for the US Preventive Services Task Force. JAMA 315(4):388–406, 2016 26813212

Ornoy A, Koren G: Selective serotonin reuptake inhibitors during pregnancy: do we have now more definite answers related to prenatal exposure? Birth Defects Res 109(12):898–908, 2017 28714608

Panchaud A, Hernandez-Diaz S, Freeman MP, et al: Use of atypical antipsychotics in pregnancy and maternal gestational diabetes. J Psychiatr Res 95:84–90, 2017 28810177

Patorno E, Huybrechts KF, Bateman BT, et al: Lithium use in pregnancy and the risk of cardiac malformations. N Engl J Med 376(23):2245–2254, 2017 28591541

Postpartum Depression: Action Towards Causes and Treatment (PACT) Consortium: Heterogeneity of postpartum depression: a latent class analysis. Lancet Psychiatry 2(1):59–67, 2015 26359613

Raffi E, Freeman M: The etiology of premenstrual dysphoric disorder: 5 interwoven pieces. Curr Psychiatr 16(9):20–28, 2017

Rai D, Lee BK, Dalman C, et al: Antidepressants during pregnancy and autism in offspring: population based cohort study. BMJ 358:j2811, 2017 28724519

Rasmussen MH, Strøm M, Wohlfahrt J, et al: Risk, treatment duration, and recurrence risk of postpartum affective disorder in women with no prior psychiatric history: a population-based cohort study. PLoS Med 14(9):e1002392, 2017 28949960

Ross LE, Grigoriadis S, Mamisashvili L, et al: Selected pregnancy and delivery outcomes after exposure to antidepressant medication: a systematic review and meta-analysis. JAMA Psychiatry 70(4):436–443, 2013 23446732

Sachs HC, Committee on Drugs: The transfer of drugs and therapeutics into human breast milk: an update on selected topics. Pediatrics 132(3):e796–e809, 2013 23979084

Salisbury AL, O'Grady KE, Battle CL, et al: The roles of maternal depression, serotonin reuptake inhibitor treatment, and concomitant benzodiazepine use on infant neurobehavioral functioning over the first postnatal month. Am J Psychiatry 173(2):147–157, 2016 26514656

Schmidt PJ, Martinez PE, Nieman LK, et al: Premenstrual dysphoric disorder symptoms following ovarian suppression: triggered by change in ovarian steroid levels but not continuous stable levels. Am J Psychiatry 174(10):980–989, 2017 28427285

Smith DJ, Nicholl BI, Cullen B, et al: Prevalence and characteristics of probable major depression and bipolar disorder within UK biobank: cross-sectional study of 172,751 participants. PLoS One 8(11):e75362, 2013 24282498

Stuenkel CA, Davis SR, Gompel A, et al: Treatment of symptoms of the menopause: an Endocrine Society clinical practice guideline. J Clin Endocrinol Metab 100(11):3975–4011, 2015 26444994

Sujan AC, Rickert ME, Öberg AS, et al: Associations of maternal antidepressant use during the first trimester of pregnancy with preterm birth, small for gestational age, autism spectrum disorder, and attention-deficit/hyperactivity disorder in offspring. JAMA 317(15):1553–1562, 2017 28418479

Suri R, Stowe ZN, Cohen LS, et al: Prospective longitudinal study of predictors of postpartum-onset depression in women with a history of major depressive disorder. J Clin Psychiatry 78(8):1110–1116, 2017 28297589

U.S. Food and Drug Administration: FDA Drug Safety Communication: Selective serotonin reuptake inhibitor (SSRI) antidepressant use during pregnancy and reports of a rare heart and lung condition in newborn babies. December 14, 2011. Available at: https://www.fda.gov/Drugs/DrugSafety/ucm283375.htm. Accessed November 12, 2018.

U.S. Food and Drug Administration: FDA Drug Safety Communication: Updated information about the risk of blood clots in women taking birth control pills containing drospirenone. April 10, 2012. Available at: https://www.fda.gov/Drugs/DrugSafety/ucm299305.htm. Accessed November 12, 2018.

Vigod SN, Wilson CA, Howard LM: Depression in pregnancy. BMJ 352:i1547, 2016 27013603

Viktorin A, Uher R, Reichenberg A, et al: Autism risk following antidepressant medication during pregnancy. Psychol Med 47(16):2787–2796, 2017 28528584

Wesseloo R, Kamperman AM, Munk-Olsen T, et al: Risk of postpartum relapse in bipolar disorder and postpartum psychosis: a systemic review and meta-analysis. Am J Psychiatry 173(2):117–127, 2016 26514657

Wesseloo R, Wierdsma AI, van Kamp IL, et al: Lithium dosing strategies during pregnancy and the postpartum period. Br J Psychiatry 211(1):31–36, 2017 28673946

Weston J, Bromley R, Jackson CF, et al: Monotherapy treatment of epilepsy in pregnancy: congenital malformation outcomes in the child. Cochrane Database Syst Rev (11):CD010224, 2016 27819746

Yonkers KA, Simoni MK: Premenstrual disorders. Am J Obstet Gynecol 218(1):68–74, 2018 28571724

Recommended Readings

Andrade C: Antidepressant exposure during pregnancy and risk of autism in the offspring, 1: meta-review of meta-analyses. J Clin Psychiatry 78(8):e1047–e1051, 2017

Bergink V, Rasgon N, Wisner KL: Postpartum psychosis: madness, mania, and melancholia in motherhood. Am J Psychiatry 173(12):1179–1188, 2016

Cohen LS, Viguera AC, McInerney KA, et al: Reproductive safety of second-generation antipsychotics: current data from the Massachusetts General Hospital National Pregnancy Registry for Atypical Antipsychotics. Am J Psychiatry 173(3):263–270, 2016

Huybrechts KF, Palmsten K, Avorn J, et al: Antidepressant use in pregnancy and the risk of cardiac defects. N Engl J Med 370(25):2397–2407, 2014

Manson JE, Aragaki AK, Rossouw JE, et al: Menopausal hormone therapy and long-term all-cause and cause-specific mortality: the Women's Health Initiative randomized trials. JAMA 318(10):927–938, 2017

Meador KJ, Baker GA, Browning N, et al: Fetal antiepileptic drug exposure and cognitive outcomes at age 6 years (NEAD study): a prospective observational study. Lancet Neurol 12(3):244–252, 2013

Oberlander TF, Zwaigenbaum L: Disentangling maternal depression and antidepressant use during pregnancy as risks for autism in children. JAMA 317(15):1533–1534, 2017

Patorno E, Huybrechts KF, Bateman BT, et al: Lithium use in pregnancy and the risk of cardiac malformations. N Engl J Med 376(23):2245–2254, 2017

Ross LE, Grigoriadis S, Mamisashvili L, et al: Selected pregnancy and delivery outcomes after exposure to antidepressant medication: a systematic review and meta-analysis. JAMA Psychiatry 70(4):436–443, 2013

Schmidt PJ, Martinez PE, Nieman LK, et al: Premenstrual dysphoric disorder symptoms following ovarian suppression: triggered by change in ovarian steroid levels but not continuous stable levels. Am J Psychiatry 174(10):980–989, 2017

Wesseloo R, Kamperman AM, Munk-Olsen T, et al: Risk of postpartum relapse in bipolar disorder and postpartum psychosis: a systemic review and meta-analysis. Am J Psychiatry 173(2):117–127, 2016

Online Resources

LactMed: https://toxnet.nlm.nih.gov/newtoxnet/lactmed.htm. National Institutes of Health drugs and lactation database.

Massachusetts General Hospital (MGH) Center for Women's Mental Health: https://womensmentalhealth.org. Website of the MGH Perinatal and Reproductive Psychiatry Program. Provides information about psychiatric conditions in women and manages the National Pregnancy Registry for Psychiatric Medications.

MotherToBaby: https://mothertobaby.org/. Provides information about medication in pregnancy as a service of the nonprofit Organization of Teratology Information Specialists (OTIS). Detailed fact sheets can be printed to give to patients.

The North American Menopause Society: http://www.menopause.org. Nonprofit organization promoting women's health during midlife and beyond, with special focus on menopausal health.

Postpartum Support International: http://www.postpartum.net. International network of individuals and organizations whose purpose is to increase awareness among public and professionals about pregnancy- and postpartum-related psychiatric disorders. Provides information and referrals.

REPROTOX®: https://reprotox.org. A subscription database containing summaries on the effects of medications, chemicals, biologics, and physical agents on pregnancy, reproduction, lactation, and development.

CHAPTER 41

Children and Adolescents

Margery R. Johnson, M.D.

Nicholas M. Hatzis, M.D.

Amandeep Jutla, M.D.

In this chapter we focus on psychiatric treatment of children and adolescents and how it differs from treatment of adults. Expanding research has led to more specific empirically tested interventions for youth. Childhood psychopathology and disorder-specific treatments are discussed in Part II of this textbook (see, e.g., Chapter 9, "Neurodevelopmental Disorders"). Throughout this chapter, unless otherwise stated, the terms *child* and *children* include adolescents. *Parent* is used for the parent, guardian, or responsible adult. The goals of all treatments are to reduce symptoms, to improve emotional and behavioral functioning, to remedy skill deficits, and to remove obstacles to normal development. In contrast to the treatment of adults, a child is usually brought by someone else, and in each instance there are at least two persons, the parent and the child, whose perceptions of the problem and goals for treatment often conflict. Compared with adults, children have less control over their lives, and they are required to attend school.

Evaluation

The psychiatric treatment of children should be preceded by a comprehensive clinical assessment and formulation of a biopsychosocial treatment plan. Clinicians must have a clear understanding of normal development and its variations in order to distinguish normal from pathological states. Interview adaptations such as drawing or symbolic play, including a parent until the child is comfortable, or using simpler language may be required.

Information must always be obtained from both the child and the parent, because each party has a different perspective and access to different pieces of information. The parent may be the more objective reporter of a child's behavior and history, but the child may more accurately report his or her feelings, perspective on life experiences, and peer relationships. The older adolescent, in the process of the transition to adulthood, may be legally an adult but is often dependent on parents for financial and emotional support, and parents obviously still feel caring and a sense of responsibility for their child. So, with the young adult's permission, parents should be involved in the evaluation and should be kept informed of any safety concerns that may arise.

Information from the school is always useful and is essential when there is concern about learning or behavior in school or with peers. With parental consent, the clinician may talk with the teacher; obtain records of testing, grades, and attendance; and request completion of standardized rating scales, such as the Child Symptom Inventory (available for purchase at www.checkmateplus.com/index.htm) or the Vanderbilt Attention-Deficit/Hyperactivity Disorder (ADHD) Diagnostic Rating Scales (Bard et al. 2013; Wolraich et al. 2013). In some circumstances, the clinician may visit the school to observe the child, or may participate (either in person or via teleconference) in planning meetings regarding special education needs.

A referral to another specialist such as a pediatrician, pediatric neurologist, or speech and language pathologist may be necessary to complete the assessment. Psychological evaluation, including an intelligence test and achievement tests, may be obtained when there are questions about learning or cognitive ability.

Treatment Planning

Treatment planning takes into consideration the psychiatric diagnosis, the target emotional and behavioral symptoms, and the strengths and weaknesses of the patient and family. Resources and risks in the school, neighborhood, and social support network, as well as cultural factors such as ethnicity and religious group affiliation, influence the selection and sequencing of treatment strategies.

Treatments not in the repertoire of the clinician or those requiring additional staff or a different setting should be arranged by referral. Unfortunately, the practical realities of the quality and availability of community resources and the family's ability to pay for or attend treatment often force the clinician to make compromises to an ideal plan. The clinician must decide which treatment is likely to be the most efficient or to have the highest benefit/cost or risk ratio and whether treatments should be administered simultaneously or in sequence. The American Academy of Child and Adolescent Psychiatry (AACAP) has developed practice parameters as guides to the evaluation and treatment of specific disorders, and these are available online at www.aacap.org.

The clinician must collaborate with the parents in choosing among possible treatment options, with the clinician presenting the probable course of the disorder if untreated as well as the possible benefits and risks of all available treatments. The child patient is included in decision making as appropriate. The motivation and ability of the responsible adults to carry out the treatment should be considered, because there is little chance of success without the cooperation of the family. Obviously, treatment planning is an ongoing process and evolves as progress is made or as additional information about the child and family comes to light.

Informed Consent

The implementation of any treatment plan requires carefully obtained informed consent from parents. Clinicians should also strive to obtain assent from child patients, being mindful of the cognitive capacities and developmental level of the patient. The discussion of consent should include the selected therapeutic modality, its intended purpose, the availability of any alternative treatments (including no treatment), and the nature of possible adverse reactions. An open discussion, with documentation of any questions or concerns, not only meets the legal obligations of practice but also can safeguard the therapeutic alliance should undesirable effects occur. Printed materials are available to supplement discussion in educating parents and children regarding medication treatments (Dulcan and Ballard 2015). The Internet has become an important source of information about medications and treatments for consumers. Because the quality of information available is inconsistent, patients and their families benefit from guidance as to the best sources of information about mental health issues (see, e.g., the AACAP website: www.aacap.org).

Confidentiality

It is essential that the guidelines for confidentiality and for sharing information between parent and child be clear. Adolescents are usually more sensitive to this issue than younger children. Agreement about what will and will not be discussed with parents is especially important when an older adolescent is away at college or otherwise not living with the parents. Parents may have concerns about a therapist's keeping vital information about their child from them or indiscriminately revealing information to the child that was disclosed in confidence to the therapist. As a general rule, either party should be told when information will be conveyed to the other. When children are engaged in potentially dangerous activities or have serious thoughts of harming themselves or others, parents must be informed. Thus, the distinction has to be made, to both the adolescent and the parent, between casual experimentation with drugs or normal adolescent sexuality and behaviors that place the adolescent at risk of physical or mental injury. Carefully planned family sessions in which the therapist coaches and supports a parent or child in sharing information may be useful.

Psychopharmacology

Medication treatment of children is different from that of adults. U.S. Food and Drug Administration (FDA) warnings have focused the attention of patients, parents, and prescribers on the potential risks surrounding medication use in children. Two important general principles are that polypharmacy should be minimized and that medication should rarely be used as the sole treatment.

Most disorders of children and adolescents that require medication are either chronic (e.g., ADHD, autism spectrum disorder [ASD], Tourette's disorder) or likely to have recurrent episodes (e.g., mood disorders). It is important to educate the family regarding the disorder, its treatment, and changes with developmental stage. The clinician must consider the meaning of the prescription and administration of a medication to the child, the family, the school, and the child's peer group.

Special Issues for Children and Adolescents

Pharmacokinetics and Pharmacodynamics

Pharmacokinetics is the study of the movement of drugs into, around, and out of the body by the processes of absorption, distribution, metabolism, and elimination. Children differ from adults in their proportions of extracellular water volume and body fat. In younger children, a greater volume of extracellular water results in a relatively larger distribution volume for water-soluble drugs, so they may require a relatively higher dosage to achieve plasma concentrations comparable to those in adults. Hepatic metabolic activity is at its peak in childhood, related to the proportionally larger liver size of children compared with adults. This greater metabolic rate contributes to decreased drug plasma concentration levels and decreased drug half-lives in children compared with adults. Children also may be more sensitive than adults to increases or decreases in drug metabolism due to interactions with the cytochrome P450 (CYP) enzyme system.

Medication dosage also is determined by *pharmacodynamics,* or how the biological system responds to the drug. Growth and development may affect receptor number, distribution, structure, function, and sensitivity. Ideally, medication dosages in children should be derived from studies of children, but these are relatively rare. Generally, children are anticipated to require higher weight-adjusted dosages to achieve the same blood levels and therapeutic effects as adults. Clinicians should, however, remain alert to the possibility that such practice occasionally results in significant side effects if the child is genetically determined to be a relatively slow metabolizer. It is thus wise to start medications at a low dosage and titrate upward, being prepared for the possibility that the final dosage may be relatively high, especially in larger adolescents.

Side Effects

Side effects are common in children being treated with psychiatric medications. Clinicians must actively look for adverse reactions, because children often will not report them and parents may not notice. Occasionally, a child will develop an atypical or paradoxical response to a particular medication. Parents are often understandably protective and may have great difficulty tolerating even the most minor side effects in their child. This reluctance may lead to premature discontinuation of a medication due to a mild side effect that would probably resolve with continued treatment. Good communication and support from the psychiatrist can be important in getting beyond this stumbling block.

There may also be behavioral toxicity, or exacerbations of the very symptom that is the target of treatment. This phenomenon is often difficult to distinguish from the natural fluctuations in symptoms of the disorder, especially in children with tics, ASD, or severe mood disorders. Having parents keep a mood or behavior chart or a tic log is helpful in tracking both response to medication and possible side effects and may prevent repeated inadequate medication trials due to premature discontinuation.

Measurement of Outcome

Effective medication management requires the identification and monitoring of target symptoms. The clinician must obtain emotional, behavioral, and physical data at baseline and periodically during treatment. Therapeutic effects can be assessed by parent and child interviews and rating scales, direct observation, collection of data from outside sources (e.g., teachers), or specific tests evaluating attention or learning. The periodic use of rating scales is especially helpful in assessing response to treatment for ADHD and for mood and anxiety disorders.

Developmentally Disabled Patients

Medication effects are even more difficult to assess in children and adolescents with intellectual disability or ASD. Their impaired ability to verbalize symptoms is relevant to diagnosis, measurement of efficacy, and detection of side effects. These individuals are at risk of experiencing idiosyncratic or paradoxical effects and/or of attaining smaller therapeutic effects in comparison with typically developing youth.

Adherence to Medication Regimen

Taking medication as directed requires the cooperation of parent(s) and child and often school personnel as well. In a patient who has a recurrence of symptoms after an initial good response, gentle inquiry about medication adherence should be made prior to making a change in dosage. Resistance to taking medication may come from the parents, the child, or even the school, and this resistance must be thoroughly explored. Children often resist taking medication because they do not want to feel "different," because they reject the very idea that there is anything wrong with them, or because they are concerned about the reactions of peers. Adherence is inversely related to the complexity of the medication regimen (including the number of medicines used and the frequency of dosing), and administration of medication during the school day is often an issue, complicated by school rules and inadequate staffing levels in some schools. Adherence to treatment often relates to child and parental attitudes about taking medications for emotional or behavioral problems. Practically, use of a weekly pill organizer is often important for even simple medication regimens. A young child whose medication is dispensed by two parents (or by nannies, grandparents, and so forth) may easily end up with either no medication or a double dose. Pill organizers may also help parents to check on adherence of an adolescent who is responsible for taking his or her own medication. Adolescents may need more supervision in taking medication than parents assume is needed, and taking responsibility for medication is a subject that needs to be discussed repeatedly before the adolescent makes the transition from home to college, where his or her schedule will be much different and more variable.

Ethical Issues and "Off-Label" Prescribing

Physicians who treat children with pharmacotherapy face significant ethical challenges. Pharmaceutical companies often do not go to the expense and risk of testing drugs in children and adolescents, although a federal (U.S.) law was passed in 1997 to encourage such testing by extending patent protection for 6 months on drugs studied in children. In 2000, the FDA released additional guidelines to encourage the clinical investigation of drugs for use in the pediatric population. Because fewer psychotropic medications have an approved FDA indication for young children, most drugs are used "off label" in this patient group. Although FDA guidelines are not meant to restrict the clinical practice of physicians, the clinician is responsible for the careful use of these medications in young patients. Lack of knowledge about the potential effect of medications on the neural development of children further complicates the issue. A clinician must balance multiple factors: the risks of the untreated disorder, the anticipated and actual efficacy of medication, and the potential adverse outcomes or unknowns of medication use.

The interaction between pharmacotherapy and the environment is even more important for children than for adult patients, because children's immature developmental status places them in the care of adults. There is a danger of misinterpreting a child's response to the family, school, or institutional milieu as an exacerbation requiring medication or as an improvement due to a medication. Some adults may seek to use drugs to control or eliminate a child's troublesome behavior rather than instituting more time-consuming and difficult therapeutic or behavioral management strategies. The clinician must therefore evaluate and monitor the environment as well as the patient, using all available information to make therapeutic decisions.

Stimulants

There is extensive empirical support for the short-term efficacy and safety of stimulant medications in the treatment of ADHD and comorbid oppositional defiant disorder (ODD) in boys and girls from preschool age through adolescence. Therapeutic effects typically seen in stimulant responders include improved sustained attention and short-term memory, reduced impulsivity and excessive motor behavior, improved classroom behavior and work completion, reduced impulsive aggression, and improved interactions with parents, teachers, and peers.

The long-term therapeutic effect of stimulant medication is observed clinically but difficult to demonstrate in research, and most studies have been of relatively short duration. The National Institute of Mental Health (NIMH) Collaborative Multisite Multimodal Treatment Study of Children With ADHD (MTA) found after 14 months of treatment that optimally titrated stimulant treatment with supportive therapy (MTA Medication) was more effective for core ADHD symptoms than very intensive behavioral therapy without medication (MTA Cooperative Group 1999). Intensive behavioral treatment added only modestly to MTA Medication (primarily in improving comorbid anxiety, social skills, and academic performance). All of the MTA treatments were more effective than treatment as usual in the community, which typically consisted of stimulant medication administered at lower dosages and fewer doses per day for a shorter period and with less careful monitoring than with MTA Medication. The NIMH Preschool ADHD Treatment Study (PATS) found methylphenidate to be safe and effective in preschool children, although improvement was less and side effects (especially sadness, irritability, clinging, insomnia, anorexia, and repetitive behaviors) were somewhat greater than in school-age children (Greenhill et al. 2006).

Despite a positive response to stimulant medication, many youths with ADHD continue to have impairment due to learning disabilities, gaps in knowledge and skills, poor social skills, and/or family problems. Adding focused behavioral treatment may augment the stimulant effect or allow for a lower dosage of medication to be used. Unfortunately, behavioral treatment is difficult to implement and sustain, and improvements do not generalize from one setting to another. Specific skills remediation (e.g., tutoring or coaching) may also be needed.

Stimulant treatment can be useful in reducing the impact of symptoms in comorbid conditions. In ADHD plus ODD, stimulants can reduce defiance, negativism, and impulsive verbal and physical aggression. In children with intellectual disability, stimulants are effective in treating ADHD target symptoms, although therapeutic effect is less robust and side effects are more common than in those of normal intelligence. Stimulants may also be useful in reducing symptoms of inattention, impulsivity, and hyperactivity in children with ASD, although the response is less robust and side effects are more common than in children with ADHD alone.

Patients with Tourette's disorder frequently have comorbid ADHD and often are far more disabled by the ADHD than by the tics. Stimulant treatment is effective in these cases, and there is no clear evidence that there is a lasting increase in tics with stimulant treatment. Exacerbation of tics, previously attributed to stimulant treatment, may be just transient or due to the natural waxing and waning nature of tics.

Initiation and Maintenance

The decision to medicate a child or adolescent with ADHD is based on the child's inattention, impulsivity, and often hyperactivity that are not due to another treatable cause and are sufficiently severe to cause impairment at school as well as at home and with peers. Parents must be willing to monitor medication and to attend appointments. In preschool children, other interventions are generally implemented first, unless severe impulsivity and noncompliance create an emergency situation. An important part of treatment is education of the child, family, and teacher, including explicitly debunking common myths about stimulant treatment. Stimulants do not have a paradoxical sedative effect, do not lead to drug abuse, and do continue to be effective after puberty. There are no evidence-based predictors of which stimulant medication or formulation would be most effective for a specific patient. Neither neurological soft signs, electroencephalography, brain scans, nor neurochemical measures have been found to predict stimulant response. Multiple outcome measures that use more than one source and setting are essential to evaluate the effect of a medication regimen. Parent and teacher rating scales (such as the Vanderbilt scales [Bard et al. 2013; Wolraich et al. 2013] or the ADHD Rating Scale V [DuPaul et al. 2016]) should be used at baseline and during titration and maintenance treatment. The clinician should work closely with parents on dosage adjustments and obtain regular reports from teachers and the results of annual academic testing done by the school.

Prior to starting a stimulant medication, the clinician should obtain a complete patient and family cardiovascular history, including structural cardiac abnormalities, chest pain, palpitations, unexplained fainting, arrhythmias, and family history of early cardiac death or sudden unexplained death. In the absence of cardiovascular indications on history or in the physical examination, an electrocardiogram is not indicated prior to stimulant treatment.

The increasing variety of available preparations of stimulant medications gives flexibility in addressing the clinical needs of an individual child. Online resources such as The ADHD Medication Guide from the Cohen Children's Medical Center (www.adhdmedicationguide.com) and the Florida Best Practice Psychotherapeutic

Medication Guidelines for Children and Adolescents (www.medicaidmentalhealth .org) provide information on all the many preparations currently on the market. Whereas each stimulant is either a form of methylphenidate or a form of amphetamine, they vary in terms of duration of action and method of delivery of the medication, so that treatment can take into consideration the optimal duration of action and whether the child can swallow a pill. Although methylphenidate is the most commonly used and best studied, both a methylphenidate and an amphetamine may need to be tried to determine the best option, and patients may have surprisingly different responses to different preparations of the same drug. The Florida Best Practice Guidelines recommend starting with stimulant monotherapy and then, if monotherapy is ineffective, switching to another stimulant monotherapy, or just starting with an extended-release α_2 agonist. Further steps involve combining an extended-release α_2 agonist with a stimulant or use of atomoxetine. Thus, considerable time and thought often go into finding the best treatment regimen for a child with ADHD.

Stimulant medication should be started at a low dosage and titrated upward (within the recommended range) every week or two according to response and side effects. Preschool-age children or patients with ADHD (predominantly inattentive type), intellectual disability, or ASD may benefit from (and have fewer side effects with) dosages lower than those used in school-age patients with ADHD who are very hyperactive and impulsive. Starting with only a morning dose may be useful in assessing drug effect by permitting morning and afternoon school performance to be compared. The need for an after-school dose or for medication on weekends should be individually determined according to the patient's target symptoms. Although some children who experience sleep or appetite disturbance but a good clinical response to stimulants may benefit from a suspension of medication on weekends and school holidays, those who are actively involved in sports or peer activities or evening or weekend academic projects require consistent daily medication (although a lower dosage may be sufficient in some settings outside of the classroom). Results from the MTA study suggest that most children continue to benefit from maintenance medication dosages that are similar to the initial titration dosage. MTA study results also support the superiority of full-day, 7-day-per-week stimulant coverage in children with combined-type ADHD (MTA Cooperative Group 1999).

If symptoms are not severe outside of the school setting, children may have an annual medication-free trial in the summer, lasting at least 2 weeks, but longer if possible. If school behavior and academic performance are stable, a carefully monitored trial off medication during the school year (but *not* at the beginning) will provide data on whether medication is still needed.

Tolerance is reported anecdotally; however, adherence is often irregular in children, and nonadherence should be the first possibility considered when medication appears to be ineffective. Children should not be held responsible for taking their medication, because these children are impulsive and forgetful at best, and most dislike the idea of taking medication, even when they can verbalize its positive effects and cannot identify any side effects. They will often avoid, "forget," or simply refuse their medication. Lower efficacy of a generic preparation may be another possibility when tolerance is suspected. Decreased drug effect also may be a reaction to a change at home or school.

Risks and Side Effects

Most side effects are similar for all stimulants (Table 41–1). Giving medication after meals and offering evening snacks reduce effects of appetite suppression. Insomnia may be due to drug effect, ADHD or ODD symptoms, separation anxiety, rebound, or a preexisting sleep problem. Stimulants may worsen or improve irritable mood. Although alarms were raised regarding a possible association between stimulant treatment for ADHD and sudden death, subsequent studies using very large databases have found no increased risk for serious cardiovascular events in youth prescribed stimulant medications compared with unmedicated youth (Hammerness et al. 2011).

Amphetamine preparations carry a "black box" warning regarding their potential for abuse and the possibility of sudden death and serious cardiovascular events if misused. They should also be avoided in patients with structural cardiac defects. Abuse is possible, but research has not found serious cardiovascular risk when amphetamines are used as prescribed.

The possibility of stimulant-induced growth retardation remains a concern. The magnitude of growth suppression is dose related and appears to be greater with amphetamine than with methylphenidate. Weight loss or slowed velocity of weight gain is common. Slowing of height growth has been found in some studies, but findings are variable, and some youth with ADHD are above average in size prior to stimulant treatment. Measurement of height and weight at the initiation of treatment and at regular intervals throughout is recommended.

Rebound effects, consisting of increased excitability, activity, talkativeness, irritability, and insomnia that begin 4–15 hours after a dose, may be seen as the last dose of the day wears off or for up to several days after sudden withdrawal of high daily doses of stimulants. This effect may resemble a worsening of the original symptoms but also may simply represent the return of original symptoms when the medication effect wanes or a result of environmental influences in the late afternoon and evening.

If there is a concern regarding abuse or diversion of medication by the patient, family, or peers, use of Concerta, Vyvanse, or Daytrana is recommended. These formulations do not produce a "high," because they cannot be snorted or injected. Addiction has *not* been found to result from the prescription of stimulants for ADHD.

Although there is a commonly held notion that stimulants lower the seizure threshold, there is no evidence that stimulants produce an increase in seizure activity.

Alpha$_2$-Noradrenergic Agonists

Clonidine and guanfacine are α_2-noradrenergic agonists developed for the treatment of hypertension. The short-acting forms (Catapres and Tenex) have been used for some time to treat ADHD, with modest empirical support. A long-acting formulation of each (Kapvay and Intuniv) is FDA approved for the treatment of ADHD, alone or in combination with a stimulant medication (Sallee et al. 2013).

Indications and Efficacy

Attention-deficit/hyperactivity disorder.   Clonidine is useful in modulating mood and activity level and in improving cooperation and frustration tolerance in a subgroup of children with ADHD, especially those who are highly excitable, hyperactive, impulsive, and defiant, and show mood lability. A randomized controlled trial in chil-

TABLE 41–1.   Side effects of stimulant medications

Common initial side effects (try dose reduction)
  Anorexia
  Weight loss
  Irritability
  Abdominal pain
  Headaches
  Emotional oversensitivity; easy crying
Less common side effects
  Insomnia
  Dysphoria (especially at higher doses)
  Decreased social interest
  Less than expected weight gain
  Rebound overactivity and irritability (as dose wears off)
  Anxiety
  Nervous habits (e.g., picking at skin; pulling hair)
  Hypersensitivity rash, conjunctivitis, or hives
  Erythema at site of Daytrana patch
Withdrawal effects
  Rebound attention-deficit/hyperactivity disorder symptoms
  Depression (rare)
Rare but potentially serious side effects
  Motor or vocal tics
  Tourette's disorder
  Depression
  Growth retardation
  Tachycardia
  Hypertension
  Hallucinations
  Priapism
  Stereotyped activities or compulsions
  Contact sensitization to methylphenidate
  Chemical leukoderma from Daytrana patch

dren with both ADHD and a chronic tic disorder (Tourette's Syndrome Study Group 2002) found significant improvements in all treatment groups (clonidine, methylphenidate, and the combination). The greatest benefit compared with placebo was seen in the combination medication group. While clonidine and methylphenidate individually were both noted to be effective for symptoms of ADHD, methylphenidate appeared more beneficial for the inattention symptoms, whereas clonidine appeared more beneficial for the impulsivity and hyperactivity symptoms.

Two large controlled trials have demonstrated the efficacy of extended-release clonidine (Kapvay) in the treatment of children and adolescents with ADHD. In the first, extended-release clonidine at 0.2 mg/day or 0.4 mg/day was superior to placebo, with significant improvement at 5 weeks (Jain et al. 2011). In the second trial, youth with ADHD (combined or hyperactive subtype) who had experienced only a partial response to a stimulant were randomly assigned to receive the addition of either placebo or extended-release clonidine to their stimulant regimen (Kollins et al. 2011). Extended-release clonidine plus stimulant was superior to placebo plus stimulant in improving inattention and hyperactivity. Commonly reported adverse effects were somnolence, headache, and fatigue.

Extended-release guanfacine (Intuniv), taken once a day in the morning or evening, has been shown to be effective in the treatment of ADHD either as monotherapy or as an augmenting agent added to stimulant medication (Wilens et al. 2015). Studies of guanfacine in adolescents suggest that weight-based dosing provides the greatest efficacy, with about 0.1 mg/kg as the target dosage (Wilens et al. 2015).

Tic disorders.   The first-line treatment for tic disorders should be habit-reversal therapy (HRT) or Comprehensive Behavioral Intervention for Tics (CBIT). Efficacy of clonidine in reducing tics in youth who do not also have ADHD has not been consistently demonstrated. Clonidine appears to be most beneficial for subjective distress and the behavioral symptoms of hyperactivity and impulsivity that often accompany Tourette's disorder. Early studies had suggested that guanfacine might be useful in reducing tics; however, in a recent study, tic reduction with guanfacine extended release did not differ significantly from that with placebo (Murphy et al. 2017).

Initiation and Maintenance

Blood pressure and pulse should be measured before initiating α_2-noradrenergic agonist treatment and at regular intervals thereafter. An electrocardiogram may be considered in preschoolers and in children with a patient or family history of cardiovascular symptoms. Baseline laboratory blood studies (especially fasting glucose) may be considered if the patient or family history suggests increased risk.

Clonidine extended release is started at 0.1 mg/day divided into two doses and is increased by 0.1 mg/day each week to a target dosage of 0.4 mg/day divided into two doses (every 12 hours). Short-acting, or immediate-release, clonidine is started at 0.05 mg at bedtime. This low dose and timing convert the side effect of initial sedation into a benefit. An alternative strategy is to begin with 0.025 mg taken four times a day. Either way, the dosage is then increased gradually over several weeks to 0.15–0.30 mg/day (0.003–0.01 mg/kg/day) taken in three—or optimally four—divided doses. Young children (ages 5–7 years) may require even lower initial and maintenance dosages.

Guanfacine extended release is started at 1 mg/day, increasing weekly by 1 mg/day to a maximum of 4.0 mg/day in children 12 years and younger, and up to 7.0 mg/day in adolescents 13 years and older. This extended-release form is given only once per day and is not milligram-to-milligram equivalent with the immediate-release form. For guanfacine immediate release, a recommended starting regimen is 0.5 mg once or twice daily in children and 1 mg once or twice daily in adolescents, to be increased every 3 or 4 days until a therapeutic effect is noted. In the setting of ADHD, it may be useful to administer the guanfacine immediate-release daily dosage in three divided doses.

One milligram of guanfacine is equivalent to 0.1 mg of clonidine. The two medications can be gradually cross-tapered to switch between them. When clonidine or guanfacine is discontinued, it should be tapered gradually rather than stopped suddenly, to avoid a withdrawal syndrome consisting of increased motor restlessness, headache, agitation, elevated blood pressure and pulse rate, and (in patients with Tourette's disorder) exacerbation of tics.

Risks and Side Effects

Sedation and irritability are troublesome side effects of clonidine, although these tend to decrease after several weeks. Dry mouth, nausea, and photophobia have been reported, with hypotension and dizziness possible at high dosages. Glucose tolerance may decrease, especially in patients at risk of diabetes. Although guanfacine is less sedating and less hypotensive than clonidine, it shares many of clonidine's other side effects. Small mean decreases in pulse and blood pressure without clinical significance have been noted with extended-release guanfacine treatment, and headache and sedation are common.

Although there were past anecdotal reports suggesting serious adverse drug reactions (including sudden death) in children treated with clonidine, alone or in combination with methylphenidate, more recent studies (Tourette's Syndrome Study Group 2002) have found benefits without acute cardiovascular risk.

Atomoxetine

Atomoxetine, a norepinephrine reuptake inhibitor, is a nonstimulant medication approved by the FDA for use in the treatment of ADHD in children and adults.

Indications and Efficacy

The efficacy of atomoxetine in the treatment of ADHD in preschoolers through adolescents has been demonstrated consistently over time. In a meta-analysis that examined 25 randomized controlled trials, atomoxetine was found to have an overall medium effect size for ADHD (Schwartz and Correll 2014).

Initiation and Maintenance

Atomoxetine is started at 0.3 mg/kg/day taken as a single dose in the morning. If the patient experiences sedation, the dose can be taken at bedtime. If there are gastrointestinal side effects, the daily dosage can be divided into morning and evening doses and given with food. Over 1–3 weeks, the total daily dosage is increased to an initial target of 1.2 mg/kg/day. In children and adolescents weighing less than 70 kg (i.e., 154 lb), the total daily dosage should not exceed 1.4 mg/kg/day or 100 mg, whichever is less. For patients who weigh more than 70 kg, the maximum daily dosage is 100 mg. Dosages up to 1.8 mg/kg/day do not provide increased benefit, except when used in youth with comorbid ODD. It may take several weeks, or even months, for the maximum response to a given dose to be achieved.

Risks and Side Effects

Atomoxetine is generally well tolerated. The most commonly reported side effects include abdominal pain, headache, irritability or mood lability, dizziness, somnolence or fatigue, decreased appetite, and nausea and vomiting. Modest dose-related increases in pulse and blood pressure have also been noted. Most side effects appear to subside over time and only rarely result in discontinuation of treatment. There is no evidence that atomoxetine has any significant effect on height and weight. The capsules should not be opened, because the contents are caustic to the eyes. There are two FDA bolded warnings: one for extremely rare severe liver injury and one (based on limited evidence) for increased hostility and aggression or suicidal ideation. The risk for suicidal ideation has been examined further and, in comparison with placebo, was found to be not significant (Bangs et al. 2014).

Routine liver function tests are not recommended during treatment; however, parents should be instructed that the medication should be stopped and the physician contacted immediately if the patient develops jaundice; unexplained decreased appetite, nausea, or vomiting; pruritus; dark urine; or abdominal tenderness.

Atomoxetine is metabolized primarily through the hepatic CYP2D6 pathway, although it is not itself an inhibitor of this enzyme. Genetically slow metabolizers of CYP2D6 are not at increased risk of side effects, and genotyping is not indicated. Atomoxetine does not increase tics, lower the seizure threshold, or cause QTc prolongation, and it has a large margin of safety in overdose.

Selective Serotonin Reuptake Inhibitors

Controversy Surrounding Use in Children

Since the early 2000s, concern has been raised, both in the United States and in the United Kingdom, about both the safety and the effectiveness of selective serotonin reuptake inhibitors (SSRIs) in children and adolescents. In 2003, the FDA issued a public health advisory alerting clinicians to reports of increased suicidal thinking in children taking antidepressants. The advisory concluded that although "the data do not clearly establish an association between the use of these drugs and increased suicidal thoughts or actions by pediatric patients," such an association could not be ruled out (U.S. Food and Drug Administration 2003). The FDA stopped short of contraindicating the use of antidepressants in children but did mandate placement of a "black box" warning on all antidepressants, noting an increased risk of suicidality in pediatric patients. While the studies on which the warning was based have since been called into question, the clinician must inform and help parents to understand this warning. A reanalysis at the person-level of longitudinal data from all of the controlled trials of fluoxetine for pediatric depression found no evidence of increased suicidal thoughts and behaviors in youth randomly assigned to medication versus placebo (Gibbons et al. 2012). Furthermore, studies of SSRI use in children with anxiety disorders have not shown any increase in suicidal ideation or behavior.

Questions have also been raised about the effectiveness of SSRIs in children, based primarily on industry-sponsored studies with high placebo response rates. The major NIMH-funded studies, however, including the important studies of SSRI treatment in adolescents with depression (Treatment for Adolescents with Depression Study [TADS], Treatment of Adolescent Suicide Attempters [TASA], and Treatment of Resistant Depression in Adolescents [TORDIA] study) and in children with anxiety (Pediatric OCD Treatment Study [POTS]), showed very positive response rates (for a review, refer to Walkup 2017). The clinical consensus is that SSRIs are clearly beneficial for children with anxiety disorders, and probably beneficial for children with depression, but monitoring for suicidal ideation is important, especially during the first few weeks of treatment.

Indications and Efficacy

Depressive disorders.   Fluoxetine has an FDA indication for the treatment of depression in children ages 8–17 years, and escitalopram is FDA indicated for the treatment of major depressive disorder (MDD) in youth ages 12 years and older. Fluoxetine's efficacy in pediatric depression was demonstrated in randomized controlled trials. The TADS (March et al. 2006), a randomized controlled trial of 439 patients ages 12–17 years with MDD, compared the efficacy of fluoxetine (10–40 mg/day) and cognitive-behavioral therapy (CBT), either alone or in combination, with that of placebo over a 12-week period. At the conclusion of the study, fluoxetine plus CBT and fluoxetine alone were superior to both placebo and CBT alone. The results of studies of other SSRIs (i.e., sertraline, citalopram, and escitalopram) in pediatric depression have been inconsistent. In summary, although more study is needed of efficacy and safety, SSRIs can be effective in the treatment of depression in children. The results may be less predictable and less positive than with adults. With respect to pharmacological treatment of pediatric depression, SSRIs are the first- and second-line choices.

Obsessive-compulsive disorder.   Fluoxetine is FDA approved for the treatment of obsessive-compulsive disorder (OCD) in children ages 7–17 years. Other SSRIs with FDA indications for OCD in youth are fluvoxamine (ages 8 years and older) and sertraline (ages 6 years and older). A meta-analysis of controlled trials of treatment of pediatric OCD found that fluoxetine, fluvoxamine, paroxetine, and sertraline were equal in efficacy and that all were superior to placebo (Geller et al. 2003).

The POTS (March et al. 2004) examined the use of sertraline, CBT, and their combination in a 12-week randomized controlled study of 112 children and adolescents with OCD. All active treatment conditions were significantly superior to placebo. The combination of CBT and sertraline was superior to monotherapy with either CBT or sertraline. The effect size of CBT monotherapy was greater than that for sertraline monotherapy, with more children achieving remission from CBT monotherapy, although the benefit over sertraline monotherapy did not reach statistical significance. The combination of CBT and medication for relatively severe OCD thus appears to be more effective and may also be more acceptable to patients and parents. When compared with medication alone, the addition of CBT includes techniques that can address subsequent relapses in obsessive-compulsive symptoms that occur despite medication treatment or that happen after medication discontinuation.

Anxiety disorders.   Studies have demonstrated the efficacy of SSRIs (e.g., fluvoxamine, sertraline, fluoxetine) in generalized anxiety disorder, separation anxiety disorder, selective mutism, panic disorder, and social phobia.

Initiation and Maintenance

Patients and parents should be cautioned regarding the black box warning of the potential for increased suicidality. The FDA recommends weekly monitoring of children during the first 4 weeks of treatment and additional monitoring at weeks 6, 8, and 12, but the American Psychiatric Association and AACAP suggest that monitoring be tailored to the individual patient and family (American Psychiatric Association 2005). With responsible parents or a mature adolescent, phone check-ins with the physician or a nurse may be substituted for some weekly visits. If the child sees another clinician for therapy, communication with that person will provide additional monitoring.

The guidelines from the Texas Children's Medication Algorithm Project (Hughes et al. 2007) recommend fluoxetine, sertraline, or citalopram as first-line medication for the treatment of pediatric MDD. Fluoxetine is the consensus conference panel's first choice, with sertraline and citalopram as alternatives. Fluoxetine and citalopram may be started at a dosage of 5–10 mg/day, with the dosage increased as needed to 20 mg/day. Although most children will respond to 20 mg/day or less of these medications, some children may require up to 40 mg/day (citalopram) or 60 mg/day (fluoxetine for OCD). Escitalopram dosages are half those of citalopram. All three of these medications are available in a liquid formulation that may facilitate medication administration or dosage titration. Sertraline and fluvoxamine may be started at 25 mg/day and increased as necessary to 100–150 mg/day. The dosage may be increased every few days, with monitoring of therapeutic and side effects.

The shorter half-life of SSRIs in children means that discontinuation syndrome is more likely to occur, even after only one missed dose. It is therefore preferable to taper the medication over several days rather than discontinue it abruptly. Discontinuation syndrome is less likely when switching from one SSRI to another, but even then, close communication and monitoring for withdrawal symptoms can eliminate unnecessary suffering. Discontinuation syndrome is not usually observed with fluoxetine because of its active metabolites and long half-life.

Risks and Side Effects

Children and adolescents usually tolerate this class of medication well, although they may experience side effects similar to those in adults, such as gastrointestinal complaints or headache. If medication is stopped abruptly, a discontinuation syndrome, consisting of malaise, myalgia, headache, and anxiety, may ensue. "Behavioral activation," or manic symptoms, may appear within days to weeks of initiating treatment with an SSRI, even with no premorbid or family history of a cyclical mood disorder. These symptoms typically resolve within a few days of dosage reduction or medication cessation. In some cases, treatment with a mood stabilizer is necessary. Behavioral activation with physical agitation and insomnia is often difficult to distinguish from emergent mania, but symptoms such as grandiosity, increased goal-directed activity, and euphoric mood may be helpful in identifying the child with true mania or hypomania. Children being treated with an SSRI may also develop disinhibition or apathy and lack of motivation. These symptoms typically develop 6–8 weeks after initiation of treatment with an SSRI or an increase in dosage and usually subside with a decrease in dosage. Although SSRIs do not consistently affect weight or appetite, weight loss or slowing of weight gain does occasionally happen, so it is wise to ask about this side effect and check weight for the first few months of treatment. Adolescents, like adults, may experience sexual dysfunction from SSRI treatment, and this side effect may affect adherence to treatment. Movement disorders, including dystonia, akathisia, and tics, have been reported in rare cases in children taking SSRIs. Serotonin syndrome is rare but may occur in children, just as in adults, and parents should be warned of this possibility, especially if more than one serotonergic medication is being taken. Treatment, as in adults, includes stopping the SSRI and providing supportive medical interventions.

Other Antidepressants

All antidepressants share the black box warning regarding increased suicidality. Bupropion and venlafaxine are used rarely to treat depression in youth. Bupropion has been demonstrated to be effective in treatment of pediatric ADHD in controlled trials and is a third-line treatment for that disorder. Its use as an antidepressant is generally limited to adolescents who have had one or more failed trials of an SSRI and have low energy and difficulty concentrating as symptoms of depression, or who have comorbid ADHD. The most serious side effect is a decrease in the seizure threshold, seen most frequently in patients with an eating disorder. Other side effects in children include skin rash, perioral edema, nausea, increased appetite, agitation, and exacerbation of tics. Use of venlafaxine is generally limited to adolescents with major depression who have had one or more failed trials of an SSRI. In the TORDIA study, after one failed trial of an SSRI, switching to another SSRI was as effective as switching to venlafaxine, and venlafaxine produced more side effects (Brent et al. 2008).

Until the introduction of the SSRIs, tricyclic antidepressants (TCAs) were used in the pharmacological treatment of a variety of disorders in children and adolescents. However, the paucity of clinical studies demonstrating the efficacy of TCAs in pediatric depression, the cardiac side effects of this class of medication, and the availability of alternative medications have resulted in a shift away from using TCAs in children, except for clomipramine, which is used to treat OCD that has not responded to an SSRI. Children metabolize TCAs more rapidly than adults do and are prone to swings in blood levels from ineffective to toxic, requiring monitoring of baseline and follow-up electrocardiograms and divided doses to produce a more stable level. TCAs are extremely dangerous in overdose, either intentional or accidental, and parents should be advised to lock up or otherwise secure the medication for the safety of all household members.

Mood-Stabilizing Agents

Lithium

Indications and efficacy.   Although lithium received an FDA indication for adolescent mania almost 50 years ago, only in the past several years have controlled trials examined its efficacy in young people. The largest pediatric bipolar trial conducted to date found that lithium was less effective than risperidone in treating acute mania (Geller et al. 2012). However, this same study underscored risperidone's serious metabolic side effects. Because lithium is superior to placebo and is unassociated with weight gain in the pediatric population, it remains a useful treatment option for acute mania.

Initiation and maintenance.   Lithium should be started only if the family is able to administer, and the patient is able to cooperate with, multiple daily doses and regular blood draws. Sexually active girls should be specifically counseled regarding lithium's teratogenicity. They should receive a pregnancy test as part of the pretreatment workup and, if appropriate, should receive contraception during therapy. An electrocardiogram, while not strictly necessary in young patients without cardiac disease, can serve as a useful baseline should electrocardiographic abnormalities develop.

In pediatric patients weighing at least 30 kg (i.e., 66 lb), a starting dosage of 300 mg three times daily is both safe and effective (Findling et al. 2011). The dosage may be increased weekly in 300-mg increments, with trough levels monitored to target a range of 0.6–1.4 mEq/L.

Risks and side effects.   Although lithium is at least as well tolerated in children and adolescents as it is in adults, younger children may experience side effects even at low serum levels. Nausea and diarrhea are common early-onset side effects that can be addressed by slowing the rate at which the dosage is increased or by switching to a controlled-release formulation. Enuresis due to polyuria and polydipsia may limit tolerability. In developing children, the consequences of hypothyroidism are potentially more severe than in adults. Lithium's tendency to aggravate acne or cause hair loss may be especially problematic for adolescents.

Because lithium's therapeutic index is narrow, adequate salt and fluid intake are crucial to prevent levels from rising into the toxic range. The family should be instructed about the importance of preventing dehydration from heat or exercise and should be warned that erratic consumption of large amounts of salty snack foods can cause lithium levels to fluctuate. Small children are especially at risk due to the fact that they dehydrate more easily and also are not good at monitoring their own thirst and fluid intake.

Anticonvulsants

Carbamazepine and oxcarbazepine.   Evidence supporting the use of carbamazepine in children is limited to a single open-label trial of the extended-release formulation, which appeared to show positive results in pediatric mania (Findling and Ginsberg 2014). Oxcarbazepine, which has been suggested as an alternative, has not been found to be effective in multicenter trials and is not generally considered to be useful in children with bipolar disorder.

Divalproex.   *Indications and efficacy.*   Trials of divalproex in pediatric mania have shown mixed results: it may be inferior to risperidone (Geller et al. 2012) in bipolar I disorder. Disruptive behavior and extreme irritability in the context of a mood disorder may, on the other hand, be a more promising treatment target, although more research is needed. There is some evidence supporting the use of divalproex as monotherapy in children with ASD and irritability and in combination with a stimulant in children with ADHD and chronic aggression.

Initiation and maintenance.   A complete blood count with differential and platelets, as well as liver function tests, should be conducted before the patient begins taking divalproex. Divalproex not only is a teratogen but also is associated with menstrual irregularities and polycystic ovary syndrome. Its use in adolescent girls should therefore be given careful thought regardless of whether they are sexually active. Those who are should, as with lithium, receive a pregnancy test and contraception if appropriate. Monthly liver function tests during the first few months of treatment are advisable for children younger than 10 years of age.

Divalproex can be started at a low dosage (125 or 250 mg taken once or twice daily) and gradually increased on the basis of tolerability and clinical response. Trough levels can provide guidance on whether a dosage increase would be safe, but no therapeutic levels have been established specifically in children, so guidelines for adult treatment are usually used.

Risks and side effects.   Gastrointestinal distress is a common side effect of divalproex, particularly early on. It can be mitigated by slowing the rate of dosage titration or by using divalproex in its enteric-coated form. Endocrine consultation is advised if hormonal abnormalities are suspected in an adolescent female patient.

Lamotrigine.   There are limited data supporting the use of lamotrigine in pediatric bipolar disorder. Lamotrigine has the potential to induce a very rare but potentially life-threatening rash, and this adverse effect may be somewhat more common in children than in adults. The need for slow dosage titration and consistent adherence to medication may make lamotrigine especially difficult to use with children and adolescents, who can be unreliable. No placebo-controlled trials of lamotrigine monotherapy have been conducted for psychiatric conditions in the pediatric population, and there is no support for lamotrigine's use as an add-on treatment for pediatric bipolar I disorder. It is, however, used with some frequency for bipolar depression and bipolar II disorder in adolescents.

Antipsychotic Medications

Indications and Efficacy

Second-generation antipsychotics (SGAs) have been much more extensively studied than first-generation antipsychotics (FGAs) in children and adolescents; SGAs make up the overwhelming majority of antipsychotic prescriptions in the pediatric population. SGAs are used to treat a variety of psychiatric symptoms, including psychosis, mood symptoms, tics, aggression, and irritability. Seven SGAs have pediatric FDA indications: aripiprazole, asenapine, lurasidone, olanzapine, paliperidone, quetiapine, and risperidone (Table 41–2).

Psychosis.   Evidence from controlled trials supports the effectiveness of aripiprazole, olanzapine, paliperidone, risperidone, and quetiapine in schizophrenia spectrum and other psychotic disorders in youth, and any one of these agents, except olanzapine, is generally acceptable as a first-line agent. Olanzapine's labeling suggests that other drugs should be considered before olanzapine is used, given its propensity to cause weight gain, which may be even more dramatic in children than in adults. An FGA trial is warranted if treatment with one or more SGAs is unsuccessful, and a clozapine trial may be justified for patients in whom trials of antipsychotics from both generations have failed to control symptoms.

Mood symptoms.   For pediatric mania, risperidone appears to be more effective than either lithium or divalproex (Geller et al. 2012). Quetiapine, aripiprazole, and olanzapine all have demonstrated efficacy as well, although, again, olanzapine should be avoided as a first-line agent because of its metabolic effects. Although clinicians will sometimes use an SGA to augment antidepressant therapy in children with treatment-resistant unipolar depression, especially if there are some psychotic symptoms, such augmentation should be used judiciously, because no strong evidence supports this practice in the pediatric age group.

TABLE 41–2. **Second-generation antipsychotics with pediatric U.S. Food and Drug Administration indications**

Antipsychotic	Indication(s) (age range, years)
Aripiprazole	Irritability in autism (5–16)
	Mania (10–17)
	Schizophrenia (13–17)
	Tourette's disorder (6–17)
Asenapine	Mania (10–17)
Lurasidone	Schizophrenia (13–17)
Olanzapine	Schizophrenia (13–17)
	Mania (13–17)
	Bipolar depression (10–17)
Paliperidone	Schizophrenia (12–17)
Quetiapine	Schizophrenia (13–17)
	Mania (10–17)
Risperidone	Schizophrenia (13–17)
	Mania (10–17)
	Irritability in autism (5–16)

Tics. Evidence supports the efficacy of risperidone and aripiprazole in reducing tic severity in children and adolescents with Tourette's disorder. Efficacy has also been established for the FGAs haloperidol and pimozide; however, because their extrapyramidal side effects are problematic, their first-line use cannot be recommended.

Aggression and irritability. A recent high-quality meta-analysis found support for the efficacy of risperidone and aripiprazole in treating aggression and severe irritability in children and adolescents regardless of underlying diagnosis (van Schalkwyk et al. 2017). Risperidone and aripiprazole have also been specifically studied for controlling aggression, self-injury, and tantrums in children with ASD, and both medications have FDA indications for that purpose. When used in the treatment of aggression or irritability, medications should be used together with, rather than in lieu of, behavioral interventions. These medications may, however, be extremely effective and thus provide major improvements in functioning and in overall quality of life in children with ASD.

Initiation and Maintenance

Whenever possible, before initiating treatment, the clinician should obtain baseline values for weight, fasting blood sugar, and fasting lipids. These measurements should be repeated yearly, or more frequently if there is a family history of type 2 diabetes or hyperlipidemia. Abnormal movements should be measured with a standardized rating scale, such as the Abnormal Involuntary Movement Scale (AIMS), especially when treating children with ASD, who often have stereotyped movements at baseline.

Antipsychotic dosing should, as a rule, be conservative (Table 41–3). Particularly when the target of treatment is aggression or irritability, even low dosages may be effective.

TABLE 41–3.　Typical SGA dosing for children and adolescents

SGA	Typical dosage range, mg/day	Remarks
Aripiprazole	5–15	Starting dosage is 2–5 mg once daily. Some patients may prefer taking the daily dose at bedtime rather than in the morning.
Asenapine	5–20	Starting dosage is 2.5 mg every 12 hours.
Clozapine	250–500	Consider use after failed trials of at least one other SGA and at least one FGA. Use only if family and patient are willing and able to cooperate with frequent blood draws. Starting dosage is 12.5 mg once daily, given in the evening.
Lurasidone	40–80	Starting dosage is 20 mg once daily, usually given after dinner.
Olanzapine	5–15	Consider use after failed trial of at least one other SGA. Starting dosage is 2.5 mg in children or 5 mg in adolescents, given once daily in the evening.
Quetiapine	300–800	Starting dosage is 25–50 mg/day, divided into two doses; increase by 25–50 mg every 1–2 days as tolerated.
Paliperidone	3–12	Starting dosage is 3 mg once daily, usually given in the evening.
Risperidone	2–6	Starting dosage is 0.25 mg in children or 0.5 mg in adolescents, beginning with bedtime dose and increasing to both morning and bedtime doses if dosage increases do not cause undue sedation.
Ziprasidone	20–120	Starting dosage is 20 mg once daily, taken at bedtime; with subsequent dosage increases, daily dose should be divided into two doses (taken in morning and at bedtime). Doses should be taken with food. A baseline ECG scan, with repeat after dosage stabilization, is recommended because of the potential for QTc prolongation.

Note.　ECG=electrocardiography; FGA=first-generation antipsychotic; SGA=second-generation antipsychotic.

Risks and Side Effects

Extrapyramidal symptoms.   Pediatric patients are thought to be more prone to extrapyramidal symptoms than are adults, even when SGAs are used rather than FGAs. Adolescent age, male gender, higher dosages, and lack of prior antipsychotic exposure may be particular risk factors. Akathisia, which is thought to be particularly common with aripiprazole, may be difficult to identify in patients who are young or who have limited verbal abilities. When mild extrapyramidal symptoms go unrecognized by clinicians, they can interfere with age-appropriate activities, speech articulation, and ultimately medication adherence.

Tardive dyskinesia.   Because tardive dyskinesia risk is thought to be associated with total duration of antipsychotic exposure, the need for continuation of antipsychotic treatment should be periodically reevaluated with the patient and family. In some patients, brief discontinuation trials at 3- or 6-month intervals may be advisable to observe for withdrawal-emergent dyskinesia and to determine whether continued treatment is still necessary.

Cardiovascular side effects.   Ziprasidone is associated with QTc prolongation in children and adolescents. Although the clinical significance of this finding in otherwise healthy patients is unclear (Jensen et al. 2015), a baseline electrocardiogram and electrocardiographic monitoring during dosage titration are reasonable precautions.

Metabolic side effects.   The weight gain, insulin resistance, and dyslipidemia associated with SGA treatment may affect children and adolescents more severely than adults. Prudence would suggest particularly cautious use of these agents in children who are already overweight or who have a strong family history of diabetes. Calculation of body mass index at baseline and at intervals throughout treatment can help distinguish normal growth-related weight gain from weight gain due to antipsychotic use.

The importance of regular exercise and a healthy diet should be emphasized with patients and families. These lifestyle changes are often overwhelmingly difficult to implement, however, especially in children with an ASD, who often have little or no motivation to lose weight and frequently resist physical exercise. Some evidence suggests that adjunctive metformin may help counteract SGA-associated weight gain in youth with ASD (Handen et al. 2017) and may be the only option for such patients.

Hyperprolactinemia.   While SGAs, particularly risperidone, usually elevate the prolactin level early in treatment, the level often returns to normal or near-normal with prolonged treatment. In the absence of symptoms of hyperprolactinemia (i.e., galactorrhea, menstrual irregularities, or sexual dysfunction), monitoring of prolactin levels in youth receiving SGAs is not advisable and often leads to unnecessary diagnostic testing and discontinuation of an effective medication.

Other side effects.   Children are thought to be less likely than adults to experience anticholinergic side effects (e.g., hypotension, dry mouth, constipation, nasal congestion, blurred vision, and urinary retention) from antipsychotics, but they are at least as likely as adults to experience sedation, a symptom that can interfere with their ability to benefit from school. Neuroleptic malignant syndrome has been reported in children and adolescents, with a presentation similar to that seen in adults.

Anxiolytics

Benzodiazepines

Benzodiazepines are best avoided in the treatment of acute pediatric agitation or anxiety because of their propensity to cause disinhibition reactions, which can manifest as psychomotor excitation, aggression, hostility, irritability, or anxiety. Benzodiazepines with relatively longer half-lives, such as clonazepam, may be appropriate in treating adolescent panic disorder that is inadequately controlled by an SSRI alone. As with benzodiazepine use in adults, there is concern about abuse and dependence, as well as cognitive side effects, all of which may be especially problematic for a high school or college student.

Buspirone

A recent meta-analysis of randomized controlled trials found no evidence that buspirone is efficacious in pediatric anxiety (Strawn et al. 2018). There is, however, anecdotal evidence of buspirone's effectiveness alone or in conjunction with an SSRI.

Sedative-Hypnotics

Although pharmacological treatment can be appropriate, particularly in the short term, behavioral interventions and improvement of sleep hygiene are the best initial treatments for insomnia in children.

Melatonin

Melatonin has been studied both in typically developing children and in children with neurodevelopmental problems such as ASD or intellectual disability. Melatonin can be used either to shift the sleep phase forward (as a chronobiotic) or to induce sleep (as a hypnotic). As a chronobiotic, it is best administered 3–5 hours before bedtime, but as a hypnotic it should be given 30 minutes beforehand. The usual dose is 3 mg (in children weighing less than 40 kg [i.e., 88 lb]) or 5 mg (in children weighing 40 kg or more). Melatonin is available over the counter as an unregulated supplement, so parents should be cautioned to purchase a high-quality brand to assure potency and absence of impurities. There is no evidence that "controlled-release" formulations of melatonin offer improved efficacy or help with maintenance of sleep. Melatonin is available in a chewable form, which is especially appropriate for young children.

Other Agents

Clonidine, described earlier in this chapter (see subsection "Alpha$_2$-Noradrenergic Agonists"), is commonly used for insomnia, particularly in children with comorbid ADHD. The so-called Z-drugs (zolpidem, zaleplon, and eszopiclone) have not been researched in the pediatric population. SGAs such as quetiapine are not recommended as monotherapy for the treatment of insomnia, in the absence of another indication for their use, given the side-effect burden of these medications.

Somatic Treatments

Neurostimulation

Repetitive transcranial magnetic stimulation and transcranial direct current stimulation are under investigation as potential treatments for psychiatric illness in children and adolescents. Not enough is known regarding either their safety or their efficacy in the pediatric population to recommend their use at this time.

Complementary and Alternative Treatments

Despite limited evidence to support their safety or efficacy, so-called complementary and alternative treatments are in widespread use. A recent review, in fact, estimated that half of children with ASD receive such interventions (Höfer et al. 2017). Parents and, if appropriate, patients should therefore always be asked about any alternative treatments they may be taking.

Parents (and some primary care practitioners) often find alternative treatments appealing because they are more "natural" than medication. Some of these treatments may be reasonable; for example, there is some evidence that omega-3 fatty acids have a small but well-replicated benefit in treating ADHD symptoms, and there is no evidence that omega-3 fatty acids are harmful or difficult to administer. Special "elimination diets," on the other hand, are ineffective for ASD, at best only minimally effective for ADHD, and often very challenging for families to implement. Families who insist on trying such diets can be permitted to do so, provided that the diets are safe and nutritionally sound, because attempts to dissuade them may disrupt the therapeutic alliance.

Ineffective and potentially unsafe treatments against which families should be advised include herbal supplements, vitamin megadoses, chelation therapy, chlorine dioxide enemas, and avoidance of vaccination.

Psychotherapy

Recent years have seen an increasing focus on empirical studies of the efficacy of psychotherapy. Although psychotherapy for children has been shown to be effective when performed in a research setting, the results are often less favorable in the usual clinical setting. Compared with children seen in research environments, children seen in "real world" practice are often more symptomatic, have comorbid conditions, have more psychosocially stressed families, and receive less structured forms of psychotherapy. Challenges include accounting for the many influences in children's lives that affect treatment and functioning as well as determining what (or who) should be the focus of change (e.g., parent, child, style of parenting).

Psychotherapies may be classified according to theoretical model, target of intervention, duration, or goals of treatment. While there are many types of therapy employed with children, there is emerging empirical support for the use of specific forms of psychotherapy for particular disorders, especially depressive and anxiety disorders. In the following sections we describe, in very general terms, some of the more common forms of psychotherapy used in children. More thorough descriptions of models of psychotherapy as they are applied to youth and families may be found in specific treatment manuals.

In the treatment of children, it is essential to consider the patient's environment and family dynamics. In most cases, work with parents and school staff, and often pediatricians, welfare agencies, courts, or recreation leaders, must accompany individual therapy. The cooperation of parents, and often teachers, is required to maintain the child in treatment and to remove any secondary gain resulting from the symptoms. The therapist must be aware of a patient's level of physical, cognitive, and emotional development in order to understand the symptoms, set appropriate goals, and tailor effective interventions.

Communicating With Children and Adolescents

Children are less able to use abstract language than are adults. They use play to express feelings, to narrate past events, to work through trauma, and to seek comfort. It is less threatening and anxiety provoking if the therapist uses the metaphor of the play and bases questions and comments on characters in the play rather than on the child (even if the connection is clear to the therapist). Effective communications are tailored to the child's stage of language, cognitive, and affective development. The therapist must be aware that the vocabulary of some bright and precocious children exceeds their emotional understanding of events and concepts. Dramatic play with dolls or puppets and drawing, painting, or modeling with clay, as well as questions about dreams, wishes, or favorite stories or movies, can provide access to children's fantasies, emotions, and concerns. Adolescents may prefer creative writing or more complex expressive art techniques.

The Uncooperative Child or Adolescent

It is not surprising that many children or adolescents do not cooperate in therapy, because most are brought to treatment by adults. These young patients often do not wish to change themselves or their behaviors and view their parents' and teachers' complaints as unreasonable or unfair. In addition, a child or adolescent may refuse to participate in or may attempt to sabotage therapy for a variety of psychological reasons. Effective interventions are tailored to the cause of the resistance.

A child who is feeling anxious or having difficulty separating from a parent may be helped by initially permitting the parent to remain in the therapy room. When a child or adolescent does not talk, whether from anxiety or opposition, the therapist may address this reluctance, either directly or through play. Long silences generally are not helpful and tend to increase anxiety or battles for control. Attractive play materials help to make therapy less threatening and to encourage participation while the therapist builds an alliance. However, the therapist must guard against the danger of sessions becoming mere play or recreation instead of therapy. A variety of techniques incorporate therapeutic activities with storytelling, drama, and game boards. Using behavioral contingencies in therapy also may improve motivation and cooperation. An amazing amount of cooperation can be inspired by the prospect of a trip to the "treasure chest" of little toys and trinkets at the end of the session.

Individual Psychotherapy

All individual therapies have certain common themes:

- Relationship with a therapist who is perceived as helpful and understanding but who also has some authority, control, and influence
- Instillation of hope and improved morale
- Use of attention, encouragement, and suggestion
- Goals of helping the patient to achieve greater control, competence, mastery, and/or autonomy; to improve coping skills; and to abandon or modify unrealistic expectations of self or others

Supportive Therapy

The therapist provides support to the patient until a stressor resolves, a developmental crisis has passed, or the patient or environment changes sufficiently so that other adults can take on the supportive role. There is a real relationship with the therapist, who facilitates verbal expression of feelings and provides understanding and judicious advice.

Time-Limited Therapy

All of the models of time-limited therapy have in common a planned, relatively brief duration; a predominant focus on the presenting problem; a high degree of structure and attention to specific, limited goals; and active roles for both therapist and patient. Length of treatment varies from several sessions to 6 months. The short duration is used to increase patient motivation, participation, and reliance on resources within the patient's world rather than on the therapist. Time-limited treatment has been recommended both for multiproblem families in crisis who are unlikely to persist in longer-term treatment and for well-functioning children and families who have circumscribed problems of relatively recent onset. Following a course of time-limited treatment, children or families may return to the therapist for an additional "round" of treatment if other problems or symptoms develop. Or, following planned termination of therapy, one or two "booster" sessions may be used to reinforce skills and maintain improvement.

Interpersonal Psychotherapy

Interpersonal psychotherapy may be successfully adapted for depressed adolescents and has demonstrated efficacy in several controlled studies. This treatment focuses on improving interpersonal relationships in the lives of depressed adolescents through role clarification and enhanced communication. Such treatment may be especially effective when an older adolescent is struggling with changing roles and changing relationships in the period of transition to adult life.

Cognitive-Behavioral Therapy

CBT techniques adapted for children and adolescents have been shown in controlled trials to be efficacious in the treatment of anxiety disorders. Results in the treatment of depression are somewhat less consistent, but CBT is considered to be an important treatment option for depressed adolescents. Therapy manuals are available for treatment of anxiety or depression, adapted to the cognitive level of school-age children or adolescents (Chorpita and Weisz 2009). The anxiety treatment programs are based on development of a hierarchy of fears, which are to be gradually faced and conquered. The depression treatments involve techniques such as examining and changing cognitive distortions regarding the world and relationships, social problem solving, behavioral activation, and goal setting. All include significant psychoeducation for both the child and parents. Trauma-focused CBT is the preferred, empirically supported treatment approach for youth suffering from posttraumatic stress disorder. CBT using exposure and response prevention is the first-line treatment for mild to moderate OCD in children and adolescents.

Caution is needed to ensure that CBT homework assignments are not perceived as aversive when added to homework assigned in school. Prepubertal children's more concrete cognitive processes may make this model less effective, although creative adaptations and the incorporation of behavioral techniques can render this approach feasible.

Dialectical Behavior Therapy

Dialectical behavior therapy has been modified for treatment of adolescents, especially those with suicidal or self-injurious behaviors, and involves a combination of individual, group, and family treatment. Key components are development of coping skills and self-soothing techniques to help such patients modulate unstable affective states and reduce impulsive destructive behaviors. Family members must be actively involved in the treatment to improve their own coping skills and learn how to help their teen put his or her coping skills to good use. The availability of a therapist on call is an important feature of this treatment to address crises.

Motivational Interviewing

Motivational interviewing is appropriate for treatment of adolescents, especially those with drug or alcohol problems, who are poorly motivated to acknowledge their problems or try to change (Miller and Rollnick 2013). It is a semidirective therapy that seeks to resolve the patient's ambivalence about changing his or her behavior. Motivational interviewing is a nonjudgmental, nonconfrontational approach that attempts to increase the adolescent's awareness of the problems caused by and the consequences and risks of the behavior in question. The treatment also tries to help the teen see a more positive future and become more motivated to reach it. The three key elements of motivational interviewing are collaboration, not confrontation; evocation or drawing out, rather than imposing ideas on or lecturing to the adolescent; and autonomy as opposed to authority. The teen becomes more motivated to change as he or she sees that current behaviors will interfere with the accomplishment of his or her own goals.

Psychodynamic Psychotherapies

Psychoanalysis is an infrequently used treatment modality for children and adolescents because of the expense, frequency of sessions, length of treatment, and often lack of prompt symptom relief.

Psychodynamically oriented psychotherapy (see Kernberg et al. [2012] for the practice parameters for this therapy with children) is grounded in psychoanalytic theory but is more flexible and emphasizes the real relationship with the therapist and the provision of a corrective emotional experience. Frequency is typically once or twice a week, most commonly over a period of 1–2 years, although shorter, time-limited dynamic psychotherapies are also available. There is active collaboration between the parents and the therapist. Goals of therapy include symptom resolution, change in behavior, and return to normal developmental processes. The therapist forms an alliance with the child or adolescent, reassures, promotes controlled regression, identifies feelings, clarifies thoughts and events, makes interpretations, judiciously educates and advises, and acts as an advocate for the patient.

Dynamically oriented individual therapy is more likely to be effective for children and adolescents who are in emotional distress or who are struggling to deal with a stressor than for those children with behavior problems. Children and adolescents with attention-deficit, oppositional, or conduct disorders rarely acknowledge their problem behaviors and are usually better treated in family or group therapy, by parent training in behavior management, or in a structured milieu. Children with ADHD often have little insight into their behavior and its effect on others, and they may be genuinely unable to report their problems or to reflect on them. However, insight-oriented therapy may be useful for some of these youngsters to address comorbid anxiety or depression or symptoms resulting from trauma.

Parent Counseling

Parent counseling or guidance is a psychoeducational intervention. It may be conducted with a single parent or couple or in groups. Parents are taught about normal child and adolescent development. Efforts are made to help parents better understand their child and his or her problems and to modify practices that may be contributing to the current difficulties (whatever their original cause). It is essential that the therapist understand the parents' point of view and their hardships, including those that result from parenting a child with a psychiatric disorder. For some parents who have serious difficulties of their own, parent counseling may merge into or pave the way for individual treatment of the adult or conjoint couple therapy.

Virtually all parents of children with psychiatric or learning problems benefit from education in the nature of their children's disorders, support of their own emotional needs, and help in selecting treatments and managing difficult behaviors. Parents of children with chronic problems must become skilled advocates to ensure that their children receive the treatment and schooling they need. Carefully selected books and websites may be useful to parents.

Behavior Therapy

Behavior therapy is by far the most thoroughly evaluated psychological treatment for children. Maximally effective programs require home and school cooperation, focus on specific target behaviors, and ensure that contingencies follow behavior quickly and consistently. In behavior therapy, symptoms are viewed as resulting from bad habits, faulty learning, or inappropriate environmental responses to behavior. Behavioral approaches are characterized by detailed assessment of problematic emotional or behavioral responses and the environmental conditions that elicit and maintain them, the development of strategies to produce change in the environment and therefore in the patient's behavior, and repeated assessment to evaluate the success of the intervention. Behavior therapy is the most effective treatment for simple phobias, for enuresis and encopresis, and for the noncompliant behaviors seen in ODD and conduct disorder. For children with ADHD, behavior modification can improve both academic achievement and behavior if specifically targeted. Both punishment (timeout and response cost) and reward components are required. Behavior modification is more effective than medication in improving peer interactions, but skills may need to be taught first. Many youngsters require behavioral programs that are consistent, intensive, and prolonged (months to years). A wide variety of other childhood problems, such as motor and vocal tics, trichotillomania, and sleep problems, are treated by behavior modification, either alone or in combination with pharmacotherapy. Applied behavioral analysis is indicated for most youth with ASD.

The greatest weaknesses of behavior therapy are lack of maintenance of improvement over time and failure of changes to generalize to situations other than the ones in which training occurred. Generalization and maintenance can be maximized by conducting training in the settings in which behavior change is desired, at multiple times and places, facilitating transfer to naturally occurring reinforcers, and gradually fading reinforcement on an intermittent schedule.

Parent Management Training

Many effective training packages have been developed for parents of noncompliant, oppositional, and aggressive children (Barkley 2013) and delinquent adolescents. Parents are taught to give clear instructions, to positively reinforce good behavior, and to use punishment effectively. Timeout is a frequently used negative contingency for young children. The child is placed in a quiet, boring area where there is a "timeout" from attention or other positive reinforcement. Highly effective parent training programs combine instruction using multiple media with therapist modeling and coaching rehearsal of skills to be used. Families with low socioeconomic status, parental psychopathology (e.g., depression), marital conflict, and/or limited social support require maximally potent interventions, with attention to parental problems as necessary. Other families may be able to succeed with written materials only (Green 2014) or with manuals supplemented by group lectures.

Parent–child interaction therapy has been shown to be effective in reducing disruptive behaviors in children up to 7 years old. It is based on both social learning theory and attachment theory. The two phases of treatment are child-directed interaction and parent-directed interaction. In the first phase, the parents practice PRIDE skills, which include **P**raising the child's appropriate behavior, **R**eflecting on appropriate talk, **I**mitating appropriate play, **D**escribing appropriate behavior, and being **E**nthusiastic. The parent in this stage is also encouraged to avoid the use of commands, questions, or criticisms and to ignore minor misconduct but to stop play for aggressive misconduct. In the next phase, the parent is taught how to give effective commands, such as emphasizing being specific, giving one command at a time, doing so in positive terms (e.g., telling the child what to do as opposed to what not to do), using age-appropriate directions, being polite and respectful, and being direct (e.g., avoiding asking "Can you…" or "Will you…"). The therapist provides in vivo coaching, giving immediate reinforcement and feedback to the parent.

Collaborative and proactive solutions is another intervention with less emphasis on therapist- or parent-directed solutions and more emphasis on shared problem solving involving both the youth and the parent. This intervention may start with development of understanding of a child's lagging skills and of what specific unsolved problems manifest as a result. Focus is placed on the parent's approach to engaging with the child in understanding the child's concerns before formulating parent-driven solutions to unsolved problems (Ollendick et al. 2016).

Classroom Behavior Modification

Techniques for behavior modification in schools include token economies, class rules, and attention to positive behavior as well as response cost programs in which reinforcers are withdrawn in response to undesirable behavior. Reinforcers such as positive recognition or stars on a chart may be dispensed by teachers, or more tangible rewards or privileges by parents through the use of daily behavioral report cards. Even special education teachers rarely have sophisticated skills in behavior modification, and therapists may need to work closely with teachers and other school staff to develop appropriate programs. Collaboration between front-line teachers or aides and a therapist can produce very creative, personalized programs that involve incentives that the individual child really values. Interpersonal rewards, such as special time with a school staff person whom the child likes, can be especially helpful and promote positive relationships.

Family Treatment

Attempts to treat children and adolescents without considering their environment and relationships are unlikely to succeed. Any change in one family member, whether resulting from a psychiatric disorder, psychiatric treatment, a normal developmental process, or an outside event, is likely to affect family members and relationships. Family constellations vary widely, ranging from the traditional nuclear family to the single-parent family, a stepfamily, an adoptive or foster family, or a group home.

Evaluation of Families

Data should be gathered on each person living with the patient as well as on others who may be important or have been so in the past (e.g., noncustodial parents, grandparents, siblings who are no longer living at home). It is often useful to have at least one session that includes all significant family members.

A family assessment includes identifying the stage of the family life cycle, whether the family is accomplishing the basic tasks needed for all families (Table 41–4), any problematic areas of family interaction that require intervention, and aspects of the child's development that may have been at risk due to impaired communication or poor role modeling by family members. Other goals of a family assessment are to define any areas of parental problems or psychopathology, identify vulnerable family members, and determine how the family may be either maintaining or compensating for a child's disorder. Family systems have become increasingly diverse, and extensive research describes variations in normal and dysfunctional family interactions (Walsh 2012).

Family Therapy

In the most general sense, family therapy is psychological treatment conducted with an identified patient and at least one biological or functional (e.g., by marriage, adoption) family member. Related techniques include therapy with an individual patient

TABLE 41–4.	Family tasks

Forming a coalition between adults to meet the needs of those adults for intimacy, sexuality, and emotional support

Establishing a parental coalition capable of flexible relationships with the children and presenting a consistent disciplinary front

Nurturing, enculturating, and emancipating children

Coping with crisis

Source.   Adapted from Fleck 1976.

that takes a family systems perspective or therapy sessions with family members other than the identified patient, who is omitted because of refusal to participate, severity of illness, or other factors. There are an increasing number of empirically supported family-based treatments for child and adolescent emotional and behavioral problems (Sprenkle 2012). These include behavioral family therapy (based on social learning theory) and functional family therapy, both of which are used in the treatment of children and adolescents with conduct disorder. Multisystemic therapy includes energetic outreach into the home, neighborhood, and school and adds peer group and school-based interventions to family treatment of adolescent delinquents. This comprehensive treatment approach is highly effective in treating this hard-to-treat patient population but requires a great deal of resources and is unfortunately quite rare.

Family therapy may be particularly useful when there are dysfunctional interactions or impaired communication within the family, especially when these appear to be related to the presenting problem. It also may be useful when symptoms seem to have been precipitated by difficulty with a developmental stage for an individual or the family or by a change in the family such as divorce or remarriage. If more than one family member is symptomatic, family therapy may be both more efficient and more effective than multiple individual treatments. Family therapy should be considered when one family member improves with treatment but another, not in treatment, worsens. In any case, the family must have, or be induced to have, sufficient motivation to participate. When the identified patient is relatively unmotivated to participate or to change, family therapy is likely to be more effective than individual therapy. Attention to family systems issues also may be useful when progress is blocked in individual therapy or in behavior therapy.

If the family equilibrium is precarious or one or more family members are at serious risk of decompensation, family therapy may be useful in combination with other treatments, such as medication or hospitalization. Family sessions are not indicated when a parent has severe, intractable, or minimally relevant psychopathology or when the child strongly prefers individual treatment. Children should not be included in sessions in which parents persist (despite redirection) in criticizing the children or in sharing inappropriate information, when the most critical need is marital therapy, or when parents primarily need specific, concrete help with practical affairs.

Group Therapy

Group therapy offers opportunities for the clinician to model and facilitate practice of important skills. Interventions by peers may be far more acute and powerful in their effect than those by an adult therapist, especially in the treatment of adolescents with substance abuse or eating disorders. In addition, the therapist can observe in vivo behavior with peers. Target symptoms for group therapy include absent or conflictual peer relationships, anxiety, depression, and deficits in social interactive and problem-solving skills. These problems often are not accessible to intervention in individual therapy sessions.

Inpatient and Residential Treatment

Inpatient treatment is indicated in emergencies or when there are immediate safety concerns. It is also helpful for children who have not responded to outpatient treatment because of severity of the disorder, lack of motivation, refusal to cooperate with treatment, or inability of the patient and/or family to provide a structured environment for medication adherence.

Placement in a residential treatment center may be indicated for children and adolescents with chronic behavior problems such as aggression, running away, truancy, substance abuse, school phobia, or self-destructive acts that the family, foster home, and/or community cannot manage or tolerate. Children for whom returning home is not advisable—because of factors in the patient, the family, or both—may be referred to a residential treatment center following a hospital stay.

Short-term hospitalization (5–10 days) is typically an acute intervention, stemming from immediate physical danger to self or others; acute psychosis; a crisis in the environment that reduces the ability of the caregiving adults to cope with the child or adolescent; or the need for more intensive, systematic, and detailed evaluation and observation of the patient and family than is possible on an outpatient basis or in a day program. The typically brief hospital stay emphasizes rapid evaluation (including medical and neurological, when indicated), crisis intervention and stabilization, and development of a treatment plan to be implemented elsewhere. The goal is not to eliminate all psychopathology but rather to address the "focal problem" that precipitated hospitalization and then to discharge the patient to the appropriate level of care deemed clinically necessary. Inpatient or residential treatment includes multiple interventions, set in a therapeutic milieu with a structured schedule for meals, sleep, school, recreation, and self-care activities. Most settings incorporate social skills training and therapies to improve emotional regulation and self-control.

Hospitalization offers an ideal opportunity for systematic trials of medication in patients who have not responded to conventional treatment; whose illness is diagnostically puzzling; who have medical problems complicating pharmacotherapy; or whose parents are noncompliant, disorganized, or unreliable reporters of efficacy or side effects. In the hospital setting, the response to treatment can be constantly observed and side effects promptly managed. As-needed medications administered to control aggression or other behavior problems should be used only for brief periods until more effective, ongoing treatments are begun.

Regularly scheduled individual sessions with a therapist are essential in developing a more complete understanding of the patient's psychological, familial, and social dynamics and in assisting him or her to develop more adaptive methods of coping with strong emotions. In addition to general or special topic groups (e.g., 12-step models, survivors of abuse), group therapy may include community meetings in which privileges and rules are decided, social skills are practiced, and patients learn to observe their own and others' behavior and to recognize the impact of their behavior on others. Work with families is an essential part of hospital treatment, including in vivo evaluation of family functioning and deciding where the child should reside. Interventions may include family therapy, parent counseling in behavior management, and education about child development and their child's disorder.

Virtually all children who require psychiatric hospitalization have had problems in school. The small classes and highly trained teachers of a hospital unit can provide a detailed evaluation of a youngster's academic strengths and weaknesses by direct observation of classroom behavior and learning. Educational strategies can be developed and tested. Key elements of discharge planning are arranging for an appropriate educational placement and transitioning back to school.

Partial Hospitalization

Partial hospitalization (day treatment) may be best for the child who requires more intensive intervention than can be provided in outpatient visits but who is able to live at home. Partial hospitalization is less restrictive for the patient than inpatient treatment or residential placement. It can offer an opportunity for more intensive work with parents, who may attend the program on a regular basis. The daily transitions between home and the treatment program may enhance parent participation and home-based strategies. Partial hospitalization may be used as a "step-down" for a child who has been hospitalized or to avert a hospitalization.

Day treatment programs involve a full day, 5 days a week, and include a school or therapeutic nursery school program. Other programs, such as intensive outpatient or "partial day" programs, may meet in the late afternoon and evening hours after patients attend community schools. It is desirable to offer the same treatment modalities as an inpatient unit.

Innovative, intensive summer "day camp" treatment programs have been developed for children with ADHD and associated behavior and learning problems. These programs provide positive social and recreational experiences for children who otherwise would not be able to participate in camp, while teaching parents behavior modification techniques, supplementing classroom work, and rigorously assessing medication efficacy and side effects. These programs not only are highly effective but also are perceived as very enjoyable and helpful by the children and families who are able to participate in them.

Adjunctive Interventions

Parent Support Groups

The parents of children with psychiatric disorders, together with mental health professionals and teachers, have established groups that provide education and support for parents, advocacy for services, and fundraising for research. National organizations with local chapters and extensive online resources include the Autism Society, CHADD (Children and Adults with Attention-Deficit/Hyperactivity Disorder), the Learning Disabilities Association of America, and NAMI (National Alliance on Mental Illness).

Special Education Plans

Federal law entitles every child with an eligible disability (as defined by the Individuals with Disabilities Education Act) to any services they might require that would allow them to benefit from a "free and appropriate" public education in the least restrictive environment possible. Eligible disabilities include ASD; intellectual disability; a specific learning disability; impairment of hearing, vision, or speech; traumatic brain injury; orthopedic impairment; "emotional disturbance"; or "other health impairment" (which can include ADHD or chronic medical illness).

The school or parent may request an evaluation for services, and a meeting is then held to discuss the child's disabilities, capacities, and achievement and develop an Individualized Educational Plan (IEP). The IEP describes the nature of the educational or developmental disability, the short-term and annual goals of treatment, and the specific educational or therapeutic interventions to be used. These interventions may include, in order of escalating intensity, in-classroom tutoring; resource classrooms several hours per week; special classrooms in mainstream schools; public or private schools that serve only children with special educational needs; and therapeutic boarding schools.

A 504b plan (named after Section 504 of the Rehabilitation Act of 1973, the first civil rights statute for persons with disabilities) is another federally mandated option for obtaining accommodations in school for a child's disabilities.

Integration of Multiple Modalities

Sophisticated simultaneous or sequential use of different techniques offers substantial promise of improved treatment outcome. There is often a need for more power and wider coverage of symptoms than any single treatment alone provides. For many disorders, data support the potential synergistic effect of combining medication with psychotherapeutic interventions. For example, the combination of CBT and pharmacotherapy has been shown to be particularly effective in treating pediatric depression and OCD (March et al. 2004, 2006). Adding CBT improves the response rate in patients with OCD who have a partial response to a serotonin reuptake inhibitor (Franklin et al. 2011).

In the treatment of ADHD, combining medication management, behavioral interventions, parent management training, appropriate school placement and school-based interventions, and social skills training is often recommended for more severe cases and can be demonstrated to be effective in the short term. For children with ADHD who have comorbid anxiety or psychosocial impairments, supplementing pharmacotherapy with behavioral treatments appears to yield additive benefits as well as addressing symptoms not treatable by medication and perhaps permitting lower dosages of medication to achieve the same positive effect.

Children with ASD require a comprehensive therapeutic plan that may include psychoeducation of the parents and family, special education placement, speech and language therapies, behavior modification (applied behavior analysis), social skills training, and pharmacotherapy. Although families often request or implement complementary or alternative treatments, few such treatments have empirical support.

Conclusion

The treatment of psychiatric disorders in children and adolescents is both an art and a science. Research on assessment and diagnosis, biological correlates of disorders, and outcome of traditional and newly developed techniques will continue to improve the specificity and outcome of treatment. A need always will exist, however, for clinical skills and creativity in tailoring and applying therapeutic techniques to individual children and their families.

Key Clinical Points

- Treatment of pediatric psychiatric patients requires expertise in psychiatric evaluation and case formulation, effective use of complex treatment strategies, and a respect for the principles of informed consent and confidentiality.

- An understanding of human development is key to the successful treatment of pediatric psychiatric patients, to include an appreciation of the differences between children and adults as well as the developmental differences among children of all ages.

- Ideally, treatments identified specifically for children and adolescents should reflect evidence-based practices. However, many have been developed by applying known effective adult treatments to the pediatric population.

- Parents should be carefully informed of the presence or absence of scientific evidence supporting the use of a specific medication in a child, as well as that medication's possible side effects.

- Much is not known about medication treatment of child psychiatric patients, especially the effect of medication on the developing brain and the impact of medication treatment on the long-term prognosis for many disorders.

- Although each psychotherapy is based on its own theoretical constructs and therapeutic principles, all psychotherapies share the importance of the relationship with the therapist, an emphasis on hopefulness, the use of therapist attention and suggestion, and the expectation of change in one or more realms—cognition, behavior, sense of self, or emotional experience.

References

American Psychiatric Association: The Use of Medication in Treating Childhood and Adolescent Depression: Information for Physicians. PhysiciansMedGuide, 2005. Available at: http://www.parentsmedguide.org/physiciansmedguide.pdf. Accessed January 9, 2019.

Bangs ME, Wietecha LA, Wang S, et al: Meta-analysis of suicide-related behavior or ideation in child, adolescent, and adult patients treated with atomoxetine. J Child Adolesc Psychopharmacol 24(8):426–434, 2014 25019647

Bard DE, Wolraich ML, Neas B, et al: The psychometric properties of the Vanderbilt attention-deficit hyperactivity disorder diagnostic parent rating scale in a community population. J Dev Behav Pediatr 34(2):72–82, 2013 23363972

Barkley RA: Defiant Children: A Clinician's Manual for Assessment and Parent Training, 3rd Edition. New York, Guilford, 2013

Brent D, Emslie G, Clarke G, et al: Switching to another SSRI or to venlafaxine with or without cognitive behavioral therapy for adolescents with SSRI-resistant depression: the TORDIA randomized controlled trial. JAMA 299(8):901–913, 2008 18314433

Chorpita BF, Weisz JR: Modular Approach to Therapy for Children With Anxiety, Depression, Trauma, or Conduct Problems. Satellite Beach, FL, PracticeWise, 2009

Dulcan MK, Ballard R (eds): Helping Parents and Teachers Understand Medications for Behavioral and Emotional Problems: A Resource Book of Medication Information Handouts, 4th Edition. Washington, DC, American Psychiatric Publishing, 2015

DuPaul G, Power TJ, Anastopoulos AD, Reid R: ADHD Rating Scale—5 for Children and Adolescents: Checklists, Norms, and Clinical Interpretation. New York, Guilford, 2016

Findling RL, Ginsberg LD: The safety and effectiveness of open-label extended-release carbamazepine in the treatment of children and adolescents with bipolar I disorder suffering from a manic or mixed episode. Neuropsychiatr Dis Treat 10:1589–1597, 2014 25210452

Findling RL, Kafantaris V, Pavuluri M, et al: Dosing strategies for lithium monotherapy in children and adolescents with bipolar I disorder. J Child Adolesc Psychopharmacol 21(3):195–205, 2011 21663422

Fleck S: A general systems approach to severe family pathology. Am J Psychiatry 133(6):669–673, 1976 1275095

Franklin ME, Sapyta J, Freeman JB, et al: Cognitive behavior therapy augmentation of pharmacotherapy in pediatric obsessive-compulsive disorder: the Pediatric OCD Treatment Study II (POTS II) randomized controlled trial. JAMA 306(11):1224–1232, 2011 21934055

Geller B, Biederman J, Stewart ES, et al: Which SSRI? A meta-analysis of pharmacotherapy trials in pediatric obsessive compulsive disorder. Am J Psychiatry 160(11):1919–1928, 2003 14594734

Geller B, Luby JL, Joshi P, et al: A randomized controlled trial of risperidone, lithium, or divalproex sodium for initial treatment of bipolar I disorder, manic or mixed phase, in children and adolescents. Arch Gen Psychiatry 69(5):515–528, 2012 22213771

Gibbons RD, Brown CH, Hur K, et al: Suicidal thoughts and behavior with antidepressant treatment: reanalysis of the randomized placebo-controlled studies of fluoxetine and venlafaxine. Arch Gen Psychiatry 69(6):580–587, 2012 22309973

Green RW: The Explosive Child: A New Approach for Understanding and Parenting Easily Frustrated, Chronically Inflexible Children, 5th Edition. New York, HarperCollins, 2014

Greenhill L, Kollins S, Abikoff H, et al: Efficacy and safety of immediate-release methylphenidate treatment for preschoolers with ADHD. J Am Acad Child Adolesc Psychiatry 45(11):1284–1293, 2006 17023867

Hammerness PG, Perrin JM, Shelley-Abrahamson R, et al: Cardiovascular risk of stimulant treatment in pediatric attention-deficit/hyperactivity disorder: update and clinical recommendations. J Am Acad Child Adolesc Psychiatry 50(10):978–990, 2011 21961773

Handen BL, Anagnostou E, Aman MG, et al: A randomized, placebo-controlled trial of metformin for the treatment of overweight induced by antipsychotic medication in young people with autism spectrum disorder: open-label extension. J Am Acad Child Adolesc Psychiatry 56(10):849P856.e6, 2017 28942807

Höfer J, Hoffmann F, Bachmann C: Use of complementary and alternative medicine in children and adolescents with autism spectrum disorder: a systematic review. Autism 21(4):387–402, 2017 27231337

Hughes CW, Emslie GJ, Crimson ML, et al: Texas Children's Medication Algorithm Project: update from Texas Consensus Conference Panel on Medication Treatment of Childhood Major Depressive Disorder. J Am Acad Child Adolesc Psychiatry 46(6):667–686, 2007 17513980

Jain R, Segal S, Kollins SH, et al: Clonidine extended-release tablets for pediatric patients with attention-deficit/hyperactivity disorder. J Am Acad Child Adolesc Psychiatry 50(2):171–179, 2011 21241954

Jensen KG, Juul K, Fink-Jensen A, et al: Corrected QT changes during antipsychotic treatment of children and adolescents: a systematic review and meta-analysis of clinical trials. J Am Acad Child Adolesc Psychiatry 54(1):25–36, 2015 25524787

Kernberg PF, Ritvo R, Keable H; American Academy of Child an Adolescent Psychiatry Committee on Quality Issues: Practice parameter for psychodynamic psychotherapy with children. J Am Acad Child Adolesc Psychiatry 51(5):541–557, 2012 22525961

Kollins SH, Jain R, Brams M, et al: Clonidine extended-release tablets as add-on therapy to psychostimulants in children and adolescents with ADHD. Pediatrics 127(6):e1406–e1413, 2011 21555501

March JS, Foa E, Gammon P, et al: Cognitive-behavior therapy, sertraline, and their combination for children and adolescents with obsessive-compulsive disorder: the Pediatric OCD Treatment Study (POTS) randomized controlled trial. JAMA 292(16):1969–1976, 2004 15507582

March J, Silva S, Vitiello B, et al: The Treatment for Adolescents with Depression Study (TADS): methods and message at 12 weeks. J Am Acad Child Adolesc Psychiatry 45(12):1393–1403, 2006 17135984

Miller WR, Rollnick S: Motivational Interviewing: Preparing People for Change, 3rd Edition. New York, Guilford, 2013

The MTA Cooperative Group: A 14-month randomized clinical trial of treatment strategies for attention-deficit/hyperactivity disorder. The MTA Cooperative Group. Multimodal Treatment Study of Children with ADHD. Arch Gen Psychiatry 56(12):1073–1086, 1999 10591283

Murphy TK, Fernandez TV, Coffey BJ, et al: Extended-release guanfacine does not show a large effect on tic severity in children with chronic tic disorders. J Child Adolesc Psychopharmacol 27(9):762–770, 2017 28723227

Ollendick TH, Greene RW, Austin KE, et al: Parent management training and collaborative and proactive solutions: a randomized control trial for oppositional youth. J Clin Child Adolesc Psychol 45(5):591–604, 2016 25751000

Sallee FR, Connor DF, Newcorn JH: A review of the rationale and clinical utilization of alpha2-adrenoceptor agonists for the treatment of attention-deficit/hyperactivity and related disorders. J Child Adolesc Psychopharmacol 23(5):308–319, 2013 23782125

Schwartz S, Correll CU: Efficacy and safety of atomoxetine in children and adolescents with attention-deficit/hyperactivity disorder: results from a comprehensive meta-analysis and meta-regression. J Am Acad Child Adolesc Psychiatry 53(2):174–187, 2014 24472252

Sprenkle DH: Intervention research in couple and family therapy: a methodological and substantive review and an introduction to the special issue. J Marital Fam Ther 38(1):3–29, 2012 22283379

Strawn JR, Mills JA, Cornwall GJ, et al: Buspirone in children and adolescents with anxiety: a review and Bayesian analysis of abandoned randomized controlled trials. J Child Adolesc Psychopharmacol 28(1):2–9, 2018 28846022

Tourette's Syndrome Study Group: Treatment of ADHD in children with tics: a randomized controlled trial. Neurology 58(4):527–536, 2002 11865128

U.S. Food and Drug Administration: FDA Public Health Advisory: Reports of suicidality in pediatric patients being treated with antidepressant medication for major depressive disorder (MDD). October 23, 2003. No longer available online.

van Schalkwyk GI, Lewis AS, Beyer C, et al: Efficacy of antipsychotics for irritability and aggression in children: a meta-analysis. Expert Rev Neurother 17(10):1045–1053, 2017 28847182

Walkup JT: Antidepressant efficacy for depression in children and adolescents: industry- and NIMH-funded studies. Am J Psychiatry 174(5):430–437, 2017 28253735

Walsh F (ed): Normal Family Processes: Growing Diversity and Complexity, 4th Edition. New York, Guilford, 2012

Wilens TE, Robertson B, Sikirica V, et al: A randomized, placebo-controlled trial of guanfacine extended release in adolescents with attention-deficit/hyperactivity disorder. J Am Acad Child Adolesc Psychiatry 54(11):916.e2–925.e2, 2015 26506582

Wolraich ML, Bard DE, Neas B, et al: The psychometric properties of the Vanderbilt attention-deficit hyperactivity disorder diagnostic teacher rating scale in a community population. J Dev Behav Pediatr 34(2):83–93, 2013 23363973

Recommended Readings

Barkley RA: Attention-Deficit Hyperactivity Disorder: A Handbook for Diagnosis and Treatment, 3rd Edition. New York, Guilford, 2006

Dulcan MK (ed): Dulcan's Textbook of Child and Adolescent Psychiatry, 2nd Edition. Washington, DC, American Psychiatric Publishing, 2016

Dulcan MK, Ballard R (eds): Helping Parents and Teachers Understand Medications for Behavioral and Emotional Problems: A Resource Book of Medication Information Handouts, 4th Edition. Washington, DC, American Psychiatric Publishing, 2015

Dulcan MK, Ballard RR, Jha P, Sadhu J: Concise Guide to Child and Adolescent Psychiatry, 5th Edition. Washington, DC, American Psychiatric Publishing, 2018

Martin A, Scahill L, Kratochvil CJ (eds): Pediatric Psychopharmacology: Principles and Practice, 2nd Edition. New York, Oxford University Press, 2011

McVoy M, Findling RL (eds): Clinical Manual of Child and Adolescent Psychopharmacology, 3rd Edition. Washington, DC, American Psychiatric Publishing, 2017

Online Resources

American Academy of Child and Adolescent Psychiatry: www.aacap.org
Children and Adults with Attention-Deficit/Hyperactivity Disorder: www.chadd.org
Cohen Children's Medical Center: www.adhdmedicationguide.com
Florida Best Practices Psychotherapeutic Medication Guidelines for Children and Adolescents: www.medicaidmentalhealth.org

CHAPTER 42

Lesbian, Gay, Bisexual, and Transgender Patients

Jack Drescher, M.D.

Laura Weiss Roberts, M.D., M.A.

Gabrielle Termuehlen, B.A.

This chapter addresses the psychiatric care of lesbian, gay, bisexual, transgender (LGBT), and gender-nonconforming individuals. Today, psychiatric focus is on treating depression, anxiety, trauma, or other diagnoses in LGBT patients as well as addressing problems encountered in living as an LGBT or gender-nonconforming person. As a minority population facing a high degree of stress and discrimination, LGBT and gender-nonconforming individuals are at greater risk for poor mental health outcomes and may use mental health care services at higher rates compared with heterosexual cisgender patients. Mental health professionals must be sensitive to the needs of LGBT and gender-nonconforming persons.

Cultural acceptance of homosexuality—and, to a lesser degree, of transgender presentations—is increasing in many societies. The sixth edition of this textbook noted that marriage equality (same-sex or gay marriage) was legal in only 16 countries, 13 U.S. states, and the District of Columbia. At the time of this writing, same-sex marriage is legal in 25 countries. In 2015, the U.S. Supreme Court ruled that the Constitution guaranteed same-sex marriage throughout the country. In 2011, the United States repealed its "don't ask, don't tell" military policy and allowed lesbian, gay, and bisexual (LGB) citizens to serve openly in the military. Increasingly, international groups define LGBT rights as human rights (Reed et al. 2016). Attention to the health of transgender individuals has grown, and a recent rigorous epidemiological study estimated that 390 persons per 100,000 population in the United States identify as transgender, which translates to roughly 1 million adults (Meerwijk and Sevelius 2017). In medicine and psychiatry, there is a growing literature of anecdotal reports and small-sample studies of LGBT patients, prompting a report by the Institute of Medicine in 2011 calling for increased research into the health and mental health needs of these populations.

Despite the important role that sexuality and gender play in human development, psychology, and relationships, many if not most physicians and health professionals have little formal training in human sexuality and gender identity. Furthermore, the biopsychosocial model of psychiatry presumes that the self-perceived *meaning* of an individual's sexual orientation or gender identity is shaped by cultural factors. Clinicians hoping to understand the lives and mental health issues of LGBT patients must therefore embark on cross-cultural exploration.

It is the aim of this chapter to introduce clinicians to both general and specific issues encountered when a patient grows up as a member of a sexual or gender minority, to consider the mental health concerns of LGBT individuals, and to provide resources and references for further study. The appendix at the end of this chapter defines a number of colloquial and professional terms used in this chapter that can assist mental health professionals in their clinical practice with LGBT patients.

Historical Perspectives on Homosexuality and Transgender Presentations

In the nineteenth century, scientific and medical knowledge sought to replace traditional religious explanations of human behavior. These efforts were applied to homosexuality and gender expression. In 1864, Karl Heinrich Ulrichs published a political treatise arguing against German laws criminalizing male homosexuality (sodomy laws). He put forward a *third sex* theory of homosexuality, arguing that some men were born with a woman's spirit trapped in their bodies and that some women were born with a man's spirit trapped in their bodies (Drescher 2015). By the beginning of the twentieth century, Magnus Hirschfeld, an openly homosexual German psychiatrist, was the leading proponent of third sex theory (Drescher 2015). Hirschfeld is also credited with being the first person to distinguish the desires of homosexuality (erotic attraction to the same sex) from those of transsexualism (a desire to *be* the other sex), a distinction that would not gain broader recognition until decades later.

In 1886, in his book *Psychopathia Sexualis*, psychiatrist Richard von Krafft-Ebing classified homosexuality as a "degenerative" disorder, which he considered to be a congenital disease. Inspired by nineteenth-century Darwinian theory, Krafft-Ebing viewed all nonprocreative sexual behaviors, including homosexuality and masturbation, as forms of psychopathology (Drescher 2015). He also referred to transgender presentations as "homosexuality" and described cases of gender dysphoria and cases of gender-variant individuals born as one sex yet living as members of the other.

Sigmund Freud saw adult homosexuality as neither normal nor pathological, and in "Three Essays on the Theory of Sexuality" (Freud 1905/1962), he put forward a view refuting Hirschfeld and Krafft-Ebing's theories. Freud believed that humans were born with an innate biological bisexuality and that homosexuality was a normal phase in heterosexual development. He believed that expressions of homosexuality in adults could be attributed to an "arrested" psychosexual development. Freud's writing did not directly address transgender expression, in part because, like many in his time, he conflated sexual orientation and gender identity.

Psychoanalytic practitioners of the mid–twentieth century based their clinical approaches on the work of Sandor Rado, who saw homosexuality as a phobic avoidance of heterosexuality caused by inadequate early parenting (Drescher 2015). Rado's theories had a significant impact on mid-twentieth-century psychiatric thought and were a contributing factor in the inclusion of homosexuality as a disorder in the first and second editions of the American Psychiatric Association's (APA's) *Diagnostic and Statistical Manual of Mental Disorders* (DSM) (American Psychiatric Association 1952, 1968), as a subtype of "sociopathic personality disturbance" and as a "sexual deviation," respectively. Therapeutic efforts at the time focused on "curing" an individual through attempted conversion to heterosexuality. In 1973, homosexuality was removed as a disorder from DSM-II following reviews of both the psychoanalytic literature and the sex research literature. Whereas the psychoanalytic literature supported a pathologizing view of homosexuality, the sex research literature supported a normal-variant view.

Notable among sex research studies were Kinsey's reports on human sexuality (Kinsey et al. 1948, 1953), which found homosexual behavior to be more common than had been generally believed. According to Kinsey, 37% of males and 13% of females reported some overtly homosexual experience. Evelyn Hooker later published a study showing that, contrary to psychiatric beliefs at the time, nonpatient homosexual men demonstrated no more psychopathology than heterosexual control subjects (Drescher 2015). In reviewing the sex research literature, the APA concluded that there was more scientific evidence supporting a normal-variant view of homosexuality than a pathologizing view. When homosexuality was removed as a disorder from DSM-II, however, it was replaced with "sexual orientation disturbance," which applied to anyone who was distressed by their same-sex attractions and wanted to change them. The sexual orientation disturbance diagnosis legitimized conversion therapy practices, even if homosexuality itself was no longer considered an illness (Drescher 2015). In DSM-III (American Psychiatric Association 1980), sexual orientation disturbance was replaced with "ego-dystonic homosexuality," but this diagnosis was inconsistent with the growing evidence-based approach of the new diagnostic system and was removed from DSM-III-R (American Psychiatric Association 1987). It was obvious to psychiatrists at this time that neither sexual orientation disturbance nor ego-dystonic homosexuality met the definition of a disorder (Drescher 2015). Since 1973, the APA has issued numerous position statements supporting civil rights for lesbians and gay men, opposing discrimination on the basis of sexual orientation, and opposing the practice of conversion therapy (see, e.g., American Psychiatric Association 2013b).

By the middle of the twentieth century, scientific and clinical views on gender identity began to diverge from views on sexual orientation. Although physicians in Europe experimented with gender reassignment surgery (GRS) in the 1920s, transsexualism and GRS entered the popular imagination when an American, George Jorgensen, went to Denmark as a natal man and returned to the United States in 1952 as Christine Jorgensen, a transwoman (Drescher 2010). Sex researchers at the time were increasingly conducting research on gender identity in intersex (hermaphroditic) children born with ambiguous genitalia as well as in transsexual adults. Subsequent work by Harry Benjamin, John Money, Robert Stoller, and Richard Green led to increased clinical recognition of the phenomena of gender identity and gender dysphoria (Drescher 2010).

The work on gender identity and gender dysphoria took place mainly in specialized gender clinics. Many physicians and psychiatrists of that time were critical of the use of surgery and hormones to irreversibly treat people suffering from what they perceived to be either a severe neurotic or a psychotic, delusional condition in need of psychotherapy and reality testing. In a 1960s survey, 400 psychiatrists, urologists, gynecologists, and general medical practitioners were asked to give their professional opinion about what to do in the case of a transsexual individual seeking GRS:

> The majority of the responding physicians were opposed to the transsexual's request for sex reassignment even when the patient was judged nonpsychotic by a psychiatrist, had undergone two years of psychotherapy, had convinced the treating psychiatrist of the indications for surgery, and would probably commit suicide if denied sex reassignment. Physicians were opposed to the procedure because of legal, professional, and moral and/or religious reasons." (Green 1969, p. 241)

The diagnosis of "trans-sexualism" first appeared in the *International Classification of Diseases,* 9th Revision (ICD-9; World Health Organization 1977). In 1980, DSM-III adopted a neo-Kraepelinian, descriptive, symptom-based framework drawing on contemporary research findings of that time. The DSM-III authors felt that there was a large enough database to support the inclusion of transsexualism as a gender identity disorder (GID). The diagnosis of transsexualism led to growing psychiatric recognition of a patient population that could benefit from gender reassignment rather than forced conformity with the sex assigned at birth.

In DSM-IV (American Psychiatric Association 1994), transsexualism was replaced by "gender identity disorder in adolescents and adults." In anticipation of DSM-5 (American Psychiatric Association 2013a), transgender activists appealed to the APA, asking that the diagnosis of GID be removed in order to lessen the stigma that they faced (Drescher 2010). GID was replaced by "gender dysphoria" in DSM-5.

In 2012, the APA issued two position statements, one supporting access to care for transgender individuals and the other opposing discrimination against transgender individuals (American Psychiatric Association 2012a, 2012b). That same year, an APA task force on the treatment of GID found sufficient evidence to recommend that the APA draft treatment recommendations for adults with GID "in the form of an evidence-based APA Practice Guideline with gaps in the empirical data supplemented by clinical consensus" (Byne et al. 2012, p. 759).

Transgender activists also petitioned the World Health Organization, asking that diagnoses related to transgender identity be removed from the mental disorders section of the ICD-11 (Reed et al. 2016). In 2018, the World Health Organization replaced "gender identity disorders" with "gender incongruence" in the ICD-11 and moved the diagnosis to a new chapter on "conditions related to sexual health" (World Health Organization 2018).

Development of a Lesbian, Gay, Bisexual, or Transgender Identity

It is impossible to delineate a developmental line for LGBT or heterosexual patients. How a person acquires either a sexual orientation or a gender identity remains a topic of theoretical speculation. No definitive research yet explains the origins of homosexuality, heterosexuality, bisexuality, a cisgender identity, or a transgender one. It is unlikely that there is a developmental line that can be applied to all LGBT patients, even within each subgroup. Some individuals become aware of their sexual orientation or gender identity in childhood, others in adolescence, still others as young adults, and yet others in midlife or later. Individuals experiencing gender dysphoria develop these symptoms at different ages. Given that *identities* are socially constructed and can be understood as a way to make meaning of one's feelings of sexual attraction or one's sense of gender, it is likely that a variety of experiences lead individuals to call themselves "gay," "lesbian," "bisexual," or "transgender." In other words, there are myriad psychological frames of mind, interpersonal experiences, and cultural beliefs from which the diversity of modern LGBT identities is constructed.

There are developmental *themes* that recur in the retrospective accounts of LGBT adults. For example, many LGBT adults look back at their lives and say that they "knew" that they were lesbian, gay, bisexual, or transgender since childhood. In one retrospective study, a significant number of adult gay men and women recalled engaging in gender-atypical behavior (Bell et al. 1981). In one prospective study in 66 boys with the DSM-III diagnosis of GID of childhood (GIDC), 75% grew up identifying as gay men and not identifying as transgender (Green 1987). However, not all LGBT adults report atypical gender behavior in childhood, and the majority of gay men did not receive a GIDC diagnosis. Consequently, it is difficult to predict what leads a child to grow up and adopt a lesbian, gay, bisexual, or transgender identity.

In this section, we focus on developmental themes in LGBT patients. For additional information on transgender developmental themes, refer to Chapter 22 ("Gender Dysphoria") in this volume.

Childhood

A common theme in the lives of individuals who come to define themselves as lesbian, gay, or bisexual in adulthood or adolescence is an early memory of same-sex attraction, a feeling they believed set them apart from others. Some of these "children who grew up to be gay" can remember experiencing same-sex attraction or interest in members of the same sex as early as 4 years of age. Because most children are taught, either implicitly or explicitly, that they are only supposed to be attracted to the other sex, children who grow up to be LGB must come to terms with heterosexual models of relatedness. The other-sex interests of children who grow up to be heterosexual are seen as natural and validated as "normal," although acting on these feelings may be discouraged until a certain age or until marriage. By contrast, children who grow up to be LGB often lack explanations for their same-sex feelings or may be given explanations that are disparaging or stigmatizing. Although what they felt as children may not have been sexual attraction, many LGB individuals retrospectively connect adult sexual feelings to childhood curiosity about or a desire for intimacy with members of their own sex (Drescher 2001).

In children who grow up to be LGB, early same-sex attractions may cause some to question the authenticity of their assigned gender. A common, though erroneous, cultural belief is that a child grows up to be gay because she wants to be a member of the other gender. Most children with gender dysphoria, however, grow up to be adults who identify as cisgender (rather than transgender) LGB, and the proportion of the LGB population who experienced gender dysphoria as children is relatively small

(Drescher and Byne 2013). More commonly, awareness of feelings for other children of the same sex may lead a young child to question the veracity of their assigned gender. For example, it may be difficult for a young boy to believe in his male identity if he possesses a trait (attraction to boys) that he has been taught belongs only to girls (Drescher 2001).

Some gay and bisexual men report a sense of childhood "otherness" that they associate with an inability to engage in "rough-and-tumble" play with other boys. It is unclear whether a feeling of otherness can lead to an inhibition of rough-and-tumble play, or vice versa, or even whether the absence of rough-and-tumble play is in any way related to feelings of same-sex attraction. Some boys who grew up to be gay or bisexual report that they found rough-and-tumble play to be too sexually stimulating and evocative of shameful sexual feelings, leading them to avoid it altogether.

Boyhood effeminacy or gender variance can sometimes be part of the normal developmental history of gay men. The social impact of marked effeminacy in boys and men can be enormous, given pressures to conform to the male gender role. Boys may be teased not only for their perceived femininity but also for their presumed homosexuality. It is not uncommon for gay men to report in treatment that when they were children, they were bullied or teased by their teachers, peers, and even family members (O'Malley Olsen et al. 2014). These shaming experiences may also make it difficult for individuals to fully trust authority figures, including mental health professionals.

Bullying can be a problem for any gender-nonconforming child. A compelling longitudinal study of 10,655 individuals used data from the Growing Up Today Study to assess depressive symptoms from ages 12 to 30 years, prevalence of bullying victimization, and gender nonconformity before age 11 years (Roberts et al. 2013). The investigators compared depressive symptoms by gender nonconformity and explored the relationship between gender nonconformity and depressive symptoms by bullying and childhood abuse. The investigators found that individuals who reported gender nonconformity in childhood had an elevated risk of depressive symptoms, and that experiences of childhood abuse and bullying accounted for approximately one-half of increased depression symptoms among individuals who were gender nonconforming.

The numbers of transgender children in the general population are small, although the numbers presenting to gender clinics have been increasing since the beginning of the twenty-first century. The popular media attention that transgender children receive is also increasing, which in turn is increasing public awareness. Even though children as young as 2 years of age may exhibit gender-variant or atypical gender behavior, most of these children will not go on feel incongruence between their experienced gender and their assigned sex. Follow-up studies show that most gender-variant children who fulfilled DSM-III or DSM-IV criteria for GID became less variant as they approached puberty (de Vries and Cohen-Kettenis 2012). Among these children, who are referred to as *desisters*, a majority develop a homosexual orientation and LGB identities as adolescents and adults. The minority of children who experience gender dysphoria continuing into adolescence and adulthood are referred to as *persisters* (see the next section). One study of girls with GID found that GID persistence was greater among those with bisexual or homosexual sexual orientation than among other comparison populations (Drummond et al. 2008). In recent years, some in the LGBT community have questioned the reliability of these studies, and efforts to address these controversies have begun to appear in scholarly journals (Steensma and Cohen-Kettenis 2018; Temple Newhook et al. 2018; Zucker 2018).

Adolescence

Recent research suggests that same-sex attraction is stable over the period of adolescence to young adulthood, especially among females (Hu et al. 2016). For LGB youth, puberty can provoke the first public "coming out" of sexual feelings—for example, when an adolescent tells her parents about being attracted to other girls. Parents might also learn about their child's feelings from other sources—for instance, by viewing a child's Internet browser history—which may raise anxieties and lead to increased scrutiny of the adolescent or even lead to coercive attempts to change the adolescent's sexual orientation.

When LGBT children become teenagers, the difficulties they encounter may be compounded by the ordinary developmental challenges of adolescence. Adolescence in general is characterized by an increase in sexual feelings. In many cultures, there are socially sanctioned, sublimated outlets for adolescents that serve the purpose of modeling or role-playing the part of future heterosexual adults. Teenage dating and supervised coeducational activities such as high school dances are useful in developing interpersonal skills required for later life and relationships. In these interactions, an adolescent's confidence may be reinforced through their ability to conform to conventional gender roles. Because the rituals of conventional adolescence teach lessons about future adult heterosexual roles, these rituals often generate confusion, shame, and anxiety in adolescents who grow up to be LGBT. LGBT adolescents can become anxious or detached at a time when their heterosexual peers are learning social skills needed for adulthood. For example, the assumption that all youth are heterosexual leads to the separation of boys and girls during public disrobing. Yet a gay male adolescent can be sexually overstimulated in this environment, much as a heterosexual boy would be if he were required to change in the girls' locker room. For some LGBT adolescents, these repeated experiences foster connections between sexual, shameful, and anxious feelings.

Historically, the invisibility of LGBT adolescents in the developmental literature stems in part from an erroneous assumption that adolescents are too young to have a fixed sexual identity. However, many teenagers can and do identify themselves as LGBT, and by many popular and scholarly accounts (Drescher and Byne 2013; Pew Research Center 2013), LGBT individuals are coming out at much younger ages than in past generations.

Transgender adolescents are a heterogeneous group. Some were gender dysphoric in childhood, a group referred to in the literature as *persisters* and representing only a minority of transgender children. Other adolescents first experience gender dysphoria after puberty. Since the beginning of this century, gender dysphoric adolescents have been able to obtain treatment with puberty-suppressing drugs (gonadotropin-releasing hormone analogs or progestin) to prevent the development of secondary sex characteristics or to allay anxieties about developing them. Puberty suppression is done when the onset of or anticipation of puberty evokes anxiety, panic, or even suicidal ideation (Drescher and Byne 2013; Hembree et al. 2017; Kreukels and Cohen-Kettenis 2011). In the event that these adolescents eventually proceed with medical and surgical transition when legally able to do so, puberty suppression will make the process easier. If and when gender dysphoria desists following puberty suppression, the drugs are discontinued and the adolescent enters puberty, albeit later than nature intended. Some adolescents initially identify as cisgender and LGB but later become more aware of gender incongruence and identify as transgender. Some adolescents experience no discomfort with their bodies and do not meet diagnostic criteria for gender dysphoria but nevertheless engage in gender-variant behavior. These adolescents may identify as transgender, genderqueer, nonbinary, or cisgender. Thus, not all gender-variant individuals will identify as transgender, and not all individuals who identify as transgender will meet the diagnostic requirements for gender dysphoria.

Some communities are accepting of LGBT adolescents, whereas others are not. Cumulative experiences of victimization have become increasingly recognized for their mental health repercussions in LGBT youth. In one study of LGBT young adults, those who reported higher levels of family rejection during adolescence were 8.4 times more likely to report having attempted suicide, 5.9 times more likely to report high levels of depression, 3.4 times more likely to report having used illegal drugs, and 3.4 times more likely to report having engaged in unprotected sexual intercourse compared with peers who reported no or low levels of family rejection (Ryan et al. 2009). In a longitudinal study in which 248 individuals were assessed in seven waves over a 4-year period, researchers found that LGBT youth with high levels of cumulative victimization experienced significantly more symptoms of depression and posttraumatic stress disorder (Mustanski et al. 2016). Sexual minority individuals who had been victims of discrimination have also been found to be at greater risk for substance use disorders (Lee et al. 2016). Furthermore, a robust meta-analysis demonstrated that among young people, the experience of peer victimization in relation to sexual orientation and gender identity or expression was associated with greater levels of depression and diminished feelings of school belonging, which are associated with poor mental health outcomes (Collier et al. 2013).

Disclosing One's Lesbian, Gay, Bisexual, or Transgender Identity

Individuals who hide their sexual or gender identities are often referred to as "closeted" or are said to be "in the closet." LGBT children and adolescents develop techniques for hiding their identities that persist into young adulthood, middle age, and even senescence. Individuals may hide their LGBT identities out of fear of being subjected to antihomosexual or transphobic harassment, which may include teasing, ridicule, bullying, or violence. Individuals also may fear family rejection or forced attempts at conversion.

Revealing one's LGBT identity to others is referred to as "coming out" or "coming out of the closet." An individual can be "out" to some but remain closeted to others. For example, a lesbian woman could come out to acquaintances who she knows will be supportive while isolating her homosexual feelings and activities from her homophobic family and coworkers. It can be psychologically painful to hide significant aspects of the self or to vigilantly separate aspects of the self. For this reason, many individuals find that coming out reduces their anxiety.

Clinical Example 1

A 22-year-old bisexual genderqueer individual presented in treatment with depression symptoms and suicidal ideation. They explained to the therapist that they had just moved back in with their parents after graduating from college. They described their college experience as happy and supportive. Their college town was LGBT friendly, and they had many LGBT-identified friends and peers. Moving back home had been difficult, because their small hometown was not as accepting of sexual and gender minorities. They described their parents as "well meaning" but explained that their parents were very religious and had "old-fashioned views." The patient had not come out to their parents because "They just wouldn't understand. They don't even know what a gender-neutral pronoun is."

The psychiatrist initially served as a sounding board for the patient, allowing the patient to express and explore concerns and fears about returning to the small community and to their parents' home. After a few sessions, the patient moved to other topics such as strategies for communicating with family members and approaches to employment opportunities that were beginning to open up. The patient continued to feel "different" and was upset by their parents' expectations, but had found a way to "coexist" in their parents' house. The therapy shifted focus to "here and now" issues common to other young adults facing the transition to independent life after completing their education.

Some individuals are aware of their homosexuality but choose to keep their homosexual feelings hidden. For example, a homosexually self-aware man whose religion condemns homosexual behavior may never tell anyone about his feelings and may choose to live a celibate life as a way to avoid the problematic integration of his religious identity and sexual desires.

A *non-gay-identified* individual (i.e., non-gay, "ex-gay") is a person who may have once identified as lesbian, gay, or bisexual but now chooses to identify as heterosexual. Such individuals find it impossible to naturalize their same-sex attraction and thus reject their homosexual feelings. Non-gay or ex-gay individuals may believe that their homosexuality was caused by certain negative life experiences (and thus can be cured) or that their homosexual desires are a test from God. Despite the low odds of success, some may have sought to change their sexual orientation through conversion therapy (Drescher 2001).

Distinguishing Sexual Orientation From Sexual Identity

Sexual orientation is defined as the sum of the majority of an individual's sexual attractions and fantasies over a demarcated period of time. If the accumulated experiences of sexual attraction primarily involve individuals of the same sex, the orientation is *homosexual;* if the desires are primarily directed toward persons of a different sex, then the orientation is defined as *heterosexual.* If a person has significant periods of being attracted to or fantasizing about members of both sexes, that person's orientation would be defined as *bisexual.*

Sexual identity is a more subjective concept and includes one's feelings and attitudes toward one's sexual attractions. A sexual identity can change when an individual *changes perspective about their sexual feelings.* Although sexual orientation may be immutable in most people, sexual identities may show more variability across the life span (Hu et al. 2016). For example, a man with a homosexual orientation may identify first as heterosexual, then as bisexual, and later as gay, or may identify first as gay and then as ex-gay or heterosexual. An individual might identify as cisgender and hetero-sexual as an adolescent and as transgender and gay as an adult.

Prevalence and Epidemiology

The Kinsey studies (Kinsey et al. 1948, 1953) reported that up to 10% of men and 2%–6% of women had a homosexual orientation. These studies were hampered by non-random selection of participants and lack of population-based samples. More recent analyses (Copen et al. 2016) studying large U.S. population–based samples found that about 1.9% of males and about 1.3% of females report their sexual identity as homo-sexual; these analyses also found that 2% of males and 5.5% of females report their sexual identity as bisexual. However, prevalence rates have varied depending on whether homosexuality is defined as an identity or as a behavior. Sexual attraction and identity correlate closely, but not completely, with reports of sexual behavior.

A recent epidemiological study estimated that 390 young adults per 100 000 iden-tify as transgender, or almost 1 million young adults nationally (Meerwijk and Seve-lius 2017). This estimate has not been replicated; however, prior to this study, data on the proportion of transgender people in the U.S. population had been lacking, and published estimates in the past were often based on children and adults seeking treat-ment at specialty clinics for gender dysphoria. Because not all, and perhaps relatively few, transgender individuals present to specialized gender clinics, such figures likely represent an underreporting of prevalence. One review of prevalence studies (World Professional Association for Transgender Health 2011) cited estimates ranging from 1 in 11,900 to 1 in 45,000 for male-to-female individuals and from 1 in 30,400 to 1 in 200,000 for female-to-male individuals.

LGBT people may be disproportionately represented in some psychiatric popula-tions. The Institute of Medicine (2011) has highlighted some health and mental health concerns of LGBT populations, as summarized in Table 42–1.

Social stigma, discrimination, cumulative victimization, and bias have been pro-posed as risk factors contributing to mental health disparities among LGBT popula-tions, although further research is needed. Other proposed factors contributing to minority stress have included poor self-esteem due to the internalization of homopho-bic and transphobic social attitudes, and the perceived inability to lead an open life, leading to loss of protective factors for mental health such as being in a long-term re-lationship (Sandfort et al. 2006).

Diagnostic Considerations

Because all diagnostic evaluations rely on the clinical interview, the interviewer should strive to maintain an empathic, nonjudgmental stance. Important clinical in-formation necessary for proper diagnosis may otherwise be missed. Therapeutic tact is important when working with stigmatized populations. Consultation is recom-mended if and when one is aware that personal biases or limited knowledge of LGBT issues may interfere with a thorough evaluation.

TABLE 42–1.	Health and mental health concerns of lesbian, gay, bisexual, and transgender (LGBT) populations
LGBT age group	**Health and mental health concerns**
Youth	Lesbian, gay, and bisexual (LGB) youth are at increased risk for suicidal ideation and attempts as well as depression. The same may be true for transgender youth.
	Smoking, alcohol consumption, and substance use may be higher among LGB youth than among heterosexual youth. Little research exists on transgender youth.
Adults	As a group, LGB adults have higher rates of mood and anxiety disorders and of depression, and elevated risk for suicidal ideation and attempts, compared with heterosexual adults. Little research has examined mood and anxiety disorder prevalence in transgender populations.
	LGB adults may have higher rates of smoking, alcohol use, and substance use than heterosexual adults. Most research is on women, with less known about gay and bisexual men. Limited research among transgender adults indicates that substance use is a concern.
Elderly	Older LGB and transgender adults experience stigma, discrimination, and violence.

Source.　Adapted from Institute of Medicine 2011.

It is particularly important to establish a trusting relationship with LGBT patients when discussing their sexual or gender identity. They may require greater assurances of confidentiality than other patients. For example, diagnostic evaluations may require obtaining collateral information; such sources might include a same-sex partner, family members unaware of the patient's sexual identity, or LGBT-identified friends. When safety issues, as in the evaluation of a suicidal patient, require contacting a patient's family or friends, obtaining the needed information does not necessarily require disclosing the patient's sexual or gender identity (*outing*). In emergency settings, however, a discharge back to family members or other caregivers may require evaluating their sensitivity and their responses to having learned the patient's sexual or gender identity.

Sexual orientation or gender identity may play an important role in understanding some patients' presenting problems, such as suicidal feelings associated with coming out, substance abuse patterns of LGBT subgroup populations, or psychiatric comorbidity associated with general medical conditions such as HIV. For all patients, a complete evaluation should include a sexual history with information about sexual orientation, gender identity, intimate relationships, extent to which the patient is "out," and sexual practices. HIV and other sexual health risk factors should be considered for all patients. Patients may be at risk of HIV infection from male sexual partners or from other behaviors. A psychiatric evaluation performed in the setting of a trusting working relationship can help facilitate a patient's willingness to receive appropriate medical care, including HIV testing.

Sexual and/or gender identity should be part of the psychosocial evaluation, including assessment of the patient's primary support group, education, housing, and access to health care, as well as occupational, economic, and legal issues. Experiences of victimization, bullying, and partner violence should be explored. A diagnostic interview of an LGBT patient should include an assessment of support networks other than family and friends, including work, religious organizations, and community groups. For example, the patient may be estranged from her biological family and relying on a network of friends (*family of choice*). She may not feel comfortable being out at work. Her religion may be welcoming, tolerant, or intolerant. She may be involved in volunteer activities with LGBT organizations or may be receiving services from such an organization. A psychosocial assessment includes a history of relationships with partners, including children from current or past relationships. For some LGBT patients, the relationship history will include past heterosexual marriages.

Treatment Issues

LGBT individuals have greater vulnerability to a number of health conditions, including physical, mental, substance-related, and co-occurring conditions. LGBT individuals may also encounter greater barriers to competent care and discrimination in clinical settings. These circumstances place greater responsibilities on the therapist than may be initially appreciated but are important to recognize and address in order to ensure that LGBT individuals receive an appropriate standard of care.

General principles of psychotherapy can be applied to work with LGBT patients. This psychotherapeutic work sometimes involves attention to aspects of the therapy process that may be overlooked in the treatment of non-LGBT patients. Leaders in the field of psychology have developed 28 specific recommendations toward defining, measuring, and evaluating LGBT cultural competence among mental health care providers (Boroughs et al. 2015). These thoughtful and wide-ranging recommendations relate to the acquisition of basic skills needed to provide competent clinical care to LGBT individuals. Examples of themes throughout these recommendations include self-awareness, education, attunement to cultural and sociopolitical changes, knowledge of system issues, creation of training experiences that ensure understanding of the LGBT issues of clients, and requirements for continuing education. Psychiatrists will find these recommendations to be valuable. In this section we provide a brief overview of some elements for psychiatrists to keep in mind when treating LGBT patients.

Respect

All patients benefit from a therapeutic environment based on respectful principles. Individuals who are gender nonconforming or individuals with different sexual orientations can evoke uncomfortable feelings in clinicians; these feelings need to be tolerated, legitimized, and further explored by the therapist. LGBT patients often come into treatment with some history of shame about their identities. To compensate for that history, therapists themselves must be able to accept their patient's sexual or gender identity without inadvertently shaming the patient. This ability is a prerequisite for conducting psychotherapy with LGBT patients.

One means of expressing respect is to be wary of psychotherapeutic interventions intended to elucidate the presumed causes of a patient's sexual orientation or gender identity; therapists do not usually try to determine the "causes" of a patient's heterosexuality. Such "detective work" is countertherapeutic. There is little empirical evidence supporting the hypothesis that psychotherapies of any kind will reveal the "causes" of a patient's sexual orientation or gender identity. When a patient tries to use psychotherapy in a search for etiological explanations, the therapist can deepen the therapeutic relationship with the patient by listening supportively to the patient's reflections and hypotheses. While the search for etiological explanations may be used to reduce patient (or therapist) anxieties, it may distract from more helpful psychotherapeutic exploration of ongoing problems in living (Drescher 2001). Clinicians should also keep in mind that efforts to change an individual's sexual or gender identity are unlikely to be successful and are potentially harmful. At the time of this writing, 14 U.S. states, the Canadian province of Ontario, and many local municipalities have banned conversion therapies for LGBT minors younger than 18 years (Drescher et al. 2016).

Another means of expressing respect is to avoid imposing medicalized terminology on the patient and to respect patient preferences regarding identifiers. Referring to a self-identified gay man or lesbian as "a homosexual" will be experienced as offensive. Transgender and gender-nonconforming patients should be directly asked which pronouns they prefer to use when referring to themselves (e.g., she/her, he/him, they/them). An individual who identifies as male, even if preoperative, and even in the early stages of transitioning, should be referred to with masculine pronouns unless other pronouns are explicitly preferred. Transgender patients should also be asked if they have a preferred name other than their given or legal name. Knowledge of a person's gender identity indicates nothing about that person's sexual orientation; transgender individuals might identify as lesbian, gay, or bisexual, and their sexual identities ought to be respected.

Finally, many LGBT individuals internalize the antihomosexual and transphobic attitudes of the dominant culture. In times of stress, regardless of where they are in their own coming-out process, LGBT individuals may become highly self-critical or self-condemning. This pattern may lead them to regard their sexual or gender identity, rather than particular life circumstances, as being the cause of their distress.

Talking About Sex

A therapist would do well not to assume anything about the sexual practices of a particular LGBT patient, or of any patient for that matter. Even with heterosexual patients, talking about sexual practices that differ from those of the therapist can generate shame or other uncomfortable feelings in a patient and countertransferential anxieties in the therapist. Similarly, LGBT patients may evoke a range of countertransference responses in the therapist when they reveal their sexual selves. It is one thing for a therapist to accept a patient's sexuality in the abstract. It is another thing for a therapist to feel sufficiently comfortable and nonjudgmental to listen and take a sexual history in a way that respects the patient's subjectivity and avoids shaming the patient.

When conducting psychotherapy, therapists should be aware of their own judgments, including beliefs about what constitutes "normal" human sexual behavior and "normal" gender expression. Because most psychiatrists and other health and mental health professionals have little or no training in human sexuality, it is not uncommon for clinicians to offer professional opinions based on personal belief systems. Therapists should be aware of the extent to which judgments about "normal" and "abnormal" sexuality are embedded in any theory they have learned (Drescher 2001). Do therapists believe in a gender binary (man vs. woman), a homosexual versus heterosexual binary, or a cisgender versus transgender binary? And do these binary beliefs come with moral underpinnings about what is normal or appropriate and what is not?

Clinical Example 2

A 35-year-old lesbian woman had anxiety symptoms consistent with a DSM diagnosis of generalized anxiety disorder. She quickly experienced a reduction in symptoms after treatment with a combination of benzodiazepines taken as needed and supportive dynamically oriented psychotherapy. As treatment proceeded, the therapeutic focus shifted to interpersonal stressors that exacerbated her anxiety. These stressors included difficulties accepting the authority of her male employer, negative interactions with coworkers related to her sexual orientation, and anxieties related to expressions of intimacy with her wife.

The patient's developmental history included severe physical abuse by her mother from age 5 years through adolescence. Her father was reported to have done nothing to stop the violence and made excuses that the patient experienced as rationalizations for his wife's behavior. At 16 years of age, the patient ran away from home and never contacted her parents again. Since that time, the patient has had many experiences of peer victimization, including in her current workplace. In recounting this history, the patient appeared to experience intense affective states of fear, rage, and anxiety, as well as flashbacks. Witnessing these states led the therapist to modify the patient's diagnosis to posttraumatic stress disorder, which led to a revised treatment plan involving different psychosocial interventions. The patient also responded to antidepressants added to her treatment.

In her current circumstances, the patient described her relationship as "loving" and her wife's "kindness" as enabling them to stay together despite the patient's long-term difficulties with intimacy. She spoke of an evening of intercourse in which she described herself as being "so happy, it was as though I had this out-of-body experience where I felt like I gravitated out of myself and I was watching me in a really happy movie."

Dissociating during intimacy is not unusual for an individual who has been severely traumatized. However, the patient's intense emotions generated complex responses in the therapist, a gay man who found himself reluctant to inquire too deeply or ask directly about what was going on sexually at the time that she felt herself "leave" her body.

Part of the therapist's reluctance came from sensing his patient's vulnerability to intrusions. However, the therapist privately noted internal discomfort inhibiting him from asking for descriptions of physical intimacy in his patient's lesbian relationship. He contrasted his unusual tentativeness in this case with the ease he felt in asking about intimate sexual details in gay men he treated, even those who were as traumatized as this lesbian patient. He decided to take the issue up in peer supervision, asking his colleagues, "How do therapists, in general, learn to comfortably talk about the intimate sexual activities of their patients if those sexual practices are dissimilar to their own?"

HIV and Risk-Taking Behavior

The Centers for Disease Control and Prevention reported that as of 2015, 1.1 million people in the United States were HIV positive, and nearly 15% of those people were not aware of their positive status. Although there have been increasing rates of HIV exposure worldwide due to unprotected heterosexual sex, unprotected sex between men who have sex with men remains an important risk of HIV transmission in the United States (Centers for Disease Control and Prevention 1993). A thorough assessment of

HIV risk factors includes 1) obtaining a risk history (especially high-risk behavior such as penile–vaginal intercourse without a condom or penile–anal intercourse without a condom), 2) considering the need for HIV antibody testing, 3) encouraging risk reduction practices, and 4) encouraging appropriate medical treatment.

Issues that may arise when counseling gay men about HIV testing include 1) fear of learning one has HIV, 2) fear of having exposed one's partners to HIV, 3) fear of having one's sexual "indiscretions" exposed, 4) fear of abandonment if found to be HIV positive, and 5) concerns about informing sexual partners. An assessment of suicide risk factors is important (see Chapter 4 in this volume).

Men who have unprotected sex with men and who frequently change partners may be at especially increased risk of HIV exposure. Transgender women are disproportionately affected by HIV and by other sexually transmitted infections (STIs) worldwide (Reisner et al. 2016). The presence of other STIs may increase the risk of HIV transmission; therefore, inquiring about STIs should be part of the HIV risk assessment. Appropriate treatment referrals should be made if STIs are present. Because minority populations—in particular, Latino and African American populations—are overrepresented among individuals who are HIV positive, it is especially important to ensure that minority patients receive an adequate risk assessment and counseling. LGBT individuals are more likely than heterosexuals to use substances; in the assessment of HIV risk factors, it is important to ask about the use of injection drugs as well as the use of drugs, such as crystal methamphetamine ("crystal meth"), that may make risky sexual behavior more likely (Brennan-Ing et al. 2014; Forstein et al. 2006).

Since 2012, preexposure prophylaxis (PrEP) against HIV infection has become increasingly utilized in the United States and, more importantly, has been effective in reducing the transmission rates of HIV in populations at high risk of infection. At present, Truvada, a combination of emtricitabine and tenofovir (FTC/TDF) taken orally, is the only approved agent for PrEP, although injectable forms of PrEP are currently under investigation. Because FTC/TDF does not protect against other STIs, its use with condoms is highly recommended.

Psychiatrists can play an important role both in assessing risk factors for HIV exposure and in providing education about risk reduction and HIV testing. They can also play a role in monitoring and encouraging treatment adherence to the complicated medication regimens used to treat HIV infection. Providing support for patients in this area can make a critical difference, given that comorbidity of HIV and psychiatric disorders may heighten the risk of treatment nonadherence. For example, individuals who are HIV positive and have a depressive disorder are, in general, at risk for poor outcomes, such as worsened disease or death (Forstein et al. 2006).

Middle-aged or older LGBT individuals, particularly gay men living in urban gay communities, may have experienced multiple losses of friends and acquaintances during the AIDS epidemic. Mortality from HIV infection was very high prior to the development of antiretroviral therapies. In 1992, HIV infection was the leading cause of death in the United States for men ages 25–44 years and the fourth leading cause of death for women ages 25–44 years (Centers for Disease Control and Prevention 1993). For some, HIV decimated support networks that were never reconstituted. Older gay men may present in treatment with social isolation, unresolved bereavement, and even posttraumatic stress disorder.

Clinical Example 3

A 35-year-old asymptomatic HIV-positive gay man, feeling depressed and anxious, presented for a psychiatric consultation. The patient was using crystal meth and engaging in risky sexual behaviors, including unprotected anal intercourse (colloquially referred to as "barebacking"). As the psychiatrist took a sexual history, the patient blandly described his unsafe sexual activities, making no direct connection between those behaviors and his depressive and anxious symptoms. The psychiatrist, feeling uncomfortable as the patient's history unfolded, said nothing about her inner responses, but just listened and asked neutral questions.

Toward the session's end, the patient reported feeling dread that kept him awake the night before, although he could not locate its source. The therapist responded that she, too, had experienced feelings of dread earlier in the session during the patient's account of his self-damaging activities. She felt frightened and out of control and expressed this directly to the patient, asking whether her feelings made sense to him.

The patient responded that he, too, felt out of control. He also felt shame and guilt that he might infect others. Yet, since childhood, he had used a bland facade as a way of living with physical and verbal abuse by his alcoholic parents. He had experienced his HIV diagnosis as traumatic; by pretending that he had *no feelings* about his positive serostatus, the patient was trying to dissociate himself from thinking about anything that might remind him of HIV.

The psychiatrist listened but made no rush to judgment, allowing the patient to talk about his feelings. Her remarks had induced anxiety in the patient but nevertheless succeeded in drawing attention to his feeling that he lacked agency in controlling his own behavior. This exchange eventually allowed them to develop a treatment plan that included a harm reduction approach to crystal meth abuse and getting into a substance abuse treatment program; frank conversations about PrEP, the use of condoms, and the incentives and risks of barebacking; and, finally, treatment of his underlying depressive disorder with combined psychotherapy and pharmacotherapy.

Overlapping Sources of Vulnerability and Double-Minority Status

In American society, being black, Latino, Asian, or Native American *and* LGBT makes one a "double minority." For ethnic and racial minority LGBT patients, this double-minority status can be a significant clinical issue. These individuals may present with difficulties associated with living in a society that generally condemns homosexuality and tolerates racial and ethnic prejudice. Being a member of a "double minority" often entails interpersonal and familial issues and conflicts in "allegiances" across identities, as well as intrapsychic conflicts that can affect the successful development of an affirmative cohesive identity and self-esteem. These issues may include not feeling accepted by either the ethnic or racial minority group or LGBT culture ("No group wants all of me"); having difficulty choosing a primary group identification ("Am I ethnic minority first or gay first?"); and dealing with overt and covert racism, homophobia, and sexism (within both minority communities and the LGBT community). A therapist can help a double-minority patient uncover, identify, and resolve some of these conflicts. Individuals with double-minority identities may be especially vulnerable to discrimination and unequal treatment in health care settings. For these reasons, it is incumbent on the therapist to explore barriers to adequate care that patients may experience in physical health as well as mental health contexts.

Treatment Issues Specific to Lesbian Patients

Lesbian patients may experience discrimination and stress both as women and as members of the LGBT community. Compared with gay men, lesbian women have greater social invisibility and fewer role models. Studies using population-based samples and reports of self-identified sexual orientation (rather than sexual practices) found that, in comparison with heterosexual women, lesbian women reported higher daily alcohol intake, higher rates of depression and antidepressant medication usage, greater emotional stress as teenagers, higher rates of eating disorders, greater frequency of suicidal ideation in the past 12 months, greater frequency of suicide attempts, and more days of poor mental health within the past month (Diamant and Wold 2003; Institute of Medicine 2011; Koh and Ross 2006).

Individuals with a more masculine gender presentation or who are otherwise gender nonconforming are an important part of lesbian culture. These lesbian patients may have faced a great degree of discrimination because of their gender variance and sexual identity.

Lesbian couples or single women considering having children will need to make decisions about whether to adopt or conceive. If using donor insemination, they will have to decide whether to use known or anonymous donors. Family stresses in lesbian couples may include adoption issues, such as whether a female partner can legally adopt the biological child of her partner.

Treatment Issues Specific to Gay Male Patients

Gay men are at greater risk for poor mental health outcomes than heterosexual men. Gay men and other men who have sex with men may engage in a culture of sexual risk taking and sexualized drug use. Some gay men perceive crystal meth and similar drugs as being able to enhance sex by increasing self-esteem and libido, improving sexual endurance, and diminishing inhibition (Bryant et al. 2018). Regular use of methamphetamines may lead to physical and mental health problems such as depression.

Some gay men present in treatment with "effeminate" mannerisms, gestures, or voices. Other gay men may have been gender variant as children, even if they appear conventionally masculine as adults. As previously discussed, gender-variant children and adolescents are often bullied and may have a long history of peer victimization. No child is more despised than the "sissy." A clinician's awareness of and sensitivity to the trauma and stigma engendered by childhood bullying can be helpful when treating this population.

Gay men considering having children face many of the same decisions and legal obstacles experienced by lesbian women. Gay men wishing to have a biological child may do so through surrogacy. As with lesbian women, family stresses include adoption issues.

Treatment Issues Specific to Bisexual Patients

In comparison with lesbian, gay, and heterosexual individuals, bisexual individuals are at greater risk of poor mental health outcomes. Bisexual men and women are more likely than lesbian women or gay men to have a mood or anxiety disorder (Bostwick et al. 2010). A study that used data from the National Health Interview Survey to compare health risk factors among lesbian, gay, and bisexual adults (Gonzales et al. 2016) found that bisexual men and women were more likely to be heavy drinkers and that bisexual men were more likely to be heavy cigarette smokers than lesbian, gay, or heterosexual adults. Bisexual women were more likely to have multiple chronic conditions. The prevalence and odds of psychological distress were found to be higher among bisexual adults, likely due to stigma and discrimination.

In treatment, bisexual patients may report alienation from heterosexual and gay and lesbian communities. Both communities may exhibit "biphobic" perspectives and may discredit or belittle bisexual individuals' identities. Bisexual individuals may be told that they are "not really bisexual," just unwilling to commit to a gay, lesbian, or heterosexual label. Bisexual individuals may be told that their identity is—or their past experiences were—just a phase. For example, a bisexual woman married to a man may be told that she "must really be straight," despite her past relationships with women.

One study examining gender and sexual orientation differences in willingness to date, have sex with, and be in a relationship with bisexual individuals found that participants were less willing to be in a relationship with a bisexual individual than they were to date or have sex with such an individual (Feinstein et al. 2014). Bisexual individuals are often stigmatized as being hypersexual, highly sexually promiscuous, or unable or unwilling to engage in long-term monogamous relationships. Partners of bisexual individuals may buy into these stigmatizing characterizations and may express fears that their bisexual partner will be unfaithful or unfulfilled.

Treatment Issues Specific to Transgender Patients

Transgender patients are at high risk of adverse health outcomes worldwide (Reisner et al. 2016). According to findings from the California Health Interview Survey, transgender adults are more likely than cisgender adults to have ever thought about suicide, to have experienced serious psychological distress, and to have struggled with emotions that interfere with their relationships, social life, and work performance (Herman et al. 2017).

Transgender individuals face discrimination, violence, and harassment. As a triple minority, transgender women of color may be particularly vulnerable. One study found that transgender college students have higher odds of experiencing violence, including being in an abusive relationship, than cisgender students (Griner et al. 2017). Transgender individuals may experience discrimination on a daily basis from family, friends, government officials, employers, and even treating psychiatrists. Some people may refuse to use a transgender individual's preferred name or pronouns and may purposefully *misgender* them as an act of aggression. Transgender individuals who are just beginning the transition process, transgender individuals who are *nonpassing* (identifiably transgender), and transgender individuals who are gender nonconforming may face more discrimination and harassment than transgender people who pass as—or are perceived as belonging to—their identified gender.

Transgender individuals may require psychotherapeutic help in the process of transitioning from one gender to the other (World Professional Association for Transgender Health 2011). Transgender individuals may have greater health risks associated with surgical procedures and hormonal treatments. Psychiatrists, as physicians, may be especially helpful to their transgender patients by raising these issues and ensuring that these patients receive adequate preventive physical as well as mental health care.

Transgender individuals who want children face many of the same decisions as gay men and lesbian women, including whether to adopt or conceive. Some transgender individuals may be able to conceive after stopping hormone replacement therapies. Others may have chosen to bank sperm or eggs before transitioning.

Treatment Issues Specific to Older Lesbian, Gay, Bisexual, or Transgender Patients

Older LGBT individuals may be at greater risk for social isolation, which is linked to poor health and aging (Fredriksen-Goldsen et al. 2015). Older LGBT individuals may have a smaller social network and may rely on peer support more heavily, particularly if they do not have children or a living partner. Older individuals may feel unwelcome in or excluded from the LGBT community due to ageism. Psychiatrists should note that religious and spiritual activities may not be associated with health-related quality of life in older LGBT adults (Fredriksen-Goldsen et al. 2015). As previously mentioned, many older LGBT adults experienced great losses during the AIDS crisis and may present with unresolved bereavement issues or even posttraumatic stress disorder. LGBT seniors may have difficulty finding supportive caregivers or senior living facilities and may face discrimination, harassment, or violence.

Conclusion

As in any other clinical encounter, psychiatric care of LGBT and gender-nonconforming individuals should focus on the symptoms and sources of distress identified by the patient. LGBT and gender-nonconforming individuals may experience depression, anxiety, trauma-related mental health conditions, and other mental or physical health issues. LGBT and gender-nonconforming patients may also experience psychosocial distress due to problems in living associated with their sexual orientation and/or gender identity. Individuals in these populations have often encountered barriers to acceptance, leading to inappropriate health care. The treatment approach should address symptoms related to the patient's mental health conditions or concerns in an empathetic and nonjudgmental manner, ensuring that the patient receives high-quality and respectful care.

Key Clinical Points

- The "causes" of heterosexuality, homosexuality, bisexuality, and gender identities (cisgender or transgender) are unknown.

- *Sexual orientation* (the sex to which one is attracted) is a variable independent from *gender identity* (whether one feels like a man or a woman). *Sexual identity* reflects one's relationship (accepting or rejecting) to one's sexual orientation.

- Growing up lesbian, gay, bisexual, or transgender is a different cultural experience from growing up as a member of the heterosexual, cisgender majority.

- Expectations about heterosexual and cisgender normativity are stressful for LGBT individuals and may lead them to hide their sexual or gender identities.

- LGBT individuals are more likely to have experienced repeated victimization, and the accumulation of these traumatic experiences may lead to an increased likelihood of psychiatric symptoms.

- Some studies have found higher rates of certain psychiatric disorders, including depressive, anxiety, and substance-related disorders, among LGB individuals. LGBT individuals may be more likely to have psychiatric comorbidity and to use psychiatric services.

- Sensitivity to sexual identity and gender identity is essential to clinical interviewing and thorough psychiatric diagnosis.

- Because LGBT patients usually have a history of being shamed, therapists should approach these patients with tact and respect.

- Some LGBT patients are members of "double minorities." Working with these patients requires careful clinical attention to cultural issues.

- LGBT individuals and individuals with "double minority" status are more likely to experience discrimination and unequal treatment in health care settings; for this reason, extra efforts are needed to ensure that LGBT patients receive an appropriate standard of physical as well as mental health care.

References

American Psychiatric Association: Diagnostic and Statistical Manual: Mental Disorders. Washington, DC, American Psychiatric Association, 1952

American Psychiatric Association: Diagnostic and Statistical Manual of Mental Disorders, 2nd Edition. Washington, DC, American Psychiatric Association, 1968

American Psychiatric Association: Diagnostic and Statistical Manual of Mental Disorders, 3rd Edition. Washington, DC, American Psychiatric Association, 1980

American Psychiatric Association: Diagnostic and Statistical Manual of Mental Disorders, 3rd Edition, Revised. Washington, DC, American Psychiatric Association, 1987

American Psychiatric Association: Diagnostic and Statistical Manual of Mental Disorders, 4th Edition. Washington, DC, American Psychiatric Association, 1994

American Psychiatric Association: APA Official Actions: Position Statement on Access to Care for Transgender and Gender Variant Individuals. Arlington, VA, American Psychiatric Association, 2012a. Available at: https://www.psychiatry.org/file%20library/about-apa/organization-documents-policies/policies/position-2012-transgender-gender-variant-access-care.pdf. Accessed August 30, 2017.

American Psychiatric Association: APA Official Actions: Position Statement on Discrimination Against Transgender and Gender Variant Individuals. Washington, DC, American Psychiatric Association, 2012b. Available at: https://www.psychiatry.org/psychiatrists/practice/helping-patients-access-care/position-statements. Accessed August 30, 2017.

American Psychiatric Association: Diagnostic and Statistical Manual of Mental Disorders, 5th Edition. Arlington, VA, American Psychiatric Association, 2013a

American Psychiatric Association: APA Official Actions: Position Statement on Issues Related to Homosexuality. Arlington, VA, American Psychiatric Association, 2013b. Available at: https://www.psychiatry.org/File%20Library/About-APA/Organization-Documents-Policies/Policies/Position-2013-Homosexuality.pdf. Accessed February 1, 2018.

Bell AP, Weinberg MS, Hammersmith FK: Sexual Preference: Its Development in Men and Women. Bloomington, Indiana University Press, 1981

Boroughs MS, Andres Bedoya C, O'Cleirigh C, Safren SA: Toward defining, measuring, and evaluating LGBT cultural competence for psychologists. Clin Psychol (New York) 22(2):151–171, 2015 26279609

Bostwick WB, Boyd CJ, Hughes TL, et al: Dimensions of sexual orientation and the prevalence of mood and anxiety disorders in the United States. Am J Public Health 100(3):468–475, 2010 19696380

Brennan-Ing M, Porter KE, Seidel L, et al: Substance use and sexual risk differences among older bisexual and gay men with HIV. Behav Med 40(3):108–115, 2014 25090363

Bryant J, Hopwood M, Dowsett GW, et al: The rush to risk when interrogating the relationship between methamphetamine use and sexual practice among gay and bisexual men. Int J Drug Policy 55:242–248, 2018 29279253

Byne W, Bradley SJ, Coleman E, et al: Report of the American Psychiatric Association Task Force on Treatment of Gender Identity Disorder. Arch Sex Behav 41(4):759–796, 2012 22736225

Centers for Disease Control and Prevention: Update: Mortality attributable to HIV infection among persons aged 25–44 years—United States, 1991 and 1992. MMWR Morb Mortal Wkly Rep 42(45):869–872, 1993 8232169

Centers for Disease Control and Prevention: HIV in the United States: At a Glance. Atlanta, GA, Centers for Disease Control and Prevention, November 2017. Available at: https://www.cdc.gov/hiv/pdf/statistics/overview/cdc-hiv-us-ataglance.pdf. Accessed August 31, 2017.

Collier KL, van Beusekom G, Bos HM, Sandfort TG: Sexual orientation and gender identity/expression related peer victimization in adolescence: a systematic review of associated psychosocial and health outcomes. J Sex Res 50(3–4):299–317, 2013 23480074

Copen CE, Chandra A, Febo-Vazquez I: Sexual behavior, sexual attraction, and sexual orientation among adults aged 18–44 in the United States: data from the 2011–2013 National Survey of Family Growth. Natl Health Stat Report (88):1–14, 2016 26766410

de Vries AL, Cohen-Kettenis PT: Clinical management of gender dysphoria in children and adolescents: the Dutch approach. J Homosex 59(3):301–320, 2012 22455322

Diamant AL, Wold C: Sexual orientation and variation in physical and mental health status among women. J Womens Health (Larchmt) 12(1):41–49, 2003 12639368

Drescher J: Psychoanalytic Therapy and the Gay Man. New York, Routledge, 2001

Drescher J: Queer diagnoses: parallels and contrasts in the history of homosexuality, gender variance, and the diagnostic and statistical manual. Arch Sex Behav 39(2):427–460, 2010 19838785

Drescher J: Out of DSM: depathologizing homosexuality. Behav Sci 5(4):565–575, 2015 26690228

Drescher J, Byne W: Treating Transgender Children and Adolescents: An Interdisciplinary Discussion. New York, Routledge, 2013

Drescher J, Schwartz A, Casoy F, et al: The Growing Regulation of Conversion Therapy. J Med Regul 102(2):7–12, 2016 27754500

Drummond KD, Bradley SJ, Peterson-Badali M, et al: A follow-up study of girls with gender identity disorder. Dev Psychol 44(1):34–45, 2008 18194003

Feinstein BA, Dyar C, Bhatia V, et al: Willingness to engage in romantic and sexual activities with bisexual partners: gender and sexual orientation differences. Psychol Sex Orientat Gend Divers 1(3):255–262, 2014. Available at: https://psycnet.apa.org/record/2014-35710-007. Accessed January 18, 2019.

Forstein M, Cournos F, Douaihy A, et al: Guideline Watch: Practice Guideline for the Treatment of Patients With HIV/AIDS. Arlington, VA, American Psychiatric Association, 2006

Fredriksen-Goldsen KI, Kim HJ, Shiu C, et al: Successful aging among LGBT older adults: physical and mental health-related quality of life by age group. Gerontologist 55(1):154–168, 2015 25213483

Freud S: Three essays on the theory of sexuality (1905), in The Standard Edition of the Complete Psychological Works of Sigmund Freud, Vol 7. Translated and edited by Strachey J. London, Hogarth, 1962, pp 123–246

Gonzales G, Przedworski J, Henning-Smith C: Comparison of health and health risk factors between lesbian, gay, and bisexual adults and heterosexual adults in the United States: results from the National Health Interview Survey. JAMA Intern Med 176(9):1344–1351, 2016 27367843

Green R: Attitudes toward transsexualism and sex-reassignment procedures, in Transsexualism and Sex Reassignment. Edited by Green R, Money J. Baltimore, MD, Johns Hopkins University Press, 1969, pp 235–251

Green R: The "Sissy Boy Syndrome" and the Development of Homosexuality. New Haven, CT, Yale University Press, 1987

Griner SB, Vamos CA, Thompson EL, et al: The intersection of gender identity and violence: victimization experienced by transgender college students. J Interpers Violence August 1, 2017 [Epub ahead of print] 29294863

Hembree WC, Cohen-Kettenis PT, Gooren L, et al: Endocrine treatment of gender-dysphoric/gender-incongruent persons: an Endocrine Society Clinical Practice Guideline. J Clin Endocrinol Metab 102(11):3869–3903, 2017 28945902

Herman JL, Wilson BD, Becker T: Demographic and health characteristics of transgender adults in California: findings from the 2015–2016 California Health Interview Survey. Policy Brief UCLA Cent Health Policy Res (8):1–10, 2017 29091375

Hu Y, Xu Y, Tornello SL: Stability of self-reported same-sex and both-sex attraction from adolescence to young adulthood. Arch Sex Behav 45(3):651–659, 2016 26048483

Hughes IA, Houk C, Ahmed SF, et al: Consensus statement on management of intersex disorders. Arch Dis Child 91(7):554–563, 2006 16624884

Institute of Medicine: The Health of Lesbian, Gay, Bisexual and Transgender People: Building a Foundation for Better Understanding. Washington, DC, National Academies Press, 2011

Kinsey AC, Pomeroy WB, Martin CE: Sexual Behavior in the Human Male. Philadelphia, PA, WB Saunders, 1948

Kinsey AC, Pomeroy WB, Martin CE, et al: Sexual Behavior in the Human Female. Philadelphia, PA, WB Saunders, 1953

Koh AS, Ross LK: Mental health issues: a comparison of lesbian, bisexual and heterosexual women. J Homosex 51(1):33–57, 2006 16893825

Kreukels BP, Cohen-Kettenis PT: Puberty suppression in gender identity disorder: the Amsterdam experience. Nat Rev Endocrinol 7(8):466–472, 2011 21587245

Lee JH, Gamarel KE, Bryant KJ, et al: Discrimination, mental health, and substance use disorders among sexual minority populations. LGBT Health 3(4):258–265, 2016 27383512

Meerwijk EL, Sevelius JM: Transgender population size in the United States: a meta-regression of population-based probability samples. Am J Public Health 107(2):e1–e8, 2017 28075632

Mustanski B, Andrews R, Puckett JA: The effects of cumulative victimization on mental health among lesbian, gay, bisexual, and transgender adolescents and young adults. Am J Public Health 106(3):527–533, 2016 26794175

O'Malley Olsen E, Kann L, Vivolo-Kantor A, et al: School violence and bullying among sexual minority high school students, 2009–2011. J Adolesc Health 55(3):432–438, 2014 24768163

Pew Research Center: A Survey of LGBT Americans: Social and Demographic Trends, June 13, 2013. Available at: http://www.pewsocialtrends.org/2013/06/13/a-survey-of-lgbt-americans/. Accessed August 31, 2017.

Reisner SL, Poteat T, Keatley J, et al: Global health burden and needs of transgender populations: a review. Lancet 388(10042):412–436, 2016 27323919

Reed GM, Drescher J, Krueger RB, et al: Disorders related to sexuality and gender identity in the ICD-11: revising the ICD-10 classification based on current scientific evidence, best clinical practices, and human rights considerations. World Psychiatry 15(3):205–221, 2016 27717275

Roberts AL, Rosario M, Slopen N, et al: Childhood gender nonconformity, bullying victimization, and depressive symptoms across adolescence and early adulthood: an 11-year longitudinal study. J Am Acad Child Adolesc Psychiatry 52(2):143–152, 2013 23357441

Ryan C, Huebner D, Diaz RM, et al: Family rejection as a predictor of negative health outcomes
in white and Latino lesbian, gay, and bisexual young adults. Pediatrics 123(1):346–352,
2009 19117902

Sandfort TG, Bakker F, Schellevis FG, et al: Sexual orientation and mental and physical health
status: findings from a Dutch population survey. Am J Public Health 96(6):1119–1125, 2006
16670235

Steensma TD, Cohen-Kettenis PT: A critical commentary on "A critical commentary on follow-up
studies and 'desistence' theories about transgender and gender non-conforming children."
International Journal of Transgenderism 19(2):225–230, 2018. Available at: https://www
.tandfonline.com/doi/full/10.1080/15532739.2018.1468292. Accessed January 18, 2019.

Temple Newhook J, Pyne J, Winters K, et al: A critical commentary on follow-up studies and "desistance" theories about transgender and gender-nonconforming children. International Journal of Transgenderism 19(2):212–224, 2018. Available at: https://www.tandfonline.com/doi/
abs/10.1080/15532739.2018.1456390. Accessed January 18, 2019.

World Health Organization: International Classification of Diseases, 9th Revision. Geneva,
Switzerland, World Health Organization, 1977

World Health Organization: Classifying disease to map the way we live and die. June 18, 2018.
Available at: https://www.who.int/health-topics/international-classification-of-diseases.
Accessed January 11, 2019.

World Professional Association for Transgender Health: Standards of Care for the Health of
Transsexual, Transgender, and Gender Nonconforming People, 7th Version. Minneapolis,
MN, World Professional Association for Transgender Health, 2011. Available at: https://
www.wpath.org/media/cms/Documents/SOC%20v7/SOC%20V7_English.pdf. Accessed December 11, 2018.

Zucker KJ: The myth of persistence: response to "A critical commentary on follow-up studies and
'desistance' theories about transgender and gender non-conforming children" by Temple
Newhook et al. (2018). International Journal of Transgenderism 19(2):231–245, 2018. Available at: https://www.tandfonline.com/doi/full/10.1080/15532739.2018.1468293. Accessed
January 18, 2019.

Recommended Readings

D'Ercole A, Drescher J (eds): Uncoupling Convention: Psychoanalytic Approaches to Same-Sex
Couples and Families. New York, Routledge, 2004

Diamond LM: Sexual Fluidity: Understanding Women's Love and Desire. Cambridge, MA,
Harvard University Press, 2008

Drescher J: Psychoanalytic Therapy and the Gay Man. New York, Routledge, 2001

Drescher J, Byne W: Treating Transgender Children and Adolescents: An Interdisciplinary Discussion. New York, Routledge, 2013

Drescher J, Merlino JP (eds): American Psychiatry and Homosexuality: An Oral History. New
York, Routledge, 2007

Kosman KA, AhnAllen CG, Fromson JA: A call to action: the need for integration of transgender topics in psychiatry education. Acad Psychiatry 43(1):82–88, 2019 30105575

Levay S: Gay, Straight, and the Reason Why: The Science of Sexual Orientation. Oxford, UK,
Oxford University Press, 2011

Levounis P, Drescher J, Barber ME (eds): The LGBT Casebook. Washington, DC, American Psychiatric Publishing, 2012

Weinberg MS, Williams CJ, Pryor DW: Dual Attraction: Understanding Bisexuality. New York,
Oxford University Press, 1994

Yarbrough E: Transgender Mental Health. Washington, DC, American Psychiatric Association
Publishing, 2018.

Online Resources

AGLP (The Association of LGBTQ Psychiatrists): http://www.aglp.org
GLMA (Health Professionals Advancing LGBT Equality): http://www.glma.org
Group for the Advancement of Psychiatry's (GAP) LGBT Mental Health Syllabus: http://www.aglp.org/gap
Journal of Gay and Lesbian Mental Health: http://www.tandfonline.com/toc/wglm20/current
Journal of Homosexuality: http://www.tandfonline.com/loi/wjhm20
LAGCAPA (Lesbian and Gay Child and Adolescent Psychiatric Association): http://www.lagcapa.org
LGBT Health: http://www.liebertpub.com/overview/lgbt-health/618/
Transgender Health: http://www.liebertpub.com/overview/transgender-health/634/
WPATH (World Professional Association for Transgender Health): http://wpath.org

Appendix: Definitions of Commonly Used Terms

SMALL CAPS indicate terms defined in this appendix.

Agender   A colloquial term used to describe a person who does not identify as having a particular GENDER and may describe themselves as genderless or lacking gender. Compare with GENDERQUEER.

Androphilic   Attracted to men; can describe men or women.

Antigay violence   Physical violence directed at people because they are gay or thought by attackers to be gay. Colloquially referred to as "gay bashing"; the latter term can describe antigay verbal abuse as well.

Antihomosexual attitudes   Attitudes that are antigay, such as HETEROSEXISM, HOMO-PHOBIA, and MORAL CONDEMNATIONS OF HOMOSEXUALITY.

Asexual   The absence of erotic attraction; the term refers to a SEXUAL IDENTITY and may or may not refer to a behavior.

Barebacking   A colloquial term for unprotected anal sex.

Bisexual   Erotically attracted to both men and women; the term can refer to SEXUAL IDENTITY and/or SEXUAL BEHAVIOR.

Cisgender (cis)   A term used to describe individuals whose gender identities align with their assigned sex at birth (not TRANSGENDER).

Closeted   A colloquial term describing individuals who hide their HOMOSEXUALITY or GENDER IDENTITY from others. Being "in the closet" or "closeted" involves a range of psychological and behavioral activities intended to keep an individual's sexual or gender identity a secret.

Coming out   A colloquial term describing a process in which a LESBIAN, GAY, BISEXUAL, or TRANSGENDER person accepts their SEXUAL IDENTITY or GENDER IDENTITY ("coming out to oneself") and/or discloses that identity to others ("coming out to others").

Down low (DL)   A colloquial term that originated in the African American community to describe men who have sex with men. Men "on the down low" engage in homosexual or bisexual behavior without adopting a gay or bisexual identity.

Gay   Colloquial, affirmative term for HOMOSEXUAL; refers to men or women, although some women may identify more with the term LESBIAN.

Gaydar   A colloquial play on "radar" referring to a presumed capacity to sense another person's SEXUAL IDENTITY, ostensibly by relying on outward appearance, behaviors, and other cues.

Gay-friendly   Fostering an environment accepting of and open to LGBT people; can describe institutions or individuals.

Gender   A cultural concept based on some combination of social, psychological, and emotional traits associated with masculinity or femininity; compare with SEX.

Gender dysphoria   Discomfort with one's assigned sex at birth. Also, a DSM-5 diagnostic category replacing DSM-IV's *gender identity disorder* diagnosis.

Gender expression   How individuals demonstrate their gender to others via manner of dress, behaviors, and appearance.

Gender identity   A person's self-identification as male, female, or other gender (e.g., GENDERQUEER); often erroneously conflated with SEXUAL ORIENTATION.

Gender incongruence   Diagnosis that will replace *transsexualism* and *gender identity disorder of childhood* in ICD-11 (Reed et al. 2016).

Gender-neutral pronouns   Pronouns used instead of *she/her* or *he/him* to describe individuals who are neither male nor female or whose gender is unknown. GENDERQUEER and NONBINARY individuals may prefer singular *they* (*they/them*) or newly coined pronouns such as *zie/hir, e/em,* or *xe/xem.*

Genderqueer   A colloquial term to describe a GENDER IDENTITY of a person whose internal sense is of being neither gender, both genders, or between the male and female genders. Compare with AGENDER.

Gender reassignment surgery (GRS)   The surgical procedures used in treating individuals with GENDER DYSPHORIA; also known as *gender confirmation surgery.* Historically referred to as *sex reassignment surgery* (SRS).

Gender role   The presentation and behaviors deemed acceptable or appropriate for one's assigned sex, as determined by cultural norms.

Gender variant; gender variance   Nonpathologizing ways to describe individuals with gender-atypical behavior or self-presentations.

Gynephilic   Attracted to women; can describe men or women.

Heterosexism   A belief system that naturalizes and idealizes heterosexuality and either dismisses or ignores LGB subjectivities.

Heterosexual   Refers to SEXUAL BEHAVIORS between individuals of different sexes; a SEXUAL ORIENTATION, and/or a SEXUAL IDENTITY.

Homophobia, external   The irrational fear and hatred that HETEROSEXUAL individuals may feel toward LGB people.

Homophobia, internal   The self-hatred LGB people may feel toward themselves; also known as *internalized* or *interiorized* homophobia.

Homosexual   As an adjective, denotes either same-sex SEXUAL BEHAVIOR or a same-sex SEXUAL ORIENTATION. Historic usage of HOMOSEXUAL as a psychopathological term in medicine and psychiatry makes its contemporary usage as a noun offensive to many LGB people.

Homosexuality   A broad term encompassing same-sex behaviors, orientation, attractions, and identities.

Intersex   Historically known as *hermaphroditism;* more recent usage refers to diverse presentations of ambiguous or atypical genitals, or *disorder of sex development* (the currently used term replacing *intersex* [Hughes et al. 2006], which is also used in

DSM-5 as a specifier for the GENDER DYSPHORIA diagnosis); sometimes confused with transsexualism.

Lesbian   Refers to women erotically attracted to women; a SEXUAL IDENTITY.

Men who have sex with men (MSM)   An epidemiological and public health term describing men who may not have adopted a gay identity but whose behavior includes sex with other men.

Misgender   A colloquial term used to describe the action of referring to a TRANSGENDER person by a pronoun or form of address that does not reflect their GENDER IDENTITY.

Moral condemnations of homosexuality   Beliefs that regard HOMOSEXUAL acts as intrinsically harmful to the individual, the individual's spirit, and the social fabric. Such beliefs are often religious in nature, although some are secular.

Nonbinary   A colloquial term used to describe a GENDER IDENTITY outside of the GENDER BINARY (man versus woman). See GENDERQUEER and AGENDER.

Outing   Colloquial term for an unwanted revelation by a third party of a CLOSETED individual's HOMOSEXUALITY or GENDER IDENTITY to others; often intended to inflict harm on the person being "outed."

Pansexual   Erotically attracted to individuals of all sexes and genders or regardless of SEX, GENDER, or GENDER IDENTITY. A colloquial term used in place of BISEXUAL to indicate inclusivity.

Passing   A colloquial term. A GAY person may "pass" for straight (HETEROSEXUAL). A TRANSGENDER person passes if others perceive them as belonging to the gender they identify as (and do not perceive them as being TRANSGENDER). Passing individuals are said to have "passing privilege" because they are less likely to be harassed or discriminated against. Some individuals may rigorously conform to cultural GENDER ROLES in order to pass. Other individuals may not be interested in passing and may prefer to present as gender nonconforming.

Queer   Historically, a derogatory term for LGBT people; reclaimed as a SEXUAL IDENTITY in the 1990s by younger gay men and lesbians. The term is now used within the LGBT community as a catch-all self-identifier for a variety of individuals with a nonheterosexual and/or noncisgender experience. LGBT individuals may prefer to self-identify as queer because it is more inclusive than other terms. Also a descriptive term used in academia (queer theory, queer studies).

Sex   The biological attributes of being male or female; compare with GENDER.

Sexual behavior   An individual's sexual activities (HOMOSEXUAL, HETEROSEXUAL, BISEXUAL), irrespective of SEXUAL ORIENTATION or SEXUAL IDENTITY.

Sexual identity (sexual orientation identity)   The subjective experience of one's SEXUAL ORIENTATION. Although sexual orientation is usually immutable, sexual identity is not. Calling oneself GAY or LESBIAN is a subjective affirmation of a HOMOSEXUAL orientation.

Sexual orientation   An individual's innate attraction to members of the same sex (HOMOSEXUAL), the other sex (HETEROSEXUAL), or both sexes (BISEXUAL). Recognition of one's homosexual orientation does not necessarily or automatically lead to acceptance of a gay or lesbian SEXUAL IDENTITY.

Transceiver   A colloquial term describing a presumed capacity to see someone presenting as conventionally male or female as being TRANSGENDER. Analogous with GAYDAR (see above).

Transgender (trans)   Someone whose GENDER IDENTITY and SEX are discordant or not conforming to social norms. GENDER IDENTITY and SEXUAL ORIENTATION are independent variables insofar as one's gender identity does not automatically reveal one's sexual attractions.

Trans man (transman, female to male [FTM])   Someone assigned at birth as a female (assigned female, natal female) but identifying as a man.

Transphobia   The irrational fear and hatred that CISGENDER individuals may feel toward TRANSSEXUAL or TRANSGENDER individuals.

Transsexual   An individual who has undergone GRS, either male to female or female to male. The term TRANSGENDER is preferred within the LGBT community.

Trans woman (transwoman, male to female [MTF])   Someone assigned at birth as a male (assigned male, natal male) but identifying as a woman.

CHAPTER 43

Older Adults

Dan G. Blazer, M.D., Ph.D.

David C. Steffens, M.D., M.H.S.

In comparison with those who work with younger adult and middle-age patients, psychiatrists who work with older adults face an added degree of complexity when they engage in the diagnosis and treatment of problems. Most older patients with psychiatric disorders do not fit easily into the diagnostic categories of DSM-5 (American Psychiatric Association 2013) because they typically experience multiple symptoms that affect both physical and psychiatric functioning. Therefore, a focus on patient functioning is critical. In this chapter, we follow a syndromal approach by identifying seven psychiatric syndromes that are most prevalent among older individuals—acute confusion, memory loss, insomnia, anxiety, suspiciousness and agitation, depression, and substance use—and describing these syndromes within the context of managing the resultant impairment. Because the psychiatric disorders that contribute to these syndromes are described in greater detail elsewhere in this volume (i.e., Chapters 9 through 27), we focus on the aspects of the syndromes that are unique to late life and on the management of these syndromes in older adults.

Acute Confusion

Acute confusion, or delirium, is a transient neurocognitive disorder (NCD) characterized by acute onset and global impairment of cognitive function. The older person with acute confusion exhibits a decreased ability to maintain attention to environmental stimuli and has difficulty shifting attention from one set of stimuli to another. Thinking is disorganized, speech becomes rambling, sleep is disrupted, and a decreased level of consciousness is exhibited. Emotional disturbances often, but not always, accompany acute confusion and may be the presenting problem in late life. These emotional disturbances include anxiety, fear, irritability, and anger. Some older persons, in contrast, are apathetic and withdrawn during an episode of delirium and thus are much more difficult to diagnose. Acute confusion, by definition, is brief, usually lasting a few hours but possibly lasting weeks, such as in the case of confusion secondary to medications, and merges into the much less common chronic state (Blazer and van Nieuwenhuizen 2012). The Confusion Assessment Method (CAM) is the most frequently used brief screening tool to detect delirium (Wei et al. 2008). Acute confusion can lead to permanent cognitive impairment.

Prevalence and Etiology

Estimates of delirium incidence range from 15% to 25% among patients on medical and surgical wards (Inouye 2006). When delirium is diagnosed in a hospitalized older patient, the hospitalization is usually prolonged, and both in-hospital and posthospital mortality rates are increased. Mortality at 2-year follow-up approaches 50%. Acute confusion is especially a risk for patients with NCD due to Alzheimer's disease, and half of those who are hospitalized become confused.

Acute confusion in late life is the common outcome of a cascade of biological, cognitive, and environmental contributors. Biological brain function declines with age, although functional capacity varies greatly within age groups. Challenges to the aging brain include drug intoxication, electrolyte disturbance, infection, dehydration, hypoalbuminemia, and hypoxia. Visual and hearing impairment may also contribute to delirium.

Cognitive contributors to delirium include a predisposition to hallucinations and delusions, such as that in an aging patient with a history of schizophrenia. Environmental contributors include the unfamiliar surroundings of a hospital or long-term-care facility and social isolation. Therefore, the hospital, where the convergence of these contributors is likely, is a high-risk environment for delirium. Additional factors that may contribute to delirium in the hospital include physical restraint and a bladder catheter (Inouye 2006).

Treatment

The treatment of acute confusion in the older adult begins with prevention. Activities that can help prevent acute confusion include the following: 1) early mobilization, 2) nonpharmacological approaches to behavioral disturbances, 3) interventions to prevent sleep deprivation, 4) communication methods to orient the patient, 5) adaptive equipment such as eyeglasses and hearing aids for vision and hearing impairment, and 6) early correction of volume depletion (Inouye et al. 1999).

General therapy for the confused older individual, to be administered in parallel with specific therapy for the underlying cause of the acute confusion, begins with medical support. Vital signs and level of consciousness should be closely monitored (Inouye et al. 1999). All medications that are not critical should be discontinued. Vasopressor agents may be needed to increase blood pressure, and excessive fever should be treated with ice baths and alcohol sponges. When the syndrome of acute confusion is recognized and the precipitant of the confusion is established through history, physical examination, and laboratory studies, the clinician can begin therapy. Laboratory tests should be ordered as indicated, including thyroid function tests, measurement of drug levels, toxicology screen, measurement of ammonia or cortisol levels, electrocardiogram, and neuroimaging (Inouye 2006). Acute confusion may present as a psychiatric emergency that threatens permanent brain damage. Severe hypoglycemia, hypoxia, and hyperthermia are examples of critical conditions that may present as acute confusion. Therefore, the initial treatment should include the establishment of an adequate airway to ensure that the patient is breathing. Level of attention should be monitored using brief bedside tests (e.g., serial 7s and digit span).

Order and simplicity in the environment are critical to the management of the confused older patient, who should be maintained in a quiet, simply furnished, and well-lit room. Lights should be left on at night. Care can best be facilitated by constant attention from familiar persons, such as family members, who should frequently orient the patient to time, place, and person. Physicians, nurses, and other hospital personnel should explain all procedures. Restraints should be kept to a minimum. Behavioral agitation generally can be managed by judicious use of antipsychotic medications, such as haloperidol (administered either intramuscularly or orally), olanzapine, or risperidone, in low dosages; yet if possible, medications should be avoided.

Memory Loss

The threat of memory loss (and other more chronic cognitive dysfunctions such as slowing of reaction time) is the most common concern of older adults. The syndrome of memory loss spans a wide range of severities, including the usual changes in cognition that accompany aging (cognitive aging), mild forms of neurocognitive impairment that may represent preclinical forms of NCDs, and more severe major NCDs. Patients with objectively measured memory loss may experience impairment in other areas of cognition, particularly if the memory impairment is moderate or severe, including language disturbances, disorientation to time and place, and disturbances in executive function, perceptual motor function, and social cognition. Late-life memory loss is typically accompanied by a more or less sustained decline in cognitive function from a previously obtained intellectual level, usually with an insidious onset. State of consciousness is usually not altered until very late in the memory loss syndrome, which is in contrast with acute confusion (delirium). However, individuals with vascular dementia may experience a fluctuating course of cognitive impairment.

Once delirium has been ruled out, the initial cognitive diagnostic task is to differentiate among usual neurocognitive function (cognitive aging), mild NCD, and major NCD. The second step is to assign an etiological category, such as NCD due to Alzheimer's disease (AD), vascular NCD, or frontotemporal NCD (Blazer et al. 2015). Individuals with cognitive aging and mild neurocognitive dysfunction may present with neurocognitive problems that do not meet criteria for a major NCD but are clearly disturbing them and/or their families. Although their symptoms and cognitive test results may not be severe enough to warrant a diagnosis, these individuals may nonetheless experience difficulty with activities of daily living (e.g., slowed reaction time that interferes with their driving) and express awareness of the problem. Cognitive aging and mild NCD are currently targets for biomedical research, including studies of biomarkers and trials of treatment and dementia prevention interventions, and as these diagnostic and treatment approaches are developed, it is imperative that our diagnostic nomenclature keep pace (Blazer 2013).

Prevalence and Etiology

Subjective cognitive complaints are common, with one study finding that more than 95% of adults ages 70–90 years or their knowledgeable informants endorsed at least one cognitive complaint (Blazer et al. 2015). Subjective memory complaints are often associated with depression and anxiety.

Disabling memory loss may begin in midlife, but it is much more frequent in persons older than 75 years than in those ages 65–74 years. Prevalence estimates of memory impairment from community samples are generally 5%–15%, with most investigators estimating memory impairment in at least 10% of persons older than 65 years in the community and in 30%–50% of institutional residents (Blazer et al. 2015). The syndrome of *mild neurocognitive impairment,* thought to be a transitional state between normal cognition and major neurocognitive impairment (dementia), particularly associated with AD, has been an intense area of study over the past two decades. The incidence of mild cognitive impairment ranges from 1% to 6% per year, while prevalence estimates range from 3% to 22% per year (Ganguli et al. 2004).

The prevalence of major NCD due to AD, the most common disorder contributing to memory loss, has been estimated to be 6%–8% in community-dwelling persons older than 65 years, and more than 30% in persons 85 years or older (Alzheimer's Association 2018). Until age 75 years, the life expectancy of persons with AD or vascular dementia is reduced by one-half. After age 75 years, life expectancy is less affected by memory loss. Recent studies find that life expectancy is decreasing among persons with AD (Centers for Disease Control and Prevention 2017). Death rates are also higher for African Americans in poverty than for the general population.

Potential causes of memory loss are listed in Table 43–1. Although the clinical presentation of memory loss does not always provide clear evidence regarding the etiology, there are some distinguishing characteristics that can provide clues, such as the increase in visual hallucinations in Lewy body disease and the sudden declines in memory with vascular disease. Even those persons who have AD may experience significant decline over a brief interval, only to enter a plateau in functioning for a subsequent interval that may last for many months. Some NCDs, however, do not inevitably lead to declines in function. For example, NCD associated with alcohol can be arrested if the person stops drinking and returns to a nutritional diet.

More than 50% of persons with chronic memory loss will, at autopsy, exhibit the changes of AD only. AD is characterized by neurofibrillary tangles, deposition of β-amyloid and tau, and brain atrophy. The next most common contributor to the syndrome is vascular disease, characterized by multiple small infarcts of the brain. Clinically and pathophysiologically, it is difficult to disaggregate these disorders. Vascular NCD often is comorbid with AD. In contrast to AD, however, vascular NCD is more common in males than in females. Many patients with Parkinson's disease develop brain changes late in the course of the disease that are similar to changes found in AD. Clinically, except for their parkinsonian symptoms, these patients cannot be distinguished from patients with AD. Approximately 5% of older persons experience memory loss as a result of chronic alcohol use. A variant of AD is Lewy body dementia, characterized by synaptophysin-containing cytoplasmic inclusions outside the substantia nigra. In addition to memory impairment, fluctuating cognitive function is characteristic of this disorder.

TABLE 43–1.	Differential diagnosis of memory loss

Mild or major neurocognitive disorder associated with:

    Alzheimer's disease

    Vascular disease

    Lewy body disease

    Parkinson's disease

    Frontotemporal disease

    Traumatic brain injury

    HIV

    Substance and medication use

    Huntington's disease

    Prion disease

Acute confusion (delirium)

The primary risk factors for AD are age and family history, with the prevalence of AD, as mentioned previously, being an exponential function of age. Other risk factors for AD include Down syndrome, head trauma, and possibly lack of education. Genetic risk factors have received much attention in recent years, especially the relationship between the disease and the ε4 allele of the apolipoprotein E gene (*APOE*) (Roses 1994). Persons who carry at least one copy of the APOE ε4 allele are at increased risk of developing AD. The deposition of β-amyloid was thought to be the major pathophysiological contributor to AD, yet failure of many medications that target amyloid has now led to an increased interest in neurofibrillary protein fragments containing tau that stabilize the neuronal microtubules under normal conditions. Much less common forms of AD have been linked to chromosomes 14 and 1 (presenilin 1 and 2 genes).

Risk factors for vascular dementia include male sex, hypertension, and possibly African American race. Alcohol use regularly over many years is the primary cause of alcohol-induced amnestic disorder.

Diagnostic Workup

The diagnostic workup of the older adult with memory loss begins with a history, the most important component of the evaluation. A history should be obtained from both the patient and the family. The nature and severity of the memory loss should be assessed in conjunction with a chronological account of the onset of the older adult's problems and specific behavioral changes. The patient and family should be asked about common problems resulting from memory loss, such as becoming lost in a familiar place, having difficulties with driving, becoming repetitive, and losing objects. Medical history should include inquiries about relevant systemic diseases, trauma, surgery, psychiatric problems, diet, and alcohol and drug use. (A thorough documentation of prescription and over-the-counter drugs is essential.) The family history should include questions about relatives who have memory loss, Down syndrome, alcohol problems, and psychiatric disorders. The physical examination should include not only a thorough neurological examination but also a general physical workup to determine the health of the patient. Genetic testing, however, is not recommended.

The nature and degree of the neurocognitive dysfunction should be assessed by both a thorough mental status examination and objective testing. Standardized mental status examinations, such as the Mini-Mental State Examination (Folstein et al. 1975) and the Montreal Cognitive Assessment (Nasreddine et al. 2005), are available and provide a useful means of quantifying and documenting memory loss at the initial evaluation.

The in-office or hospital-based initial assessment of memory and neurocognitive functioning is followed by a more in-depth evaluation of cognition, with tests of specific functions such as executive functioning, language, memory, and spatial ability (tests of constructional praxis). Performance on brief screening measures and on more in-depth neuropsychological testing provides a baseline from which decline in function and/or response to therapeutic intervention can be determined.

A routine laboratory workup is essential, with special focus on findings that could contribute to memory loss, such as hypothyroidism, anemia, and (in rarer cases) vitamin deficiencies, such as deficiency of vitamin B_{12}. Magnetic resonance imaging (MRI) or computed tomography scans are now routine in the initial evaluation of memory loss. Much interesting research is emerging to explore the association of memory loss and functional imaging (e.g., positron emission tomography and functional MRI), but the utility of these functional scans is limited to clinical scenarios in which there is a high index of suspicion for frontotemporal NCD.

Treatment

Most pharmacological therapies are based on the cholinergic hypotheses of memory and include primarily cholinesterase inhibitors, donepezil, rivastigmine, and galantamine, which are available to physicians in office-based practice. These drugs have proven moderately effective in reducing decline in memory up to 6 months after administration, but their long-term ability to retard memory loss is questioned. Memantine, an N-methyl-D-aspartate (NMDA) receptor antagonist, has been approved by the U.S. Food and Drug Administration (FDA) for the treatment of moderate to severe AD (based on the theory that glutamatergic overstimulation may cause excitotoxic neuronal changes). Patients in late life who have memory loss may be referred to specialized centers (memory disorder clinics) where they can be evaluated and, if criteria are met, enrolled in a clinical trial where they may receive a number of experimental agents, including estrogens.

Ancillary treatments for memory impairment include diet, exercise, and cognitive stimulation; careful control of blood pressure, cholesterol, blood glucose, and other measures associated with increased stroke risk; and prevention of delirium.

Psychotropic medications are used extensively in patients with memory loss, primarily because of neuropsychiatric symptoms such as verbal or physical aggression, anxiety, depression, psychosis, and severe agitation or regressive behavior (see "Suspiciousness and Agitation" section later in the chapter). Other secondary behaviors, however, such as wandering, inappropriate verbalization, repetitive activities (touching), obstinate resistance to following suggestions or commands, hoarding of materials, stealing, and inappropriate voiding, are not as amenable to medication. Therefore, the first step for the clinician treating the patient with memory loss is to assess which symptoms might be responsive to a medication.

After the clinician has determined that an emerging behavioral problem cannot be handled through nonpharmacological means and is ongoing, medication can be prescribed with caution. Decision making around pharmacological treatment has become very challenging in the past few years, with reports linking atypical antipsychotics to increased cardiovascular mortality risk, leading to the black box warning by the FDA (U.S. Food and Drug Administration 2005).

Agitation and anxiety can be treated with antianxiety agents (e.g., short-acting benzodiazepines), anticonvulsants (e.g., carbamazepine), β-blockers, lithium, and occasionally low doses of antidepressant agents (e.g., trazodone) at night. Clonazepam may be of benefit in agitated patients with vascular dementia; however, the episodic mood swings and acute confusion that often accompany such dementia are less responsive than agitation to medications.

Despite the FDA warning, most clinicians recognize that antipsychotics are effective for controlling severe agitation, aggressive behavior, and psychosis. If atypical antipsychotics are being considered for management of severe agitation, consultation with the family must be undertaken to explain the FDA warning and the benefits and risks of treatment versus no treatment, to carefully document prior treatment attempts, and to obtain the assent of the family for the proposed treatment. Most antipsychotics are effective but produce side effects; therefore, selection of a drug is usually determined by the side-effect profile least adverse for a given patient. Atypical antipsychotics, such as aripiprazole, olanzapine, quetiapine, and risperidone, are the preferred drugs at present, primarily because of the more benign immediate side-effect profile. The most troublesome side effects associated with antipsychotics are postural hypotension (and the risk of falling) and tardive dyskinesia, both of which are less frequent among users of the atypical antipsychotics.

Because depression (even the syndrome of major depressive disorder) is common among patients with chronic memory loss, use of an antidepressant is often indicated. In general, the antidepressant agent will not lead to an improvement in memory. Selective serotonin reuptake inhibitor (SSRI) agents associated with the fewest potential side effects (e.g., sertraline, escitalopram) are preferred.

Whatever medication is prescribed to the older adult with memory loss, it should be tapered slowly on a periodic basis to determine whether the medication continues to be required. Careful documentation of the target symptoms for the medication and monitoring of the effectiveness of the medication in reversing these symptoms assist the physicians and nursing staff in identifying drugs that can be discontinued.

Behavioral management of the patient with memory loss not only is useful to the patient but also provides the patient's family with a sense of accomplishment in the presence of an illness that tends to leave a family feeling helpless and bewildered. The family and the physician should develop behaviors—such as familiar routines and consistent repetition of instructions—that promote both patient and family security. The family should provide moments of fun with the patient, even if these brief moments of relief are quickly forgotten. Families can substitute for the patient's lost abilities by performing tasks such as putting out clothes in the morning. Families must also compensate for the loss of impulse control that accompanies memory loss. One means is distraction; the patient who is about to remove his or her clothes or masturbate in public can be distracted by being engaged in conversation or by being asked to walk with a family member. Patients with memory loss can usually assist in household tasks, even when the disorder is moderately severe. Although the older adult with memory loss cannot prepare a meal alone, he or she can work with the spouse or other family members in routine tasks.

Management of memory loss must include a review of the patient's environment for safety. Typical safety problems include behaviors such as becoming lost or wandering into busy traffic, using medicines erratically or accidentally, falling (secondary to poor lighting or slippery surfaces), having accidents while driving, and leaving things unattended (e.g., leaving appliances turned on).

Perhaps the most important long-term component for managing the older adult with memory loss is support of the family. With proper support, the older person can remain at home for a longer period of time, and the family can function more effectively in the midst of the devastation of the severe memory loss. Education of the family about the expected progression of memory loss, as well as the many behaviors that accompany such loss but that may not be intuitively recognized as resulting from the illness, is key to family support. Excellent educational materials are available, and support groups are located throughout the world to assist the family of the patient with memory loss. In addition, families must be monitored for caregiver stress. If the clinician is not sensitive to the potential for stress in caregivers, family members may exceed their limits and experience burnout, which could lead to neglect and/or abuse of the older adult. Respite for the caregiver, education, and therapy are essential in keeping the care system operative.

Prevention

Can cognitive decline and dementia be prevented? The National Academies recently released a thorough review of the extant literature and provided the following conclusions (National Academies 2017). Although evidence based on clinical trials is sparse, there are three areas that were considered most promising: cognitive training, blood pressure management, and increased physical activity. Cognitive training extends beyond computer-based brain games to activities such as book clubs and puzzle solving. The gains from cognitive training should be long lasting as well as transferable from the training environment to real-world activities.

Insomnia

Insomnia is more common in the elderly population than in any other age group; 28% of adults age 65 years or older report insomnia, and 48% report difficulty both falling asleep and staying asleep and use of sedative-hypnotic medications (Foley et al. 1995). Both the lack of sleep and the subsequent medication use frequently lead to deterioration in daytime alertness and functioning. The most common causes of sleep disturbances in older adults are listed in Table 43–2 (see Zdanys and Steffens 2015).

Sleep changes that are characteristic in late life include decreased total sleep time, frequent arousals, increased percentages of N1 (Stage 1) and N2 (Stage 2) sleep, decreased percentages of N3 (slow wave; formerly designated as Stages 3 and 4) sleep, decreased rapid eye movement (REM) latency, decreased absolute amounts of REM

TABLE 43–2.   Common causes of sleep disturbances in older adults

Primary sleep disorders	Neurological disorders
Insomnia disorder	Parkinson's disease
Obstructive sleep apnea	Alzheimer's disease
Central sleep apnea	Lewy body dementia
Restless leg syndrome	Other neurocognitive disorders
Medical conditions	Medications
Delirium	Cholinesterase inhibitors
Nocturia	Stimulants
Chronic obstructive pulmonary disease	Antihypertensives
Pain syndromes (acute and chronic)	Decongestants
Psychiatric and substance use disorders	Corticosteroids
Mood disorders	Stimulating antidepressants
Anxiety disorders	Diuretics
Posttraumatic stress disorder	Behavioral and environmental causes
Alcohol use disorders	Daytime napping
Tobacco and caffeine use disorders	Light, noise, and heat

sleep, and a tendency to exhibit a redistribution of sleep across the 24-hour day (e.g., napping during the day). Many of these sleep changes are similar to those that occur in depression and NCDs, although not as severe. Older persons are also more likely to phase-advance in the sleep–wake cycle, with a phase tendency toward "morningness" (see Chapter 20 in this volume, "Sleep–Wake Disorders").

Prevalence

Among elderly persons with no previously reported sleep problems, approximately 5% report new symptoms each year (Ancoli-Israel 2000). Disordered sleep and prescription of sedative-hypnotic agents are much more common among older adults living in long-term care facilities than among those living in the community. In terms of specific sleep problems, among community-dwelling older adults, more than 70% reported at least one insomnia symptom, with difficulty maintaining sleep being the most prevalent symptom in both men and women (Jaussent et al. 2011). Women more frequently reported two or three insomnia symptoms, whereas men more often reported only one insomnia symptom. In community populations, obstructive sleep apnea is found to be more prevalent in men than in women, and the respiratory disturbance index (i.e., the number of arousals per hour of sleep) is 15 or greater in 26% of males and 13% of females (Redline et al. 1994). The prevalence of periodic limb movements in sleep (PLMS; experienced most commonly as leg kicks and cold feet along with insomnia) probably ranges from 30% to 50% among healthy elderly persons in the community; polysomnography is generally required to confirm the diagnosis. Restless legs syndrome occurs in about 28% of older adults but does not require polysomnography to diagnose. Circadian rhythm sleep–wake disorders are frequently reported by elderly persons, especially in long-term-care facilities.

Diagnostic Workup

The diagnostic workup of an older person with insomnia begins with assessment of the severity of the sleep disturbance. Screening questions during the interview should include an assessment of the patient's satisfaction with his or her sleep, presence and frequency of daytime napping, fatigue during usual daily activities, and complaints by a bed partner or other observer of unusual behavior during sleep (e.g., snoring, pauses in breathing, periodic myoclonic movements). A careful medical and psychiatric history is necessary to identify or rule out serious diseases that might contribute to the sleep problem, such as depression, anxiety, and pulmonary disease. Current use of alcohol, caffeine, and tobacco should be documented, as should prior treatments (prescribed or self-administered) for sleep problems. A medication history is essential in determining the etiology of insomnia. Prescribed medications often have significant effects on sleep and also may impair cardiopulmonary function.

If a sleep–wake cycle dysfunction is suspected, patients may be asked to keep a log of napping, going to sleep, and awakening. Physical and neurological examinations are necessary, especially when sleep apnea is suspected. Heavy snoring requires a thorough examination of the nose and throat, usually by an otolaryngologist. Referral to a sleep disorder specialist (often a psychiatrist or neurologist) is indicated when the sleep problem persists. Upon referral, most patients, after a thorough history and physical examination and withdrawal from medication, are evaluated by polysomnography. Polysomnographic techniques have been improved in recent years; patients can now be fitted with a portable recording instrument and returned home to sleep for two evenings. Polysomnography, followed by a multiple sleep latency test, can be used to quantify daytime sleepiness as well as to document sleep apnea.

Treatment

Two cornerstones of effective treatment of insomnia in late life are managing the underlying causes of the sleep disturbance and improving sleep hygiene. For example, a significant proportion of older adults with chronic insomnia also have treatable psychiatric disorders, especially depression and alcohol problems. Physical problems such as hypothyroidism or arthritis are also associated with sleep disturbances that may improve with treatment of the underlying disorder. Nocturnal myoclonus, or restless legs syndrome, may respond to medications such as dopamine agonists (e.g., ropinirole, pramipexole, rotigotine), anticonvulsants (e.g., gabapentin), or benzodiazepines (e.g., clonazepam).

Institution of good sleep hygiene is the next step in managing insomnia among elderly patients. First, the patient should be encouraged to initiate sleep at the same time every night, preferably at a later rather than an earlier time (to prevent early-morning wakefulness). The bedroom should be used primarily for sleeping and not for napping. Therefore, if the elderly patient has difficulty sleeping at night, the bed should be made up in the morning and the patient should be encouraged not to nap in the bed and to spend as little time as possible in the bedroom during the day. Exercising can facilitate sleep, but exercise should not be initiated after late afternoon. Alcohol and caffeine should be avoided in the evenings, and the evening meal should be moderate and at least 2–3 hours before bedtime. Fluid intake should also be limited during the 2–3 hours before bedtime (to prevent nocturia). Effective environmental approaches include maintaining a bedroom temperature between 65° and 72°F and using "white noise" to minimize disruptive sounds.

If an older person still cannot sleep at night, he or she is encouraged to get up, go to another room, and engage in some nonstimulating activity (e.g., reading, listening to music). When the elderly person again becomes drowsy, he or she should return to the bedroom and attempt to initiate sleep once again. If the individual experiences a difficult night of sleep, he or she should make extra efforts the next day to avoid napping.

Treatment beyond sleep hygiene may also include psychotherapy. In the past decade, there has been growing published evidence for the use of cognitive-behavioral therapy (CBT) in treating insomnia in older adults. In addition, CBT has been shown to be cost-effective compared with medications when one accounts for severe adverse events, particularly falls, associated with sedative-hypnotic use (Tannenbaum et al. 2015).

Despite concerns about sedative-hypnotic side effects, a number of medications are commonly used to facilitate sleep in elderly individuals (Table 43–3). Current recommendations stress that these medications should be used with care and generally not as first-line treatment, with the aforementioned approaches being preferred initially. If the elderly patient is taking medications that adversely affect sleep (e.g., long-term use of a sedative-hypnotic agent), the pharmacological approach to treatment is to discontinue that medication (usually over about 10 days for a sedative-hypnotic). If the sleep problem is secondary to a medical problem, optimal management of the medical problem with medications can assist the patient with sleep. For example, adequate treatment of arthritis with analgesics can improve sleep.

With these caveats in mind, trazodone (25–50 mg) or doxepin (25 mg) is commonly used to treat insomnia and is seen by many clinicians as preferable to using a long-term benzodiazepine when chronic use of a sedative is indicated. However, these drugs have not been proven efficacious in clinical trials, and withdrawal may lead to rebound insomnia (in addition, they reduce time spent in REM sleep). In general, short- to medium-acting benzodiazepines and nonbenzodiazepine agents are preferred over those that are more extended in length of action. Therefore, shorter-acting agents such as zolpidem (5 mg) and temazepam (15 mg) are preferred as a sedative-hypnotic. Zaleplon (5 mg) has the shortest half-life among these agents and does not appear to cause rebound insomnia or adversely affect psychomotor function (Ancoli-Israel 2000), and it may be used for individuals who wake up during the night. Eszopiclone (1–2 mg), although approved by the FDA for long-term use to improve sleep, should be used with the same caution as other hypnotics. Importantly, each agent in this class of sleep medications has only limited evidence supporting its safety and efficacy in older adults. A newer agent, the orexin receptor antagonist suvorexant, has also been shown to be safe and effective in the elderly (Herring et al. 2017). Finally, although atypical antipsychotics such as quetiapine have been used for treatment of sleep problems, this practice is not recommended.

Anxiety

Older persons with anxiety often seek treatment in the primary care setting rather than seeing a mental health professional. There are several reasons for this phenomenon. Often, anxiety may be a symptom of a physical illness such as hyperthyroidism and is

TABLE 43–3.   **Medications and dosages commonly used for treating late-life insomnia**

Medication	Dosage
Trazodone	25–50 mg qd
Doxepin	25 mg qd
Zaleplon	5 mg qd
Zolpidem	5 mg qd
Temazepam	15 mg qd
Eszopiclone	1–2 mg qd
Suvorexant	10 mg qd

Note.   qd=once per day.

therefore managed as part of treating the underlying disorder. Also, with availability of effective medications for anxiety, primary care clinicians often are comfortable with initial management of anxiety. However, it is important for psychiatrists and other mental health clinicians to know how to assess and treat anxiety; such conditions are common (e.g., generalized anxiety disorder) and often occur as a comorbidity with depression and other psychiatric disorders (Blazer 1997; see also Chapter 13, "Anxiety Disorders," in this volume). Of note, many anxiety disorders are relatively less prevalent in late life. These include phobias and panic disorder. Because generalized anxiety disorder is relatively more common, it is thus the focus of most therapy.

Prevalence and Etiology

Community surveys of individuals with anxiety symptoms estimate that approximately 5% of older persons experience such disorders (Blazer et al. 1991). Approximately 20% of older persons report some cognitive or somatic symptoms of anxiety in community surveys, with somatic symptoms being more prevalent than cognitive symptoms. In a nationally representative survey, specific phobia was found in 4.91% of persons ages 65–74 years, compared with 7.74% of persons ages 55–64 years (Reynolds et al. 2015); these phobias are generally not disabling, however, because the older adult usually finds convenient ways to avoid the phobic situation. Agoraphobia was found in 5% of individuals 65 years or older, compared with 7% of the middle-aged persons (Blazer et al. 1991). A review of geriatric mental health by the Institute of Medicine reported a social phobia prevalence of 0.9%–2.5% among community-dwelling elders (Eden et al. 2012).

Anxiety results from a number of medical and psychiatric conditions. Many medical conditions, such as hyperthyroidism, or medications for medical conditions, such as those for hypothyroidism, can cause symptoms of anxiety. Psychiatric disorders are manifested, in part, by symptoms of anxiety. Moderate to severe delirium is usually associated with anxiety and agitation, especially when the older person is in an unfamiliar place. Anxiety is a common accompaniment in major depressive disorder (MDD); older patients with MDD also meet the criteria for generalized anxiety disorder in more than 50% of cases (Blazer et al. 1989). Somatic symptom disorder and illness anxiety disorder are associated with anxiety, especially when dependency needs are not met by family and health care professionals. NCDs, especially in the early and middle stages, are associated with anxiety and agitation. In addition, late-life schizophrenia with acute paranoid ideation is usually accompanied by agitation and anxiety.

The clinician must not overlook the possibility that the anxiety symptoms may be secondary to appropriate fear. Many older persons must expose themselves daily to situations that threaten their security. Older adults living in inner cities often fear being attacked as they walk the streets. Those with memory loss who live alone may fear that they will get lost driving to the doctor's office. Individuals who have lost the acuteness of their reflexes fear driving on busy, crowded highways.

Treatment

Benzodiazepines (e.g., alprazolam, oxazepam, lorazepam) are the key class of pharmacological agents used in the management of anxiety disorders. These drugs consistently have been shown to be efficacious in treatment of anxiety when compared with placebo, and they are relatively free of side effects. While they are generally well tolerated by persons of all ages, benzodiazepines present unique problems when prescribed to older persons. For example, their half-life may be increased dramatically in late life, with diazepam (2.5–5.0 mg) having a half-life nearing 4 days in persons in their 80s. Older persons are also more susceptible to benzodiazepines' potential side effects, such as fatigue, drowsiness, motor dysfunction, falls, and memory impairment. Clinicians must be especially careful when prescribing benzodiazepines to older individuals who drive. Therefore, the shorter-acting benzodiazepines, such as alprazolam (0.25 mg), oxazepam (15 mg), and lorazepam (0.5 mg), given two or three times a day, have been the preferred agents for anxiety in late life. Nevertheless, in some older patients, short-acting drugs may lead to brief withdrawal episodes during the day and a rebound of anxiety. Finally, buspirone, a nonbenzodiazepine anxiolytic, has been shown to be efficacious in the treatment of generalized anxiety disorder (Mokhber et al. 2010).

Antidepressant medications may also have a role in treatment of anxiety. For example, escitalopram has been shown to be efficacious in the treatment of generalized anxiety disorder in older adults (Lenze et al. 2009). Other SSRIs and serotonin–norepinephrine reuptake inhibitors (SNRIs; e.g., venlafaxine, duloxetine) may likewise be effective in treating anxiety.

Other agents are generally less effective in controlling late-life anxiety. The antidepressant agents are useful in treating anxiety mixed with depression. Nevertheless, in many older persons with a mixed anxiety–depression syndrome, the depressive symptoms improve while the antidepressant is being used, yet the anxiety symptoms persist. Therefore, a combination of a benzodiazepine and an antidepressant is sometimes used.

In terms of nonpharmacological interventions, older persons without cognitive dysfunction may be good candidates for relaxation training and biofeedback. There is also a growing literature on CBT for the treatment of anxiety in older adults, particularly in combination with pharmacological approaches. Such treatment has been shown to be effective in enhancing response and preventing relapse of anxiety symptoms (Wetherell et al. 2013). In a study of older patients with panic disorder with or without agoraphobia, paroxetine and CBT individually were each efficacious versus a waitlist control condition (Hendriks et al. 2010).

Suspiciousness and Agitation

A common symptom in older adults, especially older adults experiencing cognitive impairment, is suspiciousness, which may range from increased cautiousness and distrust of family and friends to overt paranoid delusions. Among suspicious or paranoid older persons, a unique group has been described, especially in the European literature, for many years. *Late-life paraphrenia* (or, as more recently labeled, *very-late-onset schizophrenia*) has been distinguished from both chronic schizophrenia and dementia and is characterized by marked paranoid delusions in older adults who nevertheless maintain their functioning in the community for months or even years (Almeida et al. 1995). Persons experiencing paraphrenia are predominantly women and often live alone. However, marked suspiciousness and overt psychosis in conjunction with cognitive impairment are more common manifestations of the syndrome. There is sparse empirical justification for disaggregating late-life paraphrenia from other psychotic disorders.

The predominant delusions encountered in older persons are persecutory delusions and somatic delusions. Persecutory delusions often revolve around a single theme or a series of connected themes, such as family and neighbors conspiring against the older person or a delusion of sexual abuse. Somatic delusions often involve the gastrointestinal tract and frequently reflect the older person's fear that he or she is experiencing cancer. Regardless of the etiology of suspiciousness and paranoid delusions, when older persons believe they are threatened by the social environment, often because they do not understand what is happening in that environment, agitation becomes paramount. Decreased cognitive functioning is the most common cause of suspiciousness and agitation and may result from both a loss of ability to evaluate the environment and direct neuropathological changes. Agitation in the suspicious older person is an acute symptom that may require emergency management, as described later in this section (see "Treatment").

Prevalence and Etiology

Suspiciousness and paranoid behavior were found in 17% of elderly persons in one early community survey (Lowenthal 1964), and a sense of persecution was reported in 4% in a later survey (Christenson and Blazer 1984). Thus, the perception by older persons that they live in a hostile social environment is common and represents a much larger proportion of older individuals than those who would be diagnosed with schizophrenia or suspiciousness secondary to cognitive impairment. Some of these suspicions may be justified if the older person lives in an unsafe community or has been the victim of fraud. Among older persons in the community, less than 1% have schizophrenia or a paranoid disorder.

Many different disorders may lead to suspiciousness, delusions, and agitation. Chronic schizophrenia, which has its onset earlier in life and persists into late life, is perhaps the most easily identified cause of late-life suspiciousness (Vahia et al. 2012). Because schizophrenia tends to be characterized by a decline in social functioning over the life cycle and a shorter life expectancy (although the prognosis of schizophrenia varies greatly from person to person), chronic schizophrenia that persists into late life and yet leaves the older person relatively free of other symptoms is uncommon. Nevertheless, persons may experience severe symptoms of schizophrenia in early life or midlife and then enter a period of remission from which they do not relapse with further schizophrenic behavior until late life. Schizophrenia-like illness also may have its first onset in late life. Patients with this illness are less likely to experience negative symptoms and neuropsychological impairment and often respond to lower dosages of antipsychotic medication. Usually, depression and disorders related to brain dysfunction do not contribute to these late-onset schizophrenia-like states. In contrast, disorders related to brain dysfunction and late-onset depression are frequently associated with some psychotic symptoms.

Late-onset delusional disorder, with mild to moderate symptoms, is a common cause of suspiciousness in late life. Delusions, often of being persecuted by family and friends, usually center on a single theme or interconnected themes. For example, an older woman may become convinced that her daughter was instrumental in the death of her husband (or that the daughter neglected her father during a chronic illness). The mother then may not listen to reason regarding the daughter's behavior and may never forgive the daughter for the perceived abuse or neglect. These delusions may lead to withdrawal of affection, financial support, and social contact with the daughter.

Suspiciousness and agitation in late life are also commonly caused by psychotic symptoms associated with NCDs. These symptoms, in contrast to late-onset delusional disorder, wax and wane over time in severity and in content. In some cases, the older adult functions well and does not appear to be disturbed by the delusional thoughts, even though the thoughts are frequently expressed. Imagined infidelity by a marriage partner is a common example. If the delusion does not create subjective stress and/or problems in management, regular evaluation of the patient and family without the use of medications is the preferred intervention. Persecutory delusions are the most common type and often emerge when the older person's environment is changed. Suspiciousness and agitation may derive from medications or from localized brain damage (e.g., in alcohol abuse and Huntington's chorea). Suspiciousness, however, usually results from the NCDs such as AD and vascular NCD. For some persons with AD, paranoid thoughts may dominate other symptoms of the disease, especially in the early stages. Perhaps the most common encounter psychiatrists have with suspicious older persons is with patients with AD who have become a management problem because of suspiciousness and agitation. Suspiciousness and agitation are also frequent symptoms of acute confusion.

Despite the range of disorders that may lead to suspiciousness in older persons, some investigators have suggested common psychobiological contributors to the syndrome in late life. A family history of suspiciousness and delusional thought is uncommon among suspicious older persons, and therefore hereditary contributions are probably less important than at earlier stages of the life cycle. Degeneration of subcortical tissues with aging may disrupt neurotransmission and higher brain functions, which in turn contribute to a deficiency in maintaining attention and filtering information, symptoms that have been associated with psychotic thinking. That women are more likely to experience more severe syndromes of suspiciousness than men in late life (in contrast to the equal sex distribution of psychoses earlier in life) has led some investigators to suggest that menopause and the resultant decrease in estrogen binding to dopamine receptors may place women at risk who were previously protected from developing suspicious thinking. Sensory deprivation also has been identified as a potential risk factor for suspiciousness, regardless of the underlying disorder. Social isolation also may contribute to suspiciousness.

Diagnostic Workup

The key to the diagnostic workup of the suspicious older person is the psychiatric evaluation. Because delusional thinking and agitation usually render the patient's history inaccurate, family members should be interviewed to review the patient's behavior, especially any change in behavior. Previous psychotic or delusional episodes should be documented, as well as previous treatment. Clinicians evaluating the suspicious older person should remember that older adults are occasionally abused by family members and, therefore, the seemingly delusional description of family behavior by the older individual may contain some truth.

Treatment

The management of suspiciousness in older adults requires 1) ensuring a safe environment; 2) initiating a therapeutic alliance; 3) considering and, if appropriate, instituting pharmacological therapy; and 4) managing acute behavioral crises. The clinician must first decide whether hospitalization is necessary. In general, paranoid older persons do not adapt well to the hospital. Change from familiar surroundings and interactions with strange persons tend to exacerbate the suspiciousness. Nevertheless, older patients often are so disabled in their behavior secondary to suspiciousness and agitation that hospitalization is necessary.

Once the older patient is hospitalized, the clinician must initiate a therapeutic alliance, which may be accomplished by taking a medical approach to the patient and expressing concern about all of the patient's physical and emotional concerns. Most suspicious older patients are quite accepting of medical care and are trusting of physicians. It is rarely necessary for clinicians to confront patients regarding suspicions or delusional thinking; therefore, older patients' responses to questions can be supported emotionally (e.g., "I understand your concern"), and clinicians do not need to agree with or challenge statements made by patients that are known to be untrue.

The cornerstone of managing the moderately to severely suspicious older patient is medication, especially antipsychotic agents (Table 43–4). The medications most commonly used in older persons are risperidone, olanzapine, quetiapine, and haloperidol. Dosages of these agents are relatively small initially, and one-half of the daily dosage should be given during the evening. In a large controlled study, lower dosages of risperidone (1 mg/day) significantly improved symptoms of psychosis and aggressive behavior with fewer side effects compared with 2 mg/day (Katz et al. 1999). Dosages can be increased if necessary. Clinicians should be mindful of the FDA warning about atypical antipsychotics. Physicians who prescribe antipsychotic medications for the treatment of suspiciousness in an older adult should carefully monitor the success of these agents and should discuss the potential benefits and potential risks with the patient and family. If the drug is deemed not successful—for example, if the target symptoms do not change with the medication—then it should be discontinued, given the significant side effects that may result. Tardive dyskinesia is five to six times more prevalent in elderly than in younger patients (Jeste 2000).

TABLE 43–4. **Medications for the management of suspiciousness and agitation in older adults**

Medication	Dosage
Atypical antipsychotic agents	
Risperidone	1–3 mg qd
Olanzapine	5–15 mg qd
Quetiapine	50–100 mg qd
Older antipsychotic agents	
Haloperidol	0.5–2.0 mg tid

Note. qd=once per day; tid=three times per day.

TABLE 43–5. **Suggestions for preventing aggressive and violent behavior in older adults**

Psychologically disarm the patient by helping him or her to express his or her fears.

Distract the attention of the older patient.

Provide directions to the patient in simple terms.

Communicate clearly and concisely.

Communicate expectations.

Avoid arguing and defending.

Avoid threatening body language or gestures.

Remain at a safe distance from the patient until help is available.

Finally, the physician must be prepared to deal with severe agitation and violent behavior (Table 43–5). Medications alone will not control these behaviors. Physicians must work with nursing staff to prevent such behavior in patients at risk while they are in the hospital and must instruct families on methods of prevention when these patients are at home.

Periods of severe agitation are usually brief and, if managed properly, are soon forgotten by the older patient. Then the physician once more can work toward establishing a sustained therapeutic relationship with the patient.

Depression

Depression is one of the more common and the second-most disabling of the geriatric psychiatry syndromes (after memory loss) (Blazer 2003). Late-life depression that is not comorbid with physical illness and/or an NCD is characterized by symptoms similar to those experienced at earlier stages of the life cycle, with some significant differences. Depressed mood is usually apparent in the older adult but may not be a spontaneous complaint. Older persons are more likely to experience weight loss (as opposed to weight gain or no change in weight) during a major depressive episode and are less likely to report feelings of worthlessness or guilt. Although older persons experience more difficulty with cognitive performance tests during a depressive episode, they are no more likely than persons in midlife to report cognitive problems subjectively. Complaints of cognitive dysfunction are common in more severe depressive episodes, regardless of the person's age. Persistent anhedonia associated with a lack of response to pleasurable stimuli is a common and central symptom of late-life depression. Older persons are also more likely than younger persons to exhibit psychotic symptoms during a depressive episode. Studies have suggested that executive function is impaired in older adults with depression and that this impairment may be associated with a higher likelihood of relapse and recurrence of symptoms (Alexopoulos et al. 2000). Memory impairment in the context of geriatric depression may persist after successful treatment of the depressive symptoms (Lee et al. 2007).

Prevalence and Etiology

In community surveys, older adults are less likely to be diagnosed as having MDD than are persons in young adulthood or middle age. Depressive symptoms, however, are about equally prevalent across the life cycle and increase in prevalence in the oldest old. Standardized interviews reveal that 1%–3% of persons in the community are diagnosed as having dysthymia and/or MDD (Blazer et al. 1987). However, the prevalence of MDD is much higher among older persons in the hospital and in long-term-care facilities, with rates ranging from 10% to 20% (Koenig et al. 1988). In a population-representative study in the United States, overall depression prevalence was 11.19% (Steffens et al. 2009). Prevalence was similar for men (10.19%) and women (11.44%). Whites and Hispanics had nearly three times the prevalence of depression found in African Americans.

Late-life depression fits well in the biopsychosocial model of psychiatric disorders (Blazer and Hybels 2005). Although a hereditary predisposition to depression is less likely among persons in late life who are experiencing a first onset of depression, a number of biological factors are associated with late-life depression. Poor regulation of the hypothalamic-pituitary-adrenal axis, as well as disruption of the sleep cycle and other circadian rhythms, is more likely to be present among older persons than among younger persons. These problems also have been associated with MDD. In addition, considerable attention has been focused on the association of depression with lesions in subcortical structures and their frontal projections in the brain (Alexopoulos et al. 1997; Krishnan et al. 1997). Whereas most older persons are satisfied with their lives and are not psychologically predisposed to depression, some experience demoralization and despair resulting not only from incapacities due to aging but also from a sense of not having fulfilled their life expectations. Older persons must adapt to many adverse life experiences, especially the loss of relatives and friends, yet they are often more likely than younger persons to respond to these losses without difficulty. Older persons, for example, expect that they will lose family and friends through death, and those family and friends whom they do lose often have suffered chronic illnesses for some time, thus allowing older persons to grieve the loss, in part, before the actual loss.

Although MDD is relatively uncommon among older persons, it can be a challenging disorder to manage. Older persons also may experience bipolar disorder, with a first-onset manic episode after age 65 years. Psychotic depressions are more common in late life than at other stages of the life cycle (Meyers 1992). Other common types of late-life depression include depression associated with a medical condition or medication, such as a depressed mood secondary to antihypertensive medications, and depression associated with common NCDs, such as AD and vascular NCD. Medical illness, such as hypothyroidism, frequently leads to a mood disorder. An adjustment disorder with depressed mood secondary to physical disability and/or chronic illness is among the most frequent causes of depressed mood among older individuals.

Diagnostic Workup

The patient's history and a collateral history from a family member are the keys to making the diagnosis of depression in late life. Although older persons may exhibit some tendency to "mask" their depressive symptoms, a careful interview almost invariably reveals significant depression if it is present. The history should be complemented by a thorough mental status examination with attention to disturbances of motor behavior and perception, the presence or absence of hallucinations, disturbances of thinking, and thorough cognitive testing. Psychological testing may be implemented to distinguish depression from dementia but should not be performed in the midst of a severe depressive episode. The laboratory workup of the depressed older adult is presented in Table 43–6. Some tests, such as the blood count and measurement of vitamin B_{12} and folate levels, are useful in screening for medical illnesses that may present with depressive symptoms. The thyroid panel is essential in the diagnosis of the depressed older patient, given that subclinical hypothyroid disorders are often uncovered in the workup.

Although the abnormalities in sleep associated with depression often resemble those associated with normal aging, experienced polysomnographers can distinguish them. MRI is optional despite the association of subcortical white matter hyperintensities with late-life depression. The physician ordering laboratory tests for a depressed older patient also must consider the potential adverse health consequences for an older adult experiencing a severe or chronic mood disorder. For example, MDD is associated with decreased bone mineral density, placing older women with depression at greater risk for osteoporosis (Michelson et al. 1996).

Treatment

Clinical management of late-life depression can involve pharmacotherapy, electroconvulsive therapy (ECT), psychotherapy, and work with the family. The pharmacological treatment of choice at present is one of the new-generation antidepressant medications (Table 43–7). Despite the widespread use of these agents, some geriatric psychiatrists still prefer to first administer one of the secondary-amine tricyclic antidepressants (TCAs), such as nortriptyline or desipramine, in healthy older adults. Each has relatively low anticholinergic effects and is known to be an effective antidepressant. Postural hypotension is the most troublesome side effect that older individuals usually encounter when treated with TCAs. In older adults, the SSRIs fluoxetine, sertraline, paroxetine, citalopram, and escitalopram can be used at somewhat lower dosages than are prescribed at earlier stages of the life cycle (e.g., 10 mg/day for paroxetine). The most common adverse effects that limit the use of SSRIs are agitation and persistent weight loss. Paroxetine has been shown to significantly (but not dramatically) improve the symptoms of minor depression and dysthymia at dosages between 10 and 40 mg/

TABLE 43–6.   **Laboratory workup of the depressed older adult**

Routine

  Complete blood count (CBC)

  Urinalysis

  Triiodothyronine (T_3), thyroxine (T_4), free thyroxine index, thyroid-stimulating hormone (TSH)

  Venereal Disease Research Laboratory (VDRL) test

  Vitamin B_{12} and folate assays

  Chemistry screen (sodium, chlorine, potassium, blood urea nitrogen, calcium, glucose creatine)

  Electrocardiogram

Elective

  Polysomnography

  Magnetic resonance imaging or computed tomography scan

  Thyroid-releasing hormone stimulation test

  Screening for HIV

day (Williams et al. 2000). The use of antidepressant medications, primarily the SSRIs, has increased dramatically over the past 25 years, with more than 10% of elderly persons ages 75 years and older taking antidepressants at any given time (Blazer 2000). If treatment with an SSRI is not successful, then the second-choice medications are usually the SNRIs, such as venlafaxine (beginning at around 37.5 mg/day) or duloxetine (beginning at 20 mg/day) (Alexopoulos et al. 2001).

The older person who has previously responded to ECT, who does not respond to antidepressant medications, or who experiences significant side effects from these medications may be a candidate for ECT. Presence of psychotic depression is also an indication for ECT. With proper medical support, ECT is a safe and effective treatment for older adults. Despite having high levels of physical illness and cognitive impairment, even the oldest patient with severe MDD may tolerate ECT as well as younger patients do and may demonstrate similar or better acute response. Unilateral nondominant ECT is preferred (Kellner et al. 2016). If the treatment is successful, maintenance ECT at progressively extended intervals is a method of preventing relapse. Magnetic seizure therapy and repetitive transcranial magnetic stimulation may be used for treatment-resistant depression in elderly patients (George et al. 1999; Lisanby et al. 2001).

Several studies have demonstrated the effectiveness of cognitive and behavioral therapies (including interpersonal psychotherapy) in outpatient treatment of older persons who have MDD without prominent physical symptoms (Lynch and Aspnes 2004). Cognitive therapy also may be used as an adjunct for severe depressive episodes that are treated concomitantly with medications. In a large controlled trial of patients older than 59 years with MDD, maintenance treatment with interpersonal therapy and paroxetine prevented or significantly delayed recurrence (Reynolds et al. 2006). For long-term (2-year) maintenance, medications were more effective than psychotherapy. CBT is well tolerated by older people because of its limited duration and its educational orientation, as well as the active interchange between therapist and patient.

TABLE 43–7. **Antidepressant therapy for older adults, with typical starting dosages**

Medication	Dosage
Selective serotonin reuptake inhibitors	
Fluoxetine	10 mg qd
Sertraline	50 mg qd in divided doses
Paroxetine	10 mg qd
Citalopram	10 mg qd[a]
Escitalopram	10 mg qd
Serotonin–norepinephrine reuptake inhibitors	
Venlafaxine	37.5 mg qd
Duloxetine	20 mg qd or bid
Desvenlafaxine	50 mg qd
Tricyclic antidepressants	
Nortriptyline	50–75 mg hs
Desipramine	50–75 mg hs
Other medications	
Trazodone	50 mg hs
Bupropion sustained release	100 mg qd or bid

Note. bid=twice per day; hs=at bedtime; qd=once per day.
[a]Total daily dose of citalopram should not exceed 20 mg because of the risk of cardiac arrhythmia.

Any effective therapy for depression in older persons must include work with the family. Families are often the most important allies of the clinician working with depressed older patients. Families should be informed as to the danger signs, such as potential for suicide, in a severely depressed older family member. In addition, the family can provide structure for reengaging a withdrawn and depressed older person in social activities.

Substance Use

Substance use problems in later life are emerging public health concerns. Although all drugs can be abused, two categories of substance use are of particular concern: alcohol use and nonprescription use of prescription medications, especially opioids. For example, nearly one-fourth of older adults are prescribed an opioid each year, and nearly one-fourth of those who are prescribed opioids either abuse or are dependent on the drugs (Centers for Disease Control and Prevention 2018; Kuo et al. 2016). Substance use in older adults is a hidden yet emerging epidemic. As the current baby boom generation enters later life, these problems will only increase in frequency due to the already greater burden of these problems among this cohort. Not only is the frequency of substance use increasing among older adults, but these elders bring complexities to their care that challenge the usual evidence-based practices and frustrate clinicians, patients, and families. Physical health problems, comorbid mental health conditions such as depression and memory loss, and the medications prescribed to treat these problems complicate care.

Common signs and symptoms of substance use disorders are listed in Table 43–8 (Oslin and Mavandadi 2012). None may be initially associated by the clinician with a substance use problem, and therefore the underlying cause may be missed. Both the patient and the family should be asked about use. Older persons are at increased risk because lean body mass and total body water volume are decreased relative to body fat, leading to increased serum concentrations, absorption, and distribution of alcohol and drugs in the body.

Barriers to early identification and treatment include denial of substance problems by both the clinician and the patient, hurried office visits, stigma or shame about substance use, a general reluctance by elders to seek professional help, lack of financial resources or transportation, comorbid conditions that complicate diagnosis or treatment (e.g., cognitive impairment), and a shrinking social support network. Compared with younger adults, older adults are less likely to report or to perceive their alcohol or drug use as being excessive or problematic.

Prevalence and Etiology

Alcohol misuse is by far the most common substance use problem in elderly individuals. In one large study, 66% of elderly male respondents and 55% of female respondents reported alcohol use during the past year, 13% of men and 8% of women reported at-risk use, and more than 14% of men and 3% of women reported binge drinking (Blazer and Wu 2009). A small yet clinically important proportion of older adults (1.4%) reported nonprescription use of prescription pain relievers during the previous year (Wu and Blazer 2011). Combinations of acetaminophen and hydrocodone or propoxyphene were the most commonly used drugs, yet hydrocodone, oxycodone, and fentanyl are also frequently prescribed. And deaths from opioid use continue to climb for the elderly. The use of illegal substances, however, is rare in older adults.

Risk factors for substance use problems include male sex (for alcohol), loss of a spouse/partner, loss of social and occupational roles, history of substance use problems, exposure to potentially addictive substances (such as a stockpile of prescription medications in the household), and comorbid psychiatric problems (Oslin and Mavandadi 2012). In general, substance use decreases with age, although two caveats are critical. First, younger age cohorts today have a significantly higher lifetime prevalence of substance use compared with cohorts ages 65 years and older; therefore, these middle-aged persons will likely be more burdened with substance use problems in later life than current elders, placing increased pressure on an already inadequately trained and overcommitted workforce serving older adults with substance use problems (Eden et al. 2012). Second, although substance use is less prevalent among older adults, it is often more problematic, given the unique characteristics of this population. These include a greater likelihood of taking multiple prescription medications and of having one or more comorbid physical and/or psychiatric problems. Older adults are often more isolated, and this isolation is a trigger for a number of risks, such as reductions in role obligations and absence of encouragement from family and friends.

TABLE 43–8.	Common signs and symptoms of substance use disorders in older adults

Unexplained anxiety

Blackouts, dizziness

Mood swings

Falls, bruises, burns

Memory loss

Poor hygiene

Sleep problems

Treatment

The first step in treating the older adult with a substance use problem involves detoxification and withdrawal. Symptoms of alcohol withdrawal include autonomic hyperactivity (increase in blood pressure and heart rate), restlessness, and sleep problems, and, in severe withdrawal, hallucinations, delirium, and even seizures. Older adults should be withdrawn gradually with a substitute for alcohol, such as diazepam.

Evidence-based studies have demonstrated that nonpharmacological treatment of both alcohol and substance use problems in later life is effective, although the studies have been sparse and small. The least-intensive approaches to therapy should be employed initially in the office if serious withdrawal symptoms are absent. A brief intervention (such as a 10- to 15-minute discussion with the treating physician) is the recommended first step. If this is not successful, a variety of interventions may be employed. The Center for Substance Abuse Treatment (2005) recommended that any approach to treating substance use in older adults include the following components: 1) emphasis on age-specific treatment (e.g., mixed-age 12-step programs may not be appropriate for the elderly); 2) use of supportive, nonconfrontational approaches that build self-esteem (in contrast to confrontational therapies often used with younger adults); 3) focus on cognitive-behavioral approaches (as opposed to more nondirective therapies); 4) development of skills for improving social support; 5) recruitment of counselors who are trained and motivated to work with older adults; and 6) use of age-appropriate pace and content. Adherence to treatment is usually improved if the setting for treatment remains in the primary care office.

For many years, disulfiram was the only medication available for long-term treatment of alcohol dependence, but it was seldom used because of its adverse side effects. More recently, naltrexone and acamprosate have been demonstrated to be effective treatments. Buprenorphine and naloxone are the drugs of choice in treating opioid use disorder in older adults.

Conclusion

The mental health care of elders has often been neglected; physicians and other clinicians often focus on the problems of children and young adults and on crisis situations. The treatment of psychiatric syndromes in later life is complex and generally requires attention to adaptation and function longitudinally, as opposed to single-episode interventions. For these reasons, the mental health problems of older adults far too often fly beneath the attention of health care professionals. The gray tsunami is upon us, with its accompanying public health consequences, and yet, the potential for alleviating the suffering from mental health and substance use problems in older adults has never been so promising.

Key Clinical Points

- Acute confusion is much more common in hospitalized older adults than is usually recognized. Careful screening is necessary to identify these patients.

- Working with the family of a patient with memory loss is key to easing the suffering of the patient and to preventing institutionalization before it is absolutely necessary.

- Good sleep hygiene is more important than pharmacological management of insomnia in older adults.

- Generalized anxiety disorder is usually comorbid with other conditions, such as depression or physical illness. Diagnosing comorbid conditions is the first step to managing anxiety in older adults.

- Suspiciousness and agitation are the most disruptive symptoms of neurocognitive disorders.

- Uncomplicated depression is as responsive to treatment in late life as it is in midlife. Depression comorbid with physical illness or memory loss is much more difficult to treat.

- Substance use is increasing in frequency in older persons, especially opioid use, which is particularly problematic given this population's often compromised health and high use of other prescribed medications.

References

Alexopoulos GS, Meyers BS, Young RC, et al: "Vascular depression" hypothesis. Arch Gen Psychiatry 54(10):915–922, 1997 9337771

Alexopoulos GS, Meyers BS, Young RC, et al: Executive dysfunction and long-term outcomes of geriatric depression. Arch Gen Psychiatry 57(3):285–290, 2000 10711915

Alexopoulos GS, Katz IR, Reynolds CF III, et al: The Expert Consensus Guideline Series. Pharmacotherapy of depressive disorders in older patients. Postgrad Med Special Report, October 2001, pp 1–86

Almeida OP, Howard RJ, Levy R, et al: Psychotic states arising in late life (late paraphrenia) psychopathology and nosology. Br J Psychiatry 166(2):205–214, 1995 7728365

Alzheimer's Association: 2018 Alzheimer's Disease Facts and Figures. Alzheimer's & Dementia 14(3):367–429, 2018. Available at: https://www.alzheimersanddementia.com/article/S1552-5260(18)30041-4/fulltext. Accessed January 13, 2019.

American Psychiatric Association: Diagnostic and Statistical Manual of Mental Disorders, 5th Edition. Arlington, VA, American Psychiatric Association, 2013

Ancoli-Israel S: Insomnia in the elderly: a review for the primary care practitioner. Sleep 23 (suppl 1):S23–S30, discussion S36–S38, 2000 10755805

Blazer DG: Generalized anxiety disorder and panic disorder in the elderly: a review. Harv Rev Psychiatry 5(1):18–27, 1997 9385016

Blazer DG: Psychiatry and the oldest old. Am J Psychiatry 157(12):1915–1924, 2000 11097951

Blazer DG: Depression in late life: review and commentary. J Gerontol A Biol Sci Med Sci 58(3):249–265, 2003 12634292

Blazer D: Neurocognitive disorders in DSM-5. Am J Psychiatry 170(6):585–587, 2013 23732964

Blazer DG, Hybels CF: Origins of depression in later life. Psychol Med 35(9):1241–1252, 2005 16168147

Blazer DG, van Nieuwenhuizen AO: Evidence for the diagnostic criteria of delirium: an update. Curr Opin Psychiatry 25(3):239–243, 2012 22449764

Blazer DG, Wu LT: The epidemiology of at-risk and binge drinking among middle-aged and elderly community adults: National Survey on Drug Use and Health. Am J Psychiatry 166(10):1162–1169, 2009 19687131

Blazer D, Hughes DC, George LK: The epidemiology of depression in an elderly community population. Gerontologist 27(3):281–287, 1987 3609795

Blazer D, Hughes DC, Fowler N: Anxiety as an outcome symptom of depression in elderly and middle-aged adults. International Journal of Geriatric Psychiatry 4(5):273–278, 1989

Blazer DG, Hughes D, George L: Generalized anxiety disorder, in Psychiatric Disorders in America: The Epidemiologic Catchment Area Study. Edited by Robins L, Regier D. New York, Free Press, 1991, pp 180–203

Blazer DG, Yaffe K, Liverman CT (eds): Cognitive Aging: Progress in Understanding and Opportunities for Action. Washington, DC, National Academies Press, 2015

Center for Substance Abuse Treatment: Substance Abuse Relapse Prevention for Older Adults: A Group Treatment Approach. Rockville, MD, Substance Abuse and Mental Health Services Administration, U.S. Department of Health and Human Services, 2005

Centers for Disease Control and Prevention: US death rates for Alzheimer's disease increase 55% from 1999 to 2014. CDC Newsroom, May 25, 2017. Available at: https:// www.cdc.gov/media/releases/2017/p0525-alzheimer-deaths.html. Accessed July 17, 2017.

Centers for Disease Control and Prevention: 2018 Annual Surveillance Report of Drug-Related Risks and Outcomes—United States. Surveillance Special Report. Atlanta, GA, National Center for Injury Prevention and Control, Centers for Disease Control and Prevention, U.S. Department of Health and Human Services. August 31, 2018. Available at: https:// www.cdc.gov/drugoverdose/pdf/pubs/2018-cdc-drug-surveillance-report.pdf. Accessed November 22, 2018.

Christenson R, Blazer D: Epidemiology of persecutory ideation in an elderly population in the community. Am J Psychiatry 141(9):1088–1091, 1984 6235752

Eden J, Maslow K, Le M, et al (eds): The Mental Health and Substance Use Workforce for Older Adults: In Whose Hands? Washington, DC, National Academies Press, 2012

Foley DJ, Monjan AA, Brown SL, et al: Sleep complaints among elderly persons: an epidemiologic study of three communities. Sleep 18(6):425–432, 1995 7481413

Folstein MF, Folstein SE, McHugh PR: "Mini-mental state." A practical method for grading the cognitive state of patients for the clinician. J Psychiatr Res 12(3):189–198, 1975 1202204

Ganguli M, Dodge HH, Shen C, et al: Mild cognitive impairment, amnestic type: an epidemiologic study. Neurology 63(1):115–121, 2004 15249620

George MS, Lisanby SH, Sackeim HA: Transcranial magnetic stimulation: applications in neuropsychiatry. Arch Gen Psychiatry 56(4):300–311, 1999 10197824

Hendriks GJ, Keijsers GP, Kampman M, et al: A randomized controlled study of paroxetine and cognitive-behavioural therapy for late-life panic disorder. Acta Psychiatr Scand 122(1):11–19, 2010 19958308

Herring WJ, Connor KM, Snyder E, et al: Suvorexant in elderly patients with insomnia: pooled analyses of data from phase III randomized controlled clinical trials. Am J Geriatr Psychiatry 25(7):791–802, 2017 28427826

Inouye SK: Delirium in older persons. N Engl J Med 354(11):1157–1165, 2006 16540616

Inouye SK, Bogardus ST Jr, Charpentier PA, et al: A multicomponent intervention to prevent delirium in hospitalized older patients. N Engl J Med 340(9):669–676, 1999 10053175

Jaussent I, Dauvilliers Y, Ancelin ML, et al: Insomnia symptoms in older adults: associated factors and gender differences. Am J Geriatr Psychiatry 19(1):88–97, 2011 20808113

Jeste DV: Tardive dyskinesia in older patients. J Clin Psychiatry 61 (suppl 4):27–32, 2000 10739328

Katz IR, Jeste DV, Mintzer JE, et al: Comparison of risperidone and placebo for psychosis and behavioral disturbances associated with dementia: a randomized, double-blind trial. J Clin Psychiatry 60(2):107–115, 1999 10084637

Kellner CH, Husain MM, Knapp RG, et al: Right unilateral ultrabrief pulse ECT in geriatric depression: phase 1 of the PRIDE study. Am J Psychiatry 173(11):1101–1109, 2016 27418379

Koenig HG, Meador KG, Cohen HJ, et al: Depression in elderly hospitalized patients with medical illness. Arch Intern Med 148(9):1929–1936, 1988 3415405

Krishnan KR, Hays JC, Blazer DG: MRI-defined vascular depression. Am J Psychiatry 154(4):497–501, 1997 9090336

Kuo YF, Raji MA, Chen NW, et al: Trends in opioid prescriptions among Part D Medicare recipients from 2007 to 2012. Am J Med 129(2):221.e21–221.e30, 2016 [Erratum in: Am J Med 130(5):615–616, 2017] 26522794

Lee JS, Potter GG, Wagner HR, et al: Persistent mild cognitive impairment in geriatric depression. Int Psychogeriatr 19(1):125–135, 2007 16834811

Lenze EJ, Rollman BL, Shear MK, et al: Escitalopram for older adults with generalized anxiety disorder: a randomized controlled trial. JAMA 301(3):295–303, 2009 19155456

Lisanby SH, Schlaepfer TE, Fisch HU, et al: Magnetic seizure therapy of major depression. Arch Gen Psychiatry 58(3):303–305, 2001 11231838

Lowenthal M: Lives in Distress. New York, Basic Books, 1964

Lynch T, Aspnes A: Individual and group psychotherapy, in The American Psychiatric Publishing Textbook of Geriatric Psychiatry, 3rd Edition. Edited by Blazer DG, Steffens DC, Busse EW. Washington, DC, American Psychiatric Publishing, 2004, pp 443–458

Meyers BS: Geriatric delusional depression. Clin Geriatr Med 8(2):299–308, 1992 1600480

Michelson D, Stratakis C, Hill L, et al: Bone mineral density in women with depression. N Engl J Med 335(16):1176–1181, 1996 8815939

Mokhber N, Azarpazhooh MR, Khajedaluee M, et al: Randomized, single-blind, trial of sertraline and buspirone for treatment of elderly patients with generalized anxiety disorder. Psychiatry Clin Neurosci 64(2):128–133, 2010 20132529

Nasreddine ZS, Phillips NA, Bédirian V, et al: The Montreal Cognitive Assessment, MoCA: a brief screening tool for mild cognitive impairment. J Am Geriatr Soc 53(4):695–699, 2005 15817019

National Academies: Preventing Cognitive Decline and Dementia: A Way Forward. Washington, DC, National Academies Press, 2017

Oslin DW, Mavandadi S: Alcohol and drug problems, in Essentials of Geriatric Psychiatry, 2nd Edition. Edited by Blazer DG, Steffens DS. Washington, DC, American Psychiatric Publishing, 2012, pp 223–241

Redline S, Kump K, Tishler PV, et al: Gender differences in sleep disordered breathing in a community-based sample. Am J Respir Crit Care Med 149(3 Pt 1):722–726, 1994 8118642

Reynolds CF 3rd, Dew MA, Pollock BG, et al: Maintenance treatment of major depression in old age. N Engl J Med 354(11):1130–1138, 2006 16540613

Reynolds K, Pietrzak RH, El-Gabalawy R, et al: Prevalence of psychiatric disorders in U.S. older adults: findings from a nationally representative survey. World Psychiatry 14(1):74–81, 2015 25655161

Roses AD: Apolipoprotein E affects the rate of Alzheimer disease expression: beta-amyloid burden is a secondary consequence dependent on APOE genotype and duration of disease. J Neuropathol Exp Neurol 53(5):429–437, 1994 8083686

Steffens DC, Fisher GG, Langa KM, et al: Prevalence of depression among older Americans: the Aging, Demographics and Memory Study. Int Psychogeriatr 21(5):879–888, 2009 19519984

Tannenbaum C, Diaby V, Singh D, et al: Sedative-hypnotic medicines and falls in community-dwelling older adults: a cost-effectiveness (decision-tree) analysis from a US Medicare perspective. Drugs Aging 32(4):305–314, 2015 25825121

U.S. Food and Drug Administration: Public Health Advisory: Deaths with antipsychotics in elderly patients with behavioral disturbances. April 11, 2005. Available at: http://psychrights.org/drugs/FDAantipsychotics4elderlywarning.htm. Accessed December 18, 2018.

Vahia IV, Lanoutte LM, Jeste DV: Schizophrenia and paranoid disorders, in Essentials of Geriatric Psychiatry, 2nd Edition. Edited by Blazer DG, Steffens DC. Washington, DC, American Psychiatric Publishing, 2012, pp 163–174

Wei LA, Fearing MA, Sternberg EJ, et al: The Confusion Assessment Method: a systematic review of current usage. J Am Geriatr Soc 56(5):823–830, 2008 18384586

Wetherell JL, Petkus AJ, White KS, et al: Antidepressant medication augmented with cognitive-behavioral therapy for generalized anxiety disorder in older adults. Am J Psychiatry 170(7):782–789, 2013 23680817

Williams JW Jr, Barrett J, Oxman T, et al: Treatment of dysthymia and minor depression in primary care: a randomized controlled trial in older adults. JAMA 284(12):1519–1526, 2000 11000645

Wu LT, Blazer DG: Illicit and nonmedical drug use among older adults: a review. J Aging Health 23(3):481–504, 2011 21084724

Zdanys KF, Steffens DC: Sleep disturbances in the elderly. Psychiatr Clin North Am 38(4):723–741, 2015 26600105

Recommended Readings

Alexopoulos GS, Katz IR, Reynolds CF III, et al: The Expert Consensus Guideline Series. Pharmacotherapy of depressive disorders in older patients. Postgrad Med Special Report, October 2001, pp 1–86

Blazer DG: Depression in late life: review and commentary. J Gerontol A Biol Sci Med Sci 58:249–265, 2003

Steffens DC, Blazer DG, Thakur ME (eds): The American Psychiatric Publishing Textbook of Geriatric Psychiatry, 5th Edition. Washington, DC, American Psychiatric Publishing, 2015

CHAPTER 44

Culturally Diverse Patients

Mark Sullivan, M.D.

Neil Krishan Aggarwal, M.D., M.B.A., M.A.

In this chapter we discuss the role of culture in diagnostic assessment and treatment planning. In DSM-5, *culture* is defined as "systems of knowledge, concepts, rules, and practices that are learned and transmitted across generations. Culture includes language, religion and spirituality, family structures, life-cycle stages, ceremonial rituals, and customs, as well as moral and legal systems" (American Psychiatric Association 2013, p. 749). DSM-5 explains that "cultures are open, dynamic systems that undergo continuous change over time; in the contemporary world, most individuals and groups are exposed to multiple cultures, which they use to fashion their own identities and make sense of experience. These features of culture make it crucial not to overgeneralize cultural information or stereotype groups in terms of fixed cultural traits" (American Psychiatric Association 2013, p. 749). These characterizations of culture illustrate central issues in cultural psychiatry that are relevant to the practice of all clinicians: 1) all individuals, as social beings, belong to at least one culture whose interpretations about the self, others, the world, and human predicaments (Who am I? Why are we here?) are debated in relationships and institutions across the lifespan; 2) individuals use their relationships and social groupings to fashion a unique sense of self (i.e., "identity") that informs their "psychology" (their understandings of thoughts, emotions, and behaviors); and 3) clinicians cannot make assumptions about anyone's cultural affiliation(s) lest they risk assigning stereotypes that can endanger therapeutic rapport.

DSM-5's inclusion of this definition for culture comes from evidence that mental health clinicians and services improve care when a patient's systems of knowledge, concepts, rules, and practices regarding mental health and illness are incorporated within diagnostic assessment, treatment planning, and therapeutic recovery. As recently as 1973, the American Psychiatric Association considered some forms of cultural diversity as psychopathology, to the extent that homosexuality was included as a mental disorder in DSM-II (American Psychiatric Association 1968). As cultural diversity has expanded beyond race and ethnicity to include socioeconomic status, religion, sexual orientation, and other sources of social diversity, clinicians have embraced open-mindedness and a desire to learn about differences (Jenks 2011). In addition, professional guidelines for mental health clinicians have recognized the importance of conducting standardized cultural assessments. For instance, the American Board of Psychiatry and Neurology has stated that "cultural diversity includes issues of race, gender, language, age, country of origin, sexual orientation, religious/spiritual beliefs, sociocultural class, educational/intellectual levels, and physical disability" and that "working with a culturally diverse population requires knowledge about cultural factors in the delivery of health care" (American Board of Psychiatry and Neurology 2011, p. 10). Additionally, the DSM-5 "Outline for Cultural Formulation" section on cultural identity states that "other clinically relevant aspects of identity may include religious affiliation, socioeconomic background, personal and family places of birth and growing up, migrant status, and sexual orientation" (American Psychiatric Association 2013, p. 750). The DSM-5 Outline for Cultural Formulation and Cultural Formulation Interview have now been in use since 2013, building an evidence base on the training that clinicians need to conduct cultural assessments. These assessment tools, their origins, and their impacts on clinical outcomes are discussed in this chapter.

Cultural Competence

In 2016, the National Academies of Sciences, Engineering, and Medicine defined *cultural competence* as "the ability of an organization or an individual within the health care delivery system to provide effective, equitable, understandable, and respectful quality care and services that are responsive to diverse cultural health beliefs and practices, preferred languages, health literacy, and other communication needs of the patient" (p. 12). In its evaluation process for accrediting and certifying American health care organizations and programs, the independent nonprofit Joint Commission (2014) emphasized that language is "no longer considered to be simply a patient's right; effective communication is now accepted as an essential component of quality care and patient safety" (p. 1).

Why should all clinicians consider cultural competence important? First, cultural competence has become an expected professional standard in the education of all medical professionals. At the undergraduate medical level, the Association of American Medical Colleges (2015) has identified clinician cultural competence as a critical mechanism for reducing chronic health disparities:

> Culturally responsive health care is a key strategy to reduce health care disparities and promote health equity. Education and training are important, but only represent one element of the complex web of factors that advance quality health care. An integrated systems approach that involves the trainee or the health professional and patients is necessary (p. 9)

At the postgraduate residency level, the American Board of Psychiatry and Neurology (2011), in its "Psychiatry Core Competencies Outline," listed multiple areas where physicians *must* demonstrate proficiencies: obtaining a sociocultural history; developing a case formulation that incorporates neurobiological, phenomenological, psychological, and sociocultural issues involved in diagnosis and management; creating a treatment plan that addresses biological, psychological, and sociocultural domains; integrating sociocultural interventions within evidence-based individual, group, and family psychotherapies; eliciting the experience, meaning, and illness explanations of the patient and family; mastering knowledge on the sociocultural factors of illness etiologies, human development, variations in prescribing practices, and the epidemiology of substance abuse; and communicating effectively with patients and families by respecting patients' cultural backgrounds. In August 2012, the National Quality Forum endorsed 12 quality measures focused on reducing health care disparities and promoting culturally competent care for racial and ethnic minority populations. These included measures for evaluating the engagement and experiences of patients receiving mental health services (National Quality Forum 2012). For academic medical institutions, the Accreditation Council for Graduate Medical Education's (2014) Clinical Learning Environment Review Program now requires residents, fellows, and faculty to be trained and engaged in health disparity reduction, cultural competence, and quality improvement initiatives. Cultural competence is not optional; it is expected at all levels of a physician's career.

A second reason why cultural competence should be considered important is that clinical evidence demonstrates that cultural competence is not merely a form of political correctness that emerged during the American civil rights movement but also a framework for understanding culture's various manifestations in all aspects of patient care, such as patient perceptions of what is considered appropriate and inappropriate to discuss in mental health settings, clinician interpretations of patient experiences through professionalized systems of knowledge such as DSM-5, and patient *and* clinician interpretations of acceptable and unacceptable treatments (Lewis-Fernández et al. 2014). By viewing the process of medical consultation as an intercultural exchange among the cultures of the patient, clinician, and institution in which health services are being delivered, clinicians can construct treatment plans that reduce symptom burden and increase appointment retention, treatment adherence, and quality of life.

Finally, the American medical system has determined that cultural competence is essential to the organization and delivery of health services at the systemic and societal levels. In 2013, the U.S. Department of Health and Human Services Office of Minority Health published the enhanced *National Standards for Culturally and Linguistically Appropriate Services (CLAS) in Health and Health Care*, which encompass 15 standards that define culturally competent care (Table 44–1; Office of Minority Health 2013). The CLAS standards were created to foster "the development of clinician services compatible with patient cultural beliefs, practices, and languages; an organizational workforce representing the demographic diversity in local communities; culturally and linguistically competent services; and ongoing self-assessments for accountability" (Aggarwal et al. 2017, p. 856). Just 3 years after the release of the enhanced National CLAS Standards, the Office of Minority Health found that 32 of the 50 states had enacted 172 CLAS-type programs in 2014–2015, and that nine states had adopted CLAS-specific policies, procedures, and regulations (Office of Minority Health 2016).

TABLE 44–1.   National Standards for Culturally and Linguistically Appropriate Services (CLAS)

Principal Standard

1. Provide effective, equitable, understandable, and respectful quality care and services that are responsive to diverse cultural health beliefs and practices, preferred languages, health literacy, and other communication needs.

Governance, Leadership, and Workforce

2. Advance and sustain organizational governance and leadership that promotes CLAS and health equity through policy, practices, and allocated resources.

3. Recruit, promote, and support a culturally and linguistically diverse governance, leadership, and workforce that are responsive to the population in the service area.

4. Educate and train governance, leadership, and workforce in culturally and linguistically appropriate policies and practices on an ongoing basis.

Communication and Language Assistance

5. Offer language assistance to individuals who have limited English proficiency and/or other communication needs, at no cost to them, to facilitate timely access to all health care and services.

6. Inform all individuals of the availability of language assistance services clearly and in their preferred language, verbally and in writing.

7. Ensure the competence of individuals providing language assistance, recognizing that the use of untrained individuals and/or minors as interpreters should be avoided.

8. Provide easy-to-understand print and multimedia materials and signage in the languages commonly used by the populations in the service area.

Engagement, Continuous Improvement, and Accountability

9. Establish culturally and linguistically appropriate goals, policies, and management accountability, and infuse them throughout the organization's planning and operations.

10. Conduct ongoing assessments of the organization's CLAS-related activities and integrate CLAS-related measures into measurement and continuous quality improvement activities.

11. Collect and maintain accurate and reliable demographic data to monitor and evaluate the impact of CLAS on health equity and outcomes and to inform service delivery.

12. Conduct regular assessments of community health assets and needs and use the results to plan and implement services that respond to the cultural and linguistic diversity of populations in the service area.

13. Partner with the community to design, implement, and evaluate policies, practices, and services to ensure cultural and linguistic appropriateness.

14. Create conflict and grievance resolution processes that are culturally and linguistically appropriate to identify, prevent, and resolve conflicts or complaints.

15. Communicate the organization's progress in implementing and sustaining CLAS to all stakeholders, constituents, and the general public.

Source.   Office of Minority Health, U.S. Department of Health and Human Services: *National Standards for Culturally and Linguistically Appropriate Services in Health and Health Care: A Blueprint for Advancing and Sustaining CLAS Policy and Practice.* Rockville, MD, Office of Minority Health, April 2013, p. 13. Available at: https://www.thinkculturalhealth.hhs.gov/pdfs/EnhancedCLASStandardsBlueprint.pdf. Accessed August 8, 2017.

Reducing Mental Health Disparities as a Rationale for Cultural Competence

All of the guidelines referenced here have noted that clinician cultural competence can reduce racial and ethnic health disparities. The U.S. Census Bureau has estimated that by 2044, non-Latino whites will account for less than 50% of the nation's population (Colby and Ortman 2014). These statistics demonstrate that the United States is undergoing a demographic shift and indicate that clinicians must strive to become familiar with and comfortable working within a multitude of unfamiliar systems of knowledge, concepts, rules, and practices pertaining to mental health and illness. At the same time, the Association of American Medical Colleges (2014) reported that among M.D. physicians in the United States, 4.1% are black or African American, 4.4% are Hispanic or Latino, 0.4% are American Indian or Alaska Native, 11.7% are Asian, and 48.9% are white. Past policies to redress health disparities focused on racially and ethnically matching minority patients with physicians, but directives calling for such matching were criticized for overlooking the significant political and economic constraints that individuals from minority and lower-income backgrounds must overcome to acquire a medical education (Association of American Medical Colleges 2014). Moreover, the relatively higher proportion of Asian physicians compared with the Asian proportion of the general population indicates that racial and ethnic minority clinicians are now providing care to other minorities and whites.

Health Disparities in Mental Illness

A health disparity population is one for which there exists "significant disparity in the overall rate of disease incidence, prevalence, morbidity, mortality or survival" compared with the general population (U.S. Public Law 106-525, Minority Health and Health Disparities Research and Education Act of 2000).

Disparities in Mental Illness Burden

Whereas prevalence rates of specific mental disorders are mostly similar across population groups, some differences are worthy of note. For example, members of sexual minority groups—such as those from lesbian, gay, and bisexual communities—have a likelihood of lifetime suicide attempts that is between three and five times greater than that of heterosexuals (Hottes et al. 2016). Immigrants who are successfully acculturated demonstrate significantly decreased depression scores compared with unacculturated immigrants (Gupta et al. 2013). Here, we call attention to the challenges of certain groups.

Disparities in Access to and Utilization of Mental Health Care Services

Compared with white Americans, members of racial and ethnic minority groups are less likely to access and use mental health care services. Data from the Medical Expenditure Panel Surveys administered by the Agency for Healthcare Research and

Quality between 2004 and 2012 showed that despite efforts to improve the delivery of mental health services to minority groups, there are widening disparities in access to any type of mental health care (Cook et al. 2017). Several factors are responsible for this increased gap: financial disparities, lack of insurance, and limited English proficiency (Cook et al. 2017). Limited English proficiency has been shown to correlate with decreased utilization of mental health care. Asian Americans with high English proficiency are more likely to utilize mental health care (Kang et al. 2010), and Hispanics with limited English proficiency are less likely to access or utilize such care (Falgas et al. 2017).

Disparities Related to Diagnosis, Treatment, and Quality of Care

Psychiatric disorders are more likely to be underdiagnosed and misdiagnosed in racial and ethnic minority groups than in the majority population. Black patients are more likely to be diagnosed with psychotic illnesses and less likely to be diagnosed with mood disorders compared with non-Hispanic whites, even when samples are controlled for disorder prevalence (Gara et al. 2012). Non-Hispanic white youth are more likely than minority youth to be assigned a diagnosis and to receive mental health care services (Liang et al. 2016). Furthermore, patients from some backgrounds are more likely to underreport symptoms; for example, Asian Americans are more likely than whites to report symptoms only after they become severe (Cook et al. 2017).

Minority patients face additional challenges related to quality of care. African Americans are less likely to be prescribed antidepressant medications when diagnosed with depression and medications are indicated (Conner et al. 2010). In comparison with the majority population, minority groups are also more likely to receive mental health services in emergency departments or inpatient units (Cook et al. 2014). In addition, minority groups are more likely to receive either no follow-up care or inadequate follow-up after inpatient hospitalization (Carson et al. 2014).

Clinical Cultural Competence Interventions From Cultural Psychiatry

To comply with increasing professional and governmental mandates to provide culturally and linguistically appropriate services, how can clinicians develop the attitudes, knowledge, skills, and practices needed to deliver culturally competent care? Whereas a previous generation of scholarship understood cultural competence to be "a list of dos and don'ts" based on the clinician's perceptions of which racial or ethnic groups a patient belonged to (Lewis-Fernández et al. 2014), psychiatrists who work with culturally diverse populations now recognize the need for two types of competencies: 1) training in the cultural explanatory models of health and illness for patient populations that clinicians most frequently treat, and 2) general methods to elicit cultural variables that can be applied to patients from any social group (Shaw and Armin 2011). Clinicians can accumulate knowledge about specific groups by working with interpreters, cultural brokers, and advocates who facilitate access for historically disadvantaged patients and by partnering with primary care practices that serve designated populations (Kirmayer et al. 2014). Clinicians can also learn how to conduct general cultural assessments through the DSM-5 Outline for Cultural Formulation and Cultural Formulation Interview (American Psychiatric Association 2013), which are discussed in the following section.

The Outline for Cultural Formulation

DSM-IV and DSM-IV-TR provided an Outline for Cultural Formulation (OCF) and a "Glossary of Culture-Bound Syndromes" in Appendix I (American Psychiatric Association 1994, 2000). DSM-5 provided an updated version of the OCF in Section III (pp. 749–750). The OCF is a framework for cultural assessment that can be used to evaluate patients within their life contexts by inquiring about sources of identity, the relationship of identity to the presenting problem, the effects of the illness on social relationships and daily functioning, and the extent to which the personal backgrounds of the patient and clinician affect the clinical interaction. An early contribution of the OCF has been the recognition that cultural variables are dynamic and process based, not static and trait based, such that clinicians must understand how different pieces of information obtained through the OCF's four dimensions interrelate and change over time (Lewis-Fernández 1996) (Table 44–2). The OCF can also help clinicians arrive at a diagnosis for patients whose presentations may not exactly correspond to DSM diagnostic categories (American Psychiatric Association 2013).

The OCF has been called the most important contribution of anthropology to psychiatry (Kleinman 2016). Journals such as *Culture, Medicine, and Psychiatry; Transcultural Psychiatry;* and *Cultural Diversity and Ethnic Minority Psychology* have published case reports demonstrating the effects of cultural variables on diagnostic assessment, treatment planning, and service implementation across various settings. Case studies have highlighted the OCF's shortcomings, generating an evidence base for ongoing revision. The OCF has been widely used within psychiatric education to promote cultural competence among trainees, although its dissemination has been limited by the lack of social science training among clinicians (Aggarwal and Rohrbaugh 2011). The operationalization of the OCF into the Cultural Formulation Interview (CFI) (detailed ahead) in DSM-5 responds to concerns that many clinicians may not have received training in the sociomedical sciences and would benefit from a standardized series of questions with implementation guidelines to promote the adoption of cultural assessments in routine practice settings (Lewis-Fernández et al. 2014).

Ethnopsychopharmacology

Ethnopsychopharmacology is a nascent area of research that explores how the interaction between cultural and genetic variables leads to differences in the bioactivity of psychotropic drugs. In preparation of this chapter, our search of PubMed yielded only one study published in this area since 2010, a finding that shows that this subfield within cultural psychiatry would benefit from ongoing research. The advent of genetic screening tests such as those providing cytochrome P450 (CYP) genotyping from a cheek swab sample now makes it possible to assess the activity of a particular

TABLE 44–2.	Essential skills of cultural competence: DSM-5 Outline for Cultural Formulation

A. Cultural identity of the individual

B. Cultural conceptualizations of distress

C. Psychosocial stressors and cultural features of vulnerability and resilience

D. Cultural features of the relationship between the individual and the clinician

E. Overall cultural assessment

Source. American Psychiatric Association 2013.

enzyme and to adjust dosing accordingly (AssureRx 2012). For example, ethnicity may have differential effects on the *5-HTTLPR* (serotonin transporter–linked promoter region), as the I/I allele is associated with robust treatment response to escitalopram in whites but not in Han Chinese, based on a prospective multisite study of patients with major depressive disorder (Ng et al. 2013).

Cultural Adaptation of Psychotherapies

A far more researched area has been the cultural adaptation of psychotherapy. Psychotherapy rests on assumptions that individuals can cognize and articulate aspects of themselves, which further rest on conceptions of personhood derived from Euro-American practice contexts that prioritize individualism and autonomy that are not shared in many sociocentric societies (Kirmayer 2007). To overcome these problems, clinicians and researchers have sought to align formal theories of various psychotherapies with patient cultural values. Many cultural adaptations include the substitution of colloquial expressions for technical terms (e.g., "therapeutic exercise" instead of "homework" in cognitive therapy); the incorporation of local terms rather than biomedical categories to refer to illnesses; the training of therapists in local customs and metaphors to facilitate communication; the inclusion of local illness explanations such as stressful circumstances and interpersonal difficulties within treatment manuals; and modifications to psychotherapeutic techniques that allow relatives to participate (Chowdhary et al. 2014). Culturally adapted psychotherapies may demonstrate greater efficacy than standard treatments because the adaptations are compatible with the patient's explanatory models of illness (Chowdhary et al. 2014). The OCF has increasingly been used as a research tool to obtain patient explanatory models, which can then inform cultural adaptations of psychotherapies (Aggarwal et al. 2014).

Another research focus has been the extent to which patient–clinician cultural matching produces superior outcomes compared with unmatched dyads. Meta-analyses demonstrate significant variations in effect sizes when patients and clinicians are matched by race or ethnicity. A pooled analysis of 52 studies showed that patients exhibited strong preferences for therapists of their own race/ethnicity (Cohen's *d,* 0.63), and another analysis of 81 studies showed that patients perceived therapists of their own race/ethnicity more positively than therapists who were not of their race/ethnicity (Cohen's *d,* 0.32). However, a final analysis with 53 studies showed almost no benefit in treatment outcomes resulting from patient–clinician racial/ethnic matching (Cohen's *d,* 0.09) (Cabral and Smith 2011). These results suggest that patient perceptions of demographic matching with clinicians may be overvalued compared with actual outcomes in symptom reduction or improvements in quality of life.

Cultural Psychiatry in DSM-5

DSM-5 includes cultural considerations for clinicians in multiple sections:

1. Section I: the "Introduction" (pp. 14–15)
2. Section II: the descriptive text for each disorder
3. Section III: the "Cultural Formulation" chapter, including "Outline for Cultural Formulation," "Cultural Formulation Interview (CFI)," and "Cultural Concepts of Distress" (pp. 749–759)
4. Appendix: the "Glossary of Cultural Concepts of Distress" (pp. 833–837)

To address concerns that DSM does not exhibit scientific validity outside of North America and Europe, the DSM-5 Task Force involved international experts in cultural mental health right from the start of the revision process. At least one expert in cultural psychiatry participated in each disorder study group, and the Task Force convened a DSM-5 Cross-Cultural Issues Subgroup to organize literature reviews on cultural considerations across all disorder categories and a field trial of the DSM-5 CFI spanning five continents. This work is summarized in the following sections.

The DSM-5 Introduction

The "Cultural Issues" section of the "Introduction" acknowledges that culture provides "interpretive frameworks that shape the experience and expression of the symptoms, signs, and behaviors that are criteria for diagnosis" (American Psychiatric Association 2013, p. 14). This definition operationalizes a fundamental conundrum in cultural psychiatry of knowing whether presenting behaviors are normal or pathological for patients from unfamiliar cultural populations. For example, cultural factors may determine differences in catastrophic cognitions about experiences with anxiety, representing a critical psychological mechanism that explains differential prevalence rates for anxiety disorders across societies (Marques et al. 2011). The "Cultural Issues" section outlines how cultural factors influence the diagnostic and treatment process, such as in symptom presentations (e.g., alternative symptom variants), clinician assessments (e.g., diagnostic accuracy, evaluation of severity), and patients' responses (e.g., coping strategies, help-seeking choices, treatment adherence). DSM-5's "Introduction" also explains that the antiquated term *culture-bound syndrome* has been replaced by three concepts that offer greater specificity—*cultural syndromes, idioms of distress*, and *explanations*—that are described ahead.

Inclusion of Culturally Relevant Material in the Descriptive Text for Each Disorder

DSM-IV/DSM-IV-TR limited its provision of culture-related material for each disorder to a single section titled "Specific Culture, Age, and Gender Features." In contrast, DSM-5 has separated this section into three subsections on "Development," "Culture," and "Gender." Some disorder work groups used the revision process as an opportunity to conduct systematic reviews of cultural factors that are relevant to each disorder. The first step in this process was to review the quality of data on cultural variations for each DSM disorder against the following questions:

- What level of integration is needed for cultural information within DSM-5?
- Is the evidence strong enough to warrant changes to disorder criteria?
- Or, instead, should cultural data go only in the descriptive text to help the clinician apply existing criteria across cultural presentations?
- Alternatively, should nothing be changed from DSM-IV-TR?

Most reviews elicited studies that did not meet the evidentiary standards needed to propose changes to central DSM criteria on the basis of cultural variations. Nonetheless, data were robust enough at times to warrant proposed revisions. This was the case for social anxiety disorder, agoraphobia, specific phobia, posttraumatic stress disorder, and dissociative identity disorder, among others (Lewis-Fernández et al. 2010). For example, decades of cross-cultural research have shown that the fear of negative evaluation *by* others (i.e., the hallmark of social anxiety disorder) can manifest as a fear that the individual will cause offense *to* others, in addition to or instead of the fear that the person him- or herself will feel embarrassed by engaging in social behavior (Choy et al. 2008). Labeled "other-directed" or "allocentric," this type of fear is characteristic of local idioms of distress in East Asia, described as *taijin kyofusho* in Japan and *taein kong po* in Korea. The fear of offending others is also observed among individuals with social anxiety disorder in many cultural settings, including Australia and the United States (Kim et al. 2008). Across cultures, the fear of offending others and the fear of also suffering embarrassment can occur simultaneously, rather than being mutually exclusive, indicating that they are related presentations (Lewis-Fernández et al. 2010). In acknowledgement of the strength of this evidence, the Work Group on Anxiety, Obsessive-Compulsive Spectrum, Posttraumatic, and Dissociative Disorders revised the social anxiety disorder criteria to clarify this relationship and thereby reduce the potential for misdiagnosis in settings where "other-directed" fear is the primary or initial presentation. The revised social anxiety disorder Criterion B reads as follows: "The individual fears that he or she will act in a way or show anxiety symptoms that will be negatively evaluated (e.g., will be humiliating or embarrassing; will lead to rejection or offend others)" (American Psychiatric Association 2013, p. 202).

In some cases, evidence on the impact of cultural factors in diagnosis was not sufficient to warrant a revision of diagnostic criteria but was added to the text description of the disorder (under the subheadings "Diagnostic Features," "Associated Features," and "Prevalence"). These additions were intended to help clinicians and researchers identify individuals with the disorder to facilitate assessment of severity, comorbidity, prognosis, and acceptable treatment options. These cultural additions appear in several forms:

- In light of DSM's growing international use, an effort was made to document the geographical sources of studies on specific disorders. The DSM-5 Task Force has consistently reiterated its commitment to a truly international nosology that can be integrated with the World Health Organization's *International Classification of Diseases,* 11th Revision (ICD-11), now scheduled for 2019. To advance this commitment, DSM-5 clarifies limitations of existing data. For example, if information about a disorder's development and course was available only from studies in North America and Europe, that circumstance was noted in the text. These additions respond to criticisms that DSM-5 is inapplicable outside of North America and Europe while also providing a state-of-the-science assessment of the evidence base that can inform future research.

- Two subsections of the text—"Diagnostic Features" and "Prevalence"—include culture-relevant information. The "Diagnostic Features" subsection describes symptom variations in disorder presentations that have led to a revision of fundamental disorder criteria (e.g., the revision of Criterion B for social anxiety disorder mentioned earlier). The "Prevalence" subsection enumerates variations in prevalence rates by race/ethnicity in the United States and estimated prevalence ranges internationally. For instance, most of the anxiety disorders have been examined in many countries with the same instrument, the World Health Organization's Composite International Diagnostic Interview, yielding comparable values for 12-month prevalence. The values from countries with the highest and lowest prevalence estimates are reported as endpoints of a range for each disorder.

- For each DSM-5 disorder, the new subsection "Culture-Related Diagnostic Issues" provides data on explicitly cultural features of the disorder (e.g., cultural variations in disorder symptoms that did not warrant criteria revision), as well as culture-related information on development and course, risk and prognostic factors, interpretation of stressors, impairment, and severity. Fuller information on cultural, racial, and/or ethnic variations in disorder prevalence (e.g., by nativity status, by subethnicity) is also included. Finally, cultural labels, explanatory models, and/or cultural syndromes associated with the disorder are listed and cross-referenced with individual entries in the "Glossary of Cultural Concepts of Distress" in DSM-5's Appendix. For example, a complex association exists between *ataques de nervios* (attacks of nerves), a cultural syndrome common among Latinos, and several DSM-5 disorders (Lewis-Fernández and Aggarwal 2013). Individual presentations of *ataque* can be variously diagnosed as panic disorder, other specified dissociative disorder, and conversion disorder. In other words, the cultural label unifies presentations that are considered psychiatrically diverse.

DSM-5 Outline for Cultural Formulation

As mentioned earlier, DSM-5 includes an updated version of the DSM-IV/DSM-IV-TR OCF. Revisions to the DSM-IV version were made in response to criticisms that busy clinicians were not using the OCF because it took too much time; the OCF dimensions were too indistinct and overlapping; and information from the OCF elicited information that was redundant with the standard clinical assessment (Aggarwal 2012). During the revision process, the Cross-Cultural Issues Subgroup identified at least six different types of interviews that attempted to operationalize the DSM-IV OCF with concrete questions that could be implemented, preventing standardization of training and research in this area. At the same time, the OCF approach to cultural assessment has demonstrated clear clinical utility. Clinical researchers who staff McGill University's Cultural Consultation Service have demonstrated the OCF's usefulness in identifying the misdiagnosis of psychotic disorders among ethnic minority and immigrant patients with unfamiliar symptom presentations (Adeponle et al. 2012). In this study, use of the DSM-IV/DSM-IV-TR OCF for case reassessment of 323 patients referred over a 10-year period resulted in 34 (49%) of 70 cases with a referral diagnosis of a psychotic disorder being rediagnosed as a nonpsychotic disorder, and 12 (5%) of 253 cases with a referral diagnosis of a nonpsychotic disorder being rediagnosed as a psychotic disorder. The McGill Cultural Consultation Service draws upon 60 cultural and linguistic brokers (who share the patient's background and provide interpretation as necessary), 1.5-hour clinical assessments, and a 2-hour case conference in addition to the OCF (Adeponle et al. 2012). Based in part on concerns that this level of service intensity may not be reproducible, the Cross-Cultural Issues Subgroup created the DSM-5 CFI through systematic literature reviews and the consensus of experts who operationalized their own OCF-based interviews.

DSM-5 Cultural Formulation Interview

The CFI is a standardized 16-item questionnaire that can be used at the beginning of every initial patient assessment and covers the same topical areas as the OCF. The CFI includes instructions to clinicians that precede the questions and a guide to the interviewer on content designed for elicitation through each question. The CFI is organized into four sections: 1) cultural definition of the problem (questions 1–3); 2) cultural perceptions of cause, context, and support (questions 4–10); 3) cultural factors affecting self-coping and past help seeking (questions 11–13); and 4) cultural factors affecting current help seeking (questions 14–16). The American Psychiatric Association has made the CFI available free of cost in order to encourage widespread dissemination, and it is reproduced in Table 44–3.

In response to criticisms that older models of cultural assessment unintentionally stereotyped patients by starting with group-level traits (e.g., "the black patient," "the Hispanic patient," "the gay patient"), the CFI uses a person-centered approach that emphasizes the patient's experience of illness (Lewis-Fernández et al. 2014). This approach recognizes that individuals exhibit intragroup and intergroup differences. It also allows each individual's hybridized identity to inform current understandings of the illness experience, which is best assessed by asking patients directly about their identities, not by clinicians assigning identities to patients a priori (Aggarwal 2012). In recognition that multiple conceptions of culture have existed throughout the social and behavioral sciences, a pluralistic approach to culture informs use of the CFI, with culture understood in three broad ways (American Psychiatric Association 2013, p. 750):

- The values, orientations, knowledge, and practices that individuals derive from membership in diverse social groups (e.g., ethnic groups, faith communities, occupational groups, veteran groups)
- Aspects of a person's background, developmental experiences, and current social contexts that may affect his or her perspective, such as geographical origin, migration, language, religion, sexual orientation, or race/ethnicity
- The influence of family, friends, and other community members (the individual's social network) on the individual's illness experience

Consistent with DSM-5's approach to culture, the CFI is intended for use with in-dividuals from *any* background, not just those who belong to nondominant social groups such as racial, ethnic, or sexual minorities. Even patients and clinicians who appear to share the same cultural background may differ in ways that are relevant to care, such as through socioeconomic class, nativity, occupation, and language use (Aggarwal 2012). Although the CFI has been designed for use in any clinical setting, DSM-5 explains that the interview may be most helpful in the following circum-stances (American Psychiatric Association 2013, p. 751):

- Difficulty in diagnostic assessment owing to significant differences in the cultural, religious, or socioeconomic backgrounds of the clinician and individual
- Uncertainty about the fit between culturally distinctive symptoms and diagnostic criteria
- Difficulty in judging illness severity or impairment
- Disagreement between the individual and clinician on the course of care
- Limited clinical engagement and treatment adherence by the individual

DSM-5's field trials for the CFI enrolled 318 patents and 75 clinicians in six coun-tries, and found that participants considered the CFI to be feasible, acceptable, and useful, with clinician ratings for all three dimensions improving after they adminis-tered one CFI in its entirety (Lewis-Fernández et al. 2017). In addition, the field trial has provided data on optimal methods to train clinicians in the CFI, with active partic-ipation through case-based behavioral simulations named "most helpful" and passive participation through viewing videos named "least helpful"; experience may factor into training preferences, with each additional year of a clinician's age being associated with a preference for behavioral simulations (Aggarwal et al. 2016). Since DSM-5's publication, the CFI has been used to provide cultural competence training to general psychiatry residents, who have exhibited improvements in nonverbal communica-tion and cultural knowledge on a standardized cultural competence assessment tool (Mills et al. 2017). Information obtained from the CFI has been used in specialty clin-ics that treat minority patients to develop systemwide treatment plans that focus on restoring relationships, improving stigma, and addressing psychosocial needs (Díaz et al. 2017). These studies demonstrate that the CFI can inform treatment planning for patients and systems-level interventions, as recommended by the enhanced National CLAS Standards that were introduced earlier.

Supplementary modules have also been developed for use with the core CFI to help clinicians conduct a more comprehensive cultural assessment; these modules are available free of cost online (www.psychiatry.org/dsm5). Topical modules cover the patient's illness explanatory model; level of functioning; social network; psychosocial stressors; spirituality, religion, and moral traditions; cultural identity; coping and help seeking; and the patient–clinician relationship. Population-specific modules ad-dress the needs of school-age children and adolescents, older adults, immigrants and refugees, and caregivers. Clinicians may apply selected modules if they wish to ex-pand upon a particular component of the CFI. In this manner, the core CFI may be used as an initial cultural "review of systems," with supplementary modules expand-ing the clinician's inquiry as needed.

TABLE 44–3.   DSM-5 Cultural Formulation Interview (CFI)

(Supplementary modules used to expand each CFI subtopic are noted in parentheses.)

GUIDE TO INTERVIEWER	INSTRUCTIONS TO THE INTERVIEWER ARE *ITALICIZED.*
The following questions aim to clarify key aspects of the presenting clinical problem from the point of view of the individual and other members of the individual's social network (i.e., family, friends, or others involved in current problem). This includes the problem's meaning, potential sources of help, and expectations for services.	*INTRODUCTION FOR THE INDIVIDUAL:* I would like to understand the problems that bring you here so that I can help you more effectively. I want to know about *your* experience and ideas. I will ask some questions about what is going on and how you are dealing with it. Please remember there are no right or wrong answers.

CULTURAL DEFINITION OF THE PROBLEM

CULTURAL DEFINITION OF THE PROBLEM
(Explanatory Model, Level of Functioning)

Elicit the individual's view of core problems and key concerns. *Focus on the individual's own way of understanding the problem.* *Use the term, expression, or brief description elicited in question 1 to identify the problem in subsequent questions (e.g., "your conflict with your son").*	1. What brings you here today? *IF INDIVIDUAL GIVES FEW DETAILS OR ONLY MENTIONS SYMPTOMS OR A MEDICAL DIAGNOSIS, PROBE:* People often understand their problems in their own way, which may be similar to or different from how doctors describe the problem. How would *you* describe your problem?
Ask how individual frames the problem for members of the social network.	2. Sometimes people have different ways of describing their problem to their family, friends, or others in their community. How would you describe your problem to them?
Focus on the aspects of the problem that matter most to the individual.	3. What troubles you most about your problem?

CULTURAL PERCEPTIONS OF CAUSE, CONTEXT, AND SUPPORT

CAUSES
(Explanatory Model, Social Network, Older Adults)

This question indicates the meaning of the condition for the individual, which may be relevant for clinical care. *Note that individuals may identify multiple causes, depending on the facet of the problem they are considering.*	4. Why do you think this is happening to you? What do you think are the causes of your [PROBLEM]? *PROMPT FURTHER IF REQUIRED:* Some people may explain their problem as the result of bad things that happen in their life, problems with others, a physical illness, a spiritual reason, or many other causes.
Focus on the views of members of the individual's social network. These may be diverse and vary from the individual's.	5. What do others in your family, your friends, or others in your community think is causing your [PROBLEM]?

TABLE 44–3. DSM-5 Cultural Formulation Interview (CFI) *(continued)*

(Supplementary modules used to expand each CFI subtopic are noted in parentheses.)

GUIDE TO INTERVIEWER	**INSTRUCTIONS TO THE INTERVIEWER ARE** *ITALICIZED.*
STRESSORS AND SUPPORTS (Social Network, Caregivers, Psychosocial Stressors, Religion and Spirituality, Immigrants and Refugees, Cultural Identity, Older Adults, Coping and Help Seeking)	
Elicit information on the individual's life context, focusing on resources, social supports, and resilience. May also probe other supports (e.g., from co-workers, from participation in religion or spirituality).	6. Are there any kinds of support that make your [PROBLEM] better, such as support from family, friends, or others?
Focus on stressful aspects of the individual's environment. Can also probe, e.g., relationship problems, difficulties at work or school, or discrimination.	7. Are there any kinds of stresses that make your [PROBLEM] worse, such as difficulties with money, or family problems?
ROLE OF CULTURAL IDENTITY (Cultural Identity, Psychosocial Stressors, Religion and Spirituality, Immigrants and Refugees, Older Adults, Children and Adolescents)	
	Sometimes, aspects of people's background or identity can make their [PROBLEM] better or worse. By **background** or **identity**, I mean, for example, the communities you belong to, the languages you speak, where you or your family are from, your race or ethnic background, your gender or sexual orientation, or your faith or religion.
Ask the individual to reflect on the most salient elements of his or her cultural identity. Use this information to tailor questions 9–10 as needed.	8. For you, what are the most important aspects of your background or identity?
Elicit aspects of identity that make the problem better or worse. *Probe as needed (e.g., clinical worsening as a result of discrimination due to migration status, race/ ethnicity, or sexual orientation).*	9. Are there any aspects of your background or identity that make a difference to your [PROBLEM]?
Probe as needed (e.g., migration-related problems; conflict across generations or due to gender roles).	10. Are there any aspects of your background or identity that are causing other concerns or difficulties for you?

TABLE 44–3.   **DSM-5 Cultural Formulation Interview (CFI)** *(continued)*

(Supplementary modules used to expand each CFI subtopic are noted in parentheses.)

GUIDE TO INTERVIEWER	**INSTRUCTIONS TO THE INTERVIEWER ARE** *ITALICIZED.*

CULTURAL FACTORS AFFECTING SELF-COPING AND PAST HELP SEEKING

SELF-COPING

(Coping and Help Seeking, Religion and Spirituality, Older Adults, Caregivers, Psychosocial Stressors)

Clarify self-coping for the problem.	11. Sometimes people have various ways of dealing with problems like [PROBLEM]. What have you done on your own to cope with your [PROBLEM]?

PAST HELP SEEKING

(Coping and Help Seeking, Religion and Spirituality, Older Adults, Caregivers, Psychosocial Stressors, Immigrants and Refugees, Social Network, Clinician–Patient Relationship)

Elicit various sources of help (e.g., medical care, mental health treatment, support groups, work-based counseling, folk healing, religious or spiritual counseling, other forms of traditional or alternative healing). *Probe as needed (e.g., "What other sources of help have you used?").* *Clarify the individual's experience and regard for previous help.*	12. Often, people look for help from many different sources, including different kinds of doctors, helpers, or healers. In the past, what kinds of treatment, help, advice, or healing have you sought for your [PROBLEM]? *PROBE IF DOES NOT DESCRIBE USEFULNESS OF HELP RECEIVED:* What types of help or treatment were most useful? Not useful?

BARRIERS

(Coping and Help Seeking, Religion and Spirituality, Older Adults, Psychosocial Stressors, Immigrants and Refugees, Social Network, Clinician–Patient Relationship)

Clarify the role of social barriers to help seeking, access to care, and problems engaging in previous treatment. *Probe details as needed (e.g., "What got in the way?").*	13. Has anything prevented you from getting the help you need? *PROBE AS NEEDED:* For example, money, work or family commitments, stigma or discrimination, or lack of services that understand your language or background?

CULTURAL FACTORS AFFECTING CURRENT HELP SEEKING

PREFERENCES

(Social Network, Caregivers, Religion and Spirituality, Older Adults, Coping and Help Seeking)

Clarify individual's current perceived needs and expectations of help, broadly defined. *Probe if individual lists only one source of help (e.g., "What other kinds of help would be useful to you at this time?").*	Now let's talk some more about the help you need. 14. What kinds of help do you think would be most useful to you at this time for your [PROBLEM]?
Focus on the views of the social network regarding help seeking.	15. Are there other kinds of help that your family, friends, or other people have suggested would be helpful for you now?

TABLE 44–3. **DSM-5 Cultural Formulation Interview (CFI)** *(continued)*

(Supplementary modules used to expand each CFI subtopic are noted in parentheses.)

GUIDE TO INTERVIEWER	INSTRUCTIONS TO THE INTERVIEWER ARE *ITALICIZED.*

CLINICIAN–PATIENT RELATIONSHIP
(Clinician–Patient Relationship, Older Adults)

Elicit possible concerns about the clinic or the clinician–patient relationship, including perceived racism, language barriers, or cultural differences that may undermine goodwill, communication, or care delivery. *Probe details as needed (e.g., "In what way?").* *Address possible barriers to care or concerns about the clinic and the clinician–patient relationship raised previously.*	Sometimes doctors and patients misunderstand each other because they come from different backgrounds or have different expectations. 16. Have you been concerned about this and is there anything that we can do to provide you with the care you need?

Source. Reproduced from *Diagnostic and Statistical Manual of Mental Disorders,* 5th Edition. Washington, DC, American Psychiatric Association, 2013, pp. 752–754. Copyright 2013, American Psychiatric Association. Used with permission.

Cultural Concepts of Distress

As previously noted, DSM-5 revised the DSM-IV/DSM-IV-TR "Glossary of Culture-Bound Syndromes" to produce two new sections: "Cultural Concepts of Distress" in the "Cultural Formulation" chapter in Section III, and a Glossary of these concepts in the Appendix. The text in the "Cultural Formulation" chapter in Section III updated the older conceptual description of *culture-bound syndromes* with three categories that demonstrate greater clinical utility based on a review of the scientific evidence base (American Psychiatric Association 2013): 1) *cultural syndromes* are clusters of symptoms and attributions that tend to co-occur among individuals in specific cultural groups, communities, or contexts and that are recognized locally as coherent patterns of experience; 2) *cultural idioms of distress* are ways of expressing distress that may not involve specific symptoms or syndromes but provide shared ways of experiencing and talking about personal or social concerns (e.g., everyday talk about "nerves" or "depression"); 3) *cultural explanations* or *perceived causes* are labels, attributions, or features of an explanatory model that indicate culturally recognized meanings or etiologies for symptoms, illness, or distress (Hinton and Lewis-Fernández 2010).

The differences among these three categories may be elided in common practice when the same cultural term cuts across these categories. For example, the term *depression* can describe a syndrome (e.g., major depressive disorder), an idiom of distress (e.g., as in the expression "I feel depressed"), or a perceived cause (similar to "stress"). Despite this overlap, the distinctions among syndromes, idioms of distress, and explanations can help clinicians recognize patients' use of cultural concepts in their daily lives (American Psychiatric Association 2013). For instance, the CFI asks patients to describe their presenting problem to the clinician and also to reflect on how they would describe their problem to individuals within their social network. Hearing and using the patient's own words (including cultural terms used to describe the problem) allows the clinician to better evaluate the patient's presenting problem and also improves rapport and patient comfort; studies have shown that patients express higher satisfaction with clinicians who match their vocabularies (Williams and Ogden 2004).

The "Glossary of Cultural Concepts of Distress" includes nine examples of cultural concepts of distress from around the world that typify syndromes, idioms, and explanations and their interrelationships: *ataque de nervios, dhat syndrome, khyâl cap, kufungisisa, maladi moun, nervios, shenjing shuairuo, susto,* and *taijin kyofusho.* Only high-prevalence concepts with considerable research were included, and for each concept, the glossary lists related conditions across cultural contexts, including the scientific context that has produced DSM-5. These concepts may also facilitate the clinician's translation between local categories that patients use and more universalizing labels such as DSM-5 diagnoses. One way to understand the cultural concepts in the glossary is that many DSM disorders also originated as local expressions of behaviors that were deemed abnormal in early-twentieth-century Europe and eventually became disorder prototypes, based on a process of abstraction and generalization (Roelcke 1997). Indeed, many of the cultural concepts included in the glossary cut across DSM diagnoses, so that there is not a direct correspondence between cultural concepts and DSM disorders. For example, symptoms or behaviors that might be classified into discrete DSM-5 disorders exist in a single cultural concept, just as diverse presentations of a single DSM-5 disorder may belong to multiple cultural concepts of distress (American Psychiatric Association 2013).

Conclusion

In this chapter we have provided a brief introduction to the assessment and treatment of culturally diverse populations. Whereas cultural competence initiatives in mental health care originally focused on racial and ethnic minority groups in the United States, treatment of culturally diverse populations today encompasses working with individuals whose cultural identities are self-defined, fluid, and informed by an understanding that identities can be acquired as well as inherited. Every clinical encounter can be seen as a cultural encounter in which the identities of the patient, clinician, and health care setting intersect.

Key Clinical Points

- Cultural competence is an essential aspect of professionalism that includes respect for and responsiveness to differences in race/ethnicity, age, gender, gender identity, language, socioeconomic status, sexual orientation, country of origin and acculturation, religion/spirituality, abilities/disabilities, and geographic location, among other factors.

- Cultural competence is essential for competent clinical care of all patients because cultural differences always exist between the clinician and the patient that may affect assessment, diagnosis, and treatment planning.

- Cultural competence includes knowledge, attitudes, and skills that are essential for competent care that is both respectful of and responsive to the patient's cultural identity, values, and preferences.

- For psychiatric clinicians, cultural competence includes skill in use of the DSM-5 Outline for Cultural Formulation (OCF) and Cultural Formulation Interview (CFI).

- Cultural competence, at both the clinical and the systems level, is essential to reducing and eliminating mental health care disparities while increasing health equity, a key indicator of quality in health care.

References

Accreditation Council for Graduate Medical Education: Clinical Learning Environment Review (CLER) Pathways to Excellence. Chicago, IL, Accreditation Council for Graduate Medical Education, 2014. Available at: http://www.acgme.org/Portals/0/PDFs/CLER/CLER_Brochure.pdf. Accessed August 21, 2017.

Adeponle AB, Thombs BD, Groleau D, et al: Using the cultural formulation to resolve uncertainty in diagnoses of psychosis among ethnoculturally diverse patients. Psychiatr Serv 63(2):147–153, 2012 22302332

Aggarwal NK: Hybridity and intersubjectivity in the clinical encounter: impact on the cultural formulation. Transcult Psychiatry 49(1):121–139, 2012 22218399

Aggarwal NK, Rohrbaugh R: Teaching cultural competency through an experiential seminar on anthropology and psychiatry. Acad Psychiatry 35(5):331–334, 2011 22007094

Aggarwal NK, Balaji M, Kumar S, et al: Using consumer perspectives to inform the cultural adaptation of psychological treatments for depression: a mixed methods study from South Asia. J Affect Disord 163:88–101, 2014 24836093

Aggarwal NK, Lam P, Castillo EG, et al: How do clinicians prefer cultural competence training? Findings from the DSM-5 Cultural Formulation Interview field trial. Acad Psychiatry 40(4):584–591, 2016 26449983

Aggarwal NK, Cedeno K, John D, Lewis-Fernandez R: Adoption of the national CLAS standards by state mental health agencies: a nationwide policy analysis. Psychiatr Serv 68(8):856–858, 2017 28366117

American Board of Psychiatry and Neurology: Psychiatry Core Competencies Outline. Buffalo Grove, IL, ABPN Board of Directors, July 22, 2011. Available at: https://www.abpn.com/wp-content/uploads/2015/02/2011_core_P_MREE.pdf. Accessed July 29, 2017.

American Psychiatric Association: Diagnostic and Statistical Manual of Mental Disorders, 2nd Edition. Washington, DC, American Psychiatric Association, 1968

American Psychiatric Association: Diagnostic and Statistical Manual of Mental Disorders, 4th Edition. Washington, DC, American Psychiatric Association, 1994

American Psychiatric Association: Diagnostic and Statistical Manual of Mental Disorders, 4th Edition, Text Revision. Washington, DC, American Psychiatric Association, 2000

American Psychiatric Association: Diagnostic and Statistical Manual of Mental Disorders, 5th Edition. Arlington, VA, American Psychiatric Association, 2013

Association of American Medical Colleges: Diversity in the Physician Workforce: Facts and Figures 2014. Washington, DC, Association of American Medical Colleges, 2014. Available at: http://www.aamcdiversityfactsandfigures.org/section-ii-current-status-of-us-physician-workforce/index.html. Accessed December 20, 2018,

Association of American Medical Colleges: Assessing Change: Evaluating Cultural Competence Education and Training. Washington, DC, Association of American Medical Colleges, 2015. Available at: https://www.aamc.org/download/427350/data/assessingchange.pdf. Accessed August 12, 2017.

AssureRx: GeneSightRx—AssureRx, 2012. Available at: http://www.assurerxhealth.com/GeneSightRx. Accessed March 14, 2012.

Cabral RR, Smith TB: Racial/ethnic matching of clients and therapists in mental health services: a meta-analytic review of preferences, perceptions, and outcomes. J Couns Psychol 58(4):537–554, 2011 21875181

Carson NJ, Vesper A, Chen CN, et al: Quality of follow-up after hospitalization for mental illness among patients from racial-ethnic minority groups. Psychiatr Serv 65(7):888–896, 2014 24686538

Chowdhary N, Jotheeswaran AT, Nadkarni A, et al: The methods and outcomes of cultural adaptations of psychological treatments for depressive disorders: a systematic review. Psychol Med 44(6):1131–1146, 2014 23866176

Choy Y, Schneier FR, Heimberg RG, et al: Features of the offensive subtype of Taijin-Kyofu-Sho in US and Korean patients with DSM-IV social anxiety disorder. Depress Anxiety 25(3):230–240, 2008 17340609

Colby SL, Ortman JM: Current population reports, in Projections of the Size and Composition of the U.S. Population: 2014 to 2060 (Report P25-1143). Washington, DC, U.S. Census Bureau, 2014

Conner KO, Lee B, Mayers V, et al: Attitudes and beliefs about mental health among African American older adults suffering from depression. J Aging Stud 24(4):266–277, 2010 21423819

Cook BL, Zuvekas SH, Carson N, et al: Assessing racial/ethnic disparities in treatment across episodes of mental health care. Health Serv Res 49(1):206–229, 2014 23855750

Cook BL, Trinh NH, Li Z, et al: Trends in racial-ethnic disparities in access to mental health care, 2004–2012. Psychiatr Serv 68(1):9–16, 2017 27476805

Díaz E, Añez LM, Silva M, et al: Using the cultural formulation interview to build culturally sensitive services. Psychiatr Serv 68(2):112–114, 2017 27799018

Falgas I, Ramos Z, Herrera L, et al: Barriers to and correlates of retention in behavioral health treatment among Latinos in 2 different host countries: The United States and Spain. J Public Health Manag Pract 23(1):e20–e27, 2017 26910867

Gara MA, Vega WA, Arndt S, et al: Influence of patient race and ethnicity on clinical assessment in patients with affective disorders. Arch Gen Psychiatry 69(6):593–600, 2012 22309972

Gupta A, Leong F, Valentine JC, et al: A meta-analytic study: the relationship between acculturation and depression among Asian Americans. Am J Orthopsychiatry 83(2 Pt 3):372–385, 2013 23889028

Hinton DE, Lewis-Fernández R: Idioms of distress among trauma survivors: subtypes and clinical utility. Cult Med Psychiatry 34(2):209–218, 2010 20407812

Hottes TS, Bogaert L, Rhodes AE, et al: Lifetime prevalence of suicide attempts among sexual minority adults by study sampling strategies: a systematic review and meta-analysis. Am J Public Health 106(5):e1–e12, 2016 27049424

Jenks AC: From "lists of traits" to "open-mindedness": emerging issues in cultural competence education. Cult Med Psychiatry 35(2):209–235, 2011 21560030

Joint Commission: Advancing Effective Communication, Cultural Competence, and Patient- and Family Centered Care: A Roadmap for Hospitals. Oakbrook Terrace, IL, The Joint Commission, April 3, 2014. Available at: https://www.jointcommission.org/roadmap_for_hospitals/. Accessed September 15, 2018.

Kang SY, Howard D, Kim J, et al: English language proficiency and lifetime mental health service utilization in a national representative sample of Asian Americans in the USA. J Public Health (Oxf) 32(3):431–439, 2010 20202979

Kim J, Rapee RM, Ja Oh K, et al: Retrospective report of social withdrawal during adolescence and current maladjustment in young adulthood: cross-cultural comparisons between Australian and South Korean students. J Adolesc 31(5):543–563, 2008 18076980

Kirmayer LJ: Psychotherapy and the cultural concept of the person. Transcult Psychiatry 44(2):232–257, 2007 17576727

Kirmayer LJ, Guzder J, Rousseau C: Cultural Consultation: Encountering the Other in Mental Health Care. New York, Springer-Verlag, 2014

Kleinman A: Foreword, in DSM-5 Handbook on the Cultural Formulation Interview. Edited by Lewis-Fernández R, Aggarwal NK, Hinton L, et al. Washington, DC, American Psychiatric Publishing, 2016, pp xvii–xx

Lewis-Fernández R: Cultural formulation of psychiatric diagnosis. Cult Med Psychiatry 20(2):133–144, 1996 8853962

Lewis-Fernández R, Aggarwal NK: Culture and psychiatric diagnosis. Adv Psychosom Med 33:15–30, 2013 23816860

Lewis-Fernández R, Hinton DE, Laria AJ, et al: Culture and the anxiety disorders: recommendations for DSM-V. Depress Anxiety 27(2):212–229, 2010 20037918

Lewis-Fernández R, Aggarwal NK, Bäärnhielm S, et al: Culture and psychiatric evaluation: operationalizing cultural formulation for DSM-5. Psychiatry 77(2):130–154, 2014 24865197

Lewis-Fernández R, Aggarwal NK, Lam PC, et al: Feasibility, acceptability and clinical utility of the Cultural Formulation Interview: mixed-methods results from the DSM-5 international field trial. Br J Psychiatry 210(4):290–297, 2017 28104738

Liang J, Matheson B, Douglas J: Mental health diagnostic considerations in racial/ethnic minority youth. J Child Fam Stud 25(6):1926–1940, 2016 27346929

Marques L, Robinaugh DJ, LeBlanc NJ, et al: Cross-cultural variations in the prevalence and presentation of anxiety disorders. Expert Rev Neurother 11(2):313–322, 2011 21306217

Mills S, Xiao AQ, Wolitzky-Taylor K, et al: Training on the DSM-5 Cultural Formulation Interview improves cultural competence in general psychiatry residents: a pilot study. Transcult Psychiatry 54(2):179–191, 2017 28358239

National Academies of Sciences, Engineering, and Medicine: Integrating Health Literacy, Cultural Competence, and Language Access Services: Workshop Summary. Washington, DC, National Academies Press, 2016. Available at: https://www.nap.edu/catalog/23498/integrating-health-literacy-cultural-competence-and-language-access-services-workshop. Accessed September 15, 2018.

National Quality Forum: NQF Endorses Healthcare Disparities and Cultural Competency Measures. Press release, August 10, 2012. Available at: http://www.qualityforum.org/News_And_Resources/Press_Releases/2012/NQF_Endorses_Healthcare_Disparities_and_Cultural_Competency_Measures.aspx. Accessed October 21, 2012.

Ng C, Sarris J, Singh A, et al: Pharmacogenetic polymorphisms and response to escitalopram and venlafaxine over 8 weeks in major depression. Hum Psychopharmacol 28(5):516–522, 2013 24014145

Office of Minority Health: National Standards for Culturally and Linguistically Appropriate Services in Health and Health Care: A Blueprint for Advancing and Sustaining CLAS Policy and Practice. Rockville, MD, U.S. Department of Health and Human Services, Office of Minority Health, 2013. Available at: https://www.thinkculturalhealth.hhs.gov/pdfs/EnhancedCLASStandardsBlueprint.pdf. Accessed August 5, 2013.

Office of Minority Health: National Standards for Culturally and Linguistically Appropriate Services in Health and Health Care: Compendium of State-Sponsored National CLAS Standards Implementation Activities. Washington, DC, U.S. Department of Health and Human Services, 2016. Available at: https://www.thinkculturalhealth.hhs.gov/pdfs/CLASCompendium.pdf. Accessed September 15, 2018.

Roelcke V: Biologizing social facts: an early 20th century debate on Kraepelin's concepts of culture, neurasthenia, and degeneration. Cult Med Psychiatry 21(4):383–403, 1997 9492972

Shaw SJ, Armin J: The ethical self-fashioning of physicians and health care systems in culturally appropriate health care. Cult Med Psychiatry 35(2):236–261, 2011 21553151

Williams N, Ogden J: The impact of matching the patient's vocabulary: a randomized control trial. Fam Pract 21(6):630–635, 2004 15520032

Recommended Readings

Bhugra D, Bhui K (eds): Textbook of Cultural Psychiatry. Cambridge, UK, Cambridge University Press, 2007

Burt VK, Hendrick VC: Clinical Manual of Women's Mental Health, 2nd Edition. Washington, DC, American Psychiatric Publishing, 2005

Cabaj RP, Stein TS (eds): Homosexuality and Mental Health. Washington, DC, American Psychiatric Publishing, 1996

Josephson A, Peteet J (eds): Handbook of Spirituality and Worldview in Clinical Practice. Washington, DC, American Psychiatric Publishing, 2004

Lewis-Fernández R, Aggarwal NK, Hinton L, et al (eds): DSM-5 Handbook on the Cultural Formulation Interview. Washington, DC, American Psychiatric Publishing, 2016

Lim RF (ed): Clinical Manual of Cultural Psychiatry. Washington, DC, American Psychiatric Publishing, 2015

McGoldrick M, Giordano J, Garcia-Preto N (eds): Ethnicity and Family Therapy, 3rd Edition. New York, Guilford, 2005

Ruiz P, Primm A (eds): Disparities in Psychiatric Care: Clinical and Cross-Cultural Perspectives. Baltimore, MD, Lippincott Williams & Wilkins, 2010

Tseng W-S: Clinician's Guide to Cultural Psychiatry. New York, Academic Press, 2003

Index

Page numbers printed in **boldface** type refer to tables or figures.